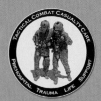
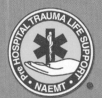

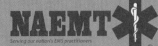

PHTLS
Prehospital Trauma Life Support
MILITARY EIGHTH EDITION

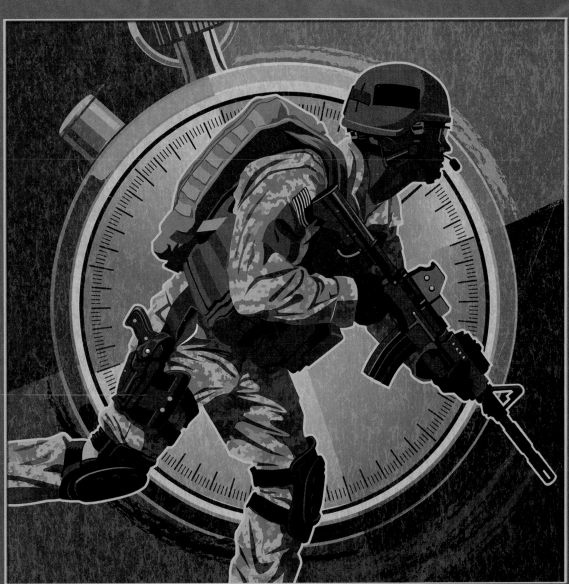

"The fate of the wounded rests in the hands of the one who applies the first dressing."

—Nicholas Senn, MD (1844–1908)
American Surgeon (Chicago, Illinois)
Founder, Association of Military Surgeons of the United States

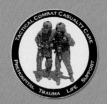
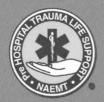
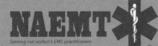

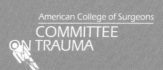
American College of Surgeons
COMMITTEE ON TRAUMA
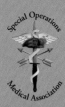

PHTLS

Prehospital Trauma Life Support

MILITARY EIGHTH EDITION

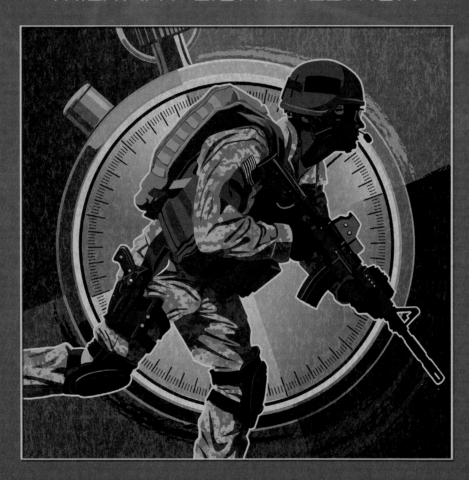

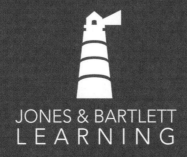
JONES & BARTLETT
LEARNING

World Headquarters
Jones & Bartlett Learning
5 Wall Street
Burlington, MA 01803
978-443-5000
info@jblearning.com
www.jblearning.com

Jones & Bartlett Learning books and products are available through most bookstores and online booksellers. To contact Jones & Bartlett Learning directly, call 800-832-0034, fax 978-443-8000, or visit our website, www.jblearning.com.

Substantial discounts on bulk quantities of Jones & Bartlett Learning publications are available to corporations, professional associations, and other qualified organizations. For details and specific discount information, contact the special sales department at Jones & Bartlett Learning via the above contact information or send an email to specialsales@jblearning.com.

08368-2

Production Credits

Chief Executive Officer: Ty Field
President: James Homer
Chief Product Officer: Eduardo Moura
Vice President, Executive Publisher: Kimberly Brophy
Executive Editor—EMS: Christine Emerton
Director—PSG Editorial Development: Carol B. Guerrero
Senior Content Developer: Jennifer Deforge-Kling
Production Editor: Jessica deMartin
Art Development Editor: Joanna Lundeen
Vice President of Marketing: Alisha Weisman

Vice President, Manufacturing and Inventory Control: Therese Connell
Vice President of Sales: Matthew Maniscalco
Director of Sales: Patricia Einstein
Composition: diacriTech
Cover Design: Kristin E. Parker
Interior Design: Michael O'Donnell
Manager of Photo Research, Rights, and Permissions: Lauren Miller
Cover Image: © NAEMT; background © feoris/iStock/Thinkstock
Printing and Binding: Courier Companies
Cover Printing: Courier Companies

Library of Congress Cataloging-in-Publication Data
PHTLS (Military edition)
  PHTLS : prehospital trauma life support. —Military eighth edition.
    p. ; cm.
  Prehospital trauma life support
  Includes bibliographical references and index.
  ISBN 978-1-284-04175-0
  I. Title. II. Title: Prehospital trauma life support.
  [DNLM: 1. Wounds and Injuries—therapy. 2. Emergencies. 3. Emergency Medical Services. 4. First Aid—methods. 5. Military Medicine—methods.
  6. Traumatology. WO 700]
  RC86.7
  616.02'5—dc23
                        2014039687
6048

Printed in the United States of America
18 17 16 15 14   10 9 8 7 6 5 4 3 2 1

Brief Table of Contents

Table of Contents

CHAPTER 6 Scene Assessment 114

CHAPTER 7 Patient Assessment and Management 136

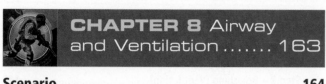

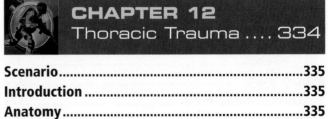

CHAPTER 18 Golden Principles of Prehospital Trauma Care 475

CHAPTER 19 Disaster Management 487

© Photos.com

CHAPTER 20
Explosions and Weapons of Mass Destruction.......... 509

DIVISION 6 Special Considerations 542

CHAPTER 21
Environmental Trauma I: Heat and Cold 542

CHAPTER 22
Environmental Trauma II: Lightning, Drowning, Diving, and Altitude 589

CHAPTER 27 Tactical Evacuation Care 726

CHAPTER 28 Scenarios 740

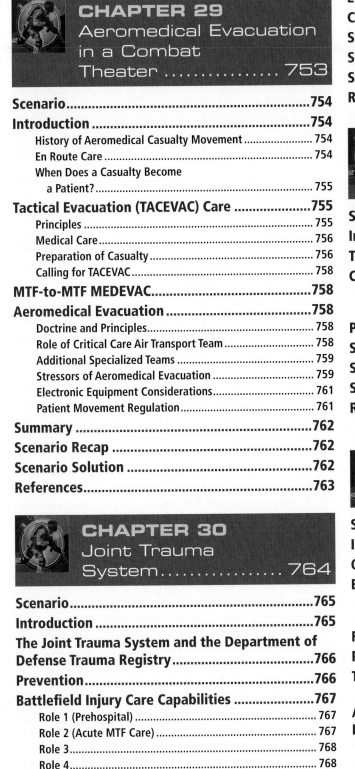

CHAPTER 33
Treatment of Burn Casualties in Tactical Combat Casualty Care ... 812

CHAPTER 34
Casualty Response Planning in Tactical Combat Casualty Care 823

CHAPTER 35 Medical Support of Urban Operations 837

CHAPTER 36 Ethical Considerations for the Combat Medic.. 848

Specific Skills Table of Contents

Acknowledgments

In 1624 John Donne wrote, "No man is an island, entire of itself." In many ways, this insight describes the process of publishing a book. Certainly, no editor is an island. Textbooks, such as *PHTLS: Prehospital Trauma Life Support*; courses, especially those that involve audiovisual materials; and instructor manuals cannot be published by editors in isolation. As a matter of fact, much, if not most, of the work involved in publishing a textbook is accomplished not by the editors and the authors whose names appear on the cover and on the inside of the book, but by the publisher's staff. The eighth edition of *PHTLS* is certainly no exception.

From the American College of Surgeons Committee on Trauma, Ronald M. Stewart, MD, FACS, the current Chairman of the Committee on Trauma, and Michael F. Rotondo, MD, FACS, the ACS Medical Director of Trauma, have provided outstanding support for this edition as well as for PHTLS.

Within Jones & Bartlett Learning, we must thank Christine Emerton for her oversight of this effort, Jennifer Deforge-Kling for her incredible work on the manuscript, Kim Brophy for her overarching support, Carol Guerrero for shepherding the art and photo program for this book, Jessica deMartin for guiding the composition of this book, and Nora Menzi for steering the production of the ancillary program.

The Editor and PHTLS Committee thank Michael Hunter, the paramedics, critical care flight medics, and flight nurses of the University of Massachusetts Memorial Medical Center Emergency Medical Services, Worcester EMS, and LifeFlight for their support and participation in preparing photos and videos for this edition.

The Editor and PHTLS Committee thank Douglas Cotanche, PhD, Director; Michael Doyle, Anatomy Labs Director; Dianne Person, Associate Director; and the donors of the Anatomical Gift Program at the University of Massachusetts Medical School for their support of this educational endeavor.

The editors also thank Kelly Lowery for her review and editing of the first draft chapter manuscripts.

The spouses, children, and significant others of the editors and authors who have tolerated the long hours in the preparation of the material are obviously the backbone of any publication.

Peter T. Pons, MD, FACEP, Editor
Norman McSwain, MD, FACS, NREMT-P, Editor-in-Chief

Contributors

Editor-in-Chief

Norman E. McSwain, Jr., MD, FACS, NREMT-P
Medical Director, PHTLS
Professor of Surgery, Tulane University
Department of Surgery
Trauma Director, Spirit of Charity
Trauma Center, Interim LSU Hospital
Police Surgeon, New Orleans Police
Department
New Orleans, Louisiana

Editor—Eighth Edition

Peter T. Pons, MD, FACEP
Associate Medical Director, PHTLS
Emergency Medicine
Denver, Colorado

Associate Editors

Will Chapleau, EMT-P, RN, TNS
Chairperson, PHTLS Committee
Director of Performance Improvement,
ATLS Program
American College of Surgeons
Chicago, Illinois

Gregory Chapman, EMT-P, RRT
Vice-Chairperson, PHTLS Committee
Center for Prehospital Medicine
Department of Emergency Medicine
Carolinas Medical Center
Charlotte, North Carolina

Editors—Military Edition

Frank K. Butler, Jr., MD
Captain, U.S. Army Retired (Hon)
Chairperson
Committee on Tactical Combat Casualty
Care
Joint Trauma System

S. D. Giebner, MD, MPH
Captain, U.S. Army Retired (Hon)
Past Chairperson
Developmental Editor
Committee on Tactical Combat
Casualty Care
Joint Trauma System

Contributors

Katherine Bakes, MD
Director of Denver Emergency Center
for Children Denver Health Medical
Center Assistant Professor, University
of Colorado SOM
Denver, Colorado

Augie Bamonti III, BA, EMT-P
Medical Officer
Chicago Heights Fire Dept. (Ret.)

Brad L. Bennett, PhD, NREMT-P, FAWM
Adjunct Assistant Professor
Military and Emergency Medicine
Department
F. Edward Hébert School of
Medicine
Uniformed Services University of the
Health Sciences
Bethesda, Maryland

David W. Callaway, MD, MPA
CEO, Operational Medicine International,
Inc.
Associate Professor of Emergency
Medicine
Carolinas Medical Center
Charlotte, North Carolina

Will Chapleau, EMT-P, RN, TNS
Chairperson, PHTLS Committee
Director of Performance Improvement,
ATLS Program
American College of Surgeons
Chicago, Illinois

Gregory Chapman, EMT-P, RRT
Vice-Chairperson, PHTLS Committee
Center for Prehospital Medicine
Department of Emergency Medicine
Carolinas Medical Center
Charlotte, North Carolina

Blaine L. Enderson, MD, MBA, FACS, FCCM
Professor of Surgery
University of Tennessee Medical Center
Knoxville, Tennessee

Jeffrey S. Guy, MD, MSc, MMHC, FACS
Chief Medical Officer
TriStar Health System/HCA
Nashville, Tennessee

Michael J. Hunter, EMT-P
Deputy Chief, Worcester EMS
UMass Memorial Medical Center—
University Campus
Worcester, Massachusetts

Craig H. Jacobus, EMT-P, BA/BS, DC
EMS Faculty Metro Community College
Fremont, Nebraska

David A. Kappel, MD, FACS
Clinical Professor of Surgery
West Virginia University
Deputy State Medical Director
West Virginia State Trauma System
Rural Emergency / Trauma Institute
Wheeling, West Virginia

Eduard Kompast
Deputy Officer
Vienna Ambulance
Instructor
Paramedic Academy
Vienna, Austria

Mark Lueder, EMT-P
PHTLS Committee
Chicago Heights Fire Department
Chicago Heights, Illinois

Norman E. McSwain, Jr., MD, FACS, NREMT-P
Medical Director, PHTLS
Professor of Surgery, Tulane University
Department of Surgery
Trauma Director, Spirit of Charity
Trauma Center, Interim LSU Hospital
Police Surgeon, New Orleans Police
Department
New Orleans, Louisiana

Jeffrey Mott, DHSc, PA-C
Assistant Professor
Physician Assistant Studies
University of North Texas Health Science
Center
Fort Worth, Texas

J. C. Pitteloud, MD
Staff Anesthesiologist
Hôpital du Valais
Sion, Switzerland

Peter T. Pons, MD, FACEP
Associate Medical Director, PHTLS
Emergency Medicine
Denver, Colorado

Jeffrey P. Salomone, MD, FACS, NREMT-P
Chief, Division of Trauma and Surgical Critical Care
Trauma Medical Director
Maricopa Medical Center
Phoenix, Arizona

Valerie Satkoske, PhD
Ethicist, Wheeling Hospital
Wheeling, West Virginia
Core Faculty
Center for Bioethics and Health Law
University of Pittsburgh
Pittsburgh, Pennsylvania

Lance E. Stuke, MD, MPH, FACS
Associate Medical Director, PHTLS
Assistant Professor of Surgery
Tulane University School of Medicine
New Orleans, Louisiana

National Association of Emergency Medical Technicians 2014 Board of Directors

Officers
President: Don Lundy
President-Elect: C. T. Kearns
Secretary: James A. Judge, II
Treasurer: Dennis Rowe
Immediate Past-President: Connie Meyer

Directors
Rod Barrett
Aimee Binning
Chris Cebollero
Ben Chlapek
Bruce Evans
Paul Hinchey, MD

Scott Matin
Chad E. McIntyre
Cory Richter
James M. Slattery
Matt Zavadsky

PHTLS—Chairpersons
1996–present: Will Chapleau, EMT-P, RN, TNS
1992–1996: Elizabeth M. Wertz, RN, BSN, MPM
1991–1992: James L. Paturas
1990–1991: John Sinclair, EMT-P
1988–1990: David Wuertz, EMT-P

1985–1988: James L. Paturas
1983–1985: Richard Vomacka, NREMT-P†
†Deceased

PHTLS—Medical Director
1983–present: Norman E. McSwain, Jr., MD, FACS, NREMT-P

PHTLS—Associate Medical Directors
2010–present: Lance E. Stuke, MD, MPH, FACS
2001–present: Jeffrey S. Guy, MD, FACS, EMT-P
2000–present: Peter T. Pons, MD, FACEP
1996–2010: Jeffrey Salomone, MD, FACS, NREMT-P
1994–2001: Scott B. Frame, MD, FACS, FCCM†
†Deceased

PHTLS Committee
Frank K. Butler, Jr., MD
Captain, U.S. Army Retired (Hon)
Chairperson
Committee on Tactical Combat Casualty Care
Joint Trauma System

Will Chapleau, EMT-P, RN, TNS
Chairperson, PHTLS Committee
Director of Performance Improvement, ATLS Program
American College of Surgeons
Chicago, Illinois

Gregory Chapman, EMT-P, RRT
Vice-Chairperson, PHTLS Committee
Center for Prehospital Medicine
Department of Emergency Medicine
Carolinas Medical Center
Charlotte, North Carolina

Jeffrey S. Guy, MD, MSc, MMHC, FACS
Associate Medical Director, PHTLS
Chief Medical Officer
TriStar Health System / HCA
Nashville, TN

Lawrence Hatfield, MEd, NREMT-P
Lead Analyst, Instructor
National Nuclear Security Administration
Emergency Operations Training Academy
Albuquerque, NM

Michael J. Hunter, EMT-P
Deputy Chief, Worcester EMS
UMass Memorial Medical Center— University Campus
Worcester, Massachusetts

Craig H. Jacobus, EMT-P, BA/BS, DC
EMS Faculty Metro Community College
Fremont, Nebraska

Mark Lueder, EMT-P
PHTLS Committee Chicago Heights Fire Department
Chicago Heights, Illinois

Norman E. McSwain, Jr., MD, FACS, NREMT-P
Medical Director, PHTLS
Professor of Surgery, Tulane University Department of Surgery
Trauma Director, Spirit of Charity Trauma Center, Interim LSU Hospital
Police Surgeon, New Orleans Police Department
New Orleans, Louisiana

Peter T. Pons, MD, FACEP
Associate Medical Director, PHTLS
Emergency Medicine
Denver, Colorado

Dennis Rowe, EMT-P
Director of Operations
Priority Ambulance
Knoxville, Tennessee

Lance E. Stuke, MD, MPH, FACS
Associate Medical Director, PHTLS
Assistant Professor of Surgery
Tulane University School of Medicine
New Orleans, Louisiana

Contributors to *PHTLS: Prehospital Trauma Life Support, Military Eighth Edition*

Special thanks and gratitude is extended to the medics, corpsmen, and pararescuers who may be called upon to risk their lives on the battlefield in order to use these Tactical Combat Casualty Care (TCCC) guidelines to save their wounded teammates.

The authors express their sincere appreciation to the many individuals, both military and civilian, who have assisted with writing the material contained in the military version of this Eighth Edition of *PHTLS: Prehospital Trauma Life Support.*

The TCCC Guidelines are the product of the Committee on Tactical Combat Casualty Care (CoTCCC). The editors extend their thanks to all of the members of the CoTCCC for the many hours that they have spent away from their primary duties in order to help keep the TCCC Guidelines updated. Thanks also to the members of the Core Board and the Trauma and Injury Subcommittee of the Defense Health Board for the critical oversight role that they play in reviewing proposed changes to the TCCC Guidelines.

Thanks also to the organizations that have supported the Committee on Tactical Combat Casualty Care in its decade of existence: The United States (U.S.) Special Operations Command, the Naval Operations Medicine Institute, and U.S. Army Institute of Surgical Research, the Bureau of Medicine and Surgery, the Office of the Surgeon General of the Army, and the Office of the Assistant Secretary of Defense for Health Affairs. Finally, thanks to the individuals who have played key roles in the establishment and or sustainment of the CoTCCC: Colonel Dave Hammer, Captain Doug Freer, Dr. John Holcomb, Ms. Ellen Embrey, and Rear Admiral Dave Smith.

Frank Butler, Jr., MD
Section Editor
Captain, U.S. Army Retired (Hon)
Chairperson
Committee on Tactical Combat Casualty Care
Joint Trauma System

Stephen D. Giebner, MD
Section Associate Editor
Captain, U.S. Army Retired (Hon)
Past Chairperson
Developmental Editor
Committee on Tactical Combat Casualty Care
Joint Trauma System

The Committee on Tactical Combat Casualty Care (CoTCCC)

CoTCCC Staff
Chairperson: Dr. Frank Butler
Developmental Editor: Dr. Steve Giebner
Senior Administrative Assistant:
   Ms. Danielle Davis

Voting Members
Dr. Jim Bagian
Col. Jeff Bailey
Cmrd. Sean Barbabella
Col. Peter Benson
Col. Lorne Blackbourne
Sgt. Maj. F. Bowling
Sgt. 1st Class Curt Conklin
Col. Jim Czarnik
Col. Joe Dubose
Col. Brian Eastridge
Col. Erin Edgar
Capt. Kyle Faudree
Dr. Doug Freer
Master Chief Hospital Corpsman
   Mike Grohman
Col. Kirby Gross
Capt. Matt Hickey
Dr. Jay Johannigman
Capt. Ken Kelly
Mr. Win Kerr
Capt. Bill Liston
Lt. Col. Bob Mabry
Lt. Col. Dave Marcozzi
Master Sgt. Harold Montgomery
Col. Al Murdock
Col. Kevin O'Connor
Lt. Cmdr. Dana Onifer

Dr. Mel Otten
Mr. Don Parsons
Mr. Gary Pesquera
Col. Todd Rasmussen
Chief Master Sgt. Tom Rich
Master Chief Petty Officer Glenn Royes
Lt. Col. Steve Rush
Col. Samual Sauer
Chief Master Sgt. Ryan Schultz
Col. Stacy Shackelford
Command Master Chief Petty
   Officer D. Eric Sine
Mr. Rick Strayer
Capt. Jeff Timby
Chief Hospital Corpsman Jeremy Torrisi
Command Master Chief Petty Officer Steve Viola

Designated Tactical Combat Casualty Care Subject Matter Experts
Dr. Frank Anders
Dr. Brad Bennett
Dr. Jeff Cain
Dr. Dave Callaway
Dr. Howard Champion
Dr. Paul Cordts
Dr. Warren Dorlac
Mr. Bill Donovan
Dr. Jim Dunne
Dr. Rocky Farr
Dr. Steve Flaherty
Dr. John Gandy
Dr. John Holcomb
Dr. Don Jenkins
Dr. Jim Kirkpatrick
Dr. Russ Kotwal
Dr. Norman McSwain
Dr. Peter Rhee

Frank Anders, MD
Colonel, U.S. Army Retired (Hon)

Frank Butler, Jr., MD
Captain, U.S. Army Retired (Hon)
Chairperson
Committee on Tactical Combat Casualty
    Care
Joint Trauma System

Col. Leopoldo Cancio, MD
U.S. Army Institute of Surgical Research
    Burn Center
San Antonio, Texas

**Howard Champion, MD, FRCS,
    FACS**
Senior Advisor in Trauma
Professor of Surgery
Uniformed Services University of
    Health Sciences
Bethesda, Maryland

Lt. Col. Kevin Chung, MD
U.S. Army Institute of Surgical Research
    Burn Center
San Antonio, Texas

Lt. Col. Peter J. Cuenca, MD
Brook Army Medical Center
San Antonio, Texas

**Col. Robert A. De Lorenzo,
    MD, MSM, MSCI**
U.S. Army Institute of Surgical
    Research
San Antonio, Texas

Col. Brian J. Eastridge, MD, FACS
Director, Joint Theater Trauma
    System
U.S. Army Institute of Surgical
    Research
San Antonio, Texas

John Gandy, MD
Uniformed Services University of the
    Health Sciences
Bethesda, Maryland

Keith S. Gates, MD, FACEP
Director, EMS Fellowship
Assistant Professor
Department of Emergency Medicine
The University of Texas
Health Science Center at Houston
Houston, Texas

Col. Robert T. Gerhardt, MD, MPH
Brook Army Medical Center
San Antonio, Texas

Maj. John Graybill
U.S. Army Institute of Surgical Research
    Burn Center
San Antonio, Texas

John Holcomb, MD, FACS
Vice Chair and Professor of Surgery
Chief, Division of Acute Care Surgery
Director, Center for Translational Injury
    Research
The University of Texas
Health Science Center at Houston
Houston, Texas

Col. Jay Johannigman, MD, FACS
Professor of Surgery
Chief, Division of Trauma and Surgical
    Critical Care
University Hospital
Cincinnati, Ohio

Col. Russ Kotwal, MD, MPH, FAAFP
Regimental Surgeon, 75th Ranger
    Regiment
Adjunct Assistant Professor, Department
    of Military and Emergency
    Medicine

Uniformed Services University of the
    Health Sciences
Bethesda, Maryland
Adjunct Assistant Professor, Department
    of Family and Community Medicine
Texas A&M Health Center
College Station, Texas

Col. Booker King
Director, U.S. Army Institute of Surgical
    Research Burn Center
San Antonio, Texas

Lt. Col. Jonathan Lundy, MD
U.S. Army Institute of Surgical Research
    Burn Center
San Antonio, Texas

Lt. Col. Robert Mabry, MD, FACEP
Physician Researcher
U.S. Army Institute of Surgical Research
San Antonio, Texas

**Master Sgt. Harold Montgomery,
    NREMT, ATP**
Regimental Senior Medic, 75th Ranger
    Regiment
U.S. Army Special Operations Command
Fort Bragg, North Carolina

Lt. Col. Wylan Peterson, MD
U.S. Army Institute of Surgical Research
    Burn Center
San Antonio, Texas

Col. Evan Ranz, MD
Commander, San Antonio Military
    Medical Center
San Antonio, Texas

**Command Master Chief Petty Officer
    D. Eric Sine, ATP, NREMT**
3d Marine Division
Okinawa, Japan

Reviewers

Linda M. Abrahamson, BA, ECRN, EMT-P, NCEE
Advocate Christ Medical Center—EMS Academy
Oak Lawn, Illinois

John Alexander, MS, NRP
Maryland Fire & Rescue Institute
University of Maryland
College Park, Maryland

Kristopher Ambrosia, FF, Paramedic, NCEE
Morton Fire Department
Morton, Illinois

Paul Arens, BS, NREMT-P
Iowa Central Community College
Fort Dodge, Iowa

William J. Armonaitis, MS, NREMT-P, NCEE
University Hospital EMS
Fairfield, New Jersey

Daniel Armstrong, DPT, MS, EMT
Queensborough Community College
Bayside, New York

Robyn M. Asher, EMT-P, IC, CC
Rural Metro of Tennessee
Knoxville, Tennessee

Juan M. Atan, MS, EMT-P
Orange County Fire Rescue
Orange County, Florida

Chuck Baird, MS, EFO, NREMT-P
Cobb County Fire and Emergency Services
Powder Springs, Georgia

Mark Baisley, MA, NREMT-P
Gold Cross Ambulance
Rochester, Minnesota

Stanley W. Baldwin
Foothill College
Los Altos Hills, California

Bruce Barry, RN, CEN, NREMT-P
Peak Paramedicine, LLC
Wilmington, New York

Ryan Batenhorst, BA, NREMT-P
Southeast Community College
Lincoln, Nebraska

John L. Beckman, AA, BS, FF/Paramedic, EMS Instructor
Addison Fire Protection District
Addison, Illinois

Deb Bell, MS, NREMT-P
Inspira Health Network—EMS
(previously Underwood-Memorial EMS)
Richland, New Jersey

Michael J. Berg, BSB/M, NREMT-P
Native Air/Air Methods
Globe, Arizona

Gerria Berryman, BS, EMT-P
Emergency Medical Training Professionals, LLC
Lexington, Kentucky

Robin E. Bishop, BA, MICP, CHS III, MEP
Crafton Hills College
Public Safety and Emergency Services Department
Yucaipa, California

Tobby Bishop, BS, NREMT-P
Spartanburg EMS
Spartanburg, South Carolina

Andy D. Booth, NREMT-P
Lanier Technical College
Oakwood, Georgia

Nick Bourdeau, RN, EMT-P I/C
Huron Valley Ambulance
Ann Arbor, Michigan

Sharon D. Boyles, BS, MEd, EMT-I
Shippensburg Area Senior High School
Shippensburg, Pennsylvania

Trent R. Brass, BS, EMT-P, RRT
SwedishAmerican Health System
Rockford, Illinois

Barbara Brennan, RN, BSN, CCRN
Hawaii PHTLS State Coordinator
Mililani, Hawaii

Lawrence D. Brewer, BA, NRP
Rogers State University
Claremore, Oklahoma

Billie Brown, BS, EMT-I, NREMT-P
Southern Alleganies, EMS Council
Saxton, Pennsylvania

Robert K. Browning, AAS, NR-P, HMC (SCW) USN
Medical Education and Training Campus
Department of Combat Medic Training
Fort Sam Houston, Texas

Cherylenn Buckley, AEMT, EMT-I
Hartford Hospital
Hartford, Connecticut

David Burdett, NREMT-P
Hamilton County EMS
Chattanooga, Tennessee

Helen E. Burkhalter, BAS, NREMT-P, RN
Atlanta Technical College
Atlanta, Georgia

Liza K. Burrill, AEMT
New Hampshire Bureau of EMS
Concord, New Hampshire

Kevin Carlisle, NREMT-P, Tactical Medic, 68W U.S. Army Reserves
Medical Center Ambulance Services
Madisonville, Kentucky

Elliot Carhart, EdD, RRT, NRP
Jefferson College of Health Sciences
Roanoke, Virginia

Greg Ceisner, EMT-P
Raleigh Fire Department
Raleigh, North Carolina

Bernadette Cekuta, BS, EMT-P, CIC
Dutchess Community College
Wappingers Falls, NY

Stacey G. Chapman, NREMT-P
Lancaster County EMS
Lancaster, South Carolina

Julie Chase, MSEd, FAWM FP-C
Immersion EMS Academy
Berryville, Virginia

Ted Chialtas, Fire Captain,
Paramedic
San Diego Fire-Rescue Department
EMSTA College
Santee, California

Patrick L. Churchwell, EMS
Instructor, EMT-P
Allen Fire Department
Allen, Texas

Jason L. Clark, NRP, CCEMT-P, FP-C,
CMTE
Erlanger Life Force
Chattanooga, Tennessee

John C. Cook, MBA, NREMT-P,
CCEMT-P, NCEE
Jefferson College of Health
Sciences
Roanoke, Virginia

Scott Cook, MS, CCEMT-P
Southern Maine Community College
South Portland, Maine

Patt Cope, MEd, NRP
Arkansas State University—Beebe
Searcy, Arkansas

Dennis L. Cosby, PM, CCP, EMS II
Lee County EMS Ambulance, Inc.
Donnellson, Iowa

Dwayne Cottel, ACP, A-EMCA,
CQIA, NCEE
Southwest Ontario Regional Base
Hospital Program
London Health Sciences Centre
London, Ontario, Canada

Shawn Crowley, MSN, RN,
CCEMT-P
Pee Dee Regional EMS
Florence, South Carolina

Lyndal M. Curry, MA, NRP
Southern Union State Community
College
Opelika, Alabama

Mark Deavers, Paramedic
Gouverneur Rescue Squad
Gouverneur, New York

James D. Dinsch, MS, NREMT-P
Indian River State College
Fort Pierce, Florida

Robert L. Ditch, EdD, MSHS, CEM,
NREMT-P
Arizona Academy of Emergency Services
Mesa, Arizona

Charles J. Dixon, NREMT-P, NCEE
Nucor Steel Berkeley EMS
Summerville, South Carolina

Stephanie Dornsife, MS, RN,
NREMT-P, CCEMT-P, I/C
Wentworth Douglass Hospital
Dover, New Hampshire

Rommie L. Duckworth, LP
New England Center for Rescue &
Emergency Medicine
Sherman, Connecticut

Michael J. Dunaway, BHS, NRP, CCP
Greenville Technical College
EMT/Paramedic Department
Greenville, South Carolina

Richard Ellis, BSOE, NRP
Central Georgia Technical College
Macon, Georgia

Erik M. Epskamp, Paramedic-IC,
Instructor II
Huron Valley Ambulance EMS
Education
Ann Arbor, Michigan

Shari Evans, RN, FP-C
Air Evac EMS. Inc,
Mineral Wells, Texas

Ronald L. Feller, Sr., MBA, NRP
Oklahoma EMS for Children
Oklahoma City Community College
Moore, Oklahoma

Tom Fitts, RN, NREMT-P, MEd
East Central College
Union, Missouri

Gustavo E. Flores, MD, EMT-P
UCC School of Medicine
Bayamón, Puerto Rico

Don Fortney, AS, NREMT-P,
CCEMT-P
EMMCO East, Inc.
Kersey, Pennsylvania

Frederick E. Fowler, BS, MPS,
Paramedic
EMS Solutions
Schuylerville, New York

Christopher Gage, AS, NRP, FP-C
Davidson County Community
College
Lexington, North Carolina

Alan Ganapol, EMT-B, EMT-I/C,
BChE, MChE
objectiveQUEST
West Tisbury, Massachusetts

Scott A. Gano, BS, NRP, FP-C,
CCEMT-P
Columbus State Community College
Columbus, Ohio

Scott C. Garrett, AHS, EFO, NRP,
CCP
Westview-Fairforest Fire Department
Spartanburg, South Carolina

William Scott Gilmore, MD, EMT-P
Washington University School of
Medicine
St. Louis Fire Department
Saint Louis, Missouri

David Glendenning, EMT-P
New Hanover Regional Medical
Center—EMS
Wilmington, North Carolina

Kathleen D. Grote, EMT-P
Anne Arundel County Fire Department
Millersville, Maryland

Anthony Guerne, BA, NREMT-P
Suffolk County Emergency Medical
    Services
Suffolk County, New York

James R. Hanley, MD, FAAP
Ochsner Clinic Foundation Hospital
Department of Emergency Medicine
New Orleans, Louisiana

Poul Anders Hansen, MD
Head of the Prehospital Care
    Organization, North Denmark Region
Chair PHTLS Denmark
Aalborg, Denmark

Anthony S. Harbour, BSN, MEd, RN,
    NRP
Southern Virginia Emergency Medical
    Services
Roanoke, Virginia

Randy Hardick, BA, NREMT-P
Saddleback College Paramedic Program
Mission Viejo, California

Richard Hayne, RN
Glendale Community College
Glendale, California

Timothy M. Hellyer, MAT, EMT-P
Ivy Tech Community College
South Bend, Indiana

Greg P. Henington, L. Paramedic,
    NREMT-P
Terlingua Fire & EMS
Terlingua, Texas

Victor Robert Hernandez, BA, EMT-P
Emergency Training & Consultations
Truckee, California

David A. Hiltbrunn, AGS, NRP, CCTP
St. Mary Corwin Pre-Hospital Education
Pueblo, Colorado

Ed Hollowell, RN, CFRN, CEN,
    NREMT-P, CCP-C, FF
Regional Fire & Rescue
Estrella Mountain Community College
Avondale, Arizona

Cathryn A. Holstein, CCEMT-P, SEI
Rural/Metro Ambulance
Seattle, Washington

Dana Hunnewell, NREMT-P,
    CCEMT-P
Chocowinity EMS
Chocowinity, North Carolina

Scott A. Jaeggi, AS, EMT-P
Mt. San Antonio College EMT &
    Paramedic Program
Walnut, California

Vanessa L. Jewett, RN, CEN,
    NREMT-P
EMSTAR Educational Facility
Elmira, New York

Michael B. Johnson, MS, NRP
Wallace State College
Hanceville, Alabama

Vincent J. Johnson, EMT-P
New York City Fire Department
New York, New York

Karen Jones, EMT-P
Mason County EMS
Point Pleasant, West Virginia

Twilla Jones, NREMT
South Bossier Parish Fire
    District Two
Elm Grove, Louisiana

Kevin F. Jura, NRP
State of Maryland Department of
    Health & Mental Hygiene
Office of Preparedness &
    Response
Baltimore, Maryland

Greg J. Kapinos, EMT-P I/C, MPH,
    SPHR
Solutions in Human Resource
    Management
Scarborough, Maine

Charmaine Kaptur, BSN, RN, NRP
Tualatin Valley Fire & Rescue
Sherwood, Oregon

Kevin Keen, AEMCA
Hamilton Fire Department
Hamilton, Ontario, Canada

David Kemper, EMT-P, FP-C, CMTE,
    NAEMSE
University of Cincinnati Medical Center
Cincinnati, Ohio

Michael Kennard, AS, Paramedic, I/C
New Hampshire Division of Fire
    Standards and Training—EMS
Concord, New Hampshire

Alan F. Kicks, BE, EMT-Instructor
Bergen County EMS Training Center
Paramus, New Jersey

Randall C. Kirby, BS/EMTP, PCC, I/C
Tennessee Technological University
Hartsville, Tennessee

Melodie J. Kolmetz, PA-C, EMT-P
Monroe Ambulance
Rochester, New York

Edward "Ted" Lee, AAS, BS, MEd,
    NREMT-P, CCEMT-P
Trident Technical College
Charleston South Carolina

William J. Leggio, Jr., EdD, MS, BS
    EMS, NREMT-P
Prince Sultan bin Abdul Aziz College
    for EMS
King Saud University
Riyadh, Kingdom of Saudi Arabia

David C. Leisten, BA, CCEMT-P,
    NREMT-P
Rochester, New York

Arthur J. Lewis II, NREMT-P
East Baton Rouge Parish
Department of Emergency Medical
    Services
Baton Rouge, Louisiana

Robert Loiselle, MA, NREMT-P,
    EMSIC
Education Training Connection
McLaren Bay Region EMS
Midland, Michigan

Elizabeth Morgan Luter, NREMT-P
O'Fallon, Missouri

Kevin M. Lynch, NYS-EMT/NYS-CLI
Greenburgh Police/EMS
Eastchester, New York

Susan M. Macklin, BS, EMT-P
Central Carolina Community College
Olivia, North Carolina

Larry Macy, NREMT-P
Western Wyoming Community College
Rock Springs, Wyoming

Jeanette S. Mann, RN, BSN,
NREMT-P
Dabney S. Lancaster Community College
Clifton Forge, Virginia

Amy Marsh, BA, NREMT-P
Sioux Falls Fire Rescue
Sioux Falls, South Dakota

Scott Matin, MBA
MONOC
Wall, New Jersey

Nancy Mayeda-Brescia, MD, OTD,
APRN, MBA, EMSI, NREMT-P
Rocky Hill EMS
Rocky Hill, Connecticut

David "Bernie" McBurnett, AAS,
NREMT-P I/C
Chattanooga Fire Department
Chattanooga, Tennessee

Randall McCargar, NREMT-P
Cherry Hill Fire Department
Cherry Hill, New Jersey

Kevin McCarthy, MPA, NREMT-P
Adjunct Faculty-Department
of Emergency Services
Utah Valley University
Orem, Utah

Candace McClain, MBA, BSN, RN,
NREMT-P, CEN, CCEMT-P
Ray County Ambulance District
Orrick, Missouri

Cliff McCollum, Chief, EMT-B, Senior
EMS Instructor
Pierce County Fire District 13
Tacoma, Washington

Joseph R. McConomy, Jr., MICP, EMT-I
Burlington County Emergency Services
Training Center
Westampton, New Jersey

Michael McDonald, RN, NRP
Loudoun County Department of Fire
Rescue and Emergency Management
Leesburg, Virginia

Gerard McEntee, MS, EMT-P
Union County College
Plainfield, New Jersey

Janis J. McManus, MS, NREMT-P
Virtua Emergency Medical Services
Mt Laurel, New Jersey

Matt McQuisten, BS, NRP
Avera Health
Sioux Falls, South Dakota

Darren S. Meador, NREMT-P
Valle Ambulance District
Desoto, Missouri

Christopher Metsgar, MS, NRP, NCEE
HealthONE EMS
Englewood, Colorado

Kelly Miyashiro, EMT
American Medical Response
Seattle, Washington

Jerry D. Morris, BA, NREMT-P
Center for Prehospital Medicine
Carolinas Medical Center
Charlotte, North Carolina

Frederick Mueller, EMTP, NREMT-P,
EMS I/C
Temple University Health System
Transport Team
Philadelphia, Pennsylvania

Daniel W. Murdock, AAS,
NREMT-P, CLI
SUNY Cobleskill Paramedic Program
Cobleskill, New York

Ivan A. Mustafa, EMT/P, MSN,
ARNP-C, CEMSO, EFO, CFO
Seminole County Fire Department
Sanford, Florida

Thomas W. Nichols, AAS,
NREMT-P
Tulsa Technology Center
Tulsa, Oklahoma

Keith Noble, Captain, MS, TX LP,
NREMT-P
Austin Travis County EMS
Kyle, Texas

Chris O'Connor, MSc, Dip EMT,
NREMT-P, NQEMT-AP
Medical Ambulance Service
Dublin, Ireland

Amiel B. Oliva, BSN, RN, R-EMT-B
EMR Healthcare & Safety Institute
Quezon City, Philippines

Chris Ottolini, EMT-P
Coast Life Support District
Gualala, California
Santa Rosa Junior College Public Safety
Training Center
Windsor, California

Norma Pancake, BS, MEP,
NREMT-P
Pierce County EMS Office
Tacoma, Washington

Sean F. Peck, MEd, EMT-P
WestMed College
Chula Vista, California

Mark Peterson, NREMT-P
Hardin County EMS
Elizabethtown, Kentucky

Rick Petrie, EMT-P
Atlantic Partners EMS
Winslow, Maine

Deborah L. Petty, BS, CICP,
EMT-P I/C
St. Charles County Ambulance
District
St. Peters, Missouri

John C. Phelps II, MAM, BS,
NREMT-P
Sutton County EMS
UTHSCSA
Sonora, Texas

Mark Podgwaite, NRAEMT,
NECEMS I/C
Vermont EMS District 5
Danville, Vermont

John Eric Powell, PhD
Walters State Community College
Morristown, Tennessee

Alice J. Quiroz, BSN, CM
Past Affiliate Faculty
349th Medical Group, Travis Air Force
    Base (2001–2008)
Gold River, California

Stephen Rea, NREMT-P, BS/HCM
Thomas Jefferson EMS Council
Charlottesville, Virginia

John Reed, MPH, BSN, RN,
    Paramedic
Birmingham Regional EMS System
Birmingham, Alabama

Timothy J. Reitz, BS, NREMT-P,
    NCEE
Conemaugh Memorial Medical Center
School of EMS
Johnstown, Pennsylvania

Les Remington, EMT-P, I/C, EMS
    Educator
Genesys Regional Medical Center
Grand Blanc, Michigan

Deborah Richeal, NREMT-P, EMS
    Educator
Capital Health System
Trenton, New Jersey

Paul Richardson, Paramedic, Lead
    Instructor
OSK St. Francis Medical Center
Peoria, Illinois

Katharine P. Rickey, BS,
    NRParamedic, EMS I/C
EMS Educator
Epsom, New Hampshire

Nicholas Russell, AAS, NREMT-P,
    EMS-I
Edgewood Fire/EMS
Edgewood, Kentucky

Thomas Russell, MS, Paramedic
CT Training & Consulting Institute
Portland, Connecticut

Christopher T. Ryther, MS, NRP
American River College
Sacramento, California

Paul Salway, Lieutenant, CCEMT-P,
    NREMT-P
South Portland Fire Department
South Portland, Maine

Ian T. T. Santee, MICT, MPA
City and County of Honolulu
Honolulu Emergency Services
    Department
Honolulu, Hawaii

Jason Scheiderer, BA, NREMT-P
Wishard EMS
IUPUI
Indianapolis EMS
Indianapolis, Indiana

Justin Schindler, NREMT-P
Brighton Volunteer Ambulance
Rochester, New York

Jared Schoenfeld, NREMT-P, CIC,
    AHA TCF
Kingsboro Community College
Brooklyn, New York

Barry M. Schyma, BSc (hons)
    Biomed, MBChB, FRCA
Department of Anaesthetics, Critical
    Care and Pain Medicine
Royal Infirmary of Edinburgh
United Kingdom

Anthony Scott, BA, NREMT-P
Montgomery County,
    Maryland Division of
    Fire/Rescue Services
Westminster, Maryland

Christopher M. Seguin, NR-P,
    EMS-I/C
Northwoods Center for Continuing
    Education
Campton, New Hampshire

William D. Shelton, AAS, BS,
    NREMT-P
Fayetteville Technical Community
    College
Benson, North Carolina

Shadrach Smith, BS Bio, NREMT-P,
    LP
Paramedic Advantage
Orange, California

Bradley L. Spratt, BS, LP, NRP, EMS-I
Salus Training Solutions
The Woodlands, Texas

Tynell N. Stackhouse, MTh, NREMT-P
Pee Dee Regional EMS, Inc.
Florence, South Carolina

Robert Stakem, Jr., CCEMT-P
Harrisburg Area Community College
Harrisburg, Pennsylvania

Andrew W. Stern, NREMT-P,
    CCEMT-P, MA, MPA
Hudson Valley Community College
Cardiorespiratory & Emergency Medicine
    Department
Troy, New York

R. E. Suarez, CCEMT-P, NCEE
Suarez, Leppert, & Associates, LLC
Cape Fear Tactical Medicine
Clermont, Florida

Daniel A. Svenson, BA, NREMT-P
Portland Fire Department
Westbrook, Maine

David M. Tauber, BS, NR-P, CCEMT-P,
    FP-C, NCEE
Yale New Haven Sponsor Hospital
New Haven, Connecticut
Advanced Life Support Institute
Conway, New Hampshire

Brent Thomas, Paramedic
Orillia Fire Department
Orillia, Ontario, Canada

Candice Thompson, BS, LAT,
    NREMT-P
Centre for Emergency Health Sciences
Spring Branch, Texas

Joshua Tilton, FF-II, NR-P, CCEMT-P,
    EMS-I, FF-I
Malta-McConnelsville Fire
    Department
Zanesville, Ohio

William F. Toon, EdD, NREMT-P
Johnson County MED-ACT
Olathe, Kansas

William Torres, Jr., NREMT-P
Marcus Daley Hospital—EMS
Hamilton, Montana

Patricia Tritt, RN, MA
HealthONE EMS
Englewood, Colorado

Brian J. Turner, NREMT-P, CCEMT-P, RN
Clinton, Iowa

Elsa Tuttle, RN, BSN, CCEMT-P
Central Jackson County Fire Protection District
Blue Springs, Missouri

Rebecca Valentine, BS, EMT-P, I/C, NCEE
Clinical Education Specialist
Natick, Massachusetts

Sara VanDusseldorp, NREMT-P, CCEMT-P, NCEE
Burlington, Wisconsin

Eric P. Victorin, MBA, EMT-I, NREMT-P
Dutchess Community College
Wappingers Falls, New York

Patricia A. Vincent, NREMT-P, MICP, BSOE
Anchorage Fire Department
Anchorage, Alaska

Carl Voskamp, LP, CCEMT-P
Victoria College
Victoria, Texas

Gary S. Walter, BA, NREMT-P
Union College
International Rescue and Relief Program
Lincoln, Nebraska

David Watson, NREMT-P, CCEMT-P
Pickens County EMS
Pickens, South Carolina

Christopher Weaver, NRP, CCEMT-P
Venture Crew 911
St. Anthony Hospital
Lakewood, Colorado

Ernie Whitener, MS, LP
Texas A&M Engineering Extension Service
Station, Texas

Charlie Williams, EMTP, EdS
Walters State Community College
Morristown, Tennessee

Jackilyn E. Williams, RN, MSN, NREMT-P
Portland Community College Paramedic Program
Portland, Oregon

Evelyn Wilson, MHS, NREMT-P
Western Carolina University
Cullowhee, North Carolina

Rich Wisniewski, BS, NREMT-P
South Carolina Department of Health and Environmental Control
Division of EMS and Trauma
Columbia, South Carolina

Andrew L. Wood, MS, NREMT-P
Emergency Medical Training Professionals, LLC
Lexington, Kentucky

Michael J. Young, BS, MEd, NREMT-P, CCEMT-P
University of Maryland Fire and Rescue Institute, ALS Division
Oxford, Maryland

Justin Yurong, BS, NRP
Yakima County Department of EMS
Yakima, Washington

Jeff Zuckernick, BS, MBA, NREMT-P
University of Hawaii—Kapiolani Community College
Honolulu, Hawaii

PHTLS Honor Roll

PHTLS continues to prosper and promote high standards of trauma care all over the world. This success would not be possible without the contributions of many dedicated and inspired individuals over the past three decades. Some of those mentioned below were instrumental in the development of our first textbook. Others were constantly "on the road" spreading the word. Still others "put out fires" and otherwise problem-solved to keep PHTLS growing. The PHTLS Committee, along with the editors and contributors of this, our eighth edition, would like to express our thanks to all of those listed below. PHTLS lives, breathes, and grows because of the efforts of those who volunteer their time to what they believe in.

Gregory H. Adkisson, MD
Melissa Alexander
Jameel Ali, MD
Stuart Alves
Augie Bamonti
J. M. Barnes
Morris L. Beard
Ann Bellows
Ernest Block, MD
Chip Boehm
Don E. Boyle, MD
Susan Brown
Susan Briggs, MD
Jonathan Busko
Alexander Butman
H. Jeannie Butman
Christain E. Callsen, Jr.
Steve Carden, MD
Edward A. Casker
Bud Caukin
Hank Christen
David Ciraulo
Victoria Cleary
Philip Coco
Frederick J. Cole
Keith Conover
Arthur Cooper, MD
Jel Coward
Michael D'Auito
Alice "Twink" Dalton
Judith Demarest
Joseph P. Dineen, MD
Leon Dontigney, MD
Joan Drake-Olsen
Mark Elcock, MD
Blaine L. Endersen, MD
Betsy Ewing
Mary E. Fallat, MD
Milton R. Fields, III
Scott B. Frame, MD†
Sheryl G. A. Gabram

Bret Gilliam
Jack Grandey
Vincent A. Greco
Nita J. Ham
Mark C. Hodges
Walter Idol
Alex Isakov, MD
Lenworth Jacobs, MD
Craig Jacobus
Lou Jordan
Richard Judd
Jon A. King
Eduard Kompast
Jon R. Krohmer, MD
Peter LeTarte, MD
Robert W. Letton, Jr.
Mark Lockhart
Dawn Loehn
Robert Loftus
Greg C. Lord
Fernando Magallenes-Negrete, MD
Paul M. Maniscalco
Scott W. Martin
Don Mauger
William McConnell, DO
Merry McSwain
John Mechtel
Claire Merrick
Bill Metcalf
George Moerkirk
Stephen Murphy
Lawrence D. Newell
Jeanne O'Brien
Dawn Orgeron
Eric Ossmann
James Paturas
Joseph Pearce
Thomas Petrich
Valerie J. Phillips, MD
James Pierce
Brian Plaisier

Mark Reading
Brian Reiselbara
Lou Romig, MD
Jeffrey S. Salomone, MD
Donald Scelza
John Sigafoos
Paul Silverston, MD
David Skinner
Dale C. Smith
Richard Sobieray
Sheila Spaid
Michael Spain
Don Stamper
Kenneth G. Swan, MD
Kenneth G. Swan, Jr., MD
David M. Tauber
Joseph J. Tepas III, MD
Brian M. Tibbs
Josh Vayer
Richard Vomacka†
Demetrios Vourvachakis, MD†
Robert K. Waddell, II
Michael Werdmann
Carl Werntz
Elizabeth Wertz
Keith Wesley, MD
David E. Wesson
Roger D. White, MD
Kenneth J. Wright
David Wuertz
Al Yellin, MD
Steven Yevich
Doug York
Alida Zamboni

Again, thanks to all of you, and thanks to everyone around the world for making PHTLS work.

PHTLS Committee
Editors and Contributors of PHTLS

†Deceased

Foreword

Prehospital personnel perform a unique service that cannot be rendered by any other individual or group. Through effective application of their knowledge and skills at the scene of an accident or illness, they are in the enviable position to be able to save lives and prevent or alleviate suffering.

Patients in the prehospital setting do not get to choose their providers. These providers accept the responsibility to deliver patient care in some of the worst situations. The scene is often chaotic, accompanied by hazard and even inclement weather. The professionalism that defines prehospital personnel ensures that patients are cared for by someone who is well trained and prepared, and who brings a passion and caring that is a unique inspiration in medicine.

All medical professionals ultimately have a bond with the public, and the public's trust in us is based on our preparedness and accountability. Prehospital Trauma Life Support (PHTLS) provides the basis for this trust in prehospital trauma care. By design, it links to Advanced Trauma Life Support (ATLS) at the hospital level. The basic premise of PHTLS is that prehospital care providers think critically, particularly under stress, and use their technical skills to deliver excellent patient care, based on an excellent foundation of knowledge.

Of all the advancements in trauma care in the last 50 years, the development of prehospital care, the training that establishes readiness, and the development of trauma centers and trauma systems have led to the greatest reductions in mortality. Dr. Norman McSwain, for over 40 years, has dedicated his life to developing prehospital care. In partnership with Will Chapleau over the last 20 years, they have developed the PHTLS program to the point that it is the standard for prehospital care in trauma throughout the world.

Their partnership has been accompanied by the contributions of many others, but their relationship and the professionalism they have engendered through their leadership have made the program what it is today. Prehospital care providers are proud individuals and carry their heads high with the utmost dedication. We would not see the amazing accomplishments that have occurred in trauma care without their participation. Their professionalism is in part due to the leadership provided by Dr. McSwain and Mr. Chapleau.

On behalf of the Eighth Edition contributors and through my honor to write this foreword, I would like to dedicate the Eighth Edition of the PHTLS program textbook to the partnerships and teamwork we see every day in prehospital care providers and the physicians and nurses they work with. This is exemplified by the leadership model and by living the values of Dr. McSwain and Mr. Chapleau. We are lucky to have the legacy created in the prehospital community and the contributions that these two leaders have provided to make this possible.

David B. Hoyt, MD, FACS
Executive Director
American College of Surgeons
Chicago, Illinois

Preface for *PHTLS: Prehospital Trauma Life Support, Military Eighth Edition*

If you are a combatant wounded on the battlefield, the most critical phase of your care is the period from the time of injury until the time that you arrive at a surgically capable medical treatment facility (MTF). Almost 90% of American service men and women who die from combat wounds do so before they arrive at an MTF, thus highlighting the importance of the battlefield trauma care that is provided by our combat medics, corpsmen, and pararescuemen (PJs), as well as by the casualties themselves and their fellow combatants.

Most of the U.S. military went to war in Afghanistan and Iraq with battlefield trauma care strategies that were not based on Tactical Combat Casualty Care (TCCC), and even in the recent past much of the U.S. military had not implemented all of the TCCC Guidelines. Only a select few Special Operations and conventional units went to war with robust TCCC capability. The 75th Ranger Regiment, for example, taught the concepts of TCCC to everyone in the Regiment as part of their TCCC-based Casualty Response Plan. The Regiment documented a preventable prehospital death rate of 0%, an unprecedented success in optimizing casualty survival on the battlefield. The overall incidence of preventable deaths among U.S. combat fatalities occurring in the prehospital phase of care is 24%.

As a result, prehospital trauma care in the military has undergone an unprecedented transformation since the beginning of the conflicts in Afghanistan and Iraq. Combat medical personnel in the U.S. military (and those of most of our coalition partners) are now trained to manage combat trauma on the battlefield using the TCCC Guidelines. TCCC started as a biomedical research project in the U.S. Special Operations Command (USSOCOM). The largely tradition-based trauma care practices that were in place in 1993 were systematically re-evaluated and found in need of revision. TCCC was introduced as a new framework on which to build trauma care guidelines customized for the battlefield. The original TCCC paper came out in Military Medicine in 1996 and provided a foundation, but TCCC has been in constant state of evolution during the last 13 years. These trauma care guidelines customized for use on the battlefield are now reviewed and updated by the Committee on TCCC (CoTCCC) on an ongoing basis. The CoTCCC is composed of trauma surgeons, emergency medicine physicians, combatant unit physicians, and combat medics, corpsmen, and PJs. There are also physician assistants and military medical educators among the members. At present the CoTCCC has representation from all of the U.S. armed services, and has the membership has 100% deployment experience. Although previously part of the Defense Health Board, the CoTCCC now functions as part of the Joint Trauma System.

Changes in TCCC are based on direct input from combat medical personnel, an ongoing review of published medical literature, new research coming from military medical research organizations, lessons learned from U.S. and allied service medical departments, and trauma conferences conducted by the Joint Trauma System and the Armed Forces Medical Examiners System.

The CoTCCC publishes its recommendations in both the *Journal of Special Operations Medicine* and the *Prehospital Trauma Life Support Manual*. The TCCC Guidelines are the only set of battlefield trauma care best-practice guidelines to have received the triple endorsement of the American College of Surgeons Committee on Trauma (ACS-COT), the National Associations of Emergency Medical Technicians (NAEMT), and the Department of Defense (DoD).

As the CoTCCC has continued to work to improve battlefield trauma care, it has formed strategic partnerships with other organizations that seek to improve prehospital trauma care in non-combat settings. TCCC began its partnership with the Prehospital Trauma Life Support (PHTLS) Committee in 1998 and continues to work with this internationally recognized group of leaders in prehospital trauma care. The PHTLS organization teaches its courses around the world and has recently established a program to provide TCCC training to law enforcement agencies and the militaries of allied countries when these groups request it.

TCCC established a critical partnership with the U.S. Army Institute of Surgical Research (USAISR) in 2004. The USAISR undertook the first preventable death analysis on fatalities from Afghanistan and Iraq, which helped to highlight the critical need for all combatants to be trained in basic TCCC interventions. The USAISR subsequently developed a research effort with a strong focus on battlefield first responder care and published breakthrough reports on items such as tourniquets, hemostatic agents, junctional tourniquets, chest seals and prehospital fluid resuscitation. This ongoing work has since firmly established USAISR as the Department of Defense leader in developing and evaluating battlefield trauma care technology and management strategies. The USAISR also led the very successful USSOCOM-sponsored TCCC Transition Initiative designed to ensure that deploying Special Operations units were equipped with the latest TCCC technologies and that feedback about both the training and the equipment was captured when the units returned from their combat deployments. It was the success of that project that provided the impetus for the eventual adoption of TCCC by conventional forces in addition to Special Operations units.

Meetings of the CoTCCC are attended by representatives from combat units, the service Surgeons Generals' offices, liaisons from allied nations, stakeholders from non-DoD government agencies, and representatives from federal law enforcement agencies. The Defense Health Agency – Medical Logistics Office is present to ensure that TCCC equipment issues, both in procurement and performance, are tracked by and discussed with the group. All of the above participants have played key roles in proposing, refining, and gaining approval for recent changes in the TCCC Guidelines. This robust interaction has helped to ensure that TCCC continues to reflect the state of the art in battlefield trauma care.

The TCCC Guidelines are best-practice trauma care guidelines customized for use on the battlefield and are updated in real time as additional combat experience is gained. **They are guidelines only – there are no rigid protocols in combat, including Tactical Combat Casualty Care**. If the recommended TCCC combat trauma management plan doesn't work for the specific tactical setting that a combat medic, corpsman, or PJ encounters, then care must be modified to best fit the tactical situation. **TCCC is a combination of good medicine and good tactics, and scenario-based planning is critical its successful application.**

Frank K Butler, Jr., MD
Captain, U.S. Army Retired (Hon)
Chairperson
Committee on Tactical Combat Casualty Care

Preface

Providers of prehospital care must accept the responsibility to provide patient care that is as close to absolutely perfect as possible. This cannot be achieved with insufficient knowledge of the subject. We must remember that the patient did not choose to be involved in a traumatic situation. On the other hand, the prehospital care provider has chosen to be there to take care of the patient. The prehospital care provider is obligated to give 100% of his or her effort during contact with every patient. The patient has had a bad day; the prehospital care provider cannot also have a bad day. The prehospital care provider must be sharp and capable in the competition between the patient and trauma and death.

The patient is the most important person at the scene of an emergency. There is no time to think about the order in which the patient assessment is performed or what treatments should take priority over others. There is no time to practice a skill before using it on a particular patient. There is no time to think about where equipment or supplies are housed within the jump kit. There is no time to think about where to transport the injured patient. All of this information and more must be stored in the prehospital care provider's mind, and all supplies and equipment must be present in the jump kit when the provider arrives on the scene. Without the proper knowledge or equipment, the prehospital care provider may neglect to do things that could increase the patient's chance of survival. The responsibilities of a prehospital care provider are too great to make such mistakes.

Those who deliver care in the prehospital setting are integral members of the trauma patient care team, as are the nurses or physicians in the emergency department, operating room, intensive care unit, ward, and rehabilitation unit. Prehospital care providers must be practiced in their skills so that they can move the patient quickly and efficiently out of the environment of the emergency and transport the patient quickly to the closest appropriate hospital.

Why PHTLS?

Course Education Philosophy

Prehospital Trauma Life Support (PHTLS) focuses on principles, not preferences. By focusing on the principles of good trauma care, PHTLS promotes critical thinking. The PHTLS Committee of the National Association of Emergency Medical Technicians (NAEMT) believes that emergency medical services (EMS) practitioners make the best decisions on behalf of their patients when given a sound foundation of key principles and evidence-based knowledge. Rote memorization of mnemonics is discouraged. Furthermore, there is no one "PHTLS way" of performing a specific skill. The principle of the skill is taught, and then one acceptable method of performing the skill that meets the principle is presented. The authors realize that no one method can apply to the myriad of unique situations encountered in the prehospital setting.

Up-to-Date Information

Development of the PHTLS program began in 1981, on the heels of the inception of the Advanced Trauma Life Support (ATLS) program for physicians. As the ATLS course is revised every 4 to 5 years, pertinent changes are incorporated into the next edition of PHTLS. This eighth edition of the PHTLS program has been revised based on the 2012 ATLS course as well as subsequent publications in the medical literature. Although following the ATLS principles, PHTLS is specifically designed for the unique requirements of caring for trauma patients in the prehospital setting. A new chapter has been added, and other chapters have been extensively revised. The new chapter includes information on the physiology of life and death. Video clips of critical skills and an eBook are available online.

Scientific Base

The authors and editors have adopted an "evidence-based" approach that includes references from medical literature supporting the key principles, and additional position papers published by national organizations are cited when applicable. Many references have been added, allowing those prehospital care providers with inquisitive minds to read the scientific data supporting our recommendations.

The PHTLS Family of Educational Offerings

Since the introduction of the PHTLS course in 1981, PHTLS has continued to expand its educational offerings to encompass all levels and types of prehospital trauma care providers.

- **PHTLS:** A 16-hour course for emergency medical responders, emergency medical technicians, paramedics, nurses, physician assistants, and physicians. The PHTLS provider course is offered in one of two formats: the traditional face-to-face format with lectures and skill stations; or a hybrid format, where a portion of the course is taken online in an interactive, web-based format, followed by one day of face-to-face classroom interaction for skill station instructions and evaluations.
- **PHTLS Refresher Course:** An 8-hour course for individuals who have successfully completed a PHTLS provider course or other approved trauma provider course within the past 4 years.

- **Trauma First Response (TFR):** An 8-hour course that teaches the principles of PHTLS to non-EMS practitioners, including first responders (emergency medical responders), police officers, fire fighters, rescue personnel, and safety officers, to help them prepare to care for trauma patients while serving as part of a transport team or awaiting a transport provider.
- **Tactical Combat Casualty Care (TCCC):** A 16-hour course that introduces evidence-based, lifesaving techniques and strategies for providing the best trauma care on the battlefield. TCCC courses are conducted under the auspices of PHTLS. The course is designed for combat EMS/military personnel, including medics, corpsmen, and pararescue personnel deploying in support of combat operations. NAEMT's TCCC courses use the *PHTLS: Prehospital Trauma Life Support, Military Edition,* textbook and are fully compliant with the Department of Defense's Committee on Tactical Combat Casualty Care (CoTCCC) guidelines. It is the only TCCC course endorsed by the American College of Surgeons.
- **Tactical Emergency Casualty Care (TECC):** A 16-hour course, derived from TCCC, that introduces evidence-based, lifesaving techniques and strategies for providing the best trauma care in the civilian tactical situation or hazardous environment. TECC courses are conducted under the auspices of PHTLS. The course is designed for civilian EMS responders deploying in support of tactical or other hazardous operations.
- **Law Enforcement and First Response Tactical Casualty Care (LEFR-TCC):** An 8-hour course that teaches public safety first responders including police, other law enforcement officers, fire fighters, and other first responders (emergency medical responders) the basic medical care interventions that will help save an injured responder's life until EMS practitioners can safely enter a tactical scene. It combines the principles of PHTLS and TCCC, and meets the recommendations of the Hartford Consensus document and TECC guidelines.
- **Bleeding Control for the Injured (BCon):** A 2-hour course that teaches lay individuals the basic steps necessary to stop external hemorrhage after a traumatic event.

PHTLS—Commitment and Mission

As we continue to pursue the potential of the PHTLS course and the worldwide community of prehospital care providers, we must remember the goals and objectives of the PHTLS program:

- To provide a description of the physiology and kinematics of injury
- To provide an understanding of the need for rapid assessment of the trauma patient
- To advance the participant's level of knowledge in regard to examination and diagnostic skills
- To enhance the participant's performance in the assessment and treatment of the trauma patient
- To advance the participant's level of competence in regard to specific prehospital trauma intervention skills
- To provide an overview and establish a management method for the prehospital care of the multisystem trauma patient
- To promote a common approach for the initiation and transition of care beginning with civilian first responders continuing up and through the levels of care until the patient is delivered to definitive medical care

It is also fitting to reprise our mission statement, which was written in a marathon session at the NAEMT conference in 1997:

> The Prehospital Trauma Life Support (PHTLS) program of the National Association of Emergency Medical Technicians (NAEMT) serves trauma victims through the global education of prehospital care providers of all levels. With medical oversight from the American College of Surgeons Committee on Trauma (ACS-COT), the PHTLS programs develop and disseminate educational materials and scientific information, and promote excellence in trauma patient management by all providers involved in the delivery of prehospital care.

The PHTLS mission also enhances the achievement of the NAEMT mission. The PHTLS program is committed to quality and performance improvement. As such, PHTLS is always attentive to changes in technology and methods of delivering prehospital trauma care that may be used to enhance the clinical and service quality of this program.

Support for NAEMT

NAEMT provides the administrative structure for the PHTLS program. All profits from the PHTLS program are channeled back into NAEMT to provide funding for issues and programs that are of prime importance to EMS professionals, such as educational conferences and advocacy efforts on behalf of prehospital care providers.

PHTLS Is a World Leader

Because of the unprecedented success of the prior editions of PHTLS, the program has continued to grow by leaps and bounds. PHTLS courses continue to proliferate across the United States, and the U.S. military has adopted it, teaching the program to U.S. Armed Forces personnel at over 100 course sites worldwide. PHTLS has been taught in more than 66 nations, and many others are expressing interest in bringing PHTLS to their countries in efforts to improve prehospital trauma care.

Prehospital care providers have the responsibility to assimilate this knowledge and these skills in order to use them for the benefit of the patients for whom they are responsible. The editors and authors of this material and the PHTLS Committee of NAEMT hope that you will incorporate this information into your practice and daily rededicate yourself to the care of those persons who cannot care for themselves—the trauma patients.

National Association of Emergency Medical Technicians

The National Association of Emergency Medical Technicians (NAEMT) was founded in 1975 to serve and represent the professional interests of EMS practitioners, including paramedics, emergency medical technicians, and emergency medical responders. NAEMT members work in all sectors of EMS, including government service agencies, fire departments, hospital-based ambulance services, private companies, industrial and special operations settings, and the military.

One of NAEMT's principal activities is EMS continuing education. The mission of NAEMT continuing education programs is to improve patient care through high-quality, cost-effective, evidence-based education that strengthens and enhances the knowledge and skills of EMS practitioners.

NAEMT strives to provide the highest quality continuing education programs. All NAEMT continuing education programs are developed by highly experienced EMS educators, clinicians, and medical directors. Course content incorporates the latest research, newest techniques, and innovative approaches in EMS learning. All NAEMT continuing education programs promote critical thinking as the foundation for providing quality care. This is based on the belief that EMS practitioners make the best decisions on behalf of their patients when given a sound foundation of evidence-based knowledge and key principles.

Once developed, continuing education programs are tested and refined to ensure that course materials are clear, accurate, and relevant to the needs of EMS practitioners. Finally, all continuing education programs are regularly updated no less than every 4 years to ensure that the content incorporates the most up-to-date research and practices.

NAEMT provides ongoing support to its instructors and the EMS training sites that hold its courses. Over 1,800 training sites, including colleges, EMS agencies, hospitals, and other training centers located in the United States and over 50 other countries, offer NAEMT continuing education programs. NAEMT headquarters staff work with the network of continuing education program volunteers from committee members; national, regional, and state coordinators; and affiliate faculty to provide administrative and educational support.

Peter T. Pons, MD, FACEP
Editor

Norman E. McSwain, Jr., MD, FACS, NREMT-P
Editor-in-Chief, PHTLS

Will Chapleau, EMT-P, RN, TNS
Gregory Chapman, EMT-P, RRT
Associate Editors

Dedication

This text is dedicated to all those individuals the world over who spend countless hours in the cold or the heat, during all hours of the day or night, in the sun or the rain or the snow, in situations that are safe or dangerous, away from their family and loved ones, to provide prehospital care to victims of trauma.

CHAPTER

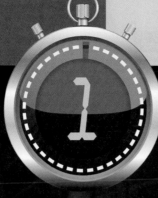

PHTLS: Past, Present, and Future

CHAPTER OBJECTIVES

At the completion of this chapter, the reader will be able to do the following:

- Recognize the magnitude of the problem both in human and financial terms caused by traumatic injury.

- Understand the three phases of trauma care.

- Understand the history and evolution of prehospital trauma care.

Introduction

Our patients did not choose us. We chose them. We could have chosen another profession, but we did not. We have accepted the responsibility for patient care in some of the worst situations: when we are tired or cold; when it is rainy and dark; when we cannot predict what conditions we will encounter. We must either accept this responsibility or surrender it. We must give to our patients the very best care that we can—not while we are daydreaming, not with unchecked equipment, not with incomplete supplies, and not with yesterday's knowledge. We cannot know what medical information is current, we cannot purport to be ready to care for our patients if we do not read and learn each day. The Prehospital Trauma Life Support (PHTLS) course provides a part of that knowledge to the working EMT, but, more important, it ultimately benefits the person who needs our all—the patient. At the end of each run, we should feel that the patient received nothing short of our very best.

Philosophy of PHTLS

PHTLS provides an understanding of anatomy and physiology, the pathophysiology of trauma, the assessment and care of the trauma patient using the ABCDE approach, and the skills needed to provide that care—no more and no less. Patients who are bleeding or breathing inadequately have a limited amount of time before their condition results in severe disability or becomes fatal. Prehospital care providers must possess and utilize critical thinking skills to make and carry out decisions that will enhance the survival of the trauma patient. PHTLS does not train prehospital care providers to memorize a "one size fits all" approach. Rather, PHTLS teaches an understanding of trauma care and critical thinking. Each prehospital care provider–patient contact involves a unique set of circumstances. If the prehospital care provider understands the basis of medical care and the specific needs of the individual patient given the circumstances at hand, then unique patient decisions can be made that ensure the greatest chance of survival for that patient.

The overarching tenets of PHTLS are that prehospital care providers must have a good foundation of knowledge, must be critical thinkers, and must have appropriate technical skills to deliver excellent patient care, even in less-than-optimal circumstances. PHTLS neither proscribes nor prescribes specific actions for the prehospital care provider, but instead supplies the appropriate knowledge and skills to enable the prehospital care provider to use critical thinking to arrive at the best management of each patient.

The opportunity for a prehospital care provider to help a patient is greater in the management of trauma victims than in any other patient encounter. The chance for survival of the trauma patient who receives excellent trauma care, in both the prehospital and the hospital setting, is probably greater than that of any other critically ill patient. The prehospital care provider can lengthen the life span and productive years of the trauma patient and benefit society by virtue of the care provided. Through effective management of the trauma patient, the prehospital care provider has a significant influence on society.

Learning, understanding, and practicing the principles of PHTLS will prove more beneficial to your patients than will completing any other educational program.[1]

The Problem

Trauma is the leading cause of death in persons between 1 and 44 years of age.[2] Over 70% of the deaths between the ages of 15 and 24 years and over 40% of deaths between the ages of 1 and 14 years are due to trauma. Trauma continues to be the eighth leading cause of death in elderly persons. Almost three times more Americans die of trauma each year than died in the entire Vietnam War and in the Iraq War through 2008.[3] Every 10 years, more Americans die of trauma than have died in all U.S. military conflicts combined. Only in the fifth decade of life do cancer and heart disease compete with trauma as a leading cause of death. About 70 times as many Americans die yearly from blunt and penetrating trauma in the United States as died yearly in the Iraq War.

Prehospital care providers can do little to increase the survival of a cancer patient; with trauma patients, however, prehospital care providers can often make the difference between life and death, between temporary disability and serious or permanent disability, or between a life of productivity and a life of dependency. It is estimated that about 60 million injuries occur each year in the United States. Of these, 40 million will require emergency department care, 2.5 million will require hospitalization, and 9 million will be disabling. About 8.7 million trauma patients will be temporarily disabled, and 300,000 will be permanently disabled.[4,5]

The cost for care of trauma patients is staggering. Billions of dollars are spent on the management of trauma patients, not including the dollars lost in wages, insurance administration costs, property damage, and employer costs. The National Safety Council estimated that the economic impact in 2007 from both fatal and nonfatal trauma was approximately $684 billion.[6] Lost productivity from disabled trauma patients is the equivalent of 5.1 million years at a cost of more than $65 billion annually. For patients who die, 5.3 million years of life are lost (34 years per person) at a cost of more than $50 billion. Comparatively, the costs per patient (measured in dollars and in years lost) for cancer and heart disease are much less (**Figure 1-1**). The prehospital care provider has an opportunity to reduce the costs of trauma. For example, proper protection of the fractured cervical spine by a prehospital care provider may make the difference between lifelong quadriplegia and a productive, healthy life of unrestricted activity. Prehospital care providers encounter many more such examples almost every day.

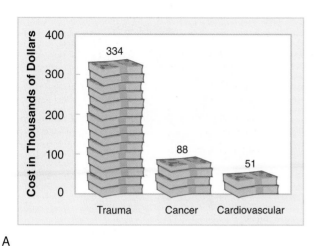

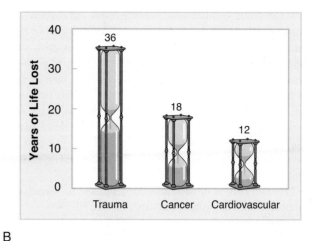

A

B

Figure 1-1 **A.** Comparative costs in thousands of dollars to U.S. victims of trauma, cancer, and cardiovascular disease each year. **B.** Comparative number of years lost as a result of trauma, cancer, and cardiovascular disease.
Source: Data from the National Safety Council.

The following data come from the World Health Organization (WHO) Road Traffic Injuries Fact Sheet No. 358:

- **Road traffic injuries are a huge public health and development problem.** Road traffic crashes kill 1.24 million people a year worldwide or an average of 3,242 people every day. They injure or disable between 20 million and 50 million people a year. Road traffic crashes rank as the ninth leading cause of death overall and the number one cause of trauma deaths, accounting for 2.2% of all deaths globally. The estimated cost of these injuries and deaths is $518 billion dollars annually.[7] WHO predicts that without improvements in prevention, 1.9 million people will be dying annually in motor vehicle crashes by the year 2020.
- **The majority of road traffic injuries affect people in low-income and middle-income countries, especially young males and vulnerable road users.** Of all road traffic deaths, over 90% occur in low-income and middle-income countries[8] (**Figure 1-2**).
- **Worldwide, over 5.8 million people die annually from trauma, both unintentional and intentional.**[9] While road traffic incidents are the most common cause of death, suicide (844,000) and homicide (600,000) are the number two and three causes, respectively.[10]

As these statistics clearly show, trauma is a worldwide problem. Although the specific events that lead to injuries and deaths differ from country to country, the consequences do not. The impact of preventable injuries is global.

We who work in the trauma community have an obligation to our patients to prevent injuries, not just to treat them after the injuries occur. An often-told story about emergency medical services (EMS) best illustrates this point. On a long, winding mountain road, there was a curve where cars would often slide off the road and plummet 100 feet to the ground below. The

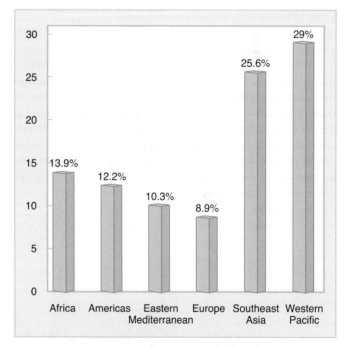

Figure 1-2 Worldwide distribution of road traffic deaths.
Source: Data from World Health Organization (WHO) Road Traffic Injuries Fact Sheet No. 358.

community decided to station an ambulance at the bottom of the cliff to care for the patients involved in these crashes. The better alternative would have been to place guardrails along the curve to prevent the incident from occurring in the first place.

The Phases of Trauma Care

Trauma is no accident, even though it is often referred to as such. An accident is defined as either "an event occurring by chance or arising from unknown causes" or "an unfortunate occurrence resulting from carelessness, unawareness, ignorance." Most trauma deaths and injuries fit the second definition but not the first and are preventable. Prevention has had a great deal of success in developed countries but has a long way to go in developing countries, with only 15% of the world's nations having traffic safety laws.[11] Traumatic incidents fall into two categories: *intentional* and *unintentional*. Intentional injury results from an act carried out on purpose with the goal of harming, injuring, or killing. Traumatic injury that occurs not as a result of a deliberate action, but rather as an unintended or accidental consequence, is considered unintentional.

Trauma care is divided into three phases: pre-event, event, and postevent. The prehospital care provider has responsibilities in each phase.

Pre-event Phase

The **pre-event phase** involves the circumstances leading up to an injury. Efforts in this phase are primarily focused on injury prevention. In working toward prevention of injuries, we must educate the public to increase the use of vehicle occupant restraint systems, promote methods to reduce the use of weapons in criminal activities, and promote nonviolent conflict resolution. In addition to caring for the trauma patient, all members of the health care delivery team have a responsibility to reduce the number of trauma victims. Currently, violence and unintentional trauma cause more deaths annually in the United States than all diseases combined.[12] Violence accounts for one-third of these deaths (**Figure 1-3**). Motor vehicles and firearms are involved in more than one-third of all trauma deaths, most of which are preventable (**Figure 1-4**).

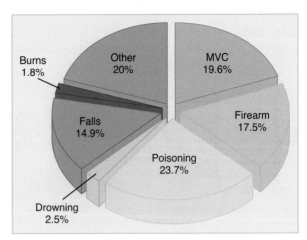

Figure 1-4   Motor vehicle trauma and firearms account for over one-third of the deaths that result from traumatic injury.
Source: Data from the National Center for Injury Prevention and Control: WISQARS. Fatal Injury Reports 1999–2010. Centers for Disease Control and Prevention. http://www.cdc.gov/injury/wisqars/fatal_injury_reports.html. Accessed January 2, 2013.

Motorcycle helmet laws are one example of legislation that has affected injury prevention. In 1966, the U.S. Congress gave the Department of Transportation the authority to mandate that states pass legislation requiring the use of motorcycle helmets. The use of helmets subsequently increased to almost 100%, and the fatality rate from motorcycle crashes decreased dramatically. The U.S. Congress rescinded this authority from the Department of Transportation in 1975. More than half the states repealed or modified their existing legislation. As states reinstated or repealed these laws, the mortality rates changed. Recently more states have repealed such laws, resulting in increased death rates in 2006 and 2007.[13]

Motorcycle deaths increased 11% in 2006.[14] The most likely explanation for this dramatic increase in mortality is the decreased use of helmets. Today, only 20 states have universal helmet laws. In states with such laws, helmet usage is 74%, whereas in states without such laws, the usage rate is 42%.[15] The decreased number of states with universal helmet laws has led to a drop in overall helmet usage from 71% in 2000 to 51% in 2006. To illustrate the effects of these trends, in Florida, a 2002 change in the law was followed by an increased death rate 24% greater than the increase in registrations would have predicted.

In August 2008, then U.S. Secretary of Transportation, Mary Peters, reported a drop in highway fatalities in automobiles while at the same time there was an increase in motorcycle fatalities. There has been major improvement in all aspects of vehicular safety except motorcycles.[16]

Another example of preventable trauma deaths involves driving while intoxicated with alcohol.[17] As a result of pressure to change state laws regarding the level of intoxication while driving and through the educational activities of such organizations as Mothers Against Drunk Driving (MADD), the number of drunk drivers involved in fatal crashes has been consistently decreasing since 1989.

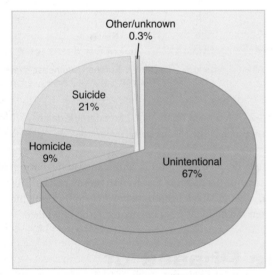

Figure 1-3   Unintentional trauma accounts for more deaths than all other causes of trauma death combined.
Source: Data from the National Center for Injury Prevention and Control: WISQARS. Fatal Injury Reports 1999–2010. Centers for Disease Control and Prevention. http://www.cdc.gov/injury/wisqars/fatal_injury_reports.html. Accessed January 2, 2013.

Another way to prevent trauma is through the use of child safety seats. Many trauma centers, law enforcement organizations, and EMS systems conduct programs to educate parents in the correct installation and use of child safety seats.

The other component of the pre-event phase is preparation by prehospital care providers for the events that are not prevented by the aforementioned efforts. Preparation includes proper and complete education with updated information to provide the most current medical care. Just as you must update your home computer or handheld device with the latest software, you must update your knowledge with current medical practices and insights. In addition, you must review the equipment on the response unit at the beginning of every shift and review with your partner the individual responsibilities and expectations of who will carry out what duties. It is just as important to review the conduct of the care when you arrive on the scene as it is to decide who will drive and who will be in the back with the patient.

Event Phase

The **event phase** is the moment of the actual trauma. Steps performed in the pre-event phase can influence the outcome of the event phase. This applies not only to our patients but also to ourselves. "Do no further harm" is the admonition for good patient care. Whether driving a personal vehicle or an emergency vehicle, prehospital care providers need to protect themselves and teach by example. You are responsible for yourself, your partner, and the patients under your care while in your ambulance vehicle; therefore prevent injury by safe and attentive driving. The same level of attention you give to your patient care must be given to your driving. Always drive safely, follow traffic laws, refrain from distracting activities such as cell phone use or texting, and use the personal protective devices available, such as vehicle restraints, in the driving compartment and in the passenger or patient care compartment.

Postevent Phase

The **postevent phase** deals with the outcome of the traumatic event. Obviously, the worst possible outcome of a traumatic event is death of the patient. Trauma surgeon Donald Trunkey, MD, has described a trimodal distribution of trauma deaths.[18] The *first phase* of deaths occurs within the first few minutes and up to an hour after an incident. These deaths would likely occur even with prompt medical attention. The best way to combat these deaths is through injury prevention and safety strategies. The *second phase* of deaths occurs within the first few hours of an incident. These deaths can often be prevented by good prehospital care and hospital care. The *third phase* of deaths occurs several days to several weeks after the incident. These deaths are generally caused by multiple organ failure. Much more needs to be learned about managing and preventing multiple organ failure; however, early and aggressive management of shock in the prehospital setting can prevent some of these deaths (**Figure 1-5**).

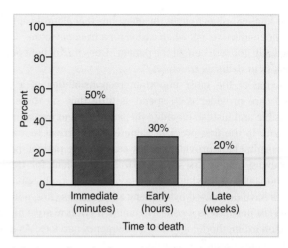

Figure 1-5 Immediate deaths can be prevented only by injury-prevention education because some patients' only chance for survival is for the incident not to have occurred. Early deaths can be prevented through timely, appropriate prehospital care to reduce mortality and morbidity. Late deaths can be prevented only through prompt transport to a hospital appropriately staffed for trauma care.

R Adams Cowley, MD, founder of the Maryland Institute of Emergency Medical Services (MIEMS), one of the first trauma centers in the United States, defined what he called the Golden Hour.[19] Based on his research, Dr. Cowley believed that patients who received definitive care soon after an injury had a much higher survival rate than those whose care was delayed. One reason for this improvement in survival is prompt treatment of hemorrhage and preservation of the body's ability to produce energy to maintain organ function. For the prehospital care provider, this translates into maintaining oxygenation and perfusion and providing rapid transport to a facility that is prepared to continue the process of resuscitation using blood and plasma (Damage Control Resuscitation) and to not elevate the blood pressure (over 90 mm Hg) by using large volumes of crystalloid.

In the United States, an average urban EMS system has a response time (from the time of notification that the incident occurred until arrival on the scene) of 6 to 8 minutes. A typical transport time to the receiving facility is another 8 to 10 minutes. Between 15 and 20 minutes of the magic Golden Hour are used just to arrive at the scene and transport the patient. If prehospital care at the scene is not efficient and well organized, an additional 30 to 40 minutes can easily be spent on the scene. With this time on the scene added to the transport time, the Golden Hour has already passed before the patient arrives at the hospital where the better resources of a well-prepared emergency department and operating suite are available for the benefit of the patient.

Research data support this concept.[20,21] One of these studies showed that critically injured patients had a significantly lower mortality rate (17.9% vs. 28.2%) when transported to the hospital by a private vehicle rather than an ambulance.[20] This unexpected finding was most likely the result of prehospital care providers spending too much time on the scene.

In the 1980s and 1990s, a trauma center documented that EMS scene times averaged 20 to 30 minutes for patients injured in motor vehicle crashes and for victims of penetrating trauma.

This finding brings to light the questions that all prehospital care providers need to ask when caring for a trauma victim: "Is what I am doing going to benefit the patient? Does that benefit outweigh the risk of delaying transport?"

One of the most important responsibilities of a prehospital care provider is to spend as little time on the scene as possible and instead expedite the field care and transport of the patient. In the first precious minutes after arrival to a scene, a prehospital care provider rapidly assesses the patient, performs lifesaving maneuvers, and prepares the patient for transport. In the 2000s, following the tenets of PHTLS, prehospital scene times have decreased by allowing all providers (fire, police, and EMS) to perform as a cohesive unit in a uniform style by having a standard methodology across emergency services. As a result, patient survival has increased.

A second responsibility is transporting the patient to an appropriate facility. The factor that is most critical to any patient's survival is the length of time that elapses between the incident and the provision of definitive care. For a cardiac arrest patient, definitive care is the restoration of a normal heart rhythm and adequate perfusion. Cardiopulmonary resuscitation (CPR) is merely a holding pattern. For a patient whose airway is compromised, definitive care is the management of the airway and restoration of adequate ventilation. The re-establishment of either ventilation or normal cardiac rhythm by defibrillation is usually easily achieved in the field. However, as critical care hospitals develop ST-elevation myocardial infarction (STEMI) programs, the amount of time from onset of cardiac symptoms until balloon dilatation of the involved cardiac vessels is becoming more important.[22-25]

While the management of trauma patients has changed, time is just as critical as ever, perhaps more so. Definitive care for the trauma patient usually involves control of hemorrhage and restoration of adequate perfusion by replacement of fluids as near to whole blood as possible. Administration of reconstituted whole blood (packed red blood cells and plasma, in a ratio of 1:1) to replace lost blood has produced impressive results by the military in Iraq and Afghanistan and now in the civilian community. These fluids replace the lost oxygen-carrying capacity, the clotting components, and the oncotic pressure to prevent fluid loss from the vascular system. They are not currently available for use in the field and are an important reason for rapid transport to the hospital. En route to the hospital, balanced resuscitation (see the Shock chapter) has proven to be important. Hemostasis (hemorrhage control) cannot always be achieved in the field or in the emergency department (ED); it must often be achieved in the operating room (OR). Therefore, when determining an appropriate facility to which a patient should be transported, it is important that the prehospital care provider utilize the critical thinking process and consider the transport time to a given facility and the capabilities of that facility.

A trauma center that has a surgeon available either before or shortly after the arrival of the patient, a well-trained and trauma-experienced emergency medicine team, and an OR team immediately available can often have a trauma patient with life-threatening hemorrhage in the OR within 10 to 15 minutes of the patient's arrival (and often faster) and make the difference between life and death.

On the other hand, a hospital without such in-house surgical capabilities must await the arrival of the surgeon and the surgical team before transporting the patient from the ED to the OR. Additional time may then elapse before the hemorrhage can be controlled, resulting in an associated increase in mortality rate (**Figure 1-6**). There is a significant increase in survival if nontrauma centers are bypassed and all severely injured patients are taken to the trauma center.[26-33]

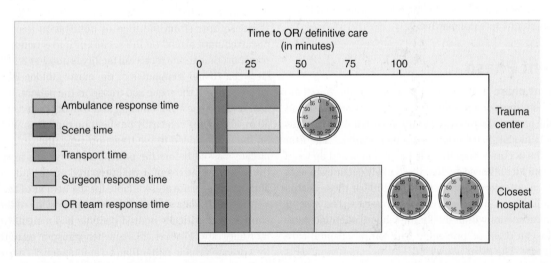

Figure 1-6 In locations in which trauma centers are available, bypassing hospitals not committed to the care of trauma patients can significantly improve patient care. In severely injured trauma patients, definitive patient care generally occurs in the OR. An extra 10 to 20 minutes spent en route to a hospital with an in-house surgeon and in-house OR staff will significantly reduce the time to definitive care in the OR. (Blue, EMS response time. Purple, on-scene time. Red, EMS transport time. Orange, surgical response from out of hospital. Yellow, OR team response from out of hospital.)

Experience, in addition to the initial training in surgery and trauma, is important. Studies have demonstrated that the more experienced surgeons in a busy trauma center have a better outcome than the less experienced trauma surgeons.[34,35]

History of Trauma Care in Emergency Medical Services

The stages and development of the management of the trauma patient can be divided roughly into four time periods as described by Norman McSwain, MD, in the Scudder Oration of the American College of Surgeons in 1999.[36] These time periods are (1) the ancient period, (2) the Larrey period, (3) the Farrington era, and (4) the modern era. This text, the entire PHTLS course, and care of the trauma patient are based on the principles developed and taught by the early pioneers of prehospital care. The list of these innovators is long; however, a few especially deserve recognition.

Ancient Period

All of the medical care that was accomplished in Egypt, Greece, and Rome, by the Israelites, and up to the time of Napoleon is classified as premodern EMS. Most of the medical care was accomplished within some type of rudimentary medical facility; little was performed by prehospital care providers in the field. The most significant contribution to our knowledge of this period is the Edwin Smith papyrus from approximately 4500 years ago, which describes the medical care in a series of case reports.

Larrey Period (Late 1700s to Approximately 1950)

In the late 1700s, Baron Dominique Jean Larrey, Napoleon's chief military physician, recognized the need for prompt prehospital care. In 1797, he noted that "... the remoteness of our ambulances deprive the wounded of the requisite attention. I was authorized to construct a carriage which I call flying ambulances."[37] He developed these horse-drawn "flying ambulances" for timely retrieval of warriors injured on the battlefield and introduced the premise that individuals working in these "flying ambulances" should be trained in medical care to provide on-scene and en-route care for patients.

By the early 1800s, he had established the basic theory of prehospital care that we continue to use to this day:

- The "flying" ambulance
- Proper medical training of medical personnel
- Movement into the field during battle for patient care and retrieval
- Field control of hemorrhage
- Transport to a nearby hospital
- Provision of care en route
- Development of frontline hospitals

He developed hospitals that were close to the front lines (much like the military of today) and stressed the rapid movement of patients from the field to medical care. Baron Larrey is now recognized as the **father of EMS in the modern era**.

Unfortunately, the type of care developed by Larrey was not used in the United States 60 years later at the beginning of the American Civil War by the Union Army. At the First Battle of Bull Run in August 1861, the wounded lay in the field—3,000 for 3 days, 600 up to a week.[36] Jonathan Letterman was appointed Surgeon General and created a separate medical corps with better organized medical care. At the Second Battle of Bull Run a year later, there were 300 ambulances, and attendants collected 10,000 wounded in 24 hours.[38]

In August 1864, the International Red Cross was created at the First Geneva Convention.[32] The convention recognized the neutrality of hospitals, of the sick and wounded, of all involved personnel, and of ambulances and guaranteed safe passage for ambulances and medical personnel to move the wounded. It also stressed the equality of medical care provided, regardless of which side of the conflict the victim was on. This convention marked the first step toward the Code of Conduct used by the U.S. military today. This Code of Conduct is an important component of the Tactical Combat Casualty Care Course (TCCC), which is now an integral part of the PHTLS program.

Hospitals, Military, and Mortuaries

In 1865, the first private ambulance service in the United States was created in Cincinnati, Ohio, at Cincinnati General Hospital.[38] Several EMS systems soon developed in the United States: Bellevue Hospital Ambulance[38] in New York in 1867; Grady Hospital Ambulance Service (the oldest continuously operating hospital-based ambulance) in Atlanta in the 1880s; Charity Hospital Ambulance Services in New Orleans, created in 1885 by a surgeon, Dr. A. B. Miles; and many other facilities in the United States. These ambulance services were run basically by hospitals, the military, or mortuaries up until 1950.[36]

In 1891, Nicholas Senn, MD, the founder of the Association of Military Surgeons, said, "The fate of the wounded rests in the hands of one who applies the first dressing." Although prehospital care was rudimentary when Dr. Senn made his statement, the words still hold true as prehospital care providers address the specific needs of the trauma patient in the field.

Some changes in medical care occurred during the various wars up until the end of World War II, but generally the system and the type of care rendered prior to arrival at the Battalion Aid Station (Echelon II) in the military or at the back door of the civilian hospital remained unchanged until the mid-1950s.

During this period, many ambulances in the major cities with teaching hospitals were staffed by interns beginning their first year of training. The last ambulance service to require physicians on the ambulance runs was Charity Hospital in New Orleans in the 1960s. Despite the fact that physicians were present, most of the trauma care was primitive. The equipment and supplies were not changed from that used during the American Civil War.[36]

Farrington Era (Approximately 1950 to 1970)

The era of J. D. "Deke" Farrington, MD (1909 to 1982), began in 1950. Dr. Farrington, the **father of EMS in the United States**, stimulated the development of improved prehospital care with his landmark article, "Death in a Ditch."[39] In the late 1960s, Dr. Farrington and other early leaders, such as Oscar Hampton, MD, and Curtis Artz, MD, brought the United States into the modern era of EMS and prehospital care.[36] Dr. Farrington was actively involved in all aspects of ambulance care. His work as chairman of the committees that produced three of the initial documents establishing the basis of EMS—the essential equipment list for ambulances of the American College of Surgeons,[40] the KKK 1822 ambulance design specifications of the U.S. Department of Transportation,[41] and the first emergency medical technician (EMT) basic training program—also propelled the idea and development of prehospital care. In addition to the efforts of Dr. Farrington, others actively helped promote the importance of prehospital care for the trauma victim. Robert Kennedy, MD, was the author of *Early Care of the Sick and Injured Patient.*[42] Sam Banks, MD, along with Dr. Farrington, taught the first prehospital training course to the Chicago Fire Department in 1957, which initiated proper care of the trauma patient.

A 1965 text edited and compiled by George J. Curry, MD, a leader of the American College of Surgeons and its Committee on Trauma, stated:

> Injuries sustained in accidents affect every part of the human body. They range from simple abrasions and contusions to multiple complex injuries involving many body tissues. This demands efficient and intelligent primary appraisal and care, on an individual basis, before transport. It is obvious that the services of trained ambulance attendants are essential. If we are to expect maximum efficiency from ambulance attendants, a special training program must be arranged.[42]

The landmark white paper, "Accidental Death and Disability: The Neglected Disease of Modern Society," further accelerated the process in 1967.[43] The National Academy of Sciences/National Research Council (NAS/NRC) issued this paper just one year after Dr. Curry's call to action.

Modern Era of Prehospital Care (Approximately 1970 to Today)

1970s

The modern era of prehospital care began with the Dunlap and Associates report to the U.S. Department of Transportation in 1968 defining the curriculum for EMT-Ambulance Training. This training became known as EMT-Basic, which is known as EMT today.

The National Registry of EMTs (NREMT) was established in 1970 and developed the standards for testing and registration of trained EMS personnel as advocated in the NAS/NRC white paper. Rocco Morando was the leader of the NREMT for many years and was associated with Drs. Farrington, Hampton, and Artz.

Dr. Curry's call for specialized training of ambulance attendants *for trauma* was initially answered by using the educational program developed by Drs. Farrington and Banks, by the publication of *Emergency Care and Transportation of the Sick and Injured* (the "Orange Book") by the American Academy of Orthopaedic Surgeons (AAOS), by the EMT training programs from the National Highway Traffic Safety Administration (NHTSA), and by the PHTLS training program during the past 25 years. The first training efforts were primitive but have progressed significantly in a relatively brief time.

The first textbook of this era was *Emergency Care and Transportation of the Sick and Injured*. This was the brainchild of Walter A. Hoyt Jr., MD, and was published in 1971 by the AAOS.[36] This text is now in its 10th edition.

During this same period, the Glasgow Coma Scale was developed in Glasgow, Scotland, by Dr. Graham Teasdale and Dr. Bryan Jennett for research purposes. Dr. Howard Champion brought it into the United States and incorporated it into the care of the trauma patient for assessment of the continued neurologic status of the patient.[44] The Glasgow Coma Scale is a very sensitive indicator of improvement or deterioration of such patients.

In 1973, federal EMS legislation was created to promote the development of comprehensive EMS systems. The legislation identified 15 individual components that were needed to have an integrated EMS system. Dr. David Boyd was placed in charge of implementing this legislation. One of these components was education. This became the basis for the development of training curricula for EMT-Basic, EMT-Intermediate, and EMT-Paramedic care throughout the United States. Today, these levels of training are called Emergency Medical Technician (EMT), Advanced Emergency Medical Technician (AEMT) and Paramedic. The curriculum was initially defined by the U.S. Department of Transportation (DOT) in the NHTSA and became known as the National Standard Curriculum or the DOT curriculum.

Dr. Nancy Caroline defined the standards and the curriculum for the first paramedic program and wrote the initial textbook, *Emergency Care in the Streets*, used in the training of paramedics. This text is now in its seventh edition.

The Blue Star of Life was designed by the American Medical Association (AMA) as the symbol of the "Medic Alert" indication that a patient had an important medical condition that EMS should note. It was given to the NREMT by the AMA as the logo of that registration and testing organization. Because the American Red Cross would not allow the "Red Cross" logo to be used on ambulances as an emergency symbol, Lew Schwartz, the chief of NHTSA's EMS branch, asked Dr. Farrington, the chairman of the NREMT board, to allow NHTSA to use the emblem for ambulances. Permission was granted by Dr. Farrington and Rocco Morando, the executive director of NREMT. It has since become an international symbol of EMS systems.[36]

The National Association of EMTs (NAEMT) was developed in 1975 by Jeffrey Harris with the financial support of NREMT. NAEMT is the nation's only organization solely dedicated to representing the professional interests of all EMS practitioners, including paramedics, EMTs, emergency medical responders, and other professionals working in prehospital emergency medicine.

1980s

In the mid-1980s it became apparent that the trauma patient was different from the cardiac patient. Trauma surgeons such as Frank Lewis, MD, and Donald Trunkey, MD, recognized the key distinction between these two groups: For the cardiac patient, all or most of the tools needed for reestablishment of cardiac output (CPR, external defibrillation, and supportive medications) were available to the properly trained paramedic in the field. For the trauma patient, however, the most important tools (surgical control of internal hemorrhage and replacement of blood) were not available in the field. The importance of moving the patient rapidly to the correct hospital became apparent to both the prehospital care providers and the medical directors. A well-prepared facility incorporated a well-trained trauma team comprised of emergency physicians, surgeons, trained nurses, and OR staff; a blood bank; registration and quality assurance processes; and all of the components necessary for the management of the trauma patient. All of these resources needed to be awaiting the arrival of the patient, with the surgical team standing by to take the patient directly into the OR. Over time, these standards were modified to include such concepts as permissive hypotension (Dr. Ken Mattox) and a transfusion ratio close to one part red blood cells for one part plasma (1:1) (Drs. John Holcomb from the U.S. military and Juan Duchesne in the civilian setting). However, the bottom line of rapid availability of a well-equipped OR has not changed.

Rapid treatment of the trauma patient depends on a prehospital care system that offers easy access to the system. This access is aided by a single emergency phone number (e.g., 9-1-1 in the United States), a good communication system to dispatch the emergency medical unit, and well-prepared and well-trained prehospital care providers. Many people have been taught that early access and early CPR save the lives of those experiencing cardiac arrest. Trauma can be approached the same way. The principles just listed are the basis for good patient care; to these basic principles has been added the importance of internal hemorrhage control, which cannot be accomplished outside of the trauma center and OR. Thus, rapid assessment, proper packaging, and rapid delivery of the patient to a facility with OR resources immediately available has become the additional principle that was not understood until the mid-1980s. These basic principles remain the bedrock of EMS care today.

The accomplishments of these great physicians, prehospital care providers, and organizations stand out; however, there are many more, too numerous to mention, who contributed to the development of EMS. To all of them, we owe a great debt of gratitude.

PHTLS—Past, Present, Future
Advanced Trauma Life Support

As happens so often in life, a personal experience brought about the changes in emergency care that resulted in the birth of the Advanced Trauma Life Support (ATLS) course and eventually the PHTLS program. ATLS started in 1978, two years after a private plane crash in a rural area of Nebraska. The ATLS course was born out of that mangled mass of metal, the injured, and the dead. The pilot, an orthopedic surgeon, his wife, and his four children were flying in their twin-engine airplane when it crashed. His wife was killed instantly. The children were critically injured. They waited for help to arrive, but it never did. After approximately 8 hours, the orthopedic surgeon walked more than half a mile along a dirt road to a highway. After two trucks passed him by, he flagged down a car. Together, they drove to the accident site, loaded the injured children into the car, and drove to the closest hospital, a few miles south of the crash site.

When they arrived at the emergency room door of the local rural hospital, they found it was locked. The on-duty nurse called the two general practitioners in the small farming community who were on call. After examining the children, one of the doctors carried one of the injured children by the shoulders and the knees to the x-ray room. Later, he returned and announced that the x-rays showed no skull fracture. An injury to the child's cervical spine had not been considered. The doctor then began suturing a laceration the child had sustained. The orthopedic surgeon called his physician partner in Lincoln, Nebraska, and told him what had happened. His partner said that he would arrange to get the surviving family to Lincoln as soon as possible.

The doctors and staff in this little rural hospital had little or no preparation for assessing and managing multiple patients with traumatic injuries. Unfortunately, there was a lack of training and experience on triage and on assessment and management of traumatic injuries. In the years that followed, the Nebraska orthopedic surgeon and his colleagues recognized that something needed to be done about the general lack of a trauma care delivery system to treat acutely injured patients in a rural setting. They decided that rural physicians needed to be trained in a systematic way on treating trauma patients. They chose to use a format similar to Advanced Cardiovascular Life Support (ACLS) and call it Advanced Trauma Life Support (ATLS).

A syllabus was created and organized into a logical approach to manage trauma. The "treat as you go" methodology was developed as well as the ABCs of trauma (airway, breathing, and circulation) to prioritize the order of assessment and treatment. In 1978, the ATLS prototype was field tested in Auburn, Nebraska, with the help of many surgeons. Next, the course was presented to the University of Nebraska and eventually to the American College of Surgeons Committee on Trauma.

Since that first ATLS course in Auburn, Nebraska, over three decades have passed and ATLS keeps spreading and growing. What was originally intended as a course for rural Nebraska has become a course for the whole world, for all types of trauma settings. It is this course that is the basis of PHTLS.

PHTLS

As Dr. Richard H. Carmona, former U.S. Surgeon General, stated in his foreword to the sixth edition of PHTLS:

> It has been said that we stand on the shoulders of giants in many apparent successes, and PHTLS is no different. With great vision and passion, as well as challenges, a small group of leaders persevered and developed PHTLS over a quarter of a century ago.

In 1958, Dr. Farrington convinced the Chicago Fire Department that fire fighters should be trained to manage emergency patients. Working with Dr. Sam Banks, Dr. Farrington started the Trauma Training Program in Chicago. Millions have been trained following the guidelines developed in this landmark program. Dr. Farrington continued to work at every level of EMS, from the field to education to legislation, to help expand and improve EMS as a profession. The principles of trauma care set forth by Dr. Farrington's work form an important part of the nucleus of PHTLS.

The first chairman of the ATLS ad hoc committee for the American College of Surgeons and Chairman of the Prehospital Care Subcommittee on Trauma for the American College of Surgeons, Dr. Norman E. McSwain, Jr., FACS, knew that ATLS would have a profound effect on the outcome of trauma patients. Moreover, he had a strong sense that an even greater effect could come from bringing this type of critical training to prehospital care providers.

Dr. McSwain, a founding member of the board of directors of the National Association of Emergency Medical Technicians (NAEMT), gained the support of the Association's president, Gary LaBeau, and began to lay plans for a prehospital version of ATLS.[44] President LaBeau directed Dr. McSwain and Robert Nelson, NREMT-P, to determine the feasibility of an ATLS-type program for prehospital care providers.

As a professor of surgery at Tulane University School of Medicine in New Orleans, Louisiana, Dr. McSwain gained the university's support in putting together the draft curriculum of what was to become Prehospital Trauma Life Support (PHTLS). With this draft in place, a PHTLS committee was established in 1983. This committee continued to refine the curriculum, and later that same year, pilot courses were conducted in Lafayette and New Orleans, Louisiana, the Marian Health Center in Sioux City, Iowa, the Yale University School of Medicine in New Haven, Connecticut, and the Norwalk Hospital in Norwalk, Connecticut.

Richard W. Vomacka (1946–2001) was a part of the task force that developed the initial PHTLS course. PHTLS became his passion as the course came together, and he traveled around the country in the early 1980s conducting pilot courses and regional faculty workshops. He worked with Dr. McSwain and the other original task force members to fine-tune the program. Mr. Vomacka was instrumental in forging a relationship between PHTLS and the U.S. military. He also worked on the first international PHTLS course sites.

National dissemination of PHTLS began with three intensive workshops taught in Denver, Colorado; Bethesda, Maryland; and Orlando, Florida, between September 1984 and February 1985. The graduates of these early PHTLS courses formed what would be the "barnstormers." These individuals were PHTLS national and regional faculty members who traveled the country training additional faculty members, spreading the word on the core PHTLS principles. Alex Butman, NREMT-P, along with Mr. Vomacka worked diligently, frequently using money out of their own pockets, to bring the first two editions of the PHTLS program to fruition.

Early courses focused on advanced life support (ALS) interventions for trauma patients in the field. In 1986, a course that encompassed basic life support (BLS) was developed. The course grew exponentially. Beginning with those first few enthusiastic faculty members, first dozens, then hundreds, and now thousands of prehospital care providers annually participate in PHTLS courses all over the world. Eventually, these two separate courses were merged into one program that teaches the complete approach to the management of the trauma victim in the prehospital setting.

As the course grew, the PHTLS committee became a division of the NAEMT. Course demand and the need to maintain course continuity and quality necessitated the building of networks of affiliate state, regional, and national faculty members. There are national coordinators for every country where PHTLS is taught. In each country, there are regional and state coordinators along with affiliate faculty members to make sure information is disseminated and courses are consistent, whether a prehospital care provider participates in a program in Chicago Heights, Illinois, or in Buenos Aires, Argentina.

Throughout the growth process, medical oversight has been provided through the American College of Surgeons Committee on Trauma. For nearly 20 years, the partnership between the American College of Surgeons and the NAEMT has ensured that PHTLS course participants receive the opportunity to help give trauma patients their best chance at survival.

More recently, Dr. Scott B. Frame, FACS, FCCM (1952–2001), was the Associate Medical Director for the PHTLS program. His major emphasis was in the development of the audiovisuals for PHTLS and its promulgation internationally. At the time of his untimely death, he had assumed the responsibility of putting together the fifth edition of the PHTLS course. This included the revision not only of the textbook but also of the instructor's manual and all of the associated teaching materials. He accepted the appointment to become Medical Director of the PHTLS course when the fifth edition was published. The PHTLS program grew tremendously under Dr. Frame's leadership, and its continuation into the future is owing to his efforts and the part of his life that he lent to PHTLS and to his patients.

It is on the shoulders of these, and many more individuals too numerous to mention, that PHTLS stands and continues to grow.

PHTLS in the Military

Beginning in 1988, the U.S. military aggressively set out to train its combat medics in PHTLS. Coordinated by the Defense Medical Readiness Training Institute (DMRTI) at Fort Sam Houston in Texas, PHTLS was taught to combat medics in the United States and stationed overseas. In 2001, the Army's 91WB program standardized the training of over 58,000 combat medics to include PHTLS.

In the fourth edition of PHTLS, a military chapter was added to better address the needs of military providers treating combat-related injuries. After the fifth edition was first published, a strong relationship was forged between the PHTLS committee and the newly established Committee on Tactical Combat Casualty Care of the Defense Health Board in the Department of Defense. As a result of this relationship, a military version of PHTLS, with an extensively revised military chapter, for a revised fifth edition was published in 2005. This collaboration between the PHTLS committee and the Committee on Tactical Combat Casualty Care led to the creation of multiple military chapters for the military edition of the sixth edition of PHTLS.

PHTLS has been taught numerous times "in theater" during the Afghanistan and Iraq Wars and has contributed to the lowest mortality rate from any armed conflict in U.S. history.

International PHTLS

The sound principles of prehospital trauma management emphasized in the PHTLS course have led prehospital care providers and physicians outside the United States to request the importation of the program to their various countries. ATLS faculty members presenting ATLS courses worldwide have assisted in this effort. This network of trauma surgeons provides medical direction and course continuity.

As PHTLS has moved across the United States and around the globe, the PHTLS committee members have been struck by the differences in our cultures and climates and also by the similarities of the people who devote their lives to caring for the sick and injured. All of us who have been blessed with the opportunity to teach overseas have experienced the fellowship with our international partners and know that we are all one people in the pursuit of caring for those who need care the most.

The PHTLS family continues to grow with over 700,000 prehospital care providers educated in 66 countries and territories since the program's inception (as of the publication of this edition). Annually, we are offering more than 3,700 courses, training approximately 43,000 students.

As of the publication of this edition, the nations and territories in the ever-growing PHTLS family include Argentina, Aruba, Australia, Austria, Barbados, Belgium, Bolivia, Brazil, Brunei, Canada, Chile, China and Hong Kong, Colombia, Costa Rica, Cyprus, Denmark, the Dominican Republic, Ecuador, Egypt, France, Georgia, Germany, Greece, Grenada, Haiti, India, Ireland, Israel, Italy, Japan, Kenya, Lebanon, Lithuania, Luxembourg, Mexico, the Netherlands, North Mariana Islands, Norway, Oman, Paraguay, Peru, Philippines, Poland, Portugal, Puerto Rico, Saudi Arabia, Serbia and Montenegro, Singapore, South Africa, Spain, Sweden, Switzerland, Trinidad and Tobago, the United Arab Emirates, the United Kingdom, the United States, and Uruguay. Demonstration courses have been held in Bulgaria, Croatia, Macedonia, New Zealand, Panama, and Venezuela, and hopefully these countries will be added to the PHTLS family in the very near future.

Translations

Our growing international family has spawned translations of the PHTLS text, which is currently available in English, Spanish, German, Greek, Portuguese, French, Dutch, Georgian, Chinese, and Italian. Negotiations are ongoing to have the text published in a number of additional languages.

Vision for the Future

The vision for the future of PHTLS is family. The father of PHTLS, Dr. McSwain, remains the foundation for the growing family that provides vital training and contributes knowledge and experience to the world. The inaugural international PHTLS Trauma Symposium was held near Chicago, Illinois, in the year 2000. In 2010, the first Pan-European PHTLS meeting was held. These programs bring the work of practitioners and researchers around the globe together to determine the standards of trauma care for the new millennium. The support of the PHTLS family worldwide, all volunteering countless hours of their lives, allows the PHTLS leadership to keep PHTLS growing.

As we continue to pursue the potential of the PHTLS course and the worldwide community of prehospital care providers, we must remember our commitment to the patient by accomplishing the following:

- Rapid and accurate assessment
- Identification of shock and hypoxemia
- Initiation of the right interventions at the right time
- Timely transport to the right place

It is also fitting to reprise our mission. The PHTLS mission continues to be to provide the highest quality prehospital trauma education to all who wish to avail themselves of this opportunity. The PHTLS program is committed to quality and performance improvement. As such, PHTLS is always attentive to changes in technology and methods of delivering prehospital trauma care that may be used to enhance the clinical and service quality of this program.

Summary

- The prehospital care of the trauma victim has undergone a profound evolution over the past 60 years and can essentially be divided into four approaches[36]:
  - *Grab and run.* No care—either in the field or en route, with rapid transport to the hospital, frequently without anyone in the patient care compartment—was the system prior to the 1950s.
  - *Field management and care.* This period began with the publication of the National Standard Curriculum and continued until the late 1970s.
  - *Stay and play.* From the mid- to late 1970s until the mid-1980s, the trauma patient and the cardiac patient were treated exactly alike; that is, attempts were made to stabilize the patient in the field, often for prolonged amounts of time.
  - *No-delay trauma care.* Beginning in the mid- to late 1980s, it was recognized that the critical trauma patient could not be "stabilized" in the field but rather required rapid assessment and intervention in an OR to control hemorrhage. This realization led to the change in prehospital management of the trauma patient of minimizing the on-scene time and rapid extrication and transport to an appropriate trauma center with most, if not all, interventions performed while en route.
- Trauma is the leading cause of death in patients younger than 44 years of age. Our efforts to provide prehospital care to trauma victims and limit death and disability have a direct effect on the future of our communities by returning young productive people to their families and their work.
- Even in older populations, people can expect to have many more productive years if they survive trauma with the least disability possible through the best care available.
- An organized, systematic approach to the care of these patients can improve patient survival. This organized approach begins initially with efforts to prevent injury from occurring. When injury does occur, the organized and systematic response of the entire health care delivery team, beginning in the prehospital setting, will help decrease the morbidity and mortality of traumatic injury.

References

1. Ali J, Adam RU, Gana TJ, et al. Effect of the Prehospital Trauma Life Support program (PHTLS) on prehospital trauma care. *J Trauma.* 1997;42(5):786–790.
2. Hoyert DL, Jiaquan X; for U.S. Department of Health and Human Services, Centers for Disease Control and Prevention, National Center for Health Statistics, National Vital Statistics System. National vital statistics report. Deaths: Preliminary data for 2011. http://www.cdc.gov/nchs/data/nvsr/nvsr61/nvsr61_06.pdf. Published October 12, 2012. Accessed January 2, 2012.
3. GlobalSecurity.org. US casualties in Iraq. http://www.globalsecurity.org/military/ops/iraq_casualties.htm. Accessed February 9, 2010.
4. US Department of Transportation (DOT), National Highway Traffic Safety Administration (NHTSA). Not-in-traffic surveillance 2007—Highlights. In: NHTSA's National Center for Statistics and Analysis: *Traffic Safety Facts,* HS 811 085. Washington, DC: DOT, NHTSA; 2009.
5. Townsend CM Jr, Beauchamp RD, Evers BM, Mattox KL, eds. *Sabiston Textbook of Surgery.* 18th ed. Philadelphia: Saunders; 2008.
6. National Safety Commission. *Highlights from Injury Facts, 2009 Edition.* http://www.nsc.org/news_resources/injury_and_death_statistics/Pages/HighlightsFromInjuryFacts.aspx. Accessed November 6, 2009.
7. World Health Organization (WHO). World report on road traffic injury prevention. Geneva, Switzerland: WHO; 2004.
8. World Health Organization. Road traffic injuries fact sheet no. 358. http://www.who.int/mediacentre/factsheets/fs358/en/index.html. Published March 2013. Accessed October 3, 2013.
9. World Health Organization (WHO). Injuries and violence: the facts. Geneva, Switzerland: WHO; 2010.
10. World Health Organization (WHO). The global burden of disease: 2004 update. Geneva, Switzerland: WHO; 2008.
11. World Health Organization. Global burden of disease: Switzerland, 2008 update. http://www.who.int/healthinfo/global_burden_disease/estimates_regional/en/index.html. Accessed January 2, 2013.
12. National Center for Injury Prevention and Control: WISQARS. Leading causes of death, 1999–2010. Centers for Disease Control and Prevention. http://www.cdc.gov/injury/wisqars/fatal_injury_reports.html. Accessed January 2, 2013.
13. US Department of Transportation (DOT), National Highway Traffic Safety Administration (NHTSA). Motorcycles. In NHTSA's National Center for Statistics and Analysis: *Traffic Safety Facts,* HS 810 990. Washington, DC: DOT, NHTSA; 2007.
14. Cars Blog. Motorcycle death rates doubled; supersport bikes the most dangerous. http://www.consumerreports.org/cro/news/2007/09/motorcycle-death-rates-doubled-supersport-bikes-the-most-dangerous/index.htm. Published September 18, 2007. Accessed October 3, 2013.
15. Krisberg K. Motorcycle safety, helmets an issue as US deaths increase: more than 5,000 US deaths in 2007. *Nation's Health.* 2008;38(9):11–20.
16. US Secretary of Transportation Mary Peters announces historic drop in highway fatalities and rate. http://www-nrd.nhtsa.dot.gov/Pubs/811017.PDF http://www.aggregateresearch.com/article.aspx?id=14468. Published August 14, 2008. Accessed October 8, 2013.

17. Mothers Against Drunk Driving. http://www.madd.org/. Accessed October 8, 2013.

18. Trunkey DD. Trauma. *Sci Am.* 1983;249(2):28–35.

19. R Adams Cowley Shock Trauma Center: tribute to R Adams Cowley, MD. http://umm.edu/programs/shock-trauma/about/history. Accessed October 8, 2013.

20. Demetriades D, Chan L, Cornwell EE, et al. Paramedic vs. private transportation of trauma patients: effect on outcome. *Arch Surg.* 1996;131(2):133–138.

21. Cornwell EE, Belzberg H, Hennigan K, et al. Emergency medical services (EMS) vs. non-EMS transport of critically injured patients: a prospective evaluation. *Arch Surg.* 2000;135(3):315–319.

22. Smith S, Hildebrandt D. Effect of workday vs. after-hours on door to balloon time with paramedic out-of-hospital catheterization laboratory activation for STEMI. *Acad Emerg Med.* 2007;14(5)(suppl 1): S126–S127.

23. Tantisiriwat W, Jiar W, Ngamkasem H, et al. Clinical outcomes of fast track managed care system for acute ST elevation myocardial infarction (STEMI) patients: Chonburi Hospital experience. *J Med Assoc Thai.* 2008;91(6):822–827.

24. So DY, Ha AC, Turek MA, et al. Comparison of mortality patterns in patients with ST-elevation myocardial infarction arriving by emergency medical services vs. self-transport (from the Prospective Ottawa Hospital STEMI Registry). *Am J Cardiol.* 2006; 97(4):458–461.

25. Bjorklund E, Stenestrand U, Lindback J, et al. Prehospital diagnosis and start of treatment reduces time delay and mortality in real-life patients with STEMI. *J Electrocardiol.* 2005;38(4)(suppl):186.

26. Bio-Medicine.org. Trauma victims' survival may depend on which trauma center treats them. http://news.bio-medicine.org/medicine -news-3/Trauma-victims-survival-may-depend-on-which -trauma-center-treats-them-8343-1/. Published October 2005. Accessed January 25, 2010.

27. Peleg K, Aharonson-Daniel L, Stein M, et al. Increased survival among severe trauma patients: the impact of a national trauma system. *Arch Surg.* 2004;139(11):1231–1236.

28. Edwards W. Emergency medical systems significantly increase patient survival rates, Part 2. *Can Doct.* 1982;48(12):20–24.

29. Haas B, Jurkovich GJ, Wang J, et al. Survival advantage in trauma centers: expeditious intervention or experience? *J Am Coll.* 2009;208(1):28–36.

30. Scheetz LJ. Differences in survival, length of stay, and discharge disposition of older trauma patients admitted to trauma centers and nontrauma center hospitals. *J Nurs Scholarsh.* 2005;37(4): 361–366.

31. Norwood S, Fernandez L, England J. The early effects of implementing American College of Surgeons level II criteria on transfer and survival rates at a rurally based community hospital. *J Trauma.* 1995;39(2):240–244; discussion 244–245.

32. Kane G, Wheeler NC, Cook S, et al. Impact of the Los Angeles county trauma system on the survival of seriously injured patients. *J Trauma.* 1992;32(5):576–583.

33. Hedges JR, Adams AL, Gunnels MD. ATLS practices and survival at rural level III trauma hospitals, 1995–1999. *Prehosp Emerg Care.* 2002;6(3):299–305.

34. Konvolinka CW, Copes WS, Sacco WJ. Institution and per-surgeon volume vs. survival outcome in Pennsylvania's trauma centers. *Am J Surg.* 1995;170(4):333–340.

35. Margulies DR, Cryer HG, McArthur DL, et al. Patient volume per surgeon does not predict survival in adult level I trauma centers. *J Trauma.* 2001;50(4):597-601; discussion 601–603.

36. McSwain NE. Prehospital care from Napoleon to Mars: the surgeon's role. *J Am Coll Surg.* 2005;200(44):487–504.

37. Larrey DJ. *Mémoires de Chirurgie Militaire, et Campagnes [Memoirs of Military Surgery and Campaigns of the French Armies].* Paris: J. Smith and F. Buisson; 1812–1817. English translation with notes by R. W. Hall of volumes 1–3 in 2 volumes, Baltimore, 1814. English translation of volume 4 by J. C. Mercer, Philadelphia, 1832.

38. Rockwood CA, Mann CM, Farrington JD, et al. History of emergency medical services in the United States. *J Trauma.* 1976;16(4): 299–308.

39. Farrington JD. Death in a ditch. *Bull Am Coll Surg.* 1967; 52(3):121–132.

40. Federal Specifications for Ambulance, KKK-A-1822D. United States General Services Administration, Specifications Section, November 1994.

41. Curry G. *Immediate Care and Transport of the Injured.* Springfield, Illinois: Charles C. Thomas Publisher; 1965.

42. Kennedy R. *Early Care of the Sick and Injured Patient.* Chicago: American College of Surgeons; 1964.

43. Committee on Trauma and Committee on Shock, Division of Medical Sciences. *Accidental Death and Disability: The Neglected Disease of Modern Society,* Washington, DC: National Academy of Sciences/ National Research Council; 1966.

44. McSwain NE. Judgment based on knowledge: a history of Prehospital Trauma Life Support, 1970–2013. *J Trauma Acute Care Surg.* 2013;75:1–7.

Suggested Reading

Callaham M. Quantifying the scanty science of prehospital emergency care. *Ann Emerg Med.* 1997;30:785.

Cone DC, Lewis RJ. Should this study change my practice? *Acad Emerg Med.* 2003;10:417.

Haynes RB, McKibbon KA, Fitzgerald D, et al. How to keep up with the medical literature: II. Deciding which journals to read regularly. *Ann Intern Med.* 1986;105:309.

Keim SM, Spaite DW, Maio RF, et al. Establishing the scope and methodological approach to out-of-hospital outcomes and effectiveness research. *Acad Emerg Med.* 2004;11:1067.

Lewis RJ, Bessen HA. Statistical concepts and methods for the reader of clinical studies in emergency medicine. *J Emerg Med.* 1991;9:221.

MacAvley D. Critical appraisal of medical literature: an aid to rational decision making. *Fam Pract.* 1995;12:98.

Reed JF III, Salen P, Bagher P. Methodological and statistical techniques: what do residents really need to know about statistics? *J Med Syst.* 2003;27:233.

Sackett DL. How to read clinical journals: V. To distinguish useful from useless or even harmful therapy. *Can Med Assoc J.* 1981;124:1156.

CHAPTER 2

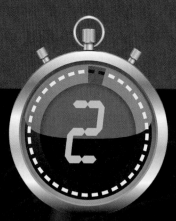

Injury Prevention

CHAPTER OBJECTIVES

At the completion of this chapter, the reader will be able to do the following:

- Describe the concept of energy as a cause of injury.

- Build a Haddon Matrix for a type of injury of interest.

- Relate the importance of accurate, attentive scene observations and documentation of data by prehospital care providers to the success of injury prevention initiatives.

- Assist in the development, implementation, and evaluation of injury prevention programs in his or her community or emergency medical services (EMS) organization.

- Describe and advocate for the role of EMS in injury prevention, to include:

  - Individual
  - Family
  - Community
  - Professional
  - Organizational
  - Coalitions of organizations

- Identify strategies that prehospital care providers can implement that will reduce the risk of injury.

SCENARIO

You and your partner are on the scene of a motor vehicle collision and are working to rapidly extricate a heavy patient from the driver's seat of his vehicle. He was unrestrained in the vehicle during the collision. You and your partner are both wearing approved safety vests over your work gear since you are near the roadway. Law enforcement is on the scene to provide traffic control, and the ambulance is parked to maximize your protection from oncoming vehicles. The patient is packaged properly and secured onto your motorized cot, which is being used due to the patient's weight. The motorized cot allows you and your partner to lift the patient safely into the ambulance without putting excess strain on your bodies.

Once inside the ambulance, you secure yourself in the rear-facing chair and continue care of the patient while your partner operates the siren and the strobe-flashing lights of the ambulance to attract other drivers' attention. She maneuvers safely into her lane and drives to the hospital. The ambulance arrives safely at the hospital, and you transfer the patient to the care of the emergency department staff.

While completing paperwork after the call, you consider the overall national injury and death statistics for prehospital care providers. You realize that thanks to the careful attention to all aspects of injury prevention that you and your partner demonstrated, the call was concluded safely for everyone involved.

- Is accident prevention a realistic approach in preventing injury and death in motor vehicle collisions and other causes of traumatic injury?
- Is there evidence that compliance with seat belt and safety seats has an impact in preventing injury and death?
- As prehospital care providers, what can we do to prevent deaths and injuries from motor vehicle collisions?

Introduction

A major impetus in the development of modern emergency medical services (EMS) systems was the publication of the 1966 white paper by the National Academy of Sciences/National Research Council (NAS/NRC), *Accidental Death and Disability: the Neglected Disease of Modern Society*. The paper spotlighted shortcomings in injury management in the United States and helped launch a formal system of on-scene care and rapid transport for patients injured as a result of "accidents." This educational initiative was instrumental in the creation of a more efficient system to deliver prehospital care to sick and injured patients.[1]

The incidence of death and disability from injury in the United States has fallen since the publication of the white paper.[2] Despite this progress, however, injury remains a major public health problem. More than 182,000 Americans die from injuries annually, and millions more are adversely affected to some degree.[3,4] Injuries remain a leading cause of death for all age groups.[5,6] For some age groups, particularly children, teenagers, and young adults, injury is the leading cause of death.

Injury is a global problem as well. Over five million people worldwide died from injuries in 2010.[5] Globally, nine people die from injuries per minute.

The desire to care for patients stricken by injury draws many into the field of EMS. The Prehospital Trauma Life Support (PHTLS) course teaches prehospital care providers to be efficient and effective in injury management. The need for well-trained prehospital care providers to care for injured patients will always exist. However, the most efficient and effective method to combat injury is to prevent it from happening in the first place. Health care providers at all levels play an active role in injury prevention to achieve the best results for not only the community at large but also for themselves.

In 1966, the authors of the NAS/NRC white paper recognized the importance of injury prevention when they wrote:

> The long-term solution to the injury problem is prevention .... Prevention of accidents involves training in the home, in the school, and at work, augmented by frequent pleas for safety in the news media; first aid courses and public meetings; and inspection and surveillance by regulatory agencies.[1]

Prevention of some diseases, such as rabies or measles, has been so effective that the occurrence of a single case makes front-page news. Public health officials recognize that prevention results in the greatest reward toward the amelioration of disease. Curricula for prehospital care providers have long included formal instruction in scene safety and personal protective equipment as a means of self-injury prevention for the emergency medical technician (EMT). To spur EMS systems to take a more active role in community prevention strategies, the *EMS Agenda for the Future*, developed by and for the EMS community, lists prevention as 1 of 14 attributes to develop further in order to "improve community health and result in more appropriate use of acute health resources."[7] To this end, the National EMS Education Standards include community injury prevention.

EMS systems are transforming themselves from a solely reactionary discipline to a broader, more effective discipline that includes more emphasis on prevention. This chapter introduces key concepts of injury prevention to the prehospital care provider.

Concepts of Injury

Definition of Injury

A discussion of injury prevention should begin with a definition of the term **injury**. Injury is now commonly defined as a harmful event that arises from the release of specific forms of physical energy or barriers to the normal flow of energy.[8] The wide variability of the causes of injury initially represented a major hurdle in its study and prevention. For example, what does a fractured hip caused by an elderly person's fall have in common with a self-inflicted gunshot wound to the head of a young adult? Furthermore, how does one compare a femur fracture from a fall in an elderly female to a femur fracture in a young male who crashed his motorcycle? All possible causes of injury—from vehicle crash, to stabbing, to suicide, to drowning—have one factor in common: the transfer of energy to the victim.

Energy exists in five physical forms: mechanical, chemical, thermal, radiation, or electrical.

- **Mechanical energy** is the energy that an object contains when it is in motion. For example, mechanical energy, the most common cause of injury, is transferred from a vehicle when an unrestrained driver collides with the windshield during a vehicle crash.
- **Chemical energy** is the energy that results from the interaction of a chemical with exposed human tissue. For instance, chemical energy results in a burn from exposure to an acid or base.
- **Thermal energy** is the energy associated with increased temperature and heat. For example, thermal energy causes injury when a cook sprays lighter fluid on actively burning charcoal in an outdoor grill, which then flashes in his face.
- **Radiation energy** is any electromagnetic wave that travels in rays (such as x-rays) and has no physical mass to it. Radiation energy produces sunburn in the teenager searching for a golden tan for the summer.
- **Electrical energy** results from the movement of electrons between two points. It is associated with direct injury as well as thermal injury and, for example, damages the skin, nerves, and blood vessels of a prehospital care provider who fails to do a proper scene assessment before touching a vehicle that hit a utility pole.

Any form of physical energy in sufficient quantity can cause tissue damage. The body can tolerate energy transfer within certain limits; however, an injury results if this threshold is exceeded.

Energy Out of Control

People harness and use all five forms of energy in many productive endeavors every day. In these situations, energy is under control and is not allowed to affect the body adversely. A person's ability to maintain control of energy depends on two factors: task performance and task demand.[9] As long as a person's ability to perform a task exceeds the demands of a task, energy is released in a controlled, usable manner.

In the following three situations, however, demand may exceed performance, leading to an uncontrolled release of energy:

1. *When the difficulty of the task suddenly exceeds the individual's performance ability.* For example, a prehospital care provider may operate an ambulance safely during normal driving conditions but loses control when the vehicle hits a sheet of black ice. The sudden increase in the demands of the task exceeds the prehospital care provider's performance capabilities and leads to a crash.
2. *When the individual's performance level falls below the demands of the task.* A person who falls asleep at the wheel of a vehicle while driving down a country road experiences a sudden drop in performance with no change in task demand, leading to a crash.
3. *When both factors change simultaneously.* Talking on a cellular phone while driving may reduce a driver's concentration on the road. If an animal darts in front of the vehicle, task demand suddenly rises. Under normal circumstances, the driver may be able to handle the increased demands of the task. A drop in concentration at the very moment when additional skill is required may lead to a crash.

Thus, injury may result when there is a release of energy in an uncontrolled manner in proximity to victims.

Injury as a Disease

The disease process has been studied for years. It is now understood that three factors must be present and interact simultaneously for an illness to occur: (1) an agent that causes the illness, (2) a host in which the agent can reside, and (3) a suitable environment in which the agent and host can come together. Once public health professionals recognized this "epidemiological triad," they discovered how to combat disease (**Figure 2-1**). Eradication of certain infectious diseases has been possible by vaccinating the host, destroying the agent with antibiotics, reducing environmental transmission through improved sanitation, or a combination of all three.

Only since the late 1940s has significant exploration of the **injury process** occurred. Pioneers in the study of injury demonstrated that despite the obviously different results, illness and injury are remarkably similar. Both require the presence of the

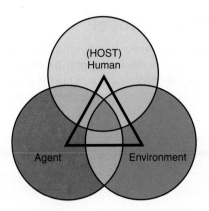

Figure 2-1 Epidemiological triad.

three elements of the epidemiological triad, and therefore, both are treated as a disease:

1. For an injury to occur, a host (i.e., the human) must exist. As with illness, susceptibility of the host does not remain constant from individual to individual; it varies as a result of internal and external factors. *Internal* factors include intelligence, gender, and reaction time. *External* factors include intoxication, anger, and social beliefs. Susceptibility also varies over time within the same person.

2. As described previously, the agent of injury is *energy.* Velocity, shape, material, and time of exposure to the object that releases the energy all play a role in whether the host's tolerance level is overwhelmed.

3. The host and agent must come together in an environment that allows the two to interact. Typically, the environment is divided into physical and social components. *Physical* environmental factors can be seen and touched. *Social* environmental factors include attitudes, beliefs, and judgments. For example, teenagers are more likely to participate in risk-taking behavior (the physical component) because they have more of a sense of invincibility (the social component) than other age groups.

The characteristics of the host, agent, and environment change with time and circumstance. Public health professionals Tom Christoffel and Susan Scavo Gallagher describe this dynamic as follows:

> To illustrate, think of the components of the Epidemiological Triad as constantly turning wheels. Inside each wheel are pie-shaped sections, one for each possible circumstantial variable—good and bad. The three wheels turn at different rates, so different characteristics interact (meet) at different times and in different combinations. Some combinations predict that no injury will occur; some predict disaster.[10]

In the case of injury, the host might be a curious, mobile 2-year-old child; the agent of injury might be a swimming pool filled with water with a beach ball floating just beyond the edge; the environment might be a pool gate left open while the babysitter runs inside to answer the telephone. With the host, agent, and environment all coming together at the same time, an unintentional injury—in this case, drowning—can occur.

Haddon Matrix

Dr. William J. Haddon, Jr., is considered the father of the science of injury prevention. Working within the concept of the epidemiological triad, in the mid-1960s, he recognized that an injury can be broken down into the following three temporal phases:

1. *Pre-event*: Before the injury.
2. *Event*: The point when harmful energy is released.
3. *Postevent*: The aftermath of the injury (see also the PHTLS: Past, Present, and Future chapter).

By examining the three factors of the epidemiological triad during each temporal phase, Haddon created a nine-cell "phase-factor" matrix (**Figure 2-2**). This grid has become known as the **Haddon Matrix**. It provides a means to depict graphically the events or actions that increase or decrease the odds that an injury will occur. It can also be used to identify prevention strategies. The Haddon Matrix demonstrates that *multiple* factors can lead to an injury, and therefore, multiple opportunities exist to prevent or reduce its severity. The matrix played a major role in dispelling the myth that injury is the result of a single cause, bad luck, or fate.

Figure 2-2 depicts a Haddon Matrix for an ambulance crash. The components in each cell of the matrix are different depending on the injury being examined. The *pre-event phase* includes factors that can contribute to the likelihood of a crash; however, energy is still under control. This phase may last from a few seconds to several years. The event phase depicts the factors that influence the severity of the injury. During this time, uncontrolled energy is released and injury occurs if energy transfer exceeds the body's tolerance. The *event phase* is typically very brief; it may last only a fraction of a second and rarely lasts more than a few minutes. Factors in the *postevent phase* affect the outcome once an injury has occurred. Depending on the type of event, it may last from a few seconds to the remaining life span of the host. (See also the PHTLS: Past, Present, and Future chapter.)

Public health programs have adopted the terminology of primary, secondary, and tertiary prevention.

■ Primary prevention is aimed at avoiding the injury before it occurs. This type of prevention activity involves education programs to help minimize risk-taking behaviors and the use of protective equipment such as helmets, child-safety seats, and vehicle restraint systems.

■ Secondary prevention refers to those actions taken to prevent the progression of an acute injury once it has occurred—for example, avoiding the occurrence of hypoxia or hypotension after a traumatic brain injury or correcting it as rapidly as possible if it already is present.

- Tertiary prevention is directed at minimizing death and the long-term disability of an injury (or disease) after it has occurred. Active and aggressive rehabilitation programs fall into this category.

Swiss Cheese Model

British psychologist James Reason proposed another way of thinking about how accidents occur.[11] He likened the process to Swiss cheese. In every situation, a hazard exists that has the potential to cause injury or allow an error to occur. There are

Figure 2-2 Haddon Matrix for an Ambulance Crash

	Epidemiological Triad		
Time Phases	**Host Factors**	**Agent Factors**	**Environment Factors**
Pre-event	Driver's visual acuity Experience and judgment Amount of time in the ambulance per shift Level of fatigue Proper nutrition Stress level Adherence to company and community driving laws Quality of driver education courses	Maintenance of brakes, tires, etc. Defective equipment Ambulance's high center of gravity Speed Ease of control	Visibility hazards Road curvature and gradient Surface coefficient of friction Narrow road shoulder Traffic signals Speed limits
Event	Safety belt use Physical conditioning Injury threshold Ejection	Speed capability Ambulance size Automatic restraints Hardness and sharpness of contact surfaces Hardness and sharpness of loose items (e.g., clipboards, flashlights) Steering column Practice of safe driving habits: speed, use of lights/siren, passing, intersections, backing Practice of good partner habits en route: watching road, clearing intersections Safe parking	Lack of guardrails Median barriers Distance between roadway and immovable objects Speed limits Other traffic Attitudes about safety belt use Maintaining an escape route Making no assumptions about an environment being safe (e.g., "nice part of town," high-income home) Weather
Postevent	Age Physical condition Type or extent of injury	Fuel system integrity Entrapment	Emergency communication capability Distance to and quality of responding EMS Training of EMS personnel Availability of extrication equipment Trauma care system of the community Rehabilitation programs in the community

usually a series of safeguards or barriers to prevent this from happening. He suggested that each of these barriers or safeguards is like a piece of Swiss cheese. The holes in the cheese are flaws or failures that increase the potential for a hazard or error to cause injury. These flaws may be the result of deficiencies in the organization or administration or may occur following oversight of the system (latent conditions), or they may occur as a result of acts of omission or commission (active failures). Reason argued that every hazard has a trajectory, and that a series of failures generally must occur in order for there to be subsequent harm, and that the trajectory must be such that it intersects with holes or failures that have aligned to allow all of the safeguards to fail and injury to occur (**Figure 2-3**).[11]

Classification of Injury

A common method to subclassify injuries is based on intent. Injury may result from either intentional or unintentional causes. Although this is a logical way to view injuries, it underscores the difficulty of injury prevention efforts.

Intentional injury is typically associated with an act of interpersonal or self-directed violence. Problems such as homicide, suicide, assault, sexual assault, domestic violence, child abuse, and war fall into this category. Previously, prevention of intentional injury was thought to be the sole responsibility of the criminal justice and mental health systems. Although these agencies are integral to reducing violent deaths, intentional injuries can best be prevented through a broad, multidisciplinary approach, which includes the medical profession.

In the past, **unintentional injuries** were called accidents. The authors of the NAS/NRC white paper appropriately referred to accidental death and disability; this was the vocabulary of the time.[1] Because it has since been understood that very specific factors must come together for an injury to occur, health care providers now realize that the term *accidental* does not describe unintentional injury resulting from events such as vehicle crashes, drownings, falls, and electrocutions. EMS systems have embraced this concept by using the term motor vehicle collisions or crashes (often abbreviated MVCs) rather than motor vehicle accidents (MVAs). However, public perception has changed much more slowly. News reporters still describe persons injured in automobile accidents or accidental shootings. The term accident suggests that a person was injured as a result of fate, divine intervention, or bad luck. It implies that the injury was random and, therefore, unavoidable. As long as this misperception exists, implementation of corrective measures will be impeded.

It is also important to note that there may be overlap between these two common classifications of injury.[12] For example, a motor vehicle collision may have resulted from a driver attempting to commit suicide. Classifying the incident as a motor vehicle crash alone implies no intent on the part of the driver to harm, whereas knowledge of the suicidal ideation of the driver clearly implies intent to cause the crash or collision.

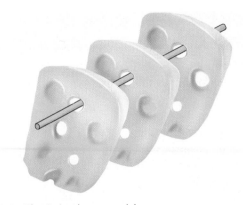

Figure 2-3 The Swiss cheese model.

Source: Reproduced from British Medical Journal. Reason, J, Human error: Models and Management, 320, p. 768, © 2000 with permission from BMJ Publishing Group Ltd.

Scope of the Problem

Death from injuries is a major health problem worldwide, resulting in more than 14,000 deaths *daily* (**Figure 2-4**), with road traffic accidents causing approximately 1.3 million, suicide 844,000, and homicide 600,000.[5] In most countries, regardless of their level of development, injuries appear among the five leading causes of death.[4] Although causes of injury deaths vary little between countries, wide variability does exist between which causes have the greatest impact on specific age groups. Because of economic, social, and developmental issues, the cause of injury-related death varies from country to country and even region to region within the same country.

For example, in low-income and middle-income countries of the western Pacific, the leading injury-related causes of death are road traffic injuries, drowning, and suicide, whereas in Africa the leading causes are road traffic injuries, war, and interpersonal violence. In high-income countries of the Americas, the leading cause of death among people between 15 and 29 years of age is road traffic injuries. For this same age group in low-income and middle-income countries of the Americas, the leading cause is interpersonal violence.[6] **Figure 2-5** demonstrates that injury plays a leading role in the global burden of disease.

In 2010, nearly 33,000 people in the United States died in motor vehicle collisions, which was the lowest number since 1949. More than 10,000 died at the hands of alcohol-impaired drivers, and nearly 2.6 million drivers and passengers were treated in the emergency department (ED) after motor vehicle collision.[3] In the United States, injuries are the overall fifth leading cause of death, accounting for more than 180,000 deaths annually or about 1 person every 3 minutes[3] (**Figure 2-6**). Injury is an especially serious problem for the youth of America as well as of most industrialized nations of the world. In the United States, injury kills more children and young adults than all diseases combined (over 32,000 in 2006).[3] Sixty-five percent of the deaths of children under 19 years of age occur due to unintentional injury.[13]

Unfortunately, deaths from injury are only the tip of the iceberg. The "injury triangle" provides a more complete picture of

Figure 2-4 Worldwide Injury-Related Statistics, 2012 Fact Sheets

Injury Overall

- The top eight injury-related causes of mortality in order were:
  1. Road traffic injuries
  2. Self-inflicted violence
  3. Interpersonal violence
  4. Drowning
  5. Poisoning
  6. War
  7. Falls
  8. Fires
- An estimated five million people die worldwide from injuries.
- Injuries accounted for 9% of the world's deaths and 16% of all disabilities.
- For persons aged 5 to 44 years, 6 of the top 10 leading causes of death were injury related.
- The burden of disease related to injuries, particularly road traffic injuries, is expected to rise dramatically by the year 2020.
- Twice as many men die from injury as women; fire-related deaths are the notable exception.
- Males in Africa have the highest injury-related mortality rates.
- More than 90% of all injury-related deaths occur in low-income and middle-income countries.
- Injury accounts for 12% of the total years of potential life lost either from premature death or from disability.

Road Traffic Injury

- An estimated 1.3 million people died as a result of road traffic injuries, and 50 million more were injured or disabled.
- Road traffic injury is the leading cause of death for children and youth aged 10 to 29 years.
- Road traffic mortality for males is almost three times higher than for females.
- Southeast Asia accounts for the highest percentage of road traffic injury deaths.

Fire-Related Burns

- Approximately 195,000 fire-related burn deaths occur annually worldwide.
- Females in Southeast Asia have the highest fire-related burn mortality rates.
- Children younger than 5 years of age and elderly persons have the highest fire-related mortality rates.
- Southeast Asia alone accounts for just over one-half of fire-related burn deaths.

Drowning

- Approximately 389,000 persons drowned in 2004.
- 97% of drowning deaths occurred in low- and middle-income countries.
- Among the various age groups, children younger than 5 years of age have the highest drowning mortality rates, accounting for more than 50%.
- Males in Africa and the western Pacific have the highest drowning mortality rates.

Falls

- It is estimated that 424,000 people die as a result of falls annually.
- A quarter of all fatal falls occurred in high-income countries.
- In all regions of the world, adults older than 65 years of age, particularly women, have the highest fall mortality rate.
- Europe and the western Pacific combined account for almost 60% of the total number of fall-related deaths.

Poisoning

- An estimated 346,000 people died from poisoning worldwide.
- More than 94% of fatal poisonings occurred in low- and middle-income countries.
- The overall poisoning rate among males in Europe is approximately three times higher than the rate in either gender in any other world region.
- The European region accounts for more than one-third of all poisoning deaths worldwide.

Interpersonal Violence

- An estimated 520,000 people died worldwide as a result of interpersonal violence.
- 95% of homicides occurred in low- and middle-income countries.
- The highest interpersonal violence rates are found in the Americas among males aged 15 to 29 years.
- Among females, Africa has the highest mortality rate from interpersonal violence.

Suicide

- 815,000 people worldwide committed suicide.
- 86% of all suicides occurred in low- and middle-income countries.
- Women in China have a suicide rate that is approximately twice that of women in other parts of the world.
- More than 50% of suicides occur in persons aged 15 to 44 years.

All figures compiled from World Health Organization (WHO) 2012 data fact sheets.

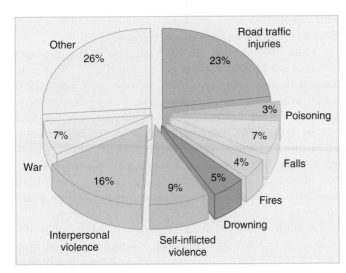

Figure 2-5 Distribution of global injury mortality by cause.

Source: Data from WHO Global Burden of Disease project, 2002, Version 1.

for more YPLL than any other cause of death. In 2006, injury stole an estimated 3.68 million years from its victims compared with 1.8 million years for cancer, even though cancer claims more lives than injury.[3]

A third measure of injury severity can be demonstrated financially. The economics of injury are felt far beyond the patient and the immediate family. The cost of injury is spread across a wide spectrum. All members of society feel the effect because the costs of injury are borne by federal and other agencies, private insurance programs that pass the expense on to other subscribers, and employers as well as the patient. As a result, everyone pays when an individual is seriously injured. Cost estimates for injury run as high as $406 billion annually, which includes the direct cost of medical care and indirect costs such as lost earnings.[4,6] Data from the World Health Organization (WHO) indicate that prevention activities are a good investment:

- Every U.S. dollar invested in motorcycle helmets results in a $32 savings of medical costs.
- Seat belts decrease the risk of ejection and of sustaining serious or fatal injury by 40% to 65% and have saved an estimated 255,000 lives between 1975 and 2008.[14]

The toll of injury in terms of morbidity, mortality, and economic stress is excessive. As stated by Maguire and colleagues:

> Injuries have always been a threat to the public's well-being, but until the mid-twentieth century, infectious diseases overshadowed the terrible contribution injury made to human morbidity and mortality. Public health's success in other areas has left injury as a major public health concern, one that has been termed "the neglected epidemic."[15]

the **public health impact of injury** (**Figure 2-7**). In the United States in 2009 more than 118,000 individuals died from injury, and another 2.8 million were hospitalized because of nonfatal injuries. Injury also resulted in more than 45.4 million ED visits.[3]

The impact can be further realized by examining the number of **years of potential life lost (YPLL)** as a result of injury. YPLL is calculated by subtracting age at death from a fixed age of the group under examination, usually 65 or 70 years or the life expectancy of the group. Injury kills or disables people of all ages, but it disproportionately affects children, youth, and young adults, especially in industrialized nations. Because injury is the leading killer of Americans between 1 and 44 years of age, it is responsible

Figure 2-6 Ranking of Causes of Injury-Related Deaths by Age Groups, 2010

	< 1	1–4	5–9	10–14	15–24	25–34	35–44	45–54	55–64	65 +	All Ages (number of deaths)
Unintentional Injury	5th	Leading	Leading	Leading	Leading	Leading	Leading	3rd	4th	9th	5th (120,859)
Intentional Injury											
Suicide	*	*	13th	3rd	3rd	2nd	4th	4th	8th	18th	10th (38,364)
Homicide	14th	3rd	4th	4th	2nd	3rd	5th	13th	17th	*	16th (16,259)

*Data not applicable or available.
Source: Extracted from National Vital Statistics System, National Center for Health Statistics, Centers for Disease Control and Prevention (CDC), Office of Statistics and Programming, National Center for Injury Prevention and Control. CDC: ranking of causes of injury-related deaths by age groups, 2010. http://www.cdc.gov/injury/wisqars/pdf/10LCID_All_Deaths_By_Age_Group_2010-a.pdf. Accessed January 11, 2013.

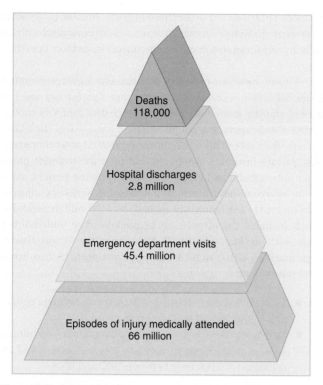

Figure 2-7 Injury triangle.

Source: Data from the US Department of Health and Human Services, Centers for Disease Control and Prevention, National Center for Health Statistics. Injury in the United States 2007 Chartbook.

Society is calling on all segments of the medical community to increase its prevention activities. With as many as 840,000 prehospital care providers in the United States alone, EMS systems can make a tremendous contribution to community-based injury prevention efforts.

Injury to EMS Personnel

EMS personnel are exposed to a wide variety of situations that can result in provider injury. Scenes are often unsecured, despite the best efforts of EMS personnel and law enforcement, because these scenes involve people in emotional and physical crisis. The very nature of the emergency work presents opportunities for injury. Just driving to the scene can be hazardous. Lifting, exposure to environmental hazards and infectious diseases, sleep deprivation, and the stress of the job also present significant opportunities for injury.

Sleep deprivation is an important factor that clearly affects prehospital care provider performance.[16] The longer a person is awake, the greater the resulting fatigue and drowsiness; the greater the impairment in reaction time, medical decision making, and judgment; and the greater the likelihood of mistakes, injury to self or others, and even fatality.[17] Sleep deprivation has been compared to alcohol intoxication, with no sleep for 18 hours approximating a blood alcohol concentration (BAC) of 0.05 and no sleep for 24 hours approximating a BAC of 0.1.

In addition, sleep deprivation can have profound effects on the health of the prehospital care provider as well as interfere with important personal and family relationships. Lack of sleep can lead to irritability, anxiety, and depression.

From 1992 through 1997, an estimated 12.7 fatalities occurred per 100,000 workers per year in EMS.[18,19] This compares with a national average fatality rate of 5.0 per 100,000 for all workers, a rate of 14.2 per 100,000 for police officers, and 16.5 for fire fighters over the same period. More than 58% of those EMS fatalities involved ambulance crashes; 9% involved assault or homicide. As with fatalities, estimating nonfatal injury can be difficult as well. However, 1 serious, disabling injury requiring hospitalization per 31,616 dispatches has been documented among urban prehospital care providers.[20]

A study published in 2011 reviewed fatal and nonfatal injuries to EMTs and paramedics during the period from 2003 to 2007.[21] The authors reviewed data from the Bureau of Labor Statistics Census of Fatal Occupational Injuries as well as the occupational portion of the National Electronic Injury Surveillance System. For that time period, they found 99,400 nonfatal injuries and 65 fatalities. Most of the fatalities were transportation related, either motor vehicle collisions (45%) or aircraft crashes (31%). Among paid EMS personnel, the fatality rate was 6.3 per 100,000, which is higher than the rate for fire fighters (6.1 per 100,000) for the same period. The only good news in this report is that the fatality figure is lower than that documented in the report from 10 years prior.

These numbers reveal a disturbing truth. According to Garrison:

> … the most dangerous times for EMS personnel are when they are inside their ambulance when it is moving or when they are working at a crash scene near other moving vehicles.[22]

It is critical that EMS personnel know and understand the concepts of injury and injury prevention so that the risks inherent in EMS can be identified and corrected. From almost the first day of training, students are taught that no one is more important at the scene than the prehospital care provider, so his or her safety must come first. Seat belt use in the ambulance is the first step of safety.

In 2009, the National EMS Advisory Council (NEMSAC) noted that the National Highway Traffic Safety Administration (NHTSA) should create a national EMS culture of safety. To accomplish this, a draft document has been developed describing the various recommended steps and actions needed to implement this concept.[23]

Prevention as the Solution

The ideal is to prevent an injury from occurring in the first place, thus obviating the need to treat it after it occurs. When injury is prevented, it spares the patient and family from suffering and economic hardship. The National Center for Injury Prevention and Control (NCIPC) of the Centers for Disease Control and Prevention (CDC) estimates the following:

- $1 spent on smoke detectors saves $69.
- $1 spent on bicycle helmets saves $29.
- $1 spent on child-safety seats saves $32.
- $1 spent on center and edge lines on roads saves $3 in medical costs alone.
- $1 spent on counseling by pediatricians to prevent injuries saves $10.
- $1 spent on poison control center services saves $7 in medical expenses.[3]

In addition to the NCIPC's findings:

- A CDC-funded evaluation study of a regional trauma care system in Portland, Oregon, found a 35% decrease in the risk of dying for severely injured patients who were treated in the system.[24]
- A smoke detector distribution program in Oklahoma reduced burn-related injuries by 80%.[25]

Because of the variability among the host, agent, and environment at any given time, health care providers cannot always predict or prevent every individual injury. However, it is possible to identify high-risk populations (which include prehospital care providers), high-risk products, and high-risk environments. Prevention efforts focused on high-risk groups or settings influence as wide a range of society as possible. Health care providers can pursue prevention in multiple ways. Some strategies have proven successful across the United States and around the world. However, other strategies work in one region but not in another. Before implementing an injury prevention strategy, efforts must focus on determining if it will work. Although it is not necessary to "reinvent the wheel," health care providers may need to modify a prevention strategy to improve its chances of success. Methods for doing this are examined in the following section.

Concepts of Injury Prevention

Goal

The goal of injury prevention programs is to bring about a change in knowledge, attitude, and behavior on the part of a previously identified segment of society. Simply providing information to potential victims is not enough to prevent injury. A program must be implemented in a manner that will influence society's attitude and—most importantly—change behavior. The hope is that any change in behavior will be long term. This task is monumental but not insurmountable.

Opportunities for Intervention

Prevention strategies can be arranged according to their effect on the injury event. They coincide with the temporal phases of the Haddon Matrix. Pre-event interventions, known as primary interventions, strive to prevent the injury from occurring. Actions intended to keep intoxicated drivers off the road, lowering speed limits, and installing traffic lights are designed to prevent crashes from occurring. Event phase interventions are intended to reduce injury severity by softening the blow of injuries that occur. Wearing safety belts, installing cushioned dashboards and air bags in vehicles, and enforcing child-safety seat laws are means to reduce the severity of injury sustained in crashes. Postevent interventions provide a means to improve the likelihood of survival for those who are injured. Encouraging physical fitness, designing fuel systems for vehicles that do not explode on impact, and implementing high-quality EMS systems are intended to reduce the recovery time for persons who are injured.

Prehospital systems have traditionally limited their community involvement to the postevent phase. Countless lives have been saved as a result. However, because of the limitations inherent in waiting until injury has occurred, the best results have not been achieved. EMS systems must explore entering the injury cycle earlier. Using the Haddon Matrix, EMS systems can identify opportunities to collaborate with other public health and public safety organizations to prevent injuries from occurring or to soften their blow.

Potential Strategies

No single strategy provides the best approach to injury prevention. The most effective option or options depends on the type of injury under study. However, Haddon developed a list of 10 generic strategies designed to break the chain of injury-producing events at numerous points (**Figure 2-8**). These strategies represent ways that the release of uncontrolled energy can be prevented or at least reduced to amounts the body can better tolerate. Figure 2-8 also presents countermeasures that can be taken in the pre-event, event, and postevent phases and that are directed toward the host, agent, or environment. This list is not complete and merely serves as a starting point to help determine the most effective options for the particular problem under study.

Most injury prevention strategies are either active or passive. **Passive strategies** require little or no action on the part of the individual; sprinkler systems and vehicle air bags are examples. **Active strategies** require the cooperation of the person being protected; examples include manual seat belts and choosing to wear a motorcycle or bicycle helmet. Passive measures are generally more effective because people do not need to consciously do anything to take advantage of the protection. Nonetheless, passive strategies are usually more difficult to implement because they can be expensive or require legislative or regulatory action. Sometimes a combination of active and passive strategies is the best option.

Strategy Implementation

Three common approaches to implementing an injury prevention strategy have become known as the Three E's of Injury

Figure 2-8 Basic Strategies for Injury Countermeasures

Strategy	Possible Countermeasures
Prevent initial creation of the hazard.	Do not produce firecrackers, three-wheeled all-terrain vehicles, or various poisons. Eliminate spearing in high school football.
Reduce amount of energy contained in the hazard.	Limit the horsepower of motor vehicle engines. Package toxic drugs in smaller, safer amounts. **Obey or reduce speed limits.** Mandate improved public transportation to reduce the number of privately owned vehicles on the road. **Encourage reduction of temperature on home hot water heaters.** Limit the muzzle velocity of guns. Limit the amount of gunpowder in firecrackers.
Prevent release of a hazard that already exists.	**Store firearms in locked containers or use gun locks.** Close pools and beaches when no lifeguard is on duty. **Encourage use of nonslip surfaces in bathtubs and showers.** **Childproof containers for all hazardous household drugs and chemicals.** **Limit cell phone use in vehicles, or use hands-free models.** Require safety shields on rotating farm machinery. Improve vehicle handling.
Modify rate or spatial distribution of the hazard.	**Require use of seat belts and child-safety seats.** Provide antilock brakes. Encourage use of short cleats on football shoes so feet rotate rather than transmit sudden force to the knees. Require vehicle air bags. Provide hydraulic bumpers on vehicles. Provide safety nets to protect workers from falls. **Encourage use of flame-retardant pajamas.**
Separate in time or space the hazard from that which is to be protected.	Provide pedestrian overpasses at high-volume crossings. Keep roadsides clear of poles and trees. Do not have play areas near unguarded bodies of water. Install bike paths. Spray pesticides at a time when people are not present. Install sidewalks. Route trucks carrying hazardous material along low-density roads. **Encourage use of smoke detectors in the home.**
Separate the hazard from that which is to be protected by a material barrier.	Install fencing around all sides of swimming pools. **Encourage use of protective eyewear for sports and occupational hazards.** Build highway medians. Build protective shields around hazardous machinery. Install guardrails between sidewalks and roads. Install reinforced panels in vehicle doors. **Require health care workers to place used needles directly into a sharps container.** **Require use of helmets for motorcyclists, bicyclists, and high-risk sporting activities.**
Modify basic nature of the hazard.	Provide air bags in motor vehicles. Provide collapsible steering columns. Provide breakaway poles. Make crib slats too narrow to strangle a baby. Adopt breakaway baseball bases. **Remove throw rugs in homes of the elderly.**

(Continues on next page)

Figure 2-8 Basic Strategies for Injury Countermeasures (*Continued*)

Strategy	Possible Countermeasures
Make what is to be protected more resistant to the hazard.	**Encourage calcium intake to reduce osteoporosis.** Encourage musculoskeletal conditioning in athletes. Prohibit alcohol sales and consumption near recreational water areas. Treat medical conditions such as epilepsy to prevent episodes that can result in burns, drownings, and falls. Check earthquake-resistant building codes in susceptible areas.
Begin to counter the damage already done by the hazard.	**Provide emergency medical care.** Employ systems to route injured persons to appropriately trained prehospital care providers. **Develop school protocols for responding to injury emergencies.** **Provide first-aid training to residents.** Install automatic sprinkler systems.
Stabilize, repair, and rehabilitate the object of the damage.	Develop rehabilitation plans at an early stage of injury treatment. Make use of occupational rehabilitation for paraplegic patients.

*The examples listed are for illustrative purposes only and are not necessarily the official recommendations of PHTLS, the National Association of EMTs, or the American College of Surgeons Committee on Trauma.
Bold = opportunities for EMS personnel to provide education and leadership.

Prevention—Education, Enforcement, and Engineering. Each of these elements is described here.

Education

Educational strategies are meant to impart information. The target audience may be individuals who engage in high-risk activities, policy makers who have the authority to enact further prevention legislation or regulation, or prehospital care providers learning to become active participants in injury prevention.

Education once was the primary means of implementing prevention programs because society believed that most injuries were simply the result of human error. Although this assumption is true to a certain extent, many failed to recognize the role that energy and the environment play in causing injury. Education is still often used, however, and is probably the easiest of the three strategies to implement.

Experience has demonstrated that educational strategies have not met with overwhelming success for several reasons. For starters, the target audience may never hear the message. If the message is heard, some may reject it outright or not embrace it enough to alter behavior. Those who embrace it may do so sporadically or with declining enthusiasm over time.[23] However, education still can be particularly useful in reducing injury in the following four areas:

1. *Teaching young children basic safety behaviors and skills that stay with them later in life.* Examples include responding appropriately when a smoke detector sounds an alarm, calling 9-1-1 for help in an emergency, or fastening seat belts.

2. *Teaching about certain types and causes of injury for certain age groups.* Education may be the only strategy available for these groups.
3. *Altering the public's perception of risk and acceptable risk to change social norms and attitudes.* This approach was used regarding drinking and driving and occurs now regarding wearing a helmet when riding a bicycle, scooter, skateboard, or rollerblades.
4. *Promoting policy change and educating consumers to demand safer products.*[18]

As a singular approach to injury prevention, educational programs have had disappointing results. Like many drugs, education needs to be "redosed" after a period of time in order to have a continued effect. However, when coupled with other forms of implementation strategies, education can be a valuable tool. Education often serves as a starting point to pave the way for enforcement and engineering strategies.

Enforcement

Enforcement seeks to tap the persuasive power of law to compel adherence to simple but effective prevention strategies. Statutory commands can either require or prohibit, and they can be directed at individual behavior (people), products (things), or environmental conditions (places), as follows:

- Legal requirements that apply to people are mandatory seat-belt, child-restraint, and helmet-use laws.
- Prohibitions that apply to people are drunk-driving laws, speed limits, and assault laws.

- Legal requirements that apply to products include design and performance standards, such as the federal Motor Vehicle Safety Standards.
- Prohibitions that apply to products include restrictions on dangerous animals and flammable fabrics.
- Legal requirements that apply to places include the installation of breakaway signposts along highways and fencing around swimming pools.
- Prohibitions that apply to places include the outlawing of rigid structures along highways and firearms in airport terminals.
- Legal requirements that apply to specific target groups and locations include the federal requirements that public safety and emergency responders wear high-visibility clothing at high-traffic crash sites.[15]

Enforcement is also an active countermeasure because people must obey the law to benefit from it. The target audiences may be less likely to comply if they believe the directive infringes on personal freedom, if they have little chance of getting caught, or if they will not face consequences of violating the law.

Because society as a whole tends to obey laws or at least stay within narrow limits around them, enforcement is often more effective than education. Enforcement in tandem with education appears to produce better results than either initiative alone. Motorcycle-helmet laws provide an interesting case study in the role of enforcement in injury prevention. In states in which helmet laws have been repealed for motorcyclists, the rate of serious injuries and fatalities has increased.[26-28]

Engineering

Often the most effective means of injury prevention are those in which destructive energy release is permanently separated from the host. Passive countermeasures accomplish this goal with little or no effort on the part of the individual. Engineering strategies strive to build injury prevention into products or environments so that the host does not have to act differently to be protected. Engineering strategies help the people who actually need them, and they do so every time. Measures such as automatic sprinkler systems in buildings, flotation hulls in boats, and backup alarms on ambulances have all proven to save lives with little or no effort on the part of the host.

Engineering seems to be the perfect answer to injury prevention. It is passive, effective, and usually the least disruptive of the Three E's. Unfortunately, it is often the most expensive to implement. Designing safety into a product usually makes it more expensive and may require legislative or regulatory initiation. The price may be more than the manufacturer is willing to absorb or the customer is willing to pay. Society dictates how much safety it wants built into a product and how much it is willing to support the endeavor financially.

Education initiatives should precede enforcement and engineering strategies. Ultimately, the most effective countermeasures may be those that incorporate all three implementation strategies.

Public Health Approach

Much has been learned about injury and injury prevention. Unfortunately, a wide discrepancy exists between what is known about injury and what is being done about it.[19] Injury is a complex problem in all societies of the world. Unfortunately, a single person or single agency, alone, will usually have little impact. A public health approach has achieved success in dealing with other diseases and is making progress with injury prevention as well. EMS agencies that have joined forces with other public and private organizations have been able to accomplish as much or more than they could on their own. Partnerships bring together a community's expertise to tackle a complex and perplexing issue.

A public health approach creates a community-based coalition to combat a community-based disease through a four-step process, as follows:

1. Surveillance
2. Risk factor identification
3. Intervention evaluation
4. Implementation

The coalition is comprised of experts from such diverse fields as epidemiology, the medical community, schools of public health, public health agencies, community advocacy programs, economics, sociology, and criminal justice. EMS systems have an important place in a public health approach to injury prevention. Participating in a coalition to improve playground safety may not have the immediate effect of providing care at the scene of a horrific vehicle crash, but the results will be much more widespread.

Surveillance

Surveillance is the process of collecting data within a community. Collection of population-based data aids in the discovery of an injury's true magnitude and effect on the community. A community can be a neighborhood, city, county, state, or even the ambulance service itself. Support for the program, proper allocation of resources, and even knowing who to include on the interdisciplinary team depend on understanding the scope of the problem.

Sources of information available within a community include the following:

- Mortality data
- Hospital admission and discharge statistics
- Medical records
- Trauma registries
- Police reports

- EMS run sheets
- Insurance reports
- Unique surveillance data collected solely for the study at hand

Risk Factor Identification

After a problem is identified and researched, it is necessary to know who is at risk to direct a prevention strategy at the correct population. "Shotgun" approaches to injury prevention are less successful than targeted ones. Identification of causes and risk factors determines who is injured; what types of injuries are sustained; and where, when, and why those injuries occur.[29] Sometimes a risk factor is obvious, such as the presence of alcohol in fatal vehicle crashes. At other times, research is required to discover the true risk factors involved in injury events. EMS systems can serve as the "eyes and ears" of public health at the scene of injuries to identify risk factors that no one else may be able to uncover. Risk factors can then be charted on a Haddon Matrix as they are properly identified.

Intervention Evaluation

As risk factors become clear, intervention strategies begin to emerge. Haddon's list of 10 injury prevention strategies serves as a starting point (see Figure 2-8). Even though communities have different characteristics, with modification, an injury prevention initiative from one community may work in another. Once a potential intervention has been selected, a pilot program using one or more of the Three E's may give indications of the success of full-scale implementation.

Implementation

The final step in the public health approach is implementation and evaluation of the intervention. Detailed implementation procedures are prepared so others interested in implementation of similar programs will have a guide to follow. Collection of evaluation data measures the effectiveness of a program. Answering the following three questions may help determine the success of a program:

1. Have attitudes, skills, or judgment changed?
2. Has behavior changed?
3. Does behavioral change lead to a favorable outcome?[8]

The public health approach provides a proven means to combat a disease such as injury. Through a multidisciplinary, community-based effort, it is possible to identify the "who, what, where, when, and why" of an injury problem and develop a plan of action. EMS systems need to play a much more substantial role in helping to close the gap between what is known about injury and what is being done about it. This approach can be thought of as a continuous loop. Continued surveillance occurs after implementation of an injury control strategy. These data are then used to modify or change the strategy. Successes in injury prevention can be broadened to wider populations at risk.

Evolving Role of EMS in Injury Prevention

Traditionally, the role of the prehospital care provider in health care focuses almost exclusively on postevent, one-on-one treatment of the individual. Little emphasis is placed on understanding the causes of the injuries or what a prehospital care provider could do to prevent them. As a result, patients may return to the same environment only to be injured again. In addition, information that could aid in the development of a community-wide prevention program to keep others from becoming injured in the first place may not be documented and, therefore, may remain unavailable to other sectors of public health.

The public health approach to injury is more proactive. It works to determine how to alter the host, agent, and environment to prevent injuries. Through coalitions that conduct surveillance and implement interventions, public health works to develop community-wide prevention programs. The Emergency Medical Services Agenda for the Future envisions closer ties between EMS systems and public health that would make both sectors of health care more effective.[7]

Prehospital care providers can take a more active role in development of community-wide injury prevention programs. EMS systems enjoy a unique position in the community. With approximately 840,000 providers in the United States alone, basic and advanced prehospital care providers are widely distributed at the community level. Prehospital care providers enjoy a credible reputation in the community, making them high-profile role models. In addition, they are readily welcomed into homes and businesses. All phases of the public health approach to injury prevention benefit from an EMS presence.

One-on-One Interventions

EMS systems do not have to give up their one-on-one approach to patient care to conduct valuable injury prevention interventions. The one-on-one approach makes EMS systems uniquely able to conduct injury prevention initiatives. Prehospital care providers can bring injury prevention messages directly to high-risk individuals. One indicator of a successful educational program is that the information is received with enough enthusiasm to change behavior. Prehospital care providers can use their role-model status to deliver important prevention messages. Implicitly, people look up to role models, listen to what they have to say, and emulate what they do.

On-scene prevention counseling takes advantage of a "teachable moment." A teachable moment is the time when a patient who does not require critical medical interventions or the patient's family members are in a state that makes them more receptive to what a role model says. The prehospital care provider may think of the on-scene time as wasted when it becomes apparent that little or no medical interventions are necessary. However, this may be the best time to deliver primary prevention.[30]

Not every call allows for injury prevention counseling. Serious and life-threatening calls require concentration on acute care. However, as many as 95% of ambulance calls are not life threatening. A significant proportion of EMS calls require minor, if any, treatment. One-on-one prevention counseling may be appropriate during these noncritical calls.

Patient interactions are typically short encounters, especially those that require little or no treatment. However, they provide enough time to discuss and demonstrate to patients and family members practices that may prevent an injury in the future. Prehospital care providers are in a unique position in that they are the only health care worker who enters the patient's environment, thereby viewing situations that may predispose to injury. A role model who discusses the importance of replacing a burned-out light bulb and removing a slippery throw rug in a dimly lit hallway may prevent a fall by an elderly resident. Prehospital care providers have an attentive audience during the ride to a hospital. Prevention is a more valuable topic to discuss than the weather or the local sports team. Teachable moments take one to two minutes to complete and do not interfere with treatment or transport.

Educational programs have been developed to train prehospital care providers to administer on-scene injury prevention counseling.[31] These types of programs must be further developed and evaluated to discover which are the most valuable and, therefore, worthy of inclusion in the primary education of a prehospital care provider.

Community-Wide Interventions

The public health approach to injury prevention is community-based and involves a multidisciplinary team. Prehospital care providers have the expertise to be valuable members of that team. Community-wide prevention strategies depend on data to address properly the "who, what, when, where, and why" of an injury problem. Multiple sources of information, as described previously, provide the needed data. Prehospital care providers, perhaps more than any other team member, have the opportunity to examine patient interaction with the environment at the time of the injury. This may allow identification of a high-risk individual, high-risk attitude, or high-risk behavior that is not present by the time the patient arrives at the ED.

The prehospital care provider can use documentation acquired en route to a medical facility in the following two ways:

1. Data can be used immediately by emergency personnel who receive the patient. Emergency physicians and nurses are also being called on to improve and increase their role in injury prevention. Their "teachable moment" can reinforce and supplement the prehospital care provider's on-scene counseling if they know what has already been discussed or demonstrated.
2. Others in public health can use injury data provided by prehospital care providers retrospectively to help develop a comprehensive, community-wide injury prevention program.

Prehospital care providers usually do not practice documentation to help support a community-wide prevention program. Knowing what to acquire and when to document information beneficial to the development of community-wide prevention programs requires opening a dialogue with other members of the public health team. Leaders in the EMS system need to build a coalition with others in public health to develop documentation policies that promote complete documentation of injuries.

EMS can be the spearhead for workable, effective injury prevention programs that make a profound impact in a community. Programs have been created out of the desire of a small group of EMS professionals to prevent childhood fatalities.[32,33] Services in Louisiana, Florida, Washington, Oregon, and Hawaii have been recognized for their efforts in designing, coordinating, and conducting injury prevention programs through the Nicholas Rosecrans Award for best practices in injury prevention in EMS.[34,35]

While opportunities exist for prehospital care providers to educate patients, one study by Dr. David Jaslow and colleagues suggests that only a minority of prehospital providers do utilize the teachable moment. They found that only 33% routinely educate their patients on how to modify injury risk behaviors, and only 19% routinely provide instruction about proper use of protective devices.[35]

Injury Prevention for EMS Providers

"Who's the most important person at an incident scene?" EMS students are always asked this question early in their training to make them think about their own safety. Invariably, one or two students will say "the patient," which is what the instructor wanted to hear. This incorrect response provides a teachable moment for the instructor to begin the course-long directive to reinforce the point that self-injury prevention is the most valuable service a prehospital care provider can provide.

Hostile environments resulting from terrorist activities or hazardous materials spills unfortunately make the news too often. However, the everyday activities of prehospital providers provide sufficient opportunity for injuries that could end a career or life. The Bureau of Labor Statistics paints an accurate picture of the "normal" dangers in EMS:

> EMTs and paramedics work both indoors and outdoors, in all types of weather. They are required to do considerable kneeling, bending, and heavy lifting. These workers risk noise-induced hearing loss from sirens and back injuries from lifting patients. In addition, EMTs and paramedics may

be exposed to diseases such as hepatitis-B and AIDS, as well as violence from drug overdose victims or mentally unstable patients. The work is not only physically strenuous but also stressful, involving life-or-death situations and suffering patients.[36]

Prehospital care providers are at substantial risk for injury or death while responding to, managing the patient at, and transporting from an emergency medical call. The risks associated with injury both on scene and in a moving ambulance can be minimized by utilizing proper preventive measures such as seat belts or reflective clothing.

Prehospital care providers can become complacent toward the everyday dangers of the job. Complacency is a feeling of security or safety in the unacknowledged face of potential danger. Compounding the situation is the idealism and invincibility of youth typical of some EMS personnel.[37] Management is needed to create a culture of injury prevention or, better, a culture of safety by instituting prevention policy, maintaining adherence to procedure, and rewarding positive performance. The prehospital care providers themselves must be equally committed to the principles of injury prevention. Failure in this initiative by either management or prehospital care providers can have potentially devastating effects.

Other factors to consider are the experience level of personnel and their degree of fatigue. Drivers must be adequately prepared and trained to operate vehicles safely, and EMS personnel must be monitored to ensure they have adequate sleep to maintain safe operations. In a study that looked at common factors in EMS personnel involved in ambulance crashes, the odds were greater that the drivers involved in emergency vehicle crashes would be younger EMS personnel and those EMS personnel reporting sleep problems.[38]

Dr. Neil Stanley, of the British Sleep Society, noted, "Nobody should be doing anything really important for 15 to 30 minutes after they wake up." This has serious implications for EMS, considering that EMS personnel must respond immediately, no matter what the time of night, whether awake or asleep, and be expected to function "normally."

In a prehospital service, employees are not only the most valuable asset but also the most expensive. The service, community, and, most importantly, the prehospital care provider benefit when the employee remains uninjured. An in-house injury prevention program is worthwhile on its own merits. When conducted through a public health approach, however, it provides valuable experience for involvement in community injury prevention initiatives as well. The community (e.g., the ambulance service) is small, there is 100% access to it, and surveillance is easier because the ambulance service has access to many of the data sources it may need. Identification of risk factors is simplified because the target audience consists of fellow employees. Gaining evaluation information should be almost immediate. Outcome data collection should be readily available as well.

Dr. Janet Kinnane and colleagues mention in-house prevention programs that utilize education, enforcement, and engineering implementation strategies.[30] The wide variability of the programs demonstrates the dangers involved in EMS systems and the need for prevention initiatives. It also demonstrates the variability among EMS communities. Even though all EMS systems are similar, individual services (communities) have different risk factors and different prevention priorities.

As described previously, education programs enhance wellness, prevent back injury, and increase awareness of the potential for violent patients. Enforcement programs introduce mandatory fitness programs and establish protocols to deal with violent patients. Engineering initiatives address increasing seat belt use in the back of the ambulance by evaluating the position of equipment and location of the seat. Preemployment screening and physical strengthening help to reduce back injury.

A small-scale, in-house injury prevention program may reap rewards beyond the most important outcome of improved employee health. Small successes lay the groundwork for participation in larger, more complicated endeavors. They provide a valuable on-the-job learning tool about injury prevention for all employees. In addition, in-house prevention programs provide an introduction of the EMS system to other public health agencies in the community that assist in in-house program implementation and evaluation.

Summary

- Trauma is the most neglected current epidemic. The health care industry has failed to measurably decrease the incidence of injuries.
- Prehospital care providers are in a unique position to influence injury morbidity and mortality rates through prevention efforts. Many opportunities exist for EMS personnel to provide public education and leadership.
- The advancement of EMS systems in injury prevention depends on the adoption of this new role by each individual prehospital care provider.
- By committing to injury prevention efforts and by recognizing injury risk factors, prehospital care providers may help prevent death and disability in their community.

SCENARIO RECAP

You and your partner are on the scene of a motor vehicle collision and are working to rapidly extricate a heavy patient from the driver's seat of his vehicle. He was unrestrained in the vehicle during the collision. You and your partner are both wearing approved safety vests over your work gear since you are near the roadway. Law enforcement is on the scene to provide traffic control, and the ambulance is parked to maximize your protection from oncoming vehicles. The patient is packaged properly and secured onto your motorized cot, which is being used due to the patient's weight. The motorized cot allows you and your partner to lift the patient safely into the ambulance without putting excess strain on your bodies.

Once inside the ambulance, you secure yourself in the rear-facing chair and continue care of the patient while your partner operates the siren and the strobe-flashing lights of the ambulance to attract other drivers' attention. She maneuvers safely into her lane and drives to the hospital. The ambulance arrives safely at the hospital, and you transfer the patient to the care of the emergency department staff.

While completing paperwork after the call, you consider the overall national injury and death statistics for prehospital care providers. You realize that thanks to the careful attention to all aspects of injury prevention that you and your partner demonstrated, the call was concluded safely for everyone involved.

- Is accident prevention a realistic approach in preventing injury and death in motor vehicle collisions and other causes of traumatic injury?
- Is there evidence that compliance with seat belt and safety seats has an impact in preventing injury and death?
- As prehospital care providers, what can we do to prevent deaths and injuries from motor vehicle collisions?

SCENARIO SOLUTION

You and your partner remained safe while at the motor vehicle collision scene because you recalled and followed your department's safety protocols. You were aware that flashing or strobe lights are not always sufficient in attracting drivers' attention, so you wore your approved reflective vests to be more visible to other drivers while operating at the scene. You also recalled and followed proper lifting techniques and safety procedures, and you ensured your safety by wearing a seat belt while in the treatment area of the ambulance.

In addition, your department recently updated the reflective chevron design on the rear of the ambulance to enhance the visibility of the ambulance from a distance. To enhance night-time visibility, red and white lights on the exterior of the ambulance were replaced by additional blue lights. These measures have all proven to be very helpful in reducing scene visibility concerns and ensuring crew member safety.

References

1. National Academy of Sciences/National Research Council (NAS/NRC). Accidental death and disability: the neglected disease of modern society, Washington, DC: NAS/NRC; 1966.
2. National Center for Health Statistics (NCHS). *Health, United States, 2000, with Adolescent Health Chartbook*, Hyattsville, MD: NCHS; 2000.
3. National Center for Injury Prevention and Control, Centers for Disease Control and Prevention. http://www.cdc.gov/injury/wisqars/index.html. Accessed August 2009.
4. Centers for Disease Control and Prevention, National Center for Injury Prevention and Control, Web-based Injury Statistics Query and Reporting System
5. World Health Organization (WHO). Injuries and violence: the facts. Geneva, Switzerland: WHO; 2010.
6. Peden M, McGee K, Sharma G. *The Injury Chart Book: A Graphical Overview of the Global Burden of Injuries*. Geneva: World Health Organization; 2002.
7. National Highway Traffic Safety Administration (NHTSA), US Department of Health and Human Services, Health Resources and Services Administration, Maternal and Child Health Bureau. Emergency Medical Services Agenda for the Future. Washington, DC: NHTSA; 1999.
8. Martinez R. Injury control: a primer for physicians. *Ann Emerg Med.* 1990;19:72-77, 1990.
9. Waller JA. *Injury Control: A Guide to the Causes and Prevention of Trauma.* Lexington, MA: Lexington Books; 1985.
10. US Department of Transportation, National Highway Traffic Safety Administration. PIER: Public Information, Education, and Relations for EMS Injury Prevention Modules. Washington, DC: DOT HS 809 520; 2002.
11. Reason J. Human error: models and management. *BMJ.* 2000;320:768-770.
12. Cohen L, Miller T, Sheppard MA, Gordon E, Gantz T, Atnafou R. Bridging the gap: bringing together intentional and unintentional injury prevention efforts to improve health and well being. *J Safety Res.* 2003;34:473-483.

13. Alterman MD, Daniel M. Considerations in pediatric trauma: epidemiology. http://emedicine.medscape.com/article/435031-overview#aw2aab6b3. Accessed March 23, 2013.

14. Centers for Disease Control and Prevention, National Center for Injury Prevention and Control. *Saving Lives and Protecting People from Injuries and Violence*. http://www.cdc.gov/injury/pdfs/NCIPC_Overview_FactSheet_Overview-a.pdf. Accessed October 4, 2013.

15. Christoffel T, Gallagher SS. *Injury Prevention and Public Health: Practical Knowledge, Skills, and Strategies*. Gaithersburg, MD: Aspen; 1999.

16. VanDale K. Sleep deprivation in EMS. http://www.fireengineering.com/articles/print/volume-166/issue-02/departments/fireems/sleep-deprivation-in-ems.html. Accessed August 1, 2013.

17. Patterson PD, Weaver MD, Frank RC, et al. Association between poor sleep, fatigue, and safety outcomes in emergency medical services providers. *Prehosp Emerg Care*. 2012;16:86-97.

18. Maguire BJ, Huntington KL, Smith GS, Levick NR. Occupational fatalities in emergency medical services: a hidden crisis. *Ann Emerg Med*. 2002;40:6.

19. Centers for Disease Control and Prevention. Ambulance crash-related injuries among emergency medical services workers—United States, 1991–2002. *MMWR*. 2003;52(8):154-156.

20. Tortella BJ, Lavery RF. Disabling job injuries among EMS providers. *Prehosp Disaster Med*. 1994;9:2120-2213.

21. Reichard A, Marsh S, Moore P. Fatal and nonfatal injuries among emergency medical technicians and paramedics. *Prehosp Emerg Care*. 2011;15(4):511-517.

22. Garrison HG. Keeping rescuers safe. *Ann Emerg Med*. 2002;40:633-635.

23. National EMS Advisory Council. Strategy for a National EMS Culture of Safety (draft). http://www.emscultureofsafety.org/wp-content/uploads/2012/12/Strategy-for-a-National-EMS-Culture-of-Safety-NEMSAC-DRAFT.pdf Accessed October 8, 2013.

24. Mullins RJ, Veum-Stone J, Helfand M, et al. Outcome of hospitalized injured patients after institution of a trauma system in an urban area. *JAMA*. 1994;271(24):1919-1924.

25. Haddix AC, Mallonee S, Waxweiler R, et al. Cost effectiveness analysis of a smoke alarm giveaway program in Oklahoma City, Oklahoma. *Inj Prev*. 2001;7:276-281.

26. Mertz KJ, Weiss HB. Changes in motorcycle-related head injury deaths, hospitalizations, and hospital charges following repeal of Pennsylvania's mandatory motorcycle helmet law. *Am J Public Health*. 2008; 98(8):1464-1467.

27. Bledsoe GH, Li G. Trends in Arkansas motorcycle trauma after helmet law repeal. *South Med J*. 22005;98(4):436-440.

28. Chenier TC, Evans L. Motorcyclist fatalities and the repeal of mandatory helmet wearing laws. *Accid Anal Prev*. 1987;19(2):133-139.

29. Todd KH. *Accidents Aren't: Proposal for Evaluation of an Injury Prevention Curriculum for EMS Providers—A Grant Proposal to the National Association of State EMS Directors*. Atlanta: Department of Emergency Medicine, Emory University School of Medicine; 1998.

30. Kinnane JM, Garrison HG, Coben JH, et al. Injury prevention: is there a role for out-of-hospital emergency medical services? *Acad Emerg Med*. 1997;4:306.

31. EPIC Medics. http://www.epicmedics.org/Conferences.html Accessed October 8, 2013.

32. Hawkins ER, Brice JH, Overby BA. Welcome to the world: findings from an emergency medical services pediatric injury prevention program. *Pediatr Emerg Care*. 2007;23(11):790-795.

33. Griffiths K. Best practices in injury prevention. *J Emerg Med Serv*. 2002;27:8.

34. Krimston J, Griffiths K. Best practices in injury prevention. *J Emerg Med Serv*. 2003;28:9.

35. Jaslow D, Ufberg J, Marsh R. Primary injury prevention in an urban EMS system. *J Emerg Med*. 2003;25(2):167-170.

36. US Department of Labor. Emergency medical technicians and paramedics. In: US Department of Labor, Bureau of Labor Statistics, eds. *Occupational Outlook Handbook, 2004–2005 Edition*. http://stats.bls.gov/oco/ocos101.htm. Accessed July 2004.

37. Federal Emergency Management Agency, US Fire Administration. *EMS Safety: Techniques and Applications*. International Association of Fire Fighters, FEMA contract EMW-91-C-3592.

38. Studnek JR, Fernandez AR. Characteristics of emergency medical technicians involved in ambulance crashes. *Prehosp Disaster Med*. 2008;23(5):432-437.

Suggested Reading

American College of Surgeons Committee on Trauma. *Advanced Trauma Life Support for Doctors, Student Course Manual*. 9th ed. Chicago: American College of Surgeons; 2012.

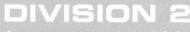
CHAPTER

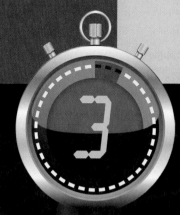

The Science, Art, and Ethics of Prehospital Care: Principles, Preferences, and Critical Thinking

CHAPTER OBJECTIVES

At the completion of this chapter, the reader will be able to do the following:

- Describe the difference between principles and preferences.

- Discuss how principles and preferences relate to decision making in the field.

- Given a trauma scenario, discuss the principles of trauma care for the specific situation, conditions, prehospital care provider knowledge and skill level, and available equipment.

- Given a trauma scenario, use critical-thinking skills to determine the preferred method for accomplishing the principles of emergency trauma care.

- Explain the relationship of ethics to prehospital trauma care.

- Relate the four principles of ethical decision making.

- Given a trauma scenario, discuss the ethical issues involved and how to address them.

- Identify the components and importance of prehospital research and literature.

SCENARIO

A prehospital crew made up of an EMT and a paramedic is called to the scene of a two-vehicle T-bone collision. This is the only available unit at the moment. In a somewhat dilapidated pickup truck, there is a young unrestrained male driver who smells strongly of alcohol and has an obviously deformed forearm. The truck has struck a small passenger sedan on the passenger's side front door, with significant intrusion into the passenger compartment. The elderly female in the front passenger seat does not appear to be breathing, and the windshield is starred directly in front of her. The female driver of the sedan is also injured but conscious and extremely anxious. In the rear seats, there are two children restrained in car seats. The child on the passenger side of the deformed compartment appears to be approximately 3 years old and is unconscious and slumped over in the car seat. On the driver's side, a 5-year-old boy is restrained in a booster seat and appears to be uninjured, though he is crying hysterically.

The driver of the pickup truck is obviously injured with an open arm fracture, but he is belligerent and verbally abusive and is refusing treatment. Meanwhile, the driver of the sedan is frantically inquiring about her children and her mother.

- How would you manage this multiple-patient incident?
- Which of these patients is of highest priority?
- What would you tell the mother of the two children about their condition?
- How would you deal with the apparently intoxicated driver of the other vehicle?
- Would you allow the apparently intoxicated driver to refuse care?

Introduction

Medicine has changed a great deal since the famous 1887 painting by Sir Luke Fildes that shows the concern and frustration of a physician sitting at the bedside of a sick child (**Figure 3-1**). At that time, there were no antibiotics, only a minimal understanding of disease and illness, and only rudimentary surgery. Medication consisted primarily of herbal remedies. For many years, it has been understood and accepted that medicine is not an exact science and that there is much art in its practice. This recognition has applied to all aspects of medicine and to all practitioners, from allied health personnel to nurses to physicians. In recent decades, our understanding of disease, technology, and electronics has advanced at a rapid rate as ever-expanding research has allowed us to provide better patient care. The practice of medicine has become more and more a science and less and less an art. However, the art remains, and medicine is still a long way from the precise science of math or physics.

It was not until the 1950s that there was thought to be any benefit to training those who encountered the patient prior to arrival to the emergency room. In those days, the emergency room was literally a "room," usually at the back of the hospital and often locked until someone came to open it. The fund of knowledge provided to prehospital care providers has significantly advanced in the years since. With this growth comes the major responsibility that each prehospital care provider must ensure that he or she is up to date with the latest knowledge and that skills are kept finely honed. Knowledge is gained from reading and continuing medical education (CME) classes, and skills

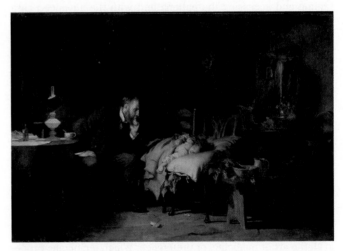

Figure 3-1 "The Doctor" by Sir Luke Fildes shows a concerned physician sitting by the bedside of an ill child. The relatively primitive state of health care offered few options for intervention beyond hopeful waiting and watching.
Source: © Tate, London 2014

improve with experience and critique, like those of a surgeon or an airplane pilot. Just as a pilot does not solo after one flight, the emergency medical technician (EMT) does not mature from using a skill only once or in only one type of situation.

The science of prehospital care involves a working knowledge of the following:

1. Anatomy—the organs, bones, muscles, arteries, nerves, and veins of the human body
2. Physiology, including how the body produces and maintains heat, Starling's law of the heart (increasing

preload increases stroke volume), and the Ficke principle (which describes cardiac output and oxygen extraction)

3. Pharmacology and the physiologic actions produced by various drugs and their interaction with each other inside the body

4. The relationship among these components

By applying one's understanding of these elements, providers can make fully correct—scientific—decisions when treating their patients.

A major improvement in the science of medicine has been in the technical components and the diagnostic equipment available. The ability to assess the condition of the patient and diagnose and treat a patient has dramatically improved with the imaging techniques of computed tomography (CT) scans, ultrasound, and magnetic resonance imaging (MRI); with sophisticated clinical laboratories that can measure almost any electrolyte, hormone, or substance produced metabolically; with the sophistication of complex medications produced by the pharmaceutical industry; with the technical advances in surgery, medicine, and invasive radiology; with the emergency medical services (EMS) communication improvements and logistic equipment such as global positioning systems (GPS) to improve finding and accessing the patient; and with the advanced care that can be provided by physicians and EMS personnel working together as part of the same medical care team. The science of medicine has become much more advanced.

Yet, with all of these advances, it is the art of medicine that continues to rely on health care providers to use their knowledge and critical-thinking skills to make appropriate judgments and decisions to identify the correct diagnostic device, the proper medication, or the most efficient procedures that will most benefit the patient. For prehospital care providers, this is the determination of which patient is potentially seriously injured; which patient needs rapid transportation to which hospital; how much should be done on the scene versus during transport; what techniques should be used to accomplish needed interventions; and what equipment is the best to use in a particular situation. This is all the art of medicine, or preference. Which technique, procedure, or device does the prehospital care provider have in his or her armamentarium that, in his or her hands, will suit the needs of the patient in the situation that exists at the time? Which is the preferred method? All of these questions must be answered based upon the critical-thinking skills of the prehospital care provider.

Principles and Preferences

The science of medicine provides the **principles** of medical care. Simply stated, principles are those things that must be present, accomplished, or ensured by the health care provider in order to optimize patient survival and outcome. How these principles are implemented by the individual provider to most efficiently manage the patient at the time of patient contact depends on

preferences, based on the situation that exists at the specific time, the clinical condition of the patient, individual training and skills, and the equipment available. This is how the *science* of medicine and the *art* of medicine come together for the good of patient care.

The importance of, and difference between, principle and preference can be illustrated by airway management. The *principle* is that air, containing oxygen, must be moved through an open airway into the lungs to provide oxygenation of the red blood cells as they course through the lungs and on to the tissue cells. This principle is true for all patients. The *preference* is in how airway management is carried out in a particular patient. In some cases, patients will manage the airway on their own; in others, the prehospital care provider will have to decide what devices are to be used, whether or not assisted ventilation is required, and so forth. In other words, the provider will determine the best way to ensure that the air passages are open to get oxygen into the lungs and, secondarily, to get carbon dioxide out. The art is how the prehospital care provider makes this determination and carries it out to achieve the principle.

The preferences of how to accomplish the principles depend upon four factors: the situation, the patient's condition, the provider's knowledge base, and the equipment available (**Figure 3-2**).

The philosophy of the Prehospital Trauma Life Support (PHTLS) program is that each situation and patient is different. PHTLS teaches the importance of having a strong understanding of the subject matter and the skills necessary to accomplish needed interventions. The judgments and decisions made on the scene should be individualized to the needs of *this* specific patient being managed at *this* specific time and in *this* specific situation. Protocols are not the final answer. Protocols are inflexible to the variability of the event. The prehospital care provider must know the scene, the situation, the abilities of the prehospital care providers involved, and the equipment available. Understanding what can and should be accomplished for a particular patient is based on this information. By understanding the principles involved and using critical-thinking skills, appropriate decisions can be made.

Figure 3-2 Principles Versus Preferences

Principle—what is necessary for patient improvement or survival

Preference—how the principle is achieved in the time given and by the prehospital care provider available

The preference used to accomplish the principle depends upon four factors:

- Situation that exists
- Condition of the patient
- Fund of knowledge of the prehospital care provider
- Equipment available

Preferences describe the way that an individual prehospital care provider can best accomplish the principle. The principle will not be accomplished the same way in every situation or for every condition of every patient. Not all prehospital care providers have skill mastery in every available technique. The tools to carry out these techniques are not necessarily available at the site of all emergencies. Just because one instructor, lecturer, or physician director prefers one technique does not mean it is the best technique for *every* prehospital care provider in *every* situation. The important point is to achieve the principle. How this is done and how the care is provided to the patient depend on the four factors listed in Figure 3-2 and described in more detail in the following sections.

Situation

The situation involves all of the factors at a scene that can affect what care is provided to a patient. These factors include, but are certainly not limited to, the following:

- Hazards on the scene
- Number of patients involved
- Location of the patient
- Position of the vehicle
- Contamination or hazardous materials concerns
- Fire or chance of fire
- Weather
- Scene control and security by law enforcement
- Time/distance to medical care, including the capabilities of the closest hospital versus the nearest trauma center
- Number of prehospital care providers and other possible helpers on the scene
- Bystanders
- Transportation available on the scene
- Other transportation available at a distance (i.e., helicopters, additional ambulances)

All of these conditions and circumstances, as well as many others, may be constantly changing and will affect the way that you, as a prehospital care provider, can respond to the needs of the patient.

Take for example the following situation: a single-vehicle crash into a tree on a rural road in a wooded area. The weather is clear and dark (time 0200 hours). The transport time by ground to the trauma center is 35 minutes. A medical helicopter can be dispatched by prehospital care providers on the scene with approval of medical control. Startup time for the helicopter is 5 minutes, and travel time is 15 minutes; a nontrauma center hospital is 15 minutes away and has a helistop. Do you transport by ground, stop at the helistop, or stay on scene, and wait for the helicopter?

Some examples of how the situation affects a procedure such as spinal immobilization include the following:

Situation 1:

- Automobile crash
- Bull's-eye fracture of the windscreen
- Warm, sunny day
- No traffic on the road

Management:

- Patient examined in the car
- Cervical collar applied
- Patient secured to the short backboard
- Rotated onto the long backboard
- Removed from the car
- Placed on the stretcher
- Physical assessment completed
- Patient transported to the hospital

Situation 2:

- Same as above except gasoline is dripping from the gas tank
- Concern for fire

Management:

- Rapid extraction techniques used
- Patient moved significant distance from the vehicle
- Physical assessment completed
- Patient transported to the hospital

Situation 3:

- House fully involved in flames
- Patient unable to move

Management:

- No assessment
- Patient dragged from the fire
- Placed on backboard
- Moved quickly to a safe distance away from the fire
- Patient assessment completed
- Patient transported quickly to the hospital depending on the patient's condition

Situation 4:

- Combat situation with nearby perpetrator or enemy combatants actively shooting (police or military action)
- Officer (or soldier) with gunshot wound to the knee and significant bleeding

Management:

- Assessment from a distance (binoculars)
- Presence of other wounds
- Patient still able to fire his weapon
- Tell patient to apply tourniquet on upper leg
- Tell patient to crawl to a protected position
- Rescue the patient when conditions permit

Condition of the Patient

This component of the decision-making process concerns the medical condition of the patient. The major question that will affect decision making is "How sick is the patient?" Some examples of issues that will facilitate this determination include the cause of the medical condition, the age of the patient, physiologic factors that affect energy production (blood pressure, pulse, ventilatory rate, skin temperature, etc.), the etiology of the trauma, the patient's medical condition prior to the event, medication that the patient is using, illicit drug use, and alcohol use. All of these factors, and others, will require critical thinking to decide when and how to transport the patient, what needs to be done to prepare for transport, and what needs to be done on the scene versus while en route.

Let's return to the scenario of the single-vehicle crash with a tree: The patient is breathing with difficulty at a rate of 30 breaths per minute, his heart rate is 110 beats per minute, blood pressure is 90 mm Hg by palpation, and his Glasgow Coma Scale score is 11 (E3V3M5); he is in his mid-20s, he was not wearing a seat belt, and his position is against the dash away from the driver-side air bag; he has a deformed right leg at mid-thigh and an open left ankle fracture with significant hemorrhage. There is approximately 1 liter of blood on the floorboard near the ankle.

Fund of Knowledge of the Prehospital Care Provider

The fund of knowledge of the prehospital care provider comes from several sources, including initial training, recent CME courses, experience in the field, experience with this specific condition, and skill with the available potential procedures that the patient might require.

For example, consider airway control. The level of the prehospital care provider has a significant impact on the available choices of preference. The authorized airway interventions depend on the level of the prehospital care provider at the scene. In addition, skill with a particular intervention and comfort with performing it depend a great deal on the frequency with which it has been performed. As the prehospital care provider, you might consider: When was the last time you had to actively manage an airway? What device did you use? When was the last time you performed an intubation? How comfortable are you with the laryngoscope? How many times have you done a cricothyrotomy

on a live patient or even an animal training model? Without the appropriate skills and experience, the patient would likely be better off and the prehospital care provider would be more comfortable choosing an oral airway plus bag-mask device rather than a more advanced intervention such as endotracheal intubation or a surgical airway as the preference for management.

Returning to the example of the patient in the single-vehicle crash, the responding prehospital care providers have been working together for 2 years. Both are nationally registered paramedics (NRPs). Their last update training for endotracheal use was 1 year ago. One paramedic last placed an endotracheal (ET) tube 2 months ago; his partner placed one a month ago. They are not authorized to use paralytic drugs for ET insertion, but they can use sedation if necessary. They were just trained on hemorrhage control using tourniquets and hemostatic agents. How will their training impact what will be done to manage the patient in the field?

Equipment Available

The experience of any prehospital care provider with the most sophisticated equipment in the world does no good if that sophisticated equipment is not available. The prehospital care provider must use the equipment or supplies that are available. As an example, blood may be the best resuscitation fluid for trauma victims. However, this is not available in the field; therefore, the resuscitation fluid at hand (crystalloid) is the best available choice, depending on the situation. Another consideration is whether hypotensive resuscitation (permissive hypotension) would be a better choice given the nature of the patient's injuries. This particular issue is discussed in more detail in the Shock chapter.

Let's return to the patient in the single-vehicle crash once again: There is complete paramedic equipment that was checked at the beginning of the shift. It includes ET tubes, laryngoscopes, tourniquets, and other equipment and supplies as indicated by the American College of Surgeons/American College of Emergency Physicians (ACS/ACEP) equipment list. The paramedics have all the appropriate drugs including hemostatic agents. They apply manual pressure to the bleeding ankle and are able to control the hemorrhage. They splint the patient's femur and transport him to the nearby trauma center.

The foundation of PHTLS is to teach the prehospital care provider to make appropriate decisions for patient care based on knowledge, not based on protocol. The goal of patient care is to achieve the principle. How this is achieved (that is, the decision made by the prehospital care provider to manage the patient) is the preference based on the situation, patient condition, fund of knowledge and skill, and equipment available at the time—the four components outlined above.

For example, when a nonbreathing patient is encountered, the *principle* is that the airway must be opened and oxygen delivered to the lungs. The *preference* chosen depends on the four preference factors (situation, patient condition, fund of knowledge and experience/skill, equipment available). A bystander on the street with only cardiopulmonary resuscitation (CPR) training may perform mouth-to-mask ventilation; the EMT may choose an oral airway and bag-mask ventilation; the paramedic may choose to place an ET tube or may decide that it is more advantageous to use the bag-mask device with rapid transport; the corpsman in combat may choose a cricothyroidotomy or nothing at all if the enemy fire is too intense; and the physician in the emergency department (ED) may choose paralytic drugs or fiber-optic–guided ET tube placement. None of the choices are wrong at a specific point in time for a given patient, and, applying the same logic, none are correct all of the time.

This concept of principle and preference for the care of the trauma patient has its most dramatic application in the combat situation in the military. For this reason, the Tactical Combat Casualty Care Committee (TCCC) wrote the military component of the PHTLS program. For the military provider, the scene situation will include whether or not there is active combat, the location of the enemy, the tactical situation, the weapons currently (or potentially) being used, and protection available for sheltering the wounded. Although this critical difference in the situation leading to alterations in preference for patient care is most apparent in combat, similar considerations exist in the civilian setting for tactical emergency medical support providers and those prehospital care providers who work in hazardous environments such as fire scenes. For example, in the middle of a house that is fully involved in fire, a fire fighter–paramedic discovering a patient who is down cannot stop to check the basic principles of patient assessment, such as airway and cardiac output. The first step is to get the patient outside and away from the immediate danger of the fire and then to check for airway and pulse.

For the military medic potentially involved in combat, the three-step process for casualty management developed by the Tactical Combat Causality Care (TCCC) is:

1. **Care Under Fire**—management in the middle of a fire fight
2. **Tactical Field Care**—management after the shooting is over but danger still exists
3. **Tactical Evacuation Care**—treatment of the casualty once the situation has been controlled and is considered safe

While the principles of patient care are not changed, the preferences of patient care may be dramatically different due to one or more of these factors. For other discussion, details, and clarification, refer to the Civilian Tactical Emergency Medical Support (TEMS) chapter or the military version of PHTLS. (These situational differences are described in more detail in the Scene Assessment chapter.)

Critical Thinking

To successfully accomplish the principle needed for a particular patient and to choose the best preference to implement the principle, critical-thinking skills are as important as—and may be

even more important than—the manual skills that will be used to perform an intervention. Critical thinking in medicine is a process in which the health care provider assesses the situation, the patient, and all of the resources that are available (**Figure 3-3**). This information is then rapidly analyzed and integrated to provide the best care possible to the patient. The critical-thinking process requires that the health care provider develop a plan of action, initiate this plan, reassess the plan as the process of caring for the patient moves forward, and make adjustments in the plan as the patient's condition changes until that phase of care is completed (**Figure 3-4**). Critical thinking is a learned skill that improves with use and experience.[1] If prehospital care providers are to function successfully, they must be equipped with the lifelong learning and critical-thinking skills necessary to acquire and process information in a rapidly and ever-changing world.[2]

For the prehospital care provider, this process begins with the initial information provided at the time of dispatch and continues until the handoff in the hospital to the next component in the chain of patient care. This critical-thinking process first requires that the prehospital care provider assess and reassess the situation in which the patient is encountered. Then, the patient's condition must be assessed and frequently reassessed during the time on the scene and while en route to the best/appropriate facility. Critical thinking is also involved in the selection of best/appropriate facility for the patient, the resources available, and the transport time to the various facilities in the vicinity. All of these critical decisions are based upon the situation, the patient condition, the fund of knowledge of the prehospital care provider, and the equipment available.

By analyzing and integrating all of this information, the prehospital care provider will develop an initial treatment plan to care for the injured trauma victim and will move that

---

Figure 3-3 Components of Critical Thinking in Emergency Medical Care

1. Assess the situation.
2. Assess the patient.
3. Assess the available resources.
4. Analyze the possible solutions.
5. Select the best answer to manage the situation and patient.
6. Develop the plan of action.
7. Initiate the plan of action.
8. Reassess the response of the patient to the plan of action.
9. Make any needed adjustments or changes to the plan of action.
10. Continue with steps 8 and 9 until this phase of care is completed.

plan forward. For each step along the way, the prehospital care provider must reassess exactly how the patient has responded to this process. Prehospital care providers must either continue the treatment plan or take steps to change the process as additional information becomes available. All of this depends on the critical-thinking skills used by prehospital care providers to carry out their responsibilities. Critical thinking is based on

accepting nothing at face value and always asking the question "Why?" as taught by Socrates.[3]

The critical-thinking process cannot be dogmatic or gullible; it must be open-minded with skepticism.[4] The prehospital care provider must question the scientific accuracy of all approaches. This is the reason why the prehospital care provider must have a strong, well-grounded fund of knowledge that can be used to

Figure 3-4 Steps in Critical Thinking

Assessment
What is going on? What needs to be done? What are the resources to achieve the goal? Analysis will involve:
- Scene assessment
- Identification of any hazards to either the patient or the prehospital care provider
- Condition of the patient
- Rapidity required for resolution
- Location of the care (in the field, during transport, and after arrival to the hospital)
- Number of patients on the scene
- Number of transport vehicles required
- Need for more rapid transport (aero-medical)
- Destination of the patient for the appropriate care

Analysis
Each of the above-described conditions must be individually and rapidly analyzed, and they must be cross-referenced with the prehospital care provider's fund of knowledge and the resources available. Steps must be defined to provide the best care.

Construction of a Plan
The plan to achieve the best outcome for the patient is developed and critically reviewed. Is any step false? Are the planned steps all achievable? Are the resources available that will allow the plan to move forward? Will they, more likely than not, lead to a successful outcome?

Action
The plan is enacted and put in motion. This is done decisively and with strength of command so that there is no doubt or hesitation from any of the individuals involved as to what needs to be accomplished, who is in command, and who is making the decisions. If the decisions are incorrect, incomplete, or causing difficulties or complications, the prehospital care provider in command must make appropriate changes. The input for change can come from observations of the commander or from other available sources.

Reassessment
Is the process moving correctly? Has the situation on scene changed? Does anything in the action plan need to be changed? What is the patient's condition? How has the treatment plan changed the patient's condition?

Changes Along the Way
Any changes that are identified by the prehospital care provider are assessed and analyzed as above and alterations made as appropriate so as to continue the best possible care for the patient. Decision making and reassessment of the patient must proceed without the worry of, "If I change, is that a sign of weakness or poor decision making initially?" Change based on patient need is not weakness, but rather strength. Once a decision is made, as the process continues and the situation and patient respond, the prehospital care provider reassesses and makes appropriate changes as required to provide the best possible care to the patient.

make appropriate decisions. However, the questioning cannot be taken too far. Aristotle suggested that one should not require more certainty than the subject allows.[5] When a prehospital care provider is assessing and caring for a patient, withholding action in hopes of securing absolute certainty in the patient's diagnosis would be foolish; such certainty is impossible, and seeking it would only delay needed interventions. A prehospital care provider must make the most informed assessment and decision possible given the information available at the time.

In other words, critical thinking involves determining how to best provide the principles of patient care needed by the patient based on the current circumstances that the prehospital care provider has noted. It relies upon the basis of appropriate medical care advocated by PHTLS: "Judgment based on knowledge." Robert Carroll described critical thinking as based on concepts and principles, not hard-and-fast rules or step-by-step procedures.[4] The emphasis throughout PHTLS education is that protocols involving robotic recall are not beneficial for patient management. Guidelines for patient care must be flexible. Critical thinking requires that flexibility. Protocols should simply serve as guidelines to assist the prehospital care provider in aligning the thought process. They are not the definitive, be-all-end-all steps that cannot be violated by thoughtful, insightful analysis of the situation and application of appropriate steps to ensure the best possible patient care in each unique situation.

Using Critical Thinking to Control Biases

All health care providers have biases that can affect the critical-thinking process and decision making about the patient. These biases must be recognized and not allowed to intrude during the patient care process. Biases usually arise from previous experiences that resulted in either a significant positive or negative impact. By becoming aware of and controlling biases, all conditions are taken into consideration and action is based on the admonition of "Assume the worst possible injury is present and prove that it is not there" as well as "Do no further harm." The patient's treatment plan is designed regardless of the attitudes of the prehospital care provider regarding the "apparent" conditions that might have led to the current circumstances. For example, the initial impression that a driver is intoxicated may be correct, but other conditions may exist as well. Because a patient is found to be intoxicated does not mean he or she is not injured too. Because the patient is intoxicated with impaired mental facilities does not mean that some of that impairment might not be due to brain injury or decreased cerebral perfusion because of shock.

Frequently, the complete picture cannot be seen until the patient arrives at the hospital (or maybe even several days thereafter); therefore, the critical thinking and response of the prehospital care provider must be based on a worst-case scenario.

Judgments must be made on the best information available. The critical thinker is constantly looking for "other information" as it becomes available and acting on it. The critical-thinking process must continue throughout the assessment of the patient, the situation, and the conditions. The brain of the critical thinker is always looking for new information, making and revising judgments, and planning two to three steps beyond the current activity.

Using Critical Thinking in Rapid Decision Making

EMS is a field of quick action and reliance on the innate ability of the prehospital care provider to respond decisively to varying presentations and varying diseases. These quick actions require the skill of critical thinking and the ability to decide, based on the current knowledge, which steps provide the best chance for patient survival—preference, not rigidity.

Critical thinking at the site of an emergency must be swift, thorough, flexible, and objective. The prehospital care provider at the site of an emergency may have only seconds to assess the situation, the condition of the patient(s), and the resources in order to make decisions and commence patient care. Critical thinking encompasses the processes of discernment, analysis, evaluation, judgment, re-evaluation, and making new decisions until the patient finally arrives at the hospital. That said, critical thinking may at times involve recognizing that you can take your time to come to a decision, take your time and stay on scene a bit longer to perform a key meaningful intervention, or take another moment to look at the entire scene prior to transporting a patient.

By way of comparison, the critical-care thinking process of an administrator may allow for several days, weeks, or even months to work through the decision-making process. In EMS, a strong fund of knowledge possessed by the prehospital care provider and the ability to communicate these judgments with strength and conviction to all involved in the response to the patient are the foundation for critical thinking.

Using Critical Thinking in Data Analysis

As taught in the Patient Assessment and Management chapter, information is gathered using all of the prehospital care provider's senses—vision, smell, touch, hearing—and simultaneously fed into the "computer" inside the brain. The prehospital care provider then analyzes the data obtained based on the predetermined priorities of the primary assessment (airway, ventilation, and circulation), resuscitation, and rapid transport to the appropriate medical facility to select the appropriate management steps for the individual needs of that particular patient.

Typically, the process of evaluating a trauma patient begins with the ABCDE priorities (airway, breathing, circulation, disability, exposure), but critical thinking guides the prehospital care provider to the most critical condition first. If the patient is in shock because of severe ongoing external hemorrhage, then a pressure dressing (and tourniquet if that fails) over the site of severe hemorrhage is the appropriate initial step after assessment. Critical thinking is the recognition that following the standard ABCDE priority may lead to a patient who has an airway but who has now exsanguinated; so, instead of attention to the airway, control of the bleeding was the appropriate first step. Critical thinking is the process of recognizing that if direct pressure and the pressure dressing are not working, something more needs to be done, and application of a tourniquet is the next best step to stop the hemorrhage. How the brain of the prehospital care provider functionally arrived at this decision is *critical thinking*. It is based on the assessment of the situation, the condition of the patient, the fund of knowledge of the prehospital care provider, the skills of the prehospital care provider, and the equipment available. As stated by Banning.

> Critical thinking is a pervasive skill that involves scrutinizing, differentiating, and appraising information and reflecting on the information gained in order to make judgments and inform clinical decisions.[6]

Using Critical Thinking Throughout the Phases of Patient Care

The art and science of medicine, the knowledge of principles, and the appropriate application of preferences will lead to the anticipated outcome of the very best care possible for the patient in the circumstances in which the care is provided. There are essentially four phases in the process of caring for patients with acute injuries:

- The prehospital phase
- The initial (resuscitative) phase in the hospital
- The stabilization and definitive care phase
- The long-term resolution and rehabilitation to return the patient to a functional status

All of these phases use the same principles of patient care in each step. All of the health care providers throughout the phases of the patient's care must use critical thinking. Critical thinking continues from the time of the injury until the time that the patient goes home. The end result of each critical-thinking step along the way varies according to the resources that are available to provide the needed care and the response of the patient to the prior decisions made. Therefore, understanding the principles of management, the options available, the reassessment as the situation and the conditions change, and the modification of the management plan throughout the patient's entire care requires use of the critical-thinking process.

EMS personnel are directly involved in the initial (prehospital) phase of care but must use critical thinking and be aware of the entire process in order to produce seamless patient care as the patient moves through the system. The prehospital care provider must think beyond the current situation to the definitive care needs and the patient's ultimate outcome. The goal is to manage the patient's injuries so that they heal and the patient can be discharged from the hospital in the best possible condition. For example, critical thinking involves recognizing that while splinting the fractured forearm of a multisystem trauma patient is not one of the initial priorities of care, when considering the definitive outcome of the patient and his or her ability to lead a productive life, the preservation of limb function (and thus splinting of the limb) is an important concern in the patient's prehospital treatment.

Ethics

Prehospital professionals face many ethically challenging scenarios that are both emergent and time sensitive. However, the lack of prehospital-specific ethics education can leave prehospital care providers feeling both unprepared and unsupported when confronted with ethically confusing or conflicting situations.[7] Critical-thinking skills can provide a sound basis for making many of the difficult ethical decisions required of prehospital care providers.

The goal of this section is to use bioethical principles and concepts to begin to develop ethical awareness and ethical reasoning skills, and to provide common frameworks and vocabulary to think through and discuss even the most ethically challenging and difficult cases. This section will rely upon the traditional elements of basic bioethics education, which are familiar to most health care providers, but will use prehospital examples and cases to provide content that is authentic, practical, and applicable to the field setting. Additionally, by exposing prehospital care providers to common bioethics principles and concepts, ethics conversations across health care disciplines and settings will be encouraged and promoted.

Ethical Principles

Everyone uses some set(s) of values, beliefs, or societal rules and laws to make decisions about right and wrong. These rules, generally accepted beliefs about moral behavior, are often referred to as principles. Ethics is using an agreed-upon set of moral principles to assist in determining what is the right thing to do. In medicine one set of principles that is often relied upon to ensure ethically appropriate behavior, to guide clinical practice, and to assist in ethical decision making includes **autonomy**, **nonmaleficence**, **beneficence**, and **justice**. The use of these four principles, often referred to as **principlism** (**Figure 3-5**), provides a framework within which one can weigh and balance benefits and burdens, generally within the context of treating a specific patient, in order to do what is in the patient's best interest.[8]

Figure 3-5 Principlism: Guide to Ethical Decision Making

- Autonomy
- Nonmaleficence
- Beneficence
- Justice

Autonomy

Autonomy is from the Greek *auto nomos*, meaning "self-rule." In medicine, it refers to the patient's right to direct his or her own health care free from interference or undue influence.[8] In other words, competent adults get to make their own health care decisions. Autonomy is the principle from which many important ethical concepts such as informed consent, privacy, confidentiality, and truth telling spring. However, the uncontrolled and time-limited (urgent) nature of emergency medicine, especially in the prehospital setting, can challenge the ability of a prehospital care provider to know how to best support patient autonomy and decision making.

Informed consent is a process through which a medical practitioner provides a patient who has decision-making capacity, or a surrogate decision maker (a person who is chosen to make health care decisions on the patient's behalf if the patient is not able to make decisions for himself or herself),[8] with the information necessary to make a fully informed consent for, or refusal of, the medical treatment being offered. While many think of informed consent as a legal form, that form is, in reality, only a record of the consent conversation. There is an ethical obligation on the part of health care providers to provide patients with the appropriate medical information to allow them to make health decisions based upon their own values, beliefs, and wishes.

In order for an informed consent to be valid, patients:

1. Must have decision-making capacity
2. Must have the ability to communicate their understanding of their diagnosis, prognosis, and treatment options
3. Must be able to give consent or refusal voluntarily
4. Must actually give a refusal or consent to treatment[8,9,10]

Assessing any one of these elements can be hard enough to accomplish in a controlled clinical setting, but in an emergency situation, it is especially difficult. Although many people use the terms competence and decision-making capacity interchangeably, **competence** is a legal term referring to a person's general ability to make good decisions for himself or herself, and decision-making capacity refers to a patient's ability to make decisions regarding a specific set of medical treatment options or therapies.

Assessing the capacity of a patient is particularly difficult in an emergency situation. There is rarely a baseline knowledge of the patient or a preassessment relationship, and the assessment must often be made when the patient is sick, scared, and/or in pain. When assessing the decision-making capacity of adult patients, it is necessary to try to determine if they understand the medical options and can weigh the risks and benefits associated with those options. Patients should also have the capacity to appreciate the anticipated outcomes of their choices as well as be able to express their wishes to the health care provider. While the informed consent process respects the rights of patients to make their own decision, the informed consent requirement may be overridden in emergency situations under certain conditions:

1. The patient lacks decision-making capacity due to unconsciousness or significant cognitive impairment and there is no surrogate available
2. The condition is life or health threatening and the patient may suffer irreversible damage in the absence of treatment
3. A reasonable person would consent to the treatment, in which case a health care provider may proceed with treatment in the absence of an autonomous consent from the patient or a surrogate[9]

Privacy and Confidentiality

Just as important as providing the patient or surrogate with the necessary information to make medical decisions is understanding the concepts of privacy and confidentiality. In the health care context, **privacy** refers to the right of patients to control who has access to their personal health information. **Confidentiality** refers to the obligation of health care providers to not share patient information that is disclosed to them within the patient–provider relationship to anyone other than those the patient has authorized, other medical professionals involved in the patient's care, and agencies responsible for processing state and/or federally mandated reporting, such as in cases of child or elder abuse.

Depending upon the circumstances, prehospital care providers may need to rely upon and interact with people other than an incapacitated patient—family, friends, neighbors—in order to gain the information necessary to care for the patient. However, great effort should be made to protect patient information from non-health care providers, such as observers or news media who may be at the scene of an event involving traumatic injury or loss of life, and to limit information given to others until an appropriate surrogate decision maker is identified.

Truth Telling

Truth telling can also present ethical challenges.[10] Truthfulness is both an expectation and a necessary part of building a trusting patient–provider relationship. Communicating honestly shows respect for the patient and enables decision making based upon truthful information. However, especially in the prehospital setting, there are situations in which telling a patient the truth has the potential to cause great harm, such as in cases of multivictim trauma in which survivors are inquiring about the condition of nonsurvivors or critically injured loved ones. At such times, the immediate obligation to tell the truth may sometimes be outweighed by the obligation to do no harm, depending upon the level of injury and the condition of the patient who is asking.[7]

Advance Directives

The right of patients to make their own health decisions does not necessarily cease to exist when they become incapacitated or can no longer make good decisions for themselves. Similarly, children and adults who have never been competent have the right to have their medical best interests protected by a competent decision maker. Protecting these rights is the role of advance directives (living will and medical power of attorney), out-of-hospital medical orders such as the physician's order for life-sustaining treatment (POLST), and surrogate decision makers. In order to protect and respect the rights of incompetent patients, it is important to have a working knowledge of these resources.

Advance directives are declarations, usually written, that describe end-of-life medical treatment wishes and appoint medical decision makers in the event that a once-competent patient is unable to make a medical decision for himself or herself.[11] The two types of written advance directives most often encountered in a medical situation are a living will and a medical power of attorney. A **living will** is a document that expresses end-of-life treatment wishes, such as whether a person would want mechanical ventilation, CPR, dialysis, or other types of life-prolonging or life-sustaining treatments. While advance directive law varies from state to state, living wills do not generally go into effect unless the patient lacks decision-making capacity and has been certified by a health care professional, usually a doctor, to be either terminally ill or permanently unconscious. Because prehospital care providers often lack an extensive knowledge of a patient's medical history and are reacting to an emergent medical situation, it is difficult to determine if a living will is operative, and therefore the prehospital care provider may be unable to rely on it to provide medical direction.

A **medical power of attorney (MPOA)** is an advance directive document used by competent adults to appoint someone to make medical decisions for them in the event that they are unable to make such decisions for themselves. Unlike living wills, MPOAs go into effect immediately anytime a patient is incapable of making his or her own decision, regardless of pre-existing condition, and become inactive again when/if the patient regains decision-making capacity. The person designated by the MPOA is authorized to make only medical decisions on the patient's behalf. These two advance directives, a living will and an MPOA, attempt to protect and respect the rights and wishes of formerly competent patients when they are no longer able to speak for themselves.

An **out-of-hospital medical order**, or **do-not-resuscitate (DNR) order**, is an order given by a physician to ensure that paramedics or other emergency personnel do not perform CPR on a terminally ill patient at home, or in some other community or nonclinical setting, against the patient's previously expressed wishes. The DNR order must be completed on the form specified by the state where the emergency occurs. Each state has its own DNR forms, and most states do not recognize DNR orders from other states. Unlike advance directives, DNR orders go into effect immediately upon being signed by a doctor or authorized health care professional and remain valid regardless of setting.[12]

While the DNR form addresses only the withholding of CPR, a **physician's order for life-sustaining treatment (POLST)** is broader in scope and is meant "to improve the quality of care people receive at the end of life. It is based on effective communication of patient wishes, documentation of medical orders on a brightly colored form and a promise by health care professionals to honor these wishes."[13] The POLST allows for the acceptance or refusal of a wide variety of life-sustaining treatments, such as CPR, medical nutrition and hydration, and ventilator support, and allows prehospital care providers to access an active physician order regarding the end-of-life wishes of the terminally ill and frail elderly. Note that different states may use different names and abbreviations for this form, such as medical orders on scope of treatment (MOST) and physician's orders on scope of treatment (POST).

Nonmaleficence

Just as health care providers are legally and ethically obligated to respect the decision-making rights of those for whom they care, there is also an obligation to avoid putting patients at risk. The principle of nonmaleficence obligates the medical practitioner not to take actions that may harm the patient. The maxim "do no harm," often attributed to the Greek physician Hippocrates and reflected in the Hippocratic Oath, is the essence of the principle of nonmaleficence.[8] If a patient tells a prehospital care provider that she is allergic to a particular drug and the prehospital care provider disregards the patient's warning and gives the drug anyway, and the patient has an allergic reaction, the prehospital care provider has physically harmed the patient.

Additionally, prehospital care providers have an obligation to not only "do no harm," but to avoid putting patients in harm's way. When transporting a patient between a skilled nursing facility and a doctor's office, the principle of nonmaleficence would dictate that the driver not place the patient in danger by driving recklessly or sending text messages while driving.

Beneficence

Beneficence involves taking an action to benefit another. Beneficence means "to do good" and requires prehospital care providers to act in a manner that maximizes the benefits and minimizes the risks to the patient. For example, a prehospital care provider may have to start an intravenous line to administer medications or fluids. The needlestick inflicts pain but is necessary to benefit the patient. Additionally, when done carefully, prehospital care providers can reduce the risk of additional harms such as bruising, swelling, or multiple needlesticks.

Beneficence can also include going above and beyond what is required by professional practice standards to benefit the patient. For example, making sure the patient is transported at a comfortable temperature and providing extra blankets to keep the patient comfortable may not be included in a prehospital protocol but is done to care for and benefit the patient. Thus, beneficence is maximizing the good done on behalf of a patient and minimizing the risk, and nonmaleficence is an obligation not to harm a patient or put at unnecessary risk.[8]

Justice

Justice, commonly thought of as that which is fair or just, usually refers to how we distribute medical resources when it is discussed with regard to health care. Distributive justice is the fair distribution of goods or services based on a socially agreed-upon set of moral guidelines or rules.[8] While many assume justice, or treating others fairly, means to treat all people equally regardless of age, race, gender, or ability to pay, treating everyone equally is not always ethically justifiable. For example, when triaging in the usual emergency situation, those with the greatest medical needs are prioritized over those with less critical needs. Thus, the most vulnerable are often given a greater portion of health care goods and services based upon a shared community value of caring for the sick and marginalized.

Conversely, in a mass-casualty incident, triage is based on probability of survival, and those with the best chance of survival may receive resources before the sickest or most vulnerable. Therefore, what is most just in a particular situation may depend upon the availability of resources and the most fair and beneficial way of using and distributing those resources in that specific case.[14]

Research

While historically there has been a lack of meaningful research specific to prehospital care, in recent years that has begun to change. Many of our most established prehospital standards of care are being challenged by evidence-based research. The use of advanced airways, rigid backboards, and cervical collars has been challenged in the literature. While some of the proposals are controversial, we are beginning to see increased emphasis on the evidence that does or does not support what prehospital care providers do in the field and new thoughts on how to best care for patients. Throughout this text, the evidence from these studies will be described and discussed to enable you to make the best choices for your patients based on your training, your skills, and the tools available to you.

Reading the EMS Literature

A major goal of PHTLS has been to ensure that the practice recommendations presented in this text accurately represent the best medical evidence available at the time of publication. PHTLS began this process with the sixth edition and has continued it with subsequent editions. We continue to add, as References and Suggested Readings, those manuscripts, sources, and resources that are fundamental to the topics covered and the recommendations made in each chapter. (See the Suggested Readings at the end of this chapter for further information on evaluating EMS literature.) Every medical practitioner and health care provider should obtain, read, and critically evaluate the publications and sources that make up the basis for all the components of daily practice.

To make optimal use of available reference material, an understanding of exactly what constitutes medical literature and of how to interpret the various sources of information is essential. In many cases the first source that is accessed for information about a particular topic is a medical textbook. As our level of interest and sophistication grows, a search is undertaken to find the specific references that are referred to in those textbook chapters or to find what, if any, primary research studies have been performed and published. Then, after reviewing and analyzing the various sources, a decision can be made about the quality and strength of the evidence that will guide our decision making and patient care interventions.

Types of Evidence

There are a number of different systems for rating the quality and strength of medical evidence. Regardless of the exact rating system used, several common assessments can be found among them. The process of evaluation begins by reading the "methods" section of the article to determine what study type is being reported. The study type alone has very important implications in terms of the strength of the recommendations in the conclusion of the study.

The highest-quality source that leads to the strongest recommendation about the treatment under study is the randomized, double-blind controlled study. Studies of this type are usually referred to as Class I evidence. This type of study is considered the best type of study because (1) all patients entered into the study are randomized (meaning each patient has an equal chance of assignment to whatever type of treatment is being studied), (2) neither the researchers nor the patients know which type of treatment the subject is receiving (double blinding), and (3) investigators are controlling and accounting for as many other aspects of the study as possible. These factors minimize the chances of any bias entering into the study or affecting the results or interpretation of the results.

Class II evidence generally includes the other types of studies that can be found in the medical literature, including nonrandomized, nonblinded studies; retrospective case-control series; and cohort studies.

Finally, Class III evidence consists of case studies, case reports, consensus documents, textbook material, and medical opinion. Class III evidence is the weakest source of evidence, although often the easiest to obtain.

Unfortunately, if the literature related to prehospital care is critically reviewed, the majority of the published research qualifies as Class III evidence. There has been remarkably little research that would qualify as Class I. Much of the practice of medicine that has been applied to the prehospital setting has been adopted from and adapted to the out-of-hospital environment from the in-hospital delivery of emergency care. The result is that most of the prehospital care provided today is based on Class III evidence. However, more and more Class I and II studies related to prehospital care are being conducted. Unfortunately, Class I studies are limited in the United States by rigid informed-consent regulations. Specifically, with few exceptions, the medical practice of prehospital care is based on "expert" opinion usually found in textbook chapters, the credentials and qualifications of the individual offering that opinion, and the forcefulness and "volume" of the delivery of that opinion.

Recently, consensus has been building to utilize a formal system for grading the quality of evidence and the strength of a resulting clinical practice recommendation.[1,15-17] Several different grading systems have been developed; however, none has been shown to be better than another. Some grading systems have suffered from inter-rater reliability issues.

Steps in Evaluation

Every medical practitioner should read medical literature and critically evaluate every study published that might alter treatment decisions in order to distinguish useful information and therapy from that which is useless or potentially even harmful. How, then, do you go about reading and critically evaluating medical literature?

The first step in this process is to develop a list of journals that will form the foundation of a regular medical literature review. This list should comprise not only those journals with the desired specialty in their name but also those publications that address related specialties or topics and have a high likelihood of also publishing applicable studies (**Figure 3-6**).

An alternative to reviewing multiple journals is to perform a computerized medical literature search if there is a particular topic of interest. The use of computerized search engines such as PubMed or Ovid allows the computer to search a massive database of multiple medical journals and automatically develop a list of suggested studies and publications (**Figure 3-7**).

Figure 3-6 Suggested Journals for Review

- *Academic Emergency Medicine*
- *American Journal of Emergency Medicine*
- *Annals of Emergency Medicine*
- *Journal of Emergency Medicine*
- *Journal of Trauma and Acute Care Surgery*
- *Prehospital Emergency Care*

Figure 3-7 Performing a Computerized Literature Search

PubMed can be accessed through the National Library of Medicine website at the following address: http://www.ncbi.nlm.nih.gov/pubmed. To perform a journal search for articles and studies, it is necessary to enter search terms into PubMed that will be used as keywords to find appropriate articles. The more specific you can be with the terms, the more likely you are to find articles that will meet your needs. However, being too specific can occasionally exclude articles that might be of interest to you. Therefore, a good strategy is to first conduct a search using very specific terms and then do a follow-up search with more generic terms. For example, if you are interested in finding articles about cricothyroidotomy in the prehospital setting, the initial search you perform might be done using the terms "cricothyroidotomy" and "prehospital." The next search might be performed using the terms "airway management" and "emergency medical services," recognizing that "airway management" may yield articles that include not only cricothyroidotomy but other forms of airway management as well.

Narrow the Selection

The next step is to review the title of every article in the table of contents of each of the selected journals to narrow down the article choices to those that clearly relate to the topic of interest. It would be impossible to read each of the selected journals from cover to cover; nor is it necessary. By reviewing the table of contents, articles that are of no interest can be immediately dismissed.

Once the selection has been narrowed, there are still a number of preliminary actions to take before reading the text of the article. Look at the article's list of authors to see if any are already known for their work in this area. Next, read the summary or abstract of the article to see if this overview of the article fulfills the expectations generated when the title was first reviewed. Then, review the site where the study was conducted to assess the similarities, differences, and applicability to the setting in which the results of the study may subsequently be applied. It must be stressed that reading the abstract alone is not enough. It serves only as the "teaser" to determine whether the full article should be reviewed. Medical practice should never be changed based on the abstract.

Read and Assess

Once these initial points have been evaluated, the full text of the article is read and critically assessed. In doing so, several specific issues must be considered. The first issue is whether the study type and the randomization of the patients entered into the study are satisfactory. Every patient included should have had the same probability of receiving one or the other treatments or interventions being compared in the study, and that probability should be known beforehand. The method for assigning patients to their treatment should be described and should be similar to the flip of a coin.

Next, the patient population entered into the study is assessed to determine the similarities or differences with the target population for which the study conclusions will be implemented. To do so, adequate information must be provided in the text describing the clinical and sociodemographic makeup of the study population. Ideally, studies that will be used to alter the care provided in the prehospital setting should have been performed in the prehospital setting. As stated by Dan Spaite, MD.

> Strong evidence for efficacy of an intervention does not mean that it will be effective when applied in the field.[17]

The next issue for consideration is the outcome measure selected by the authors. All outcomes that are clinically relevant should be considered and reported in the study. For example, cardiac arrest studies may describe such endpoints or outcomes as cardiac rhythm conversion, return of spontaneous circulation, survival to hospital admission, or survival to discharge from the hospital.

Analysis of the results section also requires critical review. Just as it is important to evaluate the study population and entry criteria, it is equally important to see if all patients entered into the study at the beginning are accounted for at the end of the study. Specifically, the authors should describe any criteria used to exclude patients from the study analysis. Simple addition by the reader of the various treatment groups or subgroups will quickly confirm if all patients were accounted for. The authors should also describe occurrences that might introduce bias into the results. For example, the authors should report mishaps such as control patients accidentally receiving the treatment or study patients receiving other diagnostics or interventions.

In addition, the clinical, as well as the statistical, significance of the results are important to consider. Although the statistical analyses may be difficult to understand, a basic comprehension of statistical test selection and utilization will validate the statistical tests performed. Equal to and perhaps more important than the statistical significance of a result is the clinical significance of the reported result. For example, in evaluating the effect of a new antihypertensive medication, the statistical analysis may show that the new drug causes a statistically significant decrease in blood pressure of 4 mm Hg. Clinically, however, the reported decrease is insignificant. Thus, the prehospital care provider must assess not only the statistical significance of the result but also the clinical significance.

If all the prior issues have been answered satisfactorily, the last issue relates to the implementation of the study results and conclusion in the reader's health care system. To determine the practicality of applying the therapy, the authors need to describe the treatment in sufficient detail, the intervention or therapy must be available for use, and it must be clinically sensible in the planned setting.

Some differences exist in the evaluation of consensus statements, overviews, and textbook chapters. Ideally, the statement or overview should address a specific, focused question. The authors should describe the criteria used to select the articles included as references, and the reader will determine the appropriateness of these criteria. This in turn will help determine the likelihood that important studies were included and not missed. In addition, the reference list should be reviewed for known studies that should have been included.

A high-quality overview or consensus statement will include a discussion of the process by which the validity of the included studies was appraised. The validity assessment should be reproducible regardless of who actually performed the appraisal. Also, multiple studies with similar results help support the conclusions and ultimate decision about whether or not to change current practice.

Similar to the review of individual studies, the review and assessment of consensus statements, overviews, and textbook chapters include a determination of whether all clinically relevant outcomes were considered and discussed and whether the results can be applied to the reader's patient care setting. This determination also includes an analysis of the benefits versus the potential risks and harm.

Determine the Impact

The final step in evaluation is to determine when a publication should cause a change in daily medical practice. Ideally, any change in medical practice will result from a study of the highest quality, specifically a randomized, controlled, double-blind study. The conclusion of that study will be based on results that have been critically evaluated, have both statistical and clinical significance, and have been reviewed and judged to be valid. The study should be the best information currently available on the issue. In addition, the change in practice must be feasible for the system planning to make the change, and the benefit of making the change must outweigh the risks.

All medical practice in the out-of-hospital setting should be based on high-quality, Class I evidence. As noted, however, most of the EMS literature qualifies as Class III evidence.

Summary

- Principles (or the *science* of medicine) determine what the patient must have in order to optimize outcome and survival.
- Preferences (or the *art* of medicine) are the methods of achieving the principle. Considerations for choosing the method include:
  - Situation that currently exists
  - Condition of the patient
  - Knowledge and experience
  - Equipment available
- Critical thinking is the assessment of all concerns and components of the traumatic event at hand. In applying critical-thinking skills, the prehospital care provider must:
  - Use all senses to achieve assessment.
  - Review the need for additional information, equipment, and personnel.
  - Identify hospitals in the vicinity and know their capabilities.
  - Develop a plan of action and management.
  - Reassess the situation, patient, and response to the action plan.
  - Make midcourse correction(s) as necessary.
- The goal of critical thinking is successful management.
- Critical thinking is *not* following protocols. It *is* swift, flexible, and objective.
- Ethics refers to applying and balancing the four principles of biomedical ethics (autonomy, nonmaleficence, beneficence, and justice). Prehospital professionals must develop, and become comfortable with, the ethical reasoning skills and vocabulary necessary to more confidently manage ethical conflict and/or confusion in the prehospital environment.
- Research provides the foundation and basis for all medical practice, including prehospital care.
- The quality of research and the strength of the conclusions and recommendations vary depending on the type of study. The highest-quality study, which provides the strongest recommendations to guide medical practice, is the randomized, double-blind controlled study.
- Everyone who reads medical literature should know how to assess the type and quality of the study being read.

SCENARIO RECAP

A prehospital crew made up of an EMT and a paramedic is called to the scene of a two-vehicle T-bone collision. This is the only available unit at the moment. In a somewhat dilapidated pickup truck, there is a young unrestrained male driver who smells strongly of alcohol and has an obviously deformed forearm. The truck has struck a small passenger sedan on the passenger's side front door, with significant intrusion into the passenger compartment. The elderly female in the front passenger seat does not appear to be breathing, and the windshield is starred directly in front of her. The female driver of the sedan is also injured, but conscious and extremely anxious. In the rear seats, there are two children restrained in car seats. The child on the passenger side of the deformed compartment appears to be approximately 3 years old and is unconscious and slumped over in the car seat. On the driver's side, a 5-year-old boy is restrained in a booster seat and appears to be uninjured, though he is crying hysterically.

The driver of the pickup truck is obviously injured with an open arm fracture, but he is belligerent and verbally abusive and is refusing treatment. Meanwhile, the driver of the sedan is frantically inquiring about her children and her mother.

- How would you manage this multiple-patient incident?
- Which of these patients is of highest priority?
- What would you tell the mother of the two children about their condition?
- How would you deal with the apparently intoxicated driver of the other vehicle?
- Would you allow the apparently intoxicated driver to refuse care?

SCENARIO SOLUTION

In this five-victim scenario, the sole ambulance crew faces a triage situation with the patients outnumbering the prehospital care providers. It is in this type of triage situation that the concept of justice becomes immediately applicable. The available resources—two prehospital care providers—are limited and must be distributed in a manner that will do the greatest good for the greatest number of people. This involves deciding who is treated first, and by which prehospital care provider.

In this scenario, a rapid decision must be made between treating the elderly female or the unconscious child first. Frequently a child has a higher likelihood of survival than an elderly patient when both patients have suffered similar traumatic injuries. However, additional assessment and medical history may change the clinical picture and the appropriateness of triaging decisions. For example, the mother may report that the unconscious minor child has a terminal condition, so making a triage decision based solely on age may not be the *just* action in this instance. While triage protocols generally provide direction in such situations and are based on concepts of justice, triage protocols cannot account for every unique situation encountered. Therefore, a basic understanding of the principle of justice can be helpful for situations in which "in the moment" triage decisions need to be made.

The appearance of the driver and his truck may potentially lead to stereotyping behaviors and judgments on the part of the prehospital care providers. Stereotypes are a set of inaccurate, simplistic generalizations or beliefs about a group that allows others to categorize them and treat them based on those beliefs. Preconceived notions about a patient's appearance and behaviors can interfere with fair and equitable treatment.

While there is a duty to treat patients in a fair and consistent manner, prehospital care providers are a valuable resource and have no obligation to put themselves at undue risk. Prehospital care providers have the right to not only protect themselves but also to protect their ability to care for others.

In addition to justice concerns, there are several challenges to autonomy raised by this scenario. The prehospital care providers must assess the decision-making capacity of both the driver of the pickup truck and the female driver of the car. Both drivers are injured and emotionally distraught, and the male driver is potentially impaired by an intoxicant. Furthermore, the female driver may be asked to make medical decisions for herself and to act as a surrogate decision maker for her two children and her mother. If, after assessing the decision-making capacity of the two drivers, either of the drivers are found to be incapacitated, then prehospital care providers would proceed with providing emergency medical care based upon established clinical protocols and the best interests of the patients.

The weighing and balancing of benefits and burdens is an important part of medical decision making. In this case, the female driver is requesting information about her mother and children. While the prehospital care provider has an obligation to tell the truth, both to establish patient–provider trust and to help the driver to make informed consent decisions for the incapacitated occupants of her vehicle, the provider must bear in mind that this patient may be injured and is likely traumatized, with an impaired capacity to make decisions. A full and truthful disclosure about the conditions of her mother and unconscious child may further traumatize her (a harm). Her potential reactions to such information may further impair her decision capacity and could be upsetting to her 5-year-old child, who is conscious and already hysterical. Depending on the potential level of harm or burden that an action may cause—in this case, telling the female driver about the conditions of her loved ones—the principle of nonmaleficence (do no harm) and beneficence (do good) may allow for full disclosure to be postponed until the patient is in a more stable environment.

As is clear in this scenario, ethics rarely gives black and white solutions to difficult situations. Rather, ethics can provide a framework, such as the four principles discussed in this chapter—autonomy, nonmaleficence, beneficence, and justice—in which to consider and reason through ethically difficult situations in an attempt to do the right thing.

References

1. Hendricson WD, Andrieu SC, Chadwick DG, et al. Educational strategies associated with development of problem-solving, critical thinking, and self-directed learning. *J Dent Educ.* 2006;70(9): 925–936.
2. Cotter AJ. Developing critical-thinking skills. *EMS Mag.* 2007; 36(7):86.
3. Wang SY, Tsai JC, Chiang HC, et al. Socrates, problem-based learning and critical thinking—a philosophic point of view. *Kaohsiung J Med Sci.* 2008;24(3)(suppl):S6–S13.
4. Carroll RT. *Becoming a Critical Thinker: A Guide for the New Millennium.* 2nd ed. Boston, MA: Pearson Custom Publishing; 2005.
5. Aristotle. *Nichomachean Ethics* (Book I, part 3). Translation by W. D. Ross, The Internet Classics Archive, 1994–2009. http://classics .mit.edu//Aristotle/nicomachaen.html. Accessed October 5, 2013.
6. Banning M. Measures that can be used to instill critical-thinking skills in nurse prescribers. *Nurse Educ Pract.* 2006;6(2):98–105.
7. Bamonti A, Heilicser B, Stotts K. To treat or not to treat: identifying ethical dilemmas in EMS. *JEMS.* 2001;26(3):100–107.
8. Beauchamp TL, Childress JF. *Principles of Biomedical Ethics.* 6th ed. New York, NY: Oxford University Press; 2009.

9. Derse AR. Autonomy and informed consent. In: Iserson KV, Sanders AB, Mathieu D, eds. *Ethics in Emergency Medicine.* 2nd ed. Tucson, AZ: Galen Press; 1995:99–105.

10. Post LF, Bluestein J, Dubler NN. *Handbook for Health Care Ethics Committees.* Baltimore, MD: The Johns Hopkins University Press; 2007.

11. Tubbs JB. *A Handbook of Bioethics Terms.* Washington, DC: Georgetown University Press; 2009.

12. The Eldercare Team website. The out of hospital do not resuscitate (DNR). http://www.eldercareteam.com/public/606.cfm. Accessed August 31, 2012.

13. Center for Ethics in Healthcare website. Physician order for life-sustaining treatment paradigm. http://www.ohsu.edu/polst/. Accessed August 31, 2012.

14. Daniels N. *Just Health Care.* New York, NY: Cambridge University Press; 1985.

15. Atkins D, Best D, Briss PA, et al. Grading quality of evidence and strength of recommendations (GRADE). *BMJ.* 2004;328:1490.

16. Guyatt GH, Oxman AD, Vist G, et al. Rating quality of evidence and strength of recommendations GRADE: an emerging consensus on rating quality of evidence and strength of recommendations. *BMJ.* 2008;336:924.

17. Spaite D. Prehospital evidence-based guidelines (presentation). From Evidence to EMS Practice: Building the National Model, a Consensus-Building Conference sponsored by The National Highway Traffic Safety Administration, the Federal Interagency Committee on EMS and The National EMS Advisory Council. September 2008.

Suggested Reading

Adams JG, Arnold R, Siminoff L, Wolfson AB. Ethical conflicts in the prehospital setting. *Ann Emerg Med.* 1992;21(10):1259.

Beauchamp TL, Childress JF. *Principles of Biomedical Ethics.* 6th ed. New York, NY: Oxford University Press; 2009.

Buchanan AE, Brock DW. *Deciding for Others: The Ethics of Surrogate Decision Making.* New York: Cambridge University Press; 1990.

Fitzgerald DJ, Milzman DP, Sulmasy DP. Creating a dignified option: ethical consideration in the formulation of prehospital DNR protocol. *Am J Emerg Med.* 1995;13(2):223.

Iverson KV. Foregoing prehospital care: should ambulance staff always resuscitate? *J Med Ethics.* 1991;17:19.

Iverson KV. Withholding and withdrawing medical treatment: an emergency medicine perspective. *Ann Emerg Med.* 1996;28(1):51.

Marco CA, Schears RM. Prehospital resuscitation practices: a survey of prehospital providers. *Ethics Emerg Med.* 2003;24(1):101.

Mohr M, Kettler D. Ethical aspects of prehospital CPR. *Acta Anaesthesiol Scand Suppl.* 1997;111:298–301.

Sandman L, Nordmark A. Ethical conflict in prehospital emergency care. *Nurs Ethics.* 2006;13(6):592.

Travers DA, Mears G. Physicians' experiences with prehospital do-not-resuscitate orders in North Carolina. *Prehosp Disaster Med.* 1996;11(2):91.

Van Vleet LM. Between black and white. The gray area of ethics in EMS. *JEMS.* 2006;31(10):55–6, 58-63; quiz 64–65.

CHAPTER 4

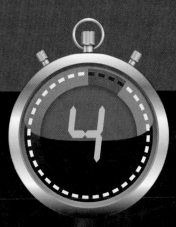

Physiology of Life and Death

CHAPTER OBJECTIVES

At the completion of this chapter, the reader will be able to do the following:

- Define shock.

- Describe how the body responds after trauma.

- Explain the method of energy production.

- Describe the Fick principle.

- Discuss the failure of energy production.

- Explain the pathophysiology of shock and its progression through phases.

- Classify shock on an etiologic basis.

- Relate shock to energy production, etiology, prevention, and treatment.

SCENARIO

It is 0218 hours on a hot summer night. You are dispatched to a report of gunshots fired outside a neighborhood bar known for frequent disturbances. As you respond to the scene, you confirm with dispatch that police are on their way as well. When you are several blocks away, dispatch reports that police have arrived and secured the scene and that there is one male victim. Upon arrival, an approximately 25-year-old male is found with a single gunshot wound to the mid-abdomen. He is noted on primary assessment to be confused, pale, diaphoretic, and somewhat cyanotic in color.

- What are the major pathologic processes occurring in this patient?
- What body systems must be addressed to ensure that they are functioning properly?
- How will you correct the pathophysiology causing this patient's presentation?

Introduction

Life depends on the complex interrelationship and interdependence of several body systems that work together to ensure that the necessary elements to sustain cellular energy production and vital metabolic processes are supplied and delivered to every cell in every organ of the body. The respiratory system, beginning with the airway and progressing to the alveoli of the lungs, and the circulatory system are crucial systems that must function together to provide and distribute the crucial component of cellular energy production: oxygen. Anything that interferes with the ability of the body to provide oxygen to the red blood cells of the circulatory system or that affects the delivery of oxygenated red blood cells to the tissues of the body will lead to cell death and ultimately patient death if not corrected promptly.

The assessment and management of the trauma patient begin with the primary assessment, which is focused on the identification and correction of problems that will affect or interfere with the critical function of the delivery of oxygen to every cell in the body. Thus, an understanding of the physiology of life and pathophysiology that can lead to death is essential for the prehospital care provider if abnormalities are to be found and addressed.

Airway and Respiratory System

The airway is the pathway that guides and conducts atmospheric air through the nose, mouth, pharynx, trachea, and bronchi to the alveoli (**Figure 4-1**). With each breath, air is drawn into the lungs. The movement of air into and out of the alveolus results from changes in intrathoracic pressure generated by the contraction and relaxation of specific muscle groups (**Figure 4-2**). The primary muscle of breathing is the diaphragm. In a healthy person, the muscle fibers of the diaphragm shorten when a stimulus is received from the brain. This flattening of the diaphragm is an active movement that creates a negative pressure inside the thoracic cavity. This negative pressure causes atmospheric air to enter the intact pulmonary tree (**Figure 4-3**).

Other muscles attached to the chest wall also contribute to the creation of this negative pressure; these include the *sternocleidomastoid* and *scalene muscles* (see Figure 4-2). The use of these secondary muscles is seen when the work of breathing increases in the trauma patient. In contrast, exhalation is normally a passive process in nature, caused by the relaxation of the diaphragm and chest wall muscles. This relaxation allows the chest to contract back to its resting position, which in the process of doing so, increases the pressure within the chest, forcing air back out. However, this process can become active as the work of breathing increases.

With each breath, the average adult takes in approximately 500 milliliters (ml) of air. The respiratory system holds up to 150 ml of air that never actually reaches the alveoli to participate in the critical gas-exchange process. The space is known as **dead space**. The air inside this dead space is not available to the body to be used for oxygenation because it never reaches the alveoli. Therefore, in order for air (and oxygen) to reach the alveoli, the inhaled volume must exceed the dead space of the airway.

When the remaining 350 ml of atmospheric air in an average breath reaches the alveoli, oxygen moves from the alveoli, across the alveolar–capillary membrane, and into the **red blood cells (RBCs)**, where it attaches to hemoglobin for

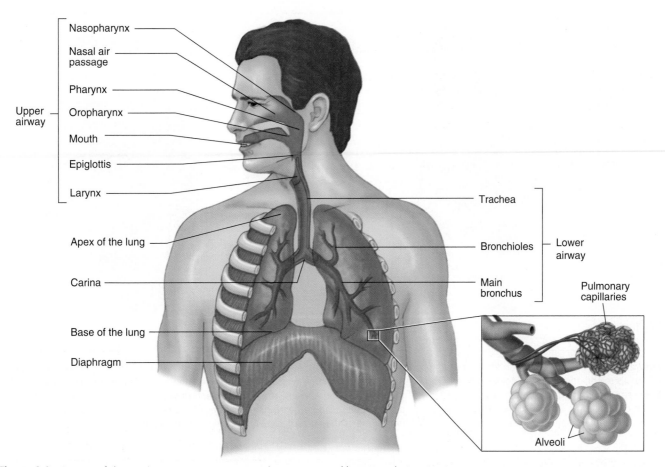

Upper airway
- Nasopharynx
- Nasal air passage
- Pharynx
- Oropharynx
- Mouth
- Epiglottis
- Larynx

Apex of the lung
Carina
Base of the lung
Diaphragm

Trachea
Bronchioles — Lower airway
Main bronchus
Pulmonary capillaries
Alveoli

Figure 4-1 Organs of the respiratory system: upper respiratory tract and lower respiratory tract.

transport (**Figure 4-4**). Then the circulatory system delivers the oxygen-carrying RBCs to the body tissues. At the cellular level, the oxygenated RBCs deliver their oxygen, which the cells then use for aerobic metabolism.

Carbon dioxide, a by-product of aerobic metabolism and energy production, is released into the blood plasma. Deoxygenated blood along with carbon dioxide–rich plasma then returns to the right side of the heart. Once again, oxygen is transferred from inside the alveoli across the cell wall and capillary *endothelium*, through the plasma, and into the RBCs. At the same time, carbon dioxide, which is carried in the plasma, in the RBCs, and as bicarbonate, moves in the opposite direction, from the bloodstream, across the alveolar–capillary membrane, and into the alveoli, where it is eliminated during exhalation. On completion of this exchange, the oxygenated RBCs and plasma with a low carbon dioxide level return to the left side of the heart to be pumped to all the cells in the body.

The alveoli must be constantly replenished with a fresh supply of air that contains an adequate amount of oxygen. This replenishment of air, known as **ventilation**, is also essential for the elimination of carbon dioxide. (See the Airway and Ventilation chapter for additional information about ventilation.)

Assessment of ventilatory function always includes an evaluation of how well a patient is taking in, diffusing, and delivering oxygen to the tissue cells. Without proper intake, delivery of oxygen to the cells, and processing of oxygen within these cells to maintain aerobic metabolism and energy production, anaerobic metabolism will begin.

Oxygenation and Ventilation of the Trauma Patient

The oxygenation process within the human body involves the following three phases:

1. **External respiration** is the transfer of oxygen molecules from air to the blood. Air contains oxygen (20.95%), nitrogen (78.1%), argon (0.93%), and carbon dioxide (0.031%). For practical purposes, consider the content of air to be 21% oxygen and 79% nitrogen. All alveolar oxygen exists as free gas; therefore, each oxygen molecule exerts pressure. Increasing the percentage of oxygen in the inspired atmosphere will increase alveolar oxygen pressure or tension. When supplemental oxygen

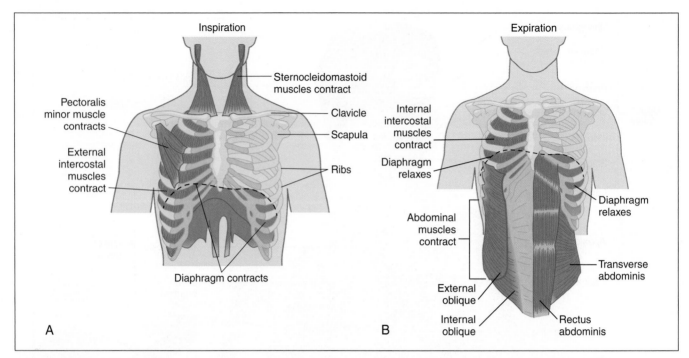

Figure 4-2   **A.** During inspiration, the diaphragm contracts and flattens. Accessory muscles of inspiration – such as the external intercostal, pectoralis minor, and sternocleidomastoid muscles – lift the ribs and sternum, which increases the diameter and volume of the thoracic cavity. **B.** In expiration during quiet breathing, the elasticity of the thoracic cavity causes the diaphragm and ribs to assume their resting positions, which decreases the volume of the thoracic cavity. In expiration during labored breathing, muscles of expiration – such as the internal intercostal and abdominal muscles – contract, causing the volume of the thoracic cavity to decrease more rapidly.

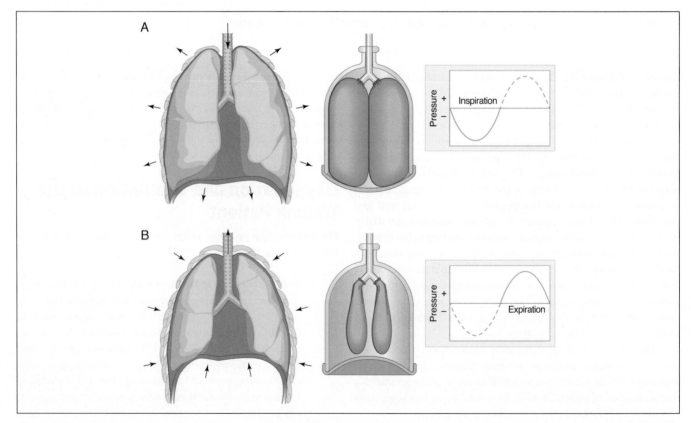

Figure 4-3   **A.** With inspiration, the diaphragm contracts and flattens, thus increasing the volume of the chest and lungs, creating a negative pressure inside the chest, which draws air into the lungs. **B.** With expiration, the diaphragm relaxes and the pressure in the chest increases forcing air out of the lungs.

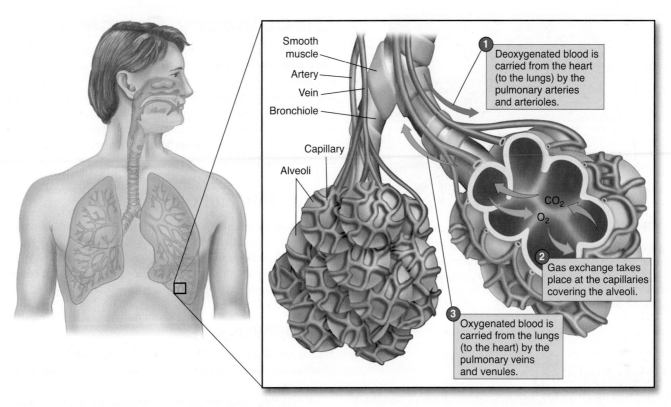

Figure 4-4 Oxygen diffuses out of the alveoli into the capillaries for transport by the red blood cells. Carbon dioxide moves in the opposite direction, entering the alveolar air to be expelled during expiration.

is provided, the percentage of oxygen in each inspiration increases, causing an increase in the amount of oxygen in each alveolus.

2. **Oxygen delivery** is the result of oxygen transfer from the atmosphere to the RBCs during ventilation and the transportation of these oxygen-rich RBCs to the tissues via the cardiovascular system. The volume of oxygen consumed by the body in 1 minute in order to maintain energy production is known as *oxygen consumption* and depends upon cardiac output and the delivery of oxygen to the cells by RBCs. One could describe the RBCs as the body's "oxygen tankers." These tankers move along the vascular system "highways" to "off-load" their oxygen supply at the body's distribution points, the capillary beds.

3. **Internal (cellular) respiration** is the movement, or diffusion, of oxygen from the RBCs into the tissue cells. Metabolism normally occurs through glycolysis and the Krebs cycle to produce energy which is stored in a molecule called adenosine triphosphate (ATP). Glucose is broken down in glycolysis to form two *pyruvate* molecules, each of which then enter the Krebs cycle to produce energy and the by-products of carbon dioxide and water. In the absence of oxygen, the pyruvate is converted to lactic acid.

Because the actual exchange of oxygen between the RBCs and the tissues occurs in the thin-walled capillaries, anything that interrupts a supply of oxygen will disrupt the body's metabolism. A major factor in this regard is the amount of fluid (or edema) located between the alveolar walls, the capillary walls, and the wall of the tissue cells (also known as the interstitial space). Overhydration of the vascular space with crystalloid, which leaks out of the vascular system into the interstitial space within 30 to 45 minutes after administration, is a major problem during resuscitation that can impair oxygen diffusion from the alveoli into the capillaries (**Figure 4-5**). Supplemental oxygen can help overcome this by increasing the amount of available oxygen to cross the alveolar–capillary membrane. The tissues and cells will not be able to consume adequate amounts of oxygen if adequate amounts of oxygen are not available.

Adequate oxygenation depends on all three of these phases. Although the ability to assess tissue oxygenation in prehospital situations is improving rapidly, ensuring adequate ventilation for all trauma patients will help to ensure that hypoxia is corrected or avoided entirely.

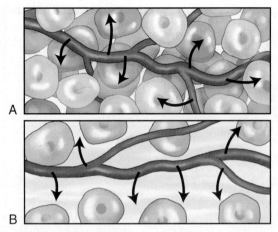

Figure 4-5   A. If the tissue cells are close to the capillary, oxygen can easily diffuse into them, and carbon dioxide can diffuse out. **B.** If tissue cells are separated from capillary walls by increased edema (interstitial fluid), it is much more difficult for the oxygen and carbon dioxide to diffuse.

Pathophysiology

Trauma can affect the respiratory system's ability to adequately provide oxygen and eliminate carbon dioxide in the following ways:

- **Hypoxemia** (decreased oxygen level in the blood) can result from decreased diffusion of oxygen across the alveolar–capillary membrane.
- **Hypoxia** (deficient tissue oxygenation) can be caused by:
  - The inability of the air to reach the capillaries, usually because the alveoli are filled with fluid or debris
  - Decreased blood flow to the alveoli
  - Decreased blood flow to the tissue cells
- **Hypoventilation** can result from:
  - Obstruction of airflow through the upper and lower airways
  - Decreased expansion of the lungs as a result of direct injury to the chest wall or lungs
  - Loss of ventilatory drive, usually because of decreased neurologic function, most often after a traumatic brain injury

Hyperventilation can cause vasoconstriction, which can be especially detrimental in the management of the traumatic brain-injured patient.

Hypoventilation results from the reduction of minute volume, which is the amount of air moved into and out of the lungs in one minute. If left untreated, hypoventilation results in carbon dioxide buildup, acidosis, and eventually death. Management involves improving the patient's ventilatory rate and depth by correcting existing airway problems and assisting ventilation as appropriate.

Circulatory System

The circulatory system is the second body system that is a crucial component in ensuring the delivery of adequate amounts of oxygen to the cells of the body while at the same time removing waste products such as carbon dioxide. Just as trauma to the respiratory system can impair ventilation and oxygenation, trauma involving the circulatory system can also affect the delivery of oxygen to the cells of the body. (See the Shock chapter for additional information.)

Circulation and Oxygenation

The circulatory system must be functioning adequately in order for oxygen to be delivered to each cell of the body (**Figure 4-6**). The heart must pump effectively, the blood vessels to each organ must be intact, and there must be an adequate amount of blood within the vascular system to reach and perfuse each organ.

Pathophysiology

Trauma can affect the circulatory system's ability to deliver oxygen to and remove carbon dioxide from the body in the following ways:

- The heart can sustain direct trauma resulting in impairment of its ability to pump effectively.
- Trauma can produce conditions such as cardiac tamponade or tension pneumothorax that compromise blood return to the heart, thus decreasing blood flow out of the heart.
- Injury to the blood vessels will result in hemorrhage and compromise of the oxygen-carrying capacity of the RBCs.

Shock

Although **shock** following trauma has been recognized for more than three centuries, its description by Samuel Gross in 1872 as a "rude unhinging of the machinery of life"[1] and by John Collins Warren as "a momentary pause in the act of death"[2] emphasizes its continuing central role in the causes of major morbidity and

Figure 4-6 Organ Tolerance to Ischemia	
Organ	**Warm Ischemia Time**
Heart, brain, lungs	4–6 minutes
Kidneys, liver, gastrointestinal tract	45–90 minutes
Muscle, bone, skin	4–6 hours

mortality in the trauma patient. Prompt diagnosis, resuscitation, and definitive management of shock resulting from trauma are all essential in determining patient outcome. The prehospital care provider faces significant challenges in accomplishing all these essential actions for shock. To improve survival from shock, a clear understanding of the definition, pathophysiology, and clinical features of shock is essential. More information about the management of shock or resuscitation has become available to the providers of trauma care in the last 5 to 10 years than in the previous 30 years. It is critical that those who care for trauma patients understand the physiology of the body process that we call life. As knowledge increases over the next 5 to 10 years, the management of these patients must continue to evolve based on a comprehensive understanding of the processes involved and not on out-of-date protocols.

This chapter defines the process of energy production and its loss, which we call "shock." It also describes the pathophysiologic changes that threaten life itself. It emphasizes the importance of energy production and the preservation of aerobic metabolism in the manufacture of energy, which is the key to life.

Definition of Shock

Probably no better definition exists today to describe the devastating impact of shock on the patient than the previously cited definition provided by Samuel Gross in 1872 as a "rude unhinging of the machinery of life."[1] More recent definitions tend to be concerned with identifying the mechanism of shock and the effects on the patient's homeostasis. These definitions are more specific and perhaps give a better picture of the particular pathophysiologic dysfunctions that take place in the body. However, it is a basic tenet of prehospital care that shock is not defined as low blood pressure, rapid pulse rates, or cool, clammy skin; these are merely systemic manifestations of the entire pathologic process called shock.

Shock is most often regarded as a state of generalized cellular function change from aerobic metabolism to anaerobic metabolism secondary to **hypoperfusion** of the tissue cells, in which the delivery of oxygen at the cellular level is inadequate to meet metabolic needs. Based on this definition, shock can be classified in terms of the determinants of cellular perfusion and oxygenation. Understanding the cellular changes arising from this state of hypoperfusion, as well as the endocrine, microvascular, cardiovascular, tissue, and end-organ effects, will also assist in directing treatment strategies.

The key to patient survival is to understand why a patient dies: lack of energy production. Energy production, which is the foundation of life, depends on aerobic metabolism. The etiology of such loss of energy production in the trauma patient is loss of blood and its oxygen-carrying capacity.

If the prehospital care provider is to understand this abnormal condition and be able to develop a treatment plan to prevent or reverse shock, it is important that he or she know and understand what is happening to the body at a cellular level.

The normal physiologic responses the body uses to protect itself from the development of shock must be understood, recognized, and interpreted. Only then can a rational approach for managing the problems of the patient in shock be developed. The critical word is "understand."

Shock can kill a patient in the field, the emergency department, the operating room, or the intensive care unit. Although actual physical death may be delayed for several hours to several weeks, the most common cause of that death is the failure of early and adequate resuscitation from shock. The lack of perfusion of cells by oxygenated blood results in anaerobic metabolism, the death of cells, and decreased energy production. Even when some cells in an organ are initially spared, death can occur later, because the fewer remaining cells are unable to carry out the organ functions indefinitely. The following section explains this phenomenon. Understanding this process is key to assisting the body in restoring aerobic metabolism and energy production.

Physiology of Shock
Metabolism: The Human Motor

The human body consists of over 100 million cells. Each one of these cells requires energy to function and glucose and oxygen to produce that energy. The cells take in oxygen and metabolize it through a complicated physiologic process that produces energy. At the same time, the metabolism of the cell requires energy, and cells must have fuel—glucose—to carry out this process. Each molecule of glucose yields 38 ATP energy storing molecules when oxygen is available. As in any combustion event, a by-product is also produced. In the body, oxygen and glucose are metabolized to produce energy, water, and carbon dioxide.

This metabolic process is similar to the process that occurs in a motor vehicle engine when gasoline and air are mixed and burned to produce energy, and carbon monoxide is created as a by-product. The motor moves the car, the heater warms the driver, and the electricity generated is used for the headlights, all powered by the burning gasoline and air mixture in the vehicle's engine.

The same is true of the human motor. Aerobic metabolism is the main "driving" system but anaerobic metabolism is the backup system. Unfortunately, it is not a strong backup. It produces much less energy than does aerobic metabolism, and it cannot produce energy for a long period of time. In fact, anaerobic metabolism only produces two ATP molecules, a 19-fold decrease in energy. However, it can assist with survival for a short time while the body repairs itself with the assistance of the prehospital care provider.

Aerobic metabolism describes the use of oxygen by cells. This form of metabolism is the body's principle combustion process. It produces energy using oxygen in the complicated processes of glycolysis and the Krebs cycle. **Anaerobic metabolism** occurs without the use of oxygen. It is the backup power system in the body and uses stored body fat as its energy source. Unfortunately, the amount of energy produced by anaerobic metabolism is significantly less than the amount produced by aerobic metabolism.

As a comparison, alternate fuel sources are available in hybrid motor vehicles; it is possible to drive a hybrid car powered only by its battery and electric starting motor if air and gasoline are not available. The hybrid car will move as long as the energy stored in the battery lasts. This movement is slower and less efficient than that powered by gasoline and air; however, the battery is able to keep the car running until it is quickly drained of its power by running all of the systems in the car, a task it was not designed to do for long periods of time.

In the body, the problems with using anaerobic metabolism to provide power are similar to the disadvantages of solely using a battery to run an automobile: It can run only for a short time, it does not produce as much energy, it produces by-products that are harmful to the body, and it may ultimately be irreversible.

The major by-product of anaerobic metabolism is excessive amounts of acid. If anaerobic metabolism is not reversed quickly, cells cannot continue to function in the increasingly acidic environment and without adequate energy, and they will die. If a sufficient number of cells in any one organ die, the entire organ ceases to function. If a large number of cells in an organ die, the organ's function will be significantly reduced and the remaining cells in that organ will have to work even harder to keep the organ functioning. These overworked cells may or may not be able to support the function of the entire organ, and the organ may still die.

A classic example is a patient who has suffered a heart attack. Blood flow and oxygen are cut off to one portion of the myocardium (heart muscle), and some cells of the heart die. This impairs cardiac function, thus decreasing cardiac output and the oxygen supply to the rest of the heart. This in turn causes a further reduction in the oxygenation of the remaining heart cells. If not enough cells remain viable or if the remaining cells are not strong enough to ensure that the heart can meet the body's blood flow needs, then heart failure can result. Unless major improvement in cardiac output occurs, the patient will not survive eventually.

Another example of this deadly process occurs in the kidneys. When the kidneys are injured or are deprived of adequate oxygenated blood, some of the kidney cells begin to die and kidney function decreases. Other cells may be compromised yet continue to function for a while before dying. If enough kidney cells die, the decreased level of kidney function results in the inadequate elimination of the toxic by-products of metabolism. The increased level of toxins further exacerbates cell death throughout the entire body. If this systemic deterioration continues, more cells and organs will die and eventually the entire organism (the human) dies.

Depending on the organ initially involved, the progression from cell death to organism death can be rapid or delayed. It can take as little as 4 to 6 minutes or as long as 2 or 3 weeks before the damage caused by hypoxia or hypoperfusion in the first minutes post-trauma results in the patient's death. The effectiveness of the prehospital care provider's actions to reverse or prevent hypoxia

and hypoperfusion in the critical prehospital period may not be immediately apparent. However, these resuscitation measures are unquestionably necessary if the patient is to ultimately survive. These initial actions are a critical component of the *Golden Hour* of trauma care described by R Adams Cowley, MD, and now called the *Golden Period* because we know that not all patients have an hour in which critical abnormalities can be corrected.

The sensitivity of cells to the lack of oxygen and the usefulness of anaerobic metabolism to cell survival varies from organ system to organ system. This sensitivity is called **ischemic sensitivity** (lack of oxygen), and it is greatest in the brain, heart, and lungs (see Figure 4-6). It may take only 4 to 6 minutes of anaerobic metabolism before one or more of these vital organs are injured beyond repair. Skin and muscle tissue have a significantly longer ischemic sensitivity—as long as 4 to 6 hours. The abdominal organs generally fall between these two groups and are able to survive 45 to 90 minutes of anaerobic metabolism.

Long-term survival of the individual organs and the body as a whole requires delivery of the two most important nutrients (oxygen and glucose) to the tissue cells. Other nutrients are also important, but because the resupply of these other materials is not a component of the prehospital emergency medical services (EMS) system, they are not discussed here. Although these factors are important, they are beyond the scope of the prehospital care provider's practice and resources. The most important supply item is oxygen.

The Fick Principle

The Fick principle is a description of the components necessary for oxygenation of the body cells. Simply stated, these three components are:

1. On-loading of oxygen to RBCs in the lung
2. Delivery of RBCs to tissue cells
3. Off-loading of oxygen from RBCs to tissue cells

A crucial part of this entire process is that the patient must have enough RBCs available to deliver adequate amounts of oxygen to tissue cells throughout the body, so that these cells can produce energy. Additionally, the patient's airway must be patent, and adequate volume and depth of respirations must be present. (See the Airway and Ventilation chapter.)

The prehospital treatment of shock is directed at ensuring that critical components of the Fick principle are maintained with the goal of preventing or reversing anaerobic metabolism, thus avoiding cellular death and, ultimately, organ death leading to patient death. These components are the major emphasis of primary assessment performed by the prehospital care provider and are implemented in the management of the trauma patient by the following actions:

- Maintaining an adequate airway and ventilation, thus providing adequate oxygen to the RBCs

- Judicious use of supplemental oxygen as part of ventilating the patient
- Maintaining adequate circulation, thus perfusing tissue cells with oxygenated blood
  - Stopping loss of additional blood to maintain as many RBCs as possible to carry oxygen

The first component (oxygenation of the lungs and RBCs) is discussed earlier in this chapter and covered in additional detail in the Airway and Ventilation chapter. The second component of the Fick principle involves perfusion, which is the delivery of blood to the tissue cells. A helpful analogy to use in describing perfusion is to think of the RBCs as transport vans, the lungs as oxygen warehouses, the blood vessels as roads and highways, and the body tissue cells as the oxygen's destination. An insufficient number of transport vans, obstructions along the roads and highways, and/or slow transport vans can all contribute to decreased oxygen delivery and the eventual starvation of the tissue cells.

The fluid component of the circulatory system—blood—contains not only RBCs but infection-fighting factors (white blood cells and antibodies), platelets and coagulation factors to support clotting in hemorrhage, protein for cellular rebuilding, nutrition in the form of glucose, and other substances necessary for metabolism and survival.

Cellular Perfusion and Shock

The prime determinants of cellular perfusion are the heart (acting as the pump or the motor of the system), fluid volume (acting as the hydraulic fluid), the blood vessels (serving as the conduits or plumbing), and, finally, the cells of the body. Based on these components of the perfusion system, shock may be classified into the following categories:

1. Hypovolemic—primarily hemorrhagic in the trauma patient, related to loss of circulating blood cells and fluid volume with oxygen-carrying capacity. This is the most common cause of shock in the trauma patient.
2. Distributive (or vasogenic)—related to abnormality in vascular tone arising from several different causes, including spinal cord injury and anaphylaxis, etc.
3. Cardiogenic—related to interference with the pump action of the heart, often occurring after a heart attack.

By far the most common cause of shock in the trauma patient is hypovolemic, resulting from hemorrhage, and the safest approach in managing the trauma patient in shock is to consider the cause of the shock as hemorrhagic until proven otherwise.

More detailed descriptions of these different types of shock follow after a discussion of the relevant anatomy and pathophysiology of shock.

Anatomy and Pathophysiology of Shock

Cardiovascular Response

Heart

The heart consists of two receiving chambers (atria) and two major pumping chambers (ventricles). The function of the atria is to accumulate and store blood so that the ventricles can fill rapidly, minimizing delay in the pumping cycle. The right atrium receives blood from the veins of the body and pumps it to the right ventricle. With each contraction of the right ventricle (**Figure 4-7**), blood is pumped through the lungs for on-loading of oxygen to the RBCs (see Figure 4-4). The oxygenated blood from the lungs is returned to the left atrium and is pumped into the left ventricle. Then, the RBCs are pumped by the contractions of the ventricle throughout the arteries of the body to the tissue cells (**Figure 4-8**).

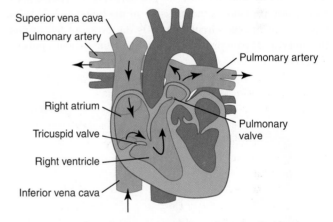

Figure 4-7 With each contraction of the right ventricle, blood is pumped through the lungs. Blood from the lungs enters the left side of the heart, and the left ventricle pumps it into the systemic vascular system.

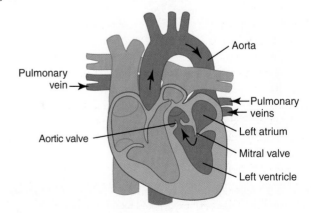

Figure 4-8 Blood returning from the lungs is pumped out of the heart and through the aorta to the rest of the body by left ventricular contraction.

Although it is one organ, the heart actually has two subsystems. The right atrium, which receives blood from the body, and the right ventricle, which pumps blood to the lungs, are referred to as the *right heart*. The left atrium, which receives oxygenated blood from the lungs, and the left ventricle, which pumps blood to the body, are referred to as the *left heart* (**Figure 4-9**). **Preload** (volume of blood entering into the heart) and **afterload** (pressure against which the blood has to push when it is squeezed out of the ventricle) of the right heart (*pulmonary*) and left heart (*systemic*) pumping systems are important concepts to understand.

Blood is forced through the circulatory system by the contraction of the left ventricle. This sudden pressure increase produces a pulse wave to push blood through the blood vessels. The peak of the pressure increase is the systolic blood pressure and represents the force of the pulse wave produced by ventricular contraction (*systole*). The resting pressure in the vessels between ventricular contractions is the diastolic blood pressure and represents the force that remains in the blood vessels that continues to move blood through the vessels while the ventricle is refilling for the next pulse of blood (**diastole**). The difference between the systolic and diastolic pressures is called **pulse pressure**. Pulse pressure is the pressure of the blood as it is being pushed out into the circulation. It is the pressure felt against the prehospital care provider's fingertip as the patient's pulse is checked.

Another term used in the discussion of blood pressure and shock but often not emphasized in the prehospital setting is **mean arterial pressure (MAP)**. This number gives a more realistic assessment of the overall pressure to produce blood flow than either the systolic or the diastolic pressures alone. The MAP is the average pressure in the vascular system and is calculated as follows:

$$\text{MAP} = \text{Diastolic pressure} + 1/3 \text{ Pulse pressure}$$

For example, the MAP of a patient with a blood pressure of 120/80 mm Hg is calculated as follows:

$$\text{MAP} = 80 + [(120-80)/3]$$
$$= 80 + (40/3)$$
$$= 80 + 13.3$$
$$= 93.3, \text{ rounded to } 93$$

Many automatic, noninvasive blood pressure devices automatically calculate and report the MAP in addition to the systolic and diastolic pressures.

The volume of fluid pumped into the circulatory system with each contraction of the ventricle is called the **stroke volume**, and the volume of blood pumped into the system over 1 minute is called the **cardiac output**. The formula for cardiac output is as follows:

$$\text{Cardiac output (CO)} = \text{Heart rate (HR)} \times \text{Stroke volume (SV)}$$

Cardiac output is reported in liters per minute (LPM, or l/min). Cardiac output is not measured in the prehospital environment. However, understanding cardiac output and its relationship to stroke volume is important in understanding shock. For the heart to work effectively, an adequate volume of blood must be present in the vena cavae and pulmonary veins to fill the ventricles.

Starling's law of the heart is an important concept that helps to explain how this relationship works. This pressure that fills the heart (*preload*) stretches the myocardial muscle fibers. The more the ventricles fill, the greater the stretch of the cardiac muscle fibers and the greater the strength of the contraction of the heart, until the point of overstretching. Significant hemorrhage or relative hypovolemia decreases cardiac preload so that a reduced volume of blood is present and the fibers are not stretched as much, resulting in a lower stroke volume; therefore blood pressure will fall. If the filling pressure of the heart is too great, the cardiac muscle fibers become overstretched and can fail to deliver a satisfactory stroke volume, and again blood pressure will decrease.

The resistance to blood flow that the left ventricle must overcome to pump blood out into the arterial system is called afterload, or **systemic vascular resistance**. As peripheral arterial vasoconstriction increases, the resistance to blood flow increases and the heart has to generate a greater force to pump blood into the arterial system. Conversely, widespread peripheral vasodilation decreases afterload.

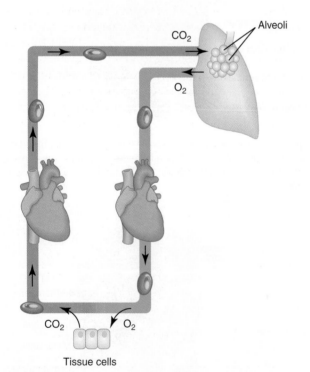

Figure 4-9 Although the heart seems to be one organ, it functions as if it were two organs. Unoxygenated blood is received into the *right heart* from the superior and inferior venae cavae and pumped through the pulmonary artery into the lungs. The blood is oxygenated in the lungs, flows back into the heart through the pulmonary vein, and is pumped out of the left ventricle.

The systemic circulation contains more capillaries and a greater length of blood vessels than the pulmonary circulation. Therefore, the left (or *left-sided*) heart system works at a higher pressure and bears a greater workload than the right (or *right-sided*) heart system. Anatomically, the muscle of the left ventricle is much thicker and stronger than that of the right ventricle.

Blood Vessels

The blood vessels contain the blood and route it to the various areas and cells of the body. They are the "highways" of the physiologic process of circulation. The single, large exit tube from the heart, the aorta, cannot, by itself, serve every individual cell in the body, and, therefore, it splits into multiple arteries of decreasing size, the smallest of which are the capillaries (**Figure 4-10**). A capillary may be only one cell wide; therefore, oxygen and nutrients carried by RBCs and plasma are able to diffuse easily through the walls of the capillary into the nearby tissue cells (**Figure 4-11**). Each tissue cell has a membranous covering called the cell membrane. Interstitial fluid is located between the cell membrane and the capillary wall. The amount of interstitial fluid varies tremendously. If little interstitial fluid is present, the cell membrane and the capillary wall are closer

together and oxygen can easily diffuse between them (see Figure 4-5A). When there is extra fluid (edema) forced into this space (such as occurs in over-resuscitation with crystalloid fluids), the cells move farther away from the capillaries, making transfer of oxygen and nutrients less efficient (see Figure 4-5B).

The size of the vascular "container" is controlled by smooth muscles in the walls of the arteries and arterioles and, to a lesser extent, by muscles in the walls of the venules and veins. These muscles respond to signals from the brain via the sympathetic nervous system, to the circulating hormones epinephrine and norepinephrine, and to other chemicals, such as nitric oxide. Depending on whether they are being stimulated to contract or allowed to relax, these muscle fibers in the walls of the vessels result in either the constriction or dilation of the blood vessels, thus changing the size of the container component of the cardiovascular system and thereby affecting the patient's blood pressure.

There are three fluid compartments: intravascular fluid (fluid that is inside the vessels), intracellular fluid (fluid that is inside the cells), and interstitial fluid (fluid that is between the cells and the vessels). Interstitial fluid in excess of normal amounts produces edema and causes the spongy, boggy feeling when the skin is compressed with a finger.

Hemodynamic Response
Blood

The fluid component of the circulatory system—the blood—contains (1) RBCs to carry oxygen, (2) infection-fighting factors (**white blood cells** [WBCs] and antibodies), and (3) platelets and clotting factors essential for blood clotting at times of vascular injury, protein for cellular rebuilding, nutrients such as glucose, and other substances necessary for metabolism and survival. The various proteins and minerals provide a high **oncotic pressure** to help keep water from leaking out through

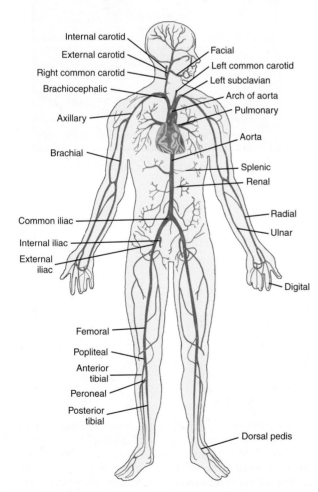

Figure 4-10 Principle arteries of the body.

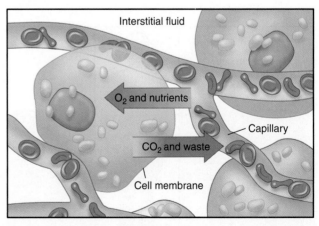

Figure 4-11 Oxygen from the RBCs and nutrients diffuse through the capillary wall, the interstitial fluid, and the cell membrane into the cell. Acid production is a by-product of cellular energy production during the Krebs cycle. By way of the buffer system of the body, this acid is converted into carbon dioxide and travels in the plasma along with the RBCs to be eliminated from the circulatory system by the lungs.

the walls of the vessels. The volume of fluid within the vascular system must equal the capacity of the blood vessels if it is to adequately fill the container and maintain perfusion. Any variance in the volume of the vascular system container compared to the volume of blood in that container will affect the flow of blood either positively or negatively.

The human body is 60% water, which is the base of all body fluids. A person who weighs 154 pounds (70kg) contains approximately 40 liters of water. Body water is present in two components: intracellular and extracellular fluid. As noted previously, each type of fluid has specific, important properties (**Figure 4-12**). **Intracellular fluid**, the fluid within the cells, accounts for approximately 45% of body weight. **Extracellular fluid**, the fluid outside the cells, can be further classified into two subtypes: interstitial fluid and intravascular fluid. **Interstitial fluid**, which surrounds the tissue cells and also includes cerebrospinal fluid (found in the brain and spinal canal) and synovial fluid (found in the joints), accounts for approximately 10.5% of body weight. Intravascular fluid, which is found in the vessels and carries the formed components of blood as well as oxygen and other vital nutrients, accounts for approximately 4.5% of body weight.

A review of some key concepts is helpful in this discussion of how fluids operate in the body. Besides movement of fluid through the vascular system, there are two major types of fluid movement: (1) movement between the plasma and interstitial fluid (across capillaries) and (2) movement between the intracellular and interstitial fluid compartments (across cell membranes).

The movement of fluid through the capillary walls is determined by (1) the difference between the *hydrostatic pressure* within the capillary (which tends to push fluid out) and the hydrostatic pressure outside the capillary (which tends to push fluid in), (2) the difference in the oncotic pressure from protein concentration within the capillary (which keeps fluid in) and the oncotic pressure outside the capillary (which pulls fluid out), and (3) the *leakiness* or permeability of the capillary (**Figure 4-13**). Hydrostatic pressure, oncotic pressure, and capillary permeability are all affected by the shock state itself, as well as by the type and volume of fluid resuscitation, leading to alterations in circulating blood volume, hemodynamics, and tissue or pulmonary edema.

Movement of fluid between the intracellular and interstitial space occurs across cellular membranes, which is determined primarily by *osmotic effects*. **Osmosis** is the process by which solutes separated by a membrane to which the solutes are impermeable govern the movement of water across that semipermeable membrane based on the concentration of the solute. Water moves from the compartment of lower solute concentration to that of higher solute concentration to maintain osmotic equilibrium across the semipermeable membrane (**Figure 4-14**).

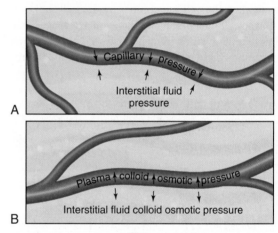

Figure 4-13 Forces governing fluid flux across capillaries.

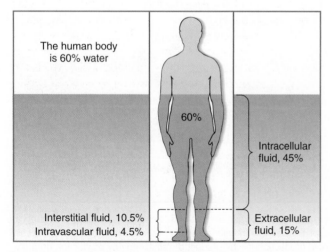

Figure 4-12 Body water represents 60% of body weight. This water is divided into intracellular and extracellular fluid. The extracellular fluid is further divided into interstitial and intravascular fluid.

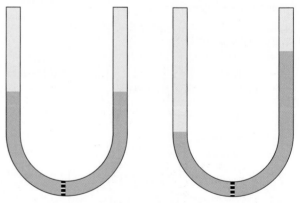

Figure 4-14 A U-tube, in which the two halves are separated by a semipermeable membrane, contains equal amounts of water and solid particles. If a solute that cannot diffuse through the semipermeable membrane is added to one side but not to the other, fluid will flow across to dilute the added particles. The pressure difference of the height of fluid in the U-tube is known as osmotic pressure.

Endocrine Response

Nervous System

The **autonomic nervous system** directs and controls the involuntary functions of the body, such as respiration, digestion, and cardiovascular function. It is divided into two subsystems—the sympathetic and parasympathetic nervous systems. These systems oppose each other to keep vital body systems in balance.

The **sympathetic nervous system** produces the fight-or-flight response. This response simultaneously causes the heart to beat faster and stronger, increases the ventilatory rate, and constricts the blood vessels to nonessential organs (skin and gastrointestinal tract) while dilating vessels and improving blood flow to muscles. The goal of this response system is to maintain sufficient amounts of oxygenated blood to critical tissues so that an individual can respond to an emergency situation while shunting blood away from nonessential areas. In contrast, the **parasympathetic nervous system** slows the heart rate, decreases the ventilatory rate, and increases gastrointestinal activity.

In patients who are hemorrhaging after sustaining trauma, the body attempts to compensate for the blood loss and to maintain energy production. The cardiovascular system is regulated by the vasomotor center in the medulla. In response to a transient fall in blood pressure, stimuli travel to the brain via cranial nerves IX and X from stretch receptors in the carotid sinus and the aortic arch. These stimuli lead to increased sympathetic nervous system activity, with increased peripheral vascular resistance resulting from arteriolar constriction and increased cardiac output from an increased rate and force of cardiac contraction. Increased venous tone enhances circulatory blood volume. Blood is diverted from the extremities, bowel, and kidney to more vital areas—the heart and brain—in which vessels constrict very little under intense sympathetic stimulation. These responses result in cold, cyanotic extremities, decreased urine output, and decreased bowel perfusion.

A decrease in the left atrial filling pressure, a fall in blood pressure, and changes in *plasma osmolality* (the total concentration of all of the chemicals in blood) cause release of antidiuretic hormone (ADH) from the pituitary gland and aldosterone from the adrenal glands, which enhances retention of sodium and water by the kidneys. This process also helps to expand the intravascular volume; however, many hours are required for this mechanism to make a clinical difference.

Types of Shock

There are three major categories of shock:

- Hypovolemic shock
  - Vascular volume smaller than normal vascular size
    - Loss of fluid and electrolytes (dehydration)
    - Loss of blood and fluid (hemorrhagic shock)
- Distributive shock
  - Vascular space larger than normal
    - Neurogenic "shock" (hypotension)
    - Psychogenic "shock"
    - Septic shock
    - Anaphylactic shock
- Cardiogenic shock
  - Pump failure

Although each of the various types of shock will be described briefly in coming sections of this chapter, not all are caused by trauma.

Hypovolemic Shock

Acute loss of blood volume, either from dehydration (loss of fluid and electrolytes) or hemorrhage (loss of plasma and RBCs), causes an imbalance in the relationship of fluid volume to the size of the container. The container retains its normal size, but the fluid volume is decreased. **Hypovolemic shock** is the most common cause of shock encountered in the prehospital environment, and blood loss is by far the most common cause of shock in trauma patients and the most dangerous for the patient.

When blood is lost from the circulation, the heart is stimulated to increase cardiac output by increasing the strength and rate of contractions. This increased output is caused by the release of epinephrine from the adrenal glands. The sympathetic nervous system releases norepinephrine to constrict the blood vessels to reduce the size of the container and bring it more into proportion with the volume of remaining fluid. Vasoconstriction results in closing of the peripheral capillaries, which reduces oxygen delivery to the affected cells, thereby forcing the switch from aerobic to anaerobic metabolism in these cells.

These compensatory defense mechanisms work well and will maintain cellular perfusion, up to a point. When the defense mechanisms can no longer compensate for the volume reduction, a patient's blood pressure will drop. A decrease in blood pressure marks the switch from compensated to decompensated shock—a sign of impending death. A patient who has signs of compensation such as tachycardia is already in shock, not "going into shock." Unless aggressive resuscitation occurs, the patient who enters decompensated shock has only one more stage of decline left—irreversible shock, leading to death.

Hemorrhagic Shock

Hemorrhagic shock (hypovolemic shock resulting from blood loss) can be categorized into four classes, depending on the severity of hemorrhage, as follows, with the proviso that the values and descriptions for the criteria listed for these classes of shock should not be interpreted as absolute determinants of the class of shock, as significant overlap exists (**Figure 4-15**):

1. *Class I hemorrhage* represents a loss of up to 15% of blood volume in the adult (up to 750 ml). This stage has

Figure 4-15 Classification of Hemorrhagic Shock

	Class I	Class II	Class III	Class IV
Blood loss (mL)	< 750	750–1500	1500–2000	> 2000
Blood loss (% blood volume)	< 15%	15–30%	30–40%	> 40%
Pulse rate	< 100	100–120	120–140	> 140
Blood pressure	Normal	Normal	Decreased	Decreased
Pulse pressure (mm Hg)	Normal or increased	Decreased	Decreased	Decreased
Respiratory rate	14–20	20–30	30–40	> 35
CNS/mental status	Slightly anxious	Mildly anxious	Anxious, confused	Confused, lethargic
Fluid replacement	Crystalloid	Crystalloid	Crystalloid and blood	Crystalloid and blood

Note: The values and descriptions for the criteria listed for these classes of shock should not be interpreted as absolute determinants of the class of shock, as significant overlap exists.
Source: From American College of Surgeons Committee on Trauma. *Advanced Trauma Life Support for Doctors, Student Course Manual.* 8th ed. Chicago: American College of Surgeons; 2008.

few clinical manifestations. Tachycardia is often minimal, and no measurable changes in blood pressure, pulse pressure, or ventilatory rate occur. Most healthy patients sustaining this amount of hemorrhage require only maintenance fluid as long as hemorrhage is controlled and no further blood loss occurs. The body's compensatory mechanisms restore the intravascular container/fluid volume ratio and assist in the maintenance of blood pressure.

2. *Class II hemorrhage* represents a loss of 15% to 30% of blood volume (750 to 1,500 ml). Most adults are capable of compensating for this amount of blood loss by activation of the sympathetic nervous system, which will maintain their blood pressure. Clinical findings include increased ventilatory rate, tachycardia, and a narrowed pulse pressure. The clinical clues to this phase are tachycardia, tachypnea, and normal systolic blood pressure. Because the blood pressure is normal, this is considered "compensated shock": The patient is in shock but is able to compensate for the time being. The patient often demonstrates anxiety or fright. Although not usually measured in the field, urine output drops slightly to between 20 and 30 ml/hour in an adult. On occasion, these patients may require blood transfusion; however, most will respond well to crystalloid infusion if hemorrhage is controlled at this point.

3. *Class III hemorrhage* represents a loss of 30% to 40% of blood volume (1,500 to 2,000 ml). When blood loss reaches this point, most patients are no longer able to compensate for the volume loss, and hypotension occurs. The classic findings of shock are obvious and include tachycardia (heart rate greater than 120 beats/minute),

tachypnea (ventilatory rate of 30 to 40 breaths/minute), and severe anxiety or confusion. Urine output falls to 5 to 15 ml/hour. Many of these patients will require blood transfusion and surgical intervention for adequate resuscitation and control of hemorrhage.

4. *Class IV hemorrhage* represents a loss of more than 40% of blood volume (greater than 2,000 ml). This stage of severe shock is characterized by marked tachycardia (heart rate greater than 140 beats/minute), tachypnea (ventilatory rate greater than 35 breaths/minute), profound confusion or lethargy, and greatly decreased systolic blood pressure, typically in the range of 60 mm Hg. These patients truly have only minutes to live. Survival depends on immediate control of hemorrhage (surgery for internal hemorrhage) and aggressive resuscitation, including blood and plasma transfusions with minimal crystalloid.

The rapidity with which a patient develops shock depends on how fast blood is lost from the circulation. Daniel Bernoulli, a Swiss mathematician, developed the mathematical physics formula that calculates the rate of fluid loss from within a tube to the outside of the tube. The details are not required for the understanding of blood loss and the production of shock, but the basics of the principle are required. From a simplistic approach, the Bernoulli principle says that the rate of fluid loss from a tube is directly proportional to the size of the hole in the wall of the tube and to the difference in pressure between the inside of the tube and the outside of the tube. These same principles apply to blood vessels.

Imagine the blood vessels as plumbing inside a home and the blood inside the vessels as water in the pipes. If the plumbing has a leak, the amount of water lost is directly related to the size of the hole and the difference in pressure inside and outside the pipe. For example, if the hole in the pipe is 1 inch (2.5 centimeters [cm]) in diameter and the pressure inside the plumbing is 100 pounds per square inch (psi, or 689 kilopascals [kPa]), more water will leak out than if the hole is 1 inch in diameter and the pressure inside the plumbing is 50 psi (345 kPa). Similarly, the blood flow from a wound in a vessel is proportional to the difference between the size of the hole in the vessel wall and the difference between *intraluminal* (inside the vessel) and *extraluminal* (outside the vessel) pressures.

The *definitive management for volume deficit* is to stop the fluid loss and replace the lost fluid. To stop the fluid loss, treat the diarrhea, vomiting, or other cause. A *dehydrated patient* needs fluid replacement with water and salt. In a conscious patient who can drink, mild to moderate dehydration can be treated with an electrolyte solution. An unconscious or severely dehydrated patient should receive the replacement intravenously. A *trauma patient* who has lost blood needs to have the source of blood loss stopped (see the Shock chapter), and if significant blood loss has occurred, blood replacement needs to be accomplished (**Figure 4-16**).

Distributive (Vasogenic) Shock

Distributive shock, or vasogenic shock, occurs when the size of the vascular container enlarges without a proportional increase in fluid volume. Although the amount of intravascular fluid has not changed, relatively less fluid is available for the now enlarged size of the container. As a result, the volume of fluid available for the heart to pump (preload) decreases and results in a decreasing cardiac output. In most situations, fluid has not been lost from the vascular system. This form of shock is not a cause of true hypovolemia, in which fluid has been lost through hemorrhage, vomiting, or diarrhea. Instead, the problem is the size of the container, which is now larger than the fluid available to fill it. For this reason, this condition is sometimes referred to as *relative hypovolemia*. Although some of the presenting signs and symptoms may closely mimic those of hypovolemic shock, the cause of the two conditions is different.

In distributive shock, resistance to blood flow is decreased because of the relatively larger size of the blood vessels. This reduced resistance causes a decrease in the diastolic blood pressure. When this reduced resistance is combined with the reduced preload and, therefore, a reduced cardiac output, the net result is a decrease in both systolic and diastolic blood pressures. Tissue oxygenation may remain adequate in the neurogenic form of shock, and blood flow remains normal although the pressure is low (neurogenic hypotension). In addition, energy production remains adequate in neurogenic hypotension.

Distributive shock can result from loss of autonomic nervous system control of the smooth muscles that control the size of the blood vessels or release of chemicals that result in peripheral vasodilation. This loss of control can stem from spinal cord trauma, simple fainting, severe infections, or allergic reactions. Management of distributive shock is directed toward improving oxygenation of the blood and improving or maintaining blood flow to the brain and vital organs.

Neurogenic "Shock"

Neurogenic "shock", or more appropriately neurogenic hypotension, occurs when a spinal cord injury interrupts the sympathetic nervous system pathway. This usually involves injury to the thoracolumbar area. Because of the loss of sympathetic control of the vascular system, which controls the smooth muscles in the walls of the blood vessels, the peripheral vessels dilate below the level of injury. The marked decrease in systemic vascular resistance and peripheral vasodilation that occurs as the container for the blood volume increases results in relative hypovolemia. The patient is not really hypovolemic, but the normal blood volume is insufficient to fill the expanded container. This decrease in blood pressure does not alter perfusion or compromise energy production and, therefore, is not shock since energy production remains unaffected. However, since there is less resistance to blood flow, the systolic and diastolic pressures are lower.

Decompensated hypovolemic shock and neurogenic "shock" both produce a decreased systolic blood pressure. However, the other vital and clinical signs, as well as the treatment for each, are different (**Figure 4-17**). Decreased systolic and diastolic pressures and a narrow pulse pressure characterize hypovolemic shock. Neurogenic "shock" also displays decreased systolic and diastolic pressures, but the pulse pressure remains normal or is widened. Hypovolemia produces cold, clammy, pale, or cyanotic skin and delayed capillary refilling time. In neurogenic "shock," the patient has warm, dry skin, especially below the area of injury. The pulse in hypovolemic shock patients is weak, thready, and rapid. In neurogenic "shock," because of unopposed parasympathetic activity on the heart, bradycardia is typically seen rather than tachycardia, but the pulse quality may be weak. Hypovolemia produces a decreased level of consciousness or at least anxiety, and often combativeness. In the absence of a traumatic brain injury, the patient with neurogenic "shock" is usually alert, oriented, and lucid when in the supine position (**Figure 4-18**).

Patients with neurogenic "shock" frequently may have associated injuries that produce significant hemorrhage. Therefore, a patient who has neurogenic "shock" and signs of hypovolemia, such as tachycardia, should be treated as if blood loss is present.

Figure 4-16 Lyophilized Plasma

At the time of this edition's preparation, *lyophilized* (freeze-dried) *plasma* is used in the field in several countries. It is under research in the United States. However, liquid plasma is being used by several EMS and helicopter EMS (HEMS) systems in the United States, and in some HEMS systems, packed RBCs are also carried.

Figure 4-17   Signs Associated With Types of Shock

Vital Sign	Hypovolemic	Neurogenic	Septic	Cardiogenic
Skin temperature	Cool, clammy	Warm, dry	Cool, clammy	Cool, clammy
Skin color	Pale, cyanotic	Pink	Pale, mottled	Pale, cyanotic
Blood pressure	Drops	Drops	Drops	Drops
Level of consciousness	Altered	Lucid	Altered	Altered
Capillary refilling time	Slowed	Normal	Slowed	Slowed

Figure 4-18   Neurogenic "Shock" Versus Spinal Shock

The term neurogenic "shock" refers to a disruption of the sympathetic nervous system, typically from injury to the spinal cord, which results in significant dilation of the peripheral arteries. If untreated, this condition may result in impaired perfusion to the body's tissues. Neurogenic "shock" should not be confused with **spinal shock**, a term that refers to an injury to the spinal cord that results in temporary loss of spinal cord function.

Psychogenic (Vasovagal) "Shock"

Psychogenic "shock" is typically mediated through the parasympathetic nervous system. Stimulation of cranial nerve X (vagus nerve) produces bradycardia. The increased parasympathetic activity may also result in transient peripheral vasodilation and hypotension. If the bradycardia and vasodilation are severe enough, cardiac output falls dramatically, resulting in insufficient blood flow to the brain. Vasovagal syncope (fainting) occurs when the patient loses consciousness. Compared to neurogenic "shock," the periods of bradycardia and vasodilation in psychogenic "shock" are generally very brief and limited to no more than a few minutes, whereas neurogenic "shock" may last up to several days. In psychogenic "shock" patients, normal blood pressure is quickly restored when the patient is placed in a horizontal position. Because it is self-limited, a vasovagal episode is unlikely to result in true shock, and the body quickly recovers before significant systemic impairment of perfusion occurs.

Septic Shock

Septic shock, seen in patients with life-threatening infections, is another condition that exhibits vascular dilation. *Cytokines*, released in response to the infection, cause damage to the walls of the blood vessels, peripheral vasodilation, and leakage of fluid from the capillaries into the interstitial space. Thus, septic shock has characteristics of both distributive shock and hypovolemic shock. Preload is diminished because of the vasodilation and loss of fluid, and hypotension occurs when the heart can no longer compensate. Septic shock is virtually never encountered within minutes of an injury; however, the prehospital care provider may be called on to care for a trauma patient in septic shock during an interfacility transfer or if a patient sustains an injury to the gastrointestinal tract and did not promptly seek medical attention.

Anaphylactic Shock

Anaphylactic shock is a severe, life-threatening allergic reaction that involves numerous body organ systems. When individuals are exposed to an allergen for the first time, they become sensitized to it. If they are later re-exposed to that same allergen, a systemic response occurs. In addition to the more common symptoms of allergic reaction such as redness of the skin (*erythema*), development of hives (*urticaria*), and itching (*pruritus*), more serious findings are noted, including respiratory distress, airway obstruction, and vasodilation leading to shock. Active airway management may be needed in some cases. Treatment involves administration of epinephrine, antihistamines, and steroids in the hospital.

Cardiogenic Shock

Cardiogenic shock, or failure of the heart's pumping activity, results from causes that can be categorized as either *intrinsic* (a result of direct damage to the heart itself) or *extrinsic* (related to a problem outside the heart).

Intrinsic Causes

Heart Muscle Damage

Any process that weakens the cardiac muscle will affect the heart's ability to pump blood. The damage may result from an acute interruption of the heart's own blood supply (as in a myocardial infarction from coronary artery disease) or from a direct bruise to the heart muscle (as in a blunt cardiac injury).

A recurring cycle will ensue: Decreased oxygenation causes decreased contractility, which results in decreased cardiac output and, therefore, decreased systemic perfusion. Decreased perfusion results in a continuing decrease in oxygenation and, thus, a continuation of the cycle. As with any muscle, the cardiac muscle does not work as efficiently when it becomes bruised or damaged.

Dysrhythmia

The development of a cardiac dysrhythmia can affect the efficiency of contractions, resulting in impaired systemic perfusion. Hypoxia may lead to myocardial ischemia and cause dysrhythmias, such as premature contractions and tachycardia. Because cardiac output is a result of the volume ejected with each contraction (stroke volume), any dysrhythmia that results in a slow rate of contractions (bradycardia) or shortens the left ventricle's filling time (tachycardia) can decrease stroke volume, and cardiac output. Blunt cardiac injury may also result in dysrhythmias, the most common of which is a mild, persistent tachycardia.

Valvular Disruption

A sudden, forceful compressing blow to the chest or abdomen (see the Kinematics of Trauma chapter) may damage the valves of the heart. Severe valvular injury results in acute heart valvular regurgitation, in which a significant amount of blood leaks back into the chamber from which it was just pumped. These patients often rapidly develop congestive heart failure (CHF), manifested by pulmonary edema and cardiogenic shock. The presence of a new heart murmur is an important clue in making this diagnosis.

Extrinsic Causes

Cardiac Tamponade

Fluid in the pericardial sac prevents the heart from refilling completely during the diastolic (relaxation) phase of the cardiac cycle. In the case of trauma, blood comes into the pericardial sac from a hole in the cardiac muscle. This mass of fluid occupies space and prevents the walls of the ventricle from expanding fully (**Figure 4-19**). This has two negative effects: (1) the ventricle cannot open fully and therefore less volume can enter the ventricle to be pumped out with each contraction, and (2) inadequate filling reduces the stretch of the cardiac muscle and results in diminished strength of the cardiac contraction. Additionally, more blood is forced out of the ventricle through the cardiac wound and occupies more space in the pericardial sac with each contraction, further compromising cardiac output. Severe shock and death may rapidly follow. (See the Shock chapter and the Thoracic Trauma chapter for more detail on recognizing and treating these conditions.)

Tension Pneumothorax

When either or both of the thoracic cavities become filled with air, the lung is compressed and is prevented from refilling with air through the nasopharynx, reducing the tidal volume with each breath. This produces multiple problems: 1) the collapsed alveoli are not available for oxygen transferal into the RBCs, 2) the pulmonary blood vessels are collapsed, reducing blood flow to the lungs and heart, 3) greater force of cardiac contraction (pulmonary hypertension) is required to force blood through the pulmonary vessels, 4) the mediastinum is pushed toward the other side of the chest producing collapse of the opposite lung, and 5) compression and kinking of the superior and inferior venae cavae producing a significant drop in preload (**Figure 4-20**). All of these components reduce cardiac output and shock rapidly ensues (see the Shock chapter and the Thoracic Trauma chapter for more detail on recognizing and treating these conditions).

Complications of Shock

The triad of death is frequently described as hypothermia, coagulopathy (discussed as follows), and acidosis. These are not causes of death but rather are symptoms indicating impending death. They are markers of anaerobic metabolism and the loss

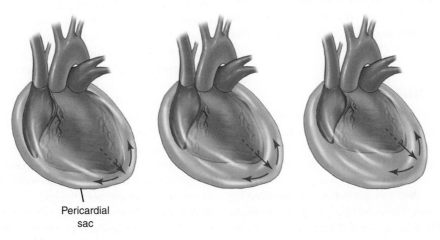

Pericardial sac

Figure 4-19 Cardiac tamponade.

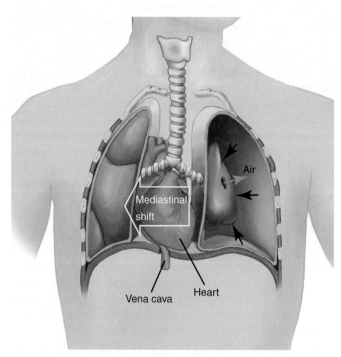

Figure 4-20 Tension pneumothorax.

of energy production and are an indicator that the interventions needed to reverse anaerobic metabolism must be provided quickly. Several complications may result in patients with persistent or inadequately resuscitated shock, which is why early recognition and aggressive management of shock are essential. The quality of care delivered in the prehospital setting can affect a patient's hospital course and outcome. *Recognizing shock and initiating proper treatment in the prehospital setting may shorten the patient's hospital length of stay and improve his or her chances for survival.* The following complications of shock are not often seen in the prehospital setting, but they are a result of shock in the field and in the emergency department. In addition, they may be encountered when transferring patients between facilities. Knowing the outcome of the process of shock helps in the understanding of the severity of the condition, the importance of rapid hemorrhage control, and appropriate fluid replacement.

Acute Renal Failure

Impaired circulation to the kidneys changes the aerobic metabolism in the kidney to anaerobic metabolism. The reduced energy production leads to renal cellular swelling, which decreases renal perfusion, thus causing additional anaerobic metabolism. The cells that make up the renal tubules are most sensitive to ischemia and may die if their oxygen delivery is impaired for more than 45 to 60 minutes. This condition, referred to as **acute tubular necrosis (ATN)** or acute renal failure, reduces the filtration process of the renal tubules. The result is decreased

renal output and reduced clearing of toxic products and electrolytes. Because the kidneys are no longer functioning, excess fluid is not excreted, and volume overload may result. Also, the kidneys lose their ability to excrete metabolic acids and electrolytes, leading to a metabolic acidosis and hyperkalemia (increased blood potassium). These patients often require dialysis for several weeks or months. Most patients who develop ATN resulting from shock will eventually recover normal renal function.

Acute Respiratory Distress Syndrome

Acute respiratory distress syndrome (ARDS) results from damage to the alveolar cells of the lung and decreased energy production to maintain the metabolism of these cells. This injury, combined with fluid overload produced by too much crystalloid administration during resuscitation, leads to leakage of fluid into the interstitial spaces and alveoli of the lungs, making it much more difficult for oxygen to diffuse across the alveolar walls and into the capillaries and bind with the RBCs. This problem was first described during World War II but was formally recognized during the Vietnam War where it was called Da Nang Lung (after the location of the hospital that saw many of these cases). Although these patients do have pulmonary edema, it is not the result of impaired cardiac function, as in congestive heart failure (*cardiogenic* pulmonary edema). ARDS represents a *noncardiogenic* pulmonary edema. The change of the resuscitative process to restricted crystalloid, permissive hypertension, and Damage Control Resuscitation (RBCs-to-plasma ratio of 1:1) has significantly reduced ARDS in the immediate trauma period (24 to 72 hours).

Hematologic Failure

The term **coagulopathy** refers to impairment in the normal clotting capabilities of blood. This abnormality may result from hypothermia (decreased body temperature), dilution of clotting factors from administration of fluids, or depletion of the clotting substances as they are used up in an effort to control bleeding (*consumptive* coagulopathy). The normal blood-clotting cascade involves several enzymes and factors that eventually result in the creation of fibrin molecules that serve as a matrix to trap platelets and form a plug in a vessel wall to stop bleeding (**Figure 4-21**). This process functions best within a narrow temperature range (i.e., near-normal body temperature). As the core temperature of the body falls (even just a few degrees) and energy production lessens, blood clotting is compromised, leading to continued hemorrhage. The blood-clotting factors may also be used up as they form blood clots in an effort to slow and control hemorrhage. The decreased body temperature worsens the clotting problems, which exacerbates hemorrhage, which further reduces the ability of the body to maintain its temperature. With inadequate resuscitation, this becomes an ever-worsening cycle. Several studies have reported fewer difficulties with coagulopathy since the increase in use of plasma for resuscitation.[3,4]

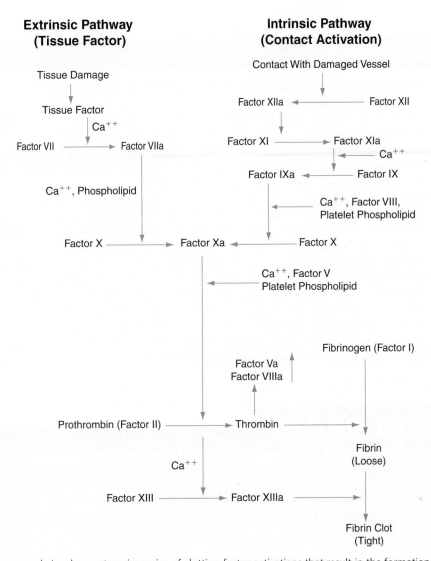

Figure 4-21 The clotting cascade involves a stepwise series of clotting factor activations that result in the formation of a blood clot.

Hepatic Failure

Severe damage to the liver may occur, although it is a less common result of prolonged shock. Evidence of damage to the liver from shock typically does not become manifest for several days, until laboratory results document elevated liver function tests. Liver failure is manifested by persistent hypoglycemia (low blood sugar), a persistent lactic acidosis, and jaundice. Because the liver produces many of the clotting factors necessary for hemostasis, a coagulopathy may accompany liver failure.

Overwhelming Infection

There is increased risk of infection associated with severe shock. This increased risk is attributed to several causes:

- A marked decrease in the number of WBCs, predisposing the shock patient to infection, is another manifestation of hematologic failure.

- The ischemia and reduction in energy production in the cells of the shock patient's bowel wall may allow bacteria to leak out into the peritoneal cavity.
- There is decreased function of the immune system in the face of ischemia and loss of energy production.

Multiple Organ Failure

Shock, if not successfully treated, can lead to dysfunction first in one organ, then in several other organs simultaneously, with sepsis as a common accompaniment, leading to multiple organ dysfunction syndrome.

Failure of one major body system (e.g., lungs, kidneys, blood-clotting cascade, liver) is associated with a mortality rate of about 40%. Cardiovascular failure, in the form of cardiogenic and septic shock, can only occasionally be reversed. By the time four organ systems fail, the mortality rate is essentially 100%.[5]

Summary

- All machines and every living animal must have energy to function. Some use external sources, while a few, such as humans, make their own energy.
- The energy that humans make is produced via a complex system, called aerobic metabolism, that uses glucose and oxygen. This entire process is dependent upon the respiratory system to provide adequate amounts of oxygen to the circulatory system, which must be able to deliver the oxygen to the cells of the body.
- The backup system to aerobic metabolism is called anaerobic metabolism. It does not require oxygen but is very inefficient and creates only a small amount of energy.
- The energy produced by aerobic metabolism is 19 times greater than that produced by anaerobic metabolism, but even so, the energy it produces will last for only a short time without a continuous supply of oxygen.
- This energy, which is stored in the form of a molecule called adenosine triphosphate, is required for all organs to function properly. Without adequate amounts of energy, the cells of the human body die.
- *Shock* is a state of generalized change in cellular function from aerobic metabolism to anaerobic metabolism secondary to hypoperfusion of the tissue cells, in which the delivery of oxygen at the cellular level is inadequate to meet metabolic needs. As a result, cellular energy production falls and, over a relatively short period of time, cellular functions become impaired, leading eventually to cell death.
- To maximize survival after trauma, prehospital providers must anticipate the development of shock, try to prevent it from occurring in the first place, and correct it when it has already occurred by taking the steps necessary to address the most critical functions first.

SCENARIO RECAP

It is 0218 hours on a hot summer night. You are dispatched to a report of gunshots fired outside a neighborhood bar known for frequent disturbances. As you respond to the scene, you confirm with dispatch that police are on their way as well. When you are several blocks away, dispatch reports that police have arrived and secured the scene and that there is one male victim. Upon arrival, an approximately 25-year-old male is found with a single gunshot wound to the mid-abdomen. He is noted on primary assessment to be confused, pale, diaphoretic, and somewhat cyanotic in color.

- What are the major pathologic processes occurring in this patient?
- What body systems must be addressed to ensure that they are functioning properly?
- How will you correct the pathophysiology causing this patient's presentation?

SCENARIO SOLUTION

You realize that this patient is in hemorrhagic shock. You know that in order for the patient's shock to be addressed, adequate oxygen must be provided to the circulatory system by the respiratory system. The fact that the patient is cyanotic indicates that he is not receiving adequate oxygen to the cells of his body. You know that if he remains hypoxic, his cellular energy production will fall as a result of anaerobic metabolism and this will lead to cell and organ death. You immediately initiate bag-mask ventilations with supplemental oxygen and note that his color improves. You know that this change indicates that aerobic metabolism can again resume if his circulatory system is intact.

Based on the location of the wound, you are concerned that he is continuing to lose blood and that he will be unable to adequately perfuse his organs and cells, so you package him for immediate transport to a trauma center. Within minutes of your arrival to the trauma center, he is taken to the operating room for repair of his intra-abdominal injury. You follow up the next day and learn that he is doing well.

References

1. Gross SD. *A System of Surgery: Pathological, Diagnostic, Therapeutic, and Operative.* Philadelphia: Blanchard and Lea; 1859.
2. Thal AP. *Shock: A Physiologic Basis for Treatment.* Chicago: Yearbook Medical Publishers; 1971.
3. Duchesne JC, Hunt JP, Wahl G, et al. Review of current blood transfusions strategies in a mature level I trauma center: were we wrong for the last 60 years? *J Trauma.* 2008;65(2):272–276; discussion 276–278.
4. Holcomb JB, Jenkins D, Rhee P, et al. Damage control resuscitation: directly addressing the early coagulopathy of trauma. *J Trauma.* 2007;62(2):307–310.
5. Marshall JC, Cook DJ, Christou NV, et al. The multiple organ dysfunction score: a reliable descriptor of a complex clinical syndrome. *Crit Care Med.* 1995;23:1638.

Suggested Reading

Shock Overview. In: Chapleau W, Burba AC, Pons PT, Page D, eds. *The Paramedic.* Updated ed. New York, NY: McGraw-Hill Publisher; 2012:259–273.
Otero RM, Nguyen HB, Rivers EP. Approach to the patient in shock. In: Tintinalli J, ed. *Emergency Medicine. A Comprehensive Study Guide.* New York, NY: McGraw-Hill Publisher; 2011:165–172.
Hypoperfusion. In: Bledsoe B, Porter RS, Cherry RA, eds. *Essentials of Paramedic Care.* 2nd ed. Upper Saddle River, NJ: Brady-Pearson Education; 2011:257–265.
Shock. In: Bledsoe B, Porter RS, Cherry RA, eds. *Essentials of Paramedic Care.* 2nd ed. Upper Saddle River, NJ: Brady-Pearson Education; 2011:837–849.

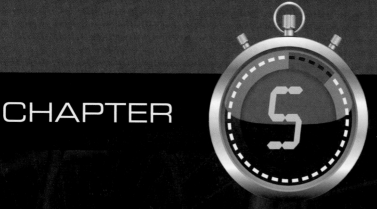

CHAPTER 5

Kinematics of Trauma

CHAPTER OBJECTIVES

At the completion of this chapter, the reader will be able to do the following:

- Define energy in the context of producing injury.

- Explain the association between the laws of motion, energy, and the kinematics of trauma.

- Describe the relationship of injury and energy exchange to speed.

- Discuss energy exchange and cavitation.

- Given the description of a motor vehicle crash, use kinematics to predict the likely injury pattern for an unrestrained occupant.

- Describe the specific injuries and their causes as related to interior and exterior vehicle damage.

- Discuss the function of restraint systems for vehicle occupants.

- Relate the laws of motion and energy to mechanisms other than motor vehicle crashes (e.g., blasts, falls).

- Define the five phases of blast injury and the injuries produced in each phase.

- Explain the differences in the production of injury with low-, medium-, and high-energy weapons.

- Discuss the relationship of the frontal surface of an impacting object to energy exchange and injury production.

- Integrate principles of kinematics into trauma patient assessment.

SCENARIO

Before first light on a cold winter morning, you and your partner are dispatched to a single-vehicle crash. On arrival, you find a single vehicle that has crashed into a tree on a rural road. The front end of the vehicle appears to have impacted the tree, and the car has spun around the tree and backed into a drainage ditch on the side of the road. The driver appears to be the only occupant. The air bag has deployed and the driver is moaning, still restrained by his safety harness. You note damage to the front end of the car where it impacted the tree as well as rear-end damage from spinning around and going into the ditch backwards.

- What is the potential for injury for this patient based on the kinematics of this event?
- How would you describe the patient's condition based upon the kinematics?
- What injuries do you expect to find?

Introduction

While road traffic deaths in the United States dropped in 2011 to levels not seen since the 1940s[1], the World Health organization (WHO) reports that nearly 1.3 million people are killed annually in car crashes around the world. That averages out to 3,562 deaths every day. In their 2009 publication, Global Status Report on Road Safety, the WHO predicts that road crashes will move from the ninth-leading cause of death to the fifth-leading cause of death worldwide by 2030. Over 90% of these deaths occur in low-income and middle-income countries.[2]

Penetrating trauma injuries from firearms are very high in the United States. In 2011, there were over 32,000 deaths from firearms. Of those deaths, over 11,000 were homicides.[3] In 2011, over 59,000 nonfatal firearm injuries were reported.[3] Blast injuries are a major cause of injuries in many countries, whereas penetrating injuries from knives are prominent in others.

Successful management of trauma patients depends on the identification of injuries or potential injuries and the use of good assessment skills. It is frequently difficult in the prehospital setting to determine the exact injury produced, but understanding the potential for injury and the potential for significant blood loss will allow the prehospital care provider to use his or her critical-thinking skills to recognize this likelihood and make appropriate triage, management, and transportation decisions.

The management of any patient begins (after initial resuscitation) with the history of the patient's injury. In trauma, the history is the story of the impact and the energy exchange that resulted from this impact.[4] An understanding of the energy exchange process will allow prehospital care providers to suspect 95% of the potential injuries.

Kinematics is the branch of mechanics that deals with the motion of objects without reference to the forces that cause the motion.[4] Any injury that results from a force applied to the body is related directly to the interaction between the host and a moving object that impacts the host. When the prehospital care provider, at any level of care, does not understand the principles of kinematics or the mechanisms involved, injuries may be missed. An understanding of these principles will increase the level of suspicion for certain injuries associated with the pattern of injuries observed at the scene on arrival. This information and the suspected injuries can be used to properly assess the patient on the scene and can be transmitted to the physicians and nurses in the emergency department (ED). At the scene and en route, these suspected injuries can be managed to provide the most appropriate patient care and "do no further harm."

Injuries that are not obvious but are still severe can be fatal if they are not managed at the scene and en route to the trauma center or appropriate hospital. Knowing where to look and how to assess for injuries is as important as knowing what to do after finding injuries. A complete, accurate history of a traumatic incident and proper interpretation of this data will provide such information. Most of a patient's injuries can be predicted by a proper survey of the scene, even before examining the patient.

This chapter discusses the general principles and mechanical principles involved in the kinematics of trauma, and the sections on the regional effects of blunt and penetrating trauma address local injury pathophysiology. The general principles are the laws of physics that govern energy exchange and the general effects of the energy exchange. Mechanical principles address the interaction of the human body with the components of a crash. A crash is the energy exchange that occurs when an object with energy, usually something solid, impacts the human body. Types of crashes include blunt trauma, penetrating trauma, and blasts. Though we often associate the word crash with a motor vehicle impact, it can also refer to the crash of a falling body onto the pavement, the impact of a bullet on the external and internal tissues of the body, and the overpressure and debris of a blast. All of these events involve energy exchange, all result in injury, all involve potentially life-threatening conditions, and all require correct management by a knowledgeable and insightful prehospital care provider.

General Principles

A traumatic event is divided into three phases: pre-event, event, and postevent. Simply stated, the *pre-event* phase is the prevention phase. The *event* phase is that portion of the traumatic event that involves the exchange of energy or the kinematics (mechanics of energy). Lastly, the *postevent* is the patient care phase.

Whether the injury results from a car crash, a weapon, a fall, or a building collapse, energy is transformed into injury when it is absorbed into the body.

Pre-event

The *pre-event phase* includes all of the events that preceded the incident. Conditions that were present before the incident occurred and that are important in the management of the patient's injuries are assessed as part of the pre-event history. These considerations include the patient's acute or pre-existing medical conditions (and medications to treat those conditions), ingestion of recreational substances (illegal and prescription drugs, alcohol, etc.), and the patient's state of mind.

Typically, young trauma patients do not have chronic illnesses. With older patients, however, medical conditions that are present before the trauma event can cause serious complications in the prehospital assessment and management of the patient and can significantly influence the outcome. For example, the elderly driver of a vehicle that has struck a utility pole may have chest pain indicative of a myocardial infarction (heart attack). Did the driver hit the utility pole and have a heart attack, or did he have a heart attack and then strike the utility pole? Does the driver take medication (e.g., beta blocker) that will prevent elevation of the pulse in shock? Most of these conditions not only directly influence the assessment and management strategies discussed in the: Scene Assessment and the Patient Assessment and Management chapters, but are important in overall patient care, even if they do not necessarily influence the kinematics of the crash.

Event

The *event phase* begins at the time of impact between one moving object and a second object. The second object can be moving or stationary and can be either an object or a person. Using a vehicle crash as an example, three impacts occur in most vehicular crashes:

1. The impact of the two objects
2. The impact of the occupants into the vehicle
3. The impact of the vital organs inside the occupants

For example, when a vehicle strikes a tree, the first impact is the collision of the vehicle with the tree. The second impact is the occupant of the vehicle striking the steering wheel or windshield. If the occupant is restrained, an impact occurs between the occupant and the seat belt. The third impact is between the occupant's internal organs and his or her chest wall, abdominal wall, or skull.

While the term crash typically brings to mind a motor vehicle incident, it does not necessarily refer to a vehicular crash. The impact of a vehicle into a pedestrian, a missile (bullet) into the abdomen, and a construction worker onto asphalt after a fall are all examples of a crash. Note that in a fall, only the second and third impacts are involved.

In all crashes, energy is exchanged between a moving object and the tissue of the human body or between the moving human body and a stationary object. The direction in which the energy exchange occurs, the amount of energy that is exchanged, and the effect that these forces have on the patient are all important considerations as assessment begins.

Postevent

During the *postevent phase*, the information gathered about the crash and pre-event phase is used to assess and manage a patient. This phase begins as soon as the energy from the crash is absorbed. The onset of the complications from life-threatening trauma can be slow or fast (or these complications can be prevented or significantly reduced), depending in part on the care provided at the scene and en route to the hospital. In the postevent phase, the understanding of the kinematics of trauma, the index of suspicion regarding injuries, and strong assessment skills all become crucial to the patient outcome.

To understand the effects of the forces that produce bodily injury, the prehospital care provider first needs to understand two components—energy exchange and human anatomy. For example, in a motor vehicle crash (MVC), what does the scene look like? Who hit what and at what speed? How long was the stopping time? Were the occupants using appropriate restraint devices such as seat belts? Did the air bag deploy? Were the children restrained properly in child seats, or were they unrestrained and thrown about the vehicle? Were occupants thrown from the vehicle? Did they strike objects? If so, how many objects and what was the nature of those objects? These and many other questions must be answered if the prehospital care provider is to understand the exchange of forces that took place and translate this information into a prediction of injuries and appropriate patient care.

The astute prehospital care provider will utilize his or her knowledge of kinematics in the process of surveying the scene to determine what forces and motion were involved and what injuries might have resulted from those forces. Because kinematics is based on fundamental principles of physics, an understanding of the pertinent laws of physics is necessary.

Energy

The initial steps in obtaining a history include evaluating the events that occurred at the time of the crash (**Figure 5-1**),

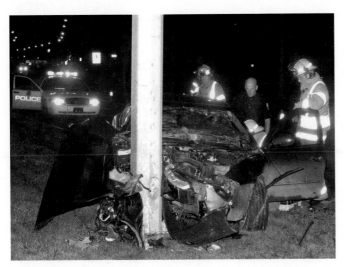

Figure 5-1 Evaluating the scene of an incident is critical. Such information as direction of impact, passenger-compartment intrusion, and amount of energy exchange provides insight into the possible injuries of the occupants.
Source: © Jack Dagley Photography/ShutterStock, Inc.

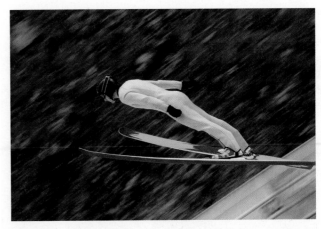

Figure 5-2 A skier was stationary until the energy from gravity moved him down the slope. Once in motion, although he leaves the ground, the momentum will keep him in motion until he hits something or returns to the ground, and the transfer of energy (friction or a collision) causes him to come to a stop.
Source: © technotr/iStockPhoto.

estimating the energy that was exchanged with the human body, and making a gross approximation of the specific conditions that resulted.

Laws of Energy and Motion

Newton's first law of motion states that a body at rest will remain at rest, and a body in motion will remain in motion unless acted on by an outside force. The skier in **Figure 5-2** was stationary until the energy from gravity moved him down the slope. Once in motion, although he leaves the ground, he will remain in motion until he hits something or returns to the ground and comes to a stop.

As previously mentioned, in any collision, when the body of the potential patient is in motion, there are three collisions:

1. The vehicle of the crash hitting an object, moving or stationary
2. The potential patient hitting the inside of the vehicle, crashing into an object, or being struck by energy in an explosion
3. The internal organs interacting with the walls of a compartment of the body or being torn loose from their supporting structures

An example is an occupant sitting in the front seat of a vehicle who is not wearing any restraint devices. When the vehicle hits a tree and stops, the unrestrained occupant continues in motion—at the same rate of speed—until he or she hits the steering column, dashboard, and windshield. The impact with these objects stops the forward motion of the torso or head, but the internal organs of the occupant remain in motion until the organs hit the inside of the chest wall, abdominal wall, or skull, halting the forward motion.

As described by the **law of conservation of energy** and **Newton's second law of motion**, energy can neither be created nor destroyed, but can be changed in form. The motion of the vehicle is a form of energy. To start the vehicle, gasoline explodes within the cylinder of the engine. This explosion moves the pistons. The motion of the pistons is transferred by a set of gears to the wheels, which grasp the road as they turn and impart motion to the vehicle. To stop the vehicle, the energy of its motion must be changed to another form, such as by heating up the brakes or crashing into an object and bending the frame. When a driver brakes, the energy of motion is converted into the heat of friction (thermal energy) by the brake pads on the brake drums/disc and by the tires on the roadway. The vehicle thus decelerates.

Newton's third law of motion is perhaps the most well-known of Newton's three laws. It states that for every action or force there is an equal and opposite reaction. As we walk across the ground, the earth is exerting a force against us equal to the force we are applying upon the earth. Those who have fired a shotgun have felt the third law as the impact of the butt of the gun against their shoulder.

Just as the mechanical energy of a vehicle that crashes into a wall is dissipated by the bending of the frame or other parts of the vehicle (**Figure 5-3**), the energy of motion of the organs and the structures inside the body must be dissipated as these organs stop their forward motion. The same concepts apply to the human body when it is stationary and comes into contact and interacts with an object in motion such as a knife, a bullet, or a baseball bat.

Kinetic energy is a function of an object's mass and velocity. Although they are not technically the same, a victim's

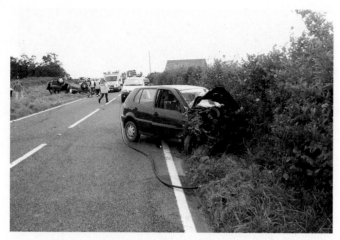

Figure 5-3 Energy is dissipated by deformation of the vehicle frame.
Source: © Peter Seyfferth/image/age fotostock.

weight is used to represent his or her mass. Likewise, speed is used to represent velocity (which really is speed and direction). The relationship between weight and speed as it affects kinetic energy is as follows:

Kinetic energy = One-half the mass times the velocity squared

$$KE = 1/2mv^2$$

Thus, the kinetic energy involved when a 150-pound (lb) (68-kilogram [kg]) person travels at 30 miles per hour (mph) (48 kilometers per hour [km/hr]) is calculated as follows:

$$KE = 150/2 \times 30^2 = 67,500 \text{ units}$$

For the purpose of this discussion, no specific physical unit of measure (e.g., foot-pounds, joules) is used. The units are used merely to illustrate how this formula affects the change in the amount of energy. As just shown, a 150-lb (68-kg) person travelling at 30 mph (48 km/hr) would have 67,500 units of energy that must be converted to another form when he or she stops. This change takes the form of damage to the vehicle and injury to the person in it unless the energy dissipation can take some less harmful form, such as on a seat belt or into an air bag.

Which factor in the formula, however, has the greatest effect on the amount of kinetic energy produced: mass or velocity? Consider adding 10 lb (4.5 kg) to the 150-lb (68-kg) person travelling at 30 mph (48 km/hr) in the prior example, making the mass equal to 160 lb (73kg):

$$KE = 160/2 \times 30^2 = 72,000 \text{ units}$$

This 10-lb increase has resulted in a 4,500-unit increase in kinetic energy. Using the initial example of a 150-lb (68-kg) person

once again, let's now see how increasing the velocity by 10 mph (16 km/hr) affects the kinetic energy:

$$KE = 150/2 \times 40^2 = 120,000 \text{ units}$$

This velocity increase has resulted in a 52,500-unit increase in kinetic energy.

These calculations demonstrate that increasing the velocity (speed) increases the kinetic energy much more than does increasing the mass. Much more energy exchange will occur (and, therefore, produce greater injury to either the occupant or the vehicle, or both) in a high-speed crash than in a crash at a slower speed. The velocity is exponential and the mass is linear, making velocity the more critical factor even when there is a great mass disparity between two objects.

In anticipating the injuries sustained during a high-speed crash, it can be helpful to bear in mind that the force involved in initiating an event is equal to the force transferred or dissipated at the end of that event.

Mass × Acceleration = Force = Mass × Deceleration

Force (energy) is required to put a structure into motion. This force (energy) is required to create a specific speed. The speed imparted is dependent on the weight (mass) of the structure. Once this energy is passed on to the structure and it is placed in motion, the motion will remain until the energy is given up (Newton's first law of motion). This loss of energy will place other components in motion (tissue particles) or be lost as heat (dissipated into the brake discs on the wheels). An example of this process is gun-related trauma. In the chamber of a gun is a cartridge that contains gunpowder. If this gunpowder is ignited, it burns rapidly creating energy that pushes the bullet out of the barrel at a great speed. This speed is equivalent to the weight of the bullet and the amount of energy produced by the burning of the gunpowder or force. To slow down (Newton's first law of motion), the bullet must give up its energy into the structure that it hits. This will produce an explosion in the tissue that is equal to the explosion that occurred in the chamber of the gun when the initial speed was given to the bullet. The same phenomenon occurs in the moving automobile, the patient falling from a building, or the explosion of an improvised explosive device.

Another important factor in a crash is the **stopping distance**. The shorter the stopping distance and the quicker the rate of that stop, the more energy transferred to the occupant and the more damage or injury done to the patient. Consider a vehicle that stops against a brick wall versus one that stops when the brakes are applied. Both dissipate the same amount of energy, just in a different manner. The rate of energy exchange (into the vehicle body or into the brake discs) is different and occurs over a different distance and time. In the first instance, the energy is absorbed in a very short distance and amount of time by the bending of the vehicle's frame. In the latter case, the energy is absorbed over a longer distance and period of time by the heat of the brakes. The forward motion of the occupant of the vehicle (energy) is absorbed in the first instance by damage to the soft tissue and bones of the occupant. In the second instance, the energy is dissipated, along with the energy of the vehicle, into the brakes.

This inverse relationship between stopping distance and injury also applies to falls. A person has a better chance of surviving a fall if he or she lands on a compressible surface, such as deep, powder snow. The same fall terminating on a hard surface, such as concrete, can produce more severe injuries. The compressible material (i.e., the snow) increases the stopping distance and absorbs at least some of the energy rather than allowing all of the energy to be absorbed by the body. The result is decreased injury and damage to the body. This principle also applies to other types of crashes. In addition, an unrestrained driver will be more severely injured than a restrained driver. The restraint system, rather than the body, will absorb a significant portion of the energy transfer.

Therefore, once an object is in motion and has energy in the form of motion, in order for it to come to a complete rest, the object must lose all of its energy by converting the energy to another form or transferring it to another object. For example, if a vehicle strikes a pedestrian, the pedestrian is knocked away from the vehicle (**Figure 5-4**). Although the vehicle is somewhat slowed by the impact, the greater force of the vehicle imparts much more acceleration to the lighter-weight pedestrian than it loses in speed because of the mass difference between the two. The softer body parts of the pedestrian versus the harder body parts of the vehicle also means more damage to the pedestrian than to the vehicle.

Energy Exchange Between a Solid Object and the Human Body

When the human body collides with a solid object, or vice versa, the number of body tissue particles that are impacted by the solid object determines the amount of energy exchange that takes place. This transfer of energy produces the amount of damage (injury) that occurs to the patient. The number of tissue particles affected is determined by (1) the density (particles per volume) of the tissue and (2) the size of the contact area of the impact.

Density

The denser the tissue (measured in particles per volume), the greater the number of particles that will be impacted by a moving object and, therefore, the greater the rate and the total amount of energy exchanged. Driving a fist into a feather pillow and driving a fist at the same speed into a brick wall will produce different effects on the hand. The fist absorbs more energy colliding with the dense brick wall than with the less dense feather pillow, thus leading to more significant injury to the hand (**Figure 5-5**).

Simplistically, the body has three different types of tissue densities: **air density** (much of the lung and some portions of the

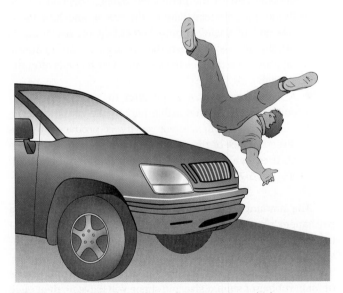

Figure 5-4 The energy exchange from a moving vehicle to a pedestrian crushes tissue and imparts speed and energy to the pedestrian to knock the victim away from the point of impact. Injury to the patient can occur both as the pedestrian is hit by the vehicle and as the pedestrian is thrown to the ground or into another vehicle.

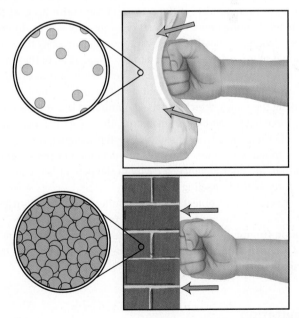

Figure 5-5 The fist absorbs more energy colliding with the dense brick wall than with the less dense feather pillow, which dissipates the force.

intestine), **water density** (muscle and most solid organs; e.g., liver, spleen), and **solid density** (bone). Therefore, the amount of energy exchange (with resultant injury) will depend on which type of organ is impacted.

Contact Area

Wind exerts pressure on a hand when it is extended out of the window of a moving vehicle. When the palm of the hand is horizontal and parallel to the direction of the flow through the wind, some backward pressure is exerted on the front of the hand (fingers) as the particles of air strike the hand. Rotating the hand 90 degrees to a vertical position places a larger surface area into the wind; thus, more air particles make contact with the hand, increasing the amount of force on it.

For trauma events, the energy imparted and the resulting damage can be modified by any change in the size of the impact surface area. Examples of this effect on the human body include the front of an automobile, a baseball bat, or a rifle bullet. The automobile's front surface contacts a large portion of the victim, a baseball bat contacts a smaller area, and a bullet contacts a very small area. The amount of energy exchange that would produce damage to the patient depends then on the energy of the object and the density of the tissue in the pathway of the energy exchange.

If all of the impact energy is in a small area and this force exceeds the resistance of the skin, the object is forced though the skin. Consider the difference between striking a wooden table with a hammer and striking a nail held to the surface of the table with that same hammer. When you strike the table with the hammer, the force of the hammer striking the table is spread out across the surface of the table and the entire head of the hammer, limiting penetration and creating only a dent. In contrast, striking the head of a nail with the hammer using the same amount of force drives the nail into the wood as all of that force is applied over a very small area. If the force is spread out over a larger area and the skin is not penetrated (like the hammer striking the table), then it fits the definition of **blunt trauma**. If the force is applied over a small area, the object can penetrate the skin and underlying tissues (like the hammer driving the nail through the table), which fits the definition of **penetrating trauma**. In either instance, a cavity in the patient is created by the force of the impacting object.

Even with an object such as a bullet, the impact surface area can be different based on such factors as bullet size, its motion (tumble) within the body, deformation ("mushroom"), and fragmentation. These factors are discussed later in this chapter.

Cavitation

The basic mechanics of energy exchange are relatively simple. The impact on the tissue particles accelerates those tissue particles away from the point of impact. These tissues then become moving objects themselves and crash into other tissue particles, producing a "falling domino" effect. Similarly, when a solid object strikes the human body or when the human body is in motion and strikes a stationary object, the tissue particles of the human body are knocked out of their normal position, creating a hole or cavity. Thus, this process is called **cavitation**. A common game that provides a visual effect of cavitation is pool.

The cue ball is driven down the length of a pool table by the force of the muscles in the arm. The cue ball crashes into the racked balls at the other end of the table. The energy from the arm into the cue ball is thus transferred onto each of the racked balls (**Figure 5-6**). The cue ball gives up its energy to the other balls. The other balls begin to move while the cue ball, which has lost its energy, slows or even stops. The other balls take on this energy as motion and move away from the impact point. A cavity has been created where the rack of balls once was. The same kind of energy exchange occurs when a bowling ball rolls down the alley, hitting the set of pins at the other end. The result of this energy exchange is a cavity. This sort of energy exchange occurs in both blunt and penetrating trauma.

Two types of cavities are created:

- A *temporary cavity* is caused by the stretching of the tissues that occurs at the time of impact. Because of the elastic properties of the body's tissues, some or all of the contents of the temporary cavity return to their previous position. The size, shape, and portions of the cavity that become part of the permanent damage depend on the tissue type, the elasticity of the tissue, and how much rebound of tissue occurs. The extent of this cavity is usually not visible when the prehospital care or hospital provider examines the patient, even seconds after the impact.

- A *permanent cavity* is left after the temporary cavity collapses and is the visible part of the tissue destruction. In addition, a crush cavity is produced by the direct impact of the object on the tissue. Both of these cavities can be seen when the patient is examined[5] (**Figure 5-7**).

The amount of the temporary cavity that remains as a permanent cavity is related to the elasticity (stretch ability) of the tissue involved. For example, forcefully swinging a baseball bat into a steel drum leaves a dent, or cavity, in its side. Swinging the same baseball bat with the same force into a mass of foam rubber of similar size and shape will leave no dent once the bat is removed (**Figure 5-8**). The difference is **elasticity**. The foam rubber is more elastic than the steel drum. The human body is more like the foam rubber than the steel drum. If a person punches another person's abdomen, he or she would feel the fist go in. However, when the person pulls the fist away,

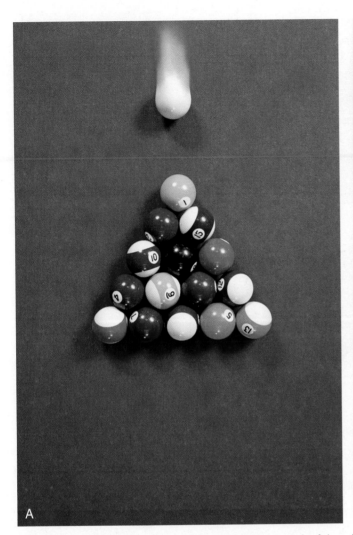

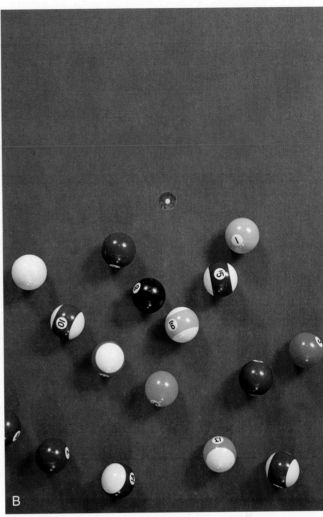

Figure 5-6   **A.** The energy of a cue ball is transferred to each of the other balls. **B.** The energy exchange pushes the balls apart to create a cavity.

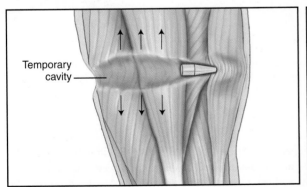

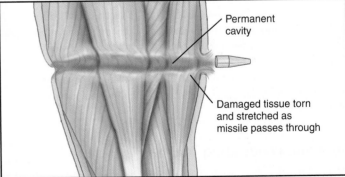

Figure 5-7   Damage to tissue is greater than the permanent cavity that remains from a missile injury. The faster or heavier the missile, the larger the temporary cavity and the greater the zone of tissue damage.

no dent is left. Similarly, a baseball bat swung into the chest will leave no obvious cavity in the thoracic wall, but it would cause damage, both from direct contact and the cavity created by the energy exchange. The history of the incident and the interpretation of energy transfer will provide the information needed to determine the potential size of the temporary cavity at the time of impact. The organs or the structures involved predict injuries.

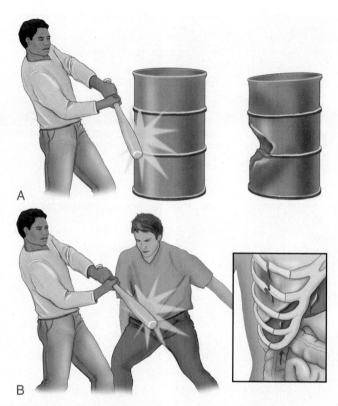

Figure 5-8 **A.** Swinging a baseball bat into a steel drum leaves a dent, or cavity, in its side. **B.** Swinging a baseball bat into a person usually leaves no visible cavity; the elasticity of the trunk usually returns the body to its normal shape even though damage has occurred.

When the trigger of a loaded gun is pulled, the firing pin strikes the cap and produces an explosion in the cartridge. The energy created by this explosion is applied to the bullet, which speeds from the muzzle of the weapon. The bullet now has energy, or force (acceleration × mass = force). Once such force is imparted, the bullet cannot slow down until acted on by an outside force (Newton's first law of motion). In order for the bullet to stop inside the human body, an explosion must occur within the tissues that is equivalent to the explosion in the weapon (acceleration × mass = force = mass × deceleration) (**Figure 5-9**). This explosion is the result of energy exchange accelerating the tissue particles out of their normal position, creating a cavity.

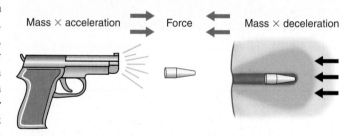

Figure 5-9 As a bullet travels through tissue, its kinetic energy is transferred to the tissue that it comes in contact with, accelerating the tissue away from the bullet.

Blunt and Penetrating Trauma

Trauma is generally classified as either blunt or penetrating. However, the energy exchanged and the injuries produced are similar in both types of trauma. Cavitation occurs in both; only the type and direction are different. The only real difference is penetration of the skin. If an object's entire energy is concentrated on one small area of skin, the skin likely will tear, and the object will enter the body and create a more concentrated energy exchange along the pathway. This can result in greater destructive power to one area. A larger object whose energy is dispersed over a much larger area of skin may not penetrate the skin. The damage will be distributed over a larger area of the body, and the injury pattern will be less localized. An example is the difference in the impact of a large truck into a pedestrian versus a gunshot impact (**Figure 5-10**).

The cavitation in blunt trauma is frequently only a temporary cavity and is directed away from the point of impact. Penetrating trauma creates both a permanent and a temporary cavity. The temporary cavity that is created will spread away from the pathway of this missile in both frontal and lateral directions.

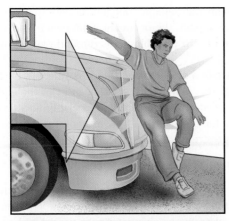

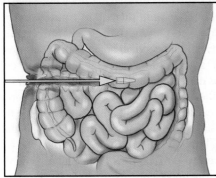

Figure 5-10 The force from a collision of a vehicle with a person is generally distributed over a large area, whereas the force of the collision between a bullet and a person is localized to a very small area and results in penetration of the body and underlying structures.

Blunt Trauma
Mechanical Principles

This section is divided into two major parts. The mechanical and structural effects on the vehicle of a crash are discussed first, and then the internal effects on the organs and body structures are addressed. Both are important and must be understood to properly assess the trauma patient and the potential injuries that exist after the crash.

The on-scene observations of the probable circumstances that led to a crash resulting in blunt trauma provide clues as to the severity of the injuries and the potential organs involved. The factors to assess are (1) direction of the impact, (2) external damage to the vehicle (type and severity),and (3) internal damage (e.g., occupant-compartment intrusion, steering wheel/column bending, bull's-eye fracture in the windshield, mirror damage, dashboard–knee impacts).

In blunt trauma, two forces are involved in the impact— shear and **compression**—both of which may result in cavitation. *Shear* is the result of one organ or structure (or part of an organ or structure) changing speed faster than another organ or structure (or part of an organ or structure). This difference in acceleration (or deceleration) causes the parts to

separate and tear. A classic example of shear force is the rupture of the thoracic aorta. The ascending aorta and aortic arch are loosely held in place within the mediastinum, whereas the descending aorta is tightly bound to the spinal column. In a sudden deceleration incident, the ascending aorta and aortic arch can continue moving while the descending aorta is held in place, leading to shearing and rupture of the aorta (see Figure 5-14).

Compression is the result of an organ or structure (or part of an organ or structure) being directly squeezed between other organs or structures. A common example of compression involves the bowel being compressed between the spinal column and the inside of the anterior abdominal wall in a patient wearing only a seat belt (see Figure 5-29). Injury can result from any type of impact, such as MVCs (vehicle or motorcycle), pedestrian collisions with vehicles, falls, sports injuries, or blast injuries. All of these mechanisms are discussed separately, followed by the results of this energy exchange on the specific anatomy in each of the body regions.

As discussed previously in this chapter, three collisions occur in blunt trauma. The first is the collision of the vehicle into another object. The second is the collision that occurs when the occupant strikes the inside of the vehicular passenger compartment, strikes the ground at the end of a fall, or is struck by the force created in an explosion. The third is when the structures within the various regions of the body (head, chest, abdomen, etc.) strike the wall of that region or are torn (shear force) from their attachment within this compartment. The first of these collisions will be discussed as it relates to MVCs, falls, and explosions. The latter two will be discussed in the specific regions involved.

Motor Vehicle Crashes

Many forms of blunt trauma occur, but MVCs (including motorcycle crashes) are the most common.[6] In 2011, 32,367 people died and an estimated 2.2 million people were injured in MVCs in the United States. While the majority of the deaths were occupants of the vehicles, over 5,000 of the deaths were pedestrians, cyclists,and other unknown nonoccupants.[1]

MVCs can be divided into the following five types:

1. Frontal impact
2. Rear impact
3. Lateral impact
4. Rotational impact
5. Rollover[7]

Although each pattern has variations, accurate identification of the five patterns will provide insight into other, similar types of crashes.

One method to estimate the potential for injury to the occupant is to look at the vehicle and determine which of the five types of collisions occurred, the energy exchange involved, and the direction of the impact. The occupant receives the same type of force as the vehicle from the same direction as the vehicle, and the potential injuries can be predicted.[7] The amount of force exchanged with the occupant, however, may be somewhat reduced by the absorption of energy by the vehicle.

Frontal Impact

In **Figure 5-11**, the vehicle has hit a utility pole in the center of the car. The impact point stopped its forward motion, but the rest of the car continued forward until the energy was absorbed by the bending of the car. The same type of motion occurs to the driver, resulting in injury. The stable steering column is impacted by the chest, perhaps in the center of the sternum. Just as the car continued in forward motion, significantly deforming the front of the vehicle, so too will the driver's chest. As the sternum stops forward motion against the dash, the posterior thoracic wall continues until the energy is absorbed by the bending and possible fracture of the ribs. This process will also crush the heart and the lungs, which are trapped between the sternum and the vertebral column and the posterior thoracic wall.

The amount of damage to the vehicle indicates the approximate speed of the vehicle at the time of impact. The greater the intrusion into the body of the vehicle, the greater the speed at the time of impact. The greater the vehicle speed, the greater the energy exchange and the more likely the occupants are to be injured.

Although the vehicle suddenly ceases to move forward in a frontal impact, the occupant continues to move and will follow one of two possible paths: up and over, or down and under.

The use of a seat belt and the deployment of an air bag or restraint system will absorb some or most of the energy, thus reducing the injury to the victim. For clarity and simplicity of discussion, the occupant in these examples will be assumed to be without restraint.

Up-and-Over Path

In this sequence, the body's forward motion carries it up and over the steering wheel (**Figure 5-12**). The head is usually the lead body portion striking the windshield, windshield frame, or roof. The head then stops its forward motion. The torso continues in motion until its energy/force is absorbed along the spine. The cervical spine is the least protected segment of the spine. The chest or abdomen then collides with the steering column, depending on the position of the torso. Impact of the chest into the steering column produces thoracic cage, cardiac, lung, and aortic injuries (see the Regional Effects of Blunt Trauma section). Impact of the abdomen into the steering column can compress and crush the solid organs, produce overpressure injuries (especially to the diaphragm), and rupture the hollow organs.

The kidneys, spleen, and liver are also subject to shear injury as the abdomen strikes the steering wheel and abruptly stops. An organ may be torn from its normal anatomic

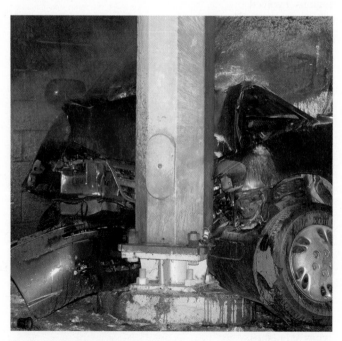

Figure 5-11 As a vehicle impacts a utility pole, the front of the car stops but the rear portion of the vehicle continues traveling forward, causing deformation of the vehicle.
Source: © Jack Dagley Photography/ShutterStock, Inc.

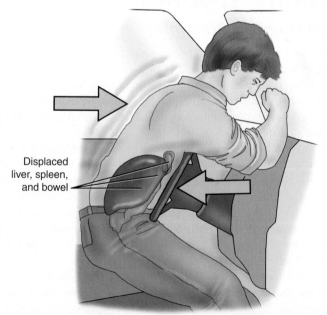

Displaced liver, spleen, and bowel

Figure 5-12 Configuration of the seat and position of the occupant can direct the initial force on the upper torso, with the head as the lead point.

restraints and supporting tissues (**Figure 5-13**). For example, the continued forward motion of the kidneys after the vertebral column has stopped moving produces shear along the attachment of the organs at their blood supply. The aorta and vena cava are tethered tightly to the posterior abdominal wall and vertebral column. The continued forward motion of the kidneys can stretch the renal vessels to the point of rupture. A similar action may tear the aorta in the chest as the unattached arch becomes the tightly adhered descending aorta (**Figure 5-14**).

Down-and-Under Path

In a down-and-under path, the occupant moves forward, downward, and out of the seat into the dashboard (**Figure 5-15**). The importance of understanding kinematics is illustrated by the injuries produced to the lower extremity in this pathway. Because many of the injuries are difficult to identify, an understanding of the mechanism of injury is very important.

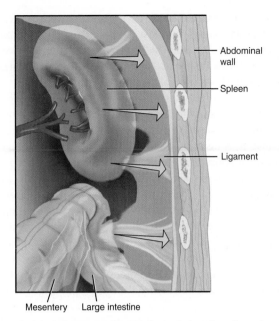

Figure 5-13 Organs can tear away from their point of attachment to the abdominal wall. The spleen, kidney, and small intestine are particularly susceptible to these types of shear forces.

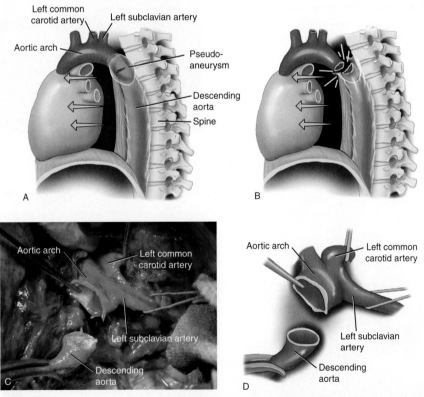

Figure 5-14 **A.** The descending aorta is a fixed structure that moves with the thoracic spine. The arch, aorta, and heart are freely movable. Acceleration of the torso in a lateral-impact collision or rapid deceleration of the torso in a frontal-impact collision produces a different rate of motion between the arch–heart complex and the descending aorta. This motion may result in a tear of the inner lining of the aorta that is contained within the outermost layer, producing a pseudo-aneurysm. **B.** Tears at the junction of the arch and descending aorta may also result in a complete rupture, leading to immediate exsanguination in the chest. **C.** and **D.** Operative photograph and drawing of a traumatic aortic tear.
Source: C., D. Courtesy Norman McSwain, MD, FACS, NREMT-P.

The foot, if planted on the floor panel or on the brake pedal with a straight knee, can twist as the continued torso motion angulates and fractures the ankle joint. More often, however, the knees are already bent, and the force is not directed to the ankle. Therefore, the knees strike the dashboard.

The knee has two possible impact points against the dashboard, the tibia and the femur (**Figure 5-16A**). If the tibia hits the dashboard and stops first, the femur remains in motion and overrides it. A dislocated knee, with torn ligaments, tendons, and other supporting structures, can result. Because the popliteal artery lies close to the knee joint, dislocation of the joint is frequently associated with injury to the vessel. The artery can be completely disrupted, or the lining alone (*intima*) may be damaged (**Figure 5-16B**). In either case, a blood clot may form in the injured vessel, resulting in significantly decreased blood flow to the leg tissues below the knee. Early recognition of the knee injury and the potential for vascular injury will alert the physicians to the need for assessment of the vessel in this area.

Early identification and treatment of such a popliteal artery injury significantly decreases the complications of distal limb ischemia. Perfusion to this tissue needs to be re-established within about 6 hours. Delays could occur because the prehospital care provider failed to consider the kinematics of the injury or overlooked important clues during assessment of the patient.

Although most of these patients have evidence of injury to the knee, an imprint on the dashboard where the knee impacted is a key indicator that significant energy was focused on this joint and adjacent structures (**Figure 5-17**). Further investigation is needed in the hospital to better eliminate the possible injuries.

When the femur is the point of impact, the energy is absorbed on the bone shaft, which can then break (**Figure 5-18**). The continued forward motion of the pelvis onto the femur that

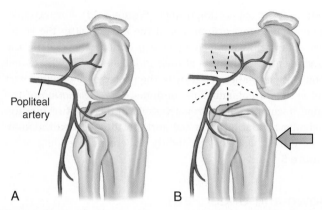

Figure 5-16 A. The knee has two possible impact points in a motor vehicle crash: the tibia and the femur. **B.** The popliteal artery lies close to the joint, tightly tied to the femur above and tibia below. Separation of these two bones stretches, kinks, and tears the artery.

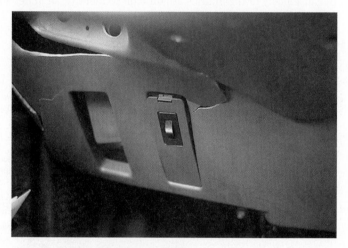

Figure 5-17 The impact point of the knee on the dashboard indicates both a down-and-under pathway and a significant absorption of energy along the lower extremity.

Source: Courtesy Norman McSwain, MD, FACS, NREMT-P.

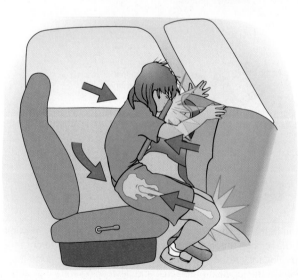

Figure 5-15 The occupant and the vehicle travel forward together. The vehicle stops, and the unrestrained occupant continues forward until something stops that motion.

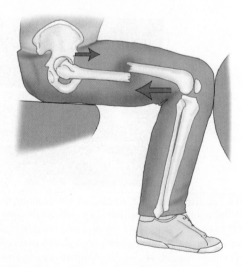

Figure 5-18 When the femur is the point of impact, the energy is absorbed on the bone shaft, which can then break.

remains intact can override the femoral head, resulting in a posterior dislocation of the acetabular joint (**Figure 5-19**).

After the knees and legs stop their forward motion, the upper body will bend forward into the steering column or dashboard. The unrestrained occupant may then sustain many of the same injuries described previously for the up-and-over pathway.

Recognizing these potential injuries and relaying the information to the ED physicians can result in long-term benefits to the patient.

Rear Impact

Rear-impact collisions occur when a slower-moving or stationary vehicle is struck from behind by a vehicle moving at a faster speed. For ease of understanding, the more rapidly moving vehicle is called the "bullet vehicle" and the slower-moving or stopped object is called the "target vehicle." In such collisions, the energy of the bullet vehicle at the moment of impact is converted to acceleration of the target vehicle and damage results to both vehicles. The greater the difference in the momentum of the two vehicles, the greater the force of the initial impact and the more energy is available to create damage and acceleration.

During a rear-impact collision, the target vehicle in front is accelerated forward. Everything that is attached to the frame will also move forward at the same speed. This includes the seats in which the occupants are riding. The unattached objects in the vehicle, including the occupants, will begin forward motion only after something in contact with the frame begins to transmit the energy of the forward motion to them. As an example, the torso is accelerated by the back of the seat after some of the energy has been absorbed by the springs in the seats. If the headrest is improperly positioned behind and below the occiput of the head, the head will begin its forward

motion after the torso, resulting in hyperextension of the neck. Shear and stretching of the ligaments and other support structures, especially in the anterior part of the neck, can result in injury (**Figure 5-20A**).

If the headrest is properly positioned, the head moves at approximately the same time as the torso without hyperextension (**Figure 5-20B** and **Figure 5-21**). If the target vehicle is allowed to move forward without interference until it slows to a stop, the occupant will probably not suffer significant injury because most of the body's motion is supported by the seat, similar to an astronaut launching into orbit.

However, if the vehicle strikes another vehicle or object or if the driver slams on the brakes and stops suddenly, the occupants will continue forward, following the characteristic pattern of a frontal-impact collision. The collision then involves two impacts—rear and frontal. The double impact increases the likelihood of injury.

Lateral Impact

Lateral-impact mechanisms come into play when the vehicle is involved in an intersection ("T-bone") collision or when the vehicle veers off the road and impacts sideways a utility pole, tree, or other obstacle on the roadside. If the collision is at an intersection, the target vehicle is accelerated from the impact in the direction away from the force created by the bullet vehicle.

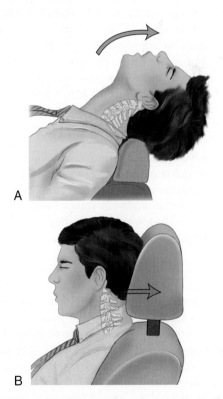

A

B

Figure 5-20 **A.** A rear-impact collision forces the torso forward. If the headrest is improperly positioned, the head is hyperextended over the top of the headrest. **B.** If the headrest is up, the head moves with the torso, and neck injury is prevented.

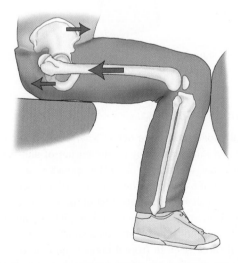

Figure 5-19 The continued forward motion of the pelvis onto the femur can override the femur's head, resulting in a posterior dislocation of the acetabular joint.

Figure 5-21 Headrests

If it can be proved that the victim's headrest was not properly positioned when the neck injury occurred, some courts consider reducing the liability of the party at fault in the crash on the grounds that the victim's negligence contributed to the injuries (contributory negligence). Similar measures have been considered in cases of failure to use occupant restraints. Elderly patients have a high frequency of neck injury, even with proper use of the headrest.[8]

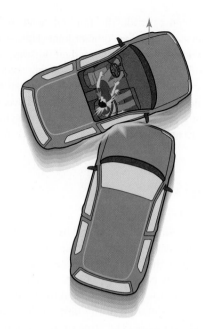

Figure 5-22 Lateral impact of the vehicle pushes the entire vehicle into the unrestrained passenger. A restrained passenger moves laterally with the vehicle.

The side of the vehicle or the door that is struck is thrust against the side of the occupant. The occupants may then be injured as they are accelerated laterally (**Figure 5-22**) or as the passenger compartment is bent inward by the door's projection (**Figure 5-23**). Injury caused by the vehicle's movement is less severe if the occupant is restrained and moves with the initial motion of the vehicle.[9]

Five body regions can sustain injury in a lateral impact:

- *Clavicle.* The clavicle can be compressed and fractured if the force is against the shoulder (**Figure 5-24A**).
- *Chest.* Compression of the thoracic wall inward can result in fractured ribs, pulmonary contusion, or compression injury of the solid organs beneath the rib cage, as well as overpressure injuries (e.g., pneumothorax) (**Figure 5-24B**). Shear injuries of the aorta can result from the lateral acceleration (25% of aortic shear injuries occur in lateral-impact collisions).[10-12]
- *Abdomen and pelvis.* The intrusion compresses and fractures the pelvis and pushes the head of the femur through the acetabulum (**Figure 5-24C**). Occupants on the driver's side are vulnerable to spleen injuries because the spleen is on the left side of the body, whereas those on the passenger side are more likely to receive an injury to the liver.
- *Neck.* The torso can move out from under the head in lateral collisions as well as in rear impacts. The attachment point of the head is posterior and inferior to the center of gravity of the head. Therefore, the motion of the head in relationship to the neck is lateral flexion and rotation. The contralateral side of the spine will be opened (distraction) and the ipsilateral side compressed. This motion can fracture the vertebrae or more likely produce jumped facets and possible dislocation as well as spinal cord injury (**Figure 5-25**).
- *Head.* The head can impact the frame of the door. Near-side impacts produce more injuries than far-side impacts.

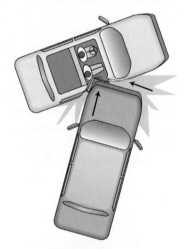

Figure 5-23 Intrusion of the side panels into the passenger compartment provides another source of injury.

Rotational Impact

Rotational-impact collisions occur when one corner of a vehicle strikes an immovable object, the corner of another vehicle, or a vehicle moving slower or in the opposite direction of the first vehicle. Following Newton's first law of motion, this corner of the vehicle will stop while the rest of the vehicle continues its forward motion until all its energy is completely transformed.

Rotational-impact collisions result in injuries that are a combination of those seen in frontal impacts and lateral collisions. The occupant continues to move forward and then is hit by the side of the vehicle (as in a lateral collision) as the vehicle rotates around the point of impact (**Figure 5-26**).

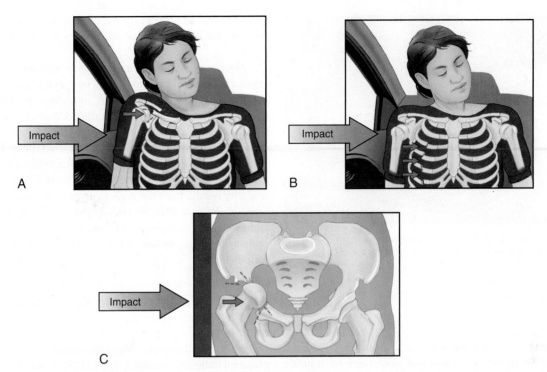

Figure 5-24 A. Compression of the shoulder against the clavicle produces midshaft fractures of this bone. **B.** Compression against the lateral chest and abdominal wall can fracture ribs and injure the underlying spleen, liver, and kidney. **C.** Lateral impact on the femur pushes the head through the acetabulum or fractures the pelvis.

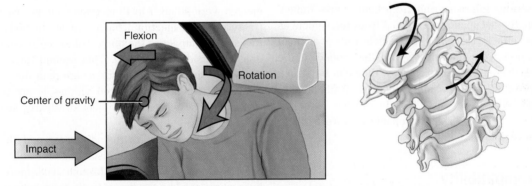

Figure 5-25 The center of gravity of the skull is anterior and superior to its pivot point between the skull and cervical spine. During a lateral impact, when the torso is rapidly accelerated out from under the head, the head turns toward the point of impact, in both lateral and anterior–posterior angles. Such motion separates the vertebral bodies from the side opposite of impact and rotates them apart. Jumped facets, ligament tears, and lateral compression fractures result.

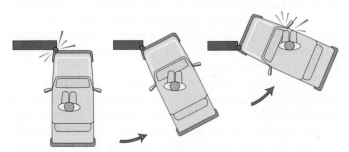

Figure 5-26 The occupant in a rotational-impact crash first moves forward and then laterally as the vehicle pivots around the impact point.

With multiple occupants, the patient closest to the point of impact will likely have the worst injuries as all of the energy of the impact is transferred into his or her body. Additional occupants may benefit from the deformation and rotation of the vehicle, which use up some of the energy before it can be absorbed by their bodies.

Rollover

During a rollover, a vehicle may undergo several impacts at many different angles, as may the unrestrained occupant's body and internal organs (**Figure 5-27**). Injury and damage

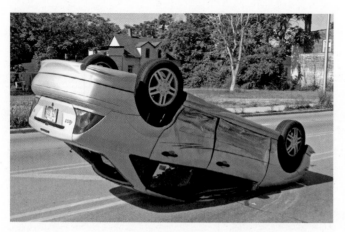

Figure 5-27 During a rollover, the unrestrained occupant can be wholly or partially ejected from the vehicle or can bounce around inside the vehicle. This action produces multiple and somewhat unpredictable injuries that are usually severe.
Source: © Rechitan Sorin/ShutterStock, Inc.

can occur with each of these impacts. In rollover collisions, a restrained occupant often sustains shearing-type injuries because of the significant forces created by a rolling vehicle. The forces are similar to the forces of a spinning carnival ride. Although the occupants are held securely by restraints, the internal organs still move and can tear at the connecting tissue areas. More serious injuries result from being unrestrained. In many cases, the occupants are ejected from the vehicle as it rolls and are either crushed as the vehicle rolls over them or sustain injuries from the impact with the ground. If the occupants are ejected onto the roadway, they can be struck by oncoming traffic. The National Highway Traffic Safety Administration (NHTSA) reports that in crashes involving fatalities in the year 2008, 77% of occupants who were totally ejected from a vehicle were killed.[13]

Vehicle Incompatibility

The types of vehicles involved in the crash play a significant role in the potential for injury and death to the occupants. For example, in a lateral impact between two cars that lack air bags, the occupants of the car struck on its lateral aspect are 5.6 times more likely to die than are the occupants in the vehicle striking that car. This disproportionate risk to the occupants of the struck vehicle can be largely explained by the relative lack of protection on the side of a car. In comparison, a large amount of deformation can occur to the front end of a vehicle before there is intrusion into the passenger compartment. When the vehicle that is struck in a lateral collision (by a car) is a sport utility vehicle (SUV), van, or pickup truck rather than a car, the risk of death to occupants in both vehicles is almost the same. This is because the passenger compartment of SUVs, vans, and

pickup trucks sits higher off the ground than does that of a car, meaning the occupants sustain less of a direct blow in a lateral impact.

More serious injuries and a greatly increased risk of death to vehicle occupants have been documented when a car is struck on its lateral aspect by a van, SUV, or pickup. In a lateral-impact collision between a van and a car, the occupants of the car struck broadside are 13 times more likely to die than are those in the van. If the striking vehicle is a pickup truck or SUV, the occupants of the car struck broadside are 25 to 30 times more likely to die than are those in the pickup truck or SUV. This tremendous disparity results from the higher center of gravity and increased mass of the van, SUV, or pickup truck. Knowledge of vehicle types in which occupants were located in a crash may lead the prehospital care provider to have a higher index of suspicion for serious injury.

Occupant Protective and Restraining Systems
Seat Belts

In the injury patterns described previously, the occupants were assumed to be unrestrained. The NHTSA reported that, in 2011, only 16% of occupants were unrestrained compared with 67% in a 1999 NHTSA report.[14] Ejection from vehicles accounted for approximately 25% of the 44,000 vehicular deaths in 2002. About 77% of passenger vehicle occupants who were totally ejected were killed; 1 in 13 ejection victims sustained a spine fracture.[13] After ejection from a vehicle, the body is subjected to a second impact as the body strikes the ground (or another object) outside the vehicle. This second impact can result in injuries that are even more severe than the initial impact. The risk of death for ejected victims is six times greater than for those who are not ejected. Clearly, seat belts save lives.[1]

The NHTSA reports that 49 states and the District of Columbia have seat belt legislation. The only exception is New Hampshire. From 2004 through 2008, more than 75,000 lives were saved by the use of these restraining devices.[15] The NHTSA estimates that over 255,000 lives have been saved in the United States alone since 1975. Also, the NHTSA reports that over 13,000 lives were saved by seat belts in the United States in 2008 and that if all occupants had worn restraints, the total lives saved would have been more than 17,000. While the Centers for Disease Control and Prevention (CDC) and NHTSA report that in 2011, 86% of motor vehicle occupants were restrained, that still leaves one in seven adults who do not wear seat belts on every trip.[16]

What occurs when the occupants are restrained? If a seat belt is positioned properly, the pressure of the impact is absorbed by the pelvis and the chest, resulting in few, if any, serious injuries (**Figure 5-28**). The proper use of restraints transfers the force of the impact from the occupant's body

forward motion of only the front-seat occupants. The air bags absorb energy slowly by increasing the body's stopping distance. They are extremely effective in the first collision of frontal and near-frontal impacts (the 65–70% of crashes that occur within 30 degrees of the headlights). However, air bags deflate immediately after the impact and, therefore, are not effective in multiple-impact or rear-impact collisions. An air bag deploys and deflates within 0.5 second. As the vehicle veers into the path of an oncoming vehicle or off the road into a tree after the initial impact, no air bag protection is left. Side air bags do add to the protection of occupants.

When air bags deploy, they can produce minor but noticeable injuries that the prehospital care provider needs to manage (**Figure 5-30**). These injuries include abrasions of the arms, chest, and face (**Figure 5-31**); foreign bodies to the face and eyes; and injuries caused by the occupant's eyeglasses (**Figure 5-32**).

Air bags that do not deploy can still be dangerous to both the patient and the prehospital care provider. Air bags can be deactivated by an extrication specialist trained to do so properly

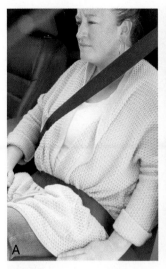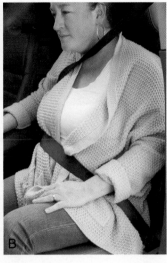

Figure 5-28 **A.** A properly positioned seat belt is located below the anterior-superior iliac spine on each side, above the femur, and is tight enough to remain in this position. The bowl-shaped pelvis protects the soft intra-abdominal organs. **B.** Improperly placed restraints can result in significant injury in the event of a crash.
Source: © Jones & Bartlett Learning. Photographed by Darren Stahlman.

to the restraint belts and restraint system. With restraints, the chance of receiving life-threatening injuries is greatly reduced.[1,15,17]

Seat belts must be worn properly to be effective. An improperly worn belt may not protect against injury in the event of a crash, and it may even cause injury. When lap belts are worn loosely or are strapped above the pelvis, compression injuries of the soft abdominal organs can occur. Injuries of the soft intra-abdominal organs (spleen, liver, and pancreas) result from compression between the seat belt and the posterior abdominal wall (**Figure 5-29**). Increased intra-abdominal pressure can cause diaphragmatic rupture and herniation of abdominal organs. Lap belts should also not be worn alone but in combination with a shoulder restraint. Anterior compression fractures of the lumbar spine can occur as the upper and lower parts of the torso pivot over the lap belt and the restrained twelfth thoracic (T12), first lumbar (L1), and second lumbar (L2) vertebrae. Many vehicle occupants place the diagonal strap under the arm and not over the shoulder, risking serious injury.

With the passage and enforcement of mandatory laws on seat belt use in the United States, the overall severity of injuries has decreased, and the number of fatal crashes has been significantly reduced.

Air Bags

Air bags (in addition to seat belts) provide supplemental protection to the vehicle occupant. Originally, front-seat driver and passenger air bag systems were designed to cushion the

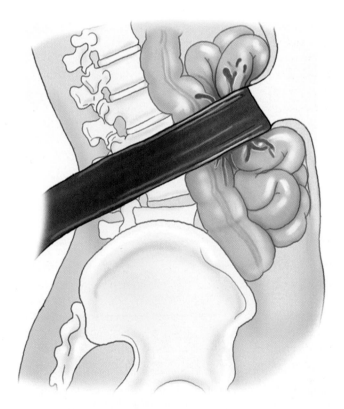

Figure 5-29 A seat belt that is incorrectly positioned above the brim of the pelvis allows the abdominal organs to be trapped between the moving posterior wall and the belt. Injuries to the pancreas and other retroperitoneal organs result, as well as blowout ruptures of the small intestine and colon.

Figure 5-30   Air Bags

Front-seat passenger air bags have been shown to be dangerous to children and small adults, especially when children are placed in incorrect positions in the front seat or in incorrectly installed child seats. Children 12 years of age and younger should always be in the proper restraint device for their size and should be in the back seat. At least one study has demonstrated that almost 99% of the parents checked did not know how to properly install child restraining systems.[3]

Drivers should always be at least 10 inches (25 cm) from the air bag cover, and front-seat passengers should be at least 18 inches (45 cm) away. In most cases, when the proper seating arrangements and distances are used, air bag injuries are limited to simple abrasions.

Air bags are now also available in many vehicles in the sides and tops of the doors.

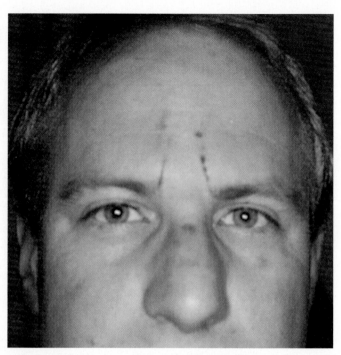

Figure 5-32   Expansion of the air bag into eyeglasses produces abrasions.
Source: Courtesy of Norman E. McSwain, JR, MD, FACS, NREMT-P

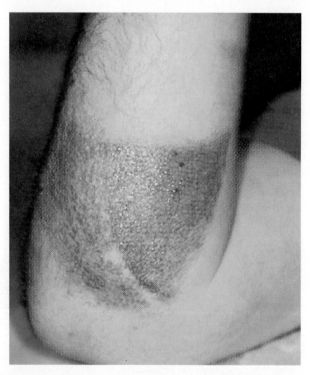

Figure 5-31   Abrasions of the forearm are secondary to rapid expansion of the air bag when the hands are tight against the steering wheel.
Source: Courtesy Norman McSwain, MD, FACS, NREMT-P.

and safely. Such deactivation should not delay patient care or extrication of the critical patient.

Air bags pose a significant hazard to infants and children if the child is either unrestrained or placed in a rear-facing child seat in the front-passenger compartment. Of the over 290 deaths from air-bag deployments, almost 70% were passengers in the front seat, and 90% of those were infants or children.

Motorcycle Crashes

Motorcycle crashes account for a significant number of the motor vehicle deaths each year. While the laws of physics for motorcycle crashes are the same, the mechanism of injury varies from automobile and truck crashes. This variance occurs in each of the following types of impacts: head-on, angular, and ejection. An additional factor that leads to increased death, disability, and injury is the lack of structural framework around the biker that is present in other motor vehicles.

Head-on Impact

A head-on collision into a solid object stops the forward motion of a motorcycle (**Figure 5-33**). Because the motorcycle's center of gravity is above and behind the front axle, which is the pivot point in such a collision, the motorcycle will tip forward, and the rider will crash into the handlebars. The rider may receive injuries to the head, chest, abdomen, or pelvis, depending on which part of the anatomy strikes the handlebars. If the rider's feet remain on the pegs of the motorcycle and the thighs hit the handlebars, the forward motion will be absorbed by the midshaft of the femur, usually resulting in bilateral femoral fractures (**Figure 5-34**). "Open-book" pelvic fractures are a common result of the interaction between the rider's pelvis and the handlebars.

Angular Impact

In an angular-impact collision, the motorcycle hits an object at an angle. The motorcycle will then collapse on the rider or cause the rider to be crushed between the motorcycle and the object that was struck. Injuries to the upper or lower extremities can occur, resulting in fractures and extensive soft-tissue injury (**Figure 5-35**). Injuries can also occur to organs of the abdominal cavity as a result of energy exchange.

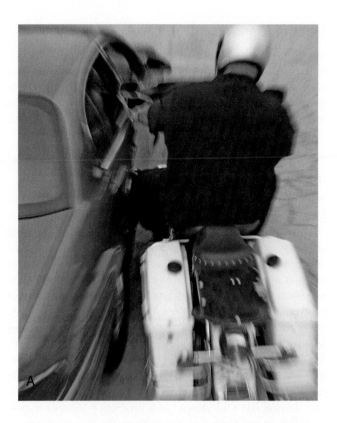

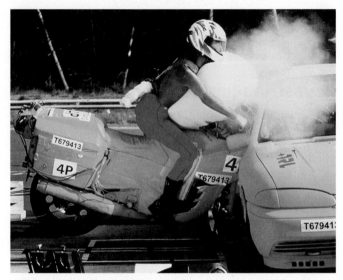

Figure 5-33 The position of a motorcycle rider is above the pivot point of the front wheel as the motorcycle impacts an object head-on.
Source: © TRL Ltd./Science Source.

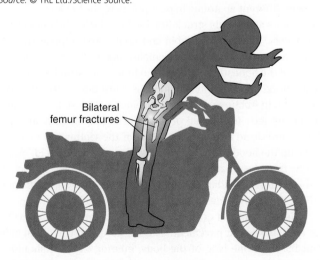

Figure 5-34 The body travels forward and over the motorcycle, and the thighs and femurs impact the handlebars. The rider can also be ejected.

Bilateral femur fractures

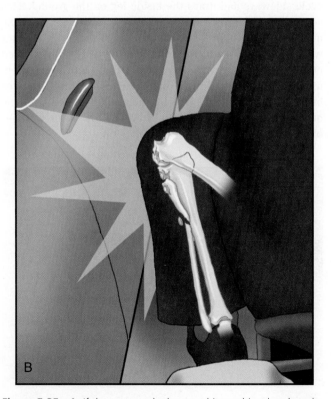

Figure 5-35 **A.** If the motorcycle does not hit an object head-on, it collapses like a pair of scissors. **B.** This collapse traps the rider's lower extremity between the object that was impacted and the motorcycle.

Ejection Impact

Because of the lack of restraint, the rider is susceptible to ejection. The rider will continue in flight until the head, arms, chest, abdomen, or legs strike another object, such as a motor vehicle, a telephone pole, or the road. Injury will occur at the point of impact and will radiate to the rest of the body as the energy is absorbed.[7]

Injury Prevention

Many motorcycle riders do not use proper protection. Protection for motorcyclists includes boots, leather clothing, and helmets. Of the three, the helmet affords the best protection. It is built similarly to the skull: strong and supportive externally and energy-absorbent internally. The helmet's structure absorbs much of the impact, thereby decreasing injury to the face, skull, and brain. Failure to use helmets has been shown to increase head injuries by more than 300%. The helmet provides only minimal protection for the neck but does not cause neck injuries. Mandatory helmet laws work. For example, Louisiana had a 60% reduction in head injuries in the first 6 years after passing a helmet law. Most states that have passed mandatory helmet legislation have found an associated reduction in motorcycle incidents.

"Laying the bike down" is a protective maneuver used by riders to separate themselves from the motorcycle in an impending crash (**Figure 5-36**). The rider turns the motorcycle sideways and drags the inside leg on the ground. This action slows the rider more than the motorcycle so that the motorcycle will move out from under the rider. The rider will then slide along on the pavement but will not be trapped between the motorcycle and any object it hits. These riders usually receive abrasions ("road rash") and minor fractures but generally avoid the severe injuries associated with the other types of impact, unless they directly strike another object (**Figure 5-37**).

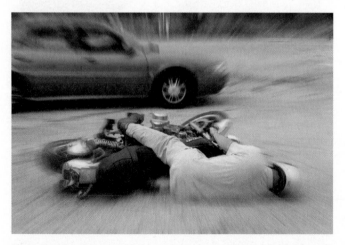

Figure 5-36   To prevent being trapped between two pieces of steel (motorcycle and vehicle), the rider "lays the bike down" to dissipate the injury. This tactic often causes abrasions ("road rash") as the rider's speed is slowed on the asphalt.

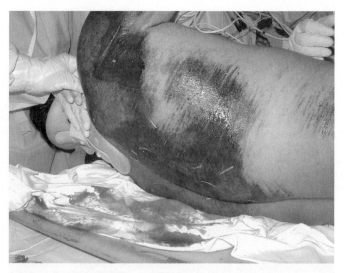

Figure 5-37   Road "burns" (abrasions) after a motorcycle crash without protective clothing.
Source: Courtesy of Dr. Jeffrey Guy.

Pedestrian Injuries

Pedestrian collisions with MVCs have three separate phases, each with its own injury pattern, as follows:

1. The initial impact is to the legs and sometimes the hips (**Figure 5-38A**).
2. The torso rolls onto the hood of the vehicle (and may strike the windshield) (**Figure 5-38B**).
3. The victim then falls off the vehicle and onto the ground, usually headfirst, with possible cervical spine trauma (**Figure 5-38C**).

The injuries produced in pedestrian crashes vary according to the height of the pedestrian and the height of the vehicle (**Figure 5-39**). A child and an adult standing in front of a vehicle present different anatomic impact points to the vehicle.

Adults are usually struck first by the vehicle's bumper in the lower legs, fracturing the tibia and fibula. As the pedestrian is impacted by the front of the vehicle's hood, depending on the height of the hood, the abdomen and thorax are struck by the top of the hood and the windshield. This substantial second strike can result in fractures of the upper femur, pelvis, ribs, and spine, producing intra-abdominal or intrathoracic crush and shear. If the victim's head strikes the hood or if the victim continues to move up the hood so that the head strikes the windshield, injury to the face, head, and cervical and thoracic spine can occur. If the vehicle has a large frontal area (such as with trucks and SUVs), the entire pedestrian is hit simultaneously.

The third impact occurs as the victim is thrown off the vehicle and strikes the pavement. The victim can receive a significant blow on one side of the body, injuring the hip, shoulder, and head. Head injury often occurs when the pedestrian strikes either the vehicle or the pavement. Similarly, because all three impacts produce sudden, violent movement of the torso, neck, and head, an unstable spine fracture may result. After falling, the

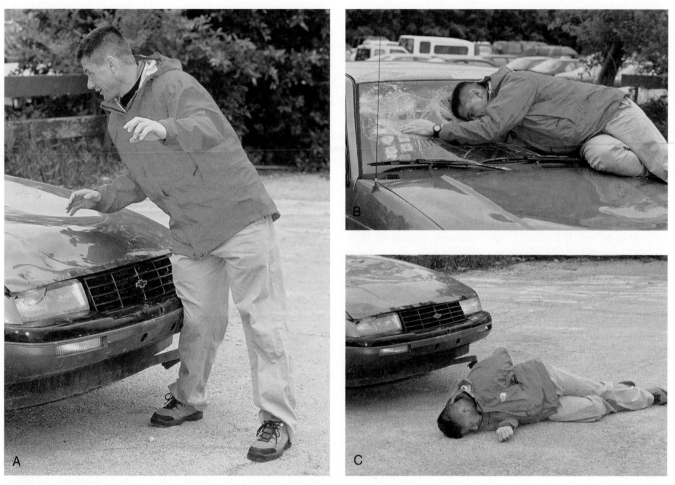

Figure 5-38 **A.** Phase 1: When a pedestrian is struck by a vehicle, the initial impact is to the legs and sometimes to the hips. **B.** Phase 2: The torso of the pedestrian rolls onto the hood of the vehicle. **C.** Phase 3: The pedestrian falls off the vehicle and hits the ground.

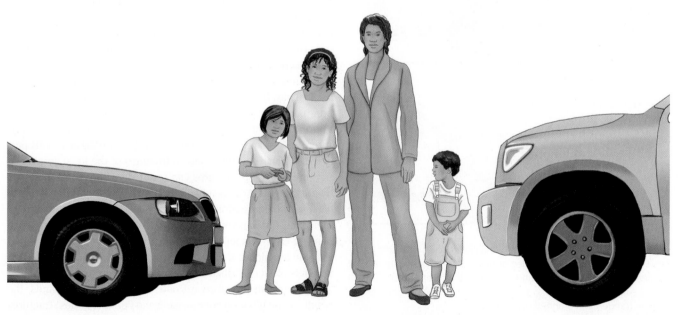

Figure 5-39 The injuries resulting from vehicle–pedestrian crashes vary according to the height of the pedestrian and the height of the vehicle.

victim may be struck by a second vehicle travelling next to or behind the first.

Because they are shorter, children are initially struck higher on the body than adults (**Figure 5-40A**). The first impact generally occurs when the bumper strikes the child's legs (above the knees) or pelvis, damaging the femur or pelvic girdle. The second impact occurs almost instantly afterward as the front of the vehicle's hood continues forward and strikes the child's thorax. Then, the head and face strike the front or top of the vehicle's hood (**Figure 5-40B**). Because of the child's smaller size and weight, the child may not be thrown clear of the vehicle, as usually occurs with an adult. Instead, the child may be dragged by the vehicle while partially under the vehicle's front end (**Figure 5-40C**). If the child falls to the side, the lower limbs may also be run over by a front wheel. If the child falls backward, ending up completely under the vehicle, almost any injury can occur (e.g., being dragged, struck by projections, or run over by a wheel).

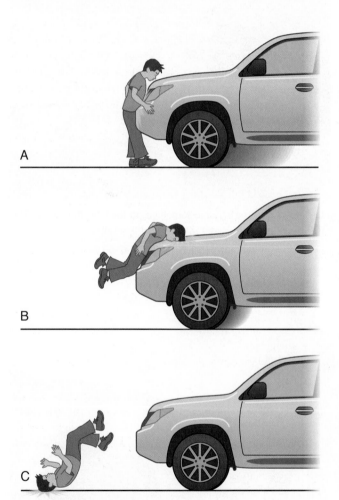

Figure 5-40 **A.** The initial impact with a child occurs when the vehicle strikes the child's upper leg or pelvis. **B.** The second impact occurs when the child's head and face strike the front or top of the vehicle's hood. **C.** A child may not be thrown clear of a vehicle but may be trapped and dragged by the vehicle.

If the foot is planted on the ground at the time of impact, the child will receive energy exchange at the upper leg, hip, and abdomen. This will force the hips and abdomen away from the impact. The upper part of the torso will come along later, as will the planted foot. The energy exchange moving the torso but not the feet will fracture the pelvis and shear the femur, producing severe angulation at the point of impact and possible spine injury as well.

To complicate these injuries further, a child will likely turn toward the car out of curiosity, exposing the anterior body and face to injuries, whereas an adult will attempt to escape and will be hit in the back or the side.

As with an adult, any child struck by a vehicle can receive some type of head injury. Because of the sudden, violent forces acting on the head, neck, and torso, cervical spine injuries are high on the suspicion list.

Knowing the specific sequence of multiple impacts in vehicle–pedestrian collision and understanding the multiple underlying injuries that they can produce are keys to making an initial assessment and determining the appropriate management of a patient.

Falls

Victims of falls can also sustain injury from multiple impacts. The estimated height from which the victim fell, the surface on which the victim landed, and the part of the body struck first are important factors to determine since they indicate the energy involved and, thus, the energy exchange that occurred. Victims who fall from greater heights have a higher incidence of injury because their velocity increases as they fall. Falls from greater than 20 feet (6.1 m) in adults and 10 feet (3.0 m) in children (two to three times the height of the child) are frequently severe.[18] The type of surface on which the victim lands and its degree of **compressibility** (ability to be deformed by the transfer of energy) also have an effect on stopping distance.

The pattern of injury in falls occurring feet first is called the **Don Juan syndrome**. Only in the movies can the character Don Juan jump from a high balcony, land on his feet, and walk painlessly away. In real life, bilateral fractures of the calcaneus (heel bone), compression or shear fractures of the ankles, and distal tibial or fibular fractures are often associated with this syndrome. After the feet land and stop moving, the legs are the next body part to absorb energy. Tibial plateau fractures of the knee, long-bone fractures, and hip fractures can result. The body is compressed by the weight of the head and torso, which are still moving, and can cause compression fractures of the spinal column in the thoracic and lumbar areas. Hyperflexion occurs at each concave bend of the S-shaped spine, producing compression injuries on the concave side and distraction injuries on the convex side. This victim is often described as breaking his or her "S."

If a victim falls forward onto the outstretched hands, the result can be bilateral compression and flexion (Colles) fractures of the wrists. If the victim did not land on the feet, the prehospital care provider will assess the part of the body that struck first, evaluate the pathway of energy displacement, and determine the injury pattern.

If the falling victim lands on the head with the body almost inline, as often occurs in shallow-water diving injuries, the entire weight and force of the moving torso, pelvis, and legs compress the head and cervical spine. A fracture of the cervical spine is a frequent result, as with the up-and-over pathway of the frontal-impact vehicle collision.

Sports Injuries

Severe injury can occur during many sports or recreational activities, such as skiing, diving, baseball, and football. These injuries can be caused by sudden deceleration forces or by excessive compression, twisting, hyperextension, or hyperflexion. In recent years, various sports activities have become available to a wide spectrum of occasional, recreational participants who often lack the necessary training and conditioning or the proper protective equipment. Recreational sports and activities include participants of all ages. Sports such as downhill skiing, waterskiing, bicycling, and skateboarding are all potentially high-velocity activities. Other sports, such as trail biking, all-terrain vehicle riding, and snowmobiling, can produce velocity deceleration, collisions, and impacts similar to motorcycle crashes or MVCs. Protective equipment worn in sports can provide some protection but must also be considered for the potential to create injury, such as when a helmeted football player drives his head into another player.

The potential injuries of a victim who is in a high-speed collision and then ejected from a skateboard, snowmobile, or bicycle are similar to those sustained when an occupant is ejected from an automobile at the same speed because the amount of energy is the same. (See the specific mechanisms of MVCs and motorcycle crashes described earlier.)

The potential mechanisms associated with each sport are too numerous to list in detail. However, the general principles are the same as for MVCs. While assessing the mechanism of injury, the prehospital care provider considers the following questions to assist in the identification of injuries:

- What forces acted on the victim, and how?
- What are the apparent injuries?
- To what object or part of the body was the energy transmitted?
- What other injuries are likely to have been produced by this energy transfer?
- Was protective gear being worn?
- Was there sudden compression, deceleration, or acceleration?
- What injury-producing movements occurred (e.g., hyperflexion, hyperextension, compression, excessive lateral bending)?

When the mechanism of injury involves a high-speed collision between two participants, as in a crash between two skiers, reconstruction of the exact sequence of events from eyewitness accounts is often difficult. In such crashes, the injuries sustained by one skier are often guidelines for examination of the other. In general, knowing which part of one victim struck which part of the other victim, and what injury resulted from the energy transfer, is important. For example, if one victim sustains an impact fracture of the hip, a part of the other skier's body must have been struck with substantial force and, therefore, must have sustained a similar high-impact injury. If the second skier's head struck the first skier's hip, the prehospital care provider will suspect potentially serious head injury and an unstable spine for the second skier.

Broken or damaged equipment is also an important indicator of injury and must be included in the evaluation of the mechanism of injury. A broken sports helmet is evidence of the magnitude of the force with which it struck. Because skis are made of highly durable material, a broken ski indicates that extreme localized force came to bear, even when the mechanism of injury may appear unimpressive. A snowmobile with a severely dented front end indicates the force with which it struck a tree. The presence of a broken stick after an ice hockey skirmish raises the questions of whose body broke it, how, and, specifically, what part of the victim's body was struck by the stick or fell on it.

Victims of significant crashes who do not complain of injury must be assessed as if severe injuries exist. The steps are as follows:

1. Evaluate the patient for life-threatening injury.
2. Evaluate the patient for mechanism of injury. (What happened and exactly how did it happen?)
3. Determine how the forces that produced injury in one victim may have affected any other person.
4. Determine whether any protective gear was worn. (It may have already been removed.)
5. Assess damage to the protective equipment. (What are the implications of this damage relative to the patient's body?)
6. Assess the patient for possible associated injuries.

High-speed falls, collisions, and falls from heights without serious injury are common in many contact sports. The ability of athletes to experience incredible collisions and falls and sustain only minor injury—largely as a result of impact-absorbing equipment—may be confusing. The potential for injury in sports participants may be overlooked. The principles of kinematics and careful consideration of the exact sequence and mechanism of injury will provide insight into sports collisions in which greater forces than usual came to bear. Kinematics is an essential tool in identifying possible underlying injuries and determining which patients require further evaluation and treatment at a medical facility.

Regional Effects of Blunt Trauma

The body can be divided into several regions: head, neck, thorax, abdomen, pelvis, and extremities. Each body region is subdivided into (1) the external part of the body, usually composed of skin, bone, soft tissue, vessels, and nerves, and (2) the internal part of the body, usually vital internal organs. The injuries produced as a result of shear, cavitation, and compression forces are used to provide an overview in each component and region for potential injuries.

Head

The only external indication that compression and shear injuries have occurred to the patient's head may be a soft-tissue injury to the scalp, a contusion of the scalp, or a bull's-eye fracture of the windshield (**Figure 5-41**).

Compression

When the body is travelling forward with the head leading the way, as in a frontal vehicular crash or a headfirst fall, the head is the first structure to receive the impact and the energy exchange. The continued momentum of the torso then compresses the head. The initial energy exchange occurs on the scalp and the skull. The skull can be compressed and fractured, pushing the broken, bony segments of the skull into the brain (**Figure 5-42**).

Shear

After the skull stops its forward motion, the brain continues to move forward, compressing against the intact or fractured skull with resultant concussion, contusions, or lacerations. The brain is soft and compressible; therefore, its length is shortened. The posterior part of the brain can continue forward, pulling away from the skull, which has already stopped moving. As the brain separates from the skull, stretching or breaking (shearing) of brain tissue itself or any blood vessels in the area occurs (**Figure 5-43**). Hemorrhage into the epidural, subdural, or subarachnoid space can then result, as well as diffuse axonal injury of the brain. If the brain separates from the spinal cord, it will most likely occur at the brain stem.

Neck

Compression

The dome of the skull is fairly strong and can absorb the impact of a collision; however, the cervical spine is much more flexible.

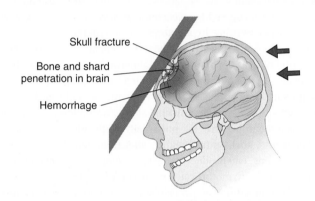

Figure 5-42 As the skull impacts an object, pieces of bone may be fractured and pushed into the brain substance.

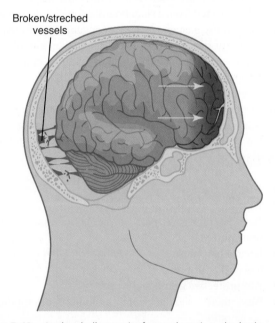

Figure 5-43 As the skull stops its forward motion, the brain continues to move forward. The part of the brain nearest the impact is compressed, bruised, and perhaps even lacerated. The portion farthest from the impact is separated from the skull, with tearing and lacerations of the vessels involved.

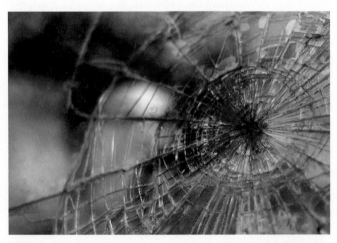

Figure 5-41 A bull's-eye fracture of the windshield is a major indication of skull impact and energy exchange to both the skull and the cervical spine.

Source: © Kristin Smith/ShutterStock, Inc.

The continued pressure from the momentum of the torso toward the stationary skull produces angulation or compression (**Figure 5-44**). Hyperextension or hyperflexion of the neck often results in fracture or dislocation of one or more vertebrae and injury to the spinal cord. The result can be jumped (dislocated) facets, potential fractures, spinal cord compression, or unstable neck fractures (**Figure 5-45**). Direct inline compression crushes the bony vertebral bodies. Both angulation and inline compression can result in an unstable spine.

Shear

The skull's center of gravity is anterior and cephalad to the point at which the skull attaches to the bony spine. Therefore, a lateral impact on the torso when the neck is unrestrained will produce lateral flexion and rotation of the neck (see Figure 5-25). Extreme flexion or hyperextension may also cause stretching injuries to the soft tissues of the neck.

Thorax

Compression

If the impact of a collision is centered on the anterior part of the chest, the sternum will receive the initial energy exchange. When the sternum stops moving, the posterior thoracic wall (muscles and thoracic spine) and the organs in the thoracic cavity continue to move forward until the organs strike and are compressed against the sternum.

The continued forward motion of the posterior thorax bends the ribs. If the tensile strength of the ribs is exceeded, fractured ribs and a flail chest can develop (**Figure 5-46**). This

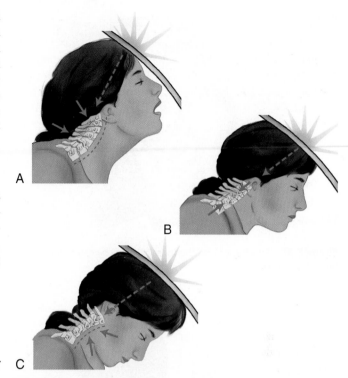

Figure 5-45 The spine can be compressed directly along its own axis or angled in hyperextension or hyperflexion.

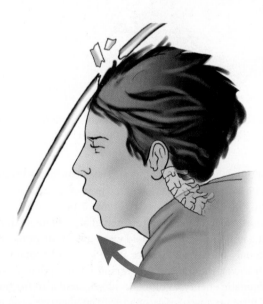

Figure 5-44 The skull frequently stops its forward motion, but the torso does not. The torso continues its forward motion until its energy is absorbed. The weakest point of this forward motion is the cervical spine.

injury is similar to what happens when a vehicle stops suddenly against a dirt embankment (see Figure 5-3). The frame of the vehicle bends, which absorbs some of the energy. The rear of the vehicle continues to move forward until the bending of the frame absorbs all the energy. In the same way, the posterior thoracic wall continues to move until the ribs absorb all the energy.

Compression of the chest wall is common with frontal and lateral impacts and produces an interesting phenomenon called the paper bag effect, which may result in a pneumothorax. A victim instinctively takes a deep breath and holds it just before impact. This closes the glottis, effectively sealing off the lungs. With a significant energy exchange on impact and compression of the chest wall, the lungs may then burst, like a paper bag full of air that is popped (**Figure 5-47**). The lungs can also become compressed and contused, compromising ventilation.

Compression injuries of the internal structures of the thorax may also include cardiac contusion, which occurs as the heart is compressed between the sternum and the spine and can result in significant dysrhythmias. Perhaps a more frequent injury is compression of the lungs leading to pulmonary contusion. Although the clinical consequences may develop over time, immediate loss of the patient's ability to properly ventilate may occur. Pulmonary contusion can have consequences in the field for the prehospital care provider and for the physicians during

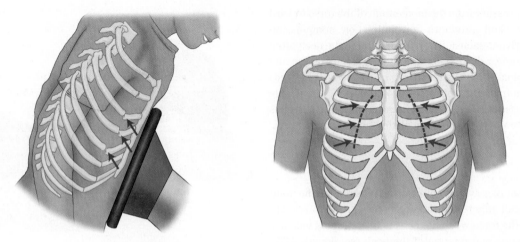

Figure 5-46   Ribs forced into the thoracic cavity by external compression usually fracture in multiple places, producing the clinical condition known as flail chest.

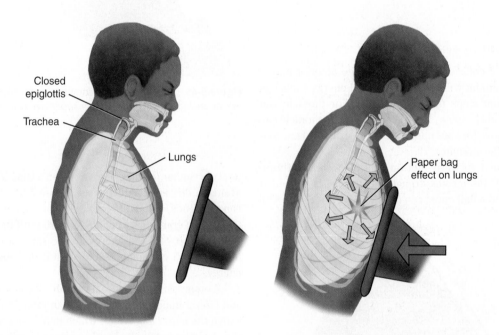

Figure 5-47   Compression of the lung against a closed glottis, by impact on either the anterior or the lateral chest wall, produces an effect similar to compressing a paper bag when the opening is closed tightly by the hands. The paper bag ruptures, as does the lung.

resuscitation after arrival in the hospital. In situations in which long transportation times are required, this condition can play a role en route.

Shear

The heart, ascending aorta, and aortic arch are relatively unrestrained within the thorax. The descending aorta, however, is tightly adhered to the posterior thoracic wall and the vertebral column. The resultant motion of the aorta is similar to holding the flexible tubes of a stethoscope just below where the rigid tubes from the earpiece end and swinging the acoustic head of the stethoscope from side to side. As the skeletal frame stops abruptly in a collision, the heart and the initial segment of the aorta continue their forward motion. The shear forces produced can tear the aorta at the junction of the portion that moves freely with the tightly bound portion (see Figure 5-14).

An aortic tear may result in an immediate, complete transection of the aorta followed by rapid exsanguination. Some aortic tears are only partial, and one or more layers of tissue remain intact. However, the remaining layers are under great pressure, and a traumatic aneurysm often develops, similar to the bubble that can form on a weak part of a tire. The aneurysm can eventually rupture within minutes, hours, or days after the original injury. Approximately 80% of these patients die on the scene at the time of the initial impact. Of the remaining 20%, one-third will die within 6 hours, one-third will die within 24 hours, and one-third will live 3 days or longer. It is important that the prehospital care provider recognize the potential for such injuries and relay this information to the hospital personnel.

Abdomen
Compression

Internal organs compressed by the vertebral column into the steering wheel or dashboard during a frontal collision may rupture. The effect of this sudden increase in pressure is similar to the effect of placing the internal organ on an anvil and striking it with a hammer. Solid organs frequently injured in this manner include the pancreas, spleen, liver, and kidneys.

Injury may also result from overpressure within the abdomen. The diaphragm is a ¼-inch (5-mm) thick muscle located across the top of the abdomen that separates the abdominal cavity from the thoracic cavity. Its contraction causes the pleural cavity to expand for ventilation. The anterior abdominal wall comprises two layers of fascia and one very strong muscle. Laterally, there are three muscle layers with associated fascia, and the lumbar spine and its associated muscles provide strength to the posterior abdominal wall. The diaphragm is the weakest of all the walls and structures surrounding the abdominal cavity. It may be torn or ruptured as the intra-abdominal pressure increases (**Figure 5-48**). This injury has four common consequences, as follows:

- The "bellows" effect that is usually created by the diaphragm is lost and ventilation is affected.
- The abdominal organs can enter the thoracic cavity and reduce the space available for lung expansion.

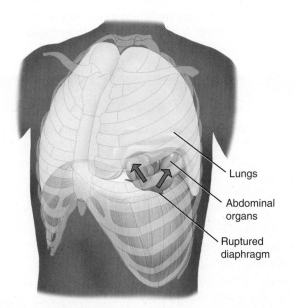

Figure 5-48 With increased pressure inside the abdomen, the diaphragm can rupture.

- The displaced organs can become ischemic from compression of their blood supply.
- If intra-abdominal hemorrhage is present, the blood can also cause a hemothorax.

Another injury caused by increased abdominal pressure is from sudden retrograde blood flow up the aorta and against the aortic valve. This force against the valve can rupture it. This injury is rare but does exist. It occurs when a collision with the steering wheel or involvement in another type of incident (e.g., ditch or tunnel cave-in) has produced a rapid increase in intra-abdominal pressure. This rapid pressure increase results in a sudden increase of aortic blood pressure. Blood is pushed back (retrograde) against the aortic valve with enough pressure to cause rupture of the valve cusps.

Shear

Injury to the abdominal organs occurs at their points of attachment to the mesentery. During a collision, the forward motion of the body stops, but the organs continue to move forward, causing tears at the points of attachment of organs to the abdominal wall. If the organ is attached by a pedicle (a stalk of tissue), the tear can occur where the pedicle attaches to the organ, where it attaches to the abdominal wall, or anywhere along the length of the pedicle (see Figure 5-13). Organs that can shear this way are the kidneys, small intestine, large intestine, and spleen.

Another type of injury that often occurs during deceleration is laceration of the liver caused by its impact with the *ligamentum teres*. The liver is suspended from the diaphragm but is only minimally attached to the posterior abdomen near the lumbar vertebrae. The ligamentum teres attaches to the anterior abdominal wall at the umbilicus and to the left lobe of the liver in the midline of the body. (The liver is not a midline structure; it lies more on the right than on the left.) A down-and-under pathway in a frontal impact or a feet first fall causes the liver to bring the diaphragm with it as it descends into the ligamentum teres (**Figure 5-49**). The ligamentum teres will fracture or transect the liver, analogous to pushing a cheese-cutting wire into a block of cheese.

Pelvic fractures are the result of damage to the external abdomen and may cause injury to the bladder or lacerations of the blood vessels in the pelvic cavity. Approximately 10% of patients with pelvic fractures also have a genitourinary injury.

Pelvic fractures resulting from compression from the side, usually due to a lateral-impact collision, have two components. One is the compression of the proximal femur into the pelvis, which pushes the head of the femur through the acetabulum itself. This frequently produces radiating fractures that involve the entire joint. Further compression of the femur and/or of the lateral walls of the pelvis produce compression fractures of the pelvic bones or the ring of the pelvis. Since a ring generally cannot be fractured in only one place, usually two fractures to the ring occur, although some of the fractures may involve the acetabulum.

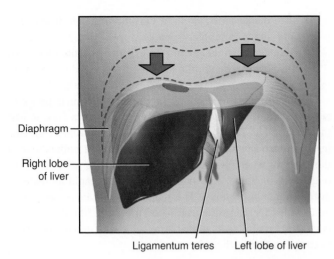

Diaphragm

Right lobe of liver

Ligamentum teres   Left lobe of liver

Figure 5-49 The liver is not supported by any fixed structure. Its major support is from the diaphragm, which moves freely. As the body travels in the down-and-under pathway, so does the liver. When the torso stops but the liver does not, the liver continues downward onto the ligamentum teres, tearing the liver. This is much like pushing a cheese-cutting wire into a block of cheese.

The other type of compression fracture occurs anteriorly when the compression force is directly over the symphysis pubis. This force will either break the symphysis by pushing in on both sides or break one side and push it back toward the sacroiliac joint. This latter mechanism opens the joint producing the so-called "open-book."

Shear fractures usually involve the ilium and the sacral area. This shearing force tears the joint open. Since the joints in a ring, such as the pelvis, generally must be fractured in two places, frequently there will be a fracture somewhere else along the pelvic ring.

For more detailed information about pelvic fractures, Andrew Burgess and his co-authors have discussed these mechanisms of injury.[19]

Penetrating Trauma
Physics of Penetrating Trauma

The principles of physics discussed earlier are equally important when dealing with penetrating injuries. Again, the kinetic energy that a striking object transfers to body tissue is represented by the following formula:

$$KE = 1/2mv^2$$

Energy can neither be created nor destroyed, but it can be changed in form. This principle is important in understanding penetrating trauma. For example, although a lead bullet is in the brass cartridge casing that is filled with explosive powder, the bullet has no force. However, when the primer explodes, the powder burns, producing rapidly expanding gases that are

transformed into force. The bullet then moves out of the gun and toward its target.

According to Newton's first law of motion, after this force has acted on the missile, the bullet will remain at that speed and force until it is acted on by an outside force. When the bullet hits something, such as a human body, it strikes the individual tissue cells. The energy (speed and mass) of the bullet's motion is exchanged for the energy that crushes these cells and moves them away (cavitation) from the path of the bullet:

Mass × Acceleration = Force = Mass × Deceleration

Factors That Affect the Size of the Frontal Area

The larger the frontal area of the moving missile, the greater the number of particles that will be hit—therefore, the greater the energy exchange that occurs and the larger the cavity that is created. The size of the frontal surface area of a projectile is influenced by three factors: profile, tumble, and fragmentation. Energy exchange or potential energy exchange can be analyzed based on these factors.

Profile

Profile describes an object's initial size and whether that size changes at the time of impact. The profile, or frontal area, of an ice pick is much smaller than that of a baseball bat, which in turn is much smaller than that of a truck. A hollow-point bullet flattens and spreads on impact (**Figure 5-50**). This change enlarges the frontal area so that it hits more tissue particles and produces greater energy exchange. As a result, a larger cavity forms and more injury occurs.

In general, a bullet should remain very aerodynamic as it travels through the air en route to the target. Low resistance while passing through the air (hitting as few air particles as possible) is a good thing. It allows the bullet to maintain most of

---

Figure 5-50   Expanding Bullets

A munitions factory in Dum Dum, India, manufactured a bullet that expanded when it hit the skin. Ballistic experts recognized this design as one that would cause more damage than is necessary in war; therefore, these bullets were prohibited in military conflicts. The Petersburg Declaration of 1868 and the Hague Convention of 1899 affirmed this principle, denouncing these "dum-dum" projectiles and other expanding missiles, such as silver tips, hollow-points, scored-lead cartridges or jackets, and partially jacketed bullets, and outlawing their use in war.

its speed. To avoid resistance, the frontal area is kept small in a conical shape. A lot of drag (resistance to travel) is a bad thing. A good bullet design would have very little drag while passing through the air but much more drag when passing through the body's tissues. If that missile strikes the skin and becomes deformed, covering a larger area and creating much more drag, then a much greater energy exchange will occur. Therefore, the ideal bullet is designed to keep its shape while in the air and only deform on impact.

Tumble

Tumble describes whether the object turns over and over and assumes a different angle inside the body than the angle it assumed as it entered the body, thus creating more drag inside the body than in the air. A wedge-shaped bullet's center of gravity is located nearer to the base than to the nose of the bullet. When the nose of the bullet strikes something, it slows rapidly. Momentum continues to carry the base of the bullet forward, with the center of gravity seeking to become the leading point of the bullet. A slightly asymmetrical shape causes an end-over-end motion, or tumble. As the bullet tumbles, the normally horizontal sides of the bullet become its leading edges, thus striking far more particles than when the bullet was in the air (**Figure 5-51**). More energy exchange is produced, and therefore, greater tissue damage occurs.

Fragmentation

Fragmentation describes whether the object breaks up to produce multiple parts or rubble and, therefore, more drag and more energy exchange. There are two types of fragmentation rounds: (1) fragmentation on leaving the weapon (e.g., shotgun pellets) (**Figure 5-52**) and (2) fragmentation after entering the body. Fragmentation inside the body can be active or passive. Active fragmentation involves a bullet that has an explosive inside it that detonates inside the body. In contrast, bullets with soft noses or vertical cuts in the nose and safety slugs that contain many small fragments to increase body damage by breaking

apart on impact are examples of passive fragmentation. The resulting mass of fragments creates a larger frontal area than a single solid bullet, and energy is dispersed rapidly into the tissue. If the missile shatters, it will spread out over a wider area, with two results: (1) More tissue particles will be struck by the larger frontal projection, and (2) the injuries will be distributed over a larger portion of the body because more organs will be struck (**Figure 5-53**). The multiple pieces of shot from a shotgun blast produce similar results. Shotgun wounds are an excellent example of the fragmentation injury pattern.

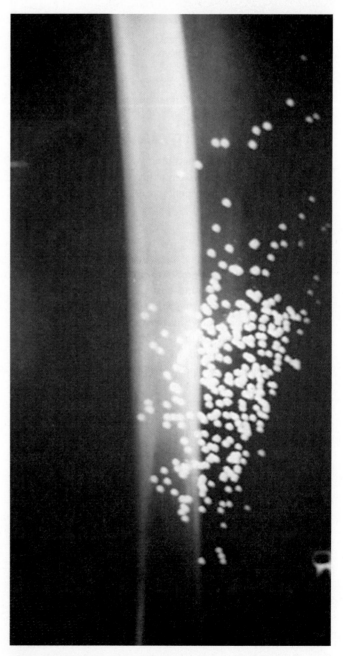

Figure 5-52 Maximum fragmentation damage is caused by a shotgun.

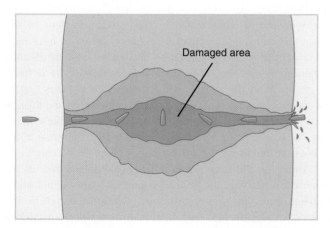

Figure 5-51 Tumble motion of a missile maximizes its damage at 90 degrees.

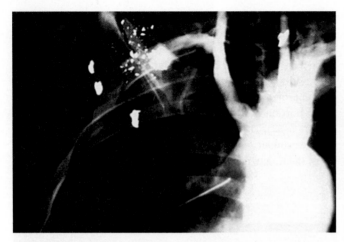

Figure 5-53 When the missile breaks up into smaller particles, this fragmentation increases its frontal area and increases the energy distribution.

Source: Courtesy Norman McSwain, MD, FACS, NREMT-P.

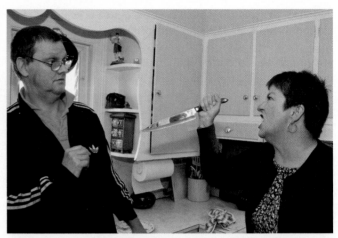

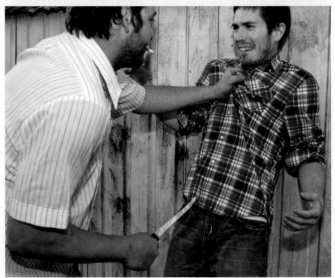

Damage and Energy Levels

The damage caused in a penetrating injury can be estimated by classifying penetrating objects into three categories according to their energy capacity: low-, medium-, and high-energy weapons.

Low-Energy Weapons

Low-energy weapons include hand-driven weapons such as a knife or an ice pick. These missiles produce damage only with their sharp points or cutting edges. Because these are low-velocity injuries, they are usually associated with less secondary trauma (i.e., less cavitation will occur). Injury in these victims can be predicted by tracing the path of the weapon into the body. If the weapon has been removed, the prehospital care provider should try to identify the type of weapon used, if time permits.

The gender of the attacker is an important factor in determining the trajectory of a knife. Men tend to thrust with the blade on the thumb side of the hand and with an upward or inward motion, whereas women tend to hold the blade on the little finger side and stab downward (**Figure 5-54**).

An attacker may stab a victim and then move the knife around inside the body. A simple-appearing entrance wound may produce a false sense of security. The entrance wound may be small, but the damage inside may be extensive. The potential scope of the movement of the inserted blade is an area of possible damage (**Figure 5-55**).

Evaluation of the patient for associated injury is important. For example, the diaphragm can reach as high as the nipple line on deep expiration. A stab wound to the lower chest can injure intra-abdominal as well as intrathoracic structures, and a wound of the upper abdomen may also involve the lower chest.

Penetrating trauma can result from impaled objects such as fence posts and street signs in vehicle crashes and falls, ski poles in snow sports, and handlebar injuries in bicycling.

Figure 5-54 The gender of an attacker often determines the trajectory of the wound in stabbing incidents. Male attackers tend to stab upwards, whereas female attackers tend to stab downwards.

Medium-Energy and High-Energy Weapons

Firearms fall into two groups: medium energy and high energy. Medium-energy weapons include handguns and some rifles whose muzzle velocity is 1,000 feet per second (ft/sec) (305 m/sec). The temporary cavity created by this weapon is three to five times the caliber of the bullet. High-energy weapons have muzzle velocity in excess of 2,000 ft/sec (610 m/sec) and significantly greater muzzle energy. They create a temporary cavity 25 times or greater than the caliber of the bullet. It is obvious that as the amount of gunpowder in the cartridge increases and the size of the bullet increases, the speed and mass of the bullet and, therefore, its kinetic energy increase (**Figure 5-56**). The mass of the bullet is an important, but smaller, component ($KE = \frac{1}{2} mv^2$).

However, the bullet mass is not to be discounted. In the American Civil War, the Kentucky long rifle 0.55-caliber Minie Ball had almost the same muzzle energy as the modern M16. The mass of the missile becomes more important when considering the damage produced by a 12-gauge shotgun at close range or an improvised explosive device (IED).

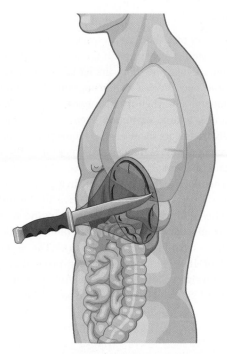

Figure 5-55 Damage produced by a knife depends on the movement of the blade inside the victim.

In general, medium-energy and high-energy weapons damage not only the tissue directly in the path of the missile, but also the tissue involved in the temporary cavity on each side of the missile's path. The variables of missile profile, tumble, and fragmentation influence the rapidity of the energy exchange and, therefore, the extent and direction of the injury. The force of the tissue particles moved out of the direct path of the missile compresses and stretches the surrounding tissue (**Figure 5-57**).

High-energy weapons discharge high-energy missiles (**Figure 5-58**). Tissue damage is much more extensive with a high-energy penetrating object than with one of medium energy. The vacuum created in the cavity created by this high-speed missile can pull clothing, bacteria, and other debris from the surface into the wound.

A consideration in predicting the damage from a gunshot wound is the range or distance from which the gun (either medium- or high-energy) is fired. Air resistance slows the bullet; therefore, increasing the distance will decrease the energy at the time of impact and will result in less injury. Most shootings are done at close range with handguns, so the probability of serious injury is related to both the anatomy involved and the energy of the weapon rather than loss of kinetic energy.

High-Energy Weapons

Cavitation

Fackler and Malinowski described the unusual injury pattern of an AK-47. Because of its eccentricity, the bullet tumbles and travels almost at a right angle to the area of entrance. During

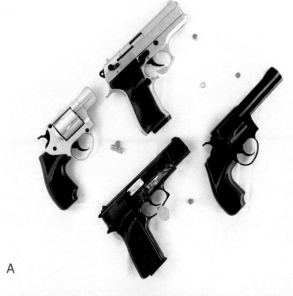

A

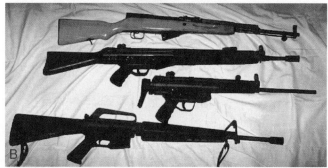

B

Figure 5-56 **A.** Medium-energy weapons are usually guns that have short barrels and contain cartridges with less power. **B.** High-energy weapons.

Source: A. © RaidenV/ShutterStock, Inc. B. Courtesy of Norman Mc Swain, MD, FACS, NREMT-P

this tumble action, the rotation carries it over and over so that there are two or sometimes even three (depending on how long the bullet stays in the body) cavitations.[20] The very high energy

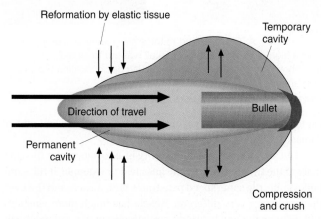

Figure 5-57 A bullet crushes tissues directly in its path. A cavity is created in the wake of the bullet. The crushed part is permanent. The temporary expansion can also produce injury.

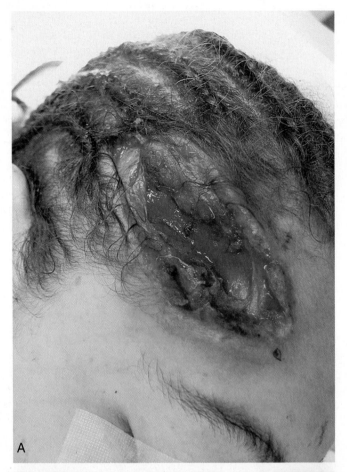

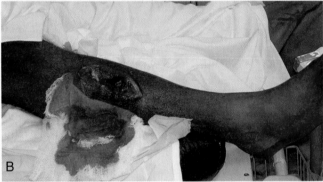

Figure 5-58 **A.** Graze wound to the scalp created by a projectile from a high-velocity weapon. The skull was not fractured.
B. High-velocity gunshot wound to the leg demonstrating the large, permanent cavity.

Source: Courtesy Norman McSwain, MD, FACS, NREMT-P.

exchange produces the cavitation and a significant amount of damage.

The size of the permanent cavity is associated with the elasticity in the tissue struck by the missile. For example, if the same bullet going the same speed penetrates both muscle and the liver, the results are very different. Muscle has much more elasticity and will expand and return to a relatively small permanent cavity. The liver, however, has very little elasticity; it develops fracture lines and a much larger permanent cavity than is produced by the same energy exchange in muscle.[21,22]

Fragmentation

The combination of a high-energy weapon with fragmentation can produce significant damage. If the high-energy missile fragments on impact (many do not), the initial entrance site may be very large and may involve significant soft-tissue injury. If the bullet fragments only when it hits a hard structure in the body (such as bone), a large cavitation occurs at this impact point and the bony fragments themselves become part of the damage-producing component. Significant destruction to the bone and nearby organs and vessels may result.[20]

Emil Theodor Kocher, a surgeon living at the latter part of the 19th century, was extremely active in the understanding of ballistics and the damage produced by the weapons. He was a strong advocate of not using the "dum-dum" bullet (produced by the arsenal in Dum Dum, India).[23] The St. Petersburg Declaration of 1868 outlawed explosive projectiles less than 400 grams in weight. This measure was followed by the Hague Convention of 1899, which outlawed the use of dum-dum bullets in war.

Anatomy

Entrance and Exit Wounds

Tissue damage will occur at the site of missile entry into the body, along the path of the penetrating object, and on exit from the body. Knowledge of the victim's position, the attacker's position, and the weapon used is helpful in determining the path of injury. If the entrance wound and the exit wound can be related, the anatomic structures that would likely be in this pathway can be approximated.

Evaluating wound sites provides valuable information to direct the management of the patient and to relay to the receiving facility. Do two holes in the victim's abdomen indicate that a single missile entered and exited or that two missiles entered and are both still inside the patient? Did the missile cross the midline (usually causing more severe injury) or remain on the same side? In what direction did the missile travel? What internal organs are likely to have been in its path?

Entrance and exit wounds usually, but not always, produce identifiable injury patterns to soft tissue. Evaluation of the apparent trajectory of a penetrating object is very helpful to the clinician. This information should be given to the physicians in the hospital. That said, prehospital care providers (and most physicians) do not have the experience or the expertise of a forensic pathologist; therefore, the assessment of which wound is an entrance and which is an exit is fraught with uncertainty. Such information is solely for patient care to try to gauge the trajectory of the missile and not for legal purposes to determine specifics about the incident. These two issues should not be confused. The prehospital care provider must have as much information as possible to determine the potential injuries sustained by the patient and to best decide how the patient is to be managed. The legal issues related to the specifics of entrance and exit wounds are best left to others.

An entrance wound from a gunshot lies against the underlying tissue, but an exit wound has no support. The former is typically a round or oval wound, depending on the entry path, and the latter is usually a **stellate (starburst) wound** (**Figure 5-59**). Because the missile is spinning as it enters the skin, it leaves a small area of abrasion (1 to 2 mm in size) that is pink (**Figure 5-60**). Abrasion is not present on the exit side. If the muzzle was placed directly against the skin at the time of discharge, the expanding gases will enter the tissue and produce crepitus on examination (**Figure 5-61**). If the muzzle is within 2 to 3 inches (5 to 7 cm), the hot gases that exit will burn the skin; at 2 to 6 inches (5 to 15 cm) the smoke will adhere to the skin; and inside 10 inches (25 cm) the burning cordite particles will tattoo the skin with small (1- to 2-mm) burned areas (**Figure 5-62**).

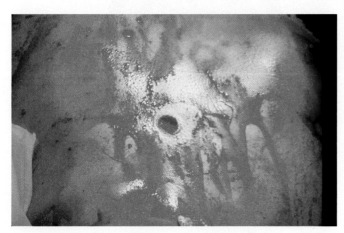

Figure 5-59 Entrance wound is round or oval in shape, and exit wound is often stellate or linear.
Source: Courtesy of Peter T. Pons, MD, FACEP.

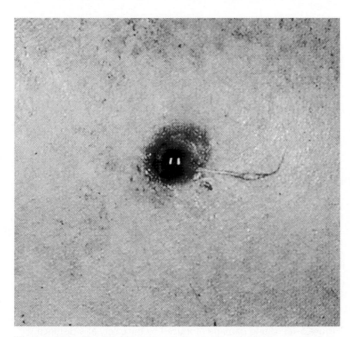

Figure 5-60 The abraded edge indicates that the bullet traveled from top right to bottom left.
Source: Courtesy Norman McSwain, MD, FACS, NREMT-P

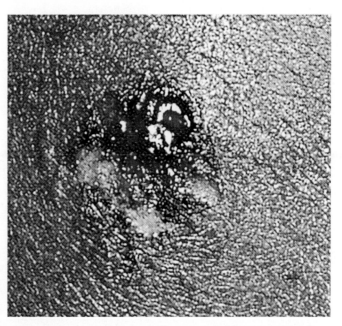

Figure 5-61 Hot gases coming from the end of a muzzle held in proximity to the skin produce partial-thickness and full-thickness burns on the skin.
Source: Courtesy Norman McSwain, MD, FACS, NREMT-P

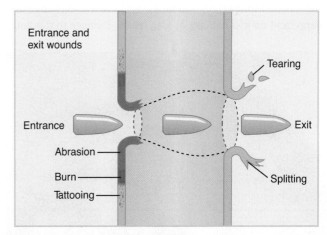

Figure 5-62 Spin and compression of the bullet on entrance produce round or oval holes. On exit, the wound is pressed open.

Regional Effects of Penetrating Trauma

This section discusses the injuries sustained by various parts of the body during penetrating trauma.

Head

After a missile penetrates the skull, its energy is distributed within a closed space. Particles accelerating away from the missile are forced against the unyielding skull, which cannot expand as can skin, muscle, or even the abdomen. Thus, the brain tissue is compressed against the inside of the skull, producing more injury than would otherwise occur if it could expand freely. It is similar to putting a firecracker in an apple and then placing the apple in a metal can. When the firecracker explodes, the apple will be destroyed against the wall of the can. In the case of a missile penetrating the skull, if the forces are strong enough, the skull may explode from the inside out (**Figure 5-63**).

A bullet may follow the curvature of the interior of the skull if it enters at an angle and has insufficient force to exit the skull. This path can produce significant damage (**Figure 5-64**). Because of this characteristic, small-caliber, medium-velocity weapons, such as the 0.22-caliber or 0.25-caliber pistol, have been called the "assassin's weapon." They go in and exchange all of their energy into the brain.

Thorax

Three major groups of structures are inside the thoracic cavity: the pulmonary system, vascular system, and gastrointestinal tract. The bones and muscles of the chest wall and spine make up the outer structure of the thorax. One or more of the anatomic structures of these systems may be injured by a penetrating object.

Pulmonary System

Lung tissue is less dense than blood, solid organs, or bone; therefore, a penetrating object will hit fewer particles, exchange less energy, and do less damage to lung tissue. Damage to the lungs can be clinically significant (**Figure 5-65**), but fewer than 15% of patients will require surgical exploration.[24]

Vascular System

Smaller vessels that are not attached to the chest wall may be pushed aside without significant damage. However, larger vessels, such as the aorta and venae cavae, are less mobile because they are tethered to the spine or the heart. They cannot move aside easily and are more susceptible to damage.

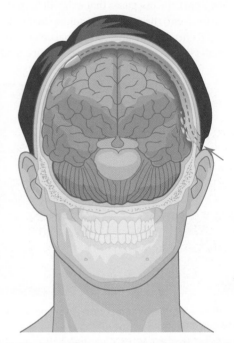

Figure 5-64   The bullet may follow the curvature of the skull.

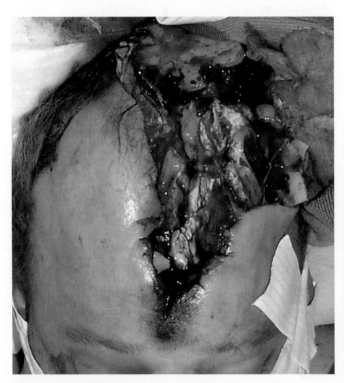

Figure 5-63   After a missile penetrates the skull, its energy is distributed within a closed space. It is like putting a firecracker in a closed container. If the forces are strong enough, the container (the skull) may explode from the inside out.
Source: Courtesy Norman McSwain, MD, FACS, NREMT-P

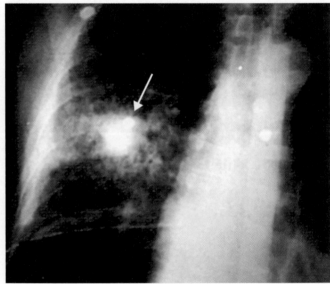

Figure 5-65   Lung damage produced by the cavity at a distance from the point of impact. The arrow shows a bullet fragment.
Source: Courtesy Norman McSwain, MD, FACS, NREMT-P

The myocardium (almost totally muscle) stretches as the bullet passes through and then contracts, leaving a smaller defect. The thickness of the muscle may control the bleeding from a low-energy penetration, such as by a knife, or even a small, medium-energy 0.22-caliber bullet. This closure can prevent immediate exsanguination and allow time to transport the victim to an appropriate facility.

Gastrointestinal Tract

The **esophagus**, the part of the gastrointestinal tract that traverses the thoracic cavity, can be penetrated and can leak its contents into the thoracic cavity. The signs and symptoms of such an injury may be delayed for several hours or several days.

Abdomen

The abdomen contains structures of three types: air-filled, solid, and bony. Penetration by a low-energy missile may not cause significant damage; only 30% of knife wounds penetrating the abdominal cavity require surgical exploration to repair damage. A medium-energy injury (e.g., handgun wound) is more damaging; 85% to 95% require surgical repair. However, in injuries caused by medium-energy missiles, the damage to solid and vascular structures frequently does not produce immediate exsanguination. This enables prehospital care providers to transport the patient to an appropriate facility in time for effective surgical intervention.

Extremities

Penetrating injuries to the extremities can include damage to bones, muscles, nerves, or vessels. When bones are hit, bony fragments become secondary missiles, lacerating surrounding tissue (**Figure 5-66**). Muscles often expand away from the path

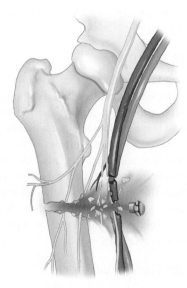

Figure 5-66 Bone fragments become secondary missiles themselves, producing damage by the same mechanism as the original penetrating object.

of the missile, causing hemorrhage. The missile may penetrate blood vessels, or a near miss may damage the lining of a blood vessel, causing clotting and obstruction of the vessel within minutes or hours.

Shotgun Wounds

Although shotguns are not high-velocity weapons, they are high-energy weapons, and, at close range, they can be more lethal than some of the highest-energy rifles. Handguns and rifles predominantly use **rifling** (grooves) on the inside of the barrel to spin a single missile in a flight pattern toward the target. In contrast, most shotguns possess a smooth, cylindrical tube barrel that directs a load of missiles in the direction of the target. Devices known as **chokes** and **diverters** can be attached to the end of a shotgun barrel to shape and form the column of missiles into specific patterns (e.g., cylindrical or rectangular). Regardless, when a shotgun is fired, a large number of missiles are ejected in a **spread**, or **spray**, pattern. The barrels may be shortened ("sawed off") to prematurely widen the trajectory of the missiles.

Although shotguns may use various types of ammunition, the structure of most shotgun shells is similar. A typical shotgun shell contains gunpowder, wadding, and projectiles. When discharged, all these individual components are propelled from the muzzle and can inflict injury on the victim. Certain types of gunpowder can **stipple** ("tattoo") the skin in close-range injuries. Wadding, which is usually lubricated paper, fibers, or plastic used to separate the shot (missiles) from the charge of gunpowder, can provide another source of infection in the wound if not removed. The missiles can vary in size, weight, and composition. A wide variety of missiles are available, from compressed metal powders to *birdshot* (small metal pellets), *buckshot* (larger metal pellets), *slugs* (a single metal missile), and more recently, plastic and rubber alternatives. The average shell is loaded with 1 to 1.5 (28 to 43 grams) ounces of shot. Fillers that are placed with the shot (polyethylene or polypropylene granules) can become embedded in the superficial layers of the skin.

An average birdshot shell may contain 200 to 2,000 pellets, whereas a buckshot shell may contain only 6 to 20 pellets (**Figure 5-67**). It is important to note that as the size of the buckshot pellets increases, they approach the wounding characteristics of 0.22-caliber missiles in regard to effective range and energy transfer characteristics. Larger or *magnum* shells are also available. These shells may contain more shot and a larger charge of gunpowder or only the larger powder charge to boost the muzzle velocity.

Categories of Shotgun Wounds

The type of ammunition used is important in gauging injuries, but the range (distance) at which the patient was shot provides the most important variable when evaluating the shotgun-injury victim. Shotguns eject a large number of missiles, most of which are spherical. These projectiles are especially susceptible

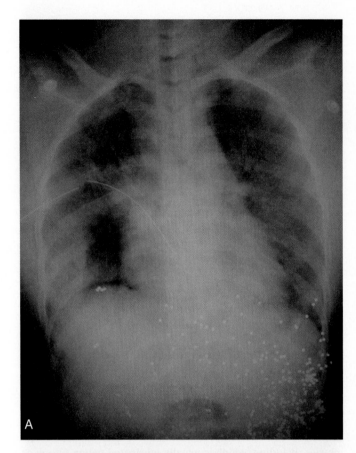

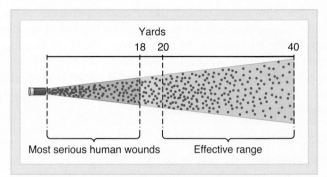

Figure 5-68 The diameter of the spread of a shot column expands as range increases.

Source: From DeMuth WE. The mechanism of gunshot wounds. *J Trauma.* 1971;11:219. Modified from Sherman RT, Parrish RA. Management of shotgun injuries: a review of 152 cases. *J Trauma.*1978;18:236.)

four major categories: contact, close-range, intermediate-range, and long-range wounds (**Figure 5-69**).

Contact Wounds

Contact wounds occur when the muzzle is touching the victim at the time the weapon is discharged. Discharge at this range typically results in circular entrance wounds, which may or may not have soot or an imprint of the muzzle (see Figure 5-61). Searing or burning of the wound edges is common, secondary to the high temperatures and the expansion of hot gases as the missiles exit the muzzle. Some contact wounds may be more stellate (star-shaped) in appearance, caused by the superheated gases from the barrel escaping from the tissue. Contact wounds usually result in widespread tissue damage and are associated with high mortality. The length of a standard shotgun barrel makes it difficult to commit suicide with this weapon, since it is difficult to reach and pull the trigger. Such attempts usually result in a split face without the shot reaching the brain.

Close-Range Wounds

Close-range wounds (less than 6 feet [1.8 m]), although still typically characterized by circular entrance wounds, will likely have more evidence of soot, gunpowder, or filler stippling around the wound margins than contact wounds. Additionally, abrasions and markings from the impact of the wadding that coincide with the wounds from the missiles may be found. Close-range wounds create significant damage in the patient; missiles fired from this range retain sufficient energy to penetrate deep structures and exhibit a slightly wider spread pattern. This pattern increases the extent of injury as missiles travel through soft tissue.

Intermediate-Range Wounds

Intermediate-range wounds are characterized by the appearance of satellite pellet holes emerging from the border around

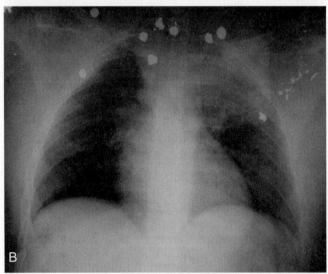

Figure 5-67 A. An average birdshot shell may contain 200 to 2,000 pellets. **B.** A buckshot shell may contain only 6 to 20 pellets.

Source: Courtesy Norman McSwain, MD, FACS, NREMT-P.

to the effects of air resistance, quickly slowing once they exit the muzzle (**Figure 5-68**). The effect of air resistance on the projectiles decreases the effective range of the weapon and changes the basic characteristics of the wounds that it generates. Consequently, shotgun wounds have been classified into

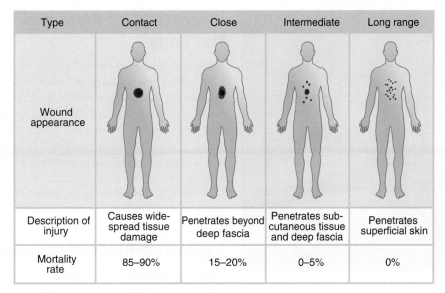

Type	Contact	Close	Intermediate	Long range
Wound appearance				
Description of injury	Causes wide-spread tissue damage	Penetrates beyond deep fascia	Penetrates sub-cutaneous tissue and deep fascia	Penetrates superficial skin
Mortality rate	85–90%	15–20%	0–5%	0%

Figure 5-69   Patterns of Shotgun Injury.

a central entrance wound. This pattern is a result of individual pellets spreading from the main column of shot and generally occurs at a range of 6 to 18 feet (1.8 to 5.5 m). These injuries are a mixture of deep, penetrating wounds and superficial wounds and abrasions. Because of the deep, penetrating components of this injury, however, victims may still have a relatively high mortality rate.

Long-Range Wounds

Long-range wounds are rarely lethal. These wounds are typically characterized by the classic spread of scattered pellet wounds and result from a range of greater than 18 feet (5.5 m). However, even at these slower velocities, the pellets can cause significant damage to certain sensitive tissues (e.g., eyes). In addition, larger buckshot pellets can retain sufficient velocity to inflict damage to deep structures, even at long range. The prehospital care provider also needs to consider the cumulative effects of many small missile wounds and their locations, focusing on sensitive tissues. *Adequate exposure* is essential when examining all patients involved in trauma, and shotgun injuries are no exception.

Assessment of Shotgun Wounds

These varying characteristics need to be taken into account when evaluating injury patterns in patients with shotgun injuries. For example, a single, circular, shotgun wound could represent a contact or close-range injury with birdshot or buckshot in which the missiles have retained a tight column or grouping. Conversely, this may also represent an intermediate-range to long-range injury with a slug or solitary missile. Only detailed examination of the wound will allow differentiation of these

injuries that will likely involve significant damage to internal structures despite strikingly different missile characteristics.

Contact and close-range wounds to the chest may result in a large, visually impressive wound resulting in an open pneumothorax, and bowel may eviscerate from such wounds to the abdomen. On occasion, a single pellet from an intermediate-range wound may penetrate deep enough to perforate the bowel, leading eventually to peritonitis, or may damage a major artery, resulting in vascular compromise to an extremity. Alternatively, a patient who exhibits multiple small wounds in a spread pattern may have dozens of entrance wounds. However, none of the missiles may have retained enough energy to penetrate through fascia, let alone produce significant damage to internal structures.

Although immediate patient care must always remain the priority, any information (e.g., shell type, suspected range of the patient from the weapon, number of shots fired) that prehospital care providers can gather from the scene and relay to the receiving facility can assist with appropriate diagnostic evaluation and treatment of the shotgun-injured patient. Furthermore, recognition of various wound types can aid prehospital care providers in maintaining a high index of suspicion for internal injury regardless of the initial impression of the injury.

Blast Injuries
Injury From Explosions

Explosive devices are the most frequently used weapons in combat and by terrorists. Explosive devices cause human injury by multiple mechanisms, some of which are exceedingly complex. The greatest challenges for clinicians at all levels of care in the

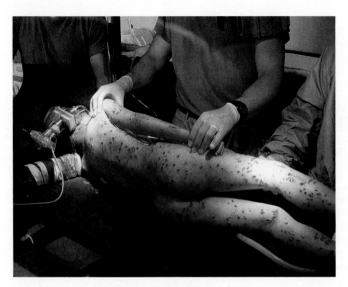

Figure 5-70 Patient with multiple fragment wounds from a bomb blast.

Source: Photo Courtesy of Maj. Scott Gering, Operation Iraqi Freedom.

aftermath of an explosion are the large numbers of casualties and multiple, penetrating injuries (**Figure 5-70**).[25]

Physics of Blast

Explosions are physical, chemical, or nuclear reactions that result in the almost instantaneous release of large amounts of energy in the form of heat and rapidly expanding, highly compressed gas, capable of projecting fragments at extremely high velocities. The energy associated with an explosion can take multiple forms: kinetic and heat energy in the **blast wave**; kinetic energy of fragments formed by the breakup of the weapon casing and surrounding debris; and electromagnetic energy.

Blast waves can travel at greater than 16,400 ft/second (5,000 m/second) and are composed of static and dynamic components. The static component (**blast overpressure**) surrounds objects in the flow field of the explosion, loading them on all sides with a discontinuous rise in pressure called the **shock front** or **shock wave** up to a **peak overpressure value**. Following the shock front, the overpressure drops down to ambient pressure, and then a partial vacuum is often formed as a result of air being sucked back (**Figure 5-71**). The dynamic component (**dynamic pressure**) is directional and is experienced as a **blast wind**. The primary significance of the blast wind is that it propels fragments at speeds in excess of several thousand meters per second (faster than standard ballistic weapons such as bullets and shells).[26] Whereas the effective range of both the static and dynamic pressure is measured in tens of feet, the fragments accelerated by the dynamic pressure will quickly outpace the blast wave to become the dominant cause of injury out to ranges of thousands of feet.

Interaction of Blast Waves With the Body

Blast waves interact with the body and other structures by transmitting energy from the blast wave into the structure. This energy causes the structure to deform in a manner dependent on the strength and the natural period of oscillation of the structure being affected. Changing density interfaces within a structure cause complex re-formations, convergences, and couplings of the transmitted blast waves. Such interactions can be seen particularly in large-density interfaces such as solid tissue to air or liquid (e.g., lung, heart, liver, and bowel).

Explosion-Related Injuries

Injuries from explosions are generally classified as primary, secondary, tertiary, quaternary, and quinary after the injury taxonomy described in Department of Defense Directive 6025.21E24 (**Figure 5-72**). Detonation of an explosive device sets off a chain of interactions in the objects and people in its path.[25] If an individual is close enough, the initial blast wave increases pressure in the body, causing stress and shear, particularly in gas-filled organs such as the ears, lungs, and (rarely) bowels (**Figure 5-73**). These primary blast injuries are more prevalent when the explosion occurs in an enclosed space because the blast wave bounces off surfaces, thus enhancing the destructive potential of the pressure waves.[27]

Immediate death from pulmonary barotrauma (blast lung) occurs more often in enclosed-space than in open-air bombings.[27-30] Most (95%) explosion injuries in Iraq and Afghanistan occur in open-space explosions.[31]

The most common form of primary blast injury is tympanic membrane rupture.[32,33] Tympanic membrane rupture, which may occur at pressures as low as 5 pounds per square inch (psi) (35 kilopascals [kPa]),[32-34] is often the only significant overpressure injury experienced. The next major injury occurs at less than 40 psi (276 kPa), a threshold known to be associated with pulmonary injuries including pneumothorax, air embolism, interstitial

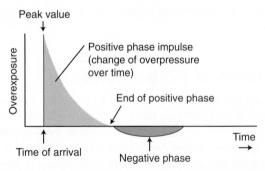

Figure 5-71 Pressure–time history of a blast wave. This graph shows the sudden massive increase in pressure (blast overpressure) following the decrease in pressure and negative pressure phase.

Source: From EXPLOSIVE BLAST 4 T - Federal Emergency Management Agency: www.fema.gov/pdf/plan/prevent/rms/428/fema428_ch4.pdf.

Figure 5-72 Blast Injury Categories

Category	Definition	Typical Injuries
Primary	<ul><li>Produced by contact of blast shockwave with body</li><li>Stress and shear waves occur in tissues</li><li>Waves reinforced/reflected at tissue density interfaces</li><li>Gas-filled organs (lungs, ears, etc.) at particular risk</li></ul>	<ul><li>Tympanic membrane rupture</li><li>Blast lung</li><li>Eye injuries</li><li>Concussion</li></ul>
Secondary	<ul><li>Ballistic wounds produced by:<ul><li>Primary fragments (pieces of exploding weapon)</li><li>Secondary fragments (environmental fragments [e.g., glass])</li></ul></li><li>Threat of fragment injury extends further than that from blast wave</li></ul>	<ul><li>Penetrating injuries</li><li>Traumatic amputations</li><li>Lacerations</li></ul>
Tertiary	<ul><li>Blast wave propels individuals onto surfaces/objects or objects onto individuals, causing whole body translocation</li><li>Crush injuries caused by structural damage and building collapse</li></ul>	<ul><li>Blunt injuries</li><li>Crush syndrome</li><li>Compartment syndrome</li></ul>
Quaternary	<ul><li>Other explosion-related injuries, illnesses, or diseases</li></ul>	<ul><li>Burns</li><li>Toxic gas and other inhalation injury</li><li>Injury or infection from environmental contamination</li></ul>
Quinary	<ul><li>Injuries resulting from specific additives such as bacteria and radiation ("dirty bombs")</li></ul>	

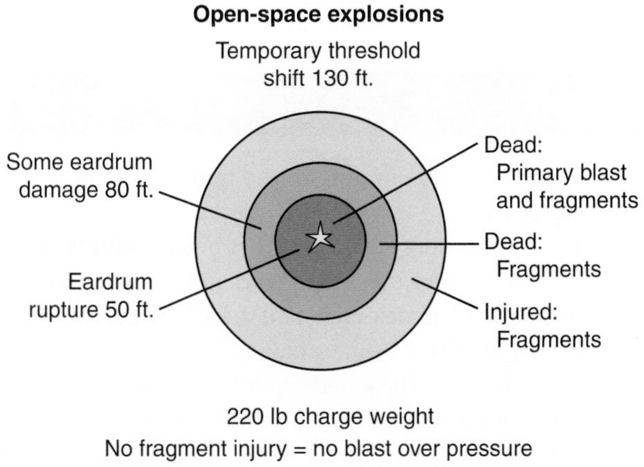

Open-space explosions

Temporary threshold
shift 130 ft.

Some eardrum
damage 80 ft.

Dead:
Primary blast
and fragments

Dead:
Fragments

Eardrum
rupture 50 ft.

Injured:
Fragments

220 lb charge weight
No fragment injury = no blast over pressure

Figure 5-73 Morbidity and mortality as a function of distance from open-space detonation of a 220-lb (100-kg) explosive.

and subcutaneous emphysema, and pneuomediastinum.[8] Data from burned soldiers from Operation Iraqi Freedom confirm that tympanic membrane rupture is not predictive of lung injury.

The shock front of the blast wave quickly dissipates and is followed by the blast wind, which propels fragments to create multiple penetrating injuries. Although these injuries are termed secondary, they are usually the predominant wounding agent.[8] The blast wind also propels large objects into people or people onto hard surfaces (whole or partial body translocation), creating blunt (tertiary blast) injuries; this category of injury also includes crush injuries caused by structural collapse.[8] Heat, flames, gas, and smoke generated during explosions cause quaternary injuries that include burns, inhalation injury, and asphyxiation.[35] Quinary injuries are produced when bacteria, chemicals, or radioactive materials are added to the explosive device and released upon detonation.

Injury From Fragments

Conventional explosive weapons are designed to maximize damage caused by fragments. With initial velocities of many thousands of feet per second, the distance that fragments may be thrown for a 50-lb (23-kg) bomb will be well over 1,000 feet (0.3 km), whereas the lethal radius of the blast overpressure is approximately 50 feet (15 m). The developers of both military and terrorist weapons, therefore, design weapons to maximize fragmentation injury so as to significantly increase the damage radius of a free-field explosive.

Very few explosive devices cause injury solely by blast overpressure, and serious primary blast injury is relatively rare compared to the predominant numbers of secondary and tertiary injuries. Thus, few patients have injuries dominated by primary blast effects. The entire array of explosion-related injuries is often referred to en masse as "blast injuries," leading to major confusion as to what constitutes a blast injury. Because energy from the blast wave dissipates rapidly, most explosive devices are constructed to cause damage primarily from fragments. These may be primary fragments generated through the breakup of the casing surrounding the explosive or secondary fragments created from debris in the surrounding environment. Regardless of whether the fragments are created from shattered munitions casing, flying debris, or embedded objects that terrorists often pack into homemade bombs, they exponentially increase the range and lethality of explosives and are the primary cause of explosion-related injury.

Multi-etiology Injury

In addition to the direct effects of an explosion, prehospital care providers must be mindful of the other causes of injury from attacks with explosions. For instance, an IED that targets a vehicle may result in minimal initial damage to the vehicle occupants. However, the vehicle itself may be displaced vertically or vectored off course resulting in occupant blunt trauma from collision, from flipping upside down as part of the vertical displacement process, or from rollover, for instance, down an embankment or culvert. In these circumstances, occupants sustain injury based on the mechanisms previously described for blunt trauma.

In the military setting, a vehicle's occupants may be afforded some protection from blunt injury by virtue of their body armor. Furthermore, the occupants of a vehicle disabled following an IED attack are subject to ambush and may be attacked with gunfire as they exit the vehicle, thus potentially becoming victims of penetrating injury.

Using Kinematics in Assessment

The assessment of a trauma patient must involve knowledge of kinematics. For example, a driver who hits the steering wheel (blunt trauma) will have a large cavity in the anterior chest at the time of impact; however, the chest rapidly returns to, or near to, its original shape as the driver rebounds from the steering wheel. If two prehospital care providers examine the patient separately— one who understands kinematics and another who does not—the one without knowledge of kinematics will be concerned only with the bruise visible on the patient's chest. The prehospital care provider who understands kinematics will recognize that a large cavity was present at the time of impact, that the ribs had to bend in for the cavity to form, and that the heart, lungs, and great vessels were compressed by the formation of the cavity. Therefore, the knowledgeable prehospital care provider will suspect injury to the heart, lungs, great vessels, and chest wall. The other prehospital care provider will not even be aware of these possibilities.

The knowledgeable prehospital care provider suspecting serious intrathoracic injuries will assess for these potential injuries, manage the patient, and initiate transport more aggressively, rather than react to what otherwise appears to be only a minor, closed, soft-tissue injury. Early identification, adequate understanding, and appropriate treatment of underlying injury will significantly influence whether a patient lives or dies.

Summary

- Integrating the principles of the kinematics of trauma into the assessment of the trauma patient is key to discovering the potential for severe or life-threatening injuries.
- Up to 95% of injuries can be anticipated by understanding the energy exchange that occurs with the human body at the time of a collision. Knowledge of kinematics allows for injuries that are not immediately apparent to be identified and treated appropriately. Left unsuspected, undetected, and therefore untreated, these injuries contribute significantly to morbidity and mortality resulting from trauma.
- Energy can be neither created nor destroyed, only changed in form. The kinetic energy of an object, expressed as a function of both velocity (speed) and mass (weight), is transferred to another object on contact.
- Damage to the object or body tissue impacted is not only a function of the amount of kinetic energy applied to it, but also a function of the tissue's ability to tolerate the forces applied to it.

Blunt Trauma

- The direction of the impact determines the pattern of and potential for injury: frontal, lateral, rear, rotational, rollover, or angular.
- Ejection from a car reduces the protection on impact afforded by the vehicle.

- Energy-absorbing protective devices are very important. These devices include seat belts, air bags, drop-down engines, and energy-absorbing auto parts, such as bumpers, collapsible steering wheels, dashboards, and helmets. The damage to the vehicles and the direction of the impact will indicate which occupants are most likely to have been more severely injured.
- Pedestrian injuries vary according to the height of the victim and which part of the patient had direct contact with the vehicle.

Falls

- Distance travelled before impact affects the severity of the injury sustained.
- Energy-absorbing capability of the target at the end of the fall (e.g., concrete versus soft snow) affects the severity of the injury.
- Victim body parts that hit the target and progression of the energy exchange through the victim's body are important.

Penetrating Trauma

- The energy varies depending on the primary injuring agent:
  - Low energy—handheld cutting devices
  - Medium energy—most handguns
  - High energy—high-powered rifles, assault weapons, etc.
- The distance of the victim to the perpetrator and the objects that the bullet might have struck will affect the amount of energy at the time of impact with the body and, therefore, the available energy to be dissipated into the patient to produce damage to the body parts.
- Organs in proximity of the pathway of the penetrating object determine the potential life-threatening conditions.
- The pathway of the penetrating trauma is determined by the wound of entrance and the wound of exit.

Blasts

- There are five types of injury in a blast:
  - Primary—over-and-under pressure
  - Secondary—projectiles (the most common source of injury from blasts)
  - Tertiary—propulsion of the body into another object
  - Quaternary—heat and flames
  - Quinary—radiation, chemicals, bacteria

SCENARIO RECAP

Before first light on a cold winter morning, you and your partner are dispatched to a single-vehicle crash. On arrival, you find a single vehicle that has crashed into a tree on a rural road. The front end of the vehicle appears to have impacted the tree, and the car has spun around the tree and backed into a drainage ditch on the side of the road. The driver appears to be the only occupant. The air bag has deployed and the driver is moaning, still restrained by his safety harness. You note damage to the front end of the car where it impacted the tree as well as rear-end damage from spinning around and going into the ditch backwards.

- What is the potential for injury for this patient based on the kinematics of this event?
- How would you describe the patient's condition based upon the kinematics?
- What injuries do you expect to find?

SCENARIO SOLUTION

As you approach the patient, your understanding of the kinematics of this event leads you to be concerned about the potential for head, neck, chest, and abdominal injuries. The patient is responsive, but his speech is slurred and he smells of alcohol. While providing manual immobilization of his head and neck, you note a small laceration on the bridge of his nose as you continue to assess him for injury. He admits that he has been drinking and is unsure of the time of day or where he was going.

Releasing the seat belt and shoulder harness, you note tenderness and an abrasion over his left clavicle. He also complains of some tenderness of his face, neck, anterior chest, and mid-abdomen. Due to his admitted alcohol use, slurred speech, and confusion, you cannot rule out more serious injuries, so you provide spinal immobilization as you remove him from the vehicle.

Continuing your exam en route to the trauma center, you note that the patient has significant tenderness to both lower abdominal quadrants, and you are concerned that there may be hollow organ injury.

References

1. U.S. Department of Transportation, National Highway Traffic Safety Administration. 2011 motor vehicle crashes: overview. http://www-nrd.nhtsa.dot.gov/Pubs/811701.pdf. Published December 2012. Accessed January 21, 2013.
2. World Health Organization. *Global Status Report on Road Safety: Time for Action.* http://whqlibdoc.who.int/publications/2009/9789241563840_eng.pdf, Published 2009. Accessed January 21, 2013.
3. Centers for Disease Control and Prevention. *National Vital Statistics Report.* Deaths: preliminary data for 2011. http://www.cdc.gov/nchs/data/nvsr/nvsr61/nvsr61_06.pdf. Published October 10, 2012. Accessed October 18,2013.
4. Hunt JP, Marr AB, Stuke LE. Kinematics. In: Mattox KL, Moore EE, Feliciano DV, eds. *Trauma.* 7th ed. New York, NY: McGraw-Hill; 2013.
5. Hollerman JJ, Fackler ML, Coldwell DM, et al. Gunshot wounds: 1. Bullets, ballistics, and mechanisms of injury. *Am J Roentgenol.* 1990;155(4):685-690.
6. Centers for Disease Control and Prevention. Leading causes of death. http://www.cdc.gov/injury/wisqars/leading_causes_death.html. Updated September 17, 2012. Accessed March 23, 2013.
7. Rogers CD, Pagliarello G, McLellan BA, et al. Mechanism of injury influences the pattern of injuries sustained by patients involved in vehicular trauma. *Can J Surg.* 1991;34(3):283–286.
8. Nixon RG, Stewart C. When things go boom: blast injuries. *Fire Engineering.* May 1, 2004.
9. Hernandez IA, Fyfe KR, Heo G, et al. Kinematics of head movement in simulated low velocity rear-end impacts. *Clin Biomech.* 2005;20(10):1011–1018.
10. Kumaresan S, Sances A, Carlin F, et al. Biomechanics of side-impact injuries: evaluation of seat belt restraint system, occupant kinematics, and injury potential. Conf Proc IEEE Eng Med Biol Soc.2006;1:87–90.
11. Siegel JH, Yang KH, Smith JA, et al. Computer simulation and validation of the Archimedes Lever hypothesis as a mechanism for aortic isthmus disruption in a case of lateral impact motor vehicle crash: a Crash Injury Research Engineering Network (CIREN) study. *J Trauma.* 2006;60(5):1072–1082.
12. Horton TG, Cohn SM, Heid MP, et al. Identification of trauma patients at risk of thoracic aortic tear by mechanism of injury. *J Trauma.* 2000; 48(6):1008–1013; discussion 1013–1014.
13. U.S. Department of Transportation, National Highway Traffic Safety Administration. Occupant restraint use in 2011: results from the National Occupant Protection Use Survey Controlled Intersection Study. http://www-nrd.nhtsa.dot.gov/Pubs/811697.pdf. Published January 2013. Accessed February 27, 2013.
14. U.S. Department of Transportation, National Highway Traffic Safety Administration. *Traffic Safety Facts.* Occupant protection. http://www-nrd.nhtsa.dot.gov/Pubs/811160.pdf. Accessed February 27, 2013.
15. U.S. Department of Transportation, National Highway Traffic Safety Administration. *Traffic Safety Facts.* Lives saved in 2008 by restraint use and minimum drinking age laws. http://www-nrd.nhtsa.dot.gov/Pubs/811153.PDF. Published May 2010. Accessed January 21, 2013.
16. Centers for Disease Control and Prevention. *Vital Signs.* Adult seat belt use in the U.S. http://www.cdc.gov/VitalSigns/SeatBeltUse/. Updated January 4, 2011. Accessed January 21, 2013.
17. U.S. Department of Transportation, National Highway Traffic Safety Administration. *Traffic Safety Facts.* Seat belt use in 2008: use rates in the states and territories. http://www-nrd.nhtsa.dot.gov/Pubs/811106.PDF. Published April 2009. Accessed October 18, 2013.
18. Centers for Disease Control and Prevention. Guidelines for field triage of injured patients: recommendations of the National Expert Panel on Field Triage. *MMWR.* 2012;61:1-20.
19. Burgess AR, Eastridge BJ, Young JW, et al. Pelvic ring disruptions: effective classification system and treatment protocols. *J Trauma.* 1990;30(7):848–856.
20. Fackler ML, Malinowski JA. Internal deformation of the AK-74: a possible cause for its erratic path in tissue. *J Trauma.* 1998;28(suppl 1) S72–S75.
21. Fackler ML, Surinchak JS, Malinowski JA, et al. Wounding potential of the Russian AK-74 assault rifle. *J Trauma.* 1984;24(3):263–266.
22. Fackler ML, Surinchak JS, Malinowski JA, et al. Bullet fragmentation: a major cause of tissue disruption. *J Trauma.* 1984;24(1):35–39.

23. Fackler ML, Dougherty PJ. Theodor Kocher and the Scientific Foundation of Wound Ballistics. *Surg Gynecol Obstet*. 1991;172(2):153–160.

24. American College of Surgeons (ACS) Committee on Trauma. *Advanced Trauma Life Support Course*. Chicago, IL:ACS; 2002.

25. Wade CE, Ritenour AE, Eastridge BJ, et al. Explosion injuries treated at combat support hospitals in the Global War on Terrorism. In: Elsayed N, Atkins J, eds. *Explosion and Blast-Related Injuries*. Burlington, MA: Elsevier; 2008.

26. Department of Defense. Directive Number 6025:21E: Medical Research for Prevention, Mitigation, and Treatment of Blast Injuries. http://www.dtic.mil/whs/directives/corres/pdf/602521p.pdf. Published July 5, 2006. Accessed October 18, 2013

27. Leibovici D, Gofrit ON, Stein M, et al. Blast injuries: bus versus open-air bombings—a comparative study of injuries in survivors of open-air versus confined-space explosions. *J Trauma*. 1996;41: 1030–1035.

28. Gutierrez de Ceballos JP, Turégano-Fuentes F, Perez-Diaz D, et al. The terrorist bomb explosions in Madrid, Spain—an analysis of the logistics, injuries sustained, and clinical management of casualties treated at the closest hospital. *Crit Care Med*. 2005;9:104–111.

29. Gutierrez de Ceballos JP, Turégano Fuentes F, Perez Diaz D, et al. Casualties treated at the closest hospital in the Madrid, March 11, terrorist bombings. *Crit Care Med*. 2005;33(1)(suppl):S107–S112.

30. Avidan V, Hersch M, Armon Y, et al. Blast lung injury: clinical manifestations, treatment, and outcome. *Am J Surg*. 2005;190:927–931.

31. Ritenour AE, Blackbourne LH, Kelly JF, et al. Incidence of primary blast injury in US military overseas contingency operations: a retrospective study. *Ann Surg*. 2010;251(6):1140–4.

32. Ritenour AE, Wickley A, Ritenour JS, et al. Tympanic membrane perforation and hearing loss from blast overpressure in Operation Enduring Freedom and Operation Iraqi Freedom wounded. *J Trauma*. 2008;64:S174–S178.

33. Zalewski T. Experimentelle Untersuchungen uber die Resistenzfahigkeit des Trommelfells. *Z Ohrenheilkd*. 1906;52:109.

34. Helling ER. Otologic blast injuries due to the Kenya embassy bombing. *Mil Med*. 2004;169:872–876.

35. National Association of Emergency Medical Technicians. Injuries from explosives. In: Butler FK, et al, eds. *PHTLS: Prehospital Trauma Life Support*. Military 7th ed. St. Louis, MO: Mosby JEMS Elsevier; 2011.

Suggested Reading

Alderman B, Anderson A. Possible effect of air bag inflation on a standing child. In: *Proceedings of 18th American Association of Automotive Medicine*. Barrington, IL: American Association of Automotive Medicine; 1974.

American College of Surgeons (ACS) Committee on Trauma. Advanced Trauma Life Support Course. Chicago, IL: ACS; 2012.

Anderson PA, Henley MB, Rivara P, et al. Flexion distraction and chance injuries to the thoracolumbar spine. *J Orthop Trauma*. 1991;5(2):153.

Anderson PA, Rivara FP, Maier RV, et al. The epidemiology of seatbelt-associated injuries. *J Trauma*. 1991;31(1):60.

Bartlett CS. Gunshot wound ballistics. *Clin Orthop*. 2003;408:28.

DePalma RG, Burris DG, Champion HR, et al. Current concepts: blast injuries. *N Engl J Med*. 2005;352:1335.

Di Maio VJM. Gunshot wounds: practical aspects of firearms, ballistics and forensic techniques. Boca Raton, FL: CRC Press; 1999.

Garrett JW, Braunstein PW. The seat belt syndrome. *J Trauma*. 1962;2:220.

Huelke DF, Mackay GM, Morris A. Vertebral column injuries and lap-shoulder belts. *J Trauma*. 1995;38:547.

Huelke DF, Moore JL, Ostrom M. Air bag injuries and occupant protection. *J Trauma*. 1992;33(6):894.

Joksch H, Massie D, Pichler R. Vehicle Aggressivity: Fleet Characterization Using Traffic Collision Data. Washington, DC: Department of Transportation; 1998.

Hunt JP, Marr AB, Stuke LE. Kinematics. In: Mattox KL, Moore EE, Feliciano DV, eds. *Trauma*. 7th ed. New York, NY: McGraw-Hill; 2013.

McSwain NE Jr, Brent CR. Trauma rounds: lipstick sign. *Emerg Med*. 1998;21:46.

McSwain NE Jr, Paturas JL. *The Basic EMT: Comprehensive Prehospital Patient Care*. 2nd ed. St. Louis, MO: Mosby; 2001.

National Safety Council (NSC). *Accident Facts 1994*. Chicago, IL: NSC; 1994.

Ordog GJ, Wasserberger JN, Balasubramaniam S. Shotgun wound ballistics. *J Trauma*. 1922;28:624.

Oreskovich MR, Howard JD, Compass MK, et al. Geriatric trauma: injury patterns and outcome. *J Trauma*. 1984;24:565.

Rutledge R, Thomason M, Oller D, et al. The spectrum of abdominal injuries associated with the use of seat belts. *J Trauma*. 1991;31(6):820.

States JD, Annechiarico RP, Good RG, et al. A time comparison study of the New York State Safety Belt Use Law utilizing hospital admission and police accident report information. *Accid Anal Prev*. 1990;22(6):509.

Swierzewski MJ, Feliciano DV, Lillis RP, et al. Deaths from motor vehicle crashes: patterns of injury in restrained and unrestrained victims. *J Trauma*. 1994;37(3):404.

Sykes LN, Champion HR, Fouty WJ. Dum-dums, hollowpoints, and devastators: techniques designed to increase wounding potential of bullets. *J Trauma*. 1988;28:618.

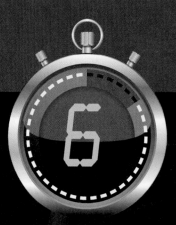
Scene Assessment

CHAPTER OBJECTIVES

At the completion of this chapter, the reader will be able to do the following:

- Identify potential threats to the safety of the patient, bystanders, and emergency personnel that are common to all emergency scenes.

- Discuss potential threats that are unique to a given scenario, such as a motor vehicle crash (MVC).

- Integrate analysis of scene safety, scene situation, and kinematics into assessment of the trauma patient to make patient care decisions.

- Describe appropriate steps to take to mitigate potential threats to safety.

- Given a mass-casualty incident (MCI) scenario (hazardous materials incident, weapon of mass destruction), discuss the use of a triage system in managing the scene, and make triage decisions based on assessment findings.

SCENARIO

You are dispatched to the scene of a domestic altercation. It is 0245 hours on a hot summer night. As you arrive on the scene of a single-family dwelling, you can hear a man and woman arguing very loudly and the sounds of children crying in the background. Police have also been dispatched to this call but have not yet arrived to the location.

- What are your concerns about the scene?
- What considerations are important before you contact the patient?

Introduction

There are a number of concerns that the prehospital care provider must consider when responding to and arriving at a scene:

1. Immediately upon being assigned to a call and receiving dispatch information, the potential issues and hazards associated with that type of call should be anticipated. Preliminary assessment of scene safety issues and the situation is initiated while en route to the scene based on information from the dispatcher. This assessment takes into consideration not only possible scene safety issues but also the need for other public safety emergency responders, such as police and fire, and preparations for patient-specific concerns.

2. The first priority for everyone arriving at a trauma incident is overall assessment of the scene. Scene assessment involves establishing that the scene is safe enough for emergency medical services (EMS) to enter and carefully considering the exact nature of the situation to ensure provider and patient safety and to determine what alterations in patient care are indicated by the current conditions. Scene safety considerations continue even after that initial scene survey and as the prehospital care providers approach the patient. Any issues identified in this evaluation must be addressed before beginning the assessment of individual patients. In some situations, such as combat or tactical situations or hazardous materials incidents, this evaluation process becomes even more critical and can alter the methods of providing patient care.

   Scene assessment is not a one-time event. Continuous attention must be paid to what is going on around the emergency responders. Scenes initially deemed safe for entry can change rapidly, and all emergency responders must be prepared to take appropriate steps to ensure their continued safety should the conditions on scene change.

3. After performing the scene assessment, the next priority is evaluating individual patients (discussed in greater detail in the Patient Assessment and Management chapter). The overall scene assessment will indicate whether the incident involves only a single patient or multiple patients.[1] If the scene involves more than one patient, the situation is classified as either a multiple-patient incident or a mass-casualty incident (MCI) (see the Disaster Management chapter). In an MCI, the number of patients exceeds available resources. The priority shifts from focusing all resources on the most injured patient to saving the maximum number of patients—that is, providing the greatest good to the greatest number of people. An initial abbreviated form of triage (discussed in the final section of this chapter) identifies the most severely injured patients to be treated first when there are multiple victims. The prioritization of patient management is (a) conditions that may result in the loss of life, (b) conditions that may result in the loss of limb, and (c) all other conditions that do not threaten life or limb.

Scene Assessment

Scene and patient assessment starts long before the prehospital care provider actually arrives to the incident location and at the patient's side. Dispatch begins the process by gathering information through questioning the caller or from information provided by other public safety or prehospital care units already on the scene and by providing that initial information about the incident and the patient to the responding EMS unit.

While travelling to the scene, taking the time to prepare mentally for a call and practicing basic communication between partners may be the difference between a well-managed scene and a hostile confrontation (or a physical assault). Good observation, perception, and communication skills are the best tools.

The on-scene information-gathering process for the prehospital care provider begins immediately upon arrival at the incident. Before making contact with the patient, the prehospital care provider should evaluate the scene by:

1. Obtaining a general impression of the situation for scene safety
2. Looking at the cause and results of the incident
3. Observing family members and bystanders

The scene's appearance creates an impression that influences the entire assessment; therefore, correct evaluation of the scene is crucial. A wealth of information is gathered by simply looking, watching, listening, and cataloguing as much information as possible, including the mechanisms of injury, the present situation, and the overall degree of safety.

Just as the patient's condition can improve or deteriorate, so can the condition of the scene. Evaluating the scene initially then failing to reassess how the scene may change can result in serious consequences to the prehospital care providers and the patient. Awareness of the situation on the scene, not just upon arrival, but as the scene evolves and unfolds over time, is crucial to the safety of all emergency responders present at the incident.

Scene assessment includes the following two major components: safety and situation.

Safety

The primary consideration when approaching any scene is the safety of *all* emergency responders. Rescue efforts should not be attempted by those untrained in the techniques required. When EMS personnel become victims, they can no longer assist other injured people and they add to the number of patients. Patient care may need to wait until the scene is safe enough that EMS can enter without undue risk. No scene is ever 100% safe and all emergency responders must maintain continued vigilance and awareness. Safety concerns vary from the exposure to body fluids that may occur on every call to rare events such as exposure to a chemical weapon of mass destruction. Clues to potential risks and hazards on scene include not only the obvious such as the sound of gunshots or the presence of blood and other body fluids, but also more subtle findings such as odors and smells or vapor clouds.

Scene safety involves both emergency responder safety and patient safety. In general, patients in a hazardous situation should be moved to a safe area before assessment and treatment begin. Threatening conditions to patient or emergency responder safety include fire, downed electrical lines, explosives, hazardous materials (including blood or body fluid, traffic, floodwater, and weapons such as guns or knives), and environmental conditions. Also, an assailant may still be on the scene and may intervene to harm the patient, emergency responders, or bystanders. However, it has been recognized that in situations involving an active shooter or assailant, having EMS work in a coordinated fashion with law enforcement to enter a scene as soon as possible improves patient survival.

The preferences employed for patient care can be drastically altered by the conditions on the scene. For example, an industrial explosion or chemical spill can produce dangerous conditions for the prehospital care providers that take precedence and alter the methods by which patient care is provided. (For more information on principle versus preference, see the chapter titled The Science, Art, and Ethics of Prehospital Care: Principles, Preferences, and Critical Thinking.)

Situation

Assessment of the situation follows the safety assessment. The situational survey includes both issues that may affect what and how the prehospital care provider manages the patient as well as incident-specific concerns related to the patient directly. Some of the issues that must be assessed based upon the individual situation include:

- What really happened at the scene? What were the circumstances that led to the injury?
- Why was help summoned and who summoned it?
- What was the mechanism of injury (kinematics), and what forces and energies led to the victims' injuries? (See the Kinematics of Trauma chapter.) A majority of patient injuries can be predicted based on evaluating and understanding the kinematics involved in the incident.
- How many people are involved, and what are their ages?
- Are additional EMS units needed for scene management, patient treatment, or victim transport?
- Is mutual aid needed? Are any other personnel or resources needed (e.g., law enforcement, fire department, power company)?
- Is special extrication or rescue equipment needed?
- Is helicopter transport necessary?
- Is a physician needed to assist with triage or on-scene medical care issues?
- Could a medical problem be the instigating factor that led to the trauma (e.g., a vehicle crash that resulted from the driver's heart attack)?

Issues related to both safety and situation have significant overlap; many safety topics are also specific to certain situations, and certain situations pose serious safety hazards. These issues are discussed in further detail in the following sections.

Safety Issues
Traffic Safety

The majority of EMS personnel who are killed or injured each year are involved in motor vehicle–related incidents (**Figure 6-1**).[2] Although most of these fatalities and injuries are related to direct ambulance collisions during the response phase, a subset occurs while working on the scene of a motor vehicle crash (MVC). In the United States, EMS responds to approximately two million MVCs annually. Many factors can result in prehospital care providers

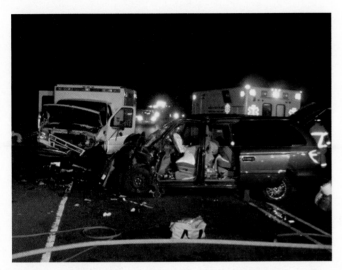

Figure 6-1 The majority of EMS personnel who are killed or injured each year are involved in motor vehicle–related incidents.
Source: Courtesy of Oregon State Police.

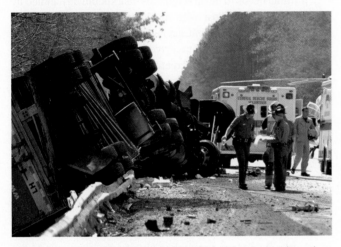

Figure 6-2 A significant number of prehospital care providers who are injured or killed are working at the scene of an MVC.
Source: © Jeff Thrower (Web Thrower)/ShutterStock, Inc.

being injured or killed on the scene of an MVC **(Figure 6-2)**. Some factors, such as weather conditions (e.g., snow, ice, rain, fog) and road design (e.g., limited-access or rural roads), cannot be changed; however, the prehospital care provider can be aware that these conditions exist and act appropriately to mitigate the dangers present at these situations. [3]

Weather/Light Conditions

Many prehospital care responses to MVCs take place in adverse weather conditions and at night. Weather conditions vary by geographic location and time of year. Prehospital care providers in many areas need to deal with ice and snow during the winter months, while those in coastal and mountainous areas often confront fog or snow, respectively. Rainstorms are common in most geographic areas, and sandstorms affect other regions.

Incoming traffic may not see or be able to stop in time to avoid emergency vehicles or EMS personnel parked on the scene.

Highway Design

High-speed, limited-access highways have made moving large amounts of traffic efficient, but when a crash occurs, the resulting traffic backup and "rubbernecking" by drivers create dangerous situations for all emergency responders. Elevated roadways and overpasses may limit an oncoming driver's vision of what lies ahead and the driver may suddenly encounter stopped vehicles and emergency responders on the road upon reaching the apex of the overpass. Law enforcement is usually reluctant to shut down a limited-access highway and strives to keep the flow of traffic moving. Although this approach may appear to produce further danger to emergency responders, it may prevent additional rear-end collisions caused by the backup of vehicles.

Rural roads present other problems. Although the volume of traffic is much less than on urban roadways, the winding, narrow, and hilly nature of these roads prevents drivers from seeing the scene of an MVC until they are dangerously close to it. Additionally, rural roads may not be as well-maintained as those in urban areas, resulting in slippery conditions long after a storm has passed and catching unsuspecting drivers off guard. Isolated areas of snow, ice, or fog that caused the original MVC may still be present, may hinder EMS arrival, and may result in suboptimal conditions for oncoming drivers.

Mitigation Strategies

It would be safest to respond to MVCs only during daylight hours on clear days; unfortunately, prehospital care providers need to respond at all times of day and in any weather condition. However, steps can be taken to reduce the risks of becoming a victim while working at the scene of an MVC. The best way is to not be there, particularly on limited-access highways. The number of people on the scene at any given time should be the number needed to accomplish the tasks at hand and no more. For example, having three ambulances and a supervisor's vehicle at a scene that has only one patient dramatically increases the risk of a prehospital care provider being hit by a passing vehicle. Although many dispatch protocols require multiple-ambulance response to limited-access highways, *all but the initial ambulance should be staged at a convenient access point nearby unless immediately needed.*

The location of equipment in the ambulance also plays a role in safety. Equipment should be placed so that it can be gathered without stepping into the traffic flow. The passenger's side of the ambulance is often toward the guardrails, and placing the equipment most often used at MVCs in these compartments will keep prehospital care providers out of the flow of traffic.

Reflective Clothing

In most cases of prehospital care providers hit by oncoming vehicles, the drivers stated that they did not see the prehospital care provider in the road. Both the National Fire Protection

Association (NFPA) and the Occupational Safety and Health Administration (OSHA) have standards for reflective warning garments to be worn when working on highways. OSHA has three levels of protection for workers on highways, with the highest level (level 3) to be used at night on a high-speed roadway. The Federal Highway Administration has mandated that all workers, including all emergency responders, wear American National Standards Institute (ANSI) Class 2 or Class 3 reflective vests when responding to an incident on a highway funded by federal aid. Common sense dictates that prehospital care providers should wear reflective clothing at all MVCs as a preventive safety measure. The ANSI standards can be met either by affixing reflective material to the outer jacket or by wearing an approved reflective vest.

Vehicle Positioning and Warning Devices

Vehicle positioning at the scene of an MVC is of the utmost importance. The incident commander or the safety officer should ensure that the responding vehicles are placed in the best positions to protect prehospital care providers. It is important for the first-arriving emergency vehicles to "take the lane" of the accident **(Figure 6-3)**. Although placement of the ambulance behind the scene will not facilitate the loading of the patient, it will protect the prehospital care providers and patient from oncoming traffic. As additional emergency vehicles arrive, they should generally be placed on the same side of the road as the incident. These vehicles should be placed farther from the incident to give increased warning time to oncoming drivers.

Headlights, especially high beams, should be turned off to avoid blinding oncoming drivers, unless the beams are needed to illuminate the scene. The number of warning lights at the scene should be evaluated; too many lights will only serve to confuse oncoming drivers. Many departments use warning signs stating "accident ahead" to give ample warning time for drivers. Flares may be arranged to warn and direct traffic flow; however, care should be used in dry conditions so as not to start grass fires. Reflective cones serve as good devices to direct traffic flow away from the lane taken up by the emergency **(Figure 6-4)**.

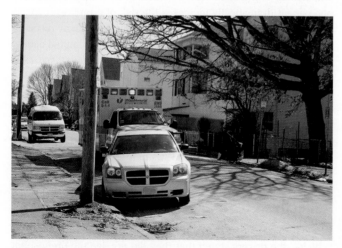

Figure 6-3 The correct positioning of an emergency vehicle.
Source: © Jones & Bartlett Learning. Photographed by Darren Stahlman.

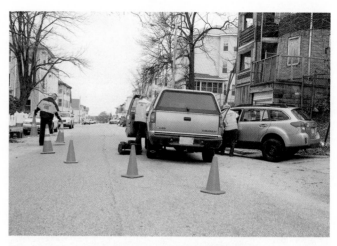

Figure 6-4 The placement of traffic delineation devices.
Source: © Jones & Bartlett Learning. Photographed by Darren Stahlman.

If traffic needs to be directed, this task should be handled by law enforcement or those with special training in traffic control so EMS can focus on patient management. Confusing or contradicting instructions given to drivers create additional safety risks. The best situations are created when traffic is not impeded and normal flow can be maintained around the emergency. Construction sites provide an example of how traffic can move smoothly around obstructions. Traffic issues at crash scenes can be handled in much the same way; prehospital care providers can observe construction sites to gain insight into how traffic flow may be directed at an MVC.

Traffic Safety Education

Several different educational programs exist that are designed to educate emergency responders about safe operations at the scene of an MVC. Each organization should check with its state EMS agency, NHTSA, or OSHA about the local availability of these programs and incorporate them into their annual required training programs.

Violence

Each call has the potential to take the prehospital care provider into an emotionally charged environment. Some EMS agencies have a policy that requires the presence of law enforcement before prehospital care providers enter a scene of violence or potential violence. Even a scene that appears benign has the potential to deteriorate into violence; therefore, prehospital care providers must always be alert to subtle clues suggesting a change in situation. The patient, family, or bystanders on the scene may not be able to perceive the situation rationally. These individuals may think the response time was too long, may be overly sensitive to words or actions, and may misunderstand the "usual" approach to patient assessment. Maintaining a confident and professional manner while demonstrating respect and concern is important to gaining the patient's trust and achieving control of the scene.

It is important that EMS personnel train themselves to *observe* the scene and not just *look* at it. EMS personnel must learn to notice the numbers and locations of individuals when arriving on the scene, the movement of bystanders into or out of the scene, any indicators of stress or tension, unexpected or unusual reactions to EMS presence, or other "gut" feelings that may develop. Watch the hands. Look for unusual bulges in waistbands, clothing that is worn out of season (e.g., an overcoat in warm weather), or oversized clothing that could easily hide a weapon.

If a developing threat is perceived, immediately begin preparing to leave the scene. An assessment or a procedure may need to be finished in the ambulance. The safety of the prehospital care providers takes priority. Consider the following situation: You and your partner are in the living room of a patient's home. While your partner is checking the patient's blood pressure, an apparently intoxicated individual enters the room from the back of the house. He looks angry, and you notice what appears to be the butt of a gun sticking out of the waistband of his pants. Your partner does not see or hear this person enter the room because he is focused on the patient. The suspicious person begins to question your presence and is extremely agitated about your uniform and your badge. His hands repeatedly move toward, then away from, his waist. He begins to pace and mumble. How can you and your partner prepare for this sort of situation?

Managing the Violent Scene

Prior to beginning the day's EMS calls, partners need to discuss and agree on methods to handle a violent or disruptive patient. Attempting to develop a process during the event is not the correct approach. Partners can use a hands-on/hands-off approach, as well as predetermined code words and hand signals, for emergencies.

- The role of the *hands-on* prehospital care provider is to take charge of the patient assessment, giving necessary attention to the patient. The *hands-off* prehospital care provider stands back (until needed) to observe the scene, interact with family or bystanders, collect necessary information, and create better access and egress. In essence, the hands-off prehospital care provider is monitoring the scene and "covering" his or her partner's back.
- A predetermined *code word* and *hand signals* allow partners to communicate a threat without alerting others of their concerns.

If both prehospital care providers have all of their attention focused on the patient, the scene can quickly become threatening, and early clues (as well as opportunities to retreat) may be missed. In many situations, patient, family, and bystander tension and anxiety are immediately reduced when an attentive prehospital care provider begins interacting with and assessing the patient.

There are various methods for dealing with a scene that has become dangerous, including the following:

1. *Don't be there.* When responding to a known violent scene, stage at a safe location until the scene has been rendered safe by law enforcement and clearance to respond has been given.
2. *Retreat.* If threats are presented when approaching the scene, tactfully retreat to the vehicle and leave the scene. Stage at a safe location and notify appropriate personnel.
3. *Defuse.* If a scene becomes threatening during patient care, use verbal defusing skills to reduce tension and aggression (while preparing to leave the scene).
4. *Defend.* As a last resort, the prehospital care provider may find it necessary to defend him- or herself. It is important that such efforts are to "disengage and get away." Do not attempt to chase or subdue an aggressive party. Ensure that law enforcement personnel have been notified and are en route. Again, the safety of the prehospital care providers is the priority.

The Active Shooter

Unfortunately, situations involving an active shooter have become all too frequent. In an effort to improve patient outcomes from injuries sustained in these sorts of incidents, there is a growing trend for EMS agencies to partner with their law enforcement colleagues to enter these scenes much sooner than would otherwise normally occur. In these cases, a contact team of officers will enter the scene to engage and neutralize the threat. They are quickly followed by a joint EMS and law enforcement team to identify and begin treating victims. (See the Civilian Tactical Emergency Medical Support [TEMS] chapter for further information.)

Hazardous Materials

Understanding the prehospital care provider's risk of exposure to hazardous materials is not as simple as recognizing environments that have obvious potential for hazardous material exposure. Hazardous materials are widespread in the modern world; vehicles, buildings, and even homes can contain hazardous materials. In addition to hazardous materials, this discussion applies equally to weapons of mass destruction. Because these dangers exist in such varied forms, all prehospital care providers must obtain a minimum of awareness-level hazardous materials training. Note that you will sometimes encounter the term hazardous materials abbreviated *hazmat* or *HazMat*.

There are four levels of hazardous materials training:

- **Awareness:** This is the first of four levels of training available to emergency responders and is designed to provide a basic level of knowledge on hazardous materials incidents.
- **Operations:** These emergency responders are trained to set up perimeters and safety zones, limiting the spread of the event. Whereas awareness represents the minimum level of training, operations-level training is helpful for all emergency responders, as it provides the training and knowledge to help control the hazardous materials event.

- **Technician**: Technicians are trained to work within the hazardous area and stop the release of hazardous materials.
- **Specialist**: This advanced level allows the emergency responder to provide command and support skills to a hazardous materials event.

Scene Safety

Prehospital care providers accept that scene safety is the first part of the approach to every patient and every scene. An important part of determining the safety of the scene is to evaluate the site for the potential of hazardous material exposure. Assessment of potential hazards should begin with dispatch. The information given by dispatch may establish a high index of suspicion. Being sent to a call that involves a large number of patients who are presenting with similar symptoms should raise the possibility of a hazardous material exposure. Additional information can be requested while en route if prehospital care providers have any concerns or questions related to the scene.

Once a scene has been determined to involve a hazardous material, the focus must shift to securing the scene and summoning appropriate help to safely isolate the involved area and remove and decontaminate exposed patients and individuals. The general simple rule is, "If the scene is not safe, make it safe." If the prehospital care provider cannot make the scene safe, help should be summoned. The *Emergency Response Guidebook* (*ERG*), produced by the U.S. Department of Transportation, or contact with an organization such as CHEMTREC, is useful to identify potential hazards **(Figure 6-5)**. The book uses a simple system that allows identification of a material by its name or identification placard number. The text then refers the reader to a guide page that provides basic information about safe distances for emergency responders, life and fire hazards, and the patient's likely complaints. CHEMTREC is available 24 hours a day, 7 days a week, and can be contacted for assistance by telephone (1-800-424-9300).

Binoculars should be used to read labels; if labels can be read without the use of viewing devices, the prehospital care provider is too close and likely to be exposed. A good rule of thumb is that if your extended thumb, held at arm's length, does not cover the entire incident scene, then you are too close.

At a hazardous materials scene, security of the site must be ensured: "Nobody in, nobody out." The staging area should be established upwind and upgrade at a safe distance from the hazard. Entry into and exit from the scene should be denied until the arrival of hazardous materials specialists. In most cases, patient care will begin when the decontaminated patient is delivered to the prehospital care provider.

It is important for the prehospital care provider to understand the command system and structure of the work zones in a hazardous materials operation **(Figure 6-6)**:

- *Hot*—The **hot zone** is the area of highest contamination, and only specially trained and protected hazardous

materials responders may enter this area. If patients are in this area, the hazardous materials team, and not the EMS personnel, will bring them out. Attempting to treat exposed victims in the hot zone prolongs the potential exposure of the rescuer, may bring the hazardous chemical directly into the patient's body by bringing the environment from the outside to the inside through either airway procedures or intravenous insertion, and contaminates all of the gear and equipment being used.

- *Warm*—A contamination reduction corridor runs through the next zone, called the **warm zone**. It is in this location that patients will be decontaminated by the hazardous materials team. From here, they will move into the cold zone.
- *Cold*—The **cold zone** is an area that is free from contamination. Patient care activities generally occur in the cold zone. The command post, treatment, and triage areas will be in the cold zone. (See the Explosions and Weapons of Mass Destruction chapter for further information.)

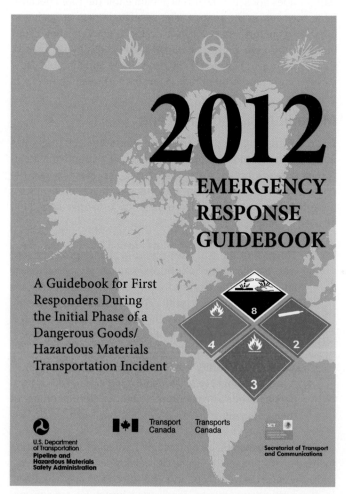

Figure 6-5 The *Emergency Response Guidebook (ERG)* produced by the U.S. Department of Transportation provides critical information at the scene of a potential hazardous materials incident. In addition to a hard copy format, the *ERG* is available as an app for smartphones.
Source: Courtesy of US DOT/ PHSMA.

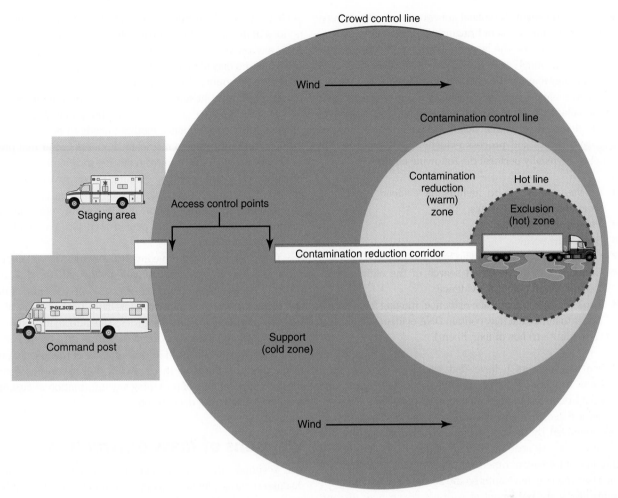

Figure 6-6 The scene of an incident involving a weapon of mass destruction or hazardous material is generally divided into hot, warm, and cold zones.

Situation Issues

There are a number of situational issues that can profoundly affect the medical care that prehospital providers are able to offer a patient.

Crime Scenes

Unfortunately, a sizable percentage of trauma patients encountered by many prehospital care providers, especially in urban settings, are injured intentionally. In addition to shootings and stabbings, patients may be victims of other types of violent crimes, including assaults with fists or blunt objects and attempted strangulation. In other cases, victims may have been intentionally struck by a vehicle or pushed from a structure or moving vehicle, resulting in significant injury. Even an MVC can be considered a crime scene if one of the drivers is thought to have been driving under the influence of alcohol or other intoxicants, driving recklessly, speeding, and, in most states, texting while driving.

When managing these types of patients, prehospital care personnel will often interact with law enforcement personnel (Figure 6-7). Although both EMS and law enforcement share

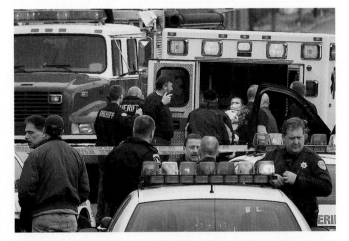

Figure 6-7 Prehospital care providers often have to manage patients at the scene of a crime and need to collaborate with law enforcement to preserve evidence.

Source: © Jason Hunt/The Coeur d'Alene Press/AP Photo.

the goal of preserving life, these parties occasionally find that their duties at a crime scene come into conflict. EMS personnel focus on the need to assess a victim for signs of life and viability, whereas law enforcement personnel are concerned with preserving evidence at a crime scene or bringing a perpetrator to justice.

With awareness of the general approach taken by law enforcement personnel at a crime scene, prehospital care providers not only may aid their patient but may better cooperate with law enforcement personnel, leading to the arrest of their patient's assailant. At the scene of a major crime (e.g., homicide, suspicious death, rape, traffic death), most law enforcement agencies will collect and process evidence. Law enforcement personnel will typically perform the following duties:

- Canvass the scene to identify all evidence, including weapons and shell casings.
- Photograph the scene.
- Sketch the scene.
- Create a log of everyone who has entered the scene.
- Conduct a more thorough search of the entire scene, looking for all potential evidence.
- Look for and collect trace evidence, ranging from fingerprints to items that may contain DNA evidence (e.g., cigarette butts, strands of hair, fibers).

Police investigators believe that everyone who enters a crime scene brings some type of evidence into a scene and unknowingly removes some evidence from the scene. To solve the crime, a detective's goal is to identify the evidence deposited and removed by the perpetrator. To accomplish this, the investigators have to account for any evidence left or removed by other law enforcement officers, EMS personnel, citizens, and anyone else who may have entered the scene. Careless behavior by prehospital care personnel at a crime scene may disrupt, destroy, or contaminate vital evidence, hampering a criminal investigation.

On occasion, prehospital care providers arrive at a potential crime scene before any law enforcement officers. If the victim is obviously dead, prehospital care providers should carefully back out of the location without touching any items and await the arrival of law enforcement. Although they would prefer that a crime scene not be disturbed, investigators realize that in some circumstances, prehospital care providers need to turn a body or move objects at a crime scene to access a patient and determine viability. If prehospital care providers needed to transport a patient or move a body or other objects in the area before the arrival of law enforcement, investigators will typically ascertain the following:

- When were the alterations made to the scene?
- What was the purpose of the movement?
- Who made the alterations?
- At what time was the victim's death identified by EMS personnel?

If prehospital care providers entered a crime scene before law enforcement personnel, investigators may want to interview and formally take a statement from the prehospital care providers regarding their actions or observations. Prehospital care providers should never be alarmed or concerned about such a request. The purpose of the interview is not to critique the actions of the prehospital care providers but to learn information that may prove helpful to the investigator in solving the case. Investigators may also request to take fingerprints of the prehospital care personnel if items in the crime scene were touched or handled by the prehospital care providers without gloves.

Proper handling of a patient's clothing may preserve valuable evidence. If a patient's clothing needs to be removed, law enforcement officers and medical examiners prefer that prehospital care providers refrain from cutting through bullet or knife holes in the clothing. If the clothing is cut, investigators may ask what alterations were made to the clothing, who made the alterations, and the reason for alterations. Any clothing that is removed should be placed in a paper (not plastic) bag and turned over to investigators.

One final important issue involving victims of violent crimes is the value of any statements made by the patient while under the care of prehospital care providers. Some patients, realizing the critical nature of their injuries, may tell prehospital care providers who inflicted their injuries. This information should be documented and passed on to investigators. If possible, prehospital care providers should inform officers of the critical nature of a patient's injuries so that a sworn officer can be present if the patient is capable of providing any information regarding the perpetrator: a "dying declaration."

Weapons of Mass Destruction

The response to a scene involving hazardous materials, as discussed earlier, includes safety and other concerns similar to the response to the scene involving a weapon of mass destruction (WMD).

Every scene that involves multiple victims or that was reported to have resulted from an explosion should trigger two questions: (1) Was a WMD was involved? and (2) Could there be a secondary device intended to harm emergency responders? In particular, when many victims complain of similar symptoms or present with similar findings, a WMD should be considered. (See the Explosions and Weapons of Mass Destruction chapter for greater detail.)

The prehospital care provider needs to approach such scenes with extreme caution and resist the urge to rush in to care for the sickest victim. This natural response of prehospital care providers only serves to increase the victim count. Instead, the prehospital care provider should approach the scene from an upwind position and take a moment to stop, look, and listen for clues indicating the possible presence of a WMD. Obvious spills of wet or dry material, visible vapors, and smoke should be avoided until the nature of the material has been ascertained. Enclosed or confined spaces should never be entered without the appropriate training and personal protective equipment (PPE). (See the Explosions and Weapons of Mass Destruction chapter for greater detail about PPE for hazardous materials and WMD incidents.)

Once a WMD has been included as a possible cause, the prehospital care provider needs to take all appropriate steps for self-protection and protection of all other responders coming to the scene. These steps include the use of PPE appropriate to the function and level of training of the individual prehospital care provider. For example, emergency responders responsible for entering the hot zone must wear the highest level of skin and respiratory protection; in the cold zone, standard precautions will suffice in most instances. Information that this may be a WMD incident should be relayed back to dispatch to alert incoming emergency responders from all services. Staging areas for additional equipment, emergency responders, and helicopters should be established upwind and at a safe distance from the site.

The scene should be secured, and zones indicating hot, warm, and cold areas should be designated. Sites for decontamination should also be determined. Once the nature of the agent has been determined (chemical, biologic, or radiologic), specific requests for antidote or antibiotics can be made.

Scene Control Zones

Just as was done at the scene of a hazardous materials incident to limit the spread of the hazardous material, the designation and use of control zones is essential at a WMD incident. Adherence to such principles reduces the likelihood of spread of contamination and injury to emergency responders and bystanders. **Figure 6-8** lists safe evacuation distances for bomb threats.

While these zones are typically illustrated as three concentric circles (see Figure 6-6), in reality, at most scenes, these zones will likely be irregularly shaped depending on the geography and wind conditions. The innermost zone, the *hot zone*, is the immediate region that contains or is adjacent to the WMD incident. The task of the properly trained emergency responders in this region is to evacuate contaminated and/or injured patients, with no provision of patient care. In order to do so, generally emergency responders must use the highest level of PPE to avoid direct exposure to the contaminant. The next zone, the *warm zone*, is where decontamination of victims, personnel, and equipment occurs. In this zone, the only patient care administered is primary assessment and spinal immobilization, as indicated. The outermost zone, the *cold zone*, is where equipment and personnel are staged. Once the patient is evacuated to the cold zone, prehospital care providers can deliver definitive patient care.

If a patient is delivered to the hospital or aid station from a hazardous materials or WMD scene, it is most prudent to re-evaluate if that patient has been decontaminated and to mimic the concepts of these zones.

Decontamination

Whether the incident involves a hazardous material or a WMD, decontamination of an exposed individual often may be required. **Decontamination** is the reduction or removal of hazardous chemical, biologic, or radiologic agents. The prehospital care provider's highest priority in the care of an exposed patient, as in any emergency, is personal and scene safety. If there is any question of a continued exposure hazard, ensuring personal safety is the first priority. Failure to do so will only produce an additional victim (the prehospital care provider) and deprive those already injured of the prehospital care provider's skills. Decontamination of the patient by appropriately trained hazardous materials technician-level personnel is the next priority. This will minimize the exposure risk to the prehospital care provider during assessment and treatment of the patient and will prevent contamination of equipment, thereby avoiding the risk of exposure of other individuals from contaminated equipment and vehicles.

OSHA provides regulatory guidelines for PPE used by prehospital care providers during the emergency care of victims in a potentially hazardous environment. Individuals providing medical care within environments of an unknown hazard must have a minimum of appropriate training and be supplied and trained with level B protection. Level B protection consists of splash-protective, chemical-resistant clothing and self-contained breathing sources. Training in advance of the need to use this level of PPE is required. (See the Explosions and Weapons of Mass Destruction chapter for greater detail about PPE for hazardous materials and WMD incidents.)

If the patient is conscious and able to assist, it is best to enlist the patient's cooperation and have the patient perform as much of the decontamination as possible to reduce the likelihood of cross-contamination to prehospital care providers. Carefully remove the patient's clothes and jewelry and place these items in plastic bags. Transfer the removed clothing carefully so as not to spread any particulate matter or splash any liquid onto noncontaminated personnel or surfaces. Brush any particulate matter off the patient, then irrigate copiously with water.

Washing with water will dilute the concentration of the potentially hazardous material and remove any remaining agent. A common axiom is, "The solution to pollution is dilution." Successful decontamination requires large amounts of water. A common mistake made by the inexperienced prehospital care provider is to irrigate (lavage) the patient with water only until the irrigating agent begins to spill onto the floor, which usually occurs after 1 or 2 liters of irrigation. This practice has two problems: The area of body contamination is increased, and the offending agent is not diluted sufficiently to render the agent harmless. Failure to provide for adequate runoff and drainage of lavage fluid may cause injury to previously unexposed areas of the body as the contaminated lavage accumulates.

Neutralizing agents for chemical burns are typically avoided. In the neutralizing process, the agents often give off heat in an exothermic reaction. Therefore, a well-meaning prehospital care provider may create a thermal burn in addition to the chemical burn. Most commercially available decontamination solutions are made for the purpose of decontaminating equipment, not people.

Secondary Devices

Within months after the bombing at the 1996 Atlanta Summer Olympics, the metropolitan area of Atlanta, Georgia, experienced

Figure 6-8   Bomb Threats: Safe Evacuation Distances

Threat Description	Explosives Capacity (TNT Capacity)	Building Evacuation Distance	Outdoor Evacuation Distance
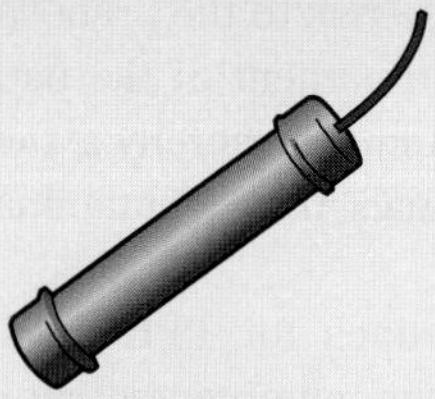 Pipe bomb	5 lb (2.3 kg)	70 ft (21.3 m)	1,200 ft (365.8 m)
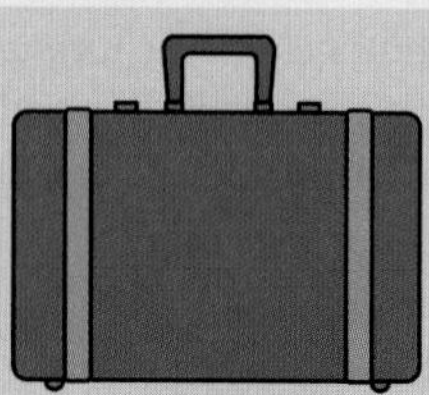 Briefcase/suitcase bomb	50 lb (22.7 kg)	150 ft (45.7 m)	1,850 ft (564 m)
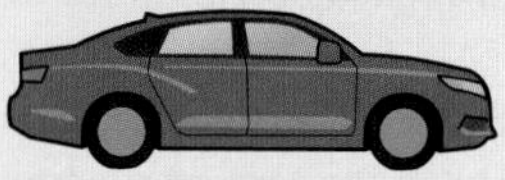 Car	500 lb (227 kg)	320 ft (97.5 m)	1,500 ft (457 m)
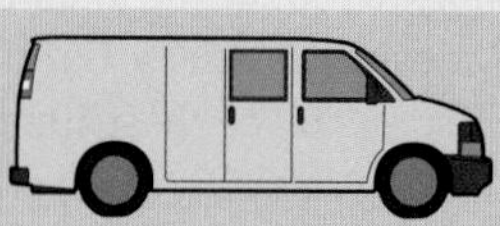 SUV/van	1,000 lb (454 kg)	400 ft (122 m)	2,400 ft (731.5 m)
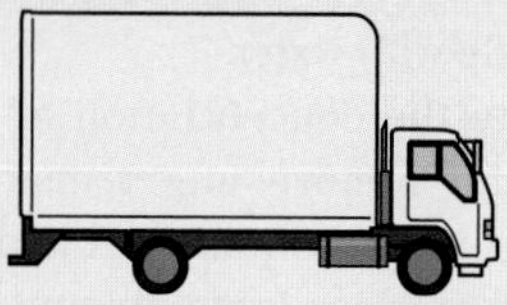 Small moving van, delivery truck	4,000 lb (1,814 kg)	640 ft (195 m)	3,800 ft (1158 m)
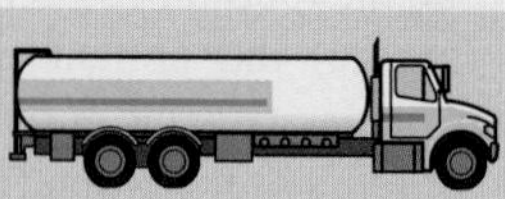 Moving van, small tank truck	10,000 lb (4,536 kg)	860 ft (262 m)	5,100 ft (1554.5 m)
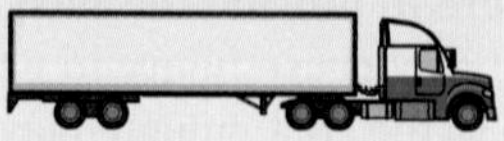 Semitrailer	60,000 lb (27216 kg)	1,570 ft (479 m)	9,300 ft (2835 m)

lb = pounds; kg = kilograms; ft = feet; m = meters.
Source: Data from U.S. Department of Homeland Security.

two additional bombings. These bombings, at an abortion clinic and a nightclub, had secondary bombs planted and represented the first time in 17 years in the United States that secondary bombs had been planted, presumably to kill or injure rescuers responding to the scene of the first blast. Unfortunately, the secondary device at the abortion clinic was not detected prior to its detonation and there were six casualties. Secondary devices have been used with regularity by terrorists in many countries. All prehospital care personnel need to be mindful of the potential presence of a secondary device.

After these incidents, the Georgia Emergency Management Agency developed the following guidelines for rescuers and prehospital care personnel responding to the scene of a bombing at which a secondary bomb might be planted:

1. *Refrain from use of electronic devices.* Sound waves from cell phones and radios may cause a secondary device to detonate, especially if used close to the bomb. Equipment used by the news media may also trigger a detonation.
2. *Ensure sufficient boundaries for the scene.* The potential zone of danger (hot zone) should extend 1,000 feet (305 meters [m]) in all directions (including vertically) from the original blast site. As more powerful bombs are created, shrapnel may travel farther. The initial bomb blast may damage infrastructure, including gas lines and power lines, which may further jeopardize the safety of emergency responders. Access to and exit from the hot zone should be carefully controlled.
3. *Provide rapid evacuation of victims from the scene and hot zone.* Because the scene of a bomb blast is considered unsafe, triage of victims should not occur in the hot zone. An EMS command post (or triage area) should be established 2,000 to 4,000 feet (610 to 1,220 m) from the scene of the initial bombing. Emergency responders can rapidly evacuate victims from the bombing site with minimal interventions until victims and emergency responders are out of the hot zone.
4. *Collaborate with law enforcement personnel on preserving and recovering evidence.* Bombing sites constitute a crime scene, and emergency responders should disrupt the scene only as necessary to evacuate victims. Any potential evidence that is inadvertently removed from the scene with a victim should be documented and turned over to law enforcement personnel to ensure proper chain of custody. Prehospital care personnel can document exactly where they were in the scene and which items they touched.

Command Structure

An ambulance responding to a call will typically have one prehospital care provider in charge (the incident commander) and another assisting in a rudimentary incident command structure. As an incident grows larger and more emergency responders from various public safety and other agencies respond to the scene, the need for a formal system and structure to oversee and control the response becomes increasingly important.

Incident Command

The **incident command system (ICS)** has developed over the years as an outgrowth of planning systems used by firefighting services for multiple-service responses to major fire situations. The program gained acceptance particularly from the experience of wildland firefighters battling expansive fire fronts, with deployment of dozens of diverse agencies. The collective experience and wisdom of their efforts resulted in FIRESCOPE, which stands for Firefighting Resources of California Organized for Potential Emergencies. In addition, the Phoenix Fire Department developed the Fire Ground Command System. Although many similarities existed between these two approaches, there were also differences, and attempts were made to combine the two systems into one comprehensive command structure.

In 1987, the NFPA published NFPA Standard 1561, the *Standard on Fire Department Incident Command Management System.* NFPA 1561 was later revised as the *Standard on Emergency Services Incident Management.* This version can be implemented and adjusted to any type or size of event by any agency managing an incident. In the 1990s, the National Fire Incident Management System (IMS) was created, which further refined the single-incident management approach.

Dealing with any incident, large or small, is enhanced by the precise command structure afforded by the ICS. At the core of the ICS are the establishment of centralized command at the scene and the subsequent buildup of divisional responsibilities. The first-arriving unit establishes the command center, and communications are established through command for the buildup of the response. The five key elements of the ICS are as follows:

1. *Command* provides overall control of the event and the communications that will coordinate the movement of resources in and patients out of the incident scene.
2. *Operations* include divisions to handle the tactical needs of the event. Fire suppression, EMS, and rescue are examples of operational divisions.
3. *Planning* is a continuous process of evaluating immediate and potential needs of the incident and planning the response. Throughout the event, this element will be used to evaluate the effectiveness of operations and to make suggested alterations in the response and tactical approach.
4. *Logistics* handles the task of acquiring resources identified by the planning section and moving them where needed. These resources include personnel, shelter, vehicles, and equipment.
5. *Finance* tracks the money. Response personnel from all involved agencies as well as contractors, personnel, and vendors brought into service in the incident will be tracked so that the cost of the event can be determined and these groups can be paid for goods, supplies, equipment, and services.

Unified Command

An expansion of the ICS is the unified command system. This expansion takes into account the needs of coordinating numerous agencies from across jurisdictional boundaries. The technical aspects of bringing resources to bear from multiple communities, counties, and states are covered by this additional coordinating structure.

National Incident Management System

On February 28, 2003, President George W. Bush directed the secretary of Homeland Security through Presidential Directive HSPD-5 to produce a National Incident Management System (NIMS). The goal of this directive is to establish a consistent, nationwide approach for federal, state, and local governments to work effectively together to prepare for, respond to, and recover from domestic incidents regardless of cause, size, or complexity. The Department of Homeland Security authorized NIMS on March 1, 2004, after collaborating with detailed working groups consisting of state and local government officials and representatives of the National Association of Emergency Medical Technicians (NAEMT), Fraternal Order of Police (FOP), International Association of Fire Chiefs (IAFC), and International Association of Emergency Managers (IAEM), as well as a wide range of other public safety organizations.[3]

NIMS focuses on the following incident management characteristics:

- Common terminology
- Modular organization
- Management by objectives
- Reliance on an incident action plan
- Manageable span of control
- Predesignated "incident mobilization center" locations and facilities
- Comprehensive resource management
- Integrated communications
- Establishment of transfer of command
- Chain of command and unity of command
- Unified command
- Accountability of resources and personnel
- Deployment
- Information and intelligence management

The key elements of NIMS are as follows:

1. ICS
2. Communications and information management
3. Preparedness
4. Joint information systems (consistent public information)
5. National Incident Management Integration Center (NIC)

Command

Command comprises the **incident commander (IC)** and command staff. Every incident should have an identified commander who oversees the response. Command staff positions to assist the IC are assigned as appropriate to the size and nature of the event and may include public information officer, safety officer, and liaison officer. Other positions can be created as deemed necessary by the IC.

As described earlier, unified command is an enhancement to incident command in situations involving multiple jurisdictions. In a single-command situation, the IC is solely responsible

for the incident management. In a unified command structure, individuals representing various jurisdictions jointly determine objectives, plans, and priorities. The unified command system seeks to solve problems involving differences in communications and operational standards **(Figure 6-9)**.

One element not included in the ICS that is added with unified command and NIMS is *intelligence*. Based on the size of the event, intelligence and information gathering related to national security may also include risk-management assessment, medical intelligence, weather information, structural design of buildings, and information on toxic containment. Although these functions are typically handled in the planning section, the IC may separate information gathering from planning in certain situations.

In NIMS, the IC can assign intelligence and information gathering as follows:

- Within the command staff
- As a unit of the planning section
- As a branch of operations
- As a separate general staff function

Incident Action Plans

Incident action plans (IAPs) include overall incident objectives and strategies established by the IC or unified command personnel. The planning section develops and documents the IAP. The IAP also addresses the tactical objectives and support activities for a designated operational period, which is generally 12 to 24 hours. The planning section also provides an ongoing critique, or "lessons learned" process, to ensure the response meets the needs of the event.

In very large incidents, multiple ICS organizations may be established. Area command may be established to manage multiple ICS organizations. Area command does not have operational responsibilities but will perform the following duties:

- Set overall incident-related priorities for the agency
- Allocate critical resources according to established priorities
- Ensure that incidents are managed properly
- Ensure effective communications
- Ensure that incident management objectives are met and do not conflict with each other or with agency policies
- Identify critical resource needs and report to the Emergency Operations Center(s)
- Ensure that short-term emergency recovery is coordinated to assist in the transition to full-recovery operations
- Provide for personnel accountability and safe operating environments

Detailed information and training programs about the ICS and NIMS can be found on the Federal Emergency Management Agency's website **(Figure 6-10)**.

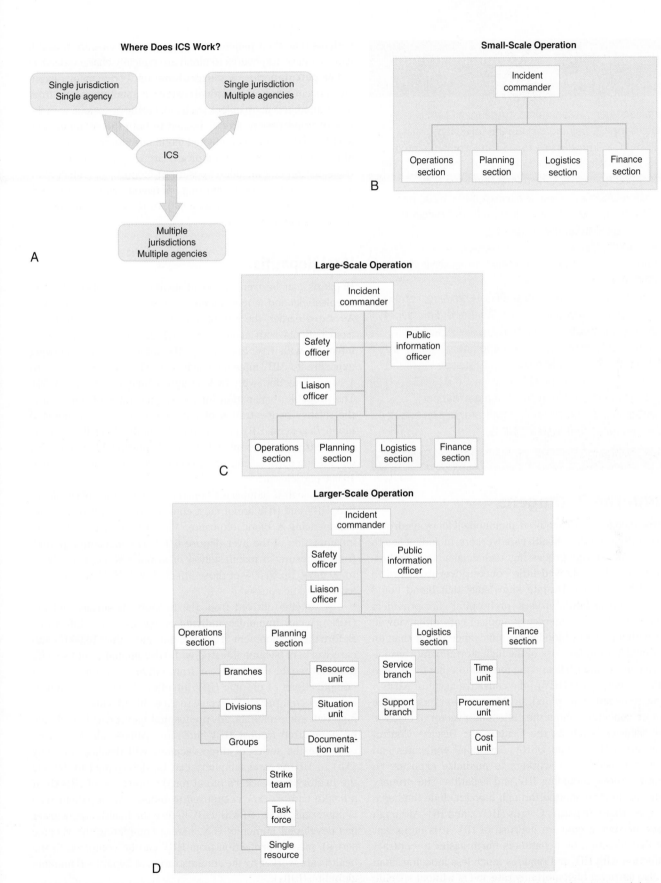

Figure 6-9 The incident command structure is flexible and can be expanded or decreased based on the number of patients and the complexity of the event. The operational functions of each of the sections under incident command are the branches. The Medical Services Branch is the operational component responsible for coordinating and providing medical services needed to meet the tactical objectives of the incident. These services include equipment and personnel management, triage, communications with medical facilities, and transport.

Figure 6-10 Incident Command Training Resources

Federal Emergency Management Agency (FEMA) resources for ICS training include the following:

- ICS-100.B, Introduction to ICS (http://training.fema .gov/EMIWeb/IS/courseOverview.aspx?code=IS-100.b)
- ICS-200.B, Basic ICS (http://training.fema.gov/ EMIWeb/IS/courseOverview.aspx?code=IS-200.b)
- ICS-700.a, NIMS, An Introduction (http://training. fema.gov/EMIWeb/IS/is700a.asp)
- ICS-800.b, National Response Framework, An Introduction (http://training.fema.gov/EMIWeb/IS/ IS800b.asp)

For information about NIMS and FEMA training, contact your state Emergency Management Agency or Emergency Management Institute and the National Fire Academy. A variety of online correspondence and onsite courses are available (http://training.fema.gov/IS/crslist.asp).

For more information on NIMS, contact the NIMS Integrations Center (http://www.fema.gov/national-incident-management-system). Data from the National Incident Management System. (NIMS)

Bloodborne Pathogens

Before the recognition of acquired immunodeficiency syndrome (AIDS) in the early 1980s, health care workers, including health care providers, sterile processing technicians, and prehospital care providers, showed little concern over exposure to blood and body fluids. Despite knowledge that blood could transmit certain hepatitis viruses, prehospital care providers and others involved in emergency medical care often viewed contact with a patient's blood as an annoyance rather than an occupational hazard. Because of the high mortality rate associated with contracting AIDS and the recognition that the human immunodeficiency virus (HIV)—the causative agent of AIDS—could be transmitted in blood, health care workers became much more concerned about the patient as a vector of disease. Federal agencies, such as the Centers for Disease Control and Prevention (CDC) and OSHA, developed guidelines and mandates for health care workers to minimize exposure to bloodborne illness, including HIV and hepatitis. The primary infectious agents transmitted through blood include the hepatitis B virus (HBV), hepatitis C virus (HCV), and HIV. Although this issue became a concern because of HIV, it is important to note that infection by hepatitis is much easier to contract than infection with HIV and requires much less inoculum than HIV. It also carries a high mortality rate and is without specific treatment.

Epidemiologic data demonstrate that health care workers are much more likely to contract bloodborne illness from their patients than their patients are to contract disease from health care workers. Exposures to blood are typically characterized as either **percutaneous** or **mucocutaneous**. Percutaneous exposures occur when an individual sustains a puncture wound from a contaminated sharp object, such as a needle or scalpel, with the risk of transmission directly related to both the contaminating agent and the volume of infected blood introduced by the injury. Mucocutaneous exposures typically are less likely to result in transmission and include exposure of blood to nonintact skin, such as a soft-tissue wound (e.g., abrasion, superficial laceration) or a skin condition (e.g., acne), or to mucous membranes (e.g., conjunctiva of eye).

Viral Hepatitis

Hepatitis can be transmitted to health care workers through needlesticks and mucocutaneous exposures on nonintact skin. As stated earlier, the rate of infection after exposure to blood from patients with hepatitis is much greater than the rate of infection with HIV. Specifically, the infection rates following exposure to HBV-infected needles is 23% to 62% (1 in 4 to 1 in 2). Infection with HCV is approximately 1.8% (1 in 50). The probable explanation for the varying rates of infection is the relative concentration of virus particles found in infected blood. In general, HBV-positive blood contains 100 million to one billion virus particles/mL, whereas HCV-positive blood contains one million particles/mL, and HIV-positive blood contains 100 to 10,000 particles/mL.

Although a number of hepatitis viruses have been identified, HBV and HCV are of most concern to health care workers experiencing a blood exposure. Viral hepatitis causes acute inflammation of the liver **(Figure 6-11)**. The incubation period, from exposure to manifestation of symptoms, is generally 60 to 90 days. Up to 30% of those infected with HBV may have an asymptomatic course.

A vaccine derived from the hepatitis B surface antigen (HBsAg) can immunize individuals against HBV infection.[4] Before the development of this vaccine, more than 10,000 health care workers became infected with HBV annually, and several hundred would die each year from either severe hepatitis or complications of chronic HBV infection. OSHA now requires employers to offer HBV vaccine to those health care workers in high-risk environments. All prehospital care providers should be immunized against HBV infection. Almost all those who complete the series of three vaccines will develop antibody (Ab) to HBsAg, and immunity can be determined by testing the health care worker's blood for the presence of HBsAb. If a health care worker is exposed to blood from a patient who is potentially infected with HBV before the health care worker has developed immunity (i.e., before completing the vaccine series), passive protection from HBV can be conferred to the health care worker by the administration of hepatitis B immune globulin (HBIG).

At present, no immune globulin or vaccine is available to protect health care workers from exposure to HCV, emphasizing the need for using standard precautions.

Figure 6-11 Hepatitis

The clinical manifestations of viral hepatitis are right upper-quadrant pain, fatigue, loss of appetite, nausea, vomiting, and alteration in liver function. Jaundice, a yellowish coloration of the skin, results from an increased level of bilirubin in the bloodstream. Although most individuals with hepatitis recover without serious problems, a small percentage of patients develop acute fulminant hepatic failure and may die. A significant number of those who recover will develop a carrier state in which their blood can transmit the virus.

As with HBV infection, infection with HCV can range from a mild, asymptomatic course to liver failure and death. The incubation period for hepatitis C is somewhat shorter than for hepatitis B, typically 6 to 9 weeks. Chronic infections with HCV are much more common than with HBV, and about 80% to 85% of those who contract HCV will develop persistently abnormal liver function, predisposing them to hepatocellular carcinoma. Hepatitis C is primarily transmitted through blood, whereas hepatitis B can be transmitted through blood or sexual contact. About two-thirds of intravenous drug abusers have been infected with HCV. Before routine testing of donated blood for presence of HBV and HCV, blood transfusion was the primary reason patients contracted hepatitis.

Figure 6-12 Human Immunodeficiency Virus

Two serotypes of HIV have been identified. HIV-1 accounts for virtually all AIDS in the United States and equatorial Africa, and HIV-2 is found almost exclusively in Western Africa. Although early victims of HIV were male homosexuals, intravenous drug users, or hemophiliacs, HIV disease is now found in many teenage and adult heterosexual populations, with the fastest-growing numbers in minority communities. The screening test for HIV is very sensitive, and false-positive tests occasionally occur. All positive screening tests should be confirmed with a more specific technique (e.g., Western blot electrophoresis).

After infection with HIV, when patients develop one of the opportunistic infections or cancers, they transition from being HIV positive to having AIDS. In the last decade, significant advances have been made in the treatment of HIV disease, primarily in developing new drugs to combat its effects. This progress has enabled many individuals with HIV infection to lead fairly normal lives because the progression of the disease is slowed dramatically.

Although health care workers typically are more concerned about contracting HIV because of its uniformly fatal prognosis, they are at greater risk of contracting HBV or HCV.

Human Immunodeficiency Virus

After infection, HIV targets the immune system of its new host. Over time, the number of certain types of white blood cells falls dramatically, leaving the individual prone to developing unusual infections or cancers **(Figure 6-12)**.

Only about 0.3% (about 1 in 300) of needlestick exposures to HIV-positive blood lead to infection. The risk of infection appears higher with exposure to a larger quantity of blood, exposure to blood from a patient with a more advanced stage of disease, a deep percutaneous injury, or an injury from a hollow-bore, blood-filled needle. HIV is primarily transmitted through infected blood or semen, but vaginal secretions and pericardial, peritoneal, pleural, amniotic, and cerebrospinal fluids are all considered potentially infected. Unless obvious blood is present, tears, urine, sweat, feces, and saliva are generally considered noninfectious.

Standard Precautions

Because clinical examination cannot reliably identify all patients who pose a potential infection threat to health care workers, standard precautions were developed to prevent health care workers from coming into direct contact with a patient's blood or body fluid (e.g., saliva, vomit). At the same time, these precautions help protect the patient from infections the prehospital care provider may have. OSHA has developed regulations that mandate employers and their employees to follow standard precautions in the workplace. Standard precautions consist of both physical barriers to blood and body fluid and exposure as well as safe-handling practices for needles and other "sharps." Because trauma patients often have external hemorrhage and because blood is an extremely high-risk body fluid, appropriate protective devices should be worn by prehospital care providers while caring for patients.

Physical Barriers
Gloves

Gloves should be worn when touching nonintact skin, mucous membranes, or areas contaminated by gross blood or other body fluids. Because perforations may readily occur in gloves while caring for a patient, gloves should be examined regularly for defects and changed immediately if a problem is noted **(Figure 6-13)**. Gloves should also be changed between contact with each patient at a multiple-casualty incident.

Masks and Face Shields

Masks serve to protect the health care worker's oral and nasal mucous membranes from exposure to infectious agents, especially in situations in which airborne pathogens are known or suspected. Masks and face shields should be changed immediately if they become wet or soiled.

Eye Protection

Eye protection must be worn in circumstances in which droplets of potentially infected fluid or blood may be splattered, such as while providing airway management to a patient with blood in the oropharynx or when dealing with any open wounds. Standard eyeglasses are not considered adequate because they lack side shields.

Gowns

Disposable gowns with impervious plastic liners offer the best protection, but they may be extremely uncomfortable and impractical in the prehospital environment. Gowns or clothing should be changed immediately if significant soilage occurs.

Resuscitation Equipment

Health care workers should have access to bag-mask devices or mouthpieces to protect them from direct contact with a patient's saliva, blood, and vomit.

Hand Washing

Hand washing is a fundamental principle of infection control. Hands should be washed with soap and running water if gross contamination with blood or body fluid occurs. Alcohol-based hand antiseptics are useful toward preventing transmission of many infectious agents but are not appropriate for situations in which obvious soiling has occurred; however, they can provide some cleansing and protective effect in situations in which running water and soap are not available. After removal of gloves, hands should be cleansed with either soap and water or an alcohol-based antiseptic.

Preventing Sharps Injury

As noted earlier, percutaneous exposure to a patient's blood or body fluid constitutes a significant manner in which viral infections could be transmitted to health care workers. Many percutaneous exposures are caused by injuries from needlesticks with contaminated needles or other sharps. Eliminate unnecessary needles and sharps, never recap a used needle, and implement safety devices such as needleless intravenous systems when possible **(Figure 6-14)**.

Management of Occupational Exposure

In the United States, OSHA mandates that every organization providing health care have a control plan for managing occupational exposures of its employees to blood and body fluids. Each exposure should be thoroughly documented, including the type of injury and estimation of the volume of inoculate. If a health care worker has a mucocutaneous or percutaneous exposure to blood or sustains an injury from a contaminated sharp, efforts are taken to prevent bacterial infection, including tetanus, HBV, and HIV infection. No prophylactic therapy to prevent HCV infection is currently approved or available. **Figure 6-15** describes a typical blood and body-fluid exposure protocol.

Patient Assessment and Triage

Once all the preceding issues have been addressed, the actual process of assessing and treating patients can begin. The greatest

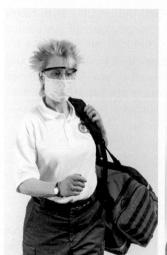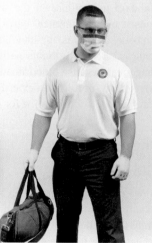

Figure 6-13 At a minimum, PPE for prehospital care providers should consist of gloves, mask, and eye protection. **A.** Goggles, face mask, and gloves. **B.** Face shield, face mask, and gloves.
Source: © Jones & Bartlett Learning. Photographed by Darren Stahlman.

Figure 6-14 Preventing Sharps Injury

Prehospital care providers are at significant risk for injury from needles and other sharps. Strategies for reducing sharps injuries include the following:

- Use safety devices, such as shielded or retracting needles and scalpels and automatically retracting lancets.
- Use "needleless" systems that allow injection of medication at ports without needles.
- Refrain from recapping needles and other sharps.
- Immediately dispose of contaminated needles into rigid sharps containers rather than setting them down or handing them to someone else for disposal.
- Use prefilled medication syringes rather than drawing medication from an ampule.
- Provide a written exposure control plan and ensure that all employees are aware of the plan.
- Maintain a sharps injury log.

challenge occurs when the prehospital care provider is faced with multiple victims.

Mass-casualty incidents (MCIs) occur in many sizes. Most emergency responders have responded to incidents with more than one victim, but large-scale events with hundreds or thousands of victims are rarely encountered.

Triage is a French word meaning "to sort." Triage is a process that is used to assign priority for treatment and transport. In the prehospital environment, triage is used in two different contexts:

1. *Sufficient resources are available to manage all patients.* In this triage situation, the most severely injured patients are treated and transported first, and those with lesser injuries are treated and transported later.
2. *The number of patients exceeds the immediate capacity of on-scene resources.* The objective in such triage situations is to ensure survival of the largest possible number of injured patients. Patients are sorted into categories for patient care. In an MCI, patient care must be rationed because the number of patients exceeds the available resources. Relatively few prehospital care providers ever experience an MCI with 50 to 100 or more simultaneously injured persons, but many will be involved in MCIs with 10 to 20 patients, and most prehospital care providers have managed an incident with 2 to 10 patients.

Incidents that involve sufficient emergency responders and medical resources allow for treatment and transport of the most severely injured patients first. In a large-scale MCI, limited resources will require that patient treatment and transport be prioritized to salvage the victims with the greatest chance of survival. These victims are prioritized for treatment and transport **(Figure 6-16)**.

The goal of patient management at the MCI scene is to do the most good for the most patients with the resources available. It is the responsibility of the prehospital care provider to make decisions about who is to be managed first. The usual rules about saving lives are different in MCIs. The decision is always to save the most lives; however, when the available resources are not sufficient for the needs of all the injured patients present, these resources should be used for the patients who have the best chance of surviving. In a choice between a patient with a catastrophic injury, such as severe brain trauma, and a patient with acute intra-abdominal hemorrhage, the proper course of action in an MCI is to manage first the salvageable patient—the patient with the abdominal hemorrhage. Treating the patient with severe head trauma first will probably result in the loss of both patients; the head trauma patient may die because he or she may not be salvageable, and the abdominal hemorrhage patient may die because time, equipment, and EMS personnel spent managing the unsalvageable patient kept this salvageable patient from receiving the simple care needed to survive until definitive surgical care was available.

Figure 6-15 Sample Exposure Protocol

After a percutaneous or mucocutaneous exposure to blood or other potentially infected body fluids, taking the appropriate actions and instituting appropriate postexposure prophylaxis (PEP) can help minimize the potential for acquiring viral hepatitis or HIV infection. Appropriate steps include:

1. Prevent bacterial infection.
    - Cleanse exposed skin thoroughly with germicidal soap and water; exposed mucous membranes (mouth, eyes) should be irrigated with copious amounts of water.
    - Administer tetanus toxoid booster, if not received in previous 5 years.
2. Perform baseline laboratory studies on both the exposed health care worker and the source patient, if known.
    - Health care worker: Hepatitis B surface antibody (HBsAb), HCV, and HIV tests.
    - Source patient: Hepatitis B and C serology and HIV test.
3. Prevent HBV infection.
    - If the health care worker has not been immunized against hepatitis B, the first dose of HBV vaccine is administered along with hepatitis B immune globulin (HBIG).

- If the health care worker has begun but not yet completed the HBV vaccine series, or if the health care worker has completed all HBV immunizations, HBIG is given if the HBsAb test fails to show the presence of protective antibodies and the source patient's tests demonstrate active infection with HBV. HBIG may be administered up to 7 days after an exposure and still be effective.
4. Prevent HIV infection.
    - PEP depends upon the route of exposure (percutaneous versus mucocutaneous) and the likelihood and severity of HIV infection in the source patient. If the source patient is known to be negative, PEP is not indicated regardless of exposure route. In the past, when recommended, PEP has generally involved a two-drug regimen. With the development of numerous antiretroviral medications, the number of drug regimen combinations has increased. In addition, three-drug treatment is warranted in specific cases involving high risk of transmission. Therefore, it is recommended that an exposed prehospital care provider be evaluated by an expert to determine the most appropriate PEP regimen, given the circumstances of the particular exposure.

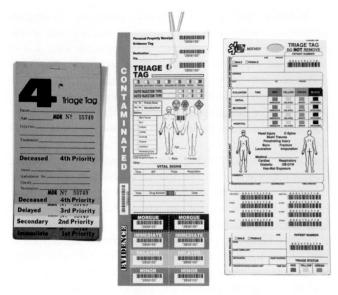

Figure 6-16 Examples of triage tags.

Source: © File of Life Foundation, Inc.

In a triage MCI situation, the catastrophically injured patient may need to be considered" "lower priority," with treatment delayed until more help and equipment become available. These are difficult decisions and circumstances, but a prehospital care provider must respond quickly and properly. EMS personnel should not make efforts to resuscitate a traumatic cardiac arrest patient with little or no chance of survival while three other patients die because of airway compromise or external hemorrhage. The "sorting scheme" most often used divides patients into five categories based on need of care and chance of survival:

1. *Immediate*—Patients whose injuries are critical, but who will require only minimal time or equipment to manage and who have a good prognosis for survival. An example is the patient with a compromised airway or massive external hemorrhage.
2. *Delayed*—Patients whose injuries are debilitating, but who do not require immediate management to salvage life or limb. An example is the patient with a long-bone fracture.
3. *Minor*—Patients, often called the "walking wounded," who have minor injuries that can wait for treatment or who may even assist in the interim by comforting other patients or helping as litter bearers.
4. *Expectant*—Patients whose injuries are so severe that they have only a minimal chance of survival. An example is the patient with a 90% full-thickness burn and thermal pulmonary injury.
5. *Dead*—Patients who are unresponsive, pulseless, and breathless. In a disaster, resources rarely allow for attempted resuscitation of cardiac arrest patients.

Figures 6-17 through **6-19** describe a commonly used triage scheme known as START, which uses only four categories: immediate, delayed, minor, and dead. (For more information on the START triage system, see the Disaster Management chapter.)

Figures 6-20 and **6-21** describe the recently published SALT triage system. [5]

Figure 6-17   START Triage

In 1983, medical personnel from Hoag Memorial Hospital and fire fighter–paramedics from the Newport Beach Fire Department created a triage process for emergency medical responders, Simple Triage and Rapid Treatment (START) (see Figure 6-18). This triage process was designed to identify critically injured patients easily and quickly. START does not establish a medical diagnosis, but instead provides a rapid and simple sorting process. START uses three simple assessments to identify those victims most at risk to die from their injuries. Typically, the process takes 30 to 60 seconds per victim. START requires no tools, specialized medical equipment, or special knowledge.

How Does START Work?

The first step is to direct anyone who can walk to a designated safe area. If the victims can walk and follow commands, their condition is categorized as minor, and they will be further triaged and tagged when more rescuers arrive. This initial sorting leads to a smaller group of presumably more seriously injured victims remaining to triage. The

mnemonic "30-2-can do" is used as the START triage prompt (see Figure 6-19). The "30" refers to the victim's respiratory rate, the "2" refers to capillary refill, and the "can do" refers to the ability of the victim to follow commands. Any victim with respirations fewer than 30 per minute, capillary refill of less than 2 seconds, and the ability to follow verbal commands and to walk is categorized as minor. When victims meet these criteria but cannot walk, they are categorized as delayed. Victims who are unconscious or have rapid breathing, or who have delayed capillary refill or absent radial pulse are categorized as immediate.

While at the victim's side, two basic lifesaving measures can be performed: opening the airway and controlling external hemorrhage. For those victims who are not breathing, the prehospital care provider should open the airway, and if breathing resumes, the victim is categorized as immediate. No cardiopulmonary resuscitation (CPR) should be attempted. If the victim does not resume breathing, the victim is categorized as dead. Bystanders or the "walking wounded" can be directed by the prehospital

(Continues on next page)

Figure 6-17 START Triage (*Continued*)

care provider to help maintain the airway and hemorrhage control.

Retriage is also needed if lack of transportation prolongs the time the victims remain at the scene. Using START criteria, significantly injured victims may be categorized as delayed. The longer they remain without treatment, the greater the chance their condition will deteriorate. Therefore, repeat evaluation and triage are appropriate over time.

Source: Courtesy of Hoag Hospital Newport Beach and the Newport Beach Fire Department.

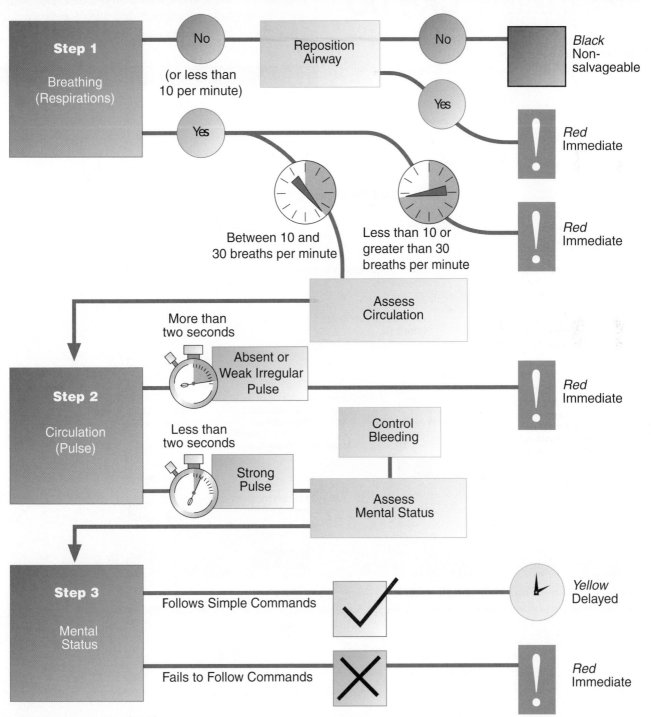

Figure 6-18 START triage algorithm.

Source: Courtesy of Hoag Hospital Newport Beach and the Newport Beach Fire Department.

Respirations **30**

Perfusion **2**

Mental status **CAN DO**

Figure 6-19 START triage algorithm.

Source: Courtesy of Hoag Hospital Newport Beach and the Newport Beach Fire Department.

Figure 6-20   SALT Triage

The SALT triage scheme was developed by the CDC in conjunction with an expert panel representing a large constituency of medical organizations. The intent of the project was to develop a triage methodology that would serve as a basis for a nationally agreed-upon triage system. This system begins by using a global sorting process: asking victims to walk or wave (follow commands). Those victims who do not respond are then assessed for life threats and subsequently categorized into immediate, delayed, minimal, or dead (see Figure 6-21).

SALT Mass Casualty Triage

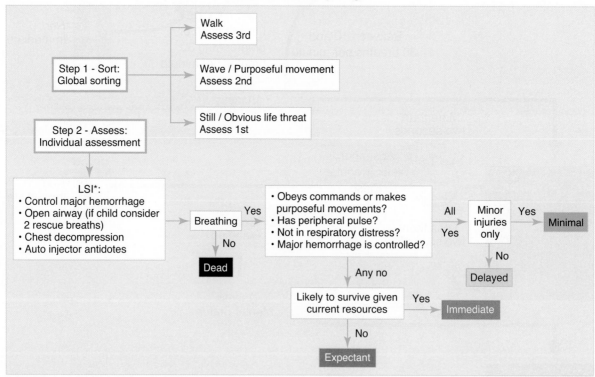

Figure 6-21 SALT triage algorithm. Note: LSI stands for life-saving interventions.

Source: Chemical Hazards Emergency Medical Management, U.S. Department of Health & Human Services, http://chemm.nlm.nih.gov/chemmimages/salt.png.

Summary

- As a part of assessing the scene for safety in each and every patient contact, it is important to assess for hazards of all types. Hazards include traffic issues, environmental concerns, violence, bloodborne pathogens, and hazardous materials.
- Assessing the scene will assure that EMS personnel and equipment are not compromised and unavailable for others and ensure that other emergency responders are protected from hazards that are not isolated or removed.
- Sometimes hazards will be ruled out quickly, but if they are not looked for, they will not be seen, and this can cause harm.
- Certain situations such as crime scenes or intentional acts including the use of weapons of mass destruction will affect how the prehospital care provider deals with the scene and the patients at that scene.
- Incidents will be managed using an incident command system (ICS) structure, and EMS is one of the components in that structure. Prehospital care providers must know and understand the ICS and their role within that system.

SCENARIO RECAP

You are dispatched to the scene of a domestic altercation. It is 0245 hours on a hot summer night. As you arrive on the scene of a single-family dwelling, you can hear a man and woman arguing very loudly and the sounds of children crying in the background. Police have also been dispatched to this call but have not yet arrived to the location.

- What are your concerns about the scene?
- What considerations are important before you contact the patient?

SCENARIO SOLUTION

Assessment of the scene reveals several potential hazards. Domestic violence incidents are among the most hazardous to emergency responders. These incidents often escalate and can lead to assault of emergency responders. Therefore the presence of law enforcement should be considered prior to entering the scene. As with all trauma cases, a bloody patient exposes prehospital care providers to the risks of bloodborne infections, and the prehospital care providers should wear physical barriers, including gloves, masks, and eye protection.

In this case, you wait until the police arrive before entering the home. Upon entering the house, you note that the female has obvious multiple bruises on her face and a small laceration over one cheek. The officers take the male into custody. You perform your primary assessment, which reveals no life-threats. The secondary assessment does not reveal any additional injuries. You transport the patient to the closest hospital without incident.

References

1. National Incident Management System. U.S. Department of Homeland Security, 2008. www.fema.gov/pdf/emergency/nims/NIMS_core.pdf. Accessed November 24, 2013.
2. Maguire BJ, Hunting KL, Smith GS, et al. Occupational fatalities in emergency medical services. *Ann Emerg Med.* 2002;40(6):625.
3. Schaeffer J. Prevent run downs: best practices for roadside incident management, 2002. www.jems.com/jems/news02/0903a.html. Accessed September 2002.
4. Poland GA, Jacobson RM. Prevention of hepatitis B with the hepatitis B vaccine. *N Engl J Med.* 2004;351:2832.
5. Lerner EB, Schwartz RB, Coule PL, et al. Mass casualty triage: an evaluation of the data and development of a proposed national guideline. *Disaster Med Public Health Prep.* 2008;2:S25–S34.

Suggested Reading

Centers for Disease Control and Prevention: See website for information on standard precautions and postexposure prophylaxis, http://www.cdc.gov.

Rinnert KJ. A review of infection control practices, risk reduction, and legislative regulations for blood-borne disease: applications for emergency medical services. *Prehosp Emerg Care.*1998;2(1):70.

Rinnert KJ, O'Connor RE, Delbridge T. Risk reduction for exposure to blood-borne pathogens in EMS: National Association of EMS Physicians. *Prehosp Emerg Care.*1998;2(1):62.

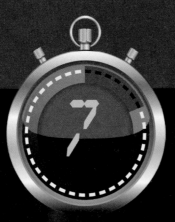

CHAPTER 7

Patient Assessment and Management

CHAPTER OBJECTIVES

At the completion of this chapter, the reader will be able to do the following:

- Relate the significance of patient assessment in the context of overall management of the trauma patient.

- Explain how assessment and management are integrated during the primary assessment.

- Describe the components of the secondary assessment and when it is used in the assessment of the trauma patient.

- Utilize the Field Triage Decision Scheme to determine destination for a trauma patient.

SCENARIO

It is a Saturday morning in early November. The weather is clear, with an outside temperature of 42°F (5.5°C). Your squad is dispatched to a residential area for a person who has fallen from the roof of a two-story building. Upon arrival at the scene, you are met by an adult family member who leads you around the house to the backyard. The family member states the patient was cleaning leaves from the rain gutters with a leaf blower when he lost his balance and fell approximately 12 feet (3.6 meters) from the roof, landing on his back. The patient initially lost consciousness for a "brief period" but was conscious by the time the family member called 9-1-1.

Approaching the patient, you observe an approximately 40-year-old man lying supine on the ground with two bystanders kneeling by his side. The patient is conscious and talking with the bystanders. As your partner provides manual stabilization to the patient's head and neck, you ask the patient where he hurts. The patient states both his upper and lower back hurt the most.

Your initial questioning serves the multiple purposes of obtaining the patient's chief complaint, determining his initial level of consciousness, and assessing his ventilatory effort. Detecting no shortness of breath, you proceed with the patient assessment. The patient answers your questions appropriately to establish that he is oriented to person, place, and time.

- Based on kinematics as they relate to this incident, what potential injuries do you anticipate finding during your assessment?
- What are your next priorities?
- How will you proceed with this patient?

Introduction

Assessment is the cornerstone of all patient care. For the trauma patient, as for other critically ill patients, assessment is the foundation on which all management and transport decisions are based. The first goal in assessment is to determine a patient's current condition. In doing so, an overall impression of a patient's status is developed and baseline values for the status of the patient's respiratory, circulatory, and neurologic systems established. When life-threatening conditions are identified, urgent intervention and resuscitation are initiated. If the patient's condition allows, a secondary assessment is conducted for injuries that are not life or limb threatening. Often this secondary assessment occurs during patient transport.

All of these steps are performed quickly and efficiently with a goal of minimizing time spent on the scene. Critical patients should not remain in the field for care other than that needed to stabilize them for transport, unless they are trapped or other complications exist that prevent early transport. By applying the principles learned in this course, on-scene delay can be minimized and patients can be moved rapidly to an appropriate medical facility. Successful assessment and intervention require a strong knowledge base of trauma physiology and a well-developed plan of management that is carried out quickly and effectively.

The trauma management literature frequently mentions the need to transport the trauma patient to definitive surgical care within an absolute minimum amount of time after the onset of the injury. This urgency is because a critical trauma patient who does not respond to initial therapy is most likely bleeding internally. This blood loss will continue until the hemorrhage is controlled. Except for the most basic external bleeding, hemorrhage control can be accomplished only in the operating room (OR).

The primary concerns for assessment and management of the trauma patient are: (1) airway, (2) oxygenation, (3) ventilation, (4) hemorrhage control, (5) perfusion, and (6) neurologic function. This sequence protects the ability of the body to oxygenate and the ability of the red blood cells (RBCs) to deliver oxygen to the tissues. Hemorrhage control, which is only temporary in the field, but permanent in the OR, depends on rapid transport by the prehospital care providers and the presence of a trauma team that is immediately available on arrival at the medical facility.

R Adams Cowley, MD, developed the concept of the "Golden Hour" of trauma. He believed that the time between injury occurrence and definitive care was critical. During this period, when bleeding is uncontrolled and inadequate tissue oxygenation is occurring because of decreased perfusion, damage occurs throughout the body. Dr. Cowley believed that if bleeding was not controlled and tissue oxygenation was not restored within one hour of the injury, the patient's chances of survival dramatically decreased.

The Golden Hour is now referred to as the "Golden Period" because this critical period of time is not necessarily one hour. Some patients have less than an hour in which to receive care, whereas others have more time. The prehospital care provider is responsible for recognizing the urgency of a given situation and transporting a patient as quickly as possible to a facility in which definitive care can be accomplished. To deliver the trauma patient to definitive care, the seriousness of the patient's life-threatening injuries must be quickly identified; only essential, lifesaving care at the scene provided; and rapid transport to an appropriate medical facility undertaken. In many urban prehospital systems, the average time between injury and arrival to the scene is 8 to 9 minutes. Usually another 8 to 9 minutes are spent transporting the patient. If the prehospital care providers spend only 10 minutes on the scene, 30 minutes of the Golden Period will have passed by the time a patient arrives at the receiving facility. Every additional minute spent on the scene is additional time that the patient is bleeding, and valuable time is ticking away from the Golden Period.

To address this critical trauma management issue, quick, efficient evaluation and management of the patient is the ultimate objective. Scene time should not exceed 10 minutes whenever possible; the shorter the scene time, the better. The longer the patient is kept on scene, the greater the potential for blood loss and death. These time parameters change as delayed extrication, delayed transport, and other unexpected circumstances arise.

This chapter covers the essentials of patient assessment and initial management in the field and is based on the approach taught to physicians in the Advanced Trauma Life Support (ATLS) program.[1] The principles described are identical to those learned in initial basic- or advanced-provider training programs, although different terminology may occasionally be used. For example, the phrase *primary survey* is used in the ATLS program to describe the patient assessment activity known as *primary assessment* in the National EMS Education Standards. For the most part, the activities performed in this phase are exactly the same; various courses simply use different terminology.

Establishing Priorities

There are three immediate priorities on arrival to a scene:

1. The first priority for everyone involved at a trauma incident is assessment of the scene. The Scene Assessment chapter discusses this in detail.

2. Responders must recognize the existence of multiple-patient incidents and mass-casualty incidents (MCIs). In an MCI, the priority shifts from focusing all resources on the most injured patient to saving the maximum number of patients (providing the greatest good to the greatest number). Factors that may impact the triage decisions when there are multiple patients include severity of the injuries and the resources (manpower and equipment) available to care for the patients. The Scene Assessment chapter and the Disaster Management chapter also discuss triage.

3. Once a brief scene assessment has been performed, attention can be turned to evaluating individual patients. The assessment and management process begins by focusing on the patient or patients who have been identified as most critical, as resources allow. Emphasis is placed on the following, in this order: (a) conditions that may result in the loss of life, (b) conditions that may result in the loss of limb, and (c) all other conditions that do not threaten life or limb. Depending on the severity of the injury, the number of injured patients, and the proximity to the receiving facility, conditions that do not threaten life or limb may never be addressed.

Most of this chapter focuses on the critical-thinking skills required to conduct a proper assessment, interpret the findings, and set priorities for proper patient care. This process will allow for the appropriate provision of needed interventions.

Primary Assessment

In the critical multisystem trauma patient, the priority for care is the rapid identification and management of life-threatening conditions (**Figure 7-1**). More than 90% of trauma patients have simple injuries that involve only one system (e.g., an isolated limb fracture). For these single-system trauma patients, there is time to be thorough in both the primary and the secondary assessment. For the critically injured patient, the prehospital care provider may not conduct more than a primary assessment.

Figure 7-1   Multisystem Versus Single-System Trauma Patient

- A **multisystem trauma patient** has injuries involving more than one body system, including the pulmonary, circulatory, neurologic, gastrointestinal, musculoskeletal, and integumentary systems. An example would be a patient involved in a motor vehicle crash who has a traumatic brain injury, pulmonary contusions, a splenic injury with shock, and a femur fracture.
- A **single-system trauma patient** has injury to only one body system. An example would be a patient with a simple ankle fracture and no evidence of blood loss or shock.

The emphasis is on rapid evaluation, initiation of resuscitation, and transport to an appropriate medical facility. This urgency does not eliminate the need for prehospital management; it means that it needs to be done faster, done more efficiently, and done en route to the receiving facility.

Quick establishment of priorities and the initial evaluation and recognition of life-threatening injuries must become ingrained in the prehospital care provider. Therefore, the components of the primary and secondary assessments need to be memorized and the logical progression of priority-based assessment and treatment understood and performed the same way every time, regardless of the severity of the injury. The prehospital care provider must think about the pathophysiology of a patient's injuries and conditions; he or she cannot waste time trying to remember which priorities are the most important.

The most common basis of life-threatening injuries is lack of adequate tissue oxygenation, which leads to anaerobic (without oxygen) metabolism (energy production). Decreased energy production that occurs with anaerobic metabolism is termed shock. Four components are necessary for normal metabolism: (1) an adequate amount of RBCs available and maintained, (2) oxygenation of RBCs in the lungs, (3) delivery of RBCs to the cells throughout the body, and (4) off-loading of oxygen to these cells. The activities involved in the primary assessment are aimed at identifying and correcting problems with the first two components.

General Impression

The primary assessment begins with a simultaneous, or global, overview of the status of a patient's respiratory, circulatory, and neurologic systems to identify obvious, significant external problems with oxygenation and circulation, hemorrhage, or gross deformities. When initially approaching a patient, the prehospital care provider observes whether the patient appears to be moving air effectively, is awake or unresponsive, is holding him- or herself up, and is moving spontaneously. Once at the patient's side, the prehospital care provider introduces him- or herself to the patient and asks the patient's name. A reasonable next step is to ask the patient, "What happened to you?" If the patient appears comfortable and answers with a coherent explanation in complete sentences, the prehospital care provider can conclude that the patient has a **patent airway**, sufficient respiratory function to support speech, adequate cerebral perfusion, and reasonable neurologic functioning; that is, there are probably no immediate threats to this patient's life.

If a patient is unable to provide such an answer or appears in distress, a detailed primary assessment to identify life-threatening problems is begun. Within a few seconds, a general impression of the patient's overall condition has been obtained. By rapidly assessing vital functions, the primary assessment serves to establish whether the patient is presently or imminently in a critical condition.

The primary assessment must proceed rapidly and in a logical order. If the prehospital care provider is alone, some key interventions may be performed as life-threatening conditions are identified. If the problem is easily correctable, such as suctioning an airway or placing a tourniquet, the prehospital care provider may opt to address the issue before moving on to the next step. Conversely, if the problem cannot be quickly addressed at the scene, such as shock resulting from suspected internal hemorrhage, the final steps of the primary assessment are expeditiously completed. If more than one prehospital care provider is present, one may complete the primary assessment while others initiate care for the problems identified. When several critical conditions are identified, the primary assessment allows the prehospital care provider to establish treatment priorities. In general, an airway issue is managed before a breathing problem, and so forth.

The same primary assessment approach is utilized regardless of the patient type. All patients, including elderly, pediatric, or pregnant patients, are assessed in a similar fashion.

While the steps of the primary assessment are taught and displayed in a sequential manner, many of the steps can, and should, be performed simultaneously. The components of the primary assessment, which are listed in order of priority for optimal patient management, are easily remembered with the ABCDE mnemonic:

- A—Airway management and cervical spine stabilization
- B—Breathing (ventilation)
- C—Circulation and bleeding
- D—Disability
- E—Expose/environment

Step A—Airway Management and Cervical Spine Stabilization

Airway

The patient's airway is quickly checked to ensure that it is **patent** (open and clear) and that no danger of obstruction exists. If the airway is compromised, it will have to be opened, initially using manual methods (trauma chin lift or trauma jaw thrust), and cleared of blood, body substances, and foreign bodies, if necessary (**Figure 7-2**). Eventually, as equipment and time become available, airway management can advance to mechanical means (oral airway, nasal airway, supraglottic airways, and endotracheal intubation or transtracheal methods). Numerous factors play a role in determining the method of airway management, including available equipment, the skill level of the prehospital care provider, and the distance from the trauma center. Some airway injuries, such as a laryngeal fracture or incomplete airway transection, can be aggravated by attempts at endotracheal intubation. Airway management is discussed in detail in the Airway and Ventilation chapter.

Cervical Spine Stabilization

Every trauma patient with a significant blunt mechanism of injury is suspected of spinal injury until spinal injury is conclusively

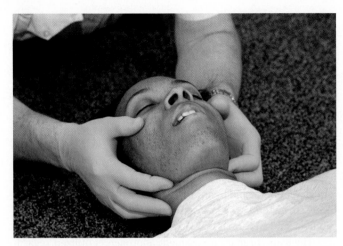

Figure 7-2 If the airway appears compromised, it must be opened while continuing to protect the spine.

ruled out. (See the Spinal Trauma chapter for a complete list of indications for spinal immobilization.) Therefore, when establishing an open airway, the possibility of cervical spine injury must always be considered. Excessive movement in any direction could either produce or aggravate neurologic damage because bony compression of the spinal cord may occur in the presence of a fractured spine. The solution is to ensure that the patient's head and neck are manually maintained (stabilized) in the neutral position during the entire assessment process, especially when opening the airway and administering necessary ventilation. This need for stabilization does not mean that necessary airway maintenance procedures cannot be applied. Instead, it means that the procedures will be performed while protecting the patient's spine from unnecessary movement. If immobilization devices that were placed need to be removed in order to reassess the patient or perform some necessary intervention, manual immobilization of the head and neck is again employed until the patient can again be fully immobilized.

Step B—Breathing (Ventilation)

The first step is to effectively deliver oxygen to a patient's lungs to help maintain the aerobic metabolic process. Hypoxia can result from inadequate ventilation of the lungs and leads to lack of oxygenation of the patient's tissues. Once the patient's airway is open, the quality and quantity of the patient's breathing (ventilation) can be evaluated as follows:

1. Check to see if the patient is breathing.
2. If the patient is not breathing (i.e., is **apneic**), immediately begin assisting ventilations with a bag-mask device with supplemental oxygen before continuing the assessment.
3. Ensure that the patient's airway is patent, continue assisted ventilation, and prepare to insert an oral, nasal, or supraglottic airway; intubate; or provide other

means of mechanical airway protection. Although commonly referred to as the "respiratory rate," a more correct term is ventilatory rate. Ventilation refers to the process of inhalation and exhalation, whereas respiration best describes the physiologic process of gas exchange between the arteries and the alveoli. This text uses the term ventilatory rate rather than respiratory rate.

4. If the patient is breathing, estimate the adequacy of the ventilatory rate and depth to determine whether the patient is moving enough air, and assess oxygenation. Ensure that the patient is not hypoxic and that the oxygen saturation is greater than 90%. Supplemental oxygen is provided as needed to maintain an adequate oxygen saturation.
5. Quickly observe the patient's chest rise, and if the patient is conscious, listen to the patient talk to assess whether he or she can speak a full sentence without difficulty.

The ventilatory rate can be divided into the following five levels:

1. *Apneic.* The patient is not breathing.
2. *Slow.* A very slow ventilatory rate may indicate ischemia (decreased supply of oxygen) of the brain. If the ventilatory rate has dropped below 10 breaths/minute (**bradypnea**), it is necessary to either assist or completely take over the patient's breathing with a bag-mask device. Assisted or total ventilatory support with the bag-mask device should include supplemental oxygen to ensure an oxygen saturation greater than 90% (**Figure 7-3**).

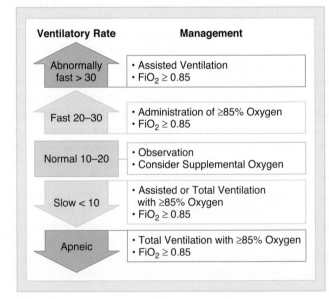

Figure 7-3 Airway management based on spontaneous ventilation rate.

3. *Normal.* If the ventilatory rate is between 10 and 20 breaths/minute (**eupnea**, a normal rate for an adult), the prehospital care provider watches the patient closely. Although the patient may appear stable, supplemental oxygen should be considered.

4. *Fast.* If the ventilatory rate is between 20 and 30 breaths/minute (**tachypnea**), the patient must be watched closely to see whether he or she is improving or deteriorating. The drive for increasing the ventilatory rate is increased accumulation of carbon dioxide in the blood or a decreased level of blood oxygen. When a patient displays an abnormal ventilatory rate, the cause must be investigated. A rapid rate indicates that not enough oxygen is reaching the body tissue. This lack of oxygen initiates anaerobic metabolism (see the Physiology of Life and Death chapter) and, ultimately, an increase in carbon dioxide. The body's detection system recognizes an increased level of carbon dioxide and tells the ventilatory system to speed up to exhale this excess. Therefore, an increased ventilatory rate may indicate that the patient needs better perfusion or oxygenation, or both. Administration of supplemental oxygen to achieve an oxygen saturation of 90% or greater is indicated for this patient—at least until the patient's overall status is determined. The prehospital care provider must remain concerned about the patient's ability to maintain adequate ventilation and alert for any deterioration in overall condition.

5. *Abnormally fast.* A ventilatory rate greater than 30 breaths/minute (severe tachypnea) indicates hypoxia, anaerobic metabolism, or both, with a resultant **acidosis**. Ventilation with supplemental oxygen must be assisted immediately with a bag-mask device as tolerated that achieves an oxygen saturation of 90% or greater. A search for the cause of the rapid ventilatory rate should begin at once to ascertain if the etiology is an oxygenation problem or an RBC delivery problem. Injuries that can produce major impairment in oxygenation and ventilation include tension pneumothorax, flail chest with pulmonary contusion, massive hemothorax, and open pneumothorax. Once the cause is identified, the intervention must occur immediately to correct the problem. (See the Thoracic Trauma chapter).

In the patient with abnormal ventilation, the chest must be exposed, observed, and palpated rapidly. Then, auscultation of the lungs will identify abnormal, diminished, or absent breath sounds. Injuries that may impede ventilation include tension pneumothorax, spinal cord injuries, and traumatic brain injuries. These injuries should be identified or suspected during the primary assessment and require that ventilatory support be initiated at once.

When assessing the trauma patient's ventilatory status, the ventilatory *depth* as well as the rate is assessed. A patient can be breathing at a normal ventilatory rate of 16 breaths/minute but have a greatly decreased ventilatory depth. Conversely, a patient can have a normal ventilatory depth but an increased or decreased ventilatory rate. The tidal volume is multiplied by the ventilatory rate to calculate the patient's minute ventilation. (See the Airway and Ventilation chapter.)

In some circumstances, it may be difficult for even experienced prehospital care providers to differentiate an airway problem from a breathing problem. In such cases, an attempt may be made to establish a secure airway. If the problem persists after management of the airway, it is most likely a breathing problem that is impairing ventilation.

Step C—Circulation and Bleeding (Perfusion and Hemorrhage)

Assessing for circulatory system compromise or failure is the next step in caring for the trauma patient. Oxygenation of the RBCs without delivery to the tissue cells is of no benefit to the patient. In the primary assessment of a trauma patient, external hemorrhage must be identified and controlled. If gross (*exsanguinating*) external hemorrhage is present, it must be controlled even before assessing the airway (or simultaneously, if adequate assistance is present at the scene). The prehospital care provider can then obtain an adequate overall estimate of the patient's cardiac output and perfusion status. Hemorrhage—either external or internal—is the most common cause of preventable death from trauma.

Hemorrhage Control

External hemorrhage is identified and controlled in the primary assessment. Hemorrhage control is included in the assessment of circulation because if gross bleeding is not controlled as soon as possible, the potential for the patient's death increases dramatically. The three types of external hemorrhage are capillary, venous, and arterial, which are described as follows:

1. *Capillary bleeding* is caused by abrasions that have scraped open the tiny capillaries just below the skin's surface. Usually capillary bleeding will have slowed or even stopped before the arrival of prehospital care.

2. *Venous bleeding* is from deeper areas within the tissue and is usually controlled with a small amount of direct pressure. Venous bleeding is usually not life threatening unless the injury is severe or blood loss is not controlled.

3. *Arterial bleeding* is caused by an injury that has lacerated an artery. This is the most important and most difficult type of blood loss to control. It is characterized by spurting blood that is bright red in color. Even a small, deep arterial puncture wound can produce life-threatening arterial blood loss.

Hemorrhage control is a priority because every red blood cell counts. Rapid control of bleeding is one of the most important goals in the care of a trauma patient. The primary assessment cannot advance unless hemorrhage is controlled.

In cases of external hemorrhage, application of direct pressure will control most major hemorrhage until the prehospital care provider can transport the patient to a hospital in which an OR and adequate equipment are available. Hemorrhage control is initiated during the primary assessment and maintained throughout transport. The prehospital care provider may require assistance to accomplish both ventilation and bleeding control.

Hemorrhage can be controlled in the following ways:

1. *Direct pressure.* Direct pressure is exactly what the name implies—applying pressure to the site of bleeding. This is accomplished by placing a dressing (e.g., 4- × 4-inch gauze) or abdominal pads directly over the site and applying pressure. The application and maintenance of direct pressure will require all of one prehospital care provider's attention, preventing the prehospital care provider from participating in other aspects of patient care. However, if assistance is limited, a pressure dressing can be fashioned out of gauze pads and an elastic bandage. If bleeding is not controlled, it will not matter how much oxygen or fluid the patient receives; perfusion will not improve in the face of ongoing hemorrhage.

2. *Tourniquets.* Tourniquets have often been described in the past as the technique of "last resort." Military experience in Afghanistan and Iraq, plus the routine and safe use of tourniquets by surgeons, has led to reconsideration of this approach.[2-4] The use of "elevation" and pressure on "pressure points" is no longer recommended because of insufficient data supporting their effectiveness.[5,6] Tourniquets are very effective in controlling severe hemorrhage and should be used if direct pressure or a pressure dressing fails to control hemorrhage from an extremity (See the Shock chapter).

The primary sites of massive internal hemorrhage include the chest (both pleural cavities), the abdomen (peritoneal cavity), the retroperitoneal space, and the long bones (primarily femur fractures). If internal hemorrhage is suspected, the thorax, abdomen, pelvis, and thighs are exposed to quickly inspect and palpate for signs of injury. These causes of hemorrhage are not easy to control outside the hospital. The prehospital treatment is rapid delivery of the patient to a facility equipped and appropriately staffed for rapid control of hemorrhage in the OR (e.g., trauma center, if available).

Perfusion

The patient's overall circulatory status can be determined by checking the pulse and the skin color, temperature, and moisture (**Figure 7-4**). Assessment of perfusion may be challenging in elderly or pediatric patients or in those who are well conditioned or on certain medications. (See the Shock chapter.)

Pulse

The pulse is evaluated for presence, quality, and regularity. The presence of a palpable peripheral pulse also provides an estimate of blood pressure. A quick check of the pulse reveals whether the patient has tachycardia, bradycardia, or an irregular rhythm. It can also reveal information about the systolic blood pressure. If a radial pulse is not palpable in an uninjured extremity, the patient has likely entered the decompensated phase of shock, a late sign of the patient's critical condition. In the primary assessment, determination of an exact pulse rate is not necessary. Instead, a gross estimate is rapidly obtained, and the assessment moves on to other gross evaluations. The actual pulse rate is obtained later in the process. If an unresponsive patient lacks a palpable carotid or femoral pulse, he or she is in cardiopulmonary arrest (see later discussion). The combination of compromised perfusion and impaired breathing should prompt the prehospital care provider to consider the presence of a tension pneumothorax. If clinical signs are present, needle decompression can be lifesaving. (See the Thoracic Trauma chapter).

Figure 7-4 Capillary Refilling Time

The capillary refilling time is checked by pressing over the nail beds and then releasing the pressure. This downward pressure removes the blood from the visible capillary bed. The rate of return of blood to the nail beds after releasing pressure (refilling time) is a tool for estimating blood flow through this most distal part of the circulation. A capillary refilling time of greater than 2 seconds may indicate that the capillary beds are not receiving adequate perfusion. However, capillary refilling time by itself is a poor indicator of shock because it is influenced by so many other factors. For example, peripheral vascular disease (arteriosclerosis), cold temperatures, the use of pharmacologic vasodilators or constrictors, or the presence of neurogenic shock can skew the results. Measuring the capillary refilling time becomes a less useful check of cardiovascular function in these cases. Capillary refilling time has a place in the evaluation of circulatory adequacy, but it should always be used in conjunction with other physical examination findings, just as the prehospital care provider uses other indicators (e.g., blood pressure).

Skin

The skin can reveal a great deal about a patient's circulatory status.

- *Color.* Adequate perfusion produces a pinkish hue to the skin. Skin becomes pale when blood is shunted away from an area. Pale coloration is associated with poor perfusion. Bluish coloration indicates incomplete oxygenation. The bluish color is caused by lack of blood or oxygen to that region of the body. Skin pigmentation can often make this determination difficult. Examination of the color of nail beds and mucous membranes helps overcome this challenge because changes in color usually first appear in the lips, gums, or fingertips.
- *Temperature.* As with overall skin evaluation, skin temperature is influenced by environmental conditions. Cool skin indicates decreased perfusion, regardless of the cause. The prehospital care provider usually assesses skin temperature by touching the patient with the back of the hand; therefore, an accurate determination can be difficult with gloves on. Normal skin temperature is warm to the touch, neither cool nor hot. Normally the blood vessels are not dilated and do not bring the heat of the body to the surface of the skin.
- *Moisture.* Dry skin indicates good perfusion. Moist skin is associated with shock and decreased perfusion. This decrease in perfusion is caused by blood being shunted to the core organs of the body as a result of vasoconstriction of peripheral vessels.

Step D—Disability

Having evaluated and corrected, to the extent possible, the factors involved in delivering oxygen to the lungs and circulating it throughout the body, the next step in the primary assessment is assessment of cerebral function, which is an indirect measurement of cerebral oxygenation. The goal is to determine the patient's level of consciousness (LOC) and ascertain the potential for hypoxia.

The prehospital care provider can infer that a confused, belligerent, combative, or uncooperative patient is hypoxic until proved otherwise. Most patients want help when their lives are medically threatened. If a patient refuses help, the reason must be questioned. Does the patient feel threatened by the presence of a prehospital care provider on the scene? If so, further attempts to establish rapport will often help to gain the patient's trust. If nothing in the situation seems to be threatening, the source of the behavior should be considered physiologic and reversible conditions identified and treated. During the assessment, the history can help determine whether the patient lost consciousness at any time since the injury occurred, whether toxic substances might be involved (and what they might be), and whether the patient has any pre-existing conditions that may produce a decreased LOC or aberrant behavior.

A decreased LOC alerts a prehospital care provider to the following four possibilities:

1. Decreased cerebral oxygenation (caused by hypoxia/hypoperfusion)
2. Central nervous system (CNS) injury
3. Drug or alcohol overdose
4. Metabolic derangement (diabetes, seizure, cardiac arrest)

The Glasgow Coma Scale (GCS) score is a tool used for determining LOC and is preferred over the AVPU classification (**Figure 7-5**).[7] It is a quick, simple method for determining cerebral function and is predictive of patient outcome, especially the best motor response. It also provides a baseline of cerebral function for serial neurologic evaluations. The GCS score is divided into three sections: (1) *eye* opening, (2) best *verbal* response, and (3) best *motor* response (EVM). The patient is assigned a score according to the *best* response to each component of the EVM (**Figure 7-6**). For example, if a patient's right eye is so severely swollen that the patient cannot open it, but the left eye opens spontaneously, the patient receives a 4 for the best eye movement. If a patient lacks spontaneous eye opening, the prehospital care provider should use a verbal command (e.g., "Open your eyes"). If the patient does not respond to a verbal stimulus, a painful stimulus, such as pressing the nail bed with a pen or squeezing the axillary tissue, can be applied.

The patient's verbal response is determined by using a question such as, "What happened to you?" If fully oriented, the patient will supply a coherent answer. Otherwise, the patient's verbal response is scored as confused, inappropriate, unintelligible, or

Figure 7-5 The AVPU System

The mnemonic AVPU is often used to describe the patient's LOC. In this system, A stands for *alert*, V for responds to *verbal* stimulus, P for responds to *painful* stimulus, and U for *unresponsive*. This approach, although very simple, fails to provide information as to specifically *how* the patient responds to verbal or painful stimuli. In other words, if the patient responds to verbal questioning, is the patient oriented, confused, or mumbling incomprehensibly? Likewise, when the patient responds to painful stimulus, does the patient localize, withdraw, or demonstrate decorticate or decerebrate posturing? Because of its lack of precision, the use of AVPU has fallen into disfavor. Although the GCS is more complicated to remember than AVPU, repeated practice will make this crucial assessment second nature.

Eye Opening	Points
Spontaneous eye opening	4
Eye opening on command	3
Eye opening to painful stimulus	2
No eye opening	1
Best Verbal Response	
Answers appropriately (oriented)	5
Gives confused answers	4
Inappropriate response	3
Makes unintelligible noises	2
Makes no verbal response	1
Best Motor Response	
Follows command	6
Localizes painful stimuli	5
Withdrawal to pain	4
Responds with abnormal flexion to painful stimuli (decorticate)	3
Responds with abnormal extension to pain (decerebrate)	2
Gives no motor response	1
Total	

Figure 7-6 Glasgow Coma Scale (GCS).

absent. If a patient is intubated, the GCS score contains only the eye and motor scales, and the letter T is added to note the inability to assess the verbal response (e.g., 8T).

The third component of the GCS is the motor score. A simple, unambiguous command, such as, "Hold up two fingers" or "Show me a hitchhiker's sign," is given to the patient. If the patient complies with the command, the highest score of 6 is given. A patient who squeezes or grasps the finger of a prehospital care provider may simply be demonstrating a grasping reflex and not purposefully following a command. If the patient fails to follow a command, a painful stimulus, as noted previously, should be used, and the patient's best motor response should be scored. A patient who attempts to push away a painful stimulus is considered to be *localizing*. Other possible responses to pain include withdrawal from the stimulus, abnormal flexion (*decorticate posturing*) or extension (*decerebrate posturing*) of the upper extremities, or absence of motor function. Recent evidence suggests that the motor component of the GCS alone is essentially as good in evaluating a patient as the entire score.[8]

The maximum GCS score is 15, indicating a patient with no disability. The lowest score of 3 is generally an ominous sign. A score of less than 8 indicates a major injury, 9 to 12 a moderate injury, and 13 to 15 a minor injury. A GCS score of 8 is an indication for considering active airway management of the patient. The prehospital care provider can easily calculate and relate the individual components of the score and will include them in the verbal report to the receiving facility as well as in the patient care report. Often times, it is preferable to communicate individual components of the GCS scale, rather than just the total score, as specific changes can then be documented. A patient care report that states that "the patient is E4, V4, M6" indicates that the patient is confused but follows commands.

If a patient is not awake, oriented, or able to follow commands, the prehospital care provider can assess the pupils quickly. Are the pupils equal and round, reactive to light (PEARRL)? Are the pupils equal to each other? Is each pupil round and of normal appearance, and does it appropriately react to light by constricting, or is it unresponsive and dilated? A GCS score of less than 14 in combination with an abnormal pupil examination can indicate the presence of a life-threatening traumatic brain injury. (See the Head Trauma chapter.)

Step E—Expose/Environment

An early step in the assessment process is to remove a patient's clothes because exposure of the trauma patient is critical to finding all injuries (**Figure 7-7**). The saying, "The one part of the body that is not exposed will be the most severely injured part," may not always be true, but it is true often enough to warrant a total body examination. Also, blood can collect in and be absorbed by clothing and go unnoticed. After seeing the patient's entire body, the prehospital care provider can then cover the patient again to conserve body heat.

Although it is important to expose a trauma patient's body to complete an effective assessment, **hypothermia** is a serious problem in the management of a trauma patient. Only what is necessary should be exposed to the outside environment. Once the patient has been moved inside the warm emergency medical services (EMS) unit, the complete examination can be accomplished and the patient covered again as quickly as possible.

The amount of the patient's clothing that should be removed during an assessment varies depending on the conditions or injuries found. A general rule is to remove as much clothing as necessary to determine the presence or absence of a condition or injury. The prehospital care provider need not

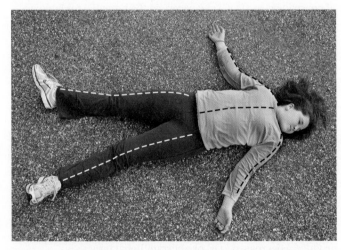

Figure 7-7 Clothing can be quickly removed by cutting, as indicated by the dotted lines.

be afraid to remove clothing if it is the only way to complete the assessment and treatment properly. On occasion, patients can sustain multiple mechanisms of injury, such as experiencing a motor vehicle crash after being shot. Potentially life-threatening injuries may be missed if the patient is inadequately examined. Injuries cannot be treated if they are not first identified.

Special care should be taken when cutting and removing clothing from a victim of a crime so as not to inadvertently destroy evidence (**Figure 7-8**).

Once the patient has been exposed for completion of the primary assessment, any exposed skin should be covered back up in an effort to help maintain body temperature. Once the patient has been moved into the ambulance, the patient care compartment should be kept warm. Maintaining the patient's body temperature is more important than the comfort of the prehospital care providers.

Simultaneous Evaluation and Management

As mentioned earlier in this chapter, while the primary assessment is presented and taught in a stepwise fashion, many steps can be assessed simultaneously. By asking follow-up questions such as, "Where do you hurt?", airway patency is further assessed and respiratory function observed. In addition, questioning can occur while the prehospital care provider is palpating the radial pulse and feeling the temperature and moistness of the skin.

Figure 7-8   Forensic Evidence

Unfortunately, some trauma patients are victims of violent crimes. In these situations, it is important to do everything possible to preserve evidence for law enforcement personnel. When cutting clothing from a crime victim, care should be taken not to cut through holes in the clothing made by bullets (projectiles), knives, or other objects because this can compromise valuable forensic evidence. If clothing is removed from a victim of a potential crime, it should be placed in a paper (not plastic) bag and turned over to law enforcement personnel on scene before patient transport. Any weapons, drugs, or personal belongings found during patient assessment should also be turned over to law enforcement personnel, as well as be thoroughly documented on the patient care report. If the patient's condition warrants transport before the arrival of law enforcement, these items are brought with the patient to the hospital, and the law enforcement agency is contacted and apprised of the destination facility.

The patient's LOC and mentation can be determined by the appropriateness of the patient's verbal responses. Then the prehospital care provider can rapidly scan the patient from head to foot looking for signs of hemorrhage or other injury. The second prehospital care provider could be directed to apply direct pressure or a tourniquet to an external hemorrhage while the first prehospital care provider continues to assess the patient's airway and breathing. By using this approach, a quick overall look at the patient is accomplished, resulting in an expeditious evaluation for life-threatening injuries. The primary assessment should be repeated frequently, especially in patients with serious injury.

Adjuncts to Primary Assessment

Several adjuncts may be useful in monitoring the patient's condition, including the following:

- *Pulse oximetry.* A pulse oximeter should be applied during the primary assessment (or at its completion). Oxygen can then be titrated to maintain oxygen saturation (SpO_2) of greater than 95%. A pulse oximeter also alerts the prehospital care provider to the patient's heart rate. Any drop in SpO_2 should prompt a repeat of the primary assessment in order to identify the underlying cause.
- *End-tidal carbon dioxide ($ETCO_2$) monitoring.* Monitoring the $ETCO_2$ can be useful in confirming intratracheal placement of an endotracheal tube as well as indirectly measuring the patient's arterial carbon dioxide level ($PaCO_2$). While $ETCO_2$ may not always correlate well with the patient's $PaCO_2$, especially in multiple trauma patients, trending of $ETCO_2$ may be useful in guiding ventilatory rate.
- *Electrocardiographic (ECG) monitoring.* ECG monitoring is less useful than monitoring pulse oximetry, as the presence of an organized cardiac electrical pattern on the monitor does not always correlate with adequate perfusion. Monitoring of the pulse and/or blood pressure is still required to assess for perfusion. An audible signal can alert the prehospital care provider of a change in the patient's heart rate.
- *Automated blood pressure monitoring.* In general, auscultating blood pressure is not part of the primary assessment; however, in a critically injured patient whose condition does not permit a more thorough secondary assessment, application of an automated blood pressure monitor during transport can provide additional information regarding the patient's degree of shock.

Resuscitation

Resuscitation describes treatment steps taken to correct life-threatening problems as identified in the primary assessment. PHTLS assessment is based on a "treat as you go" philosophy, in which treatment is initiated as each threat to life is identified or at the earliest possible moment (**Figure 7-9**).

Transport

If life-threatening conditions are identified during the primary assessment, the patient should be rapidly packaged after initiating limited field intervention. Transport of critically injured trauma patients to the closest appropriate facility should be initiated as soon as possible (**Figure 7-10**). Unless complicating circumstances exist, scene time should be limited to 10 minutes or less for these patients. Limited scene time and initiation of rapid transport to the closest appropriate facility—preferably a trauma center—are fundamental aspects of prehospital trauma resuscitation.

Fluid Therapy

Another important step in resuscitation is the restoration of the cardiovascular system to an adequate perfusing volume as quickly as possible. This step does not involve restoring blood pressure to normal but rather providing enough fluid to ensure that vital organs are being perfused. Because blood is usually not available in the prehospital setting, *lactated Ringer's* or normal saline is used for trauma resuscitation. In addition to sodium and chloride, lactated Ringer's solution contains small amounts of potassium, calcium, and lactate and is an effective volume expander. Crystalloid solutions, such as lactated Ringer's and normal saline, however, do not replace the oxygen-carrying capacity of the lost RBCs or the lost platelets that are necessary for clotting and bleeding control. Therefore, rapid transport of a severely injured patient to an appropriate facility is an absolute necessity.

En route to the receiving facility, one or two large-bore (14- or 16-gauge) intravenous (IV) catheters may be placed in the patient's forearm or antecubital veins, if possible, as time permits. In general, central IV lines (subclavian, internal jugular, or femoral) are not appropriate for the field management of trauma patients. The rate of fluid administration depends on the clinical scenario, primarily whether the patient's hemorrhage has been controlled when the IV fluid is initiated, or whether the patient has evidence of CNS injury. The Shock chapter and the Head Trauma chapter provide guidelines for fluid resuscitation.

Starting an IV line at the scene only prolongs on-scene time and delays transport. As addressed previously, the definitive treatment for the trauma patient can be accomplished only in the hospital. For example, a patient with an injury to the spleen who is losing 50 milliliters of blood per minute will continue to bleed at that rate for each additional minute that arrival in the OR is delayed. Initiating IV lines on the scene instead of early transport will not only increase blood loss but also may decrease the patient's chance of survival. Exceptions exist, such as entrapment, when a patient simply cannot be moved immediately.

External hemorrhage should be controlled prior to initiation of IV fluid. Aggressive administration of IV fluids may "pop the clot," resulting in recurrent internal hemorrhage as the blood pressure increases. More importantly, continual volume replacement is not a substitute for manual control of external hemorrhage and initiation of transport for internal hemorrhage.

Basic Versus Advanced Prehospital Care Provider Levels

The key steps in resuscitating a critically injured trauma patient are the same at both the basic and the advanced levels of prehospital care provider. They include (1) opening and maintaining the airway, (2) ensuring adequate ventilation, (3) immediately controlling major external hemorrhage, (4) rapidly packaging the patient for transport, and (5) quickly initiating rapid, but safe, transport of the patient to the closest appropriate facility. If transport time is prolonged, it may be appropriate for the basic-level prehospital care provider to call for assistance from a nearby advanced life support (ALS) service that can rendezvous with the basic unit en route. Helicopter evacuation to a trauma center is another option. Both the ALS service and the flight service will provide advanced airway management, ventilatory management, and earlier fluid replacement.

Secondary Assessment

The secondary assessment is a head-to-toe evaluation of a patient. The secondary assessment is performed only after the primary assessment is completed, all life-threatening injuries have been identified and treated, and resuscitation has been initiated. The objective of the secondary assessment is to identify injuries or problems that were not identified during the primary assessment. Because a well-performed primary assessment will identify all life-threatening conditions, the secondary assessment, by definition, deals with less serious problems. Therefore, a critical trauma patient is transported as soon as possible after conclusion of the primary assessment and not held in the field for either IV initiation or a secondary assessment.

The secondary assessment uses a "look, listen, and feel" approach to evaluate the skin and everything it contains. Rather than looking at the entire body at one time, returning to listen to all areas, and finally returning to palpate all areas, the prehospital care provider "searches" the body. The prehospital care provider identifies injuries and correlates physical findings region by region, beginning at the head and proceeding through the neck, chest, and abdomen to the extremities, concluding with a detailed neurologic examination. The following phrases capture the essence of the entire assessment process:

- *See*, don't just look.
- *Hear*, don't just listen.
- *Feel*, don't just touch (**Figure 7-11**).

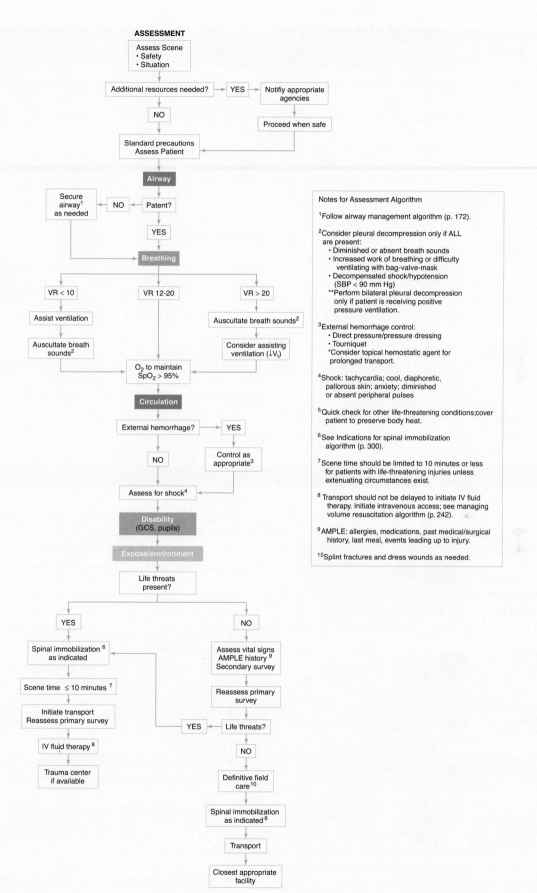

Figure 7-9 Assessment algorithm.

Figure 7-10   Critical Trauma Patient

Keep scene time as brief as possible (10 minutes or less ideally) when any of the following life-threatening conditions are present:

1. Inadequate or threatened airway
2. Impaired ventilation, as demonstrated by the following:
   - Abnormally fast or slow ventilatory rate
   - Hypoxia (SpO$_2$ < 95% even with supplemental oxygen)
   - Dyspnea
   - Open pneumothorax or flail chest
   - Suspected pneumothorax
3. Significant external hemorrhage or suspected internal hemorrhage
4. Abnormal neurologic status
   - GCS score ≤ 13
   - Seizure activity
   - Sensory or motor deficit
5. Penetrating trauma to the head, neck, or torso, or proximal to the elbow or knee in the extremities
6. Amputation or near-amputation proximal to the fingers or toes
7. Any trauma in the presence of the following:
   - History of serious medical conditions (e.g., coronary artery disease, chronic obstructive pulmonary disease, bleeding disorder)
   - Age >55 years
   - Hypothermia
   - Burns
   - Pregnancy

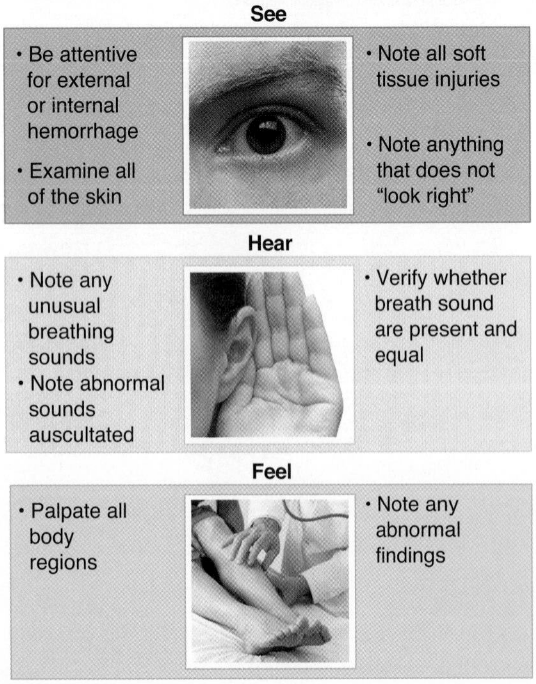

See

- Be attentive for external or internal hemorrhage
- Examine all of the skin
- Note all soft tissue injuries
- Note anything that does not "look right"

Hear

- Note any unusual breathing sounds
- Note abnormal sounds auscultated
- Verify whether breath sound are present and equal

Feel

- Palpate all body regions
- Note any abnormal findings

Figure 7-11   The physical assessment of a trauma patient involves careful observation, auscultation, and palpation.

Source: Eye photo: © iStockphoto/Thinkstock; ear photo: © iStockphoto/Thinkstock; hands photo: © Image Point Fr/ShutterStock.

While examining the patient, all available information is used to formulate a patient care plan. The prehospital care provider not only provides the patient with transport, but does everything possible to ensure his or her survival.

See

- Examine all of the skin of each region.
- Be attentive for external hemorrhage or signs of internal hemorrhage, such as distension of the abdomen, marked tenseness of an extremity, or an expanding hematoma.
- Note soft-tissue injuries, including abrasions, burns, contusions, hematomas, lacerations, and puncture wounds.
- Note any masses or swelling, or deformation of bones.
- Note abnormal indentations on the skin and the skin's color.
- Note anything that does not "look right."

Hear

- Note any unusual sounds when the patient inhales or exhales.
- Note any abnormal sounds when auscultating the chest.

- Check whether the breath sounds are equal in both lung fields.
- Auscultate over the carotid arteries and other vessels.
- Note any unusual sounds (bruits) over the vessels that would indicate vascular damage.

Feel

- Carefully move each bone in the region. Note any resulting crepitus, pain, or unusual movement.
- Firmly palpate all parts of the region. Note whether anything moves that should not, whether anything feels "squishy," whether the patient complains of tenderness, whether all pulses are present (and where they are felt), and whether pulsations are felt that should not be present.

Vital Signs

The quality of the pulse and ventilatory rates and the other components of the primary assessment are continually re-evaluated and compared to previous findings because significant changes can occur rapidly. Quantitative vital signs are measured and motor and sensory status evaluated in all four extremities as soon as possible, although this is normally not accomplished until the conclusion of the primary assessment. Depending on the situation, a second prehospital care provider may obtain vital signs while the first prehospital care provider completes the primary assessment, to avoid further delay. However, exact "numbers" for pulse rate, ventilatory rate, and blood pressure are not critical in the initial management of the patient with severe multisystem trauma. Therefore, the measurement of the exact numbers can be delayed until completion of the essential steps of resuscitation and stabilization.

A set of complete vital signs includes blood pressure, pulse rate and quality, ventilatory rate (including breath sounds), and skin color and temperature. For the critical trauma patient, a complete set of vital signs are evaluated and recorded every 3 to 5 minutes, as often as possible, or at the time of any change in condition or a medical problem. Even if an automated, non-invasive blood pressure device is available, the initial blood pressure should be taken manually. Automatic blood pressure devices may be inaccurate when the patient is significantly hypotensive; therefore, in these patients, all blood pressure measurements should be obtained manually.

SAMPLE History

A quick history is obtained on the patient. This information should be documented on the patient care report and passed on to the medical personnel at the receiving facility. The mnemonic SAMPLE serves as a reminder of the key components:

- *Symptoms:* What does the patient complain of? Pain? Trouble breathing? Numbness? Tingling?
- *Allergies:* Does the patient have any known allergies, particularly to medications?
- *Medications:* What prescription or nonprescription drugs (including vitamins, supplements, and other over-the-counter medications) does the patient regularly take?
- *Past medical and surgical history:* Does the patient have any significant medical problems requiring ongoing medical care? Has the patient undergone any prior surgeries?
- *Last meal:* How long has it been since the patient last ate? Many trauma patients will require surgery, and recent food intake increases the risk of aspiration during induction of anesthesia.
- *Events:* What events preceded the injury? Immersion in water (drowning or hypothermia) and exposure to hazardous materials should be included.

Assessing Anatomic Regions

Head

Visual examination of the head and face will reveal contusions, abrasions, lacerations, bone asymmetry, hemorrhage, bony defects of the face and supportive skull, and abnormalities of the eye, eyelid, external ear, mouth, and mandible. The following steps are included during a head examination:

- Search thoroughly through the patient's hair for any soft-tissue injuries.
- Check pupil size for reactivity to light, equality, accommodation, roundness, and irregular shape.
- Carefully palpate the bones of the face and skull to identify crepitus, deviation, depression, or abnormal mobility. (This is extremely important in the nonradiographic evaluation for head injury.) **Figure 7-12** reviews the bony anatomy of the skull.
- Care should be exercised when attempting to open and examine the eyes of an unconscious trauma patient who has evidence of facial injury. Even small amounts of pressure may further damage an eye that has a blunt or penetrating injury ("ruptured globe").

Fractures of the bones of the midface are often associated with a fracture of the portion of the skull base called the cribriform plate. If the patient has midface trauma (e.g., injury between the upper lip and orbits), a gastric tube, if utilized, should be inserted through the mouth rather than through the nose.

Neck

Visual examination of the neck for contusions, abrasions, lacerations, hematomas, and deformities will alert the prehospital care provider to the possibility of underlying injuries. Palpation may reveal subcutaneous emphysema of a laryngeal, tracheal, or pulmonary origin. Crepitus of the larynx, hoarseness, and subcutaneous emphysema constitute a triad

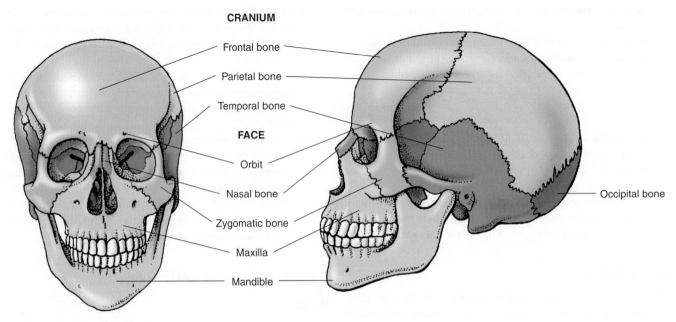

Figure 7-12 Normal anatomic structure of the face and skull.

classically indicative of laryngeal fracture. Lack of tenderness of the cervical spine may help rule out cervical spine fractures (when combined with strict criteria), whereas tenderness may frequently indicate the presence of a fracture, dislocation, or ligamentous injury. Such palpation is performed carefully, ensuring that the cervical spine remains in a neutral, in-line position. Absence of a neurologic deficit does not exclude the possibility of an unstable cervical spine injury. Re-evaluation may reveal expansion of a previously identified hematoma or shifting of the trachea. **Figure 7-13** reviews the normal anatomic structure of the neck.

Chest

Because the thorax is strong, resilient, and elastic, it can absorb a significant amount of trauma. Close visual examination of the chest for deformities, areas of paradoxical movement, contusions, and abrasions is necessary to identify underlying injuries. Other signs for which the prehospital care provider should watch closely include splinting and guarding, unequal bilateral chest excursion, and intercostal, suprasternal, or supraclavicular bulging or retraction.

A contusion over the sternum may be the only indication of an underlying cardiac injury. A stab wound near the sternum may indicate cardiac tamponade. A line traced from the fourth intercostal space anteriorly to the sixth intercostal space laterally and to the eighth intercostal space posteriorly defines the upward excursion of the diaphragm at full expiration (**Figure 7-14**). A penetrating injury that occurs below this line or with a path that may have taken it below this line should be considered to have traversed both the thoracic and abdominal cavities.

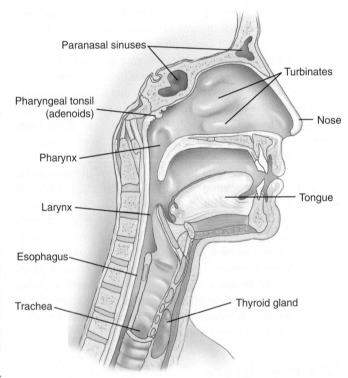

Figure 7-13 Normal anatomy of the neck.

Except for the eyes and hands, the stethoscope is the most important instrument a prehospital care provider can use for chest examination. A patient will most often be in a supine position so that only the anterior and lateral chest is available for auscultation. It is important to recognize normal and decreased breath sounds with a patient in this position. Diminished or

Lateral View of Diaphragm Position

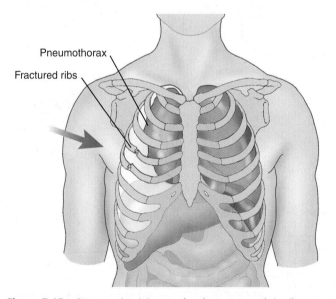

4th intercostal space

8th intercostal space

Sternum

Upper margin of diaphragm

Diaphragm

(Posterior)　　　　(Anterior)

Figure 7-14 Lateral view of diaphragm position at full expiration.

Pneumothorax

Fractured ribs

Figure 7-15 Compression injury to the chest can result in rib fracture and subsequent pneumothorax.

absent breath sounds indicate a possible pneumothorax, tension pneumothorax, or hemothorax. Crackles heard posteriorly (when the patient is logrolled) or laterally may indicate pulmonary contusion. Cardiac tamponade is characterized by distant heart sounds; however, these may be difficult to ascertain given the commotion at the scene or road noise during transport.

A small area of rib fractures may indicate a severe underlying pulmonary contusion. Any type of compression injury to the chest can result in a pneumothorax (**Figure 7-15**). The thorax is palpated for the presence of subcutaneous emphysema (air in the soft tissue).

Abdomen

The abdominal examination begins, as with the other parts of the body, by visual evaluation. Abrasions and ecchymosis indicate the possibility of underlying injury. The abdomen should be examined carefully for a telltale transverse contusion, which suggests that an incorrectly worn seat belt has caused underlying injury. Almost 50% of patients with this sign will have an intestinal injury. Lumbar spine fractures may also be associated with the "seat belt sign."

Examination of the abdomen also includes palpation of each quadrant to evaluate tenderness, abdominal muscle guarding, and masses. When palpating, the prehospital care provider notes whether the abdomen is soft or whether rigidity or guarding is present. There is no need to continue palpating after discovering abdominal tenderness or pain. Additional information will not alter prehospital management, and the only outcomes of a continued abdominal examination are further discomfort to the patient and delayed transport to the receiving facility. Similarly, auscultation of the abdomen adds virtually nothing to the assessment of a trauma patient. The peritoneal cavity can hide a large volume of blood, often with minimal or no abdominal distension.

Altered mental status resulting from a traumatic brain injury or intoxication with alcohol or other drugs often obscures evaluation of the abdomen.

Pelvis

The pelvis is evaluated by observation and palpation. The pelvis is first visually examined for abrasions, contusions, hematomas, lacerations, open fractures, and signs of distension. Pelvic fractures can produce massive internal hemorrhage, resulting in rapid deterioration of a patient's condition.

Palpation of the pelvis in the prehospital setting provides minimal information that will affect the management of the patient. When examined, the pelvis is palpated only once for tenderness and instability as part of the secondary assessment. Because palpation of the unstable pelvis can move fractured segments and disrupt any clot that has formed, thus aggravating hemorrhage, this examination step should be performed only once and not repeated. Palpation is accomplished by gently applying anterior-to-posterior pressure with the heels of the hands on the symphysis pubis and then medial pressure to the iliac crests bilaterally, evaluating for pain and abnormal movement. Any evidence of instability concludes further palpation of the pelvis and raises the likelihood of internal hemorrhage.

Genitals

In general, genitalia are not examined in the prehospital setting. However, note should be made of bleeding from the external genitalia, obvious blood at the urethral meatus, or presence of priapism in males. Additionally, clear fluid noted in the pants of a pregnant patient may represent amniotic fluid from rupture of the amniotic membranes.

Back

The back of the torso should be examined for evidence of injury. This is best accomplished when logrolling the patient for placement onto or removal from the long backboard. Breath sounds can be auscultated over the posterior thorax, and the spine palpated for tenderness and deformity.

Extremities

The examination of the extremities begins at the clavicle in the upper extremity and the pelvis in the lower extremity and then proceeds toward the most distal portion of each extremity. Each individual bone and joint is evaluated by visual inspection for deformity, hematoma, or ecchymosis and by palpation to determine the presence of crepitus, pain, tenderness, or unusual movements. Any suspected fracture should be immobilized until radiographic confirmation of its presence or absence is possible. Circulation and motor and sensory nerve function at the distal end of each extremity are also checked. If an extremity is immobilized, pulses, movement, and sensation should be rechecked after splinting.

Neurologic Examination

As with the other regional examinations described, the neurologic examination in the secondary assessment is conducted in much greater detail than in the primary assessment. Calculation of the GCS score, evaluation of motor and sensory function, and observation of pupillary response are all included. A gross examination of sensory capability and motor response will determine the presence or absence of weakness or loss of sensation in the extremities, suggesting spinal cord injury, and will identify areas that require further examination. When examining a patient's pupils, equality of response in addition to equality of size are evaluated. A small but significant portion of the population has pupils of differing sizes as a normal condition (*anisocoria*). Even in these patients, however, the pupils should react to light in a similar manner. Pupils that react at differing speeds to the introduction of light are considered to be unequal. Unequal pupils in an unconscious trauma patient may indicate increased intracranial pressure or pressure on the third cranial nerve, caused by either cerebral edema or a rapidly expanding intracranial hematoma (**Figure 7-16**). Direct eye injury can also cause unequal pupils.

Definitive Care in the Field

Included in assessment and management are the skills of packaging, transporting, and communicating. Definitive care is the

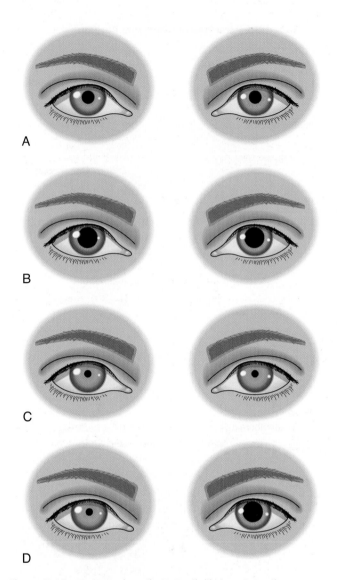

Figure 7-16 **A.** Normal pupils. **B.** Pupil dilation. **C.** Pupil constriction. **D.** Unequal pupils.
Source: © Jones & Bartlett Learning

end phase of patient care. The following are examples of definitive care:

- For a patient with cardiac arrest, definitive care is defibrillation with resultant normal rhythm; cardiopulmonary resuscitation (CPR) is just a holding pattern until defibrillation can be accomplished.
- For a patient in a diabetic hypoglycemic coma, definitive care is IV glucose and a return to normal blood glucose levels.
- For a patient with an obstructed airway, definitive care is relief of the obstruction, which may be accomplished by the trauma jaw thrust and assisted ventilation.
- For the patient with severe bleeding, definitive care is hemorrhage control and resuscitation from shock.

In general, while definitive care for some of the problems encountered in the prehospital setting can be provided in the field, definitive care for many of the injuries sustained by the critical trauma patient can be provided only in the OR. Anything that delays the administration of that definitive care will lessen the patient's chance of survival. The care given to the trauma patient in the field is similar to CPR for the cardiac arrest patient. It keeps the patient alive until something definitive can be done. For the trauma patient, the care given in the field is frequently only temporizing—buying the additional minutes needed to reach the OR.

Preparation for Transport

As discussed previously, spinal injury must be suspected in all trauma patients. Therefore, when indicated, stabilization of the spine should be an integral component of packaging the trauma patient. The entire length of the spine, and thus the entire patient, need to be immobilized, based upon the patient assessment and mechanism of injury.

If time is available, the following measures are accomplished:

- Careful stabilization of extremity fractures using specific splints
- If the patient is in critical condition, immobilization of all fractures as the patient is stabilized on a long backboard ("trauma" board)
- Bandaging of major wounds as necessary and appropriate (i.e., wounds with active hemorrhage)

Transport

Transport should begin as soon as the patient is loaded and stabilized. As discussed previously, delay at the scene to start an IV line or to complete the secondary assessment only extends the period before the receiving facility can administer blood and control hemorrhage. Continued evaluation and further resuscitation occur en route to the receiving facility. *For some critically injured trauma patients, initiation of transport is the single most important aspect of definitive care in the field.*

A patient whose condition is not critical can receive attention for individual injuries before transport, but even this patient should be transported rapidly before a hidden condition becomes critical.

Field Triage of Injured Patients

Selection of the proper destination facility for a critically injured patient can be every bit as important as other lifesaving interventions provided in the prehospital setting and is based upon the assessment of the patient's injuries or suspected injuries. For more than 40 years, numerous articles published in the medical literature have documented that facilities that have made the commitment to be prepared to care for injured patients—i.e., trauma centers—have better outcomes.[9-13] A study funded by the Centers for Disease Control and Prevention (CDC), published in 2006, demonstrated that patients were 25% more likely to survive their injuries if they received care at a level I trauma center than if they were cared for in a nontrauma center.[14] Another study, published in 2005, showed that about 90% of the population in the United States lives within an hour of a designated level I, II, or III trauma center, while a study from several years earlier noted that slightly more than half of all persons injured did not receive their care from a designated trauma center, including 36% of major trauma victims.[15,16] Thus, the data seem clear: The mortality rate from injury can be significantly reduced by transporting injured patients to designated trauma centers.

One of the more challenging decisions faced by a prehospital care provider involves determining which injured patients are best cared for in trauma centers. Proper selection of which patients to transport to a trauma center involves a balance between "overtriage" and "undertriage." Transporting all trauma patients to trauma centers may result in overtriage, meaning that a significant number of these injured patients will not need the specialized services offered by these facilities. This could result in worse care to the more seriously injured patients as the trauma center's resources are overwhelmed by those having less serious injuries, such as isolated fractures. At the opposite end of the spectrum is undertriage, where a seriously injured patient is taken to a nontrauma center. This can also result in worse patient outcomes as the facility may lack the capabilities to properly care for the patient. Some degree of undertriage seems inevitable, as some life-threatening conditions may not be identifiable in the prehospital setting. In order to minimize undertriage, experts estimate that an overtriage rate of 30% to 50% is necessary, meaning that 30% to 50% of injured patients transported to a trauma center will not need the specialized care available there.

The commonly recognized definition for a "major trauma patient" is a patient with an Injury Severity Score (ISS) of 16 or higher. Unfortunately, an ISS can be calculated only once all of the patient's injuries are diagnosed, including those found through sophisticated imaging technology (e.g., computed tomography) or surgery. Thus, the patient's ISS cannot be calculated in the prehospital setting. Alternative definitions that have been proposed include trauma patients who (1) die in the emergency department or within 24 hours of admission, (2) need massive transfusion of blood products, (3) need admission to an intensive care unit, (4) require urgent non-orthopedic surgery (i.e., surgery on their brain, chest, or abdomen), or (5) require control of internal hemorrhage using interventional angiography. While all of these definitions are useful for research purposes, like the ISS, these factors cannot generally be identified by prehospital care providers.

In an effort to identify patients who would most benefit from transport to and care at a trauma center, the American College of Surgeons Committee on Trauma (ACS-COT) has included a "Field Triage Decision Scheme" in its *Optimal Resources for the Care of the Injured Patient* for more than 25 years.[17] This algorithm has been revised over the years as new versions of the *Optimal Resources for the Care of the Injured Patient* has been published.

In 2005, the CDC teamed up with the ACS-COT and the National Highway Traffic Safety Administration to conduct an evidenced-based revision of the Field Triage Decision Scheme. These organizations assembled a National Expert Panel comprised of representatives from trauma surgery, emergency medicine, emergency medical services, public health, and the automotive industry. The ensuing revision of the scheme was published in the 2006 version of *Optimal Resources for the Care of the Injured Patient* and the sixth edition of *PHTLS: Prehospital Trauma Life Support*. The scientific evidence for the revisions was subsequently published in the CDC's *Morbidity and Mortality Weekly Report* (*MMWR*).[18] In 2011, the National Expert Panel was reassembled to consider new evidence and make revisions that were deemed appropriate. This 2011 revision appears in **Figure 7-17** and was also published in *MMWR*.[19]

The Field Triage Decision Scheme is broken down into four sections:

- *Step I:* Physiologic criteria—This section includes alteration in mental status, hypotension, and respiratory abnormalities. These criteria have been shown to best correlate with an ISS > 16.
- *Step II:* Anatomic criteria—If response times are brief, patients may not yet have developed significant alterations in physiology despite the presence of life-threatening injuries. This section lists anatomic findings that may be associated with severe injury.
- *Step III:* Mechanism of injury criteria—These criteria identify additional patients who may have occult injury not manifested with physiologic derangement or obvious external injury. In general, patients who meet one of these criteria have about a 20% chance of having an ISS > 16.
- *Step IV:* Special considerations—These criteria identify how factors such as age, use of anticoagulants, or the presence of burns or pregnancy should affect the decision to transport to a trauma center.

Patients who meet either physiologic or anatomic injury criteria should be transported to the highest level of trauma care available in a given region, while patients who meet step III and IV criteria could be transported to the closest, albeit not highest level, trauma center. The ACS-COT and the National Association of EMS Physicians have published a position statement encouraging EMS systems to adopt the Field Triage Decision Scheme as the basis for transport decisions of injured patients. As with any schematic tool, however, it should be used as a guideline and not as a replacement for good judgment.

Duration of Transport

The prehospital care provider should choose a receiving facility according to the severity of the patient's injury. In simple terms, the patient should be transported to the closest appropriate facility (i.e., the closest facility most capable of managing the patient's problems). If the patient's injuries are severe or indicate the possibility of continuing hemorrhage, the prehospital care provider can take the patient to a facility that will provide definitive care as quickly as possible (i.e., a trauma center, if available).

For example, an ambulance responds to a call in 8 minutes, and the prehospital team spends 6 minutes on the scene to package and load the patient into the transporting unit. So far 14 minutes of the Golden Period have passed. The closest hospital is 5 minutes away, and the trauma center is 14 minutes away. In scenario 1, the patient is taken to the trauma center. On arrival, the surgeon is in the emergency department (ED) with the emergency physician and the entire trauma team. The OR is staffed and ready. After 10 minutes in the ED for resuscitation, necessary radiographs, and blood work, the patient is taken to the OR. The total time since the incident is now 38 minutes. In scenario 2, the patient is taken to the closest hospital, which is 9 minutes closer than the trauma center. It has an available emergency physician, but the surgeon and OR team are out of the hospital. The patient's 10 minutes in the ED for resuscitation could stretch to 45 minutes by the time the surgeon arrives and examines the patient. Another 30 minutes could elapse while waiting for the OR team to arrive once the surgeon has examined the patient and decided to operate. The total time for scenario 2 is 94 minutes, or 2½ times longer than the trauma center scenario. The 9 minutes saved by the shorter ambulance ride to the closest hospital actually cost 56 minutes, during which time operative management could have been started and hemorrhage control achieved at the trauma center.

In a rural community, the transport time to an awaiting trauma team may be 45 to 60 minutes or even longer. In this situation, the closest hospital with an on-call trauma team is the appropriate receiving facility.

Method of Transport

Another aspect of the patient assessment and transport decision is the transportation method. Some systems have the availability of air transport. Air medical services may offer a higher level of care than ground units for critically injured trauma victims. Air transport may also be quicker and smoother than ground transport in some circumstances. As previously mentioned, if air transport is available in a community and is appropriate for the specific situation, the earlier in the assessment process that the decision is made to call for air transport, the greater the likely benefit to the patient.

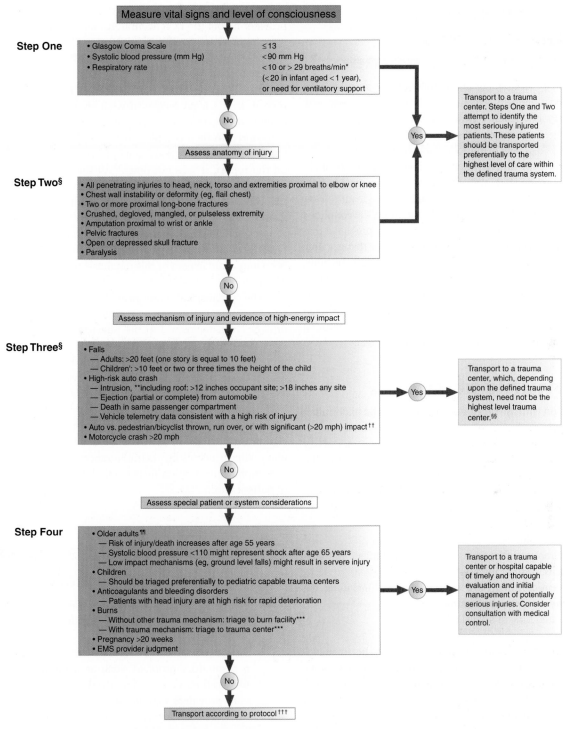

Measure vital signs and level of consciousness

Step One
- Glasgow Coma Scale   ≤13
- Systolic blood pressure (mm Hg)   <90 mm Hg
- Respiratory rate   <10 or > 29 breaths/min*
      (<20 in infant aged <1 year),
      or need for ventilatory support

Yes → Transport to a trauma center. Steps One and Two attempt to identify the most seriously injured patients. These patients should be transported preferentially to the highest level of care within the defined trauma system.

↓ No

Assess anatomy of injury

Step Two§
- All penetrating injuries to head, neck, torso and extremities proximal to elbow or knee
- Chest wall instability or deformity (eg, flail chest)
- Two or more proximal long-bone fractures
- Crushed, degloved, mangled, or pulseless extremity
- Amputation proximal to wrist or ankle
- Pelvic fractures
- Open or depressed skull fracture
- Paralysis

↓ No

Assess mechanism of injury and evidence of high-energy impact

Step Three§
- Falls
  — Adults: >20 feet (one story is equal to 10 feet)
  — Children¶: >10 feet or two or three times the height of the child
- High-risk auto crash
  — Intrusion, **including roof: >12 inches occupant site; >18 inches any site
  — Ejection (partial or complete) from automobile
  — Death in same passenger compartment
  — Vehicle telemetry data consistent with a high risk of injury
- Auto vs. pedestrian/bicyclist thrown, run over, or with significant (>20 mph) impact††
- Motorcycle crash >20 mph

Yes → Transport to a trauma center, which, depending upon the defined trauma system, need not be the highest level trauma center.§§

↓ No

Assess special patient or system considerations

Step Four
- Older adults¶¶
  — Risk of injury/death increases after age 55 years
  — Systolic blood pressure <110 might represent shock after age 65 years
  — Low impact mechanisms (eg, ground level falls) might result in servere injury
- Children
  — Should be triaged preferentially to pediatric capable trauma centers
- Anticoagulants and bleeding disorders
  — Patients with head injury are at high risk for rapid deterioration
- Burns
  — Without other trauma mechanism: triage to burn facility***
  — With trauma mechanism: triage to trauma center***
- Pregnancy >20 weeks
- EMS provider judgment

Yes → Transport to a trauma center or hospital capable of timely and thorough evaluation and initial management of potentially serious injuries. Consider consultation with medical control.

↓ No

Transport according to protocol†††

When in doubt, transport to a trauma center

Abbreviation: EMS = emergency medical services.
   * The upper limit of respiratory rate in infants is >29 breaths per minute to maintain a higher level of overtriage for infants.
   § Any injury noted in Step Two or mechanism identified in Step Three triggers a "yes" response.
   ¶ Age <15 years.
  ** Intrusion refers to interior compartment intrusion, as opposed to deformation which refers to exterior damage.
 †† Includes pedestrians or bicyclists thrown or run over by a motor vehicle or those with estimated impact >20 mph with a motor vehicle.
 §§ Local or regional protocols should be used to determine the most appropriate level of trauma center within the defined trauma system; need not be the highest-level trauma center.
 ¶¶ Age >55 years.
*** Patients with both burns and concomitant trauma for whom the burn injury poses the greatest risk for morbidity and mortality should be transferred to a burn
    center. If the nonburn trauma presents a greater immediate risk, the patient may be stabilized in a trauma center and then transferred to a burn center.
††† Patients who do not meet any of the triage criteria in Steps One through Four should be transported to the most appropriate medical facility as outlined in local EMS protocols.

Figure 7-17 Deciding where to transport a patient is critical, requiring consideration of the type and location of available facilities. Situations that will most likely require an in-house trauma team are detailed in the Field Triage Decision Scheme.

Source: Adapted from Centers for Disease Control and Prevention, Morbidity and Mortality Weekly Report (MMWR), January 13, 2012.

Monitoring and Reassessment (Ongoing Assessment)

After the primary assessment and initial care are complete, the patient must continuously be monitored, the vital signs reassessed, and the primary assessment repeated several times while en route to the receiving facility or at the scene if transport is delayed. Continuous reassessment of the components of the primary assessment will help ensure that vital functions do not deteriorate or are immediately corrected if they do. Particular attention must be paid to any significant change in a patient's condition and management re-evaluated if such a change is noted. Furthermore, the continued monitoring of a patient helps reveal conditions or problems that were overlooked during the primary assessment or that are only now presenting. Often the patient's condition will not be obvious, and looking at and listening to the patient provides much information. How the information is gathered is not as important as ensuring that all the information is gathered. Reassessment should be conducted as quickly and thoroughly as possible. Monitoring during a prolonged transport situation is described later.

Communication

Communication with the receiving facility should be undertaken as soon as possible. Early communication allows the facility to assemble the appropriate personnel and equipment necessary to best care for the patient. During transport, a member of the prehospital care team should provide a brief patient care report to the receiving facility that includes the following information:

- Patient gender and exact or estimated age
- Mechanism of injury
- Life-threatening injuries, conditions identified, and anatomic location of injuries
- Interventions that have been performed, including the patient's response to treatment
- Estimated time of arrival (ETA)

If time permits, additional information can be included, such as pertinent medical conditions and medications, other non-life-threatening injuries, characteristics of the scene, including protective gear used by the patient (seat belts, helmets, etc.), and information about additional patients.

Just as important as the radio report given before arrival is the written **patient care report (PCR)**. A good PCR is valuable for the following two reasons:

1. It gives the receiving facility staff a thorough understanding of the events that occurred and of the patient's condition should any questions arise after the prehospital care providers have left.
2. It helps ensure quality control throughout the prehospital system by making case review possible.

For these reasons, it is important that the prehospital care provider fill out the PCR accurately and completely and provide it to the receiving facility. The PCR should stay with the patient; it is of little use if it does not arrive until hours or days after the patient arrives.

The PCR often becomes a part of the patient's medical record. It is a legal record of what was found and what was done and can be used as part of a legal action. The report is considered to be a complete record of the injuries found and the actions taken. A good adage to remember is, "If it is not on the report, it was not done." All that the prehospital care provider knows, sees, and does to the patient should be recorded in the report. Another important reason for providing a copy of the PCR to the receiving facility is that most trauma centers maintain a "trauma registry," a database of all trauma patients admitted to their facility. The prehospital information is an important aspect of this database and may aid in valuable research.

The prehospital care provider also verbally transfers responsibility for a patient (often called "sign off," "report off," or "transfer over") to the physician or nurse who takes over the patient's care at the receiving facility. This verbal report is typically more detailed than the radio report and less detailed than the written PCR, providing an overview of the significant history of the incident, the action taken by the prehospital care providers, and the patient's response to this action. Both the verbal and written reports must highlight any significant changes in the patient's condition that have taken place since transmitting the radio report. Transfer of important prehospital information further emphasizes the team concept of patient care.

Special Considerations
Traumatic Cardiopulmonary Arrest

Cardiopulmonary arrest resulting from trauma differs from that caused by medical problems in three significant ways:

1. Most medical cardiac arrests are the result of either a respiratory problem, such as a foreign body airway obstruction, or a cardiac dysrhythmia that prehospital care providers may be able to treat definitively in the field. Cardiac arrest resulting from injury most often results from exsanguination or, less often, a problem incompatible with life, such as a devastating brain or spinal cord injury, and the patient cannot be appropriately resuscitated in the field.
2. Medical arrests are best managed with attempts at stabilization at the scene (e.g., removal of airway foreign body, defibrillation). In contrast, traumatic cardiopulmonary arrest is best managed with immediate transport to a facility that offers immediate blood transfusion and emergent surgery.

3. Because of the differences in etiology and management, patients with traumatic cardiopulmonary arrest in the prehospital setting have an extremely low likelihood of survival. Most studies show that less than 4% of trauma patients who require CPR in the prehospital setting survive to be discharged from the hospital, with most studies documenting that victims of penetrating trauma have a slightly increased chance of survival over those of blunt trauma. Of the small percentage of patients who are discharged from the hospital alive, many sustain significant neurologic impairment.

Resuscitation attempts in patients who are extremely unlikely to survive, aside from demonstrating very low success rates, put prehospital care providers at risk from exposure to blood and body fluids as well as injuries sustained in motor vehicle crashes during transport. Such unsuccessful attempts at resuscitation may divert resources away from patients who are viable and have a greater likelihood of survival. For these reasons, good judgment needs to be exercised regarding the decision to initiate resuscitation attempts for victims of traumatic cardiopulmonary arrest.

The National Association of EMS Physicians (NAEMSP) collaborated with the ACS-COT to develop guidelines for withholding or terminating CPR in the prehospital setting.[20] Victims of drowning, lightning strike, or hypothermia and patients in whom the mechanism of injury does not correlate with the clinical situation (suggesting a nontraumatic cause) deserve special consideration before a decision is made to withhold or terminate resuscitation. A patient found in cardiopulmonary arrest at the scene of a traumatic event may have experienced the arrest because of a medical problem (e.g., myocardial infarction), especially if the patient is elderly and evidence of injury is minimal.

Withholding CPR

If, during the primary assessment, patients are found to meet the following criteria, CPR may be withheld and the patient declared dead[21]:

- Resuscitation efforts are not indicated when the patient has sustained an obviously fatal injury (e.g., decapitation) or when evidence exists of dependent lividity, rigor mortis, and decomposition. For victims of blunt trauma, resuscitation efforts may be withheld if the patient is pulseless and apneic on arrival of prehospital care providers.
- For victims of penetrating trauma, resuscitation efforts may be withheld if there are no signs of life (no pupillary reflexes, no spontaneous movement, no organized cardiac rhythm on ECG greater than 40 beats/minute).

Extreme caution must be exercised when assessing a potentially dead victim, as the decision to withhold CPR is medically justifiable only when proper assessment has been performed.

Several times each year, a story hits the press of a trauma patient who was incorrectly presumed to be deceased only to later be discovered to have vital signs. Virtually all of these patients go on to succumb to their injuries, but such incidents can be embarrassing to both the prehospital care providers and their agencies. In the excitement of a scene with multiple patients, a prehospital care provider may not adequately assess for presence of a pulse. Dying trauma patients may be profoundly bradycardic and hypotensive, thus contributing to the difficulty in identifying a preterminal condition. Ideally, before deciding to withhold CPR, a central pulse (carotid or femoral) should be palpated for a minimum of 30 to 60 seconds. A prehospital care provider may opt to palpate for presence of a pulse at more than one location. Advanced prehospital care providers may also opt to obtain an ECG tracing in order to determine that the patient is not in pulseless electrical activity.

Basic Life Support

While many protocols include the use of closed chest compressions in algorithms for the management of traumatic cardiopulmonary arrest, many trauma surgeons question the role of CPR in the setting of exsanguination. Despite this reservation, it is reasonable to attempt CPR in patients who may be salvageable while expediting transport. As with all CPR attempts, prehospital care providers should limit interruptions to compressions.[22]

Advanced Life Support

The airway is secured with a complex airway device while simultaneously ensuring in-line stabilization of the cervical spine. Breath sounds should be auscultated and the possible presence of a tension pneumothorax ruled out. A tension pneumothorax may be present when a decrease in breath sounds is noted, with inadequate chest excursion during ventilation. If any doubt exists that the patient may have a tension pneumothorax, chest decompression is performed. Bilateral chest decompression should be performed only if the patient is receiving positive pressure ventilation.

Large-bore venous access is obtained, and isotonic crystalloid solution is delivered through a wide-open line if hypovolemic shock is a possible cause of the cardiac arrest. ECG monitoring is performed and cardiac rhythm assessed. The following dysrhythmias may be noted:

- *Pulseless electrical activity (PEA)*. A patient found in PEA should be assessed for the presence of hypovolemia, hypothermia, tension pneumothorax, and cardiac tamponade. Fluids, warming, and chest decompression should be performed if indicated. Epinephrine and atropine may be administered.
- *Bradycardia/asystole*. A patient found in this rhythm should be assessed for severe hypoxia and hypovolemia. The location of the airway should be confirmed and volume resuscitation initiated. Epinephrine and atropine may be administered.

■ *Ventricular fibrillation/pulseless ventricular tachycardia*. The primary therapy for these dysrhythmias is defibrillation. If the available defibrillator is biphasic, a shock of 120 to 200 joules is delivered. If a monophasic defibrillator is present, a shock of 360 joules is used.

Prehospital care providers should note that some trauma victims may have suffered their cardiac arrest as a result of a medical condition, such as an acute coronary syndrome, and subsequently suffered their injury, such as in a car crash. A medical cause of a cardiac arrest should be considered in older victims and those with minimal mechanism of injury or little evidence of external trauma. These patients should receive aggressive attempts at CPR and advanced cardiac life support, as their survival rate may be significantly higher than that of trauma patients who have suffered exsanguination.

Terminating CPR

The NAEMSP and the ACS-COT have published revised guidelines for termination of CPR and ALS measures in the prehospital setting.[20] Termination of resuscitation for trauma patients should be considered when there are no signs of life and no return of spontaneous circulation despite appropriate field EMS treatment that includes minimally interrupted CPR. The position statement notes that "protocols should require a specific interval of CPR that accompanies other resuscitative interventions. Past guidance has indicated that up to 15 minutes of CPR should be provided before resuscitative efforts are terminated, but the science in this regard remains unclear."

Pain Management

Pain management (*analgesia*) is often used in the prehospital setting for pain caused by angina or myocardial infarction. Traditionally, pain management has had a limited role in the management of trauma patients, primarily because of the concern that side effects (decreased ventilatory drive and vasodilatation) of narcotics may aggravate pre-existing hypoxia and hypotension. This concern has resulted in pain relief being denied to some patients with appropriate indications, such as an isolated limb injury or spinal fracture. The prehospital care provider may consider pain management in such patients, particularly if prolonged transport occurs, provided that signs of ventilatory impairment or shock are not present.

The Musculoskeletal Trauma chapter devotes a section to pain management as it relates to isolated extremity injuries and fractures. Morphine sulfate is typically the agent of choice and should be titrated intravenously in 1- to 2-milligram increments until some degree of pain relief is obtained or a change in the patient's vital signs occurs. Alternative medications for analgesia include fentanyl and ketamine.

Pulse oximetry and serial vital signs must be monitored if any narcotics are administered to a trauma patient. Sedation with an agent such as a benzodiazepine should be reserved for exceptional circumstances, such as a combative intubated patient, because the combination of a narcotic and benzodiazepine may result in respiratory arrest. Prehospital care providers can collaborate with their medical control to develop appropriate protocols.

Abuse

A prehospital care provider is often the first person on the scene, allowing the prehospital care provider to assess for a potentially abusive situation. The prehospital care provider inside a house can observe and relay the details at the scene to the receiving facility so that the appropriate social services in the area can be alerted of the concern for abuse. The prehospital care provider is often the only medically trained person to be in a position to observe, suspect, and relay information about this silent danger.

Anyone at any age can be a potential victim of abuse or an abuser. A pregnant woman, infant, toddler, child, adolescent, young adult, middle-age adult, and older adult are all at risk for abuse. Several different types of abuse exist, including physical, psychological (emotional), and financial. Abuse may occur by **commission**, in which a purposeful act results in an injury (i.e., physical abuse or sexual abuse), or by **omission** (e.g., neglectful care of a dependent). This section does not discuss types of abuse and only introduces the general characteristics and heightens a prehospital care provider's awareness and suspicion of abuse.

General characteristics of a potential abuser include dishonesty, the "story" not correlating with the injuries, a negative attitude, and abrasiveness with prehospital care providers. General characteristics of the abused patient include quietness, reluctance to elaborate on details of the incident, constant eye contact or lack of eye contact with someone at the scene, and minimization of personal injuries. Abuse, abusers, and the abused can take many different forms, and prehospital care providers need to keep their suspicion high if the scene and the story do not correlate. The prehospital care provider is required to relay suspicions and any information to the proper authorities.

Prolonged Transport

Although most urban or suburban EMS transports take 30 minutes or less, transport times may be prolonged as a result of traffic congestion, trains that block a crossing, or bridges that may be up to allow a ship to pass. These sorts of delays should be documented on the PCR to explain prolonged return times to the trauma center. Many prehospital care providers in rural and frontier settings routinely manage patients for much longer periods of time during transport. Additionally, prehospital care providers are called on to manage patients during transfer from one medical facility to another, either by ground or air. These transfers may take up to several hours.

Special preparations need to be taken when prehospital care providers are involved in the prolonged transport of a trauma patient. The issues that must be considered before undertaking such a transport can be divided into those dealing with the patient, the prehospital crew, and the equipment.

Patient Issues

Of pre-eminent importance is providing a safe, warm, and secure environment in which the patient is transported. The gurney should be appropriately secured to the ambulance, and the patient properly secured to the gurney. As emphasized throughout this text, hypothermia is a potentially deadly complication in a trauma patient, and the patient compartment must be sufficiently warm. If you, as a fully clothed prehospital care provider are comfortable with the temperature in the patient compartment, it is likely too cold for the patient who has been exposed.

The patient should be secured in a position that allows maximum access to the patient, especially the injured areas. Before transport, the security of any airway devices placed must be confirmed, and adjuncts (e.g., monitors, oxygen tanks) should be placed and secured so that they do not become projectiles in the event that the ambulance has to swerve in an evasive action or is involved in a motor vehicle crash. Adjuncts should not rest on the patient because pressure ulcers might be created during a prolonged transport. During transport, all IV lines and catheters must be securely fastened to prevent loss of the venous access.

The patient should undergo serial assessments of the primary assessment and vital signs at routine intervals. Pulse oximetry and ECG are monitored continuously for virtually all seriously injured patients, as well as $ETCO_2$, if available, in an intubated patient. The prehospital care providers accompanying the patient should be trained at a level appropriate to the anticipated needs of the patient. Critically injured patients should generally be managed by prehospital care providers with advanced training. If the patient is anticipated to require blood transfusion during transport, an individual should be in attendance whose scope of practice allows this procedure; in the United States, this generally requires a registered nurse.

Two management plans should be devised. The first, a medical plan, is developed to manage either anticipated or unexpected problems with the patient during transport. Necessary equipment, medications, and supplies should be readily available. The second plan involves identifying the most expeditious route to the receiving hospital. Weather conditions, road conditions (e.g., construction), and traffic concerns should be identified and anticipated. Additionally, the prehospital care providers should be knowledgeable about the medical facilities along the transport route in case a problem arises that cannot be managed en route to the primary destination.

Adjuncts to the care of the patient during prolonged transport may include the following:

- *Gastric catheter.* If trained in proper insertion, a naso- or orogastric tube can be inserted into the patient's stomach. Suctioning out gastric contents can decrease abdominal distension and potentially decrease the risk of vomiting and aspiration.
- *Urinary catheter.* If trained on proper insertion, a urinary catheter may be inserted into the patient's bladder. Urine output can be a sensitive measure of the patient's renal perfusion and a marker of the patient's volume status.
- *Arterial blood gas monitoring via point of care testing.* While the pulse oximeter gives valuable information regarding the oxyhemoglobin saturation, an arterial blood gas reading may give useful information regarding the patient's partial pressure of carbon dioxide (PCO_2) and the base deficit, an indicator of the severity of shock.

Crew Issues

The safety of the prehospital care crew is as important as that of the patient. The prehospital care crew needs to have appropriate safety devices, such as seat belts, and they should be utilized during transport unless an issue involving patient care prevents this. The prehospital care crew members use standard precautions and ensure that sufficient gloves and other personal protective equipment to avoid body fluids, blood, and other possible exposures are available for the trip.

Equipment Issues

Equipment issues during prolonged transport involve the ambulance, supplies, medications, monitors, and communications. The ambulance must be in good working order, including an adequate amount of fuel and a spare tire. The prehospital care crew must make sure sufficient supplies and medications are available and accessible for the transport, including gauze and pads for reinforcing dressings, IV fluids, oxygen, and pain medications. Drug supplies are based on anticipated patient needs and include sedatives, paralytic agents, analgesics, and antibiotics. A good rule of thumb is to stock the ambulance with about 50% more supplies and medications than the anticipated need in case a significant delay is encountered. Patient care equipment must be in good working order, including monitors (with functioning alarms), oxygen regulators, and suction devices. Also, success of a prolonged transport may depend on functional communications, including the ability to communicate with other crew members, medical control, and the destination facility.

The management of specific injuries during prolonged transport is discussed in the subsequent corresponding chapters of this text.

Summary

- The likelihood of survival for a patient with traumatic injuries depends on the immediate identification and mitigation of conditions that interfere with tissue perfusion.
- The identification of these conditions requires a systematic, prioritized, logical process of collecting information and acting on it. This process is referred to as patient assessment.
- Patient assessment begins with scene assessment and includes the formation of a general impression of the patient, a primary assessment, and when the patient's condition and availability of additional EMS personnel permit, a secondary assessment.
- The information obtained through this assessment process is analyzed and used as the basis for patient care and transport decisions.
- In the care of the trauma patient, a missed problem is a missed opportunity to potentially aid in an individual's survival.
- After the simultaneous determination of scene safety and general impression of the situation, the focus is on the priorities of patient assessment—on the patency of the patient's airway, the ventilatory status, and the circulatory status. This primary assessment follows the ABCDE format for evaluation of the patient's airway, breathing, circulation, disability (initial neurologic examination), and exposure (removing the patient's clothing to discover additional significant injuries). Although the sequential nature of language limits the ability to describe the simultaneity of these actions, the primary assessment of the patient is a process of actions that occur essentially at the same time.
- Immediate threats to the patient's life are quickly corrected in a "find and fix" manner. Once the prehospital care provider manages the patient's airway and breathing and controls exsanguinating hemorrhage, he or she packages the patient and begins transport without additional treatment at the scene. The limitations of field management of trauma require the safe, expedient delivery of the patient to definitive care.
- The primary and secondary assessments should be repeated frequently in order to identify any changes in the patient's condition and new problems that demand prompt intervention.

SCENARIO RECAP

It is a Saturday morning in early November. The weather is clear, with an outside temperature of 42°F (5.5°C). Your squad is dispatched to a residential area for a person who has fallen from the roof of a two-story building. Upon arrival at the scene, you are met by an adult family member who leads you around the house to the backyard. The family member states the patient was cleaning leaves from the rain gutters with a leaf blower when he lost his balance and fell approximately 12 feet (3.6 meters) from the roof, landing on his back. The patient initially lost consciousness for a "brief period" but was conscious by the time the family member called 9-1-1.

Approaching the patient, you observe an approximately 40-year-old man lying supine on the ground with two bystanders kneeling by his side. The patient is conscious and talking with the bystanders. As your partner provides manual stabilization to the patient's head and neck, you ask the patient where he hurts. The patient states both his upper and lower back hurt the most.

Your initial questioning serves the multiple purposes of obtaining the patient's chief complaint, determining his initial level of consciousness, and assessing his ventilatory effort. Detecting no shortness of breath, you proceed with the patient assessment. The patient answers your questions appropriately to establish that he is oriented to person, place, and time.

- Based on kinematics as they relate to this incident, what potential injuries do you anticipate finding during your assessment?
- What are your next priorities?
- How will you proceed with this patient?

SCENARIO SOLUTION

You have been on the scene for 1 minute, yet you have obtained much important information to guide further assessment and treatment of the patient. In the first 15 seconds of patient contact, you have developed a general impression of the patient, determining that resuscitation is not necessary. With a few simple actions, you have evaluated the A, B, C, and D of the primary assessment. The patient spoke to you without difficulty, indicating that his airway is open and he is breathing with no signs of distress. At the same time, with an awareness of the mechanism of injury, you have stabilized the cervical spine. You have noted no obvious bleeding, your partner has assessed the radial pulse, and you have observed the patient's skin color, temperature, and moisture. These findings indicate no immediate threats to the patient's circulatory status. Additionally, you have simultaneously found no initial evidence of disability because the patient is awake and alert and answers questions appropriately. This information, along with information about the fall, will help you determine the need for additional resources, the type of transport indicated, and the type of facility to which you should deliver the patient.

Now that you have completed these steps and no immediate lifesaving intervention is necessary, you will proceed with step E of the primary assessment early in the evaluation process and then obtain vital signs. You will expose the patient to look for additional injuries and bleeding that may have been concealed by clothing, then cover the patient to protect him from the environment. During this process, you will perform a more detailed examination, noting less serious injuries.

The next steps you will take are packaging the patient, including splinting the entire spine and extremity injuries and bandaging wounds if time allows; initiating transport; and communicating with medical direction and the receiving facility. During the trip to the hospital, you will continue to reevaluate and monitor the patient. Your knowledge of kinematics and the patient's witnessed loss of consciousness will generate a high index of suspicion for traumatic brain injury, lower extremity injuries, and injuries to the spine. In an ALS system, IV access will be established en route to the receiving facility.

References

1. Advanced Trauma Life Support (ATLS) Subcommittee, Committee on Trauma. Initial assessment and management. In: *Advanced Trauma Life Support Course for Doctors, Student Course Manual.* 9th ed. Chicago, IL: American College of Surgeons; 2012.
2. Kragh JF, Littrel ML, Jones JA, et al. Battle casualty survival with emergency tourniquet use to stop limb bleeding. *J Emerg Med.* 2011;41:590–597.
3. Beekley AC, Sebesta JA, Blackbourne LH, et al. Prehospital tourniquet use in Operation Iraqi Freedom: effect on hemorrhage control and outcomes. *J Trauma.* 2008;64:S28–S37.
4. Doyle GS, Taillac PP. Tourniquets: a review of current use with proposals for expanded prehospital use. *Prehosp Emerg Care.* 2008;12:241–256.
5. First Aid Science Advisory Board. First aid. *Circulation.* 2005;112(III):115.
6. Swan KG Jr, Wright DS, Barbagiovanni SS, et al. Tourniquets revisited. *J Trauma.* 2009;66:672–675.
7. Teasdale G, Jennett B. Assessment of coma and impaired consciousness: a practical scale. *Lancet.* 1974;2:81.
8. Healey C, Osler TM, Rogers FB, et al. Improving the Glasgow Coma Scale score: motor score alone is a better predictor. *J Trauma.* 2003;54:671.

9. Moylan JA, Detmer DE, Rose J, Schulz R. Evaluation of the quality of hospital care for major trauma. *J Trauma.* 1976;16(7):517–523.
10. West JG, Trunkey DD, Lim RC. Systems of trauma care. A study of two counties. *Arch Surg.* 1979;114(4):455–460.
11. West JG, Cales RH, Gazzaniga AB. Impact of regionalization. The Orange County experience. *Arch Surg.* 1983;118(6):740–744.
12. Shackford SR, Hollingworth-Fridlund P, Cooper GF, Eastman AB. The effect of regionalization upon the quality of trauma care as assessed by concurrent audit before and after institution of a trauma system: a preliminary report. *J Trauma.* 1986;26(9):812–820.
13. Waddell TK, Kalman PG, Goodman SJ, Girotti MJ. Is outcome worse in a small volume Canadian trauma centre? *J Trauma.* 1991;31(7):958–961.
14. MacKenzie EJ, Rivara FP, Jurkovich GJ, et al. A national evaluation of the effect of trauma-center care on mortality. *N Engl J Med.* 2006;354(4):366–378.
15. Branas CC, MacKenzie EJ, Williams JC, et al. Access to trauma centers in the United States. *JAMA.* 2005;293(21):2626–2633.
16. Nathens AB, Jurkovich GJ, Rivara FP, Maier RV. Effectiveness of state trauma systems in reducing injury-related mortality: a national evaluation. *J Trauma.* 2000;48(1):25–30; discussion 30–31.
17. Committee on Trauma. Resources for optimal care of the injured patient: 1999. Chicago, IL: American College of Surgeons; 1998.

18. Centers for Disease Control and Prevention. Guidelines for field triage of injured patients: recommendations of the national expert panel on field triage. *MMWR*. 2009;58:1–35.

19. Centers for Disease Control and Prevention. Guidelines for field triage of injured patients: recommendations of the national expert panel on field triage 2011. *MMWR*. 2012;61:1–21.

20. National Association of EMS Physicians and American College of Surgeons Committee on Trauma. Position Statement. Field Triage of the Injured Patient. 2010. www.naemsp.org/Documents/Position Papers/POSITION FieldTriageoftheInjuredPatient.pdf Accessed November 24, 2013.

21. National Association of EMS Physicians and American College of Surgeons Committee on Trauma. NAEMSP position statement: withholding of resuscitation for adult traumatic cardiopulmonary arrest. *Prehosp Emerg Care*. 2013;17:291.

22. American Heart Association. 2010 guidelines for cardiopulmonary resuscitation and emergency cardiovascular care. *Circulation*. 2010;122:1.

Suggested Reading

American Heart Association. Cardiac arrest associated with trauma. *Circulation*. 2010;122:S844.

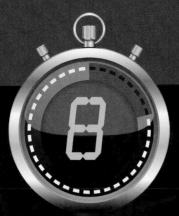

Airway and Ventilation

CHAPTER OBJECTIVES

At the completion of this chapter, the reader will be able to do the following:

- Integrate the principles of ventilation and gas exchange with the pathophysiology of trauma to identify patients with inadequate perfusion.

- Relate the concepts of minute volume and oxygenation to the pathophysiology of trauma.

- Understand the difference between ventilation and respiration.

- Explain the mechanisms by which supplemental oxygen and ventilatory support are beneficial to the trauma patient.

- Given a scenario that involves a trauma patient, select the most effective means of providing a patent airway to suit the patient's needs.

- Presented with a scenario that involves a patient who requires ventilatory support, discuss the most effective means available to suit the trauma patient's needs.

- Given situations that involve various trauma patients, formulate a plan for airway management and ventilation.

- Presented with current research, understand the risks versus benefits when discussing new invasive procedures.

- Discuss the indications and limitations of end-tidal carbon monoxide ($ETCO_2$) monitoring in the trauma patient.

SCENARIO

You and your partner are dispatched to a motorcycle crash on a curvy county road. Fellow riders report that the patient was traveling too fast to negotiate a sharp curve and was thrown over the guardrail and into a tree. They carried the patient back up the embankment to the road.

Upon your arrival, you find a police officer maintaining an open airway using a nasopharyngeal airway and administering oxygen via a nonrebreathing mask. The police officer reports that the patient has been unconscious since her arrival. You note that the patient's helmet has significant damage. You also note a deformed right humerus and an angulated lower leg.

- What indicators of airway compromise are evident in this patient?
- What other information, if any, would you seek from witnesses or the emergency medical responders?
- Describe the sequence of actions you would take to manage this patient before and during transport.

Introduction

Two of the most important prehospital maneuvers are those that provide and maintain airway patency and pulmonary ventilation. The failure to adequately ventilate a trauma patient and maintain oxygenation of ischemic sensitive organs such as the brain and heart causes additional damage, including secondary brain injury, compounding the primary brain injury produced by the initial trauma. Ensuring patency of the airway and maintaining the patient's oxygenation and supporting ventilation, when necessary, are critical steps in minimizing the overall brain injury and improving the likelihood of good outcome. To be clear on the use of terminology, *oxygenation* refers to the process by which oxygen concentration increases within a tissue, and *ventilation* refers to the mechanical exchange of air between the outside environment and the alveoli of the lungs.

Cerebral oxygenation and oxygen delivery to other parts of the body provided by adequate airway management and ventilation remain the most important components of prehospital patient care. Because techniques and adjunct devices are changing and will continue to change, keeping abreast of these changes is important. Such techniques may require active ventilation or passive observation of the patient's breathing.

The respiratory system serves two primary functions:

1. To provide oxygen to the red blood cells, which carry the oxygen to all of the body's cells
2. To remove carbon dioxide from the body

Inability of the respiratory system to provide oxygen to the cells or inability of the cells to use the oxygen supplied results in anaerobic metabolism and can quickly lead to death. Failure to eliminate carbon dioxide can lead to coma and acidosis.

Anatomy

The respiratory system is comprised of the upper airway and the lower airway, including the lungs (**Figure 8-1**). Each part of the respiratory system plays an important role in ensuring gas exchange—the process by which oxygen enters the bloodstream and carbon dioxide is removed.

Upper Airway

The upper airway consists of the nasal cavity and the oral cavity (**Figure 8-2**). Air entering the nasal cavity is warmed, humidified, and filtered to remove impurities. Beyond these cavities is the area known as the **pharynx**, which runs from the back of the soft palate to the upper end of the esophagus. The pharynx is composed of muscle lined with mucous membranes. The pharynx is divided into three discrete sections: the **nasopharynx** (upper portion), the **oropharynx** (middle portion), and the **hypopharynx** (lower or distal end of the pharynx). Below the pharynx is the **esophagus**, which leads to the stomach, and the trachea, at which point the lower airway begins. Above the trachea is the **larynx** (**Figure 8-3**), which contains the vocal cords and the muscles that make them work, housed in a strong cartilaginous box. The vocal cords are folds of tissue that meet in the midline. The false cords, or **vestibular folds**, direct the airflow through the vocal cords. Supporting the cords posteriorly is the arytenoid cartilage. Directly above the larynx is a leaf-shaped structure called the **epiglottis**. Acting as a gate or flapper valve, the epiglottis directs air into the trachea and solids and liquids into the esophagus.

Lower Airway

The lower airway consists of the trachea, its branches, and the lungs. On inspiration, air travels through the upper airway and into the lower airway before reaching the alveoli, where the actual gas exchange occurs. The trachea divides into the right

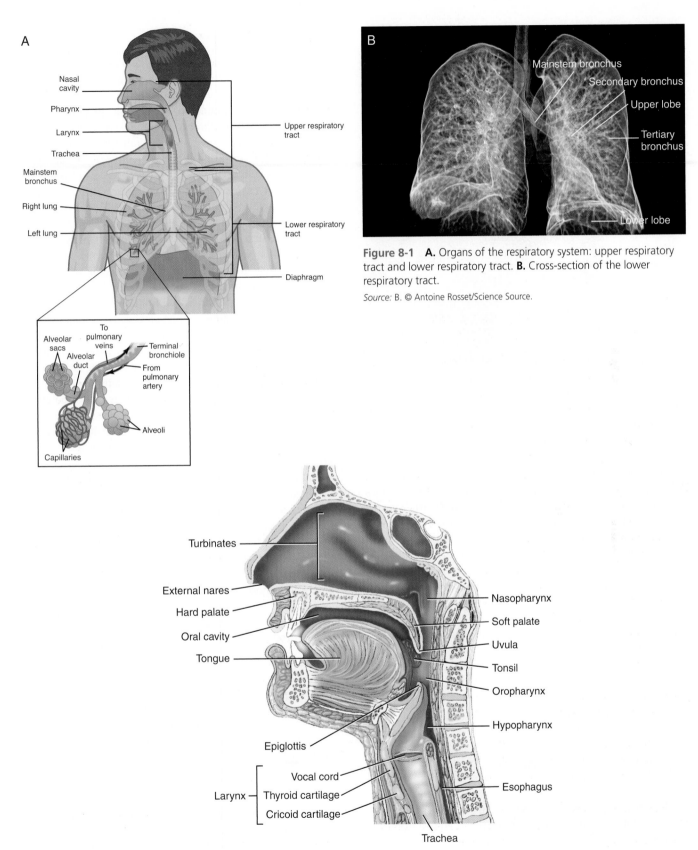

Figure 8-1 **A.** Organs of the respiratory system: upper respiratory tract and lower respiratory tract. **B.** Cross-section of the lower respiratory tract.

Source: B. © Antoine Rosset/Science Source.

Figure 8-2 Sagittal section through the nasal cavity and pharynx viewed from the medial side.

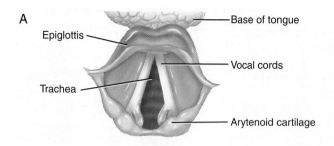

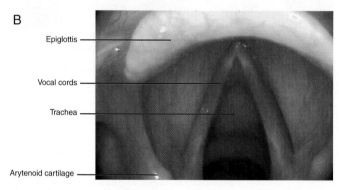

Figure 8-3 Vocal cords viewed from above, showing their relationship to the paired cartilages of the larynx and the epiglottis.
Source: Courtesy of James P. Thomas, M.D., www.voicedoctor.net

Physiology

As discussed in the Physiology of Life and Death chapter, the airway is a pathway that leads atmospheric air through the nose, mouth, pharynx, trachea, and bronchi to the alveoli. With each breath, the average 150-pound (lb) (70-kilogram [kg]) adult takes in approximately 500 milliliters (ml) of air. The airway system holds up to 150 ml of air that never actually reaches the alveoli to participate in the critical gas-exchange process. The space in which this air is held is known as *dead space*. The air inside this dead space is not available to the body to be used for oxygenation because it never reaches the alveoli.

With each breath, air is drawn into the lungs. The movement of air into and out of the alveolus results from changes in intrathoracic pressure generated by the contraction and relaxation of specific muscle groups. The primary muscle of breathing is the **diaphragm**. Normally, the muscle fibers of the diaphragm shorten when a stimulus is received from the brain. In addition to the diaphragm, the external intercostal muscles help pull the ribs forward and upward. This flattening of the diaphragm along with the action of the intercostal muscles is an active movement that creates a negative pressure inside the thoracic cavity. This negative pressure causes atmospheric air to enter the intact pulmonary tree (**Figure 8-4**). Other muscles attached to the chest wall can also contribute to the creation of this negative pressure; these include the sternocleidomastoid and scalene muscles. The use of these secondary muscles will be seen as the work of breathing increases in the trauma patient. In contrast, exhalation is normally a passive process in nature, caused by the relaxation of the diaphragm and chest wall muscles and the elastic recoil of these structures. However, exhalation can become active as the work of breathing increases.

Generating this negative pressure during inspiration requires an intact chest wall. For example, in the trauma patient, a wound that creates an open pathway between the outside atmosphere and the thoracic cavity can result in air being pulled in through the open wound rather than into the lungs. Damage to the bony structure of the chest wall may again compromise the patient's ability to generate the needed

and left main bronchi. The right main bronchus is shorter, wider, and more vertical than the left. The right main bronchus comes off the trachea at approximately a 25-degree angle, whereas the left has a 45-degree angulation. (This difference explains why right main bronchus placement of an endotracheal tube is a common complication of intubation.)

Each of the main bronchi subdivides into several primary bronchi and then into bronchioles. **Bronchioles** (very small bronchial tubes) terminate at the **alveoli**, which are tiny air sacs surrounded by capillaries. The alveoli are the site of gas exchange where the respiratory and circulatory systems meet.

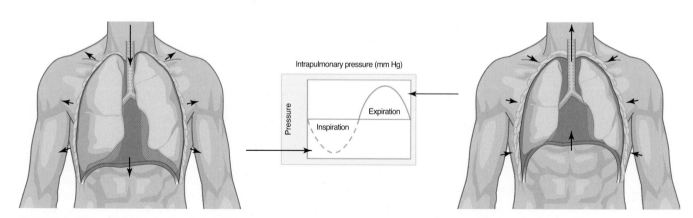

Figure 8-4 This graph shows the relationship of intrapulmonary pressure during the phases of Ventilation.

negative pressure required for adequate ventilation (see the Thoracic Trauma chapter).

When atmospheric air reaches the alveoli, oxygen moves from the alveoli, across the alveolar–capillary membrane, and into the red blood cells (RBCs) (**Figure 8-5**). The circulatory system then delivers the oxygen-carrying RBCs to the body tissues, where oxygen is used as fuel for metabolism. As oxygen is transferred from inside the alveoli across the cell wall and capillary endothelium, through the plasma, and into the RBCs, carbon dioxide is exchanged in the opposite direction, from the blood to the alveoli. Carbon dioxide, which is carried dissolved in the plasma (approximately 10%), bound to proteins (mostly hemoglobin in the RBCs [approximately 20%]), and as bicarbonate (approximately 70%), moves from the bloodstream, across the alveolar–capillary membrane, and into the alveoli, where it is eliminated during exhalation (**Figure 8-6**). On completion of this exchange, the oxygenated RBCs and plasma with a low carbon dioxide level return to the left side of the heart to be pumped to all the cells in the body.

Once at the cell, the oxygenated RBCs deliver their oxygen, which the cells then use for aerobic metabolism (see the Physiology of Life and Death chapter). Carbon dioxide, a by-product of aerobic metabolism, is released into the blood plasma. Deoxygenated blood returns to the right side of the heart. The blood is pumped to the lungs, where it is again supplied with oxygen, and the carbon dioxide is eliminated by diffusion. The oxygen is transported mostly by hemoglobin in the RBCs themselves, whereas the carbon dioxide is transported in the three ways previously mentioned: in the plasma, bound to proteins such as hemoglobin, and buffered as bicarbonate.

The alveoli must be constantly replenished with a fresh supply of air that contains an adequate amount of oxygen. This replenishment of air, known as *ventilation*, is also essential for the elimination of carbon dioxide. Ventilation is measurable. The size of each breath, called the tidal volume, multiplied by the ventilatory rate for 1 minute equals the **minute volume**:

$$\text{Minute volume} = \text{Tidal volume} \times \text{Ventilatory rate per minute}$$

During normal resting ventilation, about 500 ml of air is taken into the lungs. As mentioned previously, part of this volume, 150 ml, remains in the airway system (the trachea and bronchi) as dead space and does not participate in gas exchange. Only 350 ml is actually available for gas exchange (**Figure 8-7**). If the tidal volume is 500 ml and the ventilatory rate is 14 breaths/minute, the minute volume can be calculated as follows:

$$\text{Minute volume} = 500 \text{ ml} \times 14 \text{ breaths/minute}$$
$$= 7,000 \text{ ml/minute, or 7 liters/minute}$$

Therefore, at rest, about 7 liters of air must move in and out of the lungs each minute to maintain adequate carbon dioxide elimination and oxygenation. If the minute volume falls below normal, the patient has inadequate ventilation, a condition called *hypoventilation*. Hypoventilation leads to a buildup of carbon dioxide in the body. Hypoventilation is common when head or chest trauma causes an altered breathing pattern or an inability to move the chest wall adequately.

For example, a patient with rib fractures who is breathing quickly and shallowly because of the pain of the injury may have a

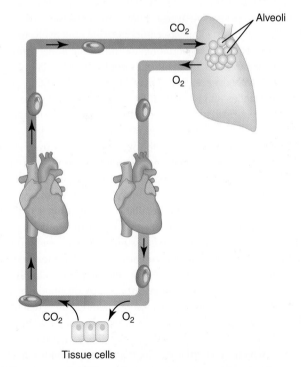

Figure 8-6 Oxygen (O_2) moves into the red blood cells from the alveoli. The O_2 is transferred to the tissue cell on the hemoglobin molecule. After leaving the hemoglobin molecule, the O_2 travels into the tissue cell. Carbon dioxide (CO_2) travels in the reverse direction, but not on the hemoglobin molecule. It travels in the plasma as CO_2.

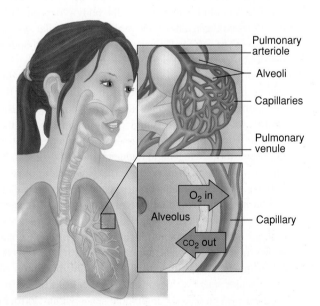

Figure 8-5 Diffusion of oxygen and carbon dioxide across the alveolar–capillary membrane of the alveoli in the lungs.

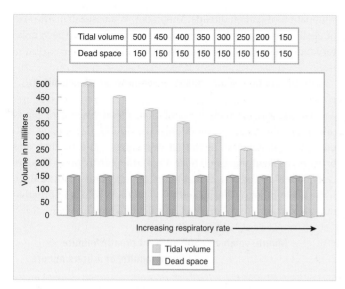

Tidal volume	500	450	400	350	300	250	200	150
Dead space	150	150	150	150	150	150	150	150

Figure 8-7 This graph shows the relationship of tidal volume to dead space with various rates of breathing.

tidal volume of 100 ml and a ventilatory rate of 40 breaths/minute. This patient's minute volume can be calculated as follows:

$$\text{Minute volume} = 100 \text{ ml} \times 40 \text{ breaths/minute}$$
$$= 4{,}000 \text{ ml/minute, or 4 liters/minute}$$

If 7 liters/minute is necessary for adequate gas exchange in a nontraumatized person at rest, 4 liters/minute is much less than the body requires to eliminate carbon dioxide effectively, indicating hypoventilation. Furthermore, 150 ml of air is necessary to overcome dead space. If the patient's tidal volume is 100 ml, oxygenated air will never reach the alveoli but instead will only get as far as the trachea and bronchi. If left untreated, this hypoventilation will quickly lead to severe respiratory distress and, ultimately, death.

In the previous example, the patient with rib fractures is hypoventilating even though the ventilatory rate is 40 breaths/minute. This patient is breathing fast (tachypneic) but at the same time is hypoventilating. Thus, respiratory rate does not, by itself, indicate the adequacy of the ventilation. Evaluating a patient's ability to exchange air involves assessing both ventilatory rate and depth. A common mistake is assuming that any patient with a fast ventilatory rate is hyperventilating. A much better measure of ventilatory status is the amount of carbon dioxide eliminated, which can be determined using carbon dioxide monitors. The effect of carbon dioxide elimination on metabolism is discussed with the Fick principle and aerobic and anaerobic metabolism in the Physiology of Life and Death and the Shock chapters.

Assessment of ventilatory function always includes an evaluation of how well a patient is taking in, diffusing, and delivering oxygen to the tissue cells. Without proper intake, delivery of oxygen to the tissue cells, and processing of oxygen within these cells to maintain aerobic metabolism and energy production, anaerobic metabolism will begin. In addition, effective

ventilation must be ensured. A patient may accomplish ventilation completely, partially, or not at all. Aggressive assessment and management of these inadequacies in both oxygenation and ventilation are paramount to a successful outcome.

Oxygenation and Ventilation of the Trauma Patient

The oxygenation process within the human body involves the following three phases:

1. *External respiration* is the transfer of oxygen molecules from air to the blood. Air contains oxygen (20.95%), nitrogen (78.1%), argon (0.93%), and carbon dioxide (0.031%), but for practical purposes, the content of air is oxygen 21% and nitrogen 79%. All alveolar oxygen exists as free gas; therefore, each oxygen molecule exerts pressure. Increasing the percentage of oxygen in the inspired atmosphere will increase alveolar oxygen pressure or tension. When supplemental oxygen is provided, the ratio of oxygen in each inspiration increases, causing an increase in the amount of oxygen in each alveolus. This, in turn, will increase the amount of gas that gets transferred to blood because the amount of gas that will enter a liquid is directly related to the pressure it exerts. The greater the pressure of the gas, the greater the amount of that gas that will be absorbed into the fluid.

2. *Oxygen delivery* is the result of oxygen transfer from the atmosphere to the RBCs during ventilation and the transportation of these RBCs to the tissues via the cardiovascular system. The volume of oxygen consumed by the body in 1 minute in order to maintain energy production is known as oxygen consumption and depends upon adequate cardiac output and the delivery of oxygen to the cells by RBCs. The RBCs could be described as the body's "oxygen tankers." These oxygen tankers move along the vascular system "highways" to "off-load" their oxygen supply at the body's distribution points, the capillary beds.

3. *Internal (cellular) respiration* is the movement, or diffusion, of oxygen from the RBCs into the tissue cells. Metabolism normally occurs through glycolysis and the Krebs cycle to produce energy. While understanding the specific details of these processes is not necessary, it is important to have a general understanding of their role in energy production. Because the actual exchange of oxygen between the RBCs and the tissues occurs in the thin-walled capillaries, any factor that interrupts a supply of oxygen will disrupt this cycle. A major factor in this regard is the amount of fluid (or edema) located between the alveolar walls, the capillary walls, and the wall of the tissue cells (also known as the interstitial space). Overhydration of the vascular space with crystalloid, which leaks out of the vascular system into the interstitial space within 30 to 45 minutes after administration, is a major problem during resuscitation. Supplemental oxygen can help overcome

some of these factors. The tissues and cells cannot consume adequate amounts of oxygen if adequate amounts are not available.

Adequate oxygenation depends on all three of these phases. Although the ability to assess tissue oxygenation in prehospital situations is improving rapidly, appropriate ventilatory support for all trauma patients begins by providing supplemental oxygen to help ensure that hypoxia is corrected or averted entirely.

Pathophysiology

Trauma can affect the respiratory system's ability to adequately provide oxygen and eliminate carbon dioxide in the following ways:

- *Hypoxemia* (decreased oxygen level in the blood) can result from decreased diffusion of oxygen across the alveolar–capillary membrane.
- *Hypoxia* (deficient tissue oxygenation) can be caused by:
  - The inability of the air to reach the capillaries, usually because the airway is obstructed or the alveoli are filled with fluid or debris
  - Decreased blood flow to the alveoli
  - Decreased blood flow to the tissue cells
- *Hypoventilation* can result from:
  - Obstruction of airflow through the upper and lower airways
  - Decreased expansion of the lungs as a result of direct injury to the chest wall or lungs
  - Loss of ventilatory drive, usually because of decreased neurologic function, most often after a traumatic brain injury

Hyperventilation can cause vasoconstriction, which can be especially detrimental in the management of the traumatic brain-injured patient.

Hypoventilation results from the reduction of minute volume. If left untreated, hypoventilation results in carbon dioxide buildup, acidosis, and eventually death. Management involves improving the patient's ventilatory rate and depth by correcting existing airway problems and assisting ventilation as appropriate.

The following sections discuss two of the causes of inadequate ventilation: decreased neurologic function and mechanical obstruction. The third cause, a reduction in minute volume as a result of decreased pulmonary expansion, is discussed in the Thoracic Trauma chapter. The remaining causes are discussed in the Shock chapter.

Decreased Neurologic Function

Decreased minute volume can be caused by two clinical conditions related to decreased neurologic function: mechanical obstruction and a decreased level of consciousness (LOC).

A common cause of decreased minute volume is mechanical airway obstruction. The source of mechanical airway obstructions may be neurologically influenced or purely mechanical in nature. Neurologic insults that alter the LOC may disrupt the "controls" that normally hold the tongue in an anatomically neutral (nonobstructing) position. If these controls are compromised, the tongue falls rearward, occluding the hypopharynx (**Figure 8-8**). This complication commonly presents as snoring with respirations. To prevent the tongue from occluding the hypopharynx or to correct the problem when it occurs, an open airway must be maintained in any supine patient with a diminished LOC, regardless of whether signs of ventilatory compromise exist. Such patients may also require periodic suctioning because secretions, saliva, blood, or vomitus may accumulate in the oropharynx.

Foreign bodies in the airway may be objects that were in the patient's mouth at the time of the injury, such as false teeth, chewing gum, tobacco, real teeth, and bone. Outside materials, such as glass from a broken windshield or any object that is near the patient's mouth on injury, may also threaten airway patency. Upper and lower airway obstructions may also be caused by bone or cartilage collapse from a fractured larynx or trachea, by mucous membrane avulsed from the hypopharynx or tongue, or by facial damage in which blood and fragments of bone and tissue create an obstruction.

Management of mechanical airway obstructions can be extremely challenging. Foreign bodies in the oral cavity may become lodged and create occlusions in the hypopharynx or the larynx. Crush injuries to the larynx and edema of the vocal cords may be present. Patients with facial injuries may present with two of the most common foreign body obstructions: blood and vomit. Direct trauma to the anterior neck can cause rupture of the trachea leading to hemoptysis and massive subcutaneous emphysema as air leaks out into the soft tissues (**Figure 8-9**). Treatment of these problems is aimed at immediate recognition of the obstruction and the steps taken to ensure airway patency.

A decreased LOC, from traumatic brain injury or associated issues such as alcohol or drug use, will also affect ventilatory

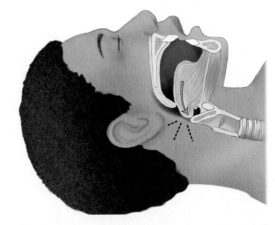

Figure 8-8 In an unconscious patient, the tongue has lost its muscle tone and falls back into the hypopharnyx, occluding the airway and preventing passage of oxygen into the trachea and lungs.

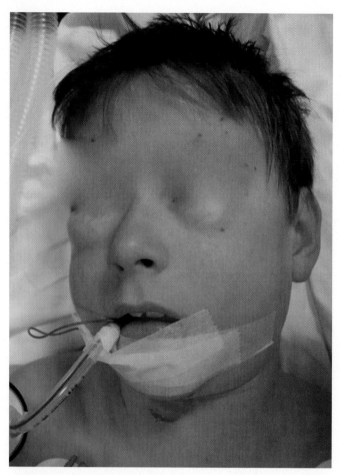

Figure 8-9   A patient who sustained trauma to the anterior neck causing rupture of the trachea and subcutaneous emphysema of the neck and face (note the markedly swollen eyelids, which are distended from air).

Source: Photograph provided courtesy of J.C. Pitteloud M.D., Switzerland.

drive and may reduce the rate of ventilation, the volume of ventilation, or both. This reduction in minute volume may be temporary or permanent.

Hyperventilation

Hyperventilation is when alveolar ventilation is so great that carbon dioxide removal exceeds its production in metabolizing cells, thus leading to *hypocapnia* (decreased amount of carbon dioxide in the arterial blood). Alveolar ventilation is usually measured by obtaining arterial blood measurements in the emergency department (ED) and intensive care unit (ICU). While we cannot obtain this lab test in the field, we do have the ability to monitor end-tidal carbon dioxide ($ETCO_2$). When carbon dioxide levels are below normal levels of 35 to 45 millimeters of mercury (mm Hg), vasoconstriction begins to occur.

Hyperventilation in the trauma patient does not usually occur without the intervention of the prehospital care provider using a **bag-mask device** at too fast a rate or too great a depth.

Evidence has shown that critical brain trauma patients in urban environments have a better outcome if managed with simple procedures rather than endotracheal intubation.[1] While there are many factors that may contribute to this outcome, including increased scene time, aspiration, and hypoxia during intubation, it is important to understand functional minute volume or the actual exchange that takes place at the alveolar level. It has been noted that as time goes on in the resuscitation process, ventilatory rate creeps up as the prehospital care provider becomes distracted.

While the ventilatory rate may increase while using the bag-mask device, the loss of a tight mask seal will cause volume leak, and thus the minute volume will remain near the normal levels. Once intubated however, a greater volume is available for gas exchange, and as the ventilatory rate increases, the combination of faster rate and greater volume causes hypocarbia (low carbon dioxide). This, in turn, causes vasoconstriction of the blood vessels within the brain. While this shrinking of the blood vessels will allow more space for expansion from bleeding or swelling of brain tissue, it causes a decreased amount of oxygenated blood to reach the brain tissue. This in turn causes more edema to develop.

Assessment of the Airway and Ventilation

The ability to assess the airway is required in order to effectively manage it. Prehospital care providers perform many aspects of assessing the airway automatically. A patient who is alert and talking as the prehospital care provider walks through the door has an open and patent airway. But when the patient's LOC is decreased, it is essential to thoroughly assess the airway prior to moving to other lower priority injuries. When examining the airway during the primary assessment, the following need to be assessed:

- Position of the airway and patient
- Any sounds emanating from the upper airway
- Airway obstructions
- Chest rise

Position of the Airway and Patient

As you make visual contact with the patient, observe the patient's position. Patients in a supine position with a decreased LOC are at risk for airway obstruction from the tongue falling back into the airway. Most trauma patients will be placed in the supine position on a backboard for spinal immobilization. Any patient exhibiting signs of decreased LOC will need constant re-examination for airway obstruction and the placement of an adjunctive device to ensure an open airway. Patients who present with an open airway while lying on their side may obstruct their airways when placed supine on a backboard. Patients with massive facial trauma and active bleeding may need to be maintained in the position in which they are found if they are maintaining their own airway. In some cases, this may mean allowing the patient to sit in an upright position as long as the airway is being maintained. Placing these patients supine on a backboard may cause obstruction to the airway and possible aspiration of blood. In such cases, if the patients are maintaining their own airways, the best course of action may be to let them continue. Suction should be available if needed to remove blood and secretions. If necessary, stabilization of the cervical spine can be accomplished by manually holding the head in the position needed to allow for maintenance of an open airway (**Figure 8-10**).

Remember that the principle is to maintain an open airway and provide stabilization for the cervical spine when indicated. This effort does not always require a full spine board and the patient lying flat.

Upper Airway Sounds

Noise coming from the upper airway is never a good sign. These noises can often be heard as you approach the patient. They are usually a result of a partial airway obstruction caused by the tongue, blood, or foreign bodies in the upper airway. Stridorous breath sounds point to a partially obstructed upper airway. This obstruction may be an anatomic obstruction, such as a tongue that has fallen back into the airway or an edematous (swollen) epiglottis or airway. It may also be caused by foreign bodies. An edematous airway is an emergent situation that demands quick action to prevent total airway obstruction. Steps must be taken immediately to alleviate the obstructions and maintain an open airway.

Examine the Airway for Obstructions

Look in the mouth for any obvious foreign matter or any gross anatomic malformations. Remove any foreign bodies found (as discussed later).

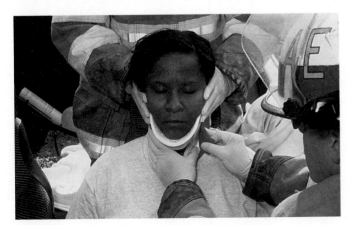

Figure 8-10 Manual stabilization of the cervical spine in a patient who is able to maintain an airway in a sitting position.
Source: © Jones & Bartlett Learning. Courtesy of MIEMSS.

Look for Chest Rise

Limited chest rise may be a sign of an obstructed airway. The use of accessory muscles and the appearance of increased work of breathing should lead to a high index of suspicion of airway compromise. Asymmetric chest rise may provide a subtle clue to the presence of a pneumothorax, although this sign is often difficult to identify in the prehospital environment.

Management
Airway Control

Ensuring a patent airway is the first priority of trauma management and resuscitation, and no action is more crucial in airway management than appropriate assessment of the airway (**Figure 8-11**). Regardless of how the airway is managed, a cervical spine injury must be considered if the mechanism of injury suggests the potential for injury. The use of any of these methods of airway control requires simultaneous manual stabilization of the cervical spine in a neutral position until the patient has been completely immobilized (see the Spinal Trauma chapter). The exception to this rule would be in penetrating trauma. Data have shown that spinal immobilization is usually not necessary in many of these patients (see the Spinal Trauma chapter).

Essential Skills

Management of the airway in trauma patients is a primary consideration because without an adequate airway, a positive outcome cannot be achieved. Management of the airway can be challenging, but in most patients, manual or simple procedures may be sufficient initially.[1] Even prehospital care providers who have been trained in more complex airway techniques need to maintain their ability to perform these essential manual and simple skills, because these methods, depending on the situation, may lead to a better patient outcome. Prehospital care providers always need to weigh the risk versus the benefit of performing highly invasive complex procedures. Such procedures require a high degree of skill proficiency and close oversight by the medical director. They should not be initiated unnecessarily.

Airway maintenance skills can be broken into three different levels. The application of these skills, as long as they are within the prehospital care provider's scope of practice, should be patient driven, dependent on the situation and the severity of the patient.

Categories for Airway Adjuncts and Procedures
Manual

Manual methods of opening the airway are the easiest to use and require no equipment other than the prehospital care provider's hands. The airway can be maintained with these methods, even

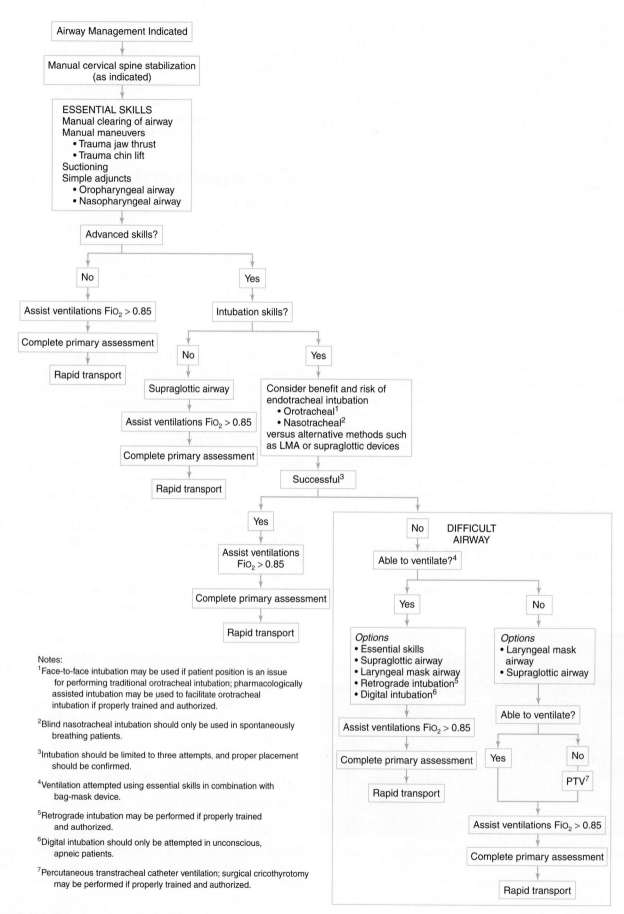

Figure 8-11 Airway management algorithm.

if the patient has a gag reflex. There are no contraindications for the use of manual techniques in airway management of the trauma patient. Examples of this type of airway management include the **trauma chin lift** and the **trauma jaw thrust**. Positioning and manual clearing of the airway also fall into this category (**Figures 8-12**).

Simple

Simple airway management involves the use of adjunctive devices that require only one piece of equipment, and the technique for inserting the device necessitates minimal training requirements. The risks associated with placement of this type of airway device are extremely low compared to the potential benefit of maintaining a patent airway. If the airway is improperly placed, it is easily recognizable and correctable. Examples of these airways include oropharyngeal and nasopharyngeal airways (**Figure 8-13**).

Complex

Complex airways include airway adjuncts that require significant initial training and then ongoing training to ensure continuing proficiency. Adjuncts that fall into this category require multiple pieces of equipment and the possible use of pharmaceuticals as well as multiple steps to insert the airway and, in some cases, direct visualization of the tracheal opening. In addition, surgical airway techniques such as cricothyroidotomy (both needle and surgical) fall into this category. The penalty for failure when using complex airways is high and may result in a less than optimal outcome for the patient. Continuous monitoring of oxygen saturation and ETCO$_2$ is also highly recommended when using this group of airways, adding to the complexity of their use. Examples of these airways include endotracheal tubes and supraglottic airways (**Figure 8-14**).

See **Figure 8-15** for a breakdown of the three methods of airway management.

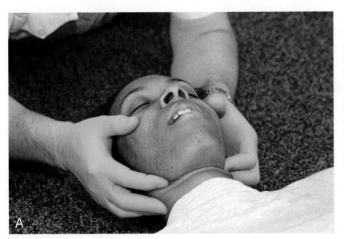
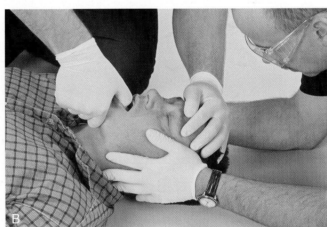

Figure 8-12 **A.** Trauma jaw thrust. The thumb is placed on each zygoma, with the index and long fingers at the angle of the mandible. The mandible is lifted superiorly. **B.** Trauma chin lift. The chin lift performs a function similar to that of the trauma jaw thrust. It moves the mandible forward by moving the tongue.

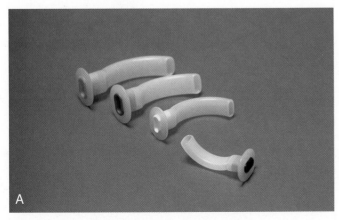
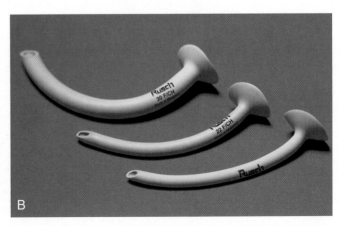

Figure 8-13 **A.** Oropharyngeal airways. **B.** Nasopharyngeal airways.
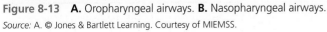
Source: A. © Jones & Bartlett Learning. Courtesy of MIEMSS.

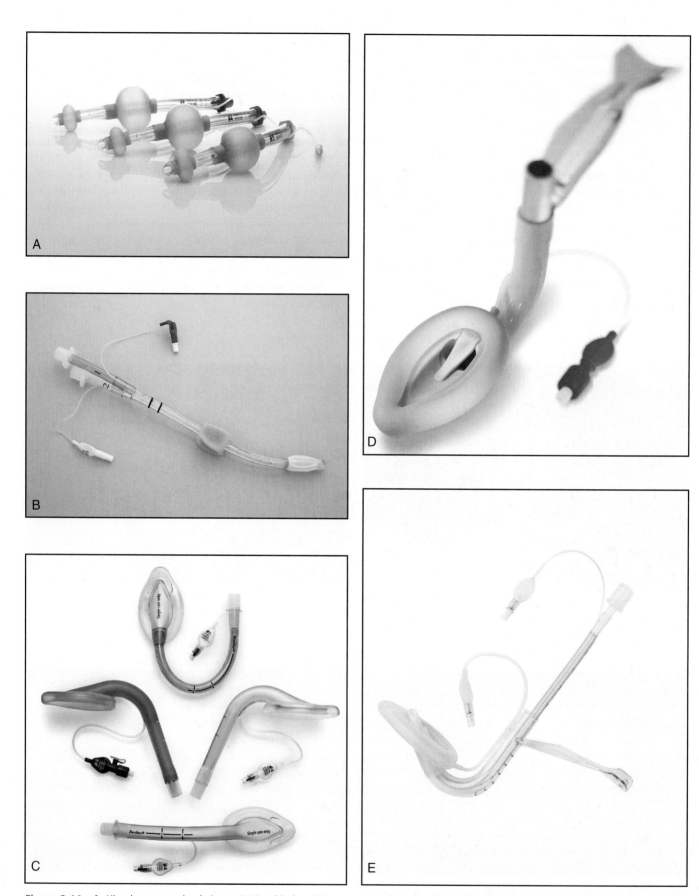

Figure 8-14   A. King laryngotracheal airway. **B.** Combitube. **C.** Laryngeal mask airway (LMA). **D.** Intubating LMA. **E.** Intubating LMA with ET tube in place.

Source: Courtesy of Ambu, Inc. (A-C) and Courtesy of Teleflex, Inc. (D, E).

Figure 8-15 Methods of Airway Management

Manual
- Hands only

Simple
- Oropharyngeal airway
- Nasopharyngeal airway

Complex
- Endotracheal intubation
- Supraglottic airways
- Pharmacologically assisted/rapid-sequence intubation
- Percutaneous airway
- Surgical airway

Manual Clearing of the Airway

The first step in airway management is a quick visual inspection of the oropharyngeal cavity. Foreign material (e.g., pieces of food) or broken teeth or dentures and blood may be found in the mouth of a trauma patient. These objects are swept out of the mouth using a gloved finger or, in the case of blood or vomitus, may be suctioned away. In addition, positioning of the patient on his or her side, when not contraindicated by possible spinal trauma, will allow for gravity-assisted clearing of secretions, blood, and vomitus.

Manual Maneuvers

In unresponsive patients, the tongue becomes flaccid, falling back and blocking the hypopharynx (see Figure 8-8). The tongue is the most common cause of airway obstruction. Manual methods to clear this type of obstruction can easily be accomplished because the tongue is attached to the mandible (jaw) and moves forward with it. Any maneuver that moves the mandible forward will pull the tongue out of the hypopharynx:

- *Trauma jaw thrust.* In patients with suspected head, neck, or facial trauma, the cervical spine is maintained in a neutral in-line position. The trauma jaw thrust maneuver allows the prehospital care provider to open the airway with little or no movement of the head and cervical spine (see Figure 8-12). The mandible is thrust forward by placing the thumbs on each zygoma (cheekbone), placing the index and long fingers on the mandible, and at the same angle, pushing the mandible forward.
- *Trauma chin lift.* The trauma chin lift maneuver is used to relieve a variety of anatomic airway obstructions in patients who are breathing spontaneously (see Figure 8-12). The chin and lower incisors are grasped and then lifted to pull the mandible forward. The prehospital care provider wears gloves to avoid body fluid contamination.

Both these techniques result in movement of the lower mandible anteriorly (upward) and slightly caudal (toward the feet), pulling the tongue forward, away from the posterior airway, and opening the mouth. The trauma jaw thrust pushes the mandible forward, whereas the trauma chin lift pulls the mandible. The trauma jaw thrust and the trauma chin lift are modifications of the conventional jaw thrust and chin lift. The modifications provide protection to the patient's cervical spine while opening the airway by displacing the tongue from the posterior pharynx.

Suctioning

A trauma patient may not be capable of effectively clearing the buildup of secretions, vomitus, blood, or foreign objects from the trachea. Providing suction is an important part of maintaining a patent airway.

The most significant complication of suctioning is that suctioning for prolonged periods will produce hypoxemia, which produces significant detrimental effects at the tissue level in many organs. The most obvious clinical clue that the patient is becoming hypoxic is a cardiac abnormality (e.g., tachycardia or dysrhythmias). Preoxygenation of the trauma patient by providing supplemental oxygen will help prevent hypoxemia. In addition, when suctioning close to or below the larynx (i.e., when suctioning an endotracheal tube), the suction catheter may stimulate either the internal branch of the superior laryngeal nerve or the recurrent laryngeal nerve that supplies the larynx above and below the cords, both of which are vagal in origin. Vagal stimulation may lead to profound bradycardia and hypotension.

The trauma patient whose airway has not yet been managed may require aggressive suctioning of the upper airway. Large amounts of blood and vomit may have already accumulated in the airway before the arrival of emergency medical services (EMS) and may have already compromised ventilation and oxygen transport into the alveoli. This accumulation may be more than a simple suction unit can quickly clear. If so, the patient may be rolled onto his or her side while maintaining cervical spine stabilization; gravity will then assist in clearing the airway. A rigid suction device is preferred to clear the oropharynx. Although hypoxia can result from prolonged suctioning, a totally obstructed airway will provide no air exchange. Aggressive suctioning and patient positioning are continued until the airway is at least partially clear. At that point, hyperoxygenation followed by repeated suctioning can be performed. Hyperoxygenation, like preoxygenation, may be accomplished with either a nonrebreathing mask on a high flow of oxygen or a bag-mask device running at 15 liters per minute. The goal when hyperoxygenating is to maintain an oxygen saturation at or above 95% at sea level.

When suctioning intubated patients through the **endotracheal (ET) tube**, the suction catheter should be made of soft material to limit trauma to the tracheal mucosa and to minimize frictional resistance. It needs to be long enough to pass the tip of the artificial airway (20 to 22 inches, or 50 to 55 centimeters [cm]) and should have smooth ends to prevent mucosal trauma. The soft catheter will probably not be effective in suctioning copious amounts of foreign material or fluid from the pharynx of a trauma patient, in which case the device of choice will be one with a tonsil-tip or

Yankauer design. Under no circumstances should a tonsil-tip or Yankauer rigid suction device be placed in the end of the ET tube.

When suctioning an intubated patient, aseptic procedures are vital. This technique includes the following steps:

1. Preoxygenate the trauma patient with 100% oxygen (fraction of inspired oxygen [FiO$_2$] of 1.0).
2. Prepare the equipment while maintaining sterility.
3. Insert the catheter without suction. Suctioning is then initiated and continued for up to 10 seconds while withdrawing the catheter.
4. Reoxygenate the patient, and ventilate for at least five assisted ventilations.
5. Repeat as necessary, allowing time for reoxygenation to take place between procedures.

Selection of Adjunctive Device

Problems found with the airway during the primary assessment require immediate action to establish and maintain a patent airway. These initial steps are the manual maneuvers such as a trauma jaw thrust or chin lift. Once opened, the airway must be maintained. The particular device should be selected based on the prehospital care provider's level of training and proficiency with that particular device and a risk–benefit analysis for the use of various types of devices and techniques that relate to the particular patient (see the chapter titled The Science, Art, and Ethics of Prehospital Care: Principles, Preferences, and Critical Thinking). The choice of the airway adjunct should be patient driven: "What is the best airway for this particular patient in this particular situation?"

During original training as well as during ongoing continuing education, prehospital care providers at various levels are exposed to a range of adjunctive devices to help maintain an open airway. The amount of training directly relates to the difficulty in placement of the device. At the emergency medical responder level, prehospital care providers are trained to place oropharyngeal airways. At the other end of the spectrum, advanced prehospital care providers have been trained to use complex airway devices, with some protocols allowing surgical airway procedures.

With complex skills such as intubation or surgical cricothyroidotomy, the more times a skill is performed, the better the chance for a successful outcome. A new paramedic who has performed these procedures only in the classroom setting has less of a chance of intubating a difficult patient successfully compared to a 10-year veteran who has performed these interventions numerous times during his or her career. The more steps there are in a procedure, the more difficult the procedure is to learn and master. These complex skills also lend themselves to a greater probability of failure as greater knowledge is required and more steps are involved in completing the intervention. As a skill increases in difficulty, so do the educational requirements, both in initial training and ongoing skills maintenance (**Figures 8-16** and **8-17**). Generally the more difficult a procedure is to perform, the greater the penalty to the patient for failure or error. With airway procedures, this is particularly true.

There are several types of airway devices that may be selected depending on the needs or potential needs of the patient (**Figure 8-18**):

- Simple Adjuncts
  - Devices that lift the tongue from the back of the pharynx only
    - ❑ Oral airway
    - ❑ Nasal airway

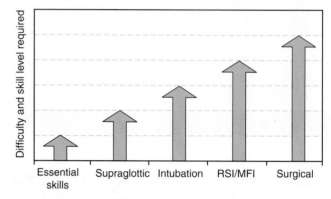

Figure 8-16 Airway skills.

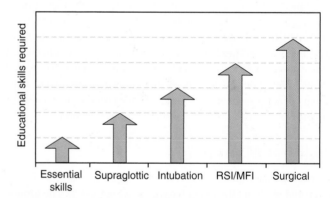

Figure 8-17 Educational skills required.

Figure 8-18 Factors in Selecting Airway Adjuncts

The prehospital care provider should choose from any of the adjuncts available in the airway toolbox based upon the particular situation. Factors influencing the decision include, but are not limited to, the following:

- Training
- Available assistance
- Transport time
- Perceived difficulty
- Ability to maintain the patient's airway with a simple adjunct

- To ventilate requires a mask (usually with bag-mask device)
- Complex Airways
  - Devices that occlude the oral pharynx
    - Supraglottic airways
      - Combitube
      - Laryngeal mask airway
      - Laryngeal tubes (LTs) (e.g., King LT)
  - Devices that isolate the trachea from the esophagus
    - ET tube
  - No mask required to ventilate

Simple Adjuncts

When manual airway maneuvers are unsuccessful or when continued maintenance of an open airway is necessary, the use of an artificial airway is the next step. After placement of a simple adjunctive device, a decision to escalate to a complex airway may be appropriate depending upon the particular patient and situation. The simple airway adjuncts are listed below.

Oropharyngeal Airway

The most frequently used artificial airway is the **oropharyngeal airway (OPA)** (see Figure 8-13). The OPA is inserted in either a direct or an inverted manner.

Indications

- Patient who is unable to maintain his or her airway
- To prevent an intubated patient from biting an ET tube

Contraindications

- Patient who is conscious or semiconscious

Complications

- Because it stimulates the gag reflex, use of the OPA may lead to gagging, vomiting, and laryngospasm in patients who are conscious

Nasopharyngeal Airway

The **nasopharyngeal airway (NPA)** is a soft, rubberlike device that is inserted through one of the nares and then along the curvature of the posterior wall of the nasopharynx and oropharynx (see Figure 8-13).

Indications

- Patient who is unable to maintain his or her airway

Contraindications

- No need for an airway adjunct
- Evidence has not supported the claim that facial/basilar skull fractures are a contraindication to placement of an NPA[2]

Complications

- Bleeding caused by insertion may be a complication

Complex Airways

Complex airway adjuncts and management techniques are appropriate when simple airway maneuvers and devices are inadequate to maintain a patent airway. Anytime a complex airway device is considered for placement in a patient, the prehospital care provider must consider the possibility that the procedure will be unsuccessful and have a backup plan in mind. Alternate methods of managing the airway should be considered and the necessary equipment prepared in the event the first choice of intervention proves unsuccessful.

Supraglottic Airways

Supraglottic airways offer a functional alternative airway to endotracheal intubation (Figures 8-14 and 8-19). Many jurisdictions allow the use of these devices because minimal training is required to achieve and retain competency. These devices are inserted without direct visualization of the vocal cords. They are also a useful backup airway when endotracheal intubation attempts are unsuccessful, even when rapid-sequence intubation has been attempted, or when, after careful evaluation of the airway, the prehospital care provider feels that the chance for successful placement is higher than for endotracheal intubation. The primary advantage of supraglottic airways is that they may be inserted independent of the patient's position, which may be especially important in trauma patients with access and extrication difficulties or a high suspicion of cervical injury.

When placed into a patient, supraglottic airways are designed to isolate the trachea from the esophagus. None of these devices provide a complete seal of the trachea; therefore, while the risk of aspiration is lowered, it is not completely prevented.

Some manufacturers have developed supraglottic airways in pediatric sizes. Prehospital care providers should ensure proper sizing according to the manufacturer's specifications if using these types of airways on pediatric patients.

Figure 8-19   Common Supraglottic Airways

- King LT airway
- Combitube
- Laryngeal mask airway
- Intubating LMA

Indications

- *Basic providers.* If the prehospital care provider is trained and authorized, a supraglottic airway is the primary airway device for an unconscious trauma patient who lacks a gag reflex and is apneic or ventilating at a rate of less than 10 breaths/minute.
- *Advanced providers.* A supraglottic airway is often the alternative airway device when the prehospital care provider is unable to perform endotracheal intubation and cannot easily ventilate the patient with a bag-mask device and an OPA or NPA.

Contraindications

- Intact gag reflex
- Nonfasting (recent meal)
- Known esophageal disease
- Recent ingestion of caustic substances

Complications

- Gagging and vomiting, if gag reflex is intact
- Aspiration
- Damage to the esophagus
- Hypoxia if ventilated using the incorrect lumen

Endotracheal Intubation

Endotracheal intubation traditionally has been the preferred method for achieving maximum control of the airway in trauma patients who are either apneic or who require assisted ventilation (**Figures 8-20** and **8-21**). Recent studies, however, have shown that in an urban environment, critically injured trauma patients with endotracheal intubation had no better outcome than those transported with a bag-mask device and OPA.[1] As a result, the role of endotracheal intubation has increasingly come under question. Few studies have demonstrated any benefit to the technique.[3] The decision to perform endotracheal intubation or use an alternative device should be made after assessment of the airway has determined the difficulty of the intubation. The risk of hypoxia from prolonged intubation attempts of a patient who has a difficult airway needs to be weighed against the need to insert the ET tube. Consideration should also be given to the effect of any increase in scene time necessary to perform the procedure.

Figure 8-21 Equipment for Endotracheal Intubation

As with any advanced life support skill, prehospital care providers need to have the proper equipment. The standard components of an intubation kit should include the following:

- Laryngoscope with adult- and pediatric-sized straight and curved blades
- Extra batteries and spare light bulbs
- Suction equipment including rigid and flexible catheters
- Adult- and pediatric-sized ET tubes
- Stylet
- Gum elastic bougie
- 10-ml syringe
- Water-soluble lubricant
- Magill forceps
- End-tidal detection device for $ETCO_2$ detection
- Wave form capnography
- Tube-securing device

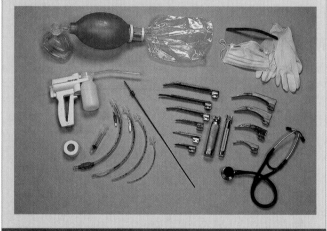

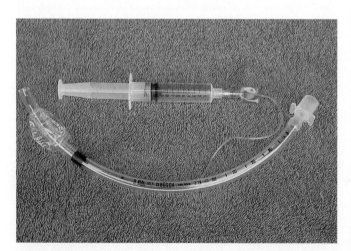

Figure 8-20 Endotracheal tube.
Source: Courtesy of AMBU

Prediction of Potentially Difficult Endotracheal Intubation

It is imperative that prior to performing endotracheal intubation an assessment of the difficulty of the intubation be done. There are many factors that can result in a difficult intubation of the trauma patient (**Figure 8-22**). Some of these are directly related to the trauma that they have sustained; others are due to anatomic anomalies of their face and upper airway.

The mnemonic LEMON has been developed to assist in the assessment of the relative difficulty that will be involved in a particular intubation (**Figures 8-23**). Although not all components of the LEMON mnemonic may be applied to the trauma patient in the field, an understanding of the components can help the prehospital care provider prepare for the difficult intubation. Other procedures or devices may be selected if the difficulty of the procedure is deemed high.

Figure 8-22 Factors That Contribute to Difficult Intubation

- Receding chin
- Short neck
- Large tongue
- Small mouth opening
- Cervical immobilization or stiff neck
- Facial trauma
- Bleeding into the airway
- Active vomiting
- Access to the patient
- Obesity

Figure 8-23 LEMON Assessment for Difficult Intubation

L = Look externally: Look for characteristics that are known to cause difficult intubation or ventilation.

E = Evaluate the 3–3–2 Rule: To allow for alignment of the pharyngeal, laryngeal, and oral axes, and therefore simple intubation, the following relationships should be observed:

- The distance between the patient's upper and lower incisor teeth should be at least 3 finger breadths (3)
- The distance between the hyoid bone and the chin should be at least 3 finger breadths (3)
- The distance between the thyroid notch and floor of the mouth should be at least 2 finger breadths (2)

M = Mallampati: The hypopharynx should be visualized adequately. This has been done traditionally by assessing the Mallampati classification.

- When possible, the patient is asked to sit upright, open the mouth fully, and protrude the tongue as far as possible. The examiner then looks into the mouth with a light to assess the degree of hypopharynx visible. In supine patients, the Mallampati score can be estimated by asking the patient to open the mouth fully and protrude the tongue; a laryngoscopy light is then shone into the hypopharynx from above.

O = Obstruction: Any condition that can cause obstruction of the airway will make laryngoscopy and ventilation difficult. Such conditions include epiglottitis, peritonsillar abscess, and trauma.

N = Neck mobility: This is a vital requirement for successful intubation. It can be assessed easily by asking the patient to place his or her chin onto the chest and then extending the neck so that he or she is looking toward the ceiling. Patients in a hard collar neck immobilizer obviously have no neck movement and are, therefore, more difficult to intubate.

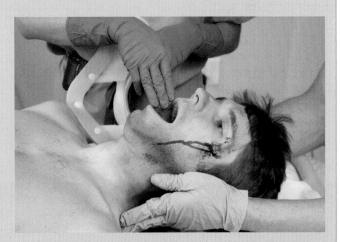

The 3–3–2 rule allows for alignment of the pharyngeal, laryngeal, and oral axes and, therefore, simple intubation. The following relationships should be observed: A. The distance between the patient's incisor teeth should be at least 3 finger breadths.

(Continues on next page)

Figure 8-23   LEMON Assessment for Difficult Intubation (Continued)

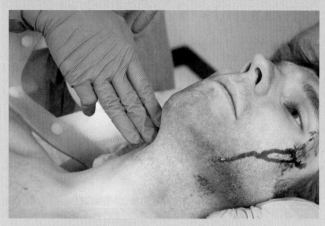

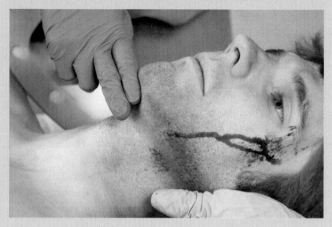

B. The distance between the hyoid bone and the chin should be at least 3 finger breadths.

C. The distance between the thyroid notch and the floor of the mouth should be at least 2 finger breadths.

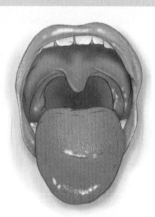 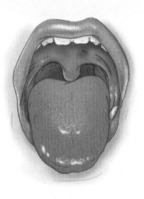 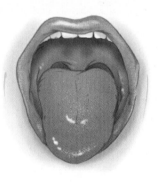 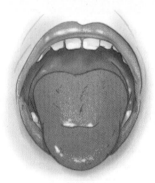

Class I	Class II	Class III	Class IV
Entire posterior pharynx is fully exposed	Posterior pharynx is partially exposed	Posterior pharynx cannot be seen; base of the uvula is exposed	No posterior pharyngeal structures can be seen

Mallampati classifications are used to visualize the hypopharynx. Class I: soft palate, uvula, fauces, pillars visible. Class II: soft palate, uvula, fauces visible. Class III: soft palate, base of uvula visible. Class IV: hard palate only visible.

Source: Modified with permission from Reed, MJ, Dunn MJG, McKeown DW. Can an airway assessment score predict difficulty at intubation in the emergency department? *Emerg Med J.* 2005;22:99–102. (In *Advanced Trauma Life Support*. Chicago: American College of Surgeons; 2008.)

Transport time may also be a factor when deciding the appropriate modality; an example may be a patient who is being maintained effectively with an OPA and bag-mask with a short transport time to the trauma center. The prehospital care provider may elect not to intubate but rather transport while maintaining the airway using simple airway techniques. Prehospital care providers need to assess the risks versus the benefits when making the decision to perform complex airway procedures.

Despite the potential challenges of this procedure, endotracheal intubation remains the preferred method of airway control because it does the following:

- Isolates the airway
- Allows for ventilation with 100% oxygen (FiO$_2$ of 1.0)
- Eliminates the need to maintain an adequate mask-to-face seal

- Significantly decreases the risk of aspiration (vomitus, foreign material, blood)
- Facilitates deep tracheal suctioning
- Prevents gastric insufflation

Indications, Contraindications, and Complications

Indications

- Patient who is unable to protect his or her airway
- Patient with significant oxygenation problem, requiring administration of high concentrations of oxygen
- Patient with significant ventilatory impairment requiring assisted ventilation

Contraindications

- Lack of training or maintenance of training in technique
- Lack of proper indications
- Proximity to receiving facility (relative contraindication)
- High probability of failed airway

Complications

- Hypoxemia from prolonged intubation attempts
- Hypercarbia from prolonged intubation attempts
- Vagal stimulation causing bradycardia
- Increased intracranial pressure
- Trauma to the airway with resultant hemorrhage and edema
- Right main bronchus intubation
- Esophageal intubation
- Vomiting leading to aspiration
- Loose or broken teeth
- Injury to the vocal cords
- Conversion of a cervical spine injury without neurologic deficit to one with neurologic deficit

As with all procedures, the prehospital care provider, along with the medical director, makes a risk–benefit judgment when using any complex procedures. Performing procedures simply because "the protocols allow it" is inappropriate. Think of the possible benefits and the possible risks, and form a plan based on the best interest of the patient in a given situation. Situations differ drastically based on transport time, location (urban vs. rural), and the prehospital care provider's level of comfort in performing a given procedure (**Figure 8-24**).

Methods of Endotracheal Intubation

Several alternative methods are available for performing endotracheal intubation. The method of choice depends on such factors as the patient's needs, the level of urgency (orotracheal vs. nasotracheal), patient positioning (face to face), or training and scope of practice (pharmacologically assisted intubation).

Figure 8-24 Practice Improves the Intubation Success Rate

Research studies have shown that practice increases the likelihood of success when intubating. Although no correlation was found between success rate and length of time as a paramedic, there was a correlation between the number of patients intubated by the paramedic and the success rate. Experience with the procedure increases the likelihood of successful performance.[4]

Regardless of the method selected, the patient's head and neck should be stabilized in a neutral position during the procedure and until spinal immobilization is completed. In general, if intubation is not successful after three attempts, consider a different technique.

Orotracheal Intubation

Orotracheal intubation involves placing an ET tube into the trachea through the mouth. The nontrauma patient is often placed in a "sniffing" position to facilitate intubation. Because this position hyperextends the cervical spine at C1–C2 (the second most common site for cervical spine fractures in the trauma patient) and hyperflexes it at C5–C6 (the most common site for cervical spine fractures in the trauma patient), it should not be used for patients with blunt trauma (**Figure 8-25**).

Nasotracheal Intubation

In conscious trauma patients or in those with an intact gag reflex, endotracheal intubation may be difficult to accomplish. If spontaneous ventilations are present, **blind nasotracheal intubation (BNTI)** may be attempted if the benefit outweighs the risk. Although nasotracheal intubation is often more difficult to perform than direct visualization and oral intubation, a 90% success rate has been reported in traumatized patients. During BNTI, the patient must be breathing to ensure that the ET tube is passed through the vocal cords. Many texts suggest that BNTI is contraindicated in the presence of midface trauma or fractures, but an exhaustive literature search reveals no documentation of an ET tube entering the cranial vault. Apnea is a contraindication specific to BNTI. In addition, no stylet is used when BNTI is performed.

Face-to-Face Intubation

Face-to-face intubation is indicated when standard trauma intubation techniques cannot be used because of the inability of the prehospital care provider to assume the standard position at the head of the trauma patient. These situations include but are not limited to the following:

- Vehicle entrapment
- Pinning of the patient in rubble

Pharmacologically Assisted Intubation

Intubation using pharmacologic agents may occasionally be required to facilitate ET tube placement in injured patients. In skilled hands, this technique can facilitate effective airway control when other methods fail or are otherwise not acceptable. To maximize the effectiveness of this procedure and ensure patient safety, personnel using drugs to assist with intubation need to be familiar with applicable local protocols, medications, and indications for use of the technique. The use of drugs to assist with intubation, particularly rapid-sequence intubation, does have risks above and beyond those of intubation alone. Pharmacologically assisted intubation is a procedure of necessity, not convenience. Intubation using drugs falls into the following two categories:

1. *Intubation using sedatives or narcotics.* Medications such as diazepam, midazolam, fentanyl, or morphine are used alone or in combination, with the goal being to relax the patient enough to permit intubation but not to abolish protective reflexes or breathing. The effectiveness of a single pharmacologic agent, such as midazolam, has been well documented.[5]
2. **Rapid-sequence intubation (RSI)** *using paralytic agents* (**Figure 8-26**). The patient is chemically paralyzed after first being sedated. This provides complete muscle paralysis but removes all protective reflexes and causes apnea. Studies of this method of airway management have demonstrated successful performance of the technique in the field, with intubation success rates reported in the mid-90% range. However, few studies have critically evaluated whether patient outcome is affected.[6] One center reported

its experience with RSI in the field and documented that patients with traumatic brain injury who underwent RSI had a poorer outcome than those who did not require RSI.[7] Subsequent analysis has shown that unrecognized hyperventilation leading to hypocarbia and unrecognized hypoxia were major contributors to the poor outcome.[8] Another study showed a better outcome at 6 months for patients with traumatic brain injury who were intubated in the field when compared to those intubated in the hospital.[9] The final answer to this important question has not yet been provided by the available research.

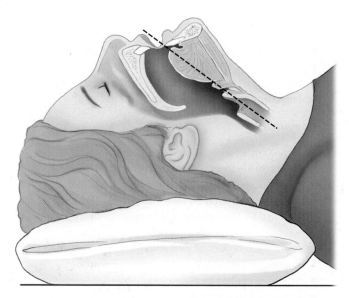

Figure 8-25 Placing the patient's head in the "sniffing" position provides ideal visualization of the larynx through the mouth. However, such positioning hyperextends the patient's neck at C1 and C2 and hyperflexes it at C5 and C6. These are the two most common points of fracture of the cervical spine.

Figure 8-26 Sample Protocol for Rapid-Sequence Intubation (RSI)

Preparation
1. Ensure availability of required equipment.
   a. Oxygen supply
   b. Bag-mask device of appropriate size and type
   c. Nonrebreathing mask
   d. Laryngoscope with blades
   e. ET tubes
   f. Gum elastic bougie
   g. Surgical and alternative airway equipment
   h. RSI medications
   i. Materials or devices to secure ET tube after placement
   j. Suction equipment
   k. Cardiac monitor
   l. Pulse oximeter
   m. Capnometer
2. Ensure that at least one (but preferably two) patent intravenous line is present.

(Continues on next page)

Figure 8-26   Sample Protocol for Rapid-Sequence Intubation (RSI) (Continued)

3. Preoxygenate the patient using a nonrebreathing mask or bag-mask device with 100% oxygen. Preoxygenation for 3 to 4 minutes is preferred.
4. Apply cardiac and pulse oximetry monitors.
5. If the patient is conscious, strongly consider the use of sedative agents.
6. Consider the administration of sedative agents and lidocaine in the presence of potential or confirmed traumatic brain injury (Figure 8-27).
7. Consider the use of analgesic medications as well since none of the medications routinely used for induction or paralysis provide pain relief.
8. After administration of paralytic agents, use the Sellick maneuver (cricoid pressure) to decrease the potential for aspiration (Figure 8-28).
9. Confirm ET tube placement immediately after intubation. Continuous cardiac and pulse oximeter monitoring is required during and after RSI. Reconfirm ET tube placement periodically throughout transport and each time the patient is moved.
10. Use repeat doses of sedation and paralytic agents as needed.

Sample Procedure

1. Assemble the required equipment.
2. Ensure the patency of the intravenous lines.
3. Preoxygenate the patient with 100% oxygen for approximately 3 to 4 minutes if possible.
4. Place the patient on cardiac and pulse oximeter monitors.

5. Administer a sedative, such as midazolam, if appropriate.
6. Administer analgesic, such as fentanyl, if appropriate
7. In the presence of confirmed or potential traumatic brain injury, administer lidocaine (1.5 mg/kg) 2 to 3 minutes before administration of a paralytic agent (See Figure 8-27).
8. For pediatric patients, prepare atropine (0.01–0.02 mg/kg) 1 to 3 minutes before paralytic administration in the event of vagal response to intubation.
9. Administer a short-acting paralytic agent intravenously, such as succinylcholine. Paralysis and relaxation should occur within 30 seconds.
   a. Adult: 1 to 2 mg/kg
   b. Pediatric: 1 to 2 mg/kg
10. Insert an ET tube. If initial attempts are unsuccessful, precede repeat attempts with preoxygenation.
11. Confirm ET tube placement.
12. If repeated attempts to achieve endotracheal intubation fail, consider placement of an alternative or surgical airway.
13. Use doses of a long-acting paralytic agent, such as vecuronium, to continue paralysis.
   a. Initial dose: 0.1 mg/kg IV push
   b. Subsequent doses: 0.01 mg/kg every 30 to 45 minutes
14. Repeat doses of sedation may also be needed.

Note: Requirements vary with individual patients.

Figure 8-27   Lidocaine for RSI

The use of lidocaine during RSI of patients with suspected traumatic brain injury has been debated for many years. The argument in favor of its use is that it blunts the rise in intracranial pressure that occurs during intubation. The evidence for this effect comes primarily from animal studies. Evidence of benefit from its administration in humans is lacking. While harm has also not been demonstrated, the final word on its use is still to come.

Figure 8-28   The Sellick Maneuver

The Sellick maneuver has been gradually falling out of favor. While it has been considered to reduce the likelihood of aspiration from regurgitated stomach contents, there is little evidence that it, in fact, does so. Several studies show that the esophagus is located to the side of the trachea and that the Sellick maneuver does little to actually compress the esophagus.[10-13] In addition, cricoid pressure may actually obscure the view of the larynx and make intubation more difficult.

Also, pharmacologically assisted intubation of any type requires time to accomplish. For every trauma patient for whom this intubation is contemplated, the benefits of securing an airway are weighed against the additional time spent on the scene to perform the procedure.

Indications

- A patient who requires a secure airway and is difficult to intubate because of uncooperative behavior (as induced by hypoxia, traumatic brain injury, hypotension, or intoxication)

Relative Contraindications

- Availability of an alternative airway (e.g., supraglottic)
- Severe facial trauma that would impair or preclude successful intubation
- Neck deformity or swelling that complicates or precludes placement of a surgical airway
- Known allergies to indicated medications
- Medical problems that would preclude use of indicated medications

Absolute Contraindications

- Inability to intubate
- Inability to maintain airway with bag-mask device and OPA

Complications

- Inability to insert the ET tube in a sedated or paralyzed patient no longer able to protect his or her airway or breathe spontaneously; patients who are medicated and then cannot be intubated require prolonged bag-mask ventilation until the medication wears off
- Development of hypoxia or hypercarbia during prolonged intubation attempts
- Aspiration
- Hypotension—virtually all the drugs have the side effect of decreasing blood pressure

Patients who are mildly or moderately hypovolemic but compensating may have a profound drop in blood pressure associated with the intravenous administration of many of these drugs. Exercise caution whenever the use of medications for intubation is considered (**Figure 8-29**).

Figure 8-29 Common Drugs Used for Pharmacologically Assisted Intubation

Drug	Dose (Adult)	Dose (Pediatric)	Indications	Complications/Side Effects
PRETREATMENT				
Oxygen	High flow; Assist ventilation as needed to achieve oxygen saturation of 100% if possible	High flow; Assist ventilation as needed to achieve oxygen saturation of 100% if possible intubation	All patients undergoing pharmacologically assisted	
Lidocaine	1–1.5 mg/kg IV	1.5 mg/kg IV	Brain injury	Seizure
Atropine	—	0.01–0.02 mg/kg IV (min. dose: 0.1 mg)	Pediatric intubation, treatment of bradycardia and excess secretions	Tachycardia
INDUCTION OF SEDATION				
Midazolam (Versed)	0.1–0.15 mg/kg up to 0.3 mg/kg intravenously (IV)	0.1–0.15 mg/kg up to 0.3 mg/kg IV	Sedation	Respiratory depression/apnea, hypotension
Fentanyl (Sublimaze)	2–3 mcg/kg IV	1–3 mcg/kg IV	Sedation, analgesia	Respiratory depression/apnea, hypotension, bradycardia
Etomidate	0.2–0.3 mg/kg IV	Not approved for patients under 10 years of age	Sedation, induced anesthesia	Apnea, hypotension, vomiting

(Continues on next page)

Drug	Dose (Adult)	Dose (Pediatric)	Indications	Complications/ Side Effects
INDUCTION OF SEDATION				
Ketamine	1–2 mg/kg IV	1–1.5 mg/kg, slow IV push	Sedation, induced anesthesia	Increased intra-ocular pressure, increased intracranial pressure
CHEMICAL PARALYSIS				
Succinylcholine	1–2 mg/kg IV	1–2 mg/kg IV	Muscle relaxation and paralysis (short duration)	Hyperkalemia, muscle fasciculations
Vecuronium (Norcuron)	0.1 mg/kg IV	0.1 mg/kg IV	Muscle relaxation and paralysis (intermediate duration)	Hypotension
Rocuronium (Zemuron)	0.6–1.2 mg/kg IV	0.6 mg/kg IV	Muscle relaxation and paralysis (intermediate duration)	Hypotension or hypertension
Pancuronium (Pavulon)	0.04–0.1 mg/kg IV	0.04–0.1 mg/kg IV	Muscle relaxation and paralysis (long duration)	Tachycardia, hypertension, salivation

Figure 8-29 Common Drugs Used for Pharmacologically Assisted Intubation (*Continued*)

Verification of Endotracheal Tube Placement

Once intubation has been performed, take specific measures to ensure that the ET tube has been properly placed in the trachea. Inadvertent esophageal placement of an ET tube, if unrecognized for only a brief period, may result in profound hypoxia, with resultant brain injury (hypoxic encephalopathy) and even death. Therefore, it is important that proper placement be confirmed. Techniques to verify intubation include the use of both clinical assessments and adjunct devices.[13] Clinical assessments include the following:

- Direct visualization of the ET tube passing through the vocal cords
- Presence of bilateral breath sounds (auscultate laterally below the axilla) and absence of air sounds over the epigastrium
- Visualization of the chest rising and falling during ventilation
- Fogging (water vapor condensation) in the ET tube on expiration

Unfortunately, none of these techniques is 100% reliable *by itself* for verifying proper ET tube placement. Therefore, prudent practice involves assessing and documenting all these clinical signs, if possible. On rare occasions, because of difficult anatomy, visualization of the ET tube passing through the vocal cords may not be possible. In a moving vehicle (ground or aeromedical), engine noise may make auscultation of breath sounds almost impossible. Obesity and chronic obstructive pulmonary disease may interfere with the ability to see chest movement during ventilation.

Monitoring devices include the following:

- ETCO$_2$ monitoring (capnography)
- Colorimetric carbon dioxide detector
- Pulse oximetry

In a patient with a perfusing rhythm, ETCO$_2$ monitoring (capnography) serves as the "gold standard" for determining ET tube placement. This technique should be used in the prehospital setting whenever available. Patients in cardiopulmonary arrest do not exhale carbon dioxide; therefore, neither colorimetric detectors nor capnography may be useful in patients who lack a perfusing cardiac rhythm.

Because none of these techniques is universally reliable, all the clinical assessments noted previously should be performed, unless impractical, followed by use of at least one of the monitoring devices. If any of the techniques used to verify proper placement suggests that the ET tube may not be properly positioned, the ET tube should be immediately removed and reinserted, with placement verified again. All the techniques used to verify ET tube placement should be noted on the patient care report.

Securing an Endotracheal Tube

Once endotracheal intubation has been performed, the ET tube must be manually held in place and proper tube placement verified; the depth of tube insertion at the central incisors (front teeth) should be noted. Next, the ET tube is secured in place. Several commercially available products may serve to secure the ET tube adequately. A recent study identified that umbilical tape held the ET tube as effectively as commercial devices; however, it needs to be tied around the ET tube using appropriate knots and technique. Ideally, if sufficient EMS personnel are present, someone should be assigned the task of manually holding the ET tube in proper position to ensure that it does not move.

Continuous pulse oximetry should be considered necessary for all patients who require endotracheal intubation. Any decline in the pulse oximetry reading (i.e., oxygen saturation [SpO$_2$]) or development of cyanosis requires reverification of ET tube placement. Additionally, an ET tube may also become dislodged during any movement of the patient. Reverify ET tube position after every move of a patient, such as logrolling to a long backboard, loading or unloading into or from the ambulance, or carrying the patient down a staircase.

Alternate Techniques

If endotracheal intubation has been unsuccessful after three attempts, consideration of airway management using the manual and simple skills described previously and ventilating with a bag-mask device is appropriate. *If the receiving facility is reasonably close, these techniques may be the most prudent option for airway management when faced with a brief transport time.* If the nearest appropriate facility is more distant, one of the following alternate techniques may be considered.

Digital Intubation

Digital, or tactile, intubation was a precursor to the current use of laryngoscopes for endotracheal intubation. Essentially, the intubator's fingers act in similar fashion to a laryngoscope blade by manipulating the epiglottis and acting as a guide for placement of the ET tube. This technique is done without direct visualization of the airway.

Indications

- Patients in whom standard endotracheal intubation failed but for whom ventilations can be assisted with a bag-mask device
- When laryngoscope is unavailable or fails

- When the airway is obscured or blocked because of large volumes of blood or vomitus
- Entrapment with inability to perform face-to-face intubation

Contraindications

- Any patient who is not comatose and may bite the intubator's fingers (dental clamp or bite stick may be used to hold the patient's mouth open)

Complications

- Esophageal intubation
- Lacerations or crush injuries to the prehospital care provider's fingers
- Hypoxia or hypercarbia during the procedure
- Damage to the vocal cords

Laryngeal Mask Airway

The **laryngeal mask airway (LMA)** is another alternative for unconscious or seriously obtunded adult and pediatric patients. The device consists of an inflatable silicone ring attached diagonally to a silicone tube (**Figure 8-30**). When inserted, the ring creates a low-pressure seal between the LMA and the glottic opening, without direct insertion of the device into the larynx itself.

Advantages of the LMA include the following:

- The LMA is designed for blind insertion. Direct visualization of the trachea and vocal cords is unnecessary.
- With proper cleaning and storage, some LMAs can be reused multiple times.

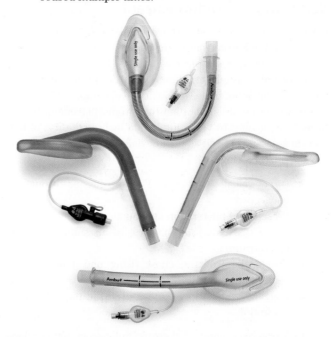

Figure 8-30 Laryngeal mask airway.
Source: Courtesy of AMBU, Inc.

- Disposable LMAs are now available.
- The LMA is available in a range of sizes to accommodate both pediatric and adult patient groups.

Prehospital use of the LMA thus far has been more prevalent in Europe than in North America. A recent development is the introduction of an "intubating LMA." This device is inserted similarly to the original LMA, but a flexible ET tube is then passed though the LMA, intubating the trachea (see Figure 8-14). This approach secures the airway without the need to visualize the vocal cords.

Indications

- May be used as a primary airway device in some EMS systems
- When unable to perform endotracheal intubation and the patient cannot be ventilated using a bag-mask device

Contraindications

- When endotracheal intubation can be performed
- Insufficient training

Complications

- Aspiration, because LMA does not completely prevent regurgitation and protect the trachea
- Laryngospasm

Needle Cricothyroidotomy

In rare cases, a trauma patient's airway obstruction cannot be relieved by the methods previously discussed. In these patients, a needle cricothyroidotomy may be performed using a percutaneously placed needle or catheter. It has been shown that adequate oxygenation can be achieved using **percutaneous transtracheal ventilation (PTV)**.[14] This technique, while it provides for oxygenation, does not support adequate ventilation for any length of time. As a result, rising levels of carbon dioxide will occur, which can be tolerated for approximately 30 minutes, after which formal airway management must be accomplished to prevent profound respiratory acidosis from developing. This technique is a temporizing measure to maintain oxygenation until a definitive airway can be obtained to provide adequate ventilation.

The advantages of PTV include the following:

- Ease of access (landmarks usually easily recognized)
- Ease of insertion
- Minimal equipment required
- No incision necessary
- Minimal training required

Indications

- When all other alternative methods of airway management fail or are impractical and the patient cannot be ventilated with a bag-mask device

Contraindications

- Insufficient training
- Lack of proper equipment
- Ability to secure airway by another technique (as described previously) or ability to ventilate with a bag-mask device

Complications

- Hypercarbia from prolonged use (carbon dioxide elimination is not as effective as with other methods of ventilation)[9]
- Damage to surrounding structures, including the larynx, thyroid gland, carotid arteries, jugular veins, and esophagus

Surgical Cricothyrotomy

Surgical cricothyrotomy involves the creation of a surgical opening in the *cricothyroid membrane*, which lies between the larynx (thyroid cartilage) and the cricoid cartilage. In most patients, the skin is very thin in this location, making it amenable to immediate access to the airway.[15] Consider this a technique of last resort in prehospital airway management.

There are a number of ways that surgical cricothyrotomy can be accomplished. The traditional method is to formally incise the skin and cricothyroid membrane using a scalpel. An alternative method is to utilize one of the several different types of commercially available cricothyrotomy kits. Learning to use these kits is easier than learning to perform a formal surgical cricothyrotomy, and generally they create an opening that is larger than that of a needle cricothyroidotomy but smaller than the surgical technique.

The use of this surgical airway in the prehospital arena is controversial. Complications are common with this procedure.[16] Proficient endotracheal intubation skills should minimize the need even to consider its use. *Surgical cricothyrotomy should never be the initial airway control method.* Insufficient data exist at this time to support a recommendation that surgical cricothyrotomy be established as a national standard for routine use in prehospital airway management.

For this technique to be successful in actual field practice, training must be done on real tissue. Current mannequins and other simulation devices do not replicate the actual tissue and feel of the anatomy of the patient. The prehospital care provider's first exposure to real tissue should not be a dying patient. In addition, this skill, perhaps more than other airway interventions, requires frequent practice in order to maintain the anatomic familiarity and skills needed to perform it correctly in only seconds during a true emergency. There is usually not a second chance to get it right. It must be done correctly the first time.

Indications

- Massive midface trauma precluding the use of a bag-mask device
- Inability to control the airway using less invasive maneuvers
- Ongoing tracheobronchial hemorrhage

Contraindications

- Any patient who can be safely intubated, either orally or nasally
- Patients with laryngotracheal injuries
- Children under 10 years of age
- Patients with acute laryngeal disease of traumatic or infectious origin
- Insufficient training

Complications

- Prolonged procedure time
- Hemorrhage
- Aspiration
- Misplacement or false passage of the ET tube
- Injury to neck structures or vessels
- Perforation of the esophagus

Continuous Quality Improvement

With the literature questioning the effectiveness of prehospital intubation of the trauma patient, it is important that the medical director or his or her designee individually review all out-of-hospital intubations or invasive airway techniques. This is even more imperative if medications have been used to facilitate the intubation attempt. Specific points include the following:

- Adherence to protocol and procedures
- Number of attempts
- Confirmation of tube placement and the procedures used for verification
- Outcome and complications
- Proper indications for the use of induction agents if used
- Proper documentation of drug dosage routes and monitoring of the patient during and after intubation

An effective continuous quality improvement (CQI) program for airway management must not be seen as a "punishment" but rather as an educational opportunity by the prehospital care providers, management, and the medical director. Since most CQI programs are self-reporting, any results that are used to discipline a particular prehospital care provider may result in misreporting. CQI should be tied directly to the continuing education program within an organization. After identifying a problem in performance, an educational component should be developed that addresses those issues. Follow-up evaluations should take place to determine if the educational component has been effective.

Ventilatory Devices

All trauma patients receive appropriate ventilatory support with supplemental oxygen to ensure that hypoxia is corrected or averted entirely. In deciding which method or equipment to use, prehospital care providers should consider the following devices and their respective oxygen concentrations (**Figure 8-31**).

Pocket Masks

Regardless of which mask is chosen to support ventilation of the trauma patient, the ideal mask has the following characteristics:

1. Is a good fit
2. Is equipped with a one-way valve
3. Is made of a transparent material
4. Has a supplemental oxygen port
5. Is available in infant, pediatric, and adult sizes

Mouth-to-mask ventilation satisfactorily delivers adequate tidal volumes by ensuring a tight face seal even when performed by those who do not use this skill often.

Bag-Mask Device

The bag-mask device consists of a self-inflating bag and a non-rebreathing device; it can be used with simple (OPA, NPA) or complex (endotracheal, nasotracheal) airway devices. Most bag-mask devices currently on the market have a volume of 1,600 ml and can deliver an oxygen concentration of 90% to 100%. Some models also have a built-in colorimetric carbon dioxide detector. However, a single prehospital care provider attempting to ventilate with a bag-mask device may create poor tidal volumes secondary to the inability to both create a tight face seal and to squeeze the bag adequately. Ongoing practice of this skill is necessary to ensure that the technique is effective and that the trauma patient receives adequate ventilatory support.

Manually Triggered (Oxygen-Powered) Devices

Manually triggered (oxygen-powered) devices can deliver oxygen concentrations of 100%. Because these devices do not permit the prehospital care provider to feel the compliance of

Figure 8-31 Ventilatory Devices and Oxygen Concentration

Device	Liter Flow (L/min)	Oxygen Concentration*
WITHOUT SUPPLEMENTAL OXYGEN		
Mouth-to-mouth	N/A	16%
Mouth-to-mask	N/A	16%
Bag-mask	N/A	21%
WITH SUPPLEMENTAL OXYGEN		
Nasal cannula	1–6	24–45%
Mouth-to-mask	10	50%
Simple face mask	8–10	40–60%
Bag-mask without reservoir	8–10	40–60%
Bag-mask with reservoir	10–15	90–100%
Nonrebreathing mask with reservoir	10–15	90–100%
Demand valve	N/A	90–100%
Ventilator	N/A	21–100%

*Percentages indicated are approximate.
N/A, Not applicable.

the chest during the ventilation process, care is taken not to overinflate the lungs. Maintaining a tight face seal with the device is easy because the trigger mechanism requires only one hand to operate. Complications may include gastric distension, overinflation of the lungs, barotrauma, and lung rupture. These devices should not be used in the field except in unusual circumstances.

Positive-Pressure Ventilators

Positive-pressure volume ventilators during prolonged transport have long been used in the aeromedical environment. However, more ground units are now adopting the use of mechanical ventilation as a means of controlling rate, depth, and minute volume in trauma patients. Importantly, only volume ventilators with appropriate alarms and pressure control/relief should be used. These ventilators do not need to be as sophisticated as those used in the hospital and only have a few simple modes of ventilation, as follows.

Assist Control Ventilation

Assist control (A/C) ventilation is probably the most widely used mode of ventilation in prehospital transport from the scene to the ED. The A/C setting delivers ventilations at a preset rate and tidal volume. If patients initiate a breath on their own, an additional ventilation of the full tidal volume is delivered, which may lead to breath-stacking and overinflation of the lungs.

Intermittent Mandatory Ventilation

Intermittent Mandatory Ventilation (IMV) delivers a set rate and tidal volume to patients. If patients initiate their own breath, only the amount that they actually pull on their own will be delivered.

Positive End-Expiratory Pressure

Positive end-expiratory pressure (PEEP) provides an elevated level of pressure at the end of expiration, thus keeping the alveolar sacs and small airways open and filled with air for a longer time. This intervention provides greater oxygenation. However, by increasing the end-expiratory pressure and, therefore, the overall intrathoracic pressure, PEEP may decrease blood return to the heart. In hemodynamically unstable patients, PEEP may further decrease blood pressure. PEEP should also be avoided in patients with traumatic brain injuries. The increase in thoracic pressure can cause an elevation in intracranial pressure.

Initial Settings for Mechanical Ventilations
Rate

The rate is set initially at between 10 and 12 breaths per minute on nonbreathing adult patients.

Tidal Volume

The tidal volume (vt) should be set using 5 to 7 ml/kg of the patient's ideal body weight. This should be used as a guide and may need to be adjusted in the trauma patient.

PEEP

PEEP should be set initially at 5 centimeters of water (cm H_2O). This setting will maintain what is known as physiologic PEEP, which is the amount of PEEP that is normally present in the airway prior to intubation. Once intubated, this positive pressure is taken away. Although increased levels of PEEP may be needed as the traumatic insult worsens, this rarely ever takes place in the first couple of hours following the traumatic event. The prehospital care provider may encounter patients requiring high levels of PEEP during a transfer of a patient from one hospital to another. The hospital staff prior to the transfer will have established these levels of PEEP. Care must be taken if PEEP is increased, as there can be adverse complications:

- Decreased blood pressure secondary to decreased thoracic return
- Increased intracranial pressure
- Increased intrathoracic pressure leading to pneumothorax or tension pneumothorax

Oxygen Concentration

The oxygen concentration should be set to maintain a saturation of 95% or greater at sea level in the trauma patient.

High-Pressure Alarm/Pop-off

The high-pressure alarm and pressure relief pop-off should be set at no more than 10 cm H_2O above the pressure needed to normally ventilate the patient (peak inspiratory pressure). Care should be taken when setting the alarm above 40 cm H_2O. Levels above this have been shown to produce barotrauma and a higher possibility of a pneumothorax. Should more than 40 cm H_2O be needed to deliver the desired tidal volume, reassessment of the airway and preset tidal volume is required. Decreasing the tidal volume and increasing the rate to maintain the same alveolar minute ventilation may be the prudent action in this case.

As with any alarm, if the high-pressure alarm continues to activate for more than a few breaths, the patient should be removed from the ventilator and manually ventilated with a bag-mask device while the ventilator circuit and ET tube are evaluated. The patient should also be re-evaluated for an increase in compliance. This increase in compliance or resistance may be caused by many factors. The most common, early in the care of the trauma patient, is either tension pneumothorax or an increasing LOC causing "bucking" on the ET tube. The tension pneumothorax should be treated with chest decompression as indicated. An increasing LOC should be treated with the administration of a sedative agent if available. Other potential problems include displacement or obstruction of the ET tube. In no case should the prehospital care provider simply continue to increase the upper pressure limit and alarm.

Low-Pressure Alarm

The low-pressure alarm alerts the prehospital care provider if the connection between the patient and the ventilator is disconnected or is losing significant volume through a leak in the ventilator circuit. In most transport ventilators, this alarm is preset and cannot be adjusted.

Evaluation
Pulse Oximetry

Over the past decades, use of pulse oximetry has increased in the prehospital environment. Appropriate use of pulse oximetry devices allows early detection of pulmonary compromise or cardiovascular deterioration before physical signs are evident. **Pulse oximeters** are particularly useful in prehospital applications because of their high reliability, portability, ease of application, and applicability across all age ranges and races (**Figure 8-32**).

Pulse oximeters provide measurements of oxygen saturation (SpO_2) and pulse rate. SpO_2 is determined by measuring the absorption ratio of red and infrared light passed through tissue. A small microprocessor correlates changes in light absorption caused by the pulsation of blood through vascular beds to determine arterial saturation and pulse rate. Normal SpO_2 is greater than 94% at sea level. When SpO_2 falls below 90%, oxygen delivery to the tissues is likely severely compromised. At higher altitudes, the acceptable levels of SpO_2 are lower than at sea level. Prehospital care providers should know what SpO_2 levels are acceptable at higher altitudes, if practicing in such settings.

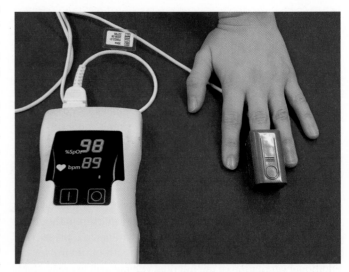

Figure 8-32 Pulse oximeter.

To ensure accurate pulse oximetry readings, the following general guidelines should be followed:

1. Use the appropriate size and type of sensor.
2. Ensure proper alignment of sensor light.
3. Ensure that sources and photodetectors are clean, dry, and in good repair.
4. Avoid sensor placement on grossly edematous (swollen) sites.
5. Remove any nail polish that may be present.

Common problems that can produce inaccurate SpO_2 measurement include the following:

- Excessive motion
- Moisture in SpO_2 sensors
- Improper sensor application and placement
- Poor patient perfusion or vasoconstriction from hypothermia
- Anemia
- Carbon monoxide poisoning

In a critical trauma patient, pulse oximetry may be less than accurate because of poor capillary perfusion status. Therefore, pulse oximetry is a valuable addition to the prehospital care provider's "toolbox" only when combined with a thorough knowledge of trauma pathophysiology and strong assessment and intervention skills.

Capnography

Capnography, or end-tidal carbon dioxide ($ETCO_2$) monitoring, has been used in critical care units for many years. Recent advances in technology have allowed smaller, more durable units to be produced for prehospital use (**Figure 8-33**). Capnography measures the partial pressure of carbon dioxide (PCO_2, or $ETCO_2$) in a sample of gas. If this sample is taken at the end of exhalation in a patient with good peripheral perfusion, it correlates closely to arterial PCO_2 ($PaCO_2$). However, in the multiple trauma patient with compromised perfusion, the correlation of $ETCO_2$ to arterial PCO_2 remains questionable.[17,18]

Most critical care units within the hospital setting use the mainstream technique. This technique places a sensor directly into the "mainstream" of the exhaled gas. In the patient being ventilated with a bag-mask device, the sensor is placed between the bag-mask device and the ET tube. In the critical patient, the $PaCO_2$ is generally 2 to 5 mm Hg higher than the $ETCO_2$. (A normal $ETCO_2$ reading in a critical trauma patient is 30 to 40 mm Hg.) Although these readings may not totally reflect the patient's $PaCO_2$, working to maintain the readings between normal levels will usually be beneficial to the patient.

Although capnography correlates closely with $PaCO_2$, certain conditions will cause variations in accuracy. These conditions are often seen in the prehospital environment and include severe

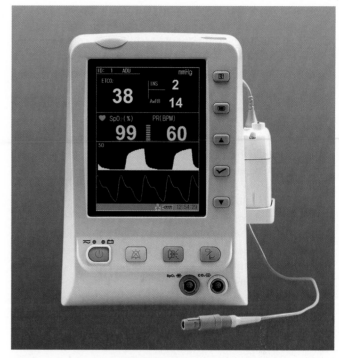

Figure 8-33   Handheld end-tidal carbon dioxide detector.
Source: Courtesy of DRE Medical Equipment.

hypotension, high intrathoracic pressure, and any increase in dead space ventilation, as with pulmonary embolism. Therefore, following trends in $ETCO_2$ levels may be more important than focusing on specific readings.

Continuous capnography provides another tool in the prehospital management of a trauma patient and must be correlated with all other information about a patient. Initial transport decisions are based on physical and environmental conditions. For example, it would be inappropriate to take time to place the patient on monitors if the patient is losing blood. Instead, capnography should be used to monitor ET tube placement and continuously monitor patient status during transport. A sudden drop in expired carbon dioxide may result either from dislodgement of the ET tube or from decreased perfusion and should prompt a re-evaluation of patient status and ET tube position.[19]

Prolonged Transport

Airway management of a patient prior to and during a prolonged transport requires complex decision making on the part of the prehospital care provider. Interventions to control and secure the airway, especially using complex techniques, depend on numerous factors, including the patient's injuries, the clinical skills of the prehospital care provider, the equipment available, and the distance and transport time to definitive care. Risks and benefits of all the airway options available should be considered prior to making a final airway decision. Both a longer distance of transport and a longer transport time lower the threshold for securing the airway with endotracheal intubation. For transports of 15 to 20 minutes, essential skills, including an oral airway and bag-mask ventilation, may be sufficient. Use of air medical transport also lowers the threshold to perform endotracheal intubation, as a cramped, noisy environment makes ongoing airway assessment and management difficult.

Any patient requiring airway management or ventilatory support requires ongoing patient monitoring. Continuous pulse oximetry should be performed on all trauma patients during transport, and capnography should be strongly considered for all intubated patients. Loss of $ETCO_2$ indicates that the ventilator circuit has become disconnected or, more importantly, the ET tube has been dislodged, or the patient's perfusion has decreased significantly. All of these possible causes require immediate action.

Serial vital signs should also be recorded on patients requiring airway or ventilation interventions. Confirmation of endotracheal intubation, as described above, should be performed each time the patient is moved or repositioned. It is also a good idea to frequently confirm the security of any airway device.

Any patient who requires increasing FiO_2 or PEEP in order to maintain oxygenation needs to be carefully re-evaluated. Possible etiologies include the development of a pneumothorax or worsening of pulmonary contusions. Any known or suspected pneumothorax must be monitored closely for the development of a tension pneumothorax, and pleural decompression should be performed if hemodynamic compromise occurs. If the patient has had an open pneumothorax sealed, the dressing should be opened to release any pressure that may have accumulated. If the patient is receiving positive pressure ventilation, the positive pressure ventilation can convert a simple pneumothorax to a tension pneumothorax.

Burn patients should receive supplemental oxygen to maintain SpO_2 greater than 95%, whereas those with known or suspected carbon monoxide poisoning should receive 100% oxygen.

Prior to embarking on a prolonged transport of a patient, potential oxygen needs should be calculated, and sufficient amounts of oxygen should be available for the transport (**Figure 8-34**). A good rule of thumb is to bring 50% more oxygen than anticipated.

Intermittent sedation may be required for an agitated intubated patient. Sedation may also decrease the work of breathing and any "fighting the ventilator" when mechanical ventilation is being used. If sedating the patient, small doses of benzodiazepines should be titrated intravenously. The use of neuromuscular blocking agents may also be considered if the patient is significantly combative, the airway is secured with an ET tube, and prehospital care personnel are properly trained and credentialed.

Figure 8-34 Oxygen Tank Size and Duration

Flow Rate (L/min)	Tank Size and Duration (in Hours)				
	D	E	M	G	H/K
2	2.5	4.4	24.7	38.2	49.7
5	1	1.8	9.9	15.3	19.9
10	0.5	0.9	4.9	7.6	9.9
15	0.3	0.6	3.3	5.1	6.6

Note: This table shows the approximate duration in hours of various sizes of oxygen tanks and flow rates. The numbers are based on the assumption that the oxygen tank is completely full at 2,100 pounds per square inch.

Summary

- The trauma patient is susceptible to various injuries that may impair ventilation and gas exchange.
- Trauma to the chest, airway obstruction, central nervous system injury, and hemorrhage can all result in inadequate tissue perfusion.
- To properly care for the trauma patient, the provider must understand and be able to do the following:
    - Integrate the principles of ventilation and gas exchange with the pathophysiology of trauma to identify patients with inadequate perfusion

- 75-90% of deaths occur before reaching treatment facility
- 3 phases of TCCC
- Point of Wounding Care
- Objectives
  - Safety
  - Treat Casualty
  - Prevent additional "
  - complete mission
- 3 Phases
  - Care Under Fire - care while being shot at Return Fire
  - Tactical Field Care - semi-safe care ABC
  - Tactical Evacuation Care - all possible care "TACEVAC Care"

Care Under Fire

- 7 Guidelines
- don't treat in Kill Zone
- Fight Fire w/ Fire
- check the hands
- only life-threatening bleeding warrents intervention in Kill zone
- Femoral Artery = death in 3 mins
- <u>Tourniquets</u>
  - Soft T
  - CAT
  - EMT - best
~ 2hrs = no side effect
   4 hrs = side effects
~ High + Die / High + Tight ~

Test

Principle
3 phases
preferred pain Morphine
GSW fluids po
IV no ASAP
moxi ASAP
motified
1L ≠ death
2.5L = death
not adv of Fentanyl = ↓RR
Combat Gauze = severe ext. bleeding control
Morphine = IV
preferred IV/Im antibiotic = Ertapenem

Tactical Field Care

- reduced hazards
- more time for care
- limited gear
- Rapid Assessment & $\overline{Tx}$
- Time to evac varies
- Address life threatening bleeding first

fty 1 • Disarm casualty w/ AMS & Secure weapon

A 2 • Airway Management
  - Chin lift / Jaw thrust
  - NPA → tape it in
  - ETT
  - Surgical Cric
    - use 6.0 ETT

3 • Breathing
  + Tension Pneumo → TD,
    - 14G, 2nd ICS, mid-clavicular line
  - Sucking Wounds
    - Occlusive dressing - burp it

C 4. Bleeding
  - #1 killer
  - Control
    - Pressure, Gauze, Tourniquet
  - Quick Clot   } see pic on phone
  - Combat Gauze   } - pack wound hold for 3 mins
  - Junctional
    - groin, butt, perineum, axilla,
      base of neck

5. IV
  - 18G
  - IO
  - Shock, Vomiting, LLOC, unable to swallow

6. TXA = Cyklokapron
   1g in 100cc NSS or LR over 10 mins
   → 3 hrs after injury
   TXA + ~~Hextend~~
       HATE each other
   SE: Hypotension = IVB
       N/V

7. Fluid Resuscitation
   - Shock only!
   Hextend 500 mL IVB
   500 cc ≠ death
   $1000 cc ≠ death
   1500 cc ≠ death
   2000 cc ≈ maybe death
   2500 cc = probably death

   500 mL of Hextend = 600 - 800 mL of volume
   1000 mL of Hextend = 7,000 mL of NSS

8. prevent hypothermia
   - leave gear on
   - remove wet & replace w/ dry
   - blankets
   🌀

9. penetrating eye trauma
   - cover injured eye
   - antibiotics ASAP

10. Monitoring
   - Pulse Ox is not accurate

Mobic 15mg k/day
Morphine
Tylenol
Toradol
Zofran
Phenergan
Fentanyl

Tactical Evacuation Care

MEDEVAC
- uses medical platforms

CASEVAC
- uses non-medical platforms

TACEVAC
- is both

- Relate the concepts of minute volume and oxygenation to the pathophysiology of trauma
- Explain the mechanisms by which supplemental oxygen and ventilatory support are beneficial to the trauma patient
- Given situations that involve various trauma patients, formulate a plan for airway management and ventilation
- Given current research, understand the risks versus benefits when discussing new, invasive procedures
- Determine by examination of the patient the relative difficulty of endotracheal intubation
- Given a scenario, develop a plan for airway management for a given patient in a given location
- Managing the airway is not without risks. When applying certain skills and modalities, the risk has to be weighed against the potential benefit for that particular patient. What may be the best choice for one patient in a certain situation may not be for another with a similar presentation.
- Sound critical-thinking skills need to be in place to make the best judgments for the trauma patient.

SCENARIO RECAP

You and your partner are dispatched to a motorcycle crash on a curvy county road. Fellow riders report that the patient was traveling too fast to negotiate a sharp curve and was thrown over the guardrail and into a tree. They carried the patient back up the embankment to the road.

Upon your arrival, you find a police officer maintaining an open airway using an NPA and administering oxygen via a nonrebreathing mask. The police officer reports that the patient has been unconscious since her arrival. You note that the patient's helmet has significant damage. You also note a deformed right humerus and an angulated lower leg.

- What indicators of airway compromise are evident in this patient?
- What other information, if any, would you seek from witnesses or the emergency medical responders?
- Describe the sequence of actions you would take to manage this patient before and during transport.

SCENARIO SOLUTION

Physical evidence at the scene suggests that the driver has likely been subjected to significant kinetic forces capable of creating life-threatening injuries. The position of the patient suggests that multiple impacts occurred.

The patient exhibits several signs of airway compromise and ventilatory insufficiency. Although his respiratory status appears within normal parameters, he has an altered LOC and requires frequent suctioning.

Emergency medical responder personnel are already administering oxygen and have managed the airway with an NPA. You continue ventilatory support and maintain cervical spine stabilization while assessing the difficulty for endotracheal intubation. You are careful to ensure that the airway remains clear and that manual ventilations are effective.

After assessing the patient's airway, you determine that it will be a difficult intubation. You decide that, due to the 12-minute transport time, the anticipated difficulty intubating the patient, and the patient supporting his own respirations, you will manage the patient's airway with the NPA and continue to monitor the airway and respirations.

After quickly moving the patient to the ambulance for transport, you place the patient on a pulse oximeter and monitor $ETCO_2$. You establish intravenous access while en route to a trauma receiving facility. You take care to maintain the effectiveness of spinal immobilization efforts and frequently reassess the patient's condition. To ensure proper activation of the receiving facility's trauma response, you notify the trauma center as early as possible during transport. On arrival at the trauma center, you concisely convey all pertinent information regarding the incident, the patient, and medical interventions to the receiving physician and other appropriate trauma team members.

References

1. Stockinger ZT, McSwain NE Jr. Prehospital endotracheal intubation for trauma does not improve survival over bag-mask ventilation. *J Trauma*. 2004;56(3):531.

2. Roberts K, Whalley H, Bleetman A. The nasopharyngeal airway: dispelling myths and establishing the facts. *Emerg Med J*. 2005;22:394-396.

3. Davis DP, Koprowicz KM, Newgard CD, et al. The relationship between out-of-hospital airway management and outcome among trauma patients with Glasgow Coma Scale Scores of 8 or less. *Prehosp Emerg Care*. 2011;15(2):184-192.

4. Garza AG, Gratton MC, Coontz D, et al. Effect of paramedic experience on orotracheal intubation success rates. *J Emerg Med*. 2003;25(3):251.

5. Dickinson ET, Cohen JE, Mechem CC. The effectiveness of midazolam as a single pharmacologic agent to facilitate endotracheal intubation by paramedics. *Prehosp Emerg Care*. 1999;3(3):191.

6. Wang HE, Davis DP, O'Connor RE, et al. Drug-assisted intubation in the prehospital setting. *Prehosp Emerg Care*. 2006;10(2):261.

7. Davis DP, Hoyt DB, Ochs M, et al. The effect of paramedic rapid sequence intubation on an outcome in patients with severe trauma brain injury. *J Trauma*. 2003;54:444.

8. Davis DP, Dunford JV, Poste JC, et al. The impact of hypoxia and hyperventilation on outcome after paramedic rapid sequence intubation of severely head-injured patient. *J Trauma*. 2004;57:1.

9. Bernard SA, Nguyen V, Cameron P, et al. Prehospital rapid sequence intubation improves functional outcome for patients with severe traumatic brain injury: a randomized controlled trial. *Ann Surg*. 2010;252(6):959-965.

10. Smith KJ, Dobranowski J, Yip G, Dauphin A, Choi PT. Cricoid pressure displaces the esophagus: an observational study using magnetic resonance imaging. *Anesthesiology*. 2003;99(1):60-64.

11. Werner SL, Smith CE, Goldstein JR, Jones RA, Cydulka RK. Pilot study to evaluate the accuracy of ultrasonography in confirming endotracheal tube placement. *Ann Emerg Med*. 2007;49(1):75-80.

12. Butler J, Sen A. Best evidence topic report. Cricoid pressure in emergency rapid sequence induction. *Emerg Med J*. Nov 2005;22(11):815-816.

13. O'Connor RE, Swor RA. Verification of endotracheal tube placement following intubation. *Prehosp Emerg Care*. 1999;3:248.

14. Frame SB, Simon JM, Kerstein MD, et al. Percutaneous transtracheal catheter ventilation (PTCV) in complete airway obstruction: a canine model. *J Trauma*. 1989;29:774.

15. American College of Surgeons (ACS) Committee on Trauma. Airway management and ventilation. In *Advanced Trauma Life Support, Student Course Manual*. 9th ed. Chicago, IL: ACS; 2012.

16. Mabry RL, Frankfurt A. An analysis of battlefield cricothyrotomy in Iraq and Afghanistan. *J Spec Oper Med*. 2012;12(1):17-23.

17. Warner KJ, Cuschieri J, Garland B, et al. The utility of early end-tidal capnography in monitoring ventilation status after severe injury. *J Trauma*. 2009;66:26-31.

18. Cooper CJ, Kraatz JJ, Kubiak DS, Kessel JW, Barnes SL. Utility of prehospital quantitative end tidal CO_2? *Prehosp Disaster Med*. 2013;28(2):87-93.

19. Silvestri S, Ralis GA, Krauss B, et al. The effectiveness of out-of-hospital use of continuous end-tidal carbon dioxide monitoring on the rate of unrecognized misplaced intubations within a regional emergency medical services system. *Ann Emerg Med*. 2005;45:497.

Suggested Reading

American College of Surgeons (ACS) Committee on Trauma. *Advanced Trauma Life Support, Student Course Manual*. 9th ed. Chicago, IL: ACS; 2012.

Brainard C. Whose tube is it? *JEMS*. 2006;31:62.

Dunford JV, David DP, Ochs M, et al. The incidence of transient hypoxia and heart rate reactivity during paramedic rapid sequence intubation. *Ann Emerg Med*. 2003;42:721.

Soubani AO. Noninvasive monitoring of oxygen and carbon dioxide. *Am J Emerg Med*. 2001;19:141.

Walls RM, Murphy MF, eds. *Manual of Emergency Airway Management*. 3rd ed. Philadelphia, PA: Lippincott Williams Wilkins Publishers/Wolters Kluwer Health; 2008.

Weitzel N, Kendal J, Pons P. Blind nasotracheal intubation for patients with penetrating neck trauma. *J Trauma*. 2004;56(5):1097.

SPECIFIC SKILLS

Airway Management and Ventilation Skills

Trauma Jaw Thrust

Principle: To open the airway without moving the cervical spine.

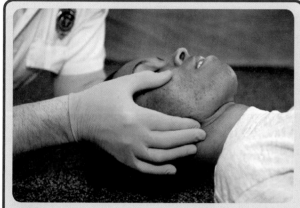

1 In both the trauma jaw thrust and the trauma chin lift, manual neutral in-line stabilization of the head and neck is maintained while the mandible is moved anteriorly (forward). This maneuver moves the tongue forward, away from the hypopharynx, and holds the mouth slightly open.

From a position above the patient's head, the prehospital care provider positions his or her hands on either side of the patient's head, fingers pointing **caudad** (toward the patient's feet).

Depending on the size of the prehospital care provider's hands, the fingers are spread across the face and around the angle of the patient's mandible.

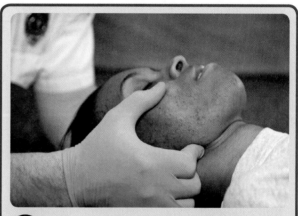

2 Gentle, equal pressure is applied with these digits to move the patient's mandible anteriorly (forward) and slightly downward (toward the patient's feet).

Airway Management and Ventilation Skills (continued)

Alternate Trauma Jaw Thrust

Principle: To open the airway without moving the cervical spine.

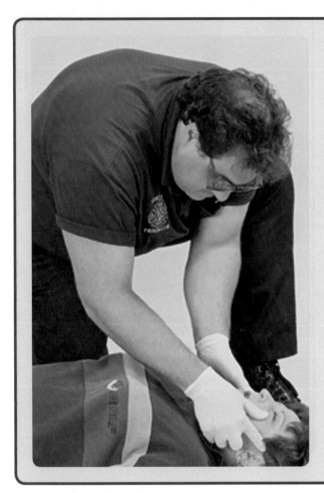

The trauma jaw thrust can also be performed while positioned beside the patient, facing the patient's head. The prehospital care provider's fingers point cephalad (toward the top of the patient's head). Depending on the size of the prehospital care provider's hands, the fingers are spread across the face and around the angle of the patient's mandible. Gentle, equal pressure is applied with these digits to move the patient's mandible anteriorly (forward) and slightly downward (toward the patient's feet).

Airway Management and Ventilation Skills (continued)

Trauma Chin Lift

Principle: To open the airway without moving the cervical spine.

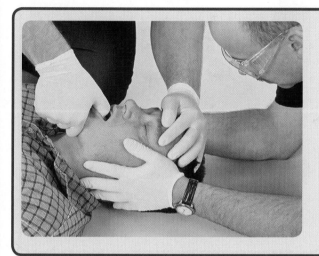

From a position above the patient's head, the patient's head and neck are moved into a neutral in-line position, and manual stabilization is maintained. The prehospital care provider is positioned at the patient's side between the patient's shoulders and hips, facing the patient's head. With the hand closest to the patient's feet, the prehospital care provider grasps the patient's teeth or the lower mandible between his or her thumb and first two fingers beneath the patient's chin. The prehospital care provider now pulls the patient's chin anteriorly and slightly caudad, elevating the mandible and opening the mouth.

Oropharyngeal Airway

Principle: An adjunct used to maintain an open airway mechanically in a patient without a gag reflex.

The oropharyngeal airway (OPA) is designed to hold the patient's tongue anteriorly out of the pharynx. The OPA is available in various sizes. Proper sizing to the patient is required to ensure a patent airway. *Placement of an OPA in the hypopharynx is contraindicated in patients who have an intact gag reflex.*

Two methods for insertion of the OPA are effective: the tongue jaw lift insertion method and the tongue blade insertion method. Regardless of which method is used, the first prehospital care provider stabilizes the patient's head and neck in a neutral in-line position while the second provider measures and inserts the OPA.

Tongue Jaw Lift Insertion Method

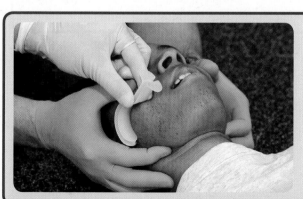

 The first provider brings the patient's head and neck into a neutral in-line position and maintains stabilization while opening the patient's airway with a trauma jaw thrust maneuver. The second provider selects and measures for a properly sized OPA. The distance from the corner of the patient's mouth to the earlobe is a good estimate for proper size.

Airway Management and Ventilation Skills (continued)

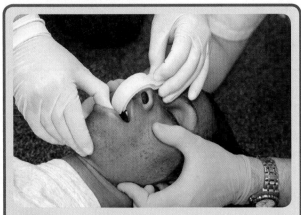

2 The patient's airway is opened with the chin lift maneuver. The OPA is turned so that the distal tip is pointing toward the top of the patient's head (flanged end pointing toward patient's head) and tilted toward the mouth opening.

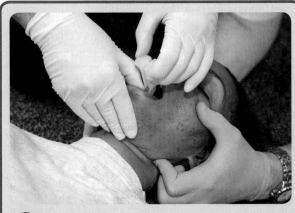

3 The OPA is inserted into the patient's mouth and rotated to fit the contours of the patient's anatomy.

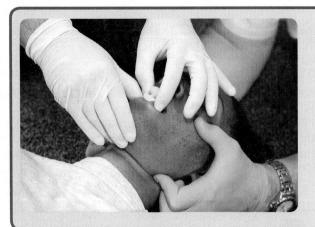

4 The OPA is rotated until the inside curve is resting against the tongue and holding it out of the posterior pharynx. The flanges of the OPA should be resting against the outside surface of the patient's teeth.

Airway Management and Ventilation Skills (continued)

Tongue Blade Insertion Method

The tongue blade insertion method is probably a safer method than the tongue jaw lift because it eliminates the accidental tearing or puncturing of gloves or skin by sharp, pointed, or broken teeth. This method also eliminates the possibility of being bitten if the patient's level of consciousness is not as deep as previously assessed or if any seizure activity occurs.

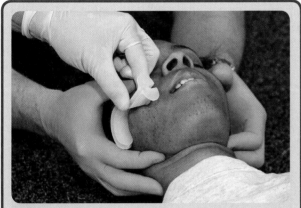

1. The first provider brings the patient's head and neck into a neutral in-line position and maintains stabilization while opening the patient's airway with the trauma jaw thrust maneuver. The second provider selects and measures for a properly sized OPA.

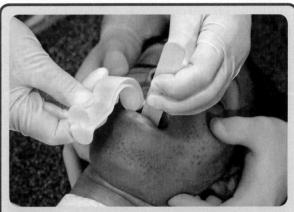

2. The second provider pulls the patient's mouth open by the chin and places a tongue blade into the patient's mouth to move the tongue forward in place and keep the airway open.

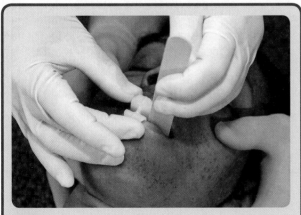

3. The device is inserted with the flanged end pointing toward the patient's feet and the distal tip pointing into the patient's mouth, following the curvature of the airway.

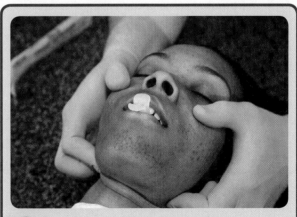

4. The OPA is advanced until the flanged end of the OPA rests against the outside surface of the patient's teeth.

Airway Management and Ventilation Skills (continued)

Nasopharyngeal Airway

Principle: An adjunct used to maintain an open airway mechanically in a patient with or without a gag reflex.

The nasopharyngeal airway (NPA) is a simple airway adjunct that provides an effective way to maintain a patent airway in patients who may still have an intact gag reflex. Most patients will tolerate the NPA if properly sized. NPAs are available in a range of diameters (internal diameters of 5–9 mm), and the length varies appropriately with the size of the diameter. NPAs are usually made of a flexible, rubberlike material. Rigid NPAs are not recommended for field use.

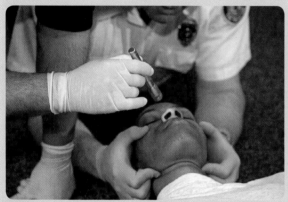

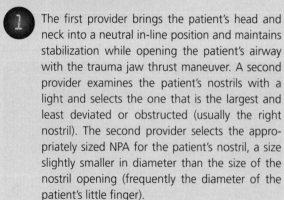

1. The first provider brings the patient's head and neck into a neutral in-line position and maintains stabilization while opening the patient's airway with the trauma jaw thrust maneuver. A second provider examines the patient's nostrils with a light and selects the one that is the largest and least deviated or obstructed (usually the right nostril). The second provider selects the appropriately sized NPA for the patient's nostril, a size slightly smaller in diameter than the size of the nostril opening (frequently the diameter of the patient's little finger).

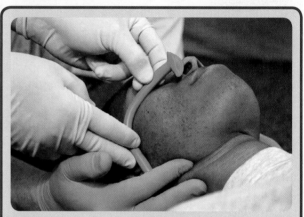

2. The length of the NPA is also important. The NPA needs to be long enough to supply an air passage between the patient's tongue and the posterior pharynx. The distance from the patient's nose to the earlobe is a good estimate for proper size.

Airway Management and Ventilation
Skills (continued)

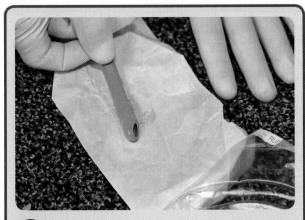
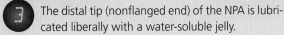

3 The distal tip (nonflanged end) of the NPA is lubricated liberally with a water-soluble jelly.

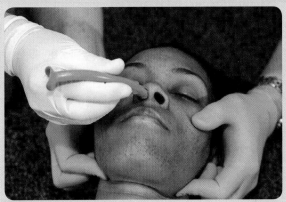

4 The NPA is slowly inserted into the nostril of choice. Insertion should be in an anterior-to-posterior direction along the floor of the nasal cavity, not in a superior-to-inferior direction. If resistance is met at the posterior end of the nostril, a gentle back-and-forth rotation of the NPA between the fingers will usually aid in passing it beyond the turbinate bones of the nasal cavity without damage. Should the NPA continue to meet with resistance, the NPA should not be forced past the obstruction but rather withdrawn, and the distal tip should be relubricated and inserted into the other nostril.

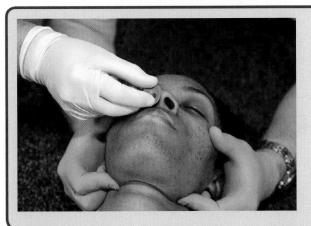

5 The second provider continues insertion until the flange end of the NPA is next to the anterior nares or until the patient gags. If the patient gags, the NPA is withdrawn slightly.

Airway Management and Ventilation Skills (continued)

Bag-Mask Ventilation

Principle: The preferred method of providing assisted ventilation.

Ventilation using a bag-mask device has an advantage over other ventilatory support systems because it gives a prehospital care provider feedback by the feel of the bag (compliance). Positive feedback ensures the operator of successful ventilations; changes in the feedback indicate a loss of mask seal, the presence of a pathologic airway, or a thoracic problem interfering with the delivery of successful ventilations. This "feel" and the control it provides also make the bag-mask device suitable for assisting ventilations. The bag-mask device's portability and readiness for immediate use make it useful for immediate delivery of ventilations on identification of the need.

Without supplemental oxygen, however, a bag-mask device provides an oxygen concentration of only 21%, or a fraction of inspired oxygen (FiO_2) of 0.21; as soon as time allows, an oxygen reservoir and high-concentration supplemental oxygen should be connected to the bag-mask. When oxygen is connected without a reservoir, the FiO_2 is limited to 0.50 or less; with a reservoir, the FiO_2 is 0.85 or greater.

If the patient being ventilated is unconscious without a gag reflex, a properly sized OPA should be inserted before attempting to ventilate with the bag-mask device. If the patient has an intact gag reflex, a properly sized NPA should be inserted before attempting to assist ventilations.

Various bag-mask devices are available, including disposable single-patient-use models that are relatively inexpensive. Different brands have varying bag, valve, and reservoir designs. All the parts used should be of the same model and brand because these parts are usually not safely interchangeable.

Bag-mask devices are available in adult, pediatric, and neonatal sizes. Although an adult bag can be used with the properly sized pediatric mask in an emergency, use of the correct bag size is recommended as a safe practice. Adequate ventilations of an adult patient are achieved when a minimum of 800 ml/breath is delivered (1,000–1,200 ml/breath is preferred).

When ventilating with any positive-pressure device, inflation should stop once the chest has risen maximally. When using the bag-mask device, the chest should be visualized for maximum inflation and the bag felt to recognize any marked increased resistance in the bag when lung expansion is at its maximum. Adequate time for exhalation is needed (1:3 ratio between time for inhalation and time for exhalation). If enough time is not allowed, "stepped or stacked breaths" occur, providing a greater volume of inspiration than expiration. Stepped breaths produce poor air exchange and result in hyperinflation, increased pressure, opening of the esophagus, and gastric distension.

Two-Provider Method

Assisting ventilation with a bag-mask device is easier with two or more prehospital care providers than with only one prehospital care provider. The first provider can focus attention on maintaining an adequate mask seal, while the second provides good delivery volume by using both hands to squeeze (deflate) the bag.

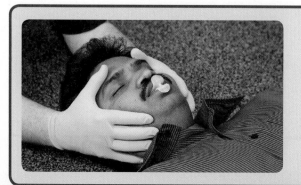

 The first provider kneels above the patient's head and maintains manual stabilization of the patient's head and neck in a neutral in-line position.

Airway Management and Ventilation Skills (continued)

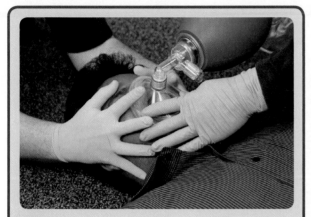

 The face mask is placed over the patient's nose and mouth, and the mask is held in place with the thumbs on the lateral portion of the mask while pulling the mandible up into the mask. The other fingers provide the manual stabilization and maintain a patent airway.

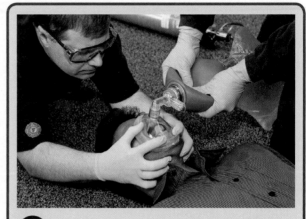

 The second provider kneels at the side of the patient and squeezes the bag with both hands to inflate the lungs.

Supraglottic Airway

Note: The Combitube and the King airways are used in the following illustrations for demonstration purposes only. Other brands of supraglottic airways may be used according to local preference.

Combitube

Principle: A mechanical device used for opening and maintaining an airway when unable to intubate.

The supraglottic airway provides prehospital care providers with a functional alternative airway. These combination airways are an acceptable prehospital field device and typically do not require extensive training to achieve competency. The airway's greatest advantage is that it can be inserted independent of the patient's position ("blindly" inserted), which may be especially important in trauma patients with high suspicion of cervical injury. The indications for placement of a supraglottic airway are the same as for the placement of any airway: the necessity of obtaining a patent airway in a patient. Each manufacturer of the supraglottic airway will identify age and size requirements pertinent to its airway. The prehospital care provider should always follow the manufacturer's recommendations for size selection, contraindications, and specific insertion procedures.

Before insertion of a supraglottic airway, as with any other invasive airway, the patient is preoxygenated with a high concentration of oxygen using a simple airway adjunct or manual airway procedure.

As with any other piece of medical equipment, the dual lumen should be inspected and each part tested before insertion. The distal end of the airway should be lubricated with a water-soluble lubricant.

Airway Management and Ventilation Skills (continued)

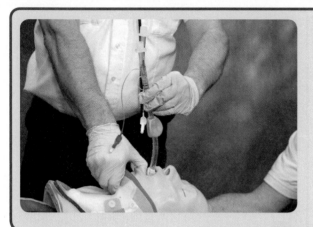

1 The prehospital care provider stops ventilations and removes all other airway adjuncts. If the patient is supine, the tongue and lower jaw are lifted upward with one hand (chin lift).

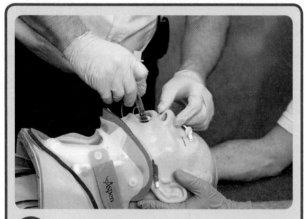

2 The end of the tube is inserted. (Tearing the cuff when inserting the airway past broken teeth or dental appliances should be avoided.) The Combitube is inserted until the marker rings line up with the patient's teeth.

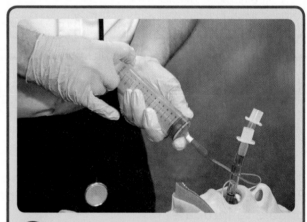

3 Using the large syringe, the pharyngeal cuff is inflated with 100 ml of air and the syringe removed. The device should seat itself in the posterior pharynx just behind the hard palate.

Airway Management and Ventilation Skills (continued)

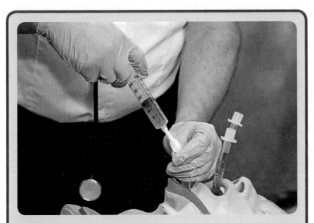

4 Using the small syringe, the distal cuff is inflated with 15 ml of air and the syringe removed. Typically the balloon will be placed (inflated) in the patient's esophagus. The prehospital care provider begins ventilation through the esophageal tube (generally marked with a #1).

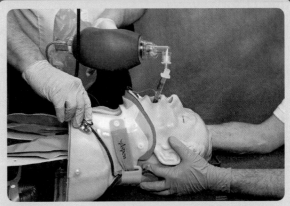

5 If auscultation of breath sounds is positive and gastric insufflation is negative, the prehospital care provider continues ventilation through the esophageal tube.

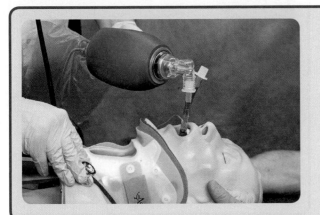

6 If auscultation of breath sounds is negative and gastric insufflation is positive, the prehospital care provider immediately ventilates with the shortened tracheal tube (generally marked with a #2), after which reauscultation of breath sounds and gastric sounds is done to affirm proper tube placement. The prehospital care provider continues to ventilate the patient and initiate immediate transport to an appropriate facility.

All esophageal airways require the patient to have no gag reflex. If the patient regains consciousness and begins to gag or vomit, these devices are removed immediately. Extubation of esophageal airways almost always causes vomiting or regurgitation. Consequently, suction equipment must be readily available when the device is removed. Due to the risk of contact with bodily fluids, observe standard precautions.

Airway Management and Ventilation Skills (continued)

King LT Airway

Principle: The King LT single-lumen airway is a blindly inserted device used to provide ventilation of the traumatized patient.

The King LT (laryngeal tube) may be used in patients over 4 feet (1.2 m) in height and in whom the risk of aspiration is considered to be low. The King LT is a single-lumen tube with both a distal and oral (proximal) cuff. Unlike dual-lumen airways, there is only one ventilatory tube and one cuff-inflation port. This design simplifies the insertion procedure of this device. It should be noted that the King LT does not provide protection from aspiration. In fact, the manufacturer lists lack of fasting as a contraindication to its use as well as "situations where gastric contents may be present [that] include, but are not limited to … multiple or massive injury, acute abdominal or thoracic injury …." Therefore, significant care must be taken to avoid aspiration when the King LT is used in these situations.

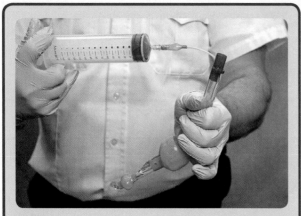

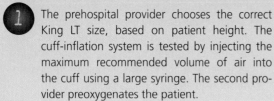

1. The prehospital provider chooses the correct King LT size, based on patient height. The cuff-inflation system is tested by injecting the maximum recommended volume of air into the cuff using a large syringe. The second provider preoxygenates the patient.

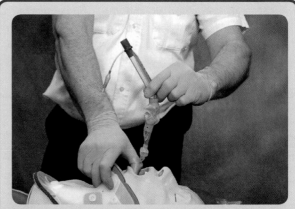

2. The first provider applies a water-based lubricant to the beveled distal tip and posterior aspect of the tube and holds the King LT with his or her dominant hand. With the nondominant hand, the first provider opens the patient's mouth and applies a chin lift. The second provider maintains cervical spine stabilization as necessary.

Airway Management and Ventilation Skills (continued)

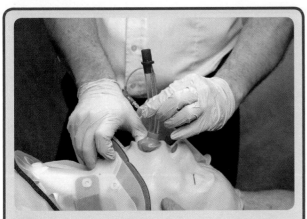

3 The first provider introduces the tip into the patient's mouth and advances it behind the base of the tongue. The first provider then rotates the tube back to the midline as the tip reaches the posterior wall of the pharynx.

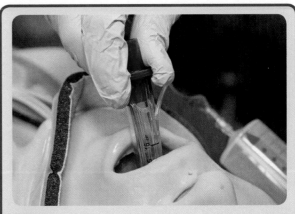

4 The first provider advances the King LT until the base of the connector is aligned with the patient's teeth.

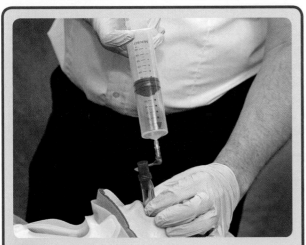

5 The first provider inflates the cuff with a large syringe. Typical inflation volumes are as follows:

- Size 3, 45–60 ml
- Size 4, 60–80 ml
- Size 5, 70–90 ml

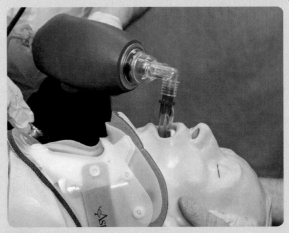

6 The first provider attaches a bag-mask device to the King LT. While gently ventilating the patient to assess ventilation, the first provider simultaneously withdraws the airway until ventilation is easy and free-flowing (large tidal volume with minimal airway pressure). Reference marks are provided at the proximal end of the King LT, which, when aligned with the upper teeth, give an indication of the depth of insertion.

Airway Management and Ventilation Skills (continued)

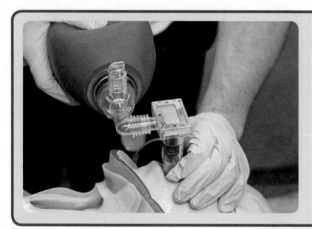

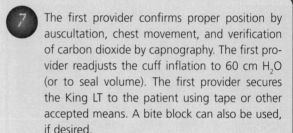

7. The first provider confirms proper position by auscultation, chest movement, and verification of carbon dioxide by capnography. The first provider readjusts the cuff inflation to 60 cm H_2O (or to seal volume). The first provider secures the King LT to the patient using tape or other accepted means. A bite block can also be used, if desired.

*Adapted from King LT manufacturer's instructions.

Laryngeal Mask Airway

Principle: A mechanical device used to maintain an open airway without direct visualization of the airway.

The laryngeal mask airway (LMA) is an airway device that can be inserted by the prehospital care provider without the need for direct visualization of the vocal cords. This blind insertion technique has advantages over endotracheal intubation, as initial training requirements are less and skill retention is easier to accomplish. The disadvantage to the LMA is that although it forms a seal around the glottic opening, this seal is not as occlusive as that of an endotracheal tube cuff. Aspiration remains a potential problem. Another potential problem is that in order to insert an LMA, it is necessary for the prehospital care provider to insert his or her fingers into the patient's mouth. This limits the usefulness of the LMA to fully unconscious patients. As with any airway in the trauma patient, cervical stabilization must be maintained for the duration of the procedure.

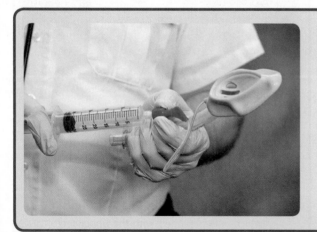

1. The prehospital care provider deflates the cuff of the mask and applies a water-soluble lubricant to the posterior surface. The LMA is held in the dominant hand, between the thumb and the other fingers, at the junction of the cuff and the tube.

Airway Management and Ventilation
Skills (continued)

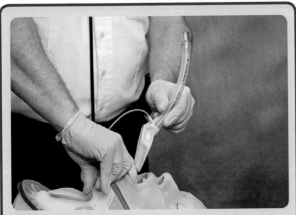

2 The prehospital care provider grasps the mandible with the other hand, opens the patient's mouth, and inserts the LMA into the patient's mouth. The prehospital care provider presses the tip of the cuff upward against the hard palate and flattens the cuff against it.

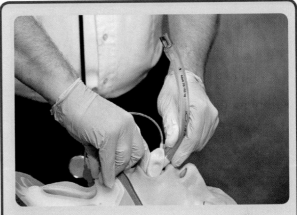

3 The LMA is guided, not forced, into the mouth and advanced it into the pharynx.

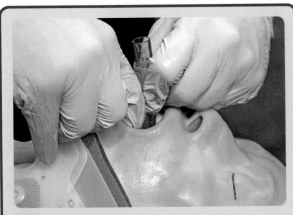

4 The prehospital care provider continues to advance the LMA into the hypopharynx until a definite resistance is felt. The end of the airway tube is held in place while the prehospital care provider removes his or her fingers from the patient's mouth.

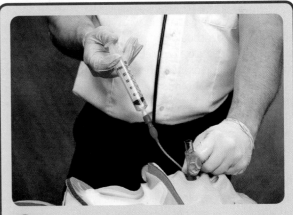

5 The prehospital care provider inflates the cuff with enough air to maintain a seal. The cuff should never be overinflated as this can cause damage to the airway structures.

Airway Management and Ventilation Skills (continued)

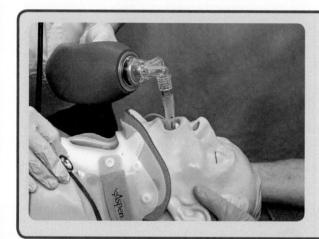

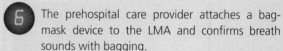

6 The prehospital care provider attaches a bag-mask device to the LMA and confirms breath sounds with bagging.

Visualized Orotracheal Intubation of the Trauma Patient

Principle: To secure a definitive airway without manipulating the cervical spine.

Visualized orotracheal intubation of the trauma patient is done with the patient's head and neck stabilized in a neutral in-line position. Orotracheal intubation while maintaining manual in-line stabilization requires additional training and practice beyond that for intubation of nontrauma patients. As with all skills, training requires observation, critique, and certification initially and at least twice a year by the medical director or designee.

In hypoxic trauma patients who are not in cardiac arrest, intubation should not be the initial airway maneuver. The prehospital care provider should perform intubation only after he or she has preoxygenated the patient with a high concentration of oxygen using a simple airway adjunct or manual maneuver. Contact with the deep pharynx when intubating a severely hypoxic patient without preoxygenation can easily produce vagal stimulation, resulting in a dangerous bradycardia.

The prehospital care provider should not interrupt ventilation for more than 20 seconds when intubating the patient. Ventilation should never be interrupted for more than 30 seconds for any reason.

Visualized orotracheal intubation is extremely difficult in conscious patients or patients with an intact gag reflex. The prehospital care provider should consider use of topical anesthesia or paralytic agents after additional training, protocol development, and approval by the EMS medical director.

For the novice prehospital care provider, the use of a straight laryngoscope blade tends to produce less rotary force (pulling the patient's head toward a "sniffing" position) than that produced by the use of a curved blade. However, because the success rate of intubation is often related to the prehospital care provider's comfort with a given design, the style of blade selection for the laryngoscope remains a matter of individual preference.

Note: The cervical collar will limit forward motion of the mandible and complete opening of the mouth. Therefore, after adequate spinal immobilization is ensured, the cervical collar is removed, manual stabilization of the cervical spine is held, and intubation is attempted. Once intubation is accomplished, the collar is reapplied.

Airway Management and Ventilation Skills (continued)

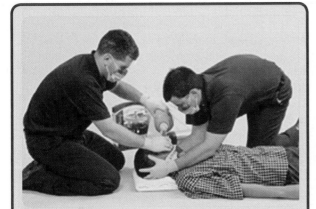

1 Before attempting intubation, the prehospital care providers should assemble and test all required equipment and follow Standard Precautions. The first provider kneels at the patient's head and ventilates the patient with a bag-mask device and high-concentration oxygen. The second provider, kneeling at the patient's side, provides manual stabilization of the patient's head and neck.

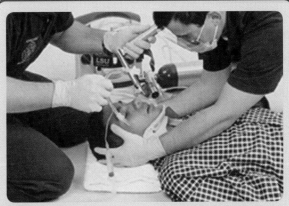

2 After preoxygenation, the first provider stops ventilations and grasps the laryngoscope in the left hand and the ET tube (with syringe attached to pilot valve) in the right hand. If a stylet is used, this should have been inserted when the equipment was inspected and tested. The distal end of the stylet should be inserted just short of the ET tube's distal opening.

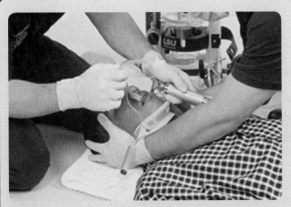

3 The laryngoscope blade is inserted into the right side of the patient's airway to the correct depth, sweeping toward the center of the airway while observing the desired landmarks.

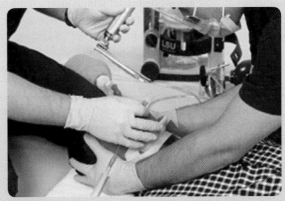

4 After identification of desired landmarks, the ET tube is inserted between the patient's vocal cords to the desired depth. The laryngoscope is then removed while holding the ET tube in place; the depth marking on the side of the ET tube is noted. If a malleable stylet has been used, it should be removed at this time.

Airway Management and Ventilation Skills (continued)

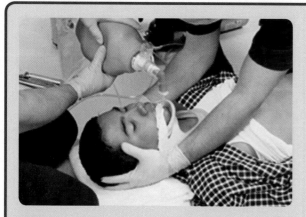

The first provider attaches the bag-valve system with a reservoir attached to the proximal end of the ET tube, and ventilation is resumed while observing the rise of the patient's chest with each delivered breath. Manual stabilization of the patient's head and neck is maintained throughout the process. Bilateral breath sounds and absence of air sounds over the epigastrium and other indications of proper ET tube placement, including wave form capnography, are checked (see the earlier discussion in this chapter, under Verification of Endotracheal Tube Placement, page 185). Once ET tube placement is confirmed, the ET tube is secured in place. Although the use of tape or other commercially available devices is adequate in controlled situations in which the patient is not moved, *the best way to guard against displacement of the ET tube in the prehospital situation is to physically hold onto the tube at all times.*

5 The pilot valve is inflated with enough air to complete the seal between the patient's trachea and the cuff of the ET tube (usually 8–10 ml of air), and the syringe is removed from the pilot valve.

Face-to-Face Orotracheal Intubation

Principle: An alternative method of securing a definitive airway when patient positioning limits use of traditional methods.

Situations may arise in the prehospital setting in which the prehospital care provider cannot take a position above the patient's head to initiate endotracheal intubation in a traditional manner. The face-to-face method for intubation is a viable option in these situations. The basic concepts of intubation still apply with face-to-face intubation: Preoxygenate the patient with a bag-mask device and high-concentration oxygen before attempting intubation, maintain manual stabilization of the patient's head and neck throughout the intubation, and do not interrupt ventilation for longer than 20 to 30 seconds at a time.

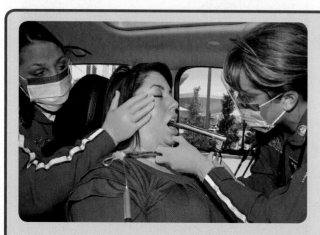

1 While manual stabilization of the patient's head and neck in a neutral in-line position is held, the prehospital care provider positions himself or herself in front of the patient, "face to face." The laryngoscope is held in the right hand with the blade on the patient's tongue. The blade moves the tongue down and out rather than up and out. The patient's airway is opened with the left hand, and the laryngoscope is placed into the patient's airway. After the laryngoscope blade is placed in the patient's airway, the desired landmarks are found. Looking into the airway from a position above the open airway provides the best view.

Airway Management and Ventilation Skills (continued)

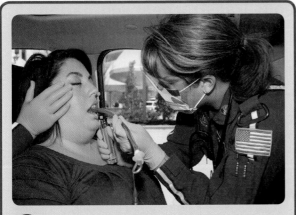

2. After identification of desired landmarks, the ET tube is passed between the patient's vocal cords to the desired depth with the left hand. The cuff is inflated with air to form the seal, and the syringe is removed. A bag-valve device is attached, and placement of the ET tube is confirmed.

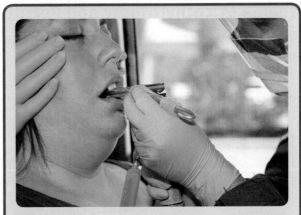

3. After confirmation of ET tube placement, the patient is ventilated while the prehospital care provider holds onto the ET tube and maintains manual stabilization of the patient's head and neck. The ET tube should then be secured into place.

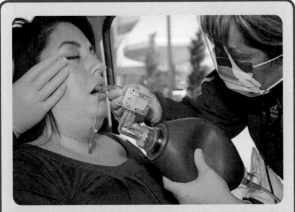

4. An alternative method for face-to-face intubation is to hold the laryngoscope in the left hand and place the ET tube with the right hand. This method may block the visualization of the lower airway as the ET tube is placed.

Airway Management and Ventilation Skills (continued)

Needle Cricothyrotomy and Percutaneous Transtracheal Ventilation

Principle: A method of providing oxygenation to a patient who cannot be intubated or ventilated with a bag-mask.

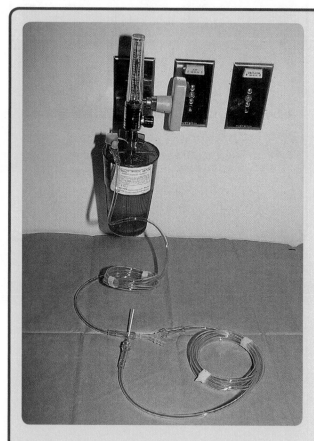

All parts except the needle, tank, and regulator should be modified as needed, preassembled, and packaged for ready availability in the field. This preparation will ensure successful assembly. When this technique is needed, time will be of the essence. The equipment should be ready to use, requiring only connection to the regulator and needle. The prehospital care provider can use a commercially available product that contains all of the necessary equipment. If this is not available, the following equipment is required:

- Syringe: 10 to 30 ml
- To allow for inflation and deflation of the lung while there is constant flow from the oxygen source, some type of bypass is necessary. The following are two examples:
  1. A hole approximately 40% of the circumference of the oxygen delivery tube, cut in the side, that can be occluded by the thumb
  2. A plastic "T" or "Y" connector of a size compatible with the oxygen tubing used and connected to the oxygen source with a length of standard universal oxygen tubing
- A short piece of tubing that will fasten over the lower end of the T or Y and snugly fit into the hub of the needle (This leaves one opening of the T or Y connector free with nothing attached to it.)
- An oxygen tank with a regulator that has a delivery pressure of 50 pounds per square inch at its supplemental oxygen nipple
- Strips of 1/2-inch adhesive tape

Airway Management and Ventilation Skills (continued)

The patient should be in the supine position while manual in-line stabilization is maintained.

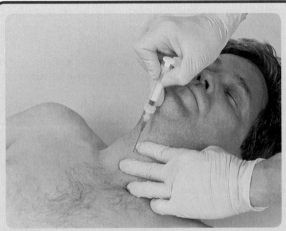

1 The larynx and trachea are stabilized with the fingers of one hand. The needle, attached to the syringe, is placed midline over the cricothyroid membrane or directly into the trachea at a slightly downward angle. As the needle is inserted into the trachea, the plunger of the syringe is withdrawn to create a negative pressure. Once the needle enters into the trachea, air will be sucked into the syringe, confirming that the tip of the needle is properly located. The needle is advanced an additional centimeter, and then the syringe is removed from the needle. The inner needle is removed, leaving the catheter in place. The prehospital care provider quickly forms a loop with adhesive tape around the needle or the hub of the catheter and places the ends of tape on the patient's neck to secure the airway. The prehospital care provider should use caution when securing the catheter to prevent kinking it.

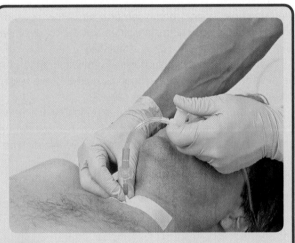

2 The oxygen delivery tube with a vent is connected to the hub of the needle while the hand that initially stabilized the trachea is moved to hold the needle in place. Ventilation is begun by occluding the opening of the tubing assembly with the thumb for 1 second. The patient's chest may or may not rise to indicate that inhalation is occurring. To stop the flow of oxygen into the lungs, the thumb is removed from the opening.

Airway Management and Ventilation
Skills (continued)

Note: The passive process of exhalation takes three to four times as long as inhalation with a normal airway. In this process, exhalation will require more time because of the smaller opening.

The patient is oxygenated by alternately closing the hole to provide the positive flow of oxygen for inhalation and opening the same hole to stop the oxygen flow and allow deflation. The proper time sequence for these maneuvers is 1 second of occlusion of the opening for inhalation and 4 seconds of leaving the hole open for passive deflation. This process is continued until a more definitive airway is established.

After percutaneous transtracheal ventilation (PTV) of 45 to 60 minutes, this technique can provide a high $PaCO_2$ level because of carbon dioxide retention as a result of the restricted expirations. Therefore, the patient should have a more definitive airway established as soon as possible.

Warning: Patients being ventilated using PTV may remain hypoxic and unstable. Prehospital care providers should initiate transport to a suitable facility without delay because the patient is in urgent need of a more definitive surgical transtracheal procedure (cricothyroidotomy) for adequate ventilation and oxygenation.

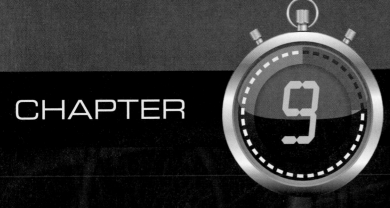

CHAPTER 9

Shock

CHAPTER OBJECTIVES

At the completion of this chapter, the reader will be able to do the following:

- Define shock.

- Explain how preload, afterload, and contractility affect cardiac output.

- Classify shock on an etiologic basis.

- Explain the pathophysiology of shock and its progression through phases.

- Relate shock to energy production, etiology, prevention, and treatment.

- Describe the physical findings in shock.

- Clinically differentiate the types of shock.

- Discuss the limitations of the field management of shock.

- Recognize the need for rapid transport and early definitive management in various forms of shock.

- Apply principles of management of shock in the trauma patient.

SCENARIO

You and your partner are dispatched to a 23-year-old man who was assaulted. Upon your arrival, you find the patient sitting on the ground in moderate distress. He states that he had just withdrawn some cash from an ATM and was returning to his car when he was robbed by two men who punched and kicked him. He complains of pain in his left lower ribs, left upper abdomen, and jaw.

The physical examination of the patient reveals pale skin color, a contusion on the left side of his mandible, and tenderness to palpation over the left lower ribs and in the left upper quadrant of the abdomen. His vital signs are pulse of 112 beats/minute, blood pressure of 100/64 millimeters of mercury (mm Hg), and ventilatory rate of 22 breaths/minute and regular. Breath sounds are present bilaterally. You transfer him to the ambulance in preparation for transport to the hospital.

- What injuries do you expect to see after this assault?
- How would you manage these injuries in the field?
- You are 15 minutes away from the nearest trauma center. How does this alter your management plans?

Introduction

As discussed in the Physiology of Life and Death chapter, and by way of brief review here, shock following trauma has been recognized for more than three centuries. It has been described by Samuel Gross in 1872 as a "rude unhinging of the machinery of life"[1] and by John Collins Warren as "a momentary pause in the act of death."[2] Shock continues to play a central role in the causes of major morbidity and mortality in the trauma patient. Prompt diagnosis, resuscitation, and definitive management of shock resulting from trauma are all essential in determining patient outcome.

In the prehospital setting, the therapeutic challenge posed by the patient in shock is compounded by the need to assess and manage such patients in a relatively austere, and sometimes dangerous, environment in which sophisticated diagnostic and management tools are either unavailable or impractical to apply. This chapter focuses on the causes of traumatic shock and describes the pathophysiologic changes present to help direct management strategies.

Physiology of Shock
Metabolism

To review, cells maintain their normal metabolic functions by producing and using energy in the form of adenosine triphosphate (ATP). The most efficient method of generating this needed energy is via *aerobic metabolism*. The cells take in oxygen and glucose and metabolize it through a complicated physiologic process that produces energy and the by-products of water and carbon dioxide.

Anaerobic metabolism, in contrast to aerobic metabolism, occurs without the use of oxygen. It is the backup power system in the body and uses stored body fat as its energy source. Unfortunately, anaerobic metabolism can run only for a short time, it produces significantly less energy, it produces by-products such as lactic acid that are harmful to the body, and it may ultimately become irreversible. However, it may afford enough energy to power the cells long enough to allow the body to restore its normal metabolism, with the assistance of the prehospital care provider.

If anaerobic metabolism is not reversed quickly, cells cannot continue to function and will die. If a sufficient number of cells in any one organ die, the entire organ ceases to function. When organs die, the patient eventually may die.

The sensitivity of cells to the lack of oxygen varies from organ system to organ system. This sensitivity is called ischemic (lack of oxygen) sensitivity, and it is greatest in the brain, heart, and lungs. It may take only 4 to 6 minutes of anaerobic metabolism before one or more of these vital organs are injured beyond repair. Skin and muscle tissue have a significantly longer ischemic sensitivity—as long as 4 to 6 hours. The abdominal organs generally fall between these two groups and are able to survive 45 to 90 minutes of anaerobic metabolism (**Figure 9-1**).

Figure 9-1 Organ Tolerance to Ischemia	
Organ	**Warm Ischemia Time**
Heart, brain, lungs	4 to 6 minutes
Kidneys, liver, gastrointestinal tract	45 to 90 minutes
Muscle, bone, skin	4 to 6 hours

Source: American College of Surgeons (ACS) Committee on Trauma: *Advanced Trauma Life Support for Doctors: Student Course Manual.* 7th ed. Chicago, IL: ACS; 2004.

Thus, maintenance of normal function of the cells of the body depends upon the crucial relationship and interaction of several body systems. The patient's airway must be patent, and respirations must be of adequate volume and depth (see the Airway and Ventilation chapter). The heart must be functioning and pumping normally. The circulatory system must have enough red blood cells (RBCs) available to deliver adequate amounts of oxygen to tissue cells throughout the body, so that these cells can produce energy.

The prehospital assessment of the trauma patient is directed at preventing or reversing anaerobic metabolism, thus avoiding cellular death and, ultimately, patient death. Ensuring that the critical systems of the body are working together correctly—namely that the patient's airway is patent and that breathing and circulation are adequate—is the major emphasis of the primary assessment. These functions are managed in the trauma patient by the following actions:

- Maintaining an adequate airway and ventilation, thus providing adequate oxygen to the RBCs (see the Airway and Ventilation chapter)
- Assisting ventilation through the judicious use of supplemental oxygen
- Maintaining adequate circulation, thus perfusing tissue cells with oxygenated blood

Definition of Shock

The major complication of disruption of the normal physiology of life is known as shock. Shock is a state of change in cellular function from aerobic metabolism to anaerobic metabolism secondary to hypoperfusion of the tissue cells. As a result, the delivery of oxygen at the cellular level is inadequate to meet the body's metabolic needs. Shock is not defined as low blood pressure, rapid pulse rates, or cool, clammy skin; these are merely systemic manifestations of the entire pathologic process called shock. The correct definition of shock is a lack of tissue perfusion (oxygenation) at the cellular level that leads to anaerobic metabolism and loss of energy production needed to support life.

Shock can kill a patient in the field, the emergency department, the operating room, or the intensive care unit. Although actual death may be delayed for several hours to several days or even weeks, the most common cause of that death is the failure of early resuscitation. The lack of perfusion of cells by oxygenated blood results in anaerobic metabolism and decreased function of cells needed for organ survival. Even when some cells are initially spared, death can occur later, because the remaining cells are unable to adequately carry out the function of that organ indefinitely.

Classification of Traumatic Shock

The prime determinants of cellular perfusion are the heart (acting as the pump or the motor of the system), fluid volume (acting as the hydraulic fluid), the blood vessels (serving as the

---

Figure 9-2   Types of Traumatic Shock

The common types of shock seen after trauma in the prehospital setting include:
- Hypovolemic shock
  - Vascular volume smaller than normal vascular size
  - Result of blood and fluid loss
    - Hemorrhagic shock
- Distributive shock
  - Vascular space larger than normal
    - Neurogenic "shock" (hypotension)
- Cardiogenic shock
  - Heart not pumping adequately
  - Result of cardiac injury

---

conduits or plumbing), and, finally, the cells of the body. Based on these components of the perfusion system, shock may be classified into the following categories (**Figure 9-2**):

1. *Hypovolemic shock* is primarily hemorrhagic in the trauma patient and is related to loss of circulating blood cells with oxygen-carrying capacity and fluid volume. This is the most common cause of shock in the trauma patient.
2. *Distributive (or vasogenic) shock* is related to abnormality in vascular tone arising from several different causes.
3. *Cardiogenic shock* is related to interference with the pump action of the heart.

By far the most common cause of shock in the trauma patient is hemorrhage, and the safest approach in managing the trauma patient in shock is to consider that the cause of the shock is hemorrhage until proven otherwise.

Types of Traumatic Shock

Hypovolemic Shock

Acute loss of blood volume from hemorrhage (loss of plasma and RBCs) causes an imbalance in the relationship of fluid volume to the size of the container. The container retains its normal size, but the fluid volume is decreased. Hypovolemic shock is the most common cause of shock encountered in the prehospital environment, and blood loss is by far the most common cause of shock in trauma patients and the most dangerous for the patient.

When blood is lost from the circulation, the heart is stimulated to increase cardiac output by increasing the strength and rate of contractions. This stimulus results from the release of **epinephrine** from the adrenal glands. At the same time, the sympathetic nervous system releases **norepinephrine** to constrict blood vessels to reduce the size of the container and bring it more into proportion with the volume of remaining fluid. Vasoconstriction results in closing of the peripheral capillaries, which reduces oxygen delivery to those affected cells and forces the switch from aerobic to anaerobic metabolism at the cellular level.

These compensatory defense mechanisms work well up to a point and will help maintain the patient's vital signs for a period of time. A patient who has signs of compensation such as tachycardia is already in shock, not "going into shock." When the defense mechanisms can no longer compensate for the amount of blood lost, a patient's blood pressure will drop. This decrease in blood pressure marks the switch from compensated to decompensated shock—a sign of impending death. Unless aggressive resuscitation occurs, the patient who enters decompensated shock has only one more stage of decline left—irreversible shock, leading to death.

Hemorrhagic Shock

The average 70-kg (150-lb) adult human has approximately 5 liters of circulating blood volume. Hemorrhagic shock (hypovolemic shock resulting from blood loss) is categorized into four classes, depending on the severity and amount of hemorrhage, as follows (**Figure 9-3**) with the proviso that the values and descriptions for the criteria listed for these classes of shock should not be interpreted as absolute determinants of the class of shock, as significant overlap exists:

1. *Class I hemorrhage* represents a loss of up to 15% of blood volume in the adult (up to 750 milliliters [ml]). This stage has few clinical manifestations. Tachycardia

is often minimal, and no measurable changes in blood pressure, pulse pressure, or ventilatory rate occur. Most healthy patients sustaining this amount of hemorrhage require only maintenance fluid as long as no further blood loss occurs. The body's compensatory mechanisms restore the intravascular container–fluid volume ratio and assist in the maintenance of blood pressure.

2. *Class II hemorrhage* represents a loss of 15% to 30% of blood volume (750 to 1,500 ml). Most adults are capable of compensating for this amount of blood loss by activation of the sympathetic nervous system, which will maintain their blood pressure. Clinical findings include increased ventilatory rate, tachycardia, and a narrowed pulse pressure. The clinical clues to this phase are tachycardia, tachypnea, and normal systolic blood pressure. Because the blood pressure is normal, this is "compensated shock"—that is, the patient is in shock but is able to compensate for the time being. The patient often demonstrates anxiety or fright. Although not usually measured in the field, urine output drops slightly to between 20 and 30 ml/hour in an adult in an effort to preserve fluid. On occasion, these patients may require blood transfusion in the hospital; however, most will respond well to crystalloid infusion if hemorrhage is controlled at this point.

3. *Class III hemorrhage* represents a loss of 30% to 40% of blood volume (1,500 to 2,000 ml). When blood loss reaches this point, most patients are no longer able to compensate for the volume loss, and hypotension occurs. The classic findings of shock are obvious and include tachycardia (heart rate greater than 120 beats/minute), tachypnea (ventilatory rate of 30 to 40 breaths/minute), and severe anxiety or confusion. Urine output

Figure 9-3 Classification of Hemorrhagic Shock

	Class I	Class II	Class III	Class IV
Blood loss (ml)	< 750	750–1500	1500–2000	> 2000
Blood loss (% blood volume)	< 15%	15–30%	30–40%	>40%
Pulse rate	< 100	100–120	120–140	> 140
Blood pressure	Normal	Normal	Decreased	Decreased
Pulse pressure (mm Hg)	Normal or increased	Decreased	Decreased	Decreased
Ventilatory rate	14 to 20	20–30	30–40	>35
CNS/mental status	Slightly anxious	Mildly anxious	Anxious, confused	Confused, lethargic
Fluid replacement	Crystalloid	Crystalloid	Crystalloid and blood	Crystalloid and blood

Note: The values and descriptions for the criteria listed for these classes of shock should not be interpreted as absolute determinants of the class of shock, as significant overlap exists.

Source: From American College of Surgeons (ACS) Committee on Trauma. *Advanced Trauma Life Support for Doctors: Student Course Manual.* 8th ed. Chicago, IL: ACS; 2008.

falls to 5 to 15 ml/hour. Many of these patients will require blood transfusion and surgical intervention for adequate resuscitation and control of hemorrhage.

4. *Class IV hemorrhage* represents a loss of more than 40% of blood volume (greater than 2,000 ml). This stage of severe shock is characterized by marked tachycardia (heart rate greater than 140 beats/minute), tachypnea (ventilatory rate greater than 35 breaths/minute), profound confusion or lethargy, and greatly decreased systolic blood pressure, typically in the range of 60 mm Hg. These patients truly have only minutes to live (**Figure 9-4**). Survival depends on immediate control of hemorrhage (surgery for internal hemorrhage) and aggressive resuscitation, including blood and plasma transfusions with minimal crystalloid.

The rapidity with which a patient develops shock depends on how fast blood is lost from the circulation. A trauma patient who has lost blood needs to have the source of blood loss stopped, and, if significant blood loss has occurred, blood replacement needs to be accomplished. The fluid that has been lost is whole blood containing all of its various components, including RBCs with oxygen-carrying capacity, clotting factors, and proteins to maintain oncotic pressure.

Whole blood replacement, or even component therapy, is usually not available in the prehospital environment; therefore, in the field, when treating trauma patients with hemorrhagic shock, providers must take measures to control external blood loss, provide minimal intravenous (IV) electrolyte solution (plasma when available), and transport rapidly to the hospital, where blood, plasma, and clotting factors are available and emergent operative steps to control blood loss can be performed, as necessary (**Figure 9-5**).

Shock research has demonstrated that for lost blood, the replacement ratio with electrolyte solution should be 3 liters

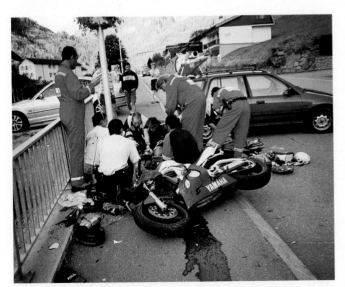

Figure 9-4 Massive blood loss such as that sustained by the victim in this motorcycle crash can rapidly lead to the onset of shock.
Source: Photograph provided courtesy of Air Glaciers, Switzerland.

Figure 9-5 Lyophilized Plasma

Lyophilized plasma is being used in the field in several countries. It is currently under study in the United States for use by emergency medical services (EMS) and is being used by several EMS systems and air medical services in the United States.

of replacement for each liter of blood lost.[3] This high ratio of replacement fluid is required because only about one-fourth to one-third of the volume of an isotonic crystalloid solution such as normal saline or lactated Ringer's solution remains in the intravascular space 30 to 60 minutes after infusing it.

Shock research has also shown that the administration of a limited volume of electrolyte solution before blood replacement is the correct approach while en route to the hospital. The result of administering too much crystalloid is increased interstitial fluid (edema), which impairs oxygen transfer to the remaining RBCs and into the tissue cells. In addition, the goal is *not* to raise the blood pressure to normal levels but to provide only enough fluid to maintain perfusion and continue to provide oxygenated RBCs to the heart, brain, and lungs. Raising the blood pressure to normal levels only serves to dilute clotting factors, disrupt any clot that has formed, and increase hemorrhage.

The best crystalloid solution for treating hemorrhagic shock is lactated Ringer's solution. Normal saline is another isotonic crystalloid solution that can be used for volume replacement, but its use may produce *hyperchloremia* (marked increase in the blood chloride level), leading to acidosis.

With significant blood loss, the optimal replacement fluid is ideally as near to whole blood as possible.[4,5] The first step is administration of packed RBCs and plasma at a ratio of 1:1 or 1:2. This intervention is currently available only in the hospital in the civilian environment. Platelets, cryoprecipitate, and other clotting factors are added as needed. Plasma contains a large number of the clotting factors and other components needed to control blood loss from small vessels. There are 13 factors in the coagulation cascade (**Figure 9-6**). In patients with massive blood loss requiring large volumes of blood replacement, most of the factors have been lost. Plasma transfusion is a reliable source of most of these factors. If major blood loss has occurred, the control of hemorrhage from large vessels requires operative management or, in some cases, endovascular placement of coils or clotting sponges.

Distributive (Vasogenic) Shock

Distributive shock, or vasogenic shock, occurs when the vascular container enlarges without a proportional increase in fluid volume. After trauma, this is typically found in patients who have sustained a spinal cord injury.

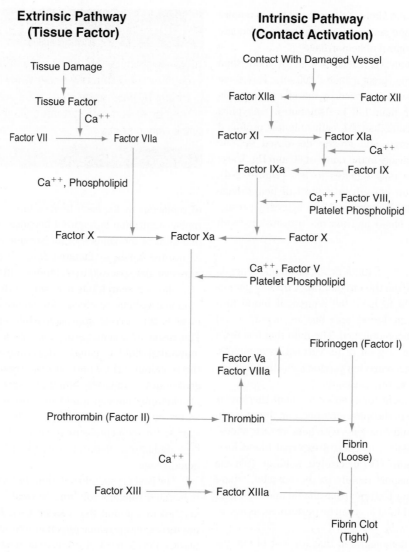

Figure 9-6 Clotting cascade.

Neurogenic "Shock"

Neurogenic "shock," or more appropriately neurogenic hypotension, occurs when a spinal cord injury interrupts the sympathetic nervous system pathway. This usually involves injury to the lower cervical, thoracolumbar, and thoracic levels. Because of the loss of sympathetic control of the vascular system, which controls the smooth muscles in the walls of the blood vessels, the peripheral vessels dilate below the level of injury. The marked decrease in systemic vascular resistance and peripheral vasodilation that occurs as the container for the blood volume increases results in relative hypovolemia. The patient is not really hypovolemic, but the ormal blood volume insufficiently fills an expanded container.

Tissue oxygenation usually remains adequate in the neurogenic form of shock, and blood flow remains normal although the blood pressure is low (neurogenic hypotension). In addition, energy production remains adequate in neurogenic hypotension. Therefore, this decrease in blood pressure is not shock since energy production remains unaffected. However, since there is less resistance to blood flow, the systolic and diastolic pressures are lower.

Decompensated hypovolemic shock and neurogenic shock both produce a decreased systolic blood pressure. However, the other vital and clinical signs, as well as the treatment for each, are different (**Figure 9-7**). Decreased systolic and diastolic pressures and a narrow pulse pressure characterize hypovolemic shock. Neurogenic shock also displays decreased systolic and diastolic pressures, but the pulse pressure remains normal or is widened. Hypovolemia produces cold, clammy, pale, or cyanotic skin and delayed capillary refilling time. In neurogenic shock the patient has warm, dry skin, especially below the area of injury. The pulse in hypovolemic shock patients is weak, thready, and rapid. In neurogenic shock, because of unopposed parasympathetic activity on the heart, bradycardia is typically seen rather than tachycardia, but the pulse quality may be weak. Hypovolemia produces a decreased level of consciousness (LOC), or, at least, anxiety and often combativeness. In the absence of a traumatic

Figure 9-7 Signs Associated With Types of Shock

Vital Sign	Hypovolemic	Neurogenic	Cardiogenic
Skin temperature/quality	Cool, clammy	Warm, dry	Cool, clammy
Skin color	Pale, cyanotic	Pink	Pale, cyanotic
Blood pressure	Drops	Drops	Drops
Level of consciousness	Altered	Lucid	Altered
Capillary refilling time	Slowed	Normal	Slowed

brain injury, the patient with neurogenic shock is usually alert, oriented, and lucid when in the supine position (**Figure 9-8**).

Patients with neurogenic shock frequently have associated injuries that produce significant hemorrhage. Therefore, a patient who has neurogenic shock and signs of hypovolemia, such as tachycardia, should be treated as if blood loss is present.

Cardiogenic Shock

Cardiogenic shock, or failure of the heart's pumping activity, results from causes that can be categorized as either *intrinsic* (a result of direct damage to the heart itself) or *extrinsic* (related to a problem outside the heart).

Intrinsic Causes

Heart Muscle Damage

Any injury that damages the cardiac muscle may affect its output. The damage may result from a direct bruise to the heart muscle (as in a blunt cardiac injury causing cardiac contusion). A recurring cycle will ensue: Decreased oxygenation causes decreased contractility, which results in decreased cardiac output and, therefore, decreased systemic perfusion. Decreased perfusion results in a continuing decrease in oxygenation and, thus, a continuation of the cycle. As with any muscle, the cardiac muscle does not work as efficiently when it becomes bruised or damaged.

Figure 9-8 Neurogenic Shock Versus Spinal Shock

As discussed in this chapter, the term neurogenic shock refers to a disruption of the sympathetic nervous system, typically from injury to the spinal cord, which results in significant dilation of the peripheral arteries. If untreated, this may result in impaired perfusion to the body's tissues. This condition should not be confused with spinal shock, a term that refers to an injury to the spinal cord that results in temporary loss of spinal cord function.

Valvular Disruption

A sudden, forceful compressing blow to the chest or abdomen (see the Kinematics of Trauma chapter and the Thoracic Trauma chapter) may damage the valves of the heart. Severe valvular injury results in acute valvular regurgitation, in which a significant amount of blood leaks back into the chamber from which it was just pumped. These patients often rapidly develop congestive heart failure, manifested by pulmonary edema and cardiogenic shock. The presence of a new heart murmur is an important clue in making this diagnosis.

Extrinsic Causes

Cardiac Tamponade

Fluid in the pericardial sac will prevent the heart from refilling completely during the diastolic (relaxation) phase of the cardiac cycle. In the case of trauma, blood leaks into the pericardial sac from a hole in the cardiac muscle. The blood that accumulates occupies space and prevents the walls of the ventricle from expanding fully. This has two negative effects on cardiac output: (1) Less volume is available for each contraction because the ventricle cannot expand fully, and (2) inadequate filling reduces the stretch of the cardiac muscle and results in diminished strength of the cardiac contraction. Additionally, more blood is forced out of the ventricle through the cardiac wound with each contraction and occupies more space in the pericardial sac, further compromising cardiac output (**Figure 9-9**). Severe shock and death may rapidly follow (see the Thoracic Trauma chapter for additional information).

Tension Pneumothorax

When either side of the thoracic cavity becomes filled with air that is under pressure, the lung becomes compressed and collapses. The involved lung is unable to refill with air from the outside through the nasopharynx. This produces at least four problems: (1) The tidal volume with each breath is reduced, (2) the collapsed alveoli are not available for oxygen transfer into the RBCs, (3) the pulmonary blood vessels are collapsed, reducing blood flow into the lung and heart, and (4) a greater force of cardiac contraction is required to force blood through the pulmonary vessels (pulmonary hypertension). If the volume

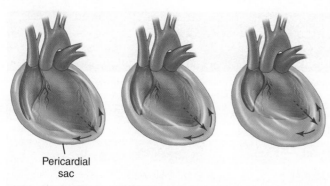

Pericardial
sac

Figure 9-9 Cardiac tamponade. As blood courses from the cardiac lumen into the pericardial space, it limits expansion of the ventricle. Therefore, the ventricle cannot fill completely. As more blood accumulates in the pericardial space, less ventricular space is available to accumulate blood, and cardiac output is reduced.

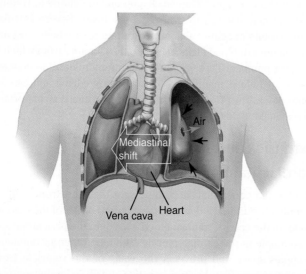

Figure 9-10 Tension pneumothorax. If the amount of air trapped in the pleural space continues to increase, not only is the lung on the affected side collapsed, but the mediastinum is also shifted to the opposite side. The mediastinal shift kinks the inferior vena cavem thus decreasing blood return to the heart and affecting cardiac output while at the same time, compressing the opposite lung.

of air and pressure inside the injured chest is great enough, the mediastinum is pushed away from the side of the injury. As the mediastinum shifts, the opposite lung becomes compressed, and compression and kinking of the superior and inferior venae cavae further impede venous return to the heart, producing a significant drop in preload (**Figure 9-10**). All of these factors reduce cardiac output, and shock rapidly ensues (see the Thoracic Trauma chapter for additional information).

Assessment

Shock is a condition resulting from decreased perfusion and diminished energy production, and heralds the potential onset of death. The loss of energy production when the body switches

from aerobic to anaerobic metabolism results in a 19-fold decrease in ATP production and the energy needed to maintain aerobic metabolism in all the cells of the body. If not quickly treated, this lack of energy production can become irreversible. The body responds to this decrease in energy production by selectively decreasing perfusion in nonessential parts of the body and increasing cardiovascular function to compensate and better perfuse other, more critical, organs of the body.

When shock develops, the physiologic response results in clinical signs that indicate the body has responded and is attempting to compensate. The body's response is identified by reduction of perfusion to nonvital organs such as the skin, which will feel cold and may look mottled, decreased pulse character in the extremities, cold cyanotic extremities with decreased capillary refill, and decreased mentation as a result of the decline in oxygenated blood perfusion to the brain. Acidosis from anaerobic metabolism produces rapid ventilations as the body attempts to blow off the carbon dioxide by-product and correct the decrease in serum pH. Decreased energy production is identified by sluggish body responses, cold skin, and decreased core temperature. The patient may be shivering in an effort to maintain body heat.

The assessment for the presence of shock must include looking for the subtle early evidence of this state of hypoperfusion. In the prehospital setting, this requires the assessment of organs and systems that are immediately accessible. Signs of hypoperfusion manifest as malfunction of these accessible organs or systems. Such systems are the brain and central nervous system (CNS), heart and cardiovascular system, respiratory system, skin and extremities, and kidneys. The signs of decreased perfusion and energy production and the body's response include the following:

- Decreased LOC, anxiety, disorientation, belligerence, bizarre behavior (brain and CNS)
- Tachycardia, decreased systolic and pulse pressure (heart and cardiovascular system)
- Rapid, shallow breathing (respiratory system)
- Cold, pale, clammy, diaphoretic or even cyanotic skin with decreased capillary refill time (skin and extremities)
- Decreased urine output (kidneys), identified only rarely in the prehospital setting in situations of prolonged or delayed transport when a urinary catheter is present

Because hemorrhage is the most common cause of shock in the trauma patient, all shock in a trauma patient should be considered to be from hemorrhage until proven otherwise. The first priority is to examine for external sources of hemorrhage and control them as quickly and completely as possible. Controlling hemorrhage may involve such techniques as application of pressure dressing, tourniquets, or splinting of extremity fractures.

If there is no evidence of external hemorrhage, internal hemorrhage should be suspected. Although definitive management of internal hemorrhage is not practical in the prehospital setting, identification of an internal source of bleeding mandates rapid transport to the definitive care institution. Internal hemorrhage can occur in the chest, abdomen, pelvis, or retroperitoneum. Evidence of blunt or penetrating chest injury, with decreased breath sounds, would suggest a thoracic source. The abdomen, pelvis, and retroperitoneum can be a source of bleeding with evidence of blunt trauma (e.g., ecchymosis) or penetrating trauma, abdominal distension or tenderness, pelvic instability, leg-length inequality, pain in the pelvic area aggravated by movement, perineal ecchymosis, and blood at the urethral meatus.

As a general rule, patients who meet National Trauma Triage Protocol criteria 1 or 2 (or both) need rapid transport to the nearest trauma center (**Figure 9-11**).

If the assessment does not suggest hemorrhage as the cause of the shock, nonhemorrhagic causes should be suspected. These include cardiac tamponade and tension pneumothorax (both evident by distended neck veins versus collapsed neck veins in hemorrhagic shock) or neurogenic hypotension. Decreased breath sounds on the side of the chest injury, subcutaneous emphysema, respiratory distress (tachypnea), and tracheal deviation (rarely seen in the field) suggest tension pneumothorax. Presence of these signs suggests the need for immediate needle decompression of the involved side of the chest.

Different sources of cardiogenic shock are suspected with blunt or penetrating chest trauma, muffled heart sounds suggesting cardiac tamponade (difficult to detect in the noisy prehospital environment), dysrhythmias, and neurogenic hypotension with signs of spinal trauma, bradycardia, and warm extremities. Most, if not all, of these features can be detected by the astute prehospital care provider, who can determine the cause of the shock and the need for appropriate intervention when feasible in the field.

Areas of patient evaluation include status of the airway, ventilation, perfusion, skin color and temperature, capillary refilling time, and blood pressure. Each is presented separately here in the context of both the primary assessment and the secondary assessment. Simultaneous evaluation is an important part of patient assessment to gather and process information from different sources expeditiously. If all systems are functioning normally, no alarm is set off.

Primary Assessment

Lord Kelvin said in a lecture he delivered in 1883, "When you can measure what you are speaking about and express it in numbers, you know something about it; but when you cannot measure it, when you cannot express it in numbers, your knowledge is of a meager and unsatisfactory kind."[6] Although this is often how we feel about vital signs, the first step in patient assessment is to get a general impression as quickly as possible of the patient's condition. It is only after that general impression that time can be taken to gather the "numbers" for a more specific assessment. The following signs identify the need for suspicion of life-threatening conditions:

- Mild anxiety, progressing to confusion or altered LOC
- Mild tachypnea, leading to rapid, labored ventilations

- Mild tachycardia, progressing to marked tachycardia
- Weakened radial pulse, progressing to an absent radial pulse
- Pale or cyanotic skin color
- Prolonged capillary refilling time
- Loss of pulses in the extremities
- Hypothermia

Any compromise or failure of the airway, breathing, or circulatory system must be managed before proceeding. The following steps are described in an ordered series; however, all of these assessments are carried out more or less simultaneously.

Airway

The airway should be evaluated initially in all patients. A patent airway is the first component in ensuring delivery of adequate amounts of oxygen to the cells of the body. Patients in need of immediate management of their airway include those with the following conditions, in order of importance:

1. Patients who are not breathing
2. Patients who have obvious airway compromise
3. Patients who have ventilatory rates greater than 20 breaths/minute
4. Patients who have noisy sounds of ventilation

Breathing

As noted in the Physiology of Life and Death chapter, the anaerobic metabolism associated with decreased cellular oxygenation produces an increase in lactic acid. The hydrogen ions produced from the acidosis are converted by the buffer system in the body into water and carbon dioxide. The brain's sensing system detects this abnormal increase in the amount of carbon dioxide and stimulates the respiratory center to increase the rate and depth of ventilation to remove the carbon dioxide. Thus, tachypnea is frequently one of the earliest signs of anaerobic metabolism and shock, even earlier than an increased pulse rate. In the primary assessment, time is not taken to measure a ventilatory rate. Instead, ventilations should be estimated to be slow, normal, fast, or very fast. A slow ventilatory rate, in conjunction with shock, generally indicates that a patient is in profound shock and may be moments away from cardiac arrest. A fast ventilatory rate is a concern and should serve as an impetus to search for the cause of shock.

A patient who tries to remove an oxygen mask, particularly when such action is associated with anxiety and belligerence, is displaying another sign of cerebral ischemia. This patient has "air hunger" and feels the need for more ventilation. The presence of a mask over the nose and mouth creates a psychological feeling of ventilatory restriction. This action should be a clue that the patient is not receiving enough oxygen and is hypoxic.

Decreased oxygen saturation, as measured by the pulse oximeter, will confirm this suspicion. Any pulse oximeter reading below 95% (at sea level) is worrisome and should serve

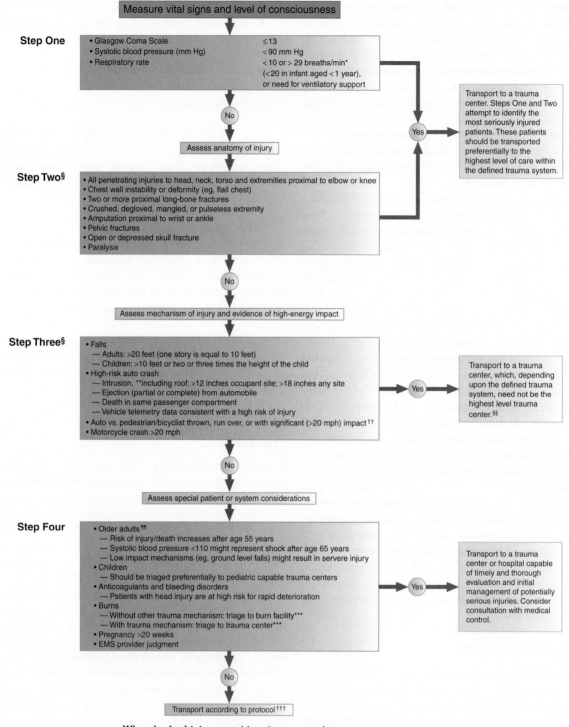

Step One

Measure vital signs and level of consciousness

- Glasgow Coma Scale — ≤13
- Systolic blood pressure (mm Hg) — <90 mm Hg
- Respiratory rate — <10 or >29 breaths/min* (<20 in infant aged <1 year), or need for ventilatory support

Yes → Transport to a trauma center. Steps One and Two attempt to identify the most seriously injured patients. These patients should be transported preferentially to the highest level of care within the defined trauma system.

No ↓

Assess anatomy of injury

Step Two§

- All penetrating injuries to head, neck, torso and extremities proximal to elbow or knee
- Chest wall instability or deformity (eg, flail chest)
- Two or more proximal long-bone fractures
- Crushed, degloved, mangled, or pulseless extremity
- Amputation proximal to wrist or ankle
- Pelvic fractures
- Open or depressed skull fracture
- Paralysis

No ↓

Assess mechanism of injury and evidence of high-energy impact

Step Three§

- Falls
  — Adults: >20 feet (one story is equal to 10 feet)
  — Children: >10 feet or two or three times the height of the child
- High-risk auto crash
  — Intrusion, **including roof: >12 inches occupant site; >18 inches any site
  — Ejection (partial or complete) from automobile
  — Death in same passenger compartment
  — Vehicle telemetry data consistent with a high risk of injury
- Auto vs. pedestrian/bicyclist thrown, run over, or with significant (>20 mph) impact††
- Motorcycle crash >20 mph

Yes → Transport to a trauma center, which, depending upon the defined trauma system, need not be the highest level trauma center.§§

No ↓

Assess special patient or system considerations

Step Four

- Older adults¶¶
  — Risk of injury/death increases after age 55 years
  — Systolic blood pressure <110 might represent shock after age 65 years
  — Low impact mechanisms (eg, ground level falls) might result in servere injury
- Children
  — Should be triaged preferentially to pediatric capable trauma centers
- Anticoagulants and bleeding disorders
  — Patients with head injury are at high risk for rapid deterioration
- Burns
  — Without other trauma mechanism: triage to burn facility***
  — With trauma mechanism: triage to trauma center***
- Pregnancy >20 weeks
- EMS provider judgment

Yes → Transport to a trauma center or hospital capable of timely and thorough evaluation and initial management of potentially serious injuries. Consider consultation with medical control.

No ↓

Transport according to protocol†††

When in doubt, transport to a trauma center

Abbreviation: EMS = emergency medical services.

  * The upper limit of respiratory rate in infants is >29 breaths per minute to maintain a higher level of overtriage for infants.
  § Any injury noted in Step Two or mechanism identified in Step Three triggers a "yes" response.
  ¶ Age <15 years.
  ** Intrusion refers to interior compartment intrusion, as opposed to deformation which refers to exterior damage.
  †† Includes pedestrians or bicyclists thrown or run over by a motor vehicle or those with estimated impact >20 mph with a motor vehicle.
  §§ Local or regional protocols should be used to determine the most appropriate level of trauma center within the defined trauma system; need not be the highest-level trauma center.
  ¶¶ Age >55 years.
  *** Patients with both burns and concomitant trauma for whom the burn injury poses the greatest risk for morbidity and mortality should be transferred to a burn center. If the nonburn trauma presents a greater immediate risk, the patient may be stabilized in a trauma center and then transferred to a burn center.
  ††† Patients who do not meet any of the triage criteria in Steps One through Four should be transported to the most appropriate medical facility as outlined in local EMS protocols.

Figure 9-11 2011 Guidelines for Field Triage of Injured Patients

Source: Adapted from Centers for Disease Control and Prevention, Morbidity and Mortality Weekly Report (MMWR), January 13, 2012.

as a stimulus to identify the cause of hypoxia. Measurement and continuous monitoring of end tidal carbon dioxide ($ETCO_2$) has become a routine practice in EMS in patients whose airway has been managed with such procedures as endotracheal intubation. While the correlation between the $ETCO_2$ and the partial pressure of carbon dioxide in arterial blood ($PaCO_2$) is good in the patient who has adequate perfusion, the correlation is poor in the patient in shock, thus limiting its utility to guide respirations. Monitoring $ETCO_2$ may still help to detect changes and trends in perfusion. It is always important to remember, however, to evaluate readings from machines in the context of the patient's appearance. If the appearance of the patient suggests hypoxia, treat the patient for hypoxia even if the machine would suggest otherwise. The clinical situation is always more important than the reading given by any device.

Circulation

There are two components in the assessment of circulation:

- Hemorrhage and the amount of blood loss
- Perfusion with oxygenated blood
  - Total body
  - Regional

The data accumulated during the circulatory assessment help to make a quick initial determination of the patient's total blood volume and perfusion status and, secondarily, provide a similar assessment of specific regions of the body. For example, when checking the capillary refilling time, the pulse, skin color, and temperature of a lower extremity may show compromised perfusion while the same signs may be normal in the upper extremity. This discrepancy does not mean the signs are inaccurate, only that one part is different from another. The immediate question that must be answered is "Why?" It is important to check for the following circulatory and perfusion findings in more than one part of the body and to remember that the assessment of the total body condition should not be based on a single part.

Hemorrhage

Assessment of circulation begins with a rapid scan for significant external hemorrhage. The patient may be lying on the major source of the hemorrhage, or it may be hidden by the patient's clothes. Efforts at restoring perfusion will be either much less effective or completely ineffective in the face of ongoing hemorrhage. The patient can lose a significant volume of blood from scalp lacerations because of the high concentration of blood vessels or from wounds that damage major blood vessels (subclavian, axillary, brachial, radial, ulnar, carotid, femoral, or popliteal). Examine the entire body to identify external hemorrhage sources.

Loss of blood means loss of RBCs, and this means a loss of oxygen-carrying capacity. Thus, while a patient who has been bleeding may have an oxygen saturation that is "normal" because what blood the patient does have is fully saturated with oxygen, this patient, in fact, has diminished total oxygen because there is just not enough blood to carry the amount of oxygen needed to supply all of the cells of the body.

Pulse

The next important assessment point for perfusion is the pulse. Initial evaluation of the pulse determines whether it is palpable at the artery being examined. In general, loss of a radial pulse indicates severe hypovolemia (or vascular damage to the arm), especially when a central pulse, such as the carotid or femoral artery, is weak, thready, and extremely fast, indicating the status of the total body circulatory system. If the pulse is palpable, its character and strength should be noted, as follows:

- Is the pulse rate strong or weak and thready?
- Is the pulse rate normal, too fast, or too slow?
- Is the pulse rate regular or irregular?

Although many prehospital care providers involved in the management of trauma patients focus on the patient's blood pressure, precious time should not be spent during the primary assessment to obtain a blood pressure. The exact level of the blood pressure is much less important in the primary assessment than other, earlier signs of shock. Significant information can be determined from the pulse rate and its character. In one series of trauma patients, a radial pulse characterized by prehospital care providers as "weak" was associated with blood pressure that averaged 26 mm Hg lower than a pulse thought to be "normal." More importantly, trauma patients with a weak radial pulse were 15 times more likely to die than those with a normal pulse.[7] Although generally obtained at the beginning of the secondary assessment, blood pressure can be palpated or auscultated earlier in the patient assessment if sufficient assistance is present, or once the primary assessment has been completed and life-threatening issues are being addressed during transport.

Level of Consciousness (LOC)

Mental status is part of the disability evaluation, but altered mental status can represent impaired cerebral oxygenation as a result of decreased perfusion. Assessment of mental status represents an assessment of end-organ perfusion and function. An anxious, belligerent patient should be assumed to have cerebral ischemia and anaerobic metabolism until another cause is identified. Drug and alcohol overdose and cerebral contusion are conditions that cannot be treated rapidly, but cerebral ischemia can be treated. Therefore, all patients in whom cerebral ischemia might be present should be managed as if it is present.

In addition to the concerns of the presence of hypoxia and poor perfusion, altered mental status also suggests traumatic brain injury (TBI). The combination of hypoxia or decreased blood pressure and TBI has a profound negative impact on patient survival; therefore, hypoxia and hypotension must be corrected if present and prevented from developing if not present.

Skin Color

Pink skin color generally indicates a well-oxygenated patient without anaerobic metabolism. Blue (cyanotic) or mottled skin indicates unoxygenated hemoglobin and a lack of adequate oxygenation to the periphery. Pale, mottled, or cyanotic skin has inadequate blood flow resulting from one of the following three causes:

1. Peripheral vasoconstriction (most often associated with hypovolemia)
2. Decreased supply of RBCs (acute anemia)
3. Interruption of blood supply to that portion of the body, such as might be found with a fracture or injury of a blood vessel supplying that part of the body

Pale skin may be a localized or generalized finding with different implications. Other findings, such as tachycardia, should be used to resolve these differences and to determine if the pale skin is a localized, regional, or systemic condition. Also, cyanosis may not develop in hypoxic patients who have lost a significant number of their RBCs from hemorrhage. In patients with dark-pigmented skin, cyanosis may be difficult to detect in the skin, but it will be noted in the lips, gums, and palms.

Skin Temperature

As the body shunts blood away from the skin to more important parts of the body, skin temperature decreases. Skin that is cool to the touch indicates vasoconstriction, decreased cutaneous perfusion, and decreased energy production and, therefore, shock. Because a significant amount of heat can be lost during the assessment phase, steps should be taken to preserve the patient's body temperature.

A good sign of adequate resuscitation is a warm, dry, pink toe. The environmental conditions in which the determination is made can affect the results, as can an isolated injury that affects perfusion; therefore the results of this assessment must be evaluated in the context of the entire situation.

Skin Quality

In addition to skin color and temperature, the skin is evaluated for dryness or moistness. The trauma patient in shock from hypovolemia typically has moist, clammy, diaphoretic skin. In contrast, the patient with hypotension from a spinal cord injury usually has dry skin.

Capillary Refilling Time

The ability of the cardiovascular system to refill the capillaries after the blood has been "removed" represents an important support system. Analyzing this support system's level of function by compressing the capillaries to remove all the blood and then measuring the refilling time provides insight into the perfusion of the capillary bed being assessed. Generally, the body shuts down circulation in the most distal parts first and restores this circulation last. Evaluation of the nail bed of the big toe or thumb provides the earliest indication that hypoperfusion is developing. Additionally, it provides a strong indication as to when resuscitation is complete. However, as with many other signs that a patient may exhibit, several conditions—both environmental and physiologic—can alter the results. A test of the capillary refilling time is a measurement of the time required to reperfuse the skin and, therefore, an indirect measurement of the actual perfusion of that part of the body. It is not a diagnostic test of any specific disease process or injury.

Capillary refilling time has been described as a poor test of shock. However, it is not a test of shock, but rather a test of perfusion of the capillary bed being analyzed. Used along with other tests and components of the assessment, it is a good indicator of perfusion and suggestive of shock, but it must be interpreted in the context of the current situation and circumstances.

Shock may be the cause of poor perfusion and delayed capillary refilling, but there are other causes, such as arterial interruption from a fracture, a vessel wounded by penetrating trauma (e.g., gunshot wound), hypothermia, and even arteriosclerosis. Another cause of poor capillary refilling is decreased cardiac output resulting from hypovolemia (other than from hemorrhage).

Capillary refilling time is a helpful diagnostic sign that can also be used to monitor the progress of resuscitation. If the resuscitation of the patient is progressing in a positive manner and the patient's condition is improving, the capillary refill time will also show improvement.

Disability

One regional body system that can be readily evaluated in the field is brain function. At least five conditions can produce an altered LOC or change in behavior (combativeness or belligerence) in trauma patients:

1. Hypoxia
2. Shock with impaired cerebral perfusion
3. TBI
4. Intoxication with alcohol or drugs
5. Metabolic processes such as diabetes, seizures, and eclampsia

Of these five conditions, the easiest to treat—and the one that will kill the patient most quickly if not treated—is hypoxia. Any patient with an altered LOC should be treated as if decreased cerebral oxygenation is the cause. An altered LOC is usually one of the first visible signs of shock.

TBI may be considered *primary* (caused by direct trauma to brain tissue) or *secondary* (caused by the effects of hypoxia, hypoperfusion, edema, loss of energy production, etc.). There is no effective treatment in the prehospital setting for the primary brain injury, but secondary brain injury can essentially be prevented or significantly reduced by maintaining oxygenation and perfusion.

The brain's ability to function decreases as perfusion and oxygenation drop and ischemia develops. This decreased function evolves through various stages as different areas of the brain become affected. Anxiety and belligerent behavior are usually the first signs, followed by a slowing of the thought processes and a decrease of the body's motor and sensory functions. The level of cerebral function is an important and measurable prehospital sign of shock. A belligerent, combative, anxious patient or one with a decreased LOC should be assumed to have a hypoxic, hypoperfused brain until another cause can be identified. Hypoperfusion and cerebral hypoxia frequently accompany brain injury and make the long-term result even worse. Even brief episodes of hypoxia and shock may worsen the original brain injury and result in poorer outcomes.

Expose/Environment

The patient's body is exposed to assess for less obvious sites of external blood loss and for clues that may indicate internal hemorrhage. The possibility of hypothermia is also considered. This exposure is best performed in the heated patient compartment of the ambulance in order to protect the patient from the environment and the prying eyes of the public.

Secondary Assessment

In some cases, the patient's injuries may be too severe for an adequate secondary assessment to be completed in the field. If time permits, the secondary assessment can be done while en route to the hospital if no other issues need to be addressed.

Vital Signs

Measurement of an accurate set of vital signs is one of the first steps in the secondary assessment or, after reassessing the primary assessment, when a few minutes are available during transport.

Ventilatory Rate

The normal ventilatory rate for an adult is 10 to 20 breaths per minute. This rate will vary depending on age (see the Pediatric Trauma chapter). A rate of 20 to 30 breaths/minute indicates a borderline abnormal rate; it suggests the onset of shock and the need for supplemental oxygen. A rate greater than 30 breaths/minute indicates a late stage of shock and the need for assisted ventilation. The physiologic drive for the increased ventilatory rate is the acidosis caused by shock, but it is usually associated with a decreased tidal volume. Both of these ventilatory rates indicate the need to look for the potential sources of impaired perfusion.

Pulse

In the secondary assessment, the pulse rate is determined more precisely. The normal pulse range for an adult is 60 to 100 beats/minute. With lower rates, except in extremely athletic individuals, an ischemic heart, or a pathologic condition such as complete heart block should be considered. A pulse in the range of 100 to 120 beats/minute identifies a patient who has early shock, with an initial cardiac response of tachycardia. A pulse above

120 beats/minute is a definite sign of shock unless it is caused by pain or fear, and a pulse over 140 beats/minute is considered extremely critical and near-death.

Blood Pressure

Blood pressure is one of the least sensitive signs of shock. Blood pressure does not begin to drop until a patient is profoundly hypovolemic (from either true fluid loss or container-enlarged relative hypovolemia). Decreased blood pressure indicates that the patient can no longer compensate for the hypovolemia and hypoperfusion. In otherwise healthy patients, blood loss must exceed 30% of blood volume before the patient's compensatory mechanisms fail and systolic blood pressure drops below 90 mm Hg. For this reason, ventilatory rate, pulse rate and character, capillary refilling time, and LOC are more sensitive indicators of hypovolemia than is blood pressure.

When the patient's pressure has begun to drop, an extremely critical situation exists, and rapid intervention is required. In the prehospital environment, a patient who is found to be hypotensive has already lost a significant volume of blood, and ongoing blood loss is likely. The development of hypotension as a first sign of shock means that earlier signs may have been overlooked.

The severity of the situation and the appropriate type of intervention vary based on the cause of the condition. For example, low blood pressure associated with neurogenic shock is not nearly as critical as low blood pressure from hypovolemic shock. **Figure 9-12** presents the signs used to assess compensated and decompensated hypovolemic shock.

One important pitfall to avoid involves equating systolic blood pressure with cardiac output and tissue perfusion.

Figure 9-12 Shock Assessment in Compensated and Decompensated Hypovolemic Shock

Vital Sign	Compensated	Decompensated
Pulse	Increased; tachycardia	Greatly increased; marked tachycardia that can progress to bradycardia
Skin	White, cool, moist	White, cold, waxy
Blood pressure range	Normal	Decreased
Level of consciousness	Unaltered	Altered, ranging from disoriented to coma

As previously emphasized, significant blood loss is typically required before the patient becomes hypotensive (Class III hemorrhage). Thus, patients will have decreased cardiac output and impaired tissue oxygenation when they have lost 15% to 30% of their blood volume, despite having a normal systolic blood pressure. Ideally, shock will be recognized and treated in the earlier stages before decompensation occurs.

Brain injuries do not cause hypotension until the brain begins to herniate through the *tentorial incisura* and *foramen magnum*. Therefore, a patient with a brain injury with hypotension should be assumed to have hypovolemia (usually blood loss) from other injuries and not from the brain injury. Young infants (less than 6 months of age) are the exception to this rule because they may bleed enough inside their head to produce hypovolemic shock as a result of open sutures and fontanelles that can spread apart and accommodate large amounts of blood.

Musculoskeletal Injuries

Significant internal hemorrhage can occur with fractures (**Figure 9-13**). Fractures of the femur and pelvis are of greatest concern. A single femoral fracture may be associated with up to 2 to 4 units (1,000 to 2,000 ml) of blood loss into a thigh. This injury alone could potentially result in the loss of 30% to 40% of an adult's blood volume, resulting in decompensated hypovolemic shock. Pelvic fractures, especially those resulting from significant falls or crushing mechanisms, can be associated with massive internal hemorrhage into the retroperitoneal space. A victim of blunt trauma can have multiple fractures and Class III or IV shock but no evidence of external blood loss, hemothoraces, intra-abdominal bleeding, or pelvic fracture. For example, an adult pedestrian struck by a vehicle and sustaining four rib fractures, a humerus fracture, a femur fracture, and bilateral tibia/fibula fractures may experience internal bleeding of 3,000 to 5,500 ml of blood. This potential

Figure 9-13	Approximate Internal Blood Loss Associated With Fractures
Type of Fracture	**Internal Blood Loss (ml)**
Rib	125
Radius or ulna	250 to 500
Humerus	500 to 750
Tibia or fibula	500 to 1000
Femur	1000 to 2000
Pelvis	1000 to massive

blood loss is enough for the patient to die from shock if it is unrecognized and inappropriately treated.

Confounding Factors

Numerous factors can confound the assessment of the trauma patient, obscuring or blunting the usual signs of shock. These factors may mislead the unwary prehospital care provider into thinking that a trauma patient is stable when in fact that is not the case.

Age

Patients at the extremes of life—the very young (neonates) and the elderly—have diminished capability to compensate for acute blood loss and other shock states. A relatively minor injury that would be tolerated without difficulty in a healthy adult may produce decompensated shock in these individuals. In contrast, children and young adults have a tremendous ability to compensate for blood loss and may appear relatively normal on a quick scan. They will often appear to be doing well until they suddenly deteriorate into decompensated shock. A closer look may reveal subtle signs of shock, such as mild tachycardia and tachypnea, pale skin with delayed capillary refilling time, and anxiety. Because of their powerful compensatory mechanisms, children found in decompensated shock represent dire emergencies. Elderly individuals may be more prone to certain complications of prolonged shock, such as acute renal failure.

Athletic Status

Well-conditioned athletes often have enhanced compensatory capabilities. Many have resting heart rates in the range of 40 to 50 beats/minute. A heart rate of 100 to 110 beats/minute or hypotension may be warning signs that indicate significant hemorrhage in a well-conditioned athlete.

Pregnancy

During pregnancy, a woman's blood volume may increase by 45% to 50%. Heart rate and cardiac output during pregnancy are also increased. Thus, a pregnant female may not demonstrate signs of shock until her blood loss exceeds 30% to 35% of her total blood volume. Also, well before a pregnant woman demonstrates signs of hypoperfusion, the fetus may be adversely affected because the placental circulation is more sensitive to the vasoconstrictive effects of *catecholamines* released in response to the shock state. During the third trimester, the gravid uterus may compress the inferior vena cava, greatly diminishing venous return to the heart and resulting in hypotension. Elevation of the pregnant patient's right side once she has been immobilized to a long backboard may alleviate this compression. Hypotension in a pregnant female that persists after performing this maneuver typically represents life-threatening blood loss.

Pre-existing Medical Conditions

Patients with serious pre-existing medical conditions, such as coronary artery disease, congestive heart failure, and chronic obstructive pulmonary disease, are typically less able to compensate for hemorrhage and shock. These patients may experience angina as their heart rate increases in an effort to maintain their blood pressure. Patients with implanted fixed-rate pacemakers are typically unable to develop the compensatory tachycardia necessary to maintain blood pressure. Patients with diabetes often have longer hospital and intensive care unit stays and more complications than patients without the underlying disease.

Medications

Numerous medications may interfere with the body's compensatory mechanisms. Beta-adrenergic blocking agents and calcium channel blockers used to treat hypertension may prevent an individual from developing a compensatory tachycardia to maintain blood pressure. Additionally, nonsteroidal anti-inflammatory drugs (NSAIDs), used in the treatment of arthritis and musculoskeletal pain, may impair platelet activity and blood clotting, and may result in increased hemorrhage. Newer anticoagulant medications may prevent clotting for several days, and there are no good antidotes to reverse the clotting abnormality. If a history of medication use can be obtained from the patient or family members, this is very important information to relay to the receiving trauma team.

Time Between Injury and Treatment

In situations in which the EMS response time has been brief, patients may be encountered who have life-threatening internal hemorrhage but have not yet lost enough blood to manifest severe shock (Class III or IV hemorrhage). Even patients with penetrating wounds to their aorta, venae cavae, or iliac vessels may arrive at the receiving facility with a normal systolic blood pressure if the EMS response, scene, and transport times are brief. The assumption that patients are not bleeding internally just because they "look good" is frequently very wrong. The patient may "look good" because he or she is in compensated shock or because not enough time has elapsed for the signs of shock to manifest. Patients should be thoroughly assessed for even the subtlest signs of shock, and internal hemorrhage should be assumed to be present until it is definitively ruled out. The possibility of late-presenting internal hemorrhage is one reason why continued reassessment of trauma patients is essential.

Management

Steps in the management of shock are as follows:

1. Ensure oxygenation (adequate airway and ventilation).
2. Identify any hemorrhaging. (Control external bleeding and recognize the likelihood of internal hemorrhage).
3. Transport the patient to definitive care.
4. Administer fluids en route as appropriate.

In addition to securing the airway and providing ventilation to maintain oxygenation, the prime goals of shock treatment include identifying the source or cause, treating the cause as specifically as possible, and supporting the circulation. By maintaining perfusion and oxygen delivery to the cells, energy production is supported and cellular function can be ensured.

In the prehospital setting, external sources of bleeding should be identified and directly controlled immediately. Internal causes of shock usually cannot be definitively treated in the prehospital setting; therefore, the approach is to transport the patient rapidly to the definitive care setting while supporting the circulation in the best way possible. Resuscitation in the prehospital setting includes the following:

- Improve oxygenation of the RBCs in the lungs through:
  - Appropriate airway management
  - Providing ventilatory support with a bag-mask device, and delivering a high concentration of supplemental oxygen (fraction of inspired oxygen [FiO_2] greater than 0.85).
- Control both external hemorrhage and internal hemorrhage, to the extent possible in the prehospital setting. *Every red blood cell counts*.
- Improve circulation to deliver the oxygenated RBCs more efficiently to the systemic tissues, and improve oxygenation and energy production at the cellular level.
- Maintain body heat by all means possible.
- Reach definitive care as soon as possible for hemorrhage control and replacement of lost RBCs, plasma, coagulation factors, and platelets.

Without appropriate measures, a patient will continue to deteriorate rapidly until he or she reaches the ultimate "stable" condition—death.

The following four questions need to be addressed when deciding what treatment to provide for a patient in shock:

1. What is the cause of the patient's shock?
2. What is the definitive care for the patient's shock?
3. Where can the patient best receive this definitive care?
4. What interim steps can be taken to support the patient and manage the condition while the patient is being transported to definitive care?

Although the first question may be difficult to answer accurately in the field, identification of the possible source of the shock assists in defining which facility is best suited to meeting the patient's needs and what measures may be necessary during transport to improve the patient's chances of survival.

Airway

Advanced techniques for securing the airway and maintaining ventilation may be required in the prehospital setting, as outlined in the Airway and Ventilation chapter. The importance of essential airway skills, especially when transport times are brief, should not be underestimated.

Breathing

Once a patent airway is ensured, patients in shock or those at risk for developing shock (almost all trauma patients) should initially receive supplemental oxygen in a concentration as close to 100% (FiO_2 of 1.0) as possible. This level of oxygenation can be achieved only with a device that has a reservoir attached to the oxygen source. Nasal prongs, a nasal cannula, or a simple face mask do not meet this requirement. *Oxygen saturation (SpO_2) should be monitored by pulse oximetry in virtually all trauma patients and maintained above 95% (at sea level) and correlated with the patient's condition.*

A nonbreathing patient, or one who is breathing without an adequate depth and rate, needs ventilatory assistance using a bag-mask device immediately. Hyperventilation during assisted ventilation produces a negative physiologic response, especially in the patient with hypovolemic shock or with TBI. Ventilating too deeply and too quickly can make the patient alkalotic. This chemical response increases the affinity of hemoglobin for oxygen, resulting in decreased oxygen delivery to the tissue. In addition, hyperventilation may increase the intrathoracic pressure, leading to impaired venous return to the heart and hypotension. Data from animal experiments utilizing a hypovolemic shock model suggest normal or higher ventilatory rates in animals with even moderate hemorrhage impaired hemodynamic functioning, as exhibited by lower systolic blood pressure and cardiac output.[8,9] The increase in intrathoracic pressure could result either from large tidal volumes (10 to 12 ml/kg body weight) or from the creation of "auto-PEEP" (positive end-expiratory pressure) when ventilated too quickly (inadequate exhalation leads to air trapping in the lungs). In the patient with TBI, inadvertent hyperventilation will lead to cerebral vasoconstriction and decreased cerebral blood flow. This will exacerbate the secondary injury occurring in the brain. For an adult patient, giving a reasonable tidal volume (350 to 500ml) at a rate of 10 ventilations/minute is probably sufficient.

End-tidal carbon dioxide ($ETCO_2$) monitoring is often used in conjunction with pulse oximetry to maintain the patient in a **eucapnic state** (normal blood carbon dioxide level) with satisfactory oxygenation; however, in the patient with compromised perfusion, the correlation of $ETCO_2$ with $PaCO_2$ is poor and cannot be relied upon to accurately judge ventilation.

Circulation: Hemorrhage Control

Control of obvious external hemorrhage immediately follows securing the airway and initiating oxygen therapy and ventilatory support, or it is performed simultaneously with these steps if sufficient assistance is present. If the hemorrhage is clearly life threatening and a rapid primary assessment reveals that the patient is breathing, then efforts to control the hemorrhage can take priority. These are critical judgments based upon knowledge. Early recognition and control of external bleeding in the trauma patient help preserve the patient's blood volume and RBCs and ensure continued perfusion of tissues. Even a small trickle of blood can add up to substantial blood loss if it is ignored for a long enough time. Thus, in the multisystem trauma patient, *no bleeding is minor, and every red blood cell counts* toward ensuring continued perfusion of the body's tissues.

External hemorrhage steps in the field management of external hemorrhage include:

- Hand-held direct pressure
- Compression dressings
- Wound packing
- Elastic wrap
- Tourniquet—extremities
- Hemostatic agent—torso

Control of external hemorrhage should proceed in a step-wise fashion, escalating if initial measures fail to control bleeding (**Figure 9-14**).

Direct Pressure

Direct hand pressure or a pressure dressing, applied directly over a bleeding site, is the initial technique employed to control external hemorrhage. This application of pressure is based upon Bernoulli's principle (see the Physiology of Life and Death chapter) and involves a number of considerations:

Fluid leak = Transmural pressure × Size of hole in vessel wall

Transmural pressure is the difference between the pressure within the vessel and the pressure outside the vessel. The pressure exerted against the inside of the blood vessel walls by the intravascular fluids and blood pressure cycle is called the **intramural (or intraluminal) pressure**. The force exerted against the wall of the blood vessel from the outside (such as by a hand or a dressing) is called the **extramural (or extraluminal) pressure**. To illustrate this relationship:

Transmural pressure = Intramural pressure − Extramural pressure

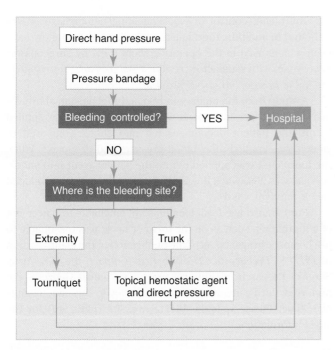

Figure 9-14 Hemorrhage control in the field.

The higher the pressure inside the vessel, the faster that blood is forced out of the hole. The more pressure that the prehospital care provider applies, the slower that blood will leak out. Direct pressure on the wound increases the extramural pressure, thus slowing the leak.

The ability of the body to respond to and control bleeding from a lacerated vessel is a function of:

- The size of the vessel
- The pressure within the vessel
- The presence of clotting factors
- The ability of the injured vessel to go into spasm and reduce the size of the hole and blood flow at the injury site
- The pressure of the surrounding tissue on the vessel at the injury site and any additional pressure provided by the prehospital care provider from the outside

Blood vessels, especially arteries, that are completely divided (transected) often retract and go into spasm. There is often less hemorrhage from the stump of an extremity with a complete amputation than from an extremity with severe trauma but with blood vessels that are damaged but not completely transected.

Direct pressure over the site of hemorrhage increases the extraluminal pressure and, therefore, reduces the transmural pressure, helping to slow or stop bleeding. Direct pressure also serves a second and equally important function. Compressing the sides of the torn vessel reduces the size (area) of the

opening and further reduces blood flow out of the vessel. Even if blood loss is not completely stemmed, it may be diminished to the point that the blood-clotting system can stop the hemorrhage. This is why direct pressure is almost always successful at controlling bleeding. Multiple studies involving hemorrhage from femoral artery puncture sites after cardiac catheterization have documented that direct pressure is an effective technique.[7,10-12]

Following a leaky pipe analogy, if there is a small hole in the pipe, simply putting one's finger over the hole will stop the leak temporarily. Tape can then be wrapped around the pipe for a short-term fix of the leak. The same concept applies to the hemorrhaging patient. Direct pressure on the open wound is followed by a pressure dressing. However, for the pressure dressing to be most effective, the pressure must be placed directly on the injury in the vessel. A simple dressing placed on the skin over the wound does not impart any direct pressure on the bleeding site itself.

To achieve the most effective use of a pressure dressing, the dressing material must be packed tightly down into the wound and then the elastic bandage placed on the outside. Packing of a wound may be accomplished with the use of a hemostatic agent such as Combat Gauze™ or Celox™ or may be performed using a plain gauze roll. The key is to place the packing material into the base of the wound, directly onto the bleeding site and then pack the entire roll into the wound. Then direct pressure over the wound should be placed for a minimum of 3 to 5 minutes if using a hemostatic dressing and for 10 minutes if using plain gauze.

From a vascular and patient perspective, this means the MAP (intraluminal pressure) and the pressure in the tissue surrounding the vessel (extraluminal pressure) have a direct relationship in controlling the rate of blood loss from the vessel as well as the size of the hole in the vessel. Of note, when a patient's blood pressure has been reduced by blood loss, it is appropriate not to increase it to back to normal levels; rather blood loss should be stopped and blood pressure maintained at a level sufficient to perfuse vital organs. This level generally occurs when the patient's systolic blood pressure is between 80 and 90 mm Hg. This means avoiding overinfusion of IV fluids into the patient and maintaining a modest degree of hypotension. Raising the blood pressure back to normal levels by administering large volumes of IV crystalloid fluids produces the exact opposite of the desired effect, increasing hemorrhage as a result of "popping" any clot that has formed over an opening in a blood vessel.

Therefore, the steps in managing hemorrhage are (1) to increase external pressure (hand-pressure dressing) which decreases the size of the hole in the lumen of the blood vessel and decreases the differential between internal and external pressure, both of which contribute to retarding blood flow out of the injured vessel; and (2) to use the technique of hypotensive resuscitation to ensure that the intraluminal pressure is not raised extensively.

Three Critical Points

Three additional points about direct pressure should be emphasized. First, when managing a wound with an impaled object, pressure should be applied on either side of the object rather than over the object. Impaled objects should not be removed in the field because the object may have damaged a vessel, and the object itself could be tamponading the bleeding. Removal of the object could result in uncontrolled internal hemorrhage.

Second, if hands are required to perform other lifesaving tasks, a pressure (compression) dressing can be created using gauze pads and an elastic roller bandage or a blood pressure cuff inflated until hemorrhage stops. This dressing is placed directly over the bleeding site.

Third, applying direct pressure to exsanguinating hemorrhage takes precedence over insertion of IV lines and fluid resuscitation. It would be a serious error to deliver a well-packaged trauma victim to the receiving facility with two IV lines inserted and neatly taped in place, but who is dying from the hemorrhage of a wound that has only trauma dressings taped in place and no direct pressure applied.

Elevation and Pressure Points

In the past, emphasis has been placed on elevation of an extremity and compression on a pressure point (proximal to the bleeding site) as intermediate steps in hemorrhage control. No research has been published on whether elevation of a bleeding extremity slows hemorrhage. If a bone in the extremity is fractured, this maneuver could potentially result in converting a closed fracture to an open one or in causing increased internal hemorrhage. Similarly, the use of pressure points for hemorrhage control has not been studied. Thus, in the absence of compelling data, these interventions can no longer be recommended for situations in which direct pressure or a pressure dressing has failed to control hemorrhage.

Tourniquets

If external bleeding from an extremity cannot be controlled by pressure, application of a tourniquet is the reasonable next step in hemorrhage control. Tourniquets had fallen out of favor because of concern about potential complications, including damage to nerves and blood vessels and potential loss of the limb if the tourniquet is left on too long. None of these concerns have been proven; in fact, data from the Iraq and Afghanistan wars have demonstrated just the opposite.[13,14] Although there is a small risk that all or part of a limb may be sacrificed, given the choice between losing a limb and saving the patient's life, the obvious decision is to preserve life. There have been no limbs lost as a result of tourniquet placement by the U.S. military. In fact, data from the military experience suggest that appropriately applied tourniquets could potentially have prevented 7 of 100 combat deaths.[15,16]

Tourniquet control of exsanguinating hemorrhage is 80% or better. In addition, tourniquets occluding arterial inflow have been widely used in the operating room (OR) by surgeons for many years with satisfactory results. *Used properly, tourniquets are not only safe, but also lifesaving.*[17]

A study from the military in Iraq and Afghanistan showed a marked difference in survival when the tourniquet was applied before the patient decompensated into shock compared to when it was applied after blood pressure had dropped.[18] When the tourniquet was applied before the patient went into shock, survival was 96%; when it was placed after the patient developed shock, survival was 4%.

For hemorrhage from locations not amenable to placement of a tourniquet, such as on the torso or neck, it is reasonable to use hemostatic agents. As of the publication of the eighth edition of *PHTLS: Prehospital Trauma Life Support*, the U.S. Army Surgical Research Institute recommends Combat Gauze as the preferred third-generation product. However, this may change over time. Please visit the PHTLS website (phtls.org) for the latest information.

Device Options

Traditionally, a tourniquet has been devised from a cravat folded into a width of about 4 inches (10 centimeters [cm]) and wrapped twice around the extremity—the "Spanish windlass." A knot is tied in the bandage, a metal or wooden rod is placed on top of the knot, and a second knot is tied. The rod is twisted until hemorrhage ceases, and the rod is then secured in place.

Tourniquets that are narrow and bandlike should be avoided. Wider tourniquets, at least 1.5 inches (4 cm) in width, are more effective at controlling bleeding, and they control hemorrhage at a lower pressure (**Figure 9-15**). An inverse relationship exists between tourniquet width and the pressure required to occlude arterial inflow. In addition, a very narrow band is more likely to result in damage to arteries and superficial nerves.

Because of the U.S. military's interest in an effective, easy-to-use tourniquet (especially one that a soldier could apply quickly with one hand should the other arm be injured), many commercial tourniquets have been developed and marketed. In a laboratory study, three products were 100% effective in occluding distal arterial blood flow: the Combat Application Tourniquet (C-A-T, Phil Durango), the Emergency Military Tourniquet (EMT, Delfi Medical Innovations), and the Special

Figure 9-15 Alternative Tourniquets

A blood pressure cuff can alternatively be used as a tourniquet in an emergency, although air may leak out of the cuff, diminishing its effectiveness.

Operations Force Tactical Tourniquet (SOFTT, Tactical Medical Solutions) (**Figure 9-16**).[19] Of these, the Committee on Tactical Combat Casualty Care (COTCCC) currently recommends use of the C-A-T. Again, this recommendation may change over time, and the latest updates from the COTCCC and PHTLS will appear on the PHTLS website (PHTLS.org).

Application Site

A tourniquet should be applied just proximal to the hemorrhaging wound. If one tourniquet does not completely stop the hemorrhage, then another one should be applied just proximal to the first. By placing two tourniquets side by side, the area of compression is doubled and successful control of hemorrhage is more likely. Once applied, the tourniquet site should not be covered so that it can be easily seen and monitored for recurrent hemorrhage.

Application Tightness

A tourniquet should be applied tight enough to block arterial flow and occlude the distal pulse. A device that only occludes venous outflow from a limb will actually increase hemorrhage from a wound. A direct relationship exists between the amount of pressure required to control hemorrhage and the size of the limb. Thus, on average, a tourniquet will need to be placed more tightly on a leg to achieve hemorrhage control than on an arm. If a tourniquet is properly applied and bleeding is not successfully controlled, a second tourniquet may be used and placed just proximal to the first. The addition of a second tourniquet provides additional compression and is usually successful in stopping bleeding in those cases where one device has proven inadequate.

Time Limit

Arterial tourniquets have been used safely for up to 120 to 150 minutes in the OR without significant nerve or muscle damage. Even in suburban or rural settings, most EMS transport times are significantly less than this period. In general, a tourniquet placed in the prehospital setting should remain in place until the patient reaches definitive care at the closest appropriate hospital. U.S. military use has not shown significant deterioration with prolonged application times.[13] If application of a tourniquet is required, the patient will most likely need emergency surgery to control hemorrhage. Thus, the ideal receiving facility for such a patient is one with surgical capabilities.

In the past, it was often recommended that a tourniquet be loosened every 10 to 15 minutes in order to allow for some blood flow back into the injured extremity with the thought being that this blood flow would help preserve the limb and prevent subsequent amputation. This practice only serves to increase the blood loss sustained by the patient and does nothing for the limb itself. Once applied, the tourniquet should be left in place until no longer needed.

A tourniquet can be painful for a conscious patient to tolerate, and pain management should be considered, provided that the patient does not have signs of Class III or IV shock. **Figure 9-17** provides a sample protocol for tourniquet application.

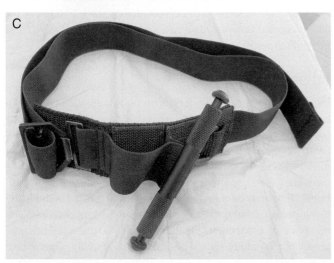
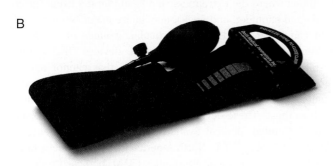

Figure 9-16   A. A CAT tourniquet. **B.** An EMT tourniquet. **C.** A SOF-T tourniquet.

Source: Parts A and C, Courtesy of Peter T. Pons, MD, FACEP. Part B Courtesy of Delhi Medical Innovations, Inc.

Figure 9-17   Protocol for Tourniquet Application

Tourniquets should be used if controlling the hemorrhage with direct pressure or pressure dressing is not possible or fails. The steps in applying a tourniquet are as follows:

1. Apply a commercially manufactured tourniquet, blood pressure cuff, or "Spanish windlass" to the extremity just proximal to the bleeding wound.
2. Tighten the tourniquet until hemorrhage ceases, then secure it in place.
3. Write the time of tourniquet application on a piece of tape and secure it to the tourniquet. For example, "TK 21:45" indicates that the tourniquet was applied at 9:45 pm.
4. Leave the tourniquet uncovered so that the site can be seen and monitored for recurrent hemorrhage. If bleeding continues after application and tightening of the initial tourniquet, a second tourniquet can be applied just above the first.
5. Consider pain management unless the patient is in Class III or IV shock.
6. Transport the patient, ideally to a facility that has surgical capability.

Hemostatic Agents

The U.S. Food and Drug Administration (FDA) has approved a number of topical hemostatic agents for use. Hemostatic agents are designed to be placed or packed into a wound, enhance clotting, and promote control of life-threatening hemorrhage that cannot be stopped with direct pressure alone in areas of the body that are not amenable to tourniquet placement. These agents generally come in two forms: (1) a powder that is poured onto the wound and (2) a gauze impregnated with the hemostatic material that is applied to or packed into the wound.

Early generations of the hemostatic agents had a number of complications associated with their use. Some of the products produced heat-generating reactions that led to significant burns in the patients to whom the material was applied. The granular powders fell out of favor because they tended to blow back into the face of the medical care provider applying them. In addition, there were studies performed in animals that showed that the granular products had the potential to embolize, leading to blood clots at locations in the circulatory system remote from the actual site of injury. Subsequent generations of these agents have preferentially gone to gauze impregnated with the active material.

It is important to note that these agents require packing the hemostatic dressing directly into the wound, not merely applying

the dressing as a cover to the open injury. Also, a minimum of 3 minutes of direct pressure must be applied to the wound site for most of the available agents. At least one manufacturer has recently offered a hemostatic product that they report does not require the application of direct pressure after the placement of the product in the wound.

As of this writing, Combat Gauze was the product recommended for use by the CoTCCC based on research done both by the U.S. Navy and Army surgical research lab. Again, this recommendation may change over time, and the latest updates from the CoTCCC and PHTLS will appear on the PHTLS website.

One study that compared a number of different hemostatic agents to plain gauze packing demonstrated no difference in blood loss or animal survival between the hemostatic agents and the plain gauze material.[20] This finding strongly suggests that, while the hemostatic agent aids in promoting clotting, the primary factor controlling hemorrhage is likely the proper packing of the dressing into the wound with the application of direct pressure onto the bleeding site.

Junctional Hemorrhage Control

Wounds located in the so-called junctional areas of the body, locations where the extremities and head join the trunk (groin, axilla and shoulder, and neck), may injure major blood vessels that can bleed profusely. In particular, wounds of the lower extremities from improvised explosive devices (IEDs) often result in high amputations and wounds that cannot accommodate tourniquet placement. The CoTCCC has approved a number of devices designed to control bleeding from wounds such as these. These devices include the Combat Ready Clamp (CRoC, Combat Medical Systems), the Junctional Emergency Treatment Tool (J.E.T.T., North America Rescue Products, LLC), and the SAM Junctional Tourniquet (SAM Medical Products). Some of these devices have been fielded by the U.S. military for use in combat theaters. The role and utility of these devices in the civilian setting has not, as yet, been studied or defined.

Internal Hemorrhage

Internal hemorrhage from fracture sites should also be considered. Rough handling of an injured extremity not only may convert a closed fracture to an open one, but also may significantly increase internal bleeding from bone ends, adjacent muscle tissue, or damaged vessels. All suspected extremity fractures should be immobilized in an effort to minimize this hemorrhage. Time may be taken to splint several fractures individually if the patient has no evidence of life-threatening conditions. If the primary assessment identifies threats to the patient's life, however, the patient should be immobilized rapidly on an appropriate device such as a long backboard or vacuum mattress, thereby immobilizing all of the extremities in an anatomic manner, and transported to a medical facility. Pelvic binders have been shown to splint and approximate the fractures of the pelvic bone, but no studies have been done to show any change in outcome if used in the prehospital setting.

Disability

There are no unique, specific interventions for altered mental status in the shock patient. If the patient's abnormal neurologic status is the result of cerebral hypoxia and poor perfusion, efforts to correct hypoxia and restore perfusion throughout the body should result in improved mental status. In assessing a patient's prognosis after TBI, an "initial" Glasgow Coma Scale (GCS) score is typically considered to be the score established following adequate resuscitation and restoration of cerebral perfusion. Assessing a patient's GCS score while still in shock may result in an overly grim prognosis.

Expose/Environment

Maintaining the patient's body temperature within a normal range is important. Hypothermia results from exposure to colder environments by convection, conduction, and other physical means (see the Environmental Trauma I: Heat and Cold chapter) and from loss of energy production with anaerobic metabolism. The greatest concern regarding hypothermia is its effect on blood clotting. As the body cools, clotting is impaired. In addition, hypothermia worsens coagulopathy, myocardial dysfunction, hyperkalemia, vasoconstriction, and a host of other problems that negatively affect a patient's chance of survival.[21] Although cold temperatures preserve tissue for a short time, the temperature drop must be very rapid and very low for preservation to occur. Such a rapid change has not been proven effective for the patient in shock after trauma.

In the prehospital setting, increasing the core temperature once hypothermia has developed can be difficult; therefore, all steps that can be taken in the field to preserve normal body temperature should be initiated. Once exposed and examined, the patient must be protected from the environment and body temperature maintained. Any wet clothing, including that saturated with blood, is removed from the patient because wet clothing increases heat loss. The patient is covered with warm blankets. The need for warming the patient can be anticipated and blankets placed near heater vents in the ambulance en route to the call. An alternative to blankets involves covering the patient with plastic sheets, such as heavy, thick garbage bags. They are inexpensive, easily stored, disposable, and effective devices for heat retention. Heated, humidified oxygen, if available, may help preserve body heat, especially in intubated patients.

Once assessed and packaged, the patient in shock is moved into the warmed patient compartment of the ambulance. Ideally, the patient compartment of an ambulance is kept at 85°F (29°C) or more when transporting a severely injured trauma patient. The patient's rate of heat loss into a cold compartment is very high. The conditions must be ideal for the patient, not for the prehospital care providers, because the patient is the most important person in any emergency. A good rule of thumb is that if the prehospital care provider is comfortable in the patient compartment, it is too cold for the patient.

Patient Transport

Effective treatment of a patient in severe hemorrhagic shock requires a surgeon with access to an OR and blood. Because neither is routinely available in the prehospital trauma setting, rapid transport to a facility that is capable of managing the patient's injuries is extremely important. Rapid transport does not mean doing the old-fashioned "scoop and run" and disregarding or neglecting the treatment modalities that are important in patient care. However, it does mean that the prehospital care provider quickly institutes key, potentially lifesaving measures, such as airway management, ventilatory support, and hemorrhage control. Time must not be wasted on an inappropriate assessment or with unnecessary immobilization maneuvers. When caring for a critically injured patient, many steps, such as warming the patient, starting IV therapy, and even performing the secondary assessment, are accomplished in the ambulance while en route.

Patient Positioning

In general, trauma patients who are in shock should be transported in the supine position, immobilized as necessary on an appropriate device such as the long backboard or vacuum mattress. Special positioning, such as the Trendelenburg position (placed on an incline with the feet elevated above the head) or the "shock" position (head and torso supine with legs elevated), although used for 150 years, has not been proven to be effective. The Trendelenburg position may aggravate already impaired ventilatory function by placing the weight of the abdominal organs on the diaphragm and may increase intracranial pressure in patients with TBI. More importantly, patients who are in severe hypovolemic shock are, generally, maximally vasoconstricted.[22,23]

Vascular Access
Intravenous Route

Intravenous access is obtained in a trauma patient who has known or suspected serious injuries so that the prehospital care provider can initiate fluid administration if appropriate. Except in unusual circumstances, such as a patient undergoing extrication from a vehicle or prehospital care providers awaiting the arrival of a helicopter, IV access should be obtained after the patient has been placed in the ambulance and transport has been initiated to the closest appropriate facility. Gaining IV access should not delay transport to the hospital for the severely injured patient.

Although volume resuscitation of a trauma patient in shock makes empiric sense, no research has demonstrated improved survival rates of critically injured trauma patients when IV fluid therapy was initiated in the prehospital setting. In fact, one physiologic computer model of prehospital IV fluid administration found that IV fluid is only beneficial when three conditions exist: (1) the patient is bleeding at a rate of 25 to 100 ml/minute, (2) the IV fluid administration rate is equal to the bleeding rate, and (3) the scene time and transport time exceed 30 minutes.[24]

Therefore, *transport of the trauma patient should never be delayed to initiate IV lines*.

One study has demonstrated that there was no benefit from the use of IV fluids before the hemorrhage was controlled.[25] Unfortunately, there have been no good studies that randomized the use of fluid resuscitation in patients with uncontrolled hemorrhage versus controlled hemorrhage. All of the studies that have been done mix both types of patients. Until such a study is done, the use of anecdotal and mixed studies will be the basis for the recommended practice.

For patients in shock or with potentially serious injuries, one or two large-bore (14- or 16-gauge), short (1-inch) IV catheters should be inserted by percutaneous puncture as time permits. The rate of fluid administration is directly proportional to the fourth power of the radius of the catheter and inversely proportional to its length (meaning more fluid will rapidly flow through a shorter, larger-diameter catheter than through a longer, smaller-diameter catheter). The preferred site for percutaneous access is a vein of the forearm. Alternative sites for IV access are the veins of the antecubital fossa, the hand, and the upper arm (cephalic vein). If two attempts at percutaneous access are unsuccessful in a child, inserting an intraosseous line should be considered. Central venous lines or venous cutdowns are not generally considered appropriate venous access in the prehospital setting and are rarely needed.

Intraosseous Route

Another alternative for vascular access in adults is the intraosseous route.[26,27] The intraosseous route of giving IV fluids is not new and was described by Dr. Walter E. Lee in 1941. This method of vascular access can be accomplished in a number of ways. It can be established via the sternal technique, using appropriately designed devices[28,29] (e.g., F.A.S.T.1, Pyng Medical Corporation). Specially designed devices such as the Bone Injection Gun ("BIG," WaisMed) and the EZ-IO (Vidacare Corp.) may also be used to establish access through sites in the distal tibia above the ankle, the proximal tibia, the distal femur, the proximal humerus, or the sternum (though an EZ-IO should not be used at the sternal site) (**Figures 9-18** and **9-19**).[30] Such techniques are becoming commonly used in the prehospital setting, but the focus should be on rapid transport rather than IV fluid administration. For delayed or prolonged transport to definitive care, intraosseous vascular access may have a role in adult trauma patients.

Volume Resuscitation

There are two general categories of fluid resuscitation products that have been used in the last 50 years for the management of trauma patients—blood and IV solutions. These products can be further subdivided as follows:

- Blood
  - Packed red blood cells (PRBCs)
  - Whole blood
  - Reconstituted whole blood as blood products

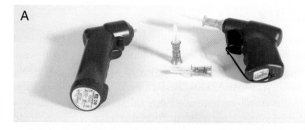

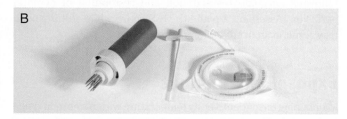

Figure 9-18 A. IO needles and IO gun for manual insertion (various sizes shown). **B.** IO sternal driver.

Source: Jones and Bratlett Learning. Photographed by Darren Stahlman.

- IV solutions
  - Large volumes of crystalloid
  - Hypertonic fluid
    - 7% saline
    - 3% saline
  - Colloid solutions
  - Hypotensive or restricted fluid
  - Blood substitutes (only investigational use)

Each of these products has both advantages and disadvantages.

Blood

Because of its ability to transport oxygen, blood or various blood products remain the fluid of choice for the resuscitation of a patient in severe hemorrhagic shock. Experience gained by the U.S. military as a result of the Iraq and Afghanistan wars has demonstrated the importance of administration of RBCs and plasma to the survival of injured soldiers. This "reconstituted" blood replaces the lost oxygen-carrying capacity, the clotting factors, and the proteins needed to maintain oncotic pressure to prevent fluid loss from the vascular system. Unfortunately, blood, for the most part, is impractical for use in the civilian prehospital setting because of issues related to blood typing and because blood and its subcomponents are perishable if not kept refrigerated or frozen until the moment of use.

Currently, *lyophilized plasma* is being used in the field in several countries. Lyophilized plasma is human plasma that has been freeze-dried. It has a stable shelflife of approximately 2 years, does not require refrigeration, and must be reconstituted prior to use. Liquid plasma is being carried by a few EMS and HEMS (helicopter EMS) systems in the United States, and research is underway to evaluate the use of plasma in the civilian prehospital setting for the resuscitation of trauma patients.

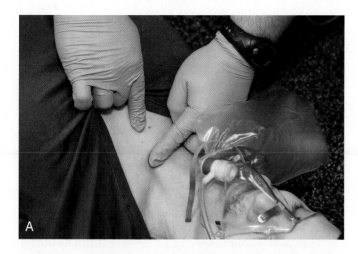

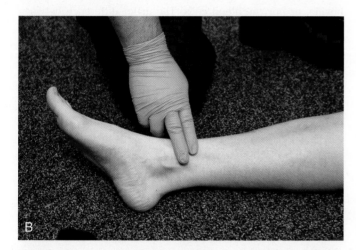

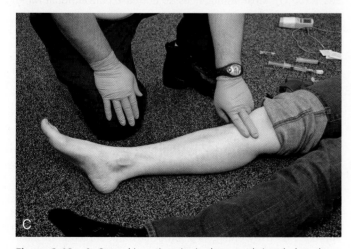

Figure 9-19 A. Sternal insertion site in the manubrium below the suprasternal notch. Note that the EZ-IO device cannot be used at the sternal site. **B.** Distal tibial insertion site above the ankle. **C.** Proximal tibial insertion site below the knee.

Intravenous Solutions

Alternative solutions for volume resuscitation fall into one of four categories: (1) isotonic crystalloids, (2) hypertonic crystalloids, (3) synthetic (artificial) colloids, and (4) blood substitutes.

Isotonic Crystalloid Solutions

Isotonic crystalloids are balanced salt solutions comprised of electrolytes (substances that separate into charged ions when dissolved in solutions). They act as effective volume expanders for a short time, but they possess no oxygen-carrying capacity. Immediately after infusion, crystalloids fill the vascular space that was depleted by blood loss, improving preload and cardiac output. **Lactated Ringer's** solution remains the isotonic crystalloid solution of choice for the management of shock because its composition is most similar to the electrolyte composition of blood plasma. It contains specific amounts of sodium, potassium, calcium, chloride, and lactate ions. **Normal saline** (0.9% sodium chloride [NaCl] solution) remains an acceptable alternative, although *hyperchloremia* (a marked increase in the blood chloride level) may occur with massive volume resuscitation with normal saline administration. Solutions of dextrose in water (e.g., D_5W) are not effective volume expanders and have no place in the resuscitation of trauma patients. In fact, administration of glucose-containing fluids only serves to increase the patient's blood glucose level, which then has a diuretic effect and will actually increase fluid loss via the kidneys.

Unfortunately, within 30 to 60 minutes after administration of a crystalloid solution, only about one-fourth to one-third of the administered volume remains in the cardiovascular system. The rest has shifted into the interstitial space because both the water and the electrolytes in the solution can freely cross the capillary membranes. The lost fluid becomes edema in the soft tissues and organs of the body. This extra fluid causes difficulties with the onloading and offloading of oxygen to the RBCs.

If possible, IV fluids should be warmed to about 102°F (39°C) before infusion. Infusion of large amounts of room temperature or cold IV fluid contributes to hypothermia and increased hemorrhage.

Hypertonic Crystalloid Solutions

Hypertonic crystalloid solutions have extremely high concentrations of electrolytes compared to blood plasma. The most commonly used experimental model is **hypertonic saline**, a 7.5% NaCl solution, which is more than eight times the concentration of NaCl in normal saline. This is an effective plasma expander, especially in that a small, 250-ml infusion often produces the same effect as infusing 2 to 3 liters of isotonic crystalloid solution.[31,32] An analysis of several studies of hypertonic saline failed, however, to demonstrate improved survival rates over the use of isotonic crystalloids.[33] This solution is not FDA approved for patient care in the United States. Lesser concentrations, such as 3.0%, are approved for patient care and are frequently used in intensive care units.

Synthetic Colloid Solutions

Proteins are large molecules produced by the body comprised of amino acids. They have countless functions. One type of protein found in the blood, albumin, helps maintain fluid in the intravascular space. Intravenous administration of human albumin is costly and has been associated with the transmission of infectious diseases, such as hepatitis. When administered to a patient in hemorrhagic shock, synthetic colloid solutions draw fluid from the interstitial and intracellular spaces into the intravascular space, thereby producing expansion of the blood volume. As with crystalloids, colloid plasma expanders do not transport oxygen.

Gelofusine is a 4% gelatin solution produced from bovine protein and is occasionally used in Europe and Australia for fluid resuscitation. It is moderately expensive and carries a risk of severe allergic reactions. A small infusion of gelofusine produces expansion of the intravascular volume for several hours.

Hetastarch (Hespan, Hextend) and dextran (Gentran) are synthetic colloids that have been created by linking numerous starch (amylopectin) or dextrose molecules together until they are similar in size to an albumin molecule. These solutions are also moderately expensive compared to crystalloids and have been associated with allergic reactions and impairment of blood typing. Two recent meta-analyses of the literature related to use of hetastarch have raised the concern about increased incidence of acute kidney injury and increased mortality related to administration of these compounds.[34,35]

The use of crystalloids versus colloids has been a long-standing debate in the management of trauma patients.[36] A study of almost 7,000 patients admitted to intensive care units demonstrated no difference in outcome when patients were resuscitated with colloid (albumin) versus normal saline.[37] A recent meta-analysis echoes this finding.[35] A single study presented at the 2009 American Association for the Surgery of Trauma (AAST) meeting identified a greater survival with Hextend than with normal saline; however, more information needs to be available before its routine use can be recommended. Hextend is a colloid solution that has been used in military situations as a volume expander. The benefits are that it is a smaller and lighter (although more expensive) package, which is more easily carried, it improves perfusion without overloading the patient with crystalloid, and it appears to be effective. However, a recent meta-analysis raises the question about possible increased mortality from acute kidney injury from this type of product.[34]

Virtually no research exists involving the use of these synthetic colloid solutions in the civilian prehospital setting, and no data exist from their use in the hospital that shows them to be superior to crystalloid solutions. These products are not recommended for the prehospital management of shock.

Blood Substitutes

Blood transfusion has several limitations as well as undesirable qualities, including the need to type and crossmatch, a short shelf life, perishability when not refrigerated, a potential for transmission of infectious disease, and an increasing shortage of donated units that limits its use in the prehospital setting. This has led to intense research in blood substitutes during the last two to three decades. The U.S. military has played a central role in this research because a blood substitute that does not need refrigeration and does not require blood typing could be carried to a wounded soldier on the battlefield and infused rapidly to combat shock.

Perfluorocarbons (PFCs) are synthetic compounds that have high oxygen solubility. These inert materials can dissolve approximately 50 times more oxygen than blood plasma can. PFCs contain no hemoglobin or protein; they are completely free of biologic materials, thereby greatly reducing the threat of infectious agents being found in them; and oxygen is transported by dissolving in the plasma portion. First-generation PFCs were of limited use because of numerous problems, including a short half-life and the need for a concurrent high-FiO_2 administration. Newer PFCs have fewer of these disadvantages, but their role as oxygen carriers remains undetermined.

Most *hemoglobin-based oxygen carriers* (HBOCs) use the same oxygen-carrying molecule (hemoglobin) found in human, bovine, or porcine blood cells. The major difference between HBOCs and human blood is that the hemoglobin in HBOCs is not contained within a cell membrane. This removes the need for conducting type and crossmatch studies because the antigen–antibody risk is removed when the hemoglobin is extracted from the cell. Additionally, many of these HBOCs can be stored for long periods, making them the ideal solution for mass-casualty incidents. Early problems with hemoglobin-based oxygen-carrying solutions included toxicity from hemoglobin. To date, none of those experimental solutions have been found to be safe or effective in humans.

Warming Intravenous Fluids

Any IV fluid given to a patient in shock should be warm, not room temperature or cold. The ideal temperature for such fluids is 102°F (39°C). Most ambulances do not have conventional rapid fluid warmers, but other steps can keep fluids at an adequate temperature. A convenient storage area for fluids is in a box in the engine compartment. Wrapping heat packs around the bag can also warm fluid. Commercially available fluid-warmer units for the patient care compartment provide an easy and reliable means to keep fluids at the correct temperature. These units are costly but justifiable for prolonged transports.

Managing Volume Resuscitation

As noted earlier, significant controversy surrounds prehospital fluid administration for a trauma patient who is in shock. When Prehospital Trauma Life Support (PHTLS) was first introduced in the United States, prehospital care providers adopted the approach used by emergency physicians and surgeons in most hospitals and trauma centers: Administer an IV crystalloid solution until the vital signs return to normal (typically, pulse less than 100 beats/minute and systolic blood pressure greater than 100 mm Hg). When sufficient crystalloid solution is infused to restore vital signs to normal, the patient's perfusion should be improved. At the time, experts believed that such rapid intervention would clear lactic acid and restore energy production in the cells of the body and also decrease the risk of developing irreversible shock and kidney failure. However, no study of trauma patients in the prehospital setting has shown that the administration of IV fluid actually does decrease complications and death.

A major contribution of PHTLS over the past two decades has been to establish the conceptual change that, in the critically injured trauma patient, *transport should never be delayed while IV lines are placed and fluid is infused.* These actions can be performed in the back of the ambulance en route to the closest appropriate facility. The critically injured trauma patient who is in shock generally requires blood transfusion and surgical intervention to control internal hemorrhage, neither of which can be accomplished in the field.

Research, primarily in experimental models of shock, has shown that IV volume resuscitation may have detrimental side effects when administered before surgical control of the source of hemorrhage. In experimental animals, internal hemorrhage often continues until the animal is hypotensive, at which point bleeding slows and a blood clot (*thrombus*) typically forms at the site of injury. In one sense, this hypotension is protective in that it is associated with a dramatic slowing or cessation of internal hemorrhage. When aggressive IV fluids were administered to the animals in an attempt to restore perfusion and blood pressure, internal hemorrhage started again, and the thrombus was disrupted.

In addition, crystalloid infusions may dilute coagulation factors. The experimental animals often had a worse outcome compared to animals that received resuscitation after surgical control of the injury site.[38-40] In a similar animal model, improved survival was noted with "hypotensive resuscitation," in which the blood pressure was purposefully kept low until hemorrhage was controlled, then resuscitation took place.[41-43]

Clearly, these studies have potential implications on fluid resuscitation in the prehospital setting. Theoretically, on one hand, aggressive volume resuscitation could return the blood pressure to normal. This, in turn, may dislodge blood clots that formed at bleeding sites in the peritoneal cavity or elsewhere and may result in renewed hemorrhage that cannot be controlled until the patient reaches the OR. On the other hand, withholding IV fluid from a patient in profound shock only leads to further tissue hypoxia and failure of energy production. A single clinical study conducted in an urban prehospital setting demonstrated a worse outcome in trauma patients who received crystalloid solutions before control of internal hemorrhage (survival rate of 62% versus 70% in the delayed-treatment group).[21] The findings of this single study have not been replicated in other prehospital systems, and the findings cannot be generalized to rural EMS systems. In a survey of trauma surgeons, fewer than 4% opted for an approach that involved withholding IV fluid from a patient in Class III shock. Almost two-thirds of the surgeons recommended that such a patient be maintained in a relatively hypotensive state during transport.[44]

Prehospital volume resuscitation should be tailored to the clinical situation as described in the following discussion (**Figure 9-20**).

Uncontrolled Hemorrhage

For patients with suspected internal hemorrhage in their chest, abdomen, or retroperitoneum (pelvis), sufficient IV crystalloid solution should be titrated to maintain a systolic blood pressure in the range of 80 to 90 mm Hg, which will provide a MAP of 60 to 65 mm Hg. This blood pressure level should maintain adequate perfusion to the kidneys with less risk of worsening internal hemorrhage. A fluid bolus should not be administered because this may "overshoot" the target blood pressure range, resulting in recurrent intrathoracic, intra-abdominal, or retroperitoneal bleeding.

The current philosophy of restricted crystalloid administration in the prehospital setting and during the initial hospital care has been called by several names, including permissive hypotension, hypotensive resuscitation, and "balanced" resuscitation, meaning that a balance must be struck between the amount of fluid administered and the degree of blood pressure elevation. Once the patient arrives at the hospital, fluid administration continues by giving plasma and blood (1:1 ratio) until the hemorrhage is controlled. Blood pressure is then returned to normal values with ongoing 1:1 (plasma to blood) transfusion with restricted crystalloid administration in most trauma centers.

Central Nervous System Injuries

Hypotension has been associated with increased mortality in the setting of TBI. Patients with certain conditions (e.g., TBIs) appear to benefit from a more aggressive fluid resuscitation.[45] Guidelines published by the Brain Trauma Foundation recommend maintaining the systolic blood pressure above 90 mm Hg in patients with suspected TBI.[46] Consensus guidelines focusing on the management of acute spinal cord injury recommend not only avoiding hypotension (systolic blood pressure less than 90 mm Hg), but also maintaining a MAP of at least 85 to 90 mm Hg in hopes of improving spinal cord perfusion. To accomplish this goal, more aggressive volume resuscitation may be required, increasing the risk of recurrent bleeding from associated internal injuries.[47]

Controlled Hemorrhage

Patients with significant external hemorrhage that has been controlled can be managed with a more aggressive volume resuscitation strategy, provided the prehospital care provider has no reason to suspect associated intrathoracic, intra-abdominal, or retroperitoneal injuries. Examples include a large scalp laceration or a wound in an extremity involving major blood vessels, but with the bleeding controlled with a pressure dressing or tourniquet. Adult patients who fall in this category and present in Class II, III, or IV shock should receive an initial rapid bolus of 1 to 2 liters of warmed crystalloid solution, preferably lactated Ringer's. Pediatric patients should receive a bolus of 20 ml/kg of warmed crystalloid solution. As noted previously, this should always occur during transport to

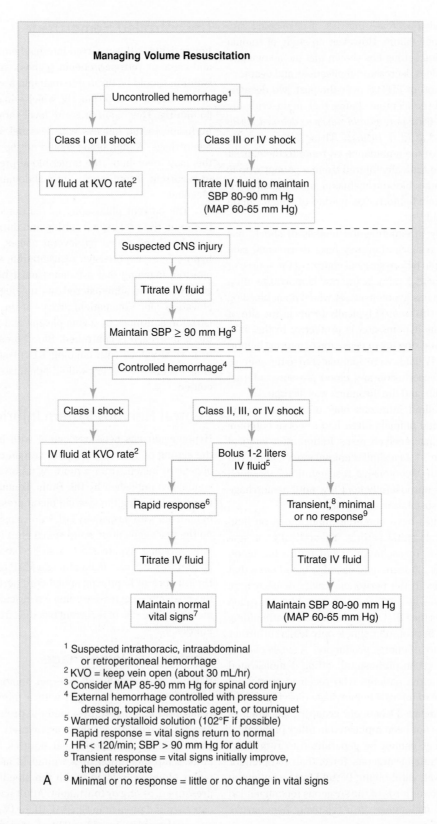

Figure 9-20   A. Algorithm for managing volume resuscitation.

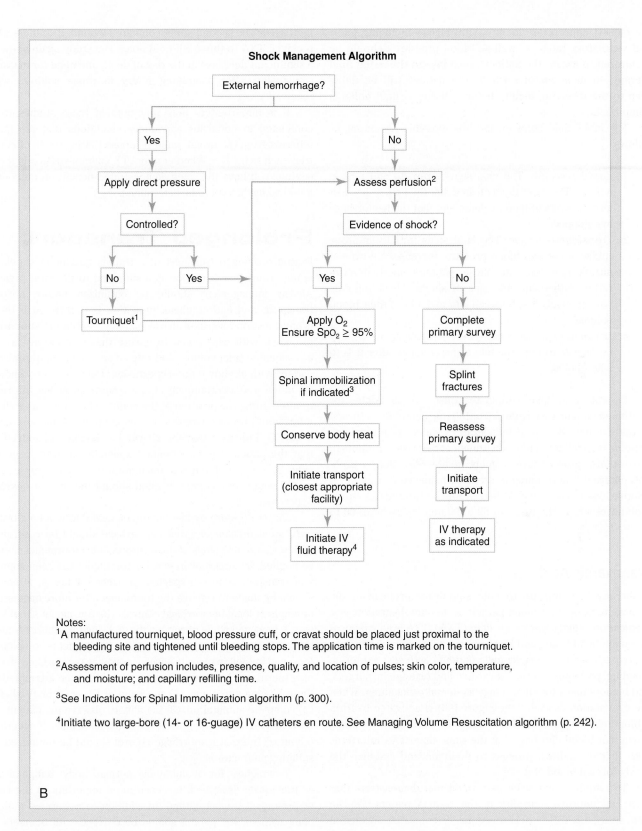

Shock Management Algorithm

Notes:
[1]A manufactured tourniquet, blood pressure cuff, or cravat should be placed just proximal to the bleeding site and tightened until bleeding stops. The application time is marked on the tourniquet.

[2]Assessment of perfusion includes, presence, quality, and location of pulses; skin color, temperature, and moisture; and capillary refilling time.

[3]See Indications for Spinal Immobilization algorithm (p. 300).

[4]Initiate two large-bore (14- or 16-guage) IV catheters en route. See Managing Volume Resuscitation algorithm (p. 242).

B

Figure 9-20 **B.** Algorithm for managing shock.

the closest appropriate facility. Vital signs—including pulse and ventilatory rates, as well as blood pressure—should be monitored to assess the patient's response to the initial fluid therapy. In most urban settings, the patient will be delivered to the receiving facility before the initial fluid bolus is completed.

The initial fluid bolus elicits three possible responses, as follows:

1. *Rapid response.* The vital signs return to and remain normal. This typically indicates that the patient has lost less than 20% of blood volume and that the hemorrhage has stopped.
2. *Transient response.* The vital signs initially improve (pulse slows and blood pressure increases); however, during reassessment, these patients show deterioration with recurrent signs of shock. These patients have typically lost between 20% and 40% of their blood volume.
3. *Minimal or no response.* These patients show virtually no change in the profound signs of shock after a 1- to 2-liter bolus.

Patients who have a rapid response are candidates for continued volume resuscitation, until vital signs have returned to normal and all clinical indicators of shock have resolved. Patients who fall into either the transient response or minimal/no response groups have ongoing hemorrhage that is probably internal. These patients are best managed in a state of relative hypotension, and IV fluid should be titrated to systolic blood pressure in the range of 80 to 90 mm Hg (MAP of 60 to 65 mm Hg).

Tranexamic Acid

A therapy that appears to hold significant promise in the management of the trauma patient is the administration of a medication called *tranexamic acid* (TXA). TXA is an analog of the amino acid lysine and has been used for many decades to decrease bleeding in gynecologic patients with severe uterine bleeding, patients undergoing cardiac and orthopedic surgery, and hemophiliacs for such things as dental procedures. When the coagulation cascade (see Figure 9-6) is activated to form a blood clot as a result of an injury, the process of breaking down that blood clot begins at the same time. TXA interferes with that breakdown process to maintain and stabilize the newly formed blood clot.

Two studies have been performed that demonstrate that TXA can improve mortality in the trauma patient.[48,49] The first study, CRASH-2, performed in 40 countries, evaluated TXA in adult trauma patients who had or could have significant hemorrhage.[48] The result was a statistically significant decrease in the risk of death in the group receiving TXA when the TXA was given within 3 hours of the time of the injury. If given at more than 3 hours postinjury, the risk of death actually

increased. The second study compared wounded soldiers who received TXA to those who did not.[49] The study again showed a significant decrease in the risk of death and need for massive transfusion after sustaining injury in those soldiers who received TXA.

It is important to note that both of these studies were conducted in countries and under conditions that are quite different from the urban, rapid response EMS systems of countries such as the U.S. Whether or not TXA administration in these settings will have the same demonstrated benefit on outcomes after trauma has yet to be determined.

Prolonged Transport

During prolonged transport of a trauma patient in shock, it is important that perfusion is maintained to the vital organs. Airway management should be optimized before a long transport, and endotracheal intubation is performed if there is any question regarding airway patency. Ventilatory support is provided, with care taken to ensure that ventilations are of a reasonable tidal volume and rate so as not to compromise a patient with already tenuous perfusion. Pulse oximetry should be monitored continuously. Capnography provides information regarding the position of the endotracheal tube, as well as information on the patient's perfusion status. A marked drop in $ETCO_2$ indicates that the airway has become dislodged or that the patient has experienced a significant drop in perfusion. A suspected tension pneumothorax is decompressed, or the equipment is kept at hand should the patient develop hypotension.

Direct pressure by hand is impractical during a long transport, so significant external hemorrhage should be controlled with pressure dressings. If these efforts fail, a tourniquet should be applied. In situations in which a tourniquet has been applied and transport time is expected to exceed 4 hours, attempts should be made to remove the tourniquet after more aggressive attempts at local hemorrhage control. The tourniquet should be slowly loosened while observing the dressing for signs of hemorrhage. If bleeding does not reoccur, the tourniquet is completely loosened but left in place in case hemorrhage recurs. Conversion of a tourniquet back to a dressing should not be attempted in the following situations: (1) presence of Class III or IV shock, (2) complete amputation, (3) inability to observe the patient for reoccurrence of bleeding, and (4) tourniquet in place longer than 6 hours.[15] Internal hemorrhage control should be optimized by splinting all fractures.

Techniques for maintaining normal body temperature, as previously described, are even more important in the case of prolonged transport time. In addition to a warmed patient compartment, the patient should be covered with blankets or materials that preserve body heat; even large, plastic garbage bags help prevent loss of heat. Intravenous fluids should be warmed before administration.

In prolonged-transport circumstances, vascular access for fluid administration may be critical, and two large-bore

IV lines should be established. For both children and adults, inability to obtain vascular percutaneous venous access may necessitate use of the intraosseous route, as described previously.

For patients with suspected ongoing hemorrhage, maintaining systolic blood pressure in the range of 80 to 90 mm Hg or MAP of 60 to 65 mm Hg can usually accomplish the goal of maintaining perfusion to vital organs with less risk of renewing internal hemorrhage. Patients with suspected TBIs or spinal cord injuries should have systolic blood pressure maintained above 90 to 100 mm Hg.

Vital signs should be reassessed frequently to monitor response to resuscitation. The following should be documented at serial intervals: ventilation rate, pulse rate, blood pressure, skin color and temperature, capillary refill, GCS score, SpO_2, and $ETCO_2$, if available.

Although insertion of a urinary catheter is not usually required in rapid transport circumstances, monitoring urine output is an important tool that can help guide decisions regarding the need for additional fluid therapy during prolonged transport. Insertion of a urinary catheter, if local protocols permit, should be considered so that urine output can be monitored. Adequate urine outputs include 0.5 ml/kg/hour for adults, 1 ml/kg/hour for pediatric patients, and 2 ml/kg/hour for infants younger than 1 year. Urine output of less than these amounts may be a key indicator that the patient requires further volume infusion.

If time and local protocols permit during prolonged transport, placement of a nasogastric catheter should be considered for all intubated patients, unless fractures of the patient's midface are suspected. If such fractures are present, placement of an orogastric catheter should be considered. Gastric distension may cause unexplained hypotension and dysrhythmias, especially in children. Placement of a nasogastric or orogastric tube may also decrease the risk of vomiting and aspiration.

During prolonged transport, assessing the patient's clinical status and response to resuscitation is key to determining outcome. There are encouraging reports supporting the use of the Life Support for Trauma and Transport (LSTAT, Integrated Medical Systems) for monitoring critically injured patients during transport. This transport bed, which contains all of the monitoring equipment to make a "mobile intensive care unit," has shown promising results in the military for transport of critically injured patients, as well as in the transfer of critically injured patients in civilian practice.[50] Disadvantages of using such devices are the cost and weight. If these obstacles could be overcome, there may be a wider application for these devices when prolonged transport of the critically injured trauma patient is necessary.

Summary

- Shock causes a state of generalized hypoperfusion, resulting in cellular hypoxia, anaerobic metabolism, loss of energy production, lactic acidosis, hypothermia, and death if not appropriately treated.
- In the trauma patient, hemorrhage is the most common cause of shock.
- Care of the patient in shock or one that may go into shock begins with appropriate and complete assessment of the patient beginning with a history of the event and a quick visual examination of the patient looking for obvious signs of shock and blood loss.
- The primary goal of therapy is to identify the likely source of hemorrhage and treat it specifically, if possible. In the prehospital setting, this approach is most effective when the bleeding source is external. Internal hemorrhage can be treated definitively only in the hospital environment, so rapid transport of the patient to the appropriate hospital is essential.
- External hemorrhage should be controlled with direct pressure, followed by application of a pressure dressing. If this is ineffective, a tourniquet may be applied to the extremity proximal to the bleeding site. On the torso, a topical hemostatic agent may be used.
- In some cases, nonhemorrhagic sources of shock in the trauma patient (e.g., tension pneumothorax) can be temporarily corrected.
- All trauma patients in shock, in addition to maintenance of adequate oxygenation, require rapid extrication and expeditious transport to a definitive care institution where the cause of the shock can be specifically identified and treated.
- Transport should not be delayed for such measures as IV access and volume infusion. These interventions should be done in the ambulance during transport.
- Overaggressive fluid infusion should be avoided to minimize further bleeding and edema formation in the patient with hemorrhagic shock after trauma.

SCENARIO RECAP

You and your partner are dispatched to a 23-year-old man who was assaulted. Upon your arrival, you find the patient sitting on the ground in moderate distress. He states that he had just withdrawn some cash from an ATM and was returning to his car when he was robbed by two men who punched and kicked him. He complains of pain in his left lower ribs, left upper abdomen, and jaw.

The physical examination of the patient reveals pale skin color, a contusion on the left side of his mandible, and tenderness to palpation over the left lower ribs and in the left upper quadrant of the abdomen. His vital signs are pulse of 112 beats/minute, blood pressure of 100/64 mm Hg, and ventilatory rate of 22 breaths/minute and regular. Breath sounds are present bilaterally. You transfer him to the ambulance in preparation for transport to the hospital.

- What injuries do you expect to see after this assault?
- How would you manage these injuries in the field?
- You are 15 minutes away from the nearest trauma center. How does this alter your management plans?

SCENARIO SOLUTION

You recognize that this patient is showing the signs of hypovolemia (increased heart rate, decreased blood pressure, and increased ventilatory rate). You are concerned about the possibility of an injury to this patient's spleen. You immediately transfer him to the ambulance and instruct your partner to begin transport to the closest trauma center.

While en route, you apply oxygen and initiate a large-bore IV line, giving only minimal fluid at this point. You notify the trauma center of your findings and concerns and that you are en route. The patient is transported uneventfully with no change in his status or vital signs.

References

1. Gross SD. *A System of Surgery: Pathological, Diagnostic, Therapeutic, and Operative*. Philadelphia, PA: Blanchard and Lea; 1859.
2. Thal AP. *Shock: A Physiologic Basis for Treatment*. Chicago, IL: Yearbook Medical Publishers; 1971.
3. McClelland RN, Shires GT, Baxter CR, et al. Balanced salt solutions in the treatment of hemorrhagic shock. *JAMA*. 1967;199:830.
4. Duchesne JC, Hunt JP, Wahl G, et al. Review of current blood transfusions strategies in a mature level I trauma center: were we wrong for the last 60 years? *J Trauma*. 2008;65(2):272–276; discussion 276–278.
5. Holcomb JB, Jenkins D, Rhee P, et al. Damage control resuscitation: directly addressing the early coagulopathy of trauma. *J Trauma*. 2007;62(2):307–310.
6. Today in Science History. Science quotes by Baron William Thomson Kelvin. http://todayinsci.com/K/Kelvin_Lord/KelvinLord-Quotations.htm, Accessed September 30, 2013.
7. Koreny M, Riedmuller E, Nikfardjam M, et al. Arterial puncture closing devices compared with standard manual compression after cardiac catheterization: systematic review and meta analysis. *JAMA*. 2004;291:350.
8. Pepe PE, Raedler C, Lurie KG, et al. Emergency ventilatory management in hemorrhagic states: elemental or detrimental? *J Trauma*. a2003;54:1048.
9. Pepe PE, Roppolo LP, Fowler RL. The detrimental effects of ventilation during low-blood-flow states. *Curr Opin Crit Care*. 2005;11:212.
10. Walker SB, Cleary S, Higgins M. Comparison of the FemoStop device and manual pressure in reducing groin puncture site complications following coronary angioplasty and coronary stent placement. *Int J Nurs Pract*. 2001;7:366.
11. Simon A, Baumgarner B, Clark K, et al. Manual versus mechanical compression for femoral artery hemostasis after cardiac catheterization. *Am J Crit Care*. 1998;7:308.
12. Lehmann KG, Heath-Lange SJ, Ferris ST. Randomized comparison of hemostasis techniques after invasive cardiovascular procedures. *Am Heart J*. 1999;138:1118.
13. Beekley AC, Sebesta JA, Blackbourne LH, et al. Prehospital tourniquet use in Operation Iraqi Freedom: effect on hemorrhage control and outcomes. *J Trauma*. 2008;64(2):S28–S37.
14. Kragh JF Jr, Walters TJ, Baer DG, et al. Practical use of emergency tourniquets to stop bleeding in major limb trauma. *J Trauma*. 2008;64(2):S38-S50.
15. Bellamy RF. The causes of death in conventional land warfare: implications for combat casualty care research. *Mil Med*. 1984;149:55.
16. Mabry RL, Holcomb JB, Baker AM, et al. United States Army Rangers in Somalia: an analysis of combat casualties on an urban battlefield. *J Trauma*. 2000;49:515.
17. Walters TJ, Mabry RL. Use of tourniquets on the battlefield: a consensus panel report. *Mil Med*. 2005;170:770.
18. Kragh JF Jr, Littrel ML, Jones JA, et al. Battle casualty survival with emergency tourniquet use to stop limb bleeding. *J Emerg Med*. 2011;41:590–597.

19. Walters TL, Wenke JC, Kauvar DS, et al. Effectiveness of self-applied tourniquets in human volunteers. *Prehosp Emerg Care.* 2005;9:416–422.

20. Littlejohn LF, Devlin JJ, Kircher SS, Lueken R, Melia MR, Johnson AS. Comparison of Celox-A, ChitoFlex, Wound Stat, and combat gauze hemostatic agents versus standard gauze dressing in control of hemorrhage in a swine model of penetrating trauma. *Acad Emerg Med.* 2011;18(4):340–350.

21. Gentilello LM. Advances in the management of hypothermia. *Surg Clin North Am.* 1995;75:2.

22. Marino PL. *The ICU Book.* 2nd ed. Baltimore, MD: Williams & Wilkins; 1998.

23. Johnson S, Henderson SO, Myth L. The Trendelenburg position improves circulation in cases of shock. *Can J Emerg Med.* 2004;6:48.

24. Lewis FR. Prehospital intravenous fluid therapy: physiologic computer modeling. *J Trauma.* 1986;26:804.

25. Bickell WH, Wall MJ Jr, Pepe PE, et al. Immediate versus delayed fluid resuscitation for hypotensive patients with penetrating torso injuries. *N Engl J Med.* 1994;331:1105.

26. Deboer S, Seaver M, Morissette C. Intraosseous infusion: not just for kids anymore. *J Emerg Med Serv.* 2005;34:54.

27. Glaeser PW, Hellmich TR, Szewczuga D, et al. Five-year experience in prehospital intraosseous infusions in children and adults. *Ann Emerg Med.* 1993;22:1119.

28. Sawyer RW, Bodai BI, Blaisdell FW, et al. The current status of intraosseous infusion. *J Am Coll Surg.* 1994;179:353.

29. Macnab A, Christenson J, Findlay J, et al. A new system for sternal intraosseous infusion in adults. *Prehosp Emerg Care.* 2000;4:173.

30. Hubble MW, Trigg DC. Training prehospital personnel in saphenous vein cut down and adult intraosseous techniques. *Prehosp Emerg Care.* 2001;5(2):181.

31. Vassar MJ, Fischer RP, Obrien PE, et al. A multicenter trial of resuscitation of injured patients with 7.5% sodium chloride: the effect of added dextran 70. *Arch Surg.* 1993;128:1003.

32. Vassar MJ, Perry CA, Holcroft JW. Prehospital resuscitation of hypotensive trauma patients with 7.5% NaCl versus 7.5% NaCl with added dextran: a controlled trial. *J Trauma.* 1993;34:622.

33. Wade CE, Kramer GC, Grady JJ. Efficacy of hypertonic 7.5% saline and 6% dextran in treating trauma: a meta analysis of controlled clinical trials. *Surgery.* 1997;122:609.

34. Zarychanski R, Abou-Setta AM, Turgeon AF, et al. Association of hydroxyethyl starch with mortality and acute kidney injury in critically ill patients requiring volume resuscitation. *JAMA.* 2013;309:678-688.

35. Perel P, Roberts I, Ker K. Are colloids more effective than crystalloids in reducing death in people who are critically ill or injured? The Cochrane Library, 2013. http://summaries.cochrane.org/CD000567/are-colloids-more-effective-than-crystalloids-in-reducing-death-in-people-who-are-critically-ill-or-injured. Accessed March 4, 2013.

36. Rizoli SB. Crystalloids and colloids in trauma resuscitation: a brief overview of the current debate. *J Trauma.* 2003;54:S82.

37. SAFE Study Investigators. A comparison of albumin and saline for fluid resuscitation in the intensive care unit. *N Engl J Med.* 2004;350:2247.

38. Solomonov E, Hirsh M, Yahiya A, et al. The effect of vigorous fluid resuscitation in uncontrolled hemorrhagic shock after massive splenic injury. *Crit Care Med.* 2000;28:749.

39. Krausz MM, Horn Y, Gross D. The combined effect of small volume hypertonic saline and normal saline solutions in uncontrolled hemorrhagic shock. *Surg Gynecol Obstet.* 1992;174:363.

40. Bickell WH, Bruttig SP, Millnamow, et al. The detrimental effects of intravenous crystalloid after aortotomy in swine. *Surgery.* 1991;110:529.

41. Kowalenko T, Stern S, Dronen SC, et al. Improved outcome with hypotensive resuscitation of uncontrolled hemorrhagic shock in a swine model. *J Trauma.* 1992;33:349.

42. Sindlinger JF, Soucy DM, Greene SP, et al. The effects of isotonic saline volume resuscitation in uncontrolled hemorrhage. *Surg Gynecol Obstet.* 1993;177:545.

43. Capone AC, Safar, Stezoski W, et al. Improved outcome with fluid restriction in treatment of uncontrolled hemorrhagic shock. *J Am Coll Surg.* 1995;180:49.

44. Salomone JP, Ustin JS, McSwain NE, et al. Opinions of trauma practitioners regarding prehospital interventions for critically injured patients. *J Trauma.* 2005;58:509.

45. York J, Abenamar A, Graham R, et al. Fluid resuscitation of patients with multiple injuries and severe closed head injury: experience with an aggressive fluid resuscitation strategy. *J Trauma.* 2000;48(3):376.

46. Brain Trauma Foundation. *Guidelines for Prehospital Management of Traumatic Brain Injury.* New York, NY: Brain Trauma Foundation; 2000.

47. American Association of Neurological Surgeons and Congress of Neurological Surgeons Joint Section on Disorders of the Spine and Peripheral Nerves. Blood pressure management after acute spinal cord injury. *Neurosurgery.* 2002;50:S58.

48. The CRASH-2 Collaborators. Effects of tranexamic acid on death, vascular occlusive events, and blood transfusion in trauma patients with significant haemorrhage (CRASH-2): a randomised, placebo-controlled trial. *Lancet.* 2010;376:23–32.

49. Morrison JJ, Dubose JJ, Rasmussen TE, Midwinter MJ. Military Application of Tranexamic Acid in Trauma Emergency Resuscitation (MATTERs) Study. *Arch Surg.* 2012;147:113–119.

50. Velmahos GC, Demetriades D, Ghilardi M, et al. Life Support for Trauma and Transport: a mobile ICU for safe in-hospital transport of critically injured patients. *J Am Coll Surg.* 2004;199:62.

Suggested Reading

Allison KP, Gosling P, Jones S, et al. Randomized trial of hydroxyethyl starch versus gelatine for trauma resuscitation. *J Trauma.* 1999;47:1114.

American College of Surgeons (ACS) Committee on Trauma. Shock. In: *Advanced Trauma Life Support for Doctors, Student Course Manual.* 9th ed. Chicago, IL: ACS; 2012.

Moore EE. Blood substitutes: the future is now. *J Am Coll Surg.* 2003;196:1.

Novak L, Shackford SR, Bourgenignon P, et al. Comparison of standard and alternative prehospital resuscitation in uncontrolled hemorrhagic shock and head injury. *J Trauma.* 1999;47(5):834.

Proctor KG. Blood substitutes and experimental models of trauma. *J Trauma.* 2003;54:S106.

Revell M, Greaves I, Porter K. Endpoints for fluid resuscitation in hemorrhagic shock. *J Trauma.* 2003;54:S637.

Trunkey DD. Prehospital fluid resuscitation of the trauma patient: an analysis and review. *Emerg Med.* 2001;30(5):93.

SPECIFIC SKILLS

Intraosseous Vascular Access

Principle: To establish a vascular access site for fluids and medications when traditional IV access is unobtainable.

This technique may be performed in both adult and pediatric patients, using a variety of commercially available devices.

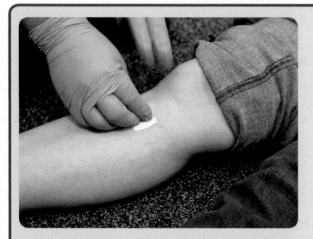

 Assemble the equipment, which includes intraosseous infusion needle, syringe filled with at least 5 ml of sterile saline, antiseptic, IV fluid and tubing, and tape. Ensure proper body substance isolation (BSI). Place the patient in a supine position.

The choice of insertion site may be the anterior tibia, in children or adults, or the sternum, which is used only in adults. For tibial insertion in adult patients, the insertion site is usually located at the anterior-medial distal tibia. For pediatric patients, the insertion site is the anterior-medial proximal tibia just below the tibial tuberosity. The prehospital care provider identifies the insertion site and landmarks. If the tibia is the insertion site, the lower extremity is stabilized by another prehospital care provider. Clean the insertion site area with an antiseptic.

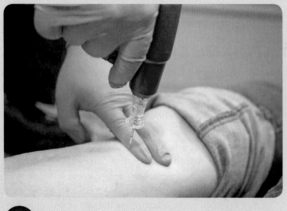

 Holding the drill and needle at a 90-degree angle to the selected bone, activate the drill and insert the rotating needle through the skin and into the bone cortex. A "pop" will be felt upon entering the bone cortex.

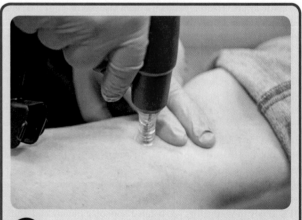

 When you feel a lack of resistance against the needle, release the trigger of the drill. While holding the needle, remove the drill from the needle.

Intraosseous Vascular Access (continued)

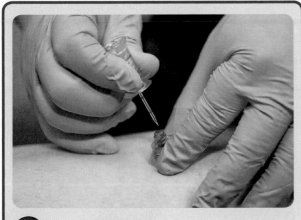

4 Release and remove the trocar from the center of the needle.

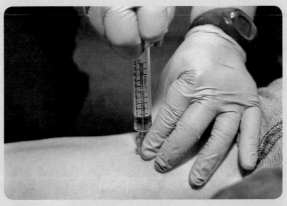

5 Attach the syringe with saline to the needle hub. Draw back with the syringe plunger slightly, looking for fluid from the marrow cavity to mix with the saline. "Dry" taps are not uncommon.

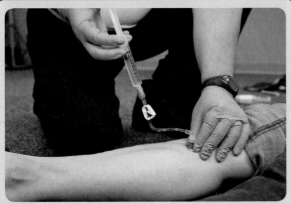

6 Next inject 5 ml of the saline, observing for signs of infiltration. If there are no signs of infiltration, remove the syringe from the needle hub, attach the IV tubing, and set the flow rate. Secure the needle and IV tubing.

Tourniquet Application

The Combat Application Tourniquet (C-A-T) is demonstrated in these photos. Any approved tourniquet may be used. Please note, the provider in the photos is not wearing gloves because he is demonstrating self-application of the C-A-T tourniquet to his own extremity. Proper PPE should always be worn during the assessment and treatment of a patient.

C-A-T Self-Application to an Upper Extremity

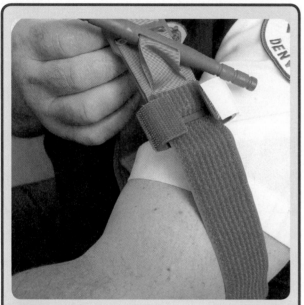

Courtesy of Peter T. Pons, MD, FACEP.

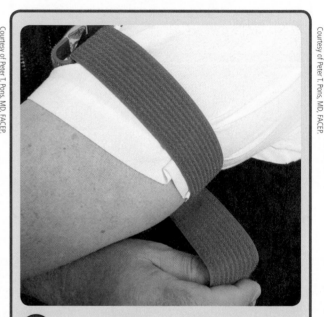

Courtesy of Peter T. Pons, MD, FACEP.

1. Insert the wounded extremity through the loop of the self-adhering band.

2. Pull the self-adhering band tight, and securely fasten it back on itself.

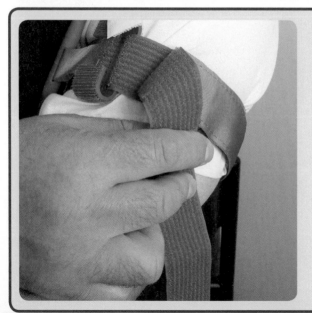

3. Adhere the band around the arm. Do not adhere the band past the clip.

Courtesy of Peter T. Pons, MD, FACEP.

Tourniquet Application (continued)

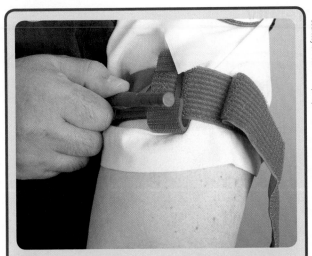

4 Twist the windlass rod until the bleeding stops (usually no more than three 180-degree turns).

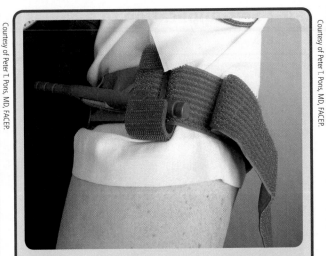

5 Lock the rod in place with the windlass clip.

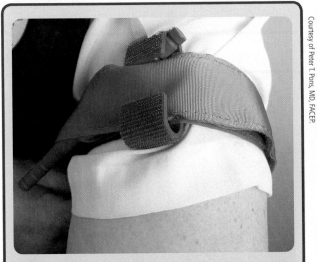

6 Adhere the band over the windlass rod. For small extremities, continue to adhere the band around the extremity.

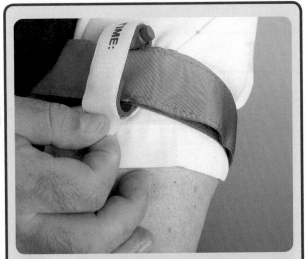

7 Secure the rod and band with the windlass strap. Grasp the strap, pull it tight, and adhere it to the opposite hook on the windlass clip.

Tourniquet Application (continued)

C-A-T Self-Application to a Lower Extremity

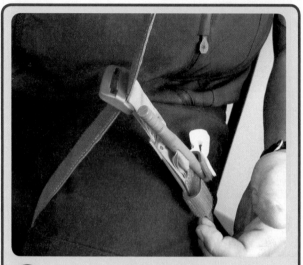

Courtesy of Peter T. Pons, MD, FACEP.

1 Pass the self-adhering band through the inside slit of the friction adapter buckle.

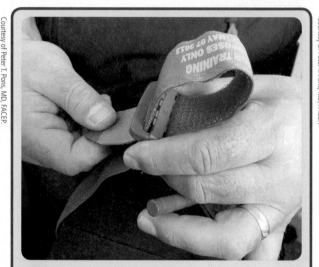

Courtesy of Peter T. Pons, MD, FACEP.

2 Pass the band through the outside slit of the friction adapter buckle, which will lock the band in place.

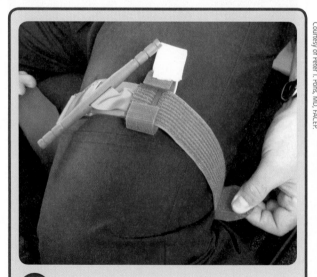

Courtesy of Peter T. Pons, MD, FACEP.

3 Pull the self-adhering band tight, and securely fasten it back on itself.

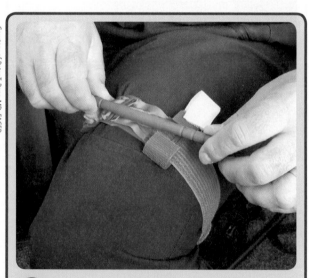

Courtesy of Peter T. Pons, MD, FACEP.

4 Twist the windlass rod until the bleeding stops (usually no more than three 180-degree turns).

Tourniquet Application (continued)

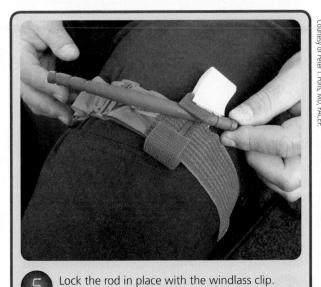

Courtesy of Peter T. Pons, MD, FACEP.

5 Lock the rod in place with the windlass clip.

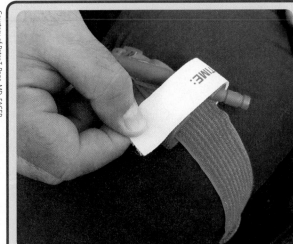

Courtesy of Peter T. Pons, MD, FACEP.

6 Secure the rod with the windlass strap. Grasp the strap, pull it tight, and adhere it to the opposite hook on the windlass clip.

Wound Packing With Topical Hemostatic Dressing or Plain Gauze

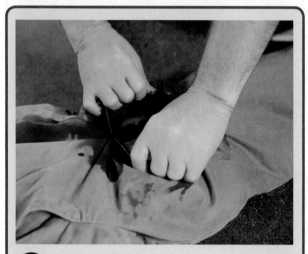

© Jones and Bartlett Learning. Photographed by Darren Stahlman.

1 Expose the wound.

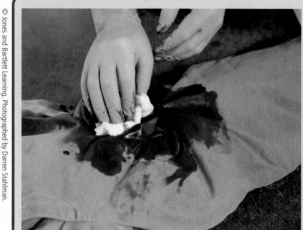

© Jones and Bartlett Learning. Photographed by Darren Stahlman.

2 Gently remove excess blood from the wound site while trying to preserve any clots that have formed. Locate the source of active bleeding in the wound (often at the base of the wound).

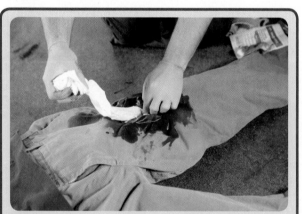

© Jones and Bartlett Learning. Photographed by Darren Stahlman.

3 Remove the selected dressing from its packaging and pack the entire dressing tightly into the wound, directly over the most active point of bleeding.

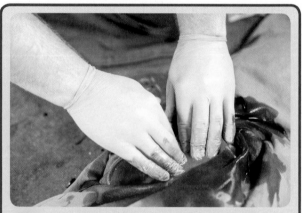

© Jones and Bartlett Learning. Photographed by Darren Stahlman.

4 Apply direct pressure onto the wound and packing for a minimum of 3 minutes or until bleeding has stopped.

Wound Packing With Topical Hemostatic Dressing or Plain Gauze (continued)

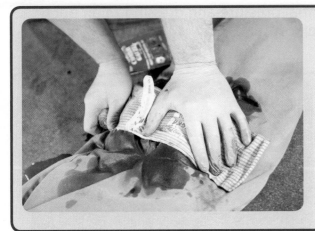

5 Reassess to ensure that bleeding has stopped. Wound may be repacked or a second dressing inserted into the wound if need to control continued bleeding. If bleeding is controlled, leave packing in place and apply a compression wrap around the wound to secure the dressing.

Pressure Dressing Using Israeli Trauma Bandage

Principle: To provide mechanical circumferential pressure and dressing to an open wound of an extremity with uncontrolled hemorrhage.

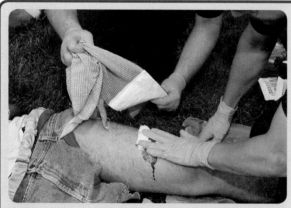
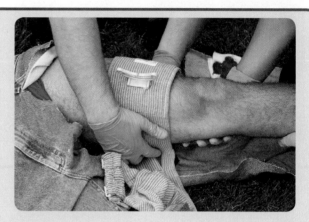

1 Ensure proper BSI and place the dressing pad over the wound.

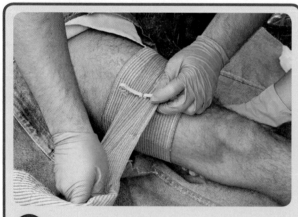
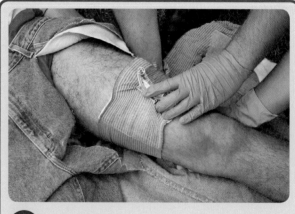

2 Wrap the elastic bandage around the extremity at least once.

3 Loop the elastic bandage through the bar.

Pressure Dressing Using Israeli Trauma Bandage (continued)

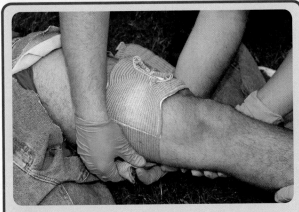

4 Wrap the bandage tightly around the wounded extremity in the opposite direction, applying enough pressure to control the bleeding.

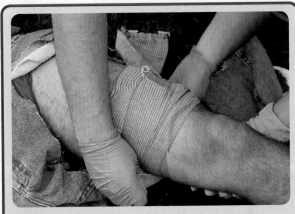

5 Continue wrapping the bandage around the extremity.

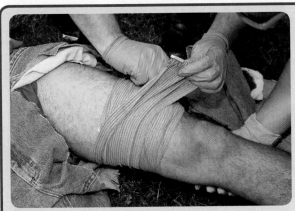

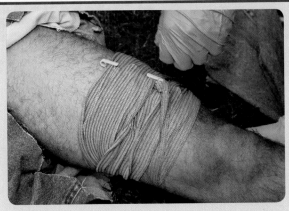

6 Secure the distal end of the bandage to maintain continued pressure to control the hemorrhage.

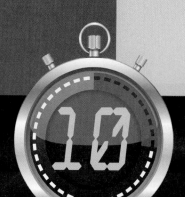

CHAPTER

Head Trauma

CHAPTER OBJECTIVES

At the completion of this chapter, the reader will be able to do the following:

- Relate the kinematics of trauma to the potential for traumatic brain injury (TBI).

- Incorporate the recognition of pathophysiologic manifestations and historical data significant for TBI into the assessment of the trauma patient to formulate a field impression.

- Formulate a plan of field intervention for both short and prolonged transport times for patients with TBI.

- Compare and contrast the pathophysiology, management, and potential consequences of specific types of primary TBI and secondary brain injury.

- Identify criteria for patient care decisions with regard to mode of transport, level of prehospital care, and hospital resources needed for the appropriate management of the TBI patient.

- Discuss the role of hyperventilation in the TBI patient.

SCENARIO

On an 85°F (29°C) summer day, you and your partner are dispatched to the finish line of a marathon race for a 30-year-old man who fell 14 feet (4.3 meters) off a ladder while attempting to secure the finish line banner. Upon your arrival, the patient is supine and unresponsive. A bystander is holding the patient's head and neck in-line.

You note an irregular breathing rate that increases and then decreases in depth. You also note that there is bloody fluid coming from both ears and both nostrils of the patient. The patient's airway is maintained with an oropharyngeal airway once absence of the gag reflex is noted. Your partner ventilates the patient with a bag-mask device at a rate of 12 breaths per minute. You notice that the patient's right pupil is dilated. The radial pulse is 54 and regular. Oxygen saturation (Spo$_2$) is 96%. The patient's skin is cool, dry, and pale. His Glasgow Coma Scale (GCS) score is calculated to be 7, with eyes = 2, verbal = 1, and motor = 4 (E2V1M4).

You rapidly prepare the patient for transport and place him into your ambulance to perform the secondary assessment while en route to the hospital. Palpation of the occiput generates a painful moan from the patient. You cover the patient with a warm blanket and measure his blood pressure, which is 184/102 mm Hg. An electrocardiogram reveals sinus bradycardia with infrequent premature ventricular beats noted. The right pupil remains widely dilated.

- What injury is most likely present given the patient's presenting signs?
- What are your management priorities at this point?
- What actions may you need to take to combat increased intracranial pressure and maintain cerebral perfusion during a prolonged transport?

Introduction

Of the 1.7 million traumatic brain injuries (TBIs) that occur annually in the United States, approximately 1.4 million patients present to the emergency department (ED).[1] Eighty percent of these patients are categorized as having only mild injuries, with about 75% of these patients diagnosed as having concussions. Approximately 275,000 patients with TBI are hospitalized annually, and about 52,000 patients with TBI die as a result of their injury.[1] TBI contributes significantly to the death of about half of *all* trauma victims. Moderate to severe brain injuries are identified in about 100,000 trauma patients annually. Mortality rates for moderate and severe brain injuries are about 10% and 30%, respectively. Of those who survive moderate or severe brain injuries, between 50% and 99% have some degree of permanent neurologic disability. Globally, it is estimated that the annual incidence of TBI is approximately 200 cases per 100,000 population (and this is likely an underestimate).[2]

Motor vehicle crashes remain the leading cause of TBI in patients between the ages of 5 and 65 years of age, and falls are the leading cause of TBI in pediatric patients up to the age of 4 years as well as in the elderly population. The head is the most frequently injured part of the body in patients with multisystem injuries. The incidence of gunshot wounds to the brain has increased in recent years in urban areas, and up to 60% of these victims die from their injury.

Patients with TBI represent some of the most challenging trauma patients to treat. They may be combative, and attempts to manage their airway can be extremely difficult because of clenched jaw muscles and vomiting. Intoxication with drugs or alcohol or the presence of shock from other injuries can hinder assessment. Occasionally, serious intracranial injuries can be present with only minimal external evidence of trauma. Skilled care in the prehospital setting focuses on ensuring the adequate delivery of oxygen and nutrients to the brain and rapidly identifying patients at risk for herniation and elevated intracranial pressure. This approach can not only decrease mortality from TBI, but also reduce the incidence of permanent neurologic disability.

Anatomy

Knowledge of head and brain anatomy is essential to understanding the pathophysiology of TBI. The scalp is the outermost covering of the head and offers some protection to the skull and brain. The scalp is comprised of several layers, including skin, connective tissue, **galea aponeurotica**, and the **periosteum** of the skull. The galea, a tough, thick fibrous tissue, is important because it provides the structural support to the scalp and is the key to its integrity. The scalp and soft tissues overlying the face are highly vascular and can bleed profusely when lacerated.

The skull, or cranium, is composed of a number of bones that fuse into a single structure during childhood (see Figure 7-12). Several small openings (**foramina**) through the base of the skull provide pathways for blood vessels and cranial nerves. One large opening, the **foramen magnum**, is located at the base of the skull and serves as a passageway for the brain stem to the spinal cord (**Figure 10-1**). In infants, "soft spots" (**fontanelles**) can often be

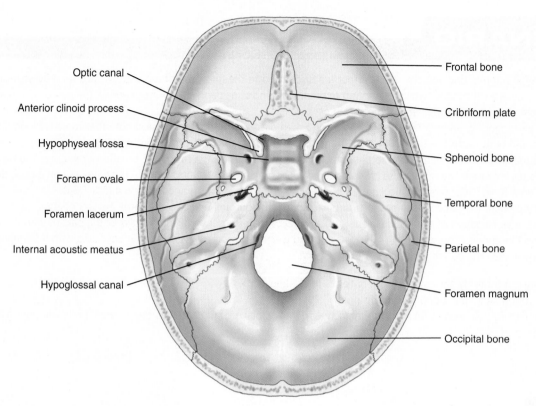

Figure 10-1   Internal view of the base of the skull.

identified between the bones. The infant has no bony protection over these portions of the brain until the bones fuse, typically by 2 years of age. In addition, because the infant's skull is not fused, hemorrhage within the skull can cause the bones to spread apart, allowing more blood to accumulate within the cranium.

The cranium provides significant protection to the brain. Although most of the bones forming the cranium are thick and strong, the skull is especially thin in the temporal and ethmoid regions; thus these locations are more prone to fracture. The bony structure of the skull is made up of two dense layers of bone separated by a layer of more porous bone. The two dense layers are referred to as the outer and inner tables of the skull. In addition, the interior surface of the skull base is rough and irregular (see Figure 10-1). When exposed to a blunt force, the brain may slide across these irregularities, producing cerebral contusions or lacerations.

Three separate membranes, the **meninges**, cover the brain (**Figure 10-2**). The outermost layer, the **dura mater**, is composed of tough fibrous tissue and is applied to the inner table, or inside, of the skull, similar to a laminate. Under normal circumstances, the space between the dura and the inside of the skull—the **epidural space**—does not exist; it is a potential space. The dura serves as a lining to the inside of the skull and, as such, there is normally no space between it and the skull. If something such as blood or an abscess were to develop between the skull and the dura, it could strip the dura away from the skull, thus creating an actual space. The middle meningeal arteries are

located in grooves in the temporal bones on either side of the head, outside the dura and just inside the inner table of the skull. A blow to the thin temporal bone can create a fracture and tear the middle meningeal artery, the common etiology for **epidural hematomas**.

Unlike the epidural space, which is a potential space, the subdural space is an actual space located beneath the dura mater and between it and the brain. This space is spanned in places by veins, which create a vascular communication between the skull and the brain. The traumatic rupture of these veins often creates **subdural hematomas**, which, unlike epidural hematomas, are venous, of lower pressure, and often associated with brain injury. Injury to these bridging veins accounts for the morbidity of subdural hematomas.

On the other side of the subdural space lies the brain, which is closely covered with two additional meningeal layers, the arachnoid and the pia. The **pia mater** is closely adhered to the brain, again similar to a laminate, and is the final brain covering. On top of the pia run cerebral blood vessels, which emerge from the base of the brain and then cover its surface. Layered on top of these blood vessels is the **arachnoid membrane**, which more loosely covers the brain and its blood vessels, giving the appearance of a "cellophane wrap" around the brain when it is viewed from the subdural space. Before cellophane existed, this covering was thought to resemble a spider web, thus the name "arachnoid." Because the cerebral blood vessels run on the surface of the brain but beneath the arachnoid membrane, their rupture

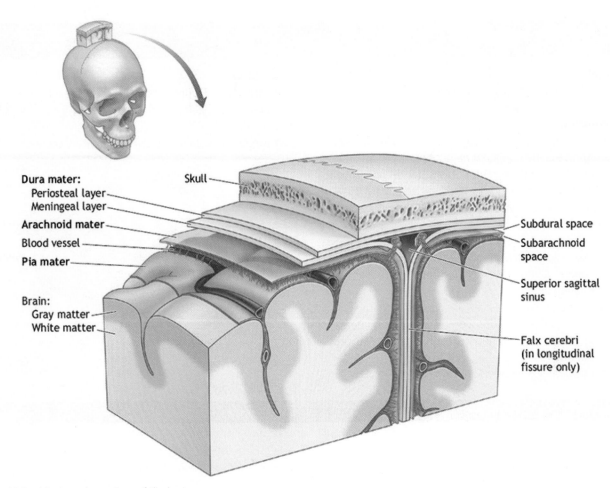

Figure 10-2 Meningeal coverings of the brain.

(usually from trauma or a ruptured cerebral aneurysm) will result in bleeding into the subarachnoid space, causing a subarachnoid bleed. This blood normally does not enter the subdural space but is contained beneath the arachnoid; it can be seen at surgery as a thin layer of blood on the surface of the brain, contained beneath this translucent membrane. Unlike epidural and subdural hematomas, subarachnoid blood does not normally create mass effect but can be symptomatic of other serious injury to the brain.

The brain occupies about 80% of the **cranial vault** and is divided into three main regions: the **cerebrum**, **cerebellum**, and **brain stem** (**Figure 10-3**). The cerebrum consists of right and left hemispheres that can be subdivided into several lobes. The cerebrum houses sensory functions, motor functions, and higher intellectual functions such as intelligence and memory. The cerebellum is located in the posterior fossa of the cranium, behind the brain stem and beneath the cerebrum, and coordinates movement. The brain stem contains the **medulla**, an area that controls many vital life functions, including breathing and heart rate. Much of the **reticular activating system**, the portion of the brain responsible for arousal and alertness, is also found in the brain stem. Blunt trauma can impair the reticular activating system, leading to a transient loss of consciousness.

The brain **parenchyma** occupies approximately 1,300 to 1,500 milliliters (ml) of volume, with an additional 100 to 150 ml of intravascular blood in the cranial vault. The brain also is surrounded by about 100 to 150 ml of **cerebrospinal fluid (CSF)**, which is produced in the ventricular system of the brain and also surrounds the spinal cord. CSF helps cushion the brain and is contained in the subarachnoid space as well. The brain tissue, blood, and CSF all combine to exert pressure against the skull. This pressure is referred to as the **intracranial pressure (ICP)**. Because the space within the cranium is fixed, anything that occupies additional space will cause the ICP to rise.

The **tentorium cerebelli**, a portion of the dura mater, lies between the cerebrum and the cerebellum and contains an opening—the **tentorial incisura**—at the level of the midbrain.

The 12 cranial nerves originate from the brain and brain stem (**Figure 10-4**). Cranial nerve III (**oculomotor nerve**) controls pupillary constriction. Cranial nerve III crosses the surface of the tentorium. Hemorrhage or edema that leads to downward herniation of the brain will compress the nerve, impairing its function, thus leading to pupil dilation. This finding is an important tool in the assessment of a patient with a suspected brain injury.

Figure 10-3   The Brain

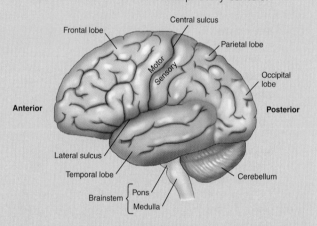

Cerebellum
Controls coordination and balance.

Cerebrum
The cerebrum is composed of the right and left cerebral hemispheres. The dominant hemisphere is the one that contains the language center. This is the left hemisphere in virtually all right-handed individuals and about 85% of left-handed individuals. The cerebrum is composed of the following lobes:

- *Frontal.* Contains emotions, motor function, and expression of speech on the dominant side.
- *Parietal.* Contains sensory function and spatial orientation.
- *Temporal.* Regulates certain memory functions; contains the area for speech reception and integration in all right-handed and the majority of left-handed individuals.
- *Occipital.* Contains vision.

Brain Stem
- **Midbrain** and upper pons. Contain the reticular activating system, which is responsible for arousal and alertness.
- *Medulla.* Contains the cardiorespiratory centers.

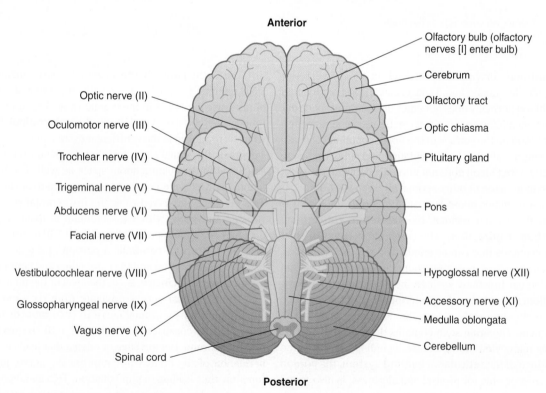

Figure 10-4   Inferior surface of the brain showing the origins of the cranial nerves.

Physiology

Cerebral Blood Flow

It is critical that the brain's neurons receive a constant flow of blood in order to provide oxygen and glucose. This constant cerebral blood flow is maintained by ensuring (1) an adequate pressure (cerebral perfusion pressure) to force blood through the brain and (2) a regulatory mechanism (autoregulation), which ensures a constant blood flow by varying the resistance to blood flow as the perfusion pressure changes.

Mean Arterial Pressure

The heart is a cyclic pump; thus the pressure created by the heart is represented by two pressure measurements. The diastolic pressure is the baseline pressure that is maintained within the circulatory system when the heart is resting and not pumping, and the **systolic pressure** is the maximum pressure generated at the peak of cardiac contraction. For the purposes of discussing cerebral blood flow and perfusion pressure, we use an average pressure for the entire cardiac cycle—the mean arterial pressure (MAP)—to characterize the pressure driving blood into the head.

Calculation of the MAP assumes that cardiac contraction (systole) takes up one-third of the cardiac cycle and that the remaining two-thirds of the cycle, the systemic pressure, remains at baseline (diastole). The pressure added to the circulatory system during systole is the pulse pressure. It is divided by three, since it is one-third of the entire cardiac cycle, and the result is added to the diastolic pressure, as follows:

Pulse pressure = Systolic pressure − Diastolic pressure

and

MAP = Diastolic pressure + 1/3 Pulse pressure

Most blood pressure monitors report the MAP with a much more accurate method of calculation that uses the actual blood pressure waveform. Because the percentage of time the heart spends in systole increases as the heart rate increases, the assumption that systole is one-third of diastole becomes less and less accurate as the patient becomes more tachycardic. Therefore, the blood pressure monitor, in the vast majority of patients being transported for neurologic injury, will more accurately represent the MAP than the preceding calculation.

Cerebral Perfusion Pressure

Cerebral perfusion pressure is the amount of pressure it takes to push blood through the cerebral circulation and, thus, maintain blood flow and oxygen and glucose delivery to the energy-demanding cells of the brain. Cerebral perfusion pressure relates directly to the patient's blood pressure and the amount of pressure inside the cranial vault, the ICP. It is expressed by the following formula:

Cerebral perfusion pressure = Mean arterial pressure − Intracranial pressure

or

CPP = MAP − ICP

Normal MAP ranges from about 85 to 95 mm Hg. In adults, ICP is normally below 15 mm Hg; in children, it is usually about 3 to 7 mm Hg; and in infants, it may range from 1.5 to 6.0 mm Hg.[1] Therefore, cerebral perfusion pressure is normally about 70 to 80 mm Hg. Sudden increases or decreases in blood pressure may affect cerebral perfusion.

As mentioned earlier in this chapter, because the space inside the skull is fixed in size, anything that occupies additional space within the cranial vault will cause the ICP to start to increase. This is termed *mass effect*. As the ICP increases, the amount of pressure needed to push blood through the brain also increases. If the MAP cannot keep up with the increase in ICP or if treatment to decrease the ICP is not rapidly instituted, the amount of blood flowing through the brain will start to decrease, leading to ischemic brain damage and impaired brain function.

Autoregulation of Cerebral Blood Flow

The most important factor for the brain, however, is not cerebral perfusion pressure itself, but rather cerebral blood flow. The brain works very hard at keeping its cerebral blood flow constant over a wide range of changing conditions. This process is known as **autoregulation**. Autoregulation is crucial to the brain's normal function.

To understand autoregulation, we need to remember that for any flowing system:

Pressure = Flow × Resistance

In the case of the brain, this translates into:

Cerebral perfusion pressure = Cerebral blood flow × Cerebral vascular resistance

or

CPP = CBF × CVR

Because the brain's principal concern is cerebral blood flow, it is useful to rewrite this equation as:

CBF = CPP/CVR

Looking at this equation, it is evident how the brain keeps blood flow constant. If a person changes position from lying down to standing up, the cerebral perfusion pressure will fall. The only way to keep the cerebral blood flow constant is to have the **cerebral vascular resistance** drop as well. The brain accomplishes this decline in cerebral vascular resistance by dilating the cerebral vasculature. The process of changing the caliber of the cerebral blood vessels to adjust cerebral vascular resistance to compensate for changes in cerebral perfusion pressure is how the brain accomplishes its autoregulation.

In people who stand up too quickly and faint, their autoregulatory mechanisms simply did not react quickly enough to their change in position, resulting in a temporary but dramatic loss of cerebral blood flow and, therefore, brain function.

To function normally, the autoregulatory mechanism must have a certain minimum pressure. Clearly, at a pressure of 0 mm Hg, no amount of vasodilation will cause blood to flow, and there are limits to how much the blood vessels in the head can dilate. Therefore, below a cerebral perfusion pressure of about 50 mm Hg, the autoregulatory mechanisms can no longer compensate for the decreased cerebral perfusion pressure, and cerebral blood flow starts to decrease. A reduction in cerebral blood flow can be compensated for by extracting more oxygen from the blood that is passing through the brain. The clinical signs and symptoms of ischemia (dizziness and altered mental status) will not be noticed until the diminished perfusion has exceeded the ability of increased oxygen extraction to meet the brain's metabolic needs.[3] Cerebral function, therefore, declines as cerebral blood flow begins to fall, and the risk of permanent cerebral injury from ischemia increases.

To make matters worse, injured brains often require higher-than-normal cerebral perfusion pressures to activate the autoregulatory mechanisms and keep cerebral blood flow adequate. Although each individual patient probably has his or her own cerebral perfusion pressure threshold above which cerebral blood flow is adequate, there is no way to determine this threshold in the field. Therefore, the best estimate of an adequate cerebral perfusion pressure is 60 to 70 mm Hg.

Unfortunately, the best ways to measure cerebral blood flow are not very convenient; therefore, cerebral perfusion pressure is used to estimate the adequacy of cerebral blood flow. Measuring cerebral perfusion pressure requires both a blood pressure monitor and an ICP monitor. In the absence of an ICP monitor, the best practice is simply to try to maintain a high normal MAP. Because most literature on outcomes from TBI has used systolic blood pressure instead of MAP to measure blood pressure, systolic blood pressure is the value used to monitor the adequacy of cerebral perfusion in settings without ICP monitoring. Best evidence currently suggests that a systolic blood pressure greater than 90 mm Hg is desirable for neurologically injured patients.[4-8]

Carbon Dioxide and Cerebral Blood Flow

The cerebral blood vessels respond to changes in arterial carbon dioxide levels by constricting or dilating. Decreased levels of carbon dioxide result in vasoconstriction, and elevated levels allow the vessels to dilate. Hyperventilation has been used to reduce ICP but also impacts cerebral blood flow. In fact, data suggest that hyperventilation more reliably reduces cerebral blood flow than ICP. Hyperventilation reduces the arterial carbon dioxide partial pressure ($PaCO_2$) by increasing the rate at which carbon dioxide is blown off by the lungs. This reduced $PaCO_2$ (hypocapnia) changes the acid–base balance in the brain, resulting in vasoconstriction. This cerebral vasoconstriction reduces the intravascular volume of the brain, reducing cerebral blood volume and, therefore, often ICP.[9,10]

Under normal circumstances, autoregulation ensures adequate cerebral blood flow by making sure that cerebral vascular resistance is correct for the available cerebral perfusion pressure to ensure continuing adequate cerebral blood flow. However, hyperventilation of a patient bypasses the autoregulation mechanisms of the brain. Thus, hyperventilation causes cerebral vasoconstriction, which may reduce cerebral blood volume enough to reduce ICP, but it also increases cerebral vascular resistance, regardless of whether cerebral perfusion pressure is adequate to maintain cerebral blood flow. As a result, hyperventilation can reduce cerebral blood flow, placing the injured brain at greater risk for ischemic injury. A $PaCO_2$ less than 35 mm Hg increases the risk of cerebral ischemia, and a $PaCO_2$ greater than the normal range of 35 to 45 mm Hg (hypercapnia) leads to dilation of cerebral arterioles, thus increasing cerebral blood flow while at the same time potentially increasing ICP. (Management of TBI using hyperventilation is discussed later in this chapter.)

Pathophysiology

TBI can be divided into two categories: primary and secondary.

Primary Brain Injury

Primary brain injury is the direct trauma to the brain and associated vascular structures that occurs at the time of the original insult. It includes contusions, hemorrhages, and lacerations and other direct mechanical injury to the brain, its vasculature, and its coverings. Because neural tissue does not regenerate well, there is minimal expectation of recovery of the structure and function lost due to primary injury. Also, little possibility exists for repair.

Secondary Brain Injury

Secondary brain injury refers to the ongoing injury processes that are set in motion by the primary injury. At the time of injury, pathophysiologic processes are initiated that continue to injure the brain for hours, days, and weeks after the initial insult. The primary focus in the prehospital (and hospital) management of TBI is to identify and limit or stop these secondary injury mechanisms. The secondary effects are insidious in nature. In most cases, there can be significant, ongoing damage occurring that is not immediately apparent or appreciated. By understanding what secondary injury is likely to occur as a result of the primary trauma, we can prepare for and intervene to correct or prevent these complications from occurring.

Before computed tomography (CT) was available, the principal secondary injury mechanism was "unidentified intracranial bleeds." The literature referred to "talk and die" patients, or those who were initially lucid after a traumatic insult but then lapsed into a coma and died as an unidentified intracranial hematoma expanded, leading to fatal herniation of the brain. Clearly, in these patients, if the initiated pathologic process could be recognized and interrupted, the patient's life could be saved.[11-13]

Pathologic mechanisms related to intracranial mass effect, elevated ICP, and herniation still are major concerns as causes of secondary injury, but their management has been revolutionized by CT, ICP monitoring, and immediate surgery. In the prehospital environment, the identification of patients at high risk for herniation from mass effect and their rapid transport to a hospital with the facilities to address these issues are still the key priorities.

With the advent of CT, it became easier to identify and treat these hematomas. However, it also became clear that other mechanisms besides hemorrhage or direct trauma were present and continued to injure the brain after injury. Large studies in the late 1980s demonstrated that unrecognized and untreated hypoxia and hypotension were as damaging to the injured brain as elevated ICP. Subsequent observations have shown that impaired delivery of oxygen or energy substrate (e.g., glucose) to the injured brain has a much more devastating impact than in the normal brain. Therefore, in addition to hematoma, two other sources of secondary injury are hypoxia and hypotension.[7,8,14-16]

Ongoing research in the laboratory is revealing a fourth class of secondary injury mechanisms—those occurring at the cellular level. Studies have identified multiple destructive cellular mechanisms that are initiated by injury. The ability to understand, manipulate, and stop these mechanisms may lead to new therapies to limit brain injury. At present, the study of these mechanisms is limited to the laboratory.

Secondary injury mechanisms include the following:

1. Mass effect and the subsequent elevated ICP and mechanical shifting of the brain, which can lead to herniation and significant morbidity and mortality if not addressed.
2. Hypoxia, which results from inadequate delivery of oxygen to the injured brain caused by ventilatory or circulatory failure or mass effect.
3. Hypotension and inadequate cerebral blood flow, which can cause inadequate oxygen delivery to the brain. Low cerebral blood flow also reduces delivery of energy substrate (e.g., glucose) to the injured brain and results in inadequate substrate (e.g., glucose).
4. Cellular mechanisms, including energy failure, inflammation, and "suicide" cascades, which can be triggered at the cellular level and can lead to cell death, called **apoptosis**.

Intracranial Causes of Secondary Brain Injury
Mass Effect and Herniation

The secondary injury mechanisms most often recognized are those related to mass effect. These mechanisms are the result of the complex interactions described by the Monro-Kellie doctrine.[17] The brain is encased within a space that is fixed in size once the fontanelles are closed, usually by age 2 years. All of the space within the cranium is taken up by brain, blood, or CSF. If any other mass, such as a hematoma, cerebral swelling, or a tumor, occupies space within the cranial vault, some other structure needs to be forced out (**Figure 10-5**).

The dynamics of forcing blood, CSF, and eventually brain out of the cranial vault in response to an expanding mass effect are the second part of the Monro-Kellie doctrine. At first, in response to the expanding mass, the volume of CSF surrounding the brain is reduced. The CSF naturally circulates within and around the brain, brain stem, and spinal cord; however, as the mass expands, more CSF is forced out of the head, and the total CSF volume within the skull is reduced. Blood volume in the cranial vault is also reduced in a similar manner, with venous blood the principal volume reduced in the head since it is low pressure.

As a result of the reduction of CSF and blood volumes, the pressure in the head does not rise during the early phases of the expansion of intracranial masses. During this phase, if the growing mass is the only intracranial pathology, patients can appear to be asymptomatic. Once the ability to force out CSF and blood has been exhausted, however, the pressure inside the cranium—the ICP—starts to rise rapidly and causes brain shift and various herniation syndromes, which can compress vital centers and jeopardize arterial blood supply to the brain (**Figure 10-6A**). The consequences of this movement toward the foramen magnum are described as the various herniation syndromes (**Figure 10-6B**).

If the expanding mass is along the convexity of the brain, as in the typical position for a temporal lobe epidural hematoma, the temporal lobe will be forced toward the center of the brain at the tentorial opening. This movement forces the medial portion of the temporal lobe, the **uncus**, into the third cranial nerve, the motor tract, and the brain stem and reticular activating system on that side. This condition is called **uncal herniation** and results in malfunction of the third cranial nerve, causing a dilated or blown pupil on the side of the herniation (**Figure 10-7**). It also results in loss of function of the motor tract on the same side, which causes weakness on the side of the body opposite from the lesion. In the last stages of uncal herniation, the reticular activating system is affected, and the patient lapses into coma, an event associated with a much poorer prognosis.

Some convexity masses lead to **cingulate herniation**, either in isolation or in conjunction with uncal herniation. In cingulate herniation, the cingulate gyrus located along the medial surface of the cerebral hemispheres is forced under the **falx**, the dural divider between the two hemispheres. This can cause injury to the medial cerebral hemispheres and the midbrain.

Another type of herniation, called **tonsillar herniation**, occurs as the brain is pushed down toward the foramen magnum

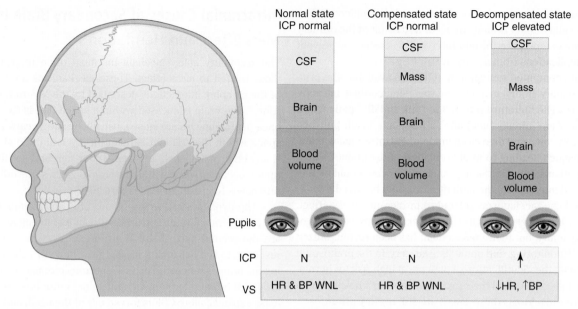

Figure 10-5 Monro-Kellie doctrine: intracranial compensation for expanding mass. The volume of the intracranial contents remains constant. If the addition of a mass such as a hematoma results in the squeezing out of an equal volume of CSF and venous blood, the ICP remains normal. However, when this compensatory mechanism is exhausted, an exponential increase occurs in ICP for even a small additional increase in the volume of the hematoma.

and pushes the cerebellum and medulla ahead of it. This can ultimately result in the most caudal (posterior) part of the cerebellum, the cerebellar tonsils, and the medulla becoming wedged in the foramen magnum, with the medulla subsequently being crushed. Injury to the lower medulla results in cardiac and respiratory arrest, a common final event for patients with herniation. The process of forcing the posterior fossa contents into the foramen magnum is referred to as "coning"[18] (**Figure 10-8**).

Clinical Herniation Syndromes

Clinical features of the herniation syndromes can help identify a patient who is herniating. Traditionally, as just mentioned, uncal herniation will often result in dilation or sluggishness of the **ipsilateral** pupil, referred to as a blown pupil. Abnormal motor findings can also accompany herniation. Contralateral weakness may be associated with uncal herniation due to compression of the pyramidal tract. This herniation may also lead to a positive finding in the adult of the Babinski reflex (extension of the great toe and fanning out of the other toes when the sole of the foot is stroked). More extensive herniation can result in destruction of structures in the brain stem known as the red nucleus or the **vestibular nuclei**. This can result in **decorticate posturing**, which involves flexion of the upper extremities and rigidity and extension of the lower extremities. A more ominous finding is **decerebrate posturing**, in which all extremities are extended and arching of the spine may occur. Decerebrate posturing occurs with injury and damage to the brain stem. After herniation, a terminal event may ensue and the extremities become flaccid, and motor activity is absent.[19,20]

In the final stages, herniation often produces abnormal ventilatory patterns or apnea, with worsening hypoxia and

significantly altered blood carbon dioxide levels. *Cheyne-Stokes ventilations* are a repeating cycle of slow, shallow breaths that become deeper and more rapid and then return to slow, shallow breaths. Brief periods of apnea may occur between cycles. **Central neurogenic hyperventilation** refers to consistently rapid, deep breaths, and ataxic breathing refers to erratic ventilatory efforts that lack any discernible pattern. Spontaneous respiratory function ceases with compression of the brain stem, a common final pathway for herniation (**Figure 10-9**).[18]

As tissue hypoxia develops in the brain, reflexes are activated in an effort to maintain cerebral oxygen delivery. To overcome rising ICP, the autonomic nervous system is activated to increase systemic blood pressure, and therefore the MAP, in an effort to maintain a normal cerebral perfusion pressure. Systolic pressures can reach up to 250 mm Hg. However, as the baroreceptors in the carotid arteries and aortic arch sense a greatly increased blood pressure, messages are sent to the brain stem to activate the parasympathetic nervous system. A signal then travels via the 10th cranial nerve, the vagus nerve, to slow the heart rate. **Cushing's phenomenon** refers to this ominous combination of greatly increased arterial blood pressure and the resultant bradycardia that can occur with severely increased ICP.

Ischemia and Herniation

The herniation syndromes describe how the swelling brain, because it is contained in a fully enclosed space, can sustain mechanical damage. However, elevated ICP from cerebral swelling can also cause injury to the brain by creating cerebral ischemia as well as the resulting decreased oxygen delivery. As cerebral swelling increases, ICP also increases. Because CPP = MAP − ICP, as ICP increases, cerebral perfusion pressure decreases. Increases

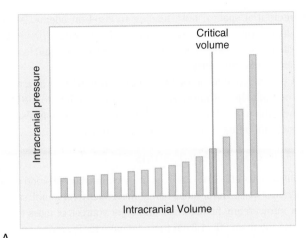

A

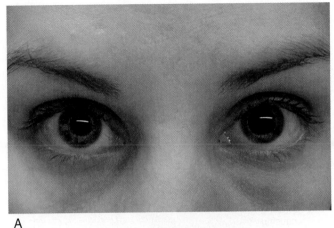

A

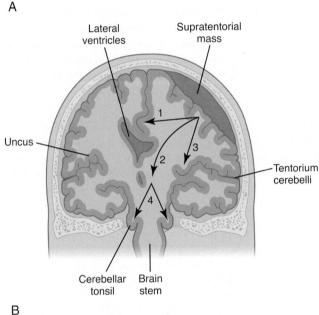

B

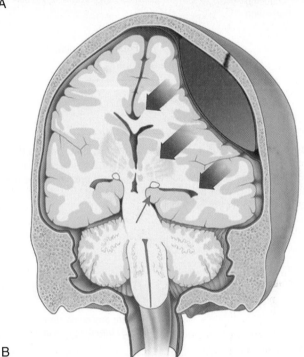

B

Figure 10-6 **A.** This graph demonstrates the relationship between intracranial volume and ICP. As the volume increases, the pressure remains relatively constant as CSF and blood are forced out. Finally a point is reached when no additional compensation can occur and ICP rises dramatically. **B.** This image demonstrates the various herniation syndromes that can result from mass effect and increased intracranial pressure. (1) Cingulate herniation (2) Central herniation (3) Uncal or transtentorial herniation (4) Cerebellotonsillar herniation.

Figure 10-7 **A.** Suspect injury to the brain whenever a patient's pupils are unequal in size. **B.** The pathophysiology of uncal herniation—as the hematoma expands, it pushes the uncus of the brain down against the tentorium, which in turn compresses cranial nerve III leading to pupillary dilation.

Source: A. Courtesy of Deborah Austin. B. Courtesy of the American College of Surgeons.

in ICP, therefore, threaten cerebral blood flow. In addition to mechanical injury to the brain, cerebral swelling also can cause ischemic injury to the brain, compounding the ischemic insults the brain might sustain from other causes, such as systemic hypotension.

To complicate matters further, as these mechanical and ischemic insults create injury to the brain, they create more cerebral swelling. In this way, cerebral edema can cause injury that creates more cerebral edema, which in turn leads to further injury and edema in a downward spiral that can lead to herniation and

death if not interrupted. Limiting this secondary injury and breaking this cycle of injury is the principal goal of TBI management.

Cerebral Edema

Cerebral edema (brain swelling) often occurs at the site of a primary brain injury. Injury to the neuronal cell membranes allows intracellular fluid to collect within damaged neurons, leading to cerebral edema. In addition, injury can lead to inflammatory responses that injure the neurons and the cerebral capillaries, leading to fluid collection within the neurons as well as within

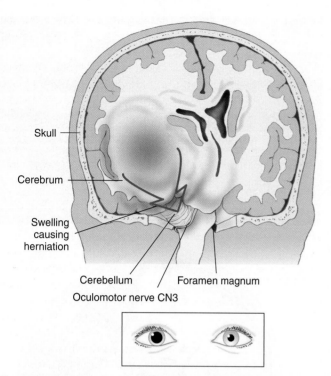

Figure 10-8 The skull is a large, bony structure that contains the brain. The brain cannot escape the skull if it expands because of edema or if there is hemorrhage in the skull that presses on the brain.

the interstitial spaces, both leading to cerebral edema. As the edema develops, the mechanical and ischemic injury previously described occurs, which aggravates these processes and leads to further edema and injury.

Cerebral edema can occur in association with or as a result of intracranial hematomas, as a result of direct injury to the brain parenchyma in the form of cerebral contusion, or as a result of diffuse brain injury from hypoxia or hypotension.

Intracerebral Hematomas

In trauma, mass effect results from the accumulation of blood in the intracranial space. Intracranial hematomas, such as epidural, subdural, or intracerebral hematomas, are major sources of mass effect. Because the mass effect from these hematomas is caused by their size, rapid removal of these hematomas can break the cycle of edema and injury described earlier. Unfortunately, these hematomas often have associated cerebral edema, and other interventions in addition to removing the hematoma are required to stop the cycle of injury and edema. (Specific cerebral hematomas are described later.)

Intracranial Hypertension

Intracranial hypertension results because cerebral edema occurs in an enclosed space. ICP is measured as a way to quantify and assess the degree of cerebral edema. ICP monitors are placed in the hospital to allow health care providers to quantify the

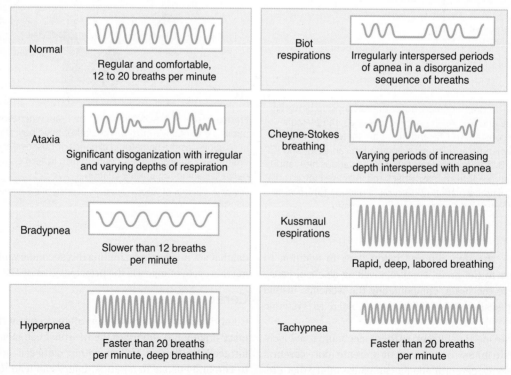

Figure 10-9 This image demonstrates the various types of breathing patterns that may occur after head and brain trauma.
Source: Modified from Mosby's Guide to Physical Examination, Seidel HM, Ball JW, Dains JE, et al. Copyright Elsevier (Mosby) 1999.

cerebral swelling, assess the risk of herniation, and monitor the effectiveness of therapies designed to combat cerebral edema. In this sense, elevated ICP is a sign of cerebral swelling.

Because elevated ICP, or intracranial hypertension, is part of the cycle previously described, it also causes cerebral injury in the form of mechanical compression of the brain and ischemic and hypoxic injury to the brain. For this reason, ICP is often discussed, correctly, both as a symptom and as a cause of cerebral edema.

ICP monitoring is not routinely available in the prehospital environment, but understanding it and the reasons for its control can help prehospital care providers with decision making for the brain-injured patient.

Extracranial Causes of Secondary Brain Injury

Hypotension

As has long been known, brain ischemia is common in head injury. Evidence of cerebral ischemia is found in 90% of the patients who die of TBI, and even many of the survivors have evidence of ischemic injury.[21] Therefore, the impact of low cerebral blood blow on the outcome from TBI has been a primary focus for limiting secondary injury after TBI.

In the national TBI database, the two most significant predictors of poor outcome from TBI were the amount of time spent with an ICP greater than 20 mm Hg and the time spent with a systolic blood pressure less than 90 mm Hg. In fact, a single episode of systolic blood pressure less than 90 mm Hg can lead to a poorer outcome.[22] Several studies have confirmed the profound impact of low systolic blood pressure on the outcome after TBI.

Many patients with TBI sustain other injuries, often involving hemorrhage and subsequent low blood pressure. Fluid resuscitation of these injuries in a focused effort to maintain systolic blood pressure between 90 and 100 mm Hg is essential to limiting the secondary injury to the brain that can result from failing to meet this goal.

In addition to hemorrhage, a second factor threatens cerebral blood flow after TBI, especially in the most severe injuries. A typical cortical cerebral blood flow is 50 ml per 100 grams (g) per minute (or 50 ml/100 g/minute) for each 100 g of brain tissue. After severe TBI, this value can drop to 30 ml or even as low as 20 ml/100 g/minute in the most severe injuries. Exactly why this decline in cerebral blood flow occurs is not clear. It may be caused by loss of autoregulation, or it may be a protective mechanism to try to downregulate the entire brain in response to injury. Whatever the cause, this effect—added to the impact of hemorrhagic shock—compounds the ischemic threat to the brain.[10,22,23]

In addition, as noted earlier, autoregulation in the injured brain is deranged. As a result, higher cerebral perfusion pressure is required to maintain adequate cerebral blood flow. Severely injured areas of the brain can lose almost all ability to autoregulate. In these areas, the blood vessels become dilated, causing hyperemia and shunting of blood toward the most severely injured brain areas and possibly away from areas that could still be saved by adequate perfusion.[24,25] Lastly, aggressive hyperventilation can further threaten cerebral blood flow and compound the ischemic threat by constricting blood vessels to compromised and unaffected areas of the brain.

This combination of physiologic downregulation, shunting, and hemorrhagic shock creates multiple ischemic threats to the salvageable areas of the brain and makes the aggressive management of hypotension an essential part of the management of TBI. For this reason, an aggressive approach in the prehospital environment, with fluid resuscitation aimed at keeping the systolic blood pressure above 90 mm Hg, is essential to limit secondary injury in the brain-injured patient.

Hypoxia

One of the most critical substrates delivered to the injured brain by the circulation is oxygen. Irreversible brain damage can occur after only 4 to 6 minutes of cerebral anoxia. Studies have also demonstrated a profound impact of an oxygen saturation of hemoglobin (SpO_2) less than 90% in TBI patients.[4,7,16] A significant number of TBI patients are not adequately resuscitated in the field.[16] In addition, several studies have demonstrated that significant numbers of TBI victims present with low or inadequate SpO_2, which in many cases is not easily recognized clinically unless measured with a pulse oximeter.[15] The emphasis on prehospital airway management and oxygen delivery for brain-injured patients has partly been the result of these studies.

Elegant work with brain-tissue-oxygen monitors has demonstrated the impact of hemorrhagic shock on oxygen delivery to the brain. Limiting hypotension is a key component in ensuring that the brain receives an adequate supply of oxygen during the postinjury phase.[26] Hemorrhage is common in patients with TBI, resulting not only in shock but also in loss of blood and, therefore, hemoglobin.

For oxygenated blood to be delivered to the brain, the lungs must be functioning properly, which often is not the case after trauma. Patients with an inadequate airway, aspiration of blood or gastric contents, pulmonary contusions, or hemopneumothoraces have pathology that will interfere with good respiratory function and the ability to transfer oxygen from the air to the blood. In addition to ensuring oxygen transport to the brain by minimizing blood loss and maintaining circulation, prehospital care providers must ensure adequate oxygenation through a patent airway and adequate ventilation.

As with hypotension, aggressive limitation of cerebral hypoxia with appropriate management of airway, breathing, and circulation is essential for limiting secondary brain injury.

Anemia

Also critical to the delivery of oxygen to the brain is the oxygen-carrying capacity of the blood, which is determined by the amount of hemoglobin it contains. A 50% drop in hemoglobin has a much more profound effect on oxygen delivery to the brain than a 50% drop in the partial pressure of oxygen (PO_2). For this reason, anemia from blood loss can impact the outcome of TBI.

Hypocapnia and Hypercapnia

As discussed earlier in this chapter, both hypocapnia (decreased $PaCO_2$) and hypercapnia (increased $PaCO_2$) can worsen brain injury. When cerebral blood vessels constrict, as results from significant hypocapnia, cerebral blood flow is compromised, leading to a decrease in oxygen delivery to the brain. Hypercapnia can result from hypoventilation from many causes, including drug or alcohol intoxication and abnormal ventilation patterns seen in patients with increased ICP. Hypercapnia causes cerebral vasodilation, which can further increase ICP.

Hypoglycemia and Hyperglycemia

Hypotension makes it highly likely that cerebral blood flow is also low. As cerebral blood flow falls, oxygen delivery to the brain also falls, as does delivery of glucose and other necessary brain metabolites. The effects of low systolic blood pressure and the physiology of low oxygen delivery to the brain have been well studied. However, the injured brain's use of glucose and the impact of glucose utilization and delivery on the injured brain are still the subjects of research.

The research available, however, offers a fascinating look into the brain's response to injury. It appears that after head injury, cerebral glucose metabolism can become deranged in complex ways. Some compelling evidence indicates that glucose metabolism and, therefore, cerebral glucose requirements actually increase after severe head injury, threatening a mismatch between glucose delivery and utilization.[27-29] On the other hand, good clinical and laboratory data in stroke patients show that patients whose serum glucose is allowed to remain elevated for long periods in the intensive care unit may have larger areas of infarction and less effective resuscitation of salvageable brain than patients whose glucose is better controlled. Limited studies seem to indicate that these same factors are present in the ischemia that occurs after head injury. Elevated blood glucose levels in patients with TBI have also been associated with poorer neurologic outcome.

Both elevations (hyperglycemia) and decreases (hypoglycemia) in blood sugar can jeopardize ischemic brain tissue. The disastrous impact of significant hypoglycemia on the nervous system, during injury and at other times, is well known. Neurons are unable to store sugar and require a continual supply of glucose to carry out cellular metabolism. In the absence of glucose, ischemic neurons can be permanently damaged. However, it is also true that a prolonged serum glucose level greater than 150 mg/dl, and probably greater than 200 mg/dl, may be harmful to the injured brain and should be avoided.[30,31]

In the prehospital environment, the emphasis should be on avoiding hypoglycemia because the physiologic threat from low sugar is much more immediate than the danger from elevated serum glucose. Blood-glucose measurement should be performed in the field, if available, in all patients with altered mentation and, if found to be below normal values, treated with glucose administration. In addition, any induced hyperglycemia is likely to be transient, and the tight glucose control required to manage these patients properly will be established upon admission to the hospital.

Seizures

A patient with acute TBI is at risk for seizures for several reasons. Hypoxia from either airway or breathing problems can induce generalized seizure activity, as can hypoglycemia and electrolyte abnormalities. Ischemic or damaged brain tissue can serve as an irritable focus to produce **grand mal seizures** or **status epilepticus**. Seizures, in turn, can aggravate pre-existing hypoxia caused by impairment of respiratory function. Additionally, the massive neuronal activity associated with generalized seizures rapidly depletes oxygen and glucose levels, further worsening cerebral ischemia.

Assessment

A quick survey of the kinematics of the injury, combined with a rapid primary assessment, will help identify potential life-threatening problems in a patient with a suspected TBI. Because the pathophysiology of TBI is a dynamic process, so too must the assessment and management be. It is critical to continually reassess the TBI patient, perhaps more often than usual, because the examination findings may fluctuate significantly as the condition of the patient changes over time.

Kinematics

As with all trauma patients, assessment must include consideration of the mechanism of injury. Because many patients with severe TBI have an altered level of consciousness (LOC), key data about the kinematics will frequently come from observation of the scene or from bystanders. The windshield of the patient's vehicle may have a "spider web" pattern, suggesting an impact with the patient's head, or a bloody object may be present that was used as a weapon during an assault. A lateral impact on the side of the head can cause fracture of the temporal bone of the skull with injury to the underlying middle meningeal artery leading to epidural hematoma, or it may cause a **coup or contrecoup injury** with venous damage and subdural hemorrhage. This important information should be reported to personnel at the receiving facility because it may be essential for proper diagnosis and management of the patient, not only as it relates to possible brain injury but also for other injuries.

Primary Assessment
Airway

The patency of the patient's airway should be examined and ensured. In unconscious individuals, the tongue may completely occlude the airway. Noisy ventilations indicate partial obstruction by either the tongue or foreign material. Emesis, hemorrhage, and swelling from facial trauma are common causes of airway compromise in patients with TBI.

Breathing

Evaluation of respiratory function must include an assessment of the rate, depth, and adequacy of breathing. As noted previously, several different breathing patterns can result from severe brain injury. In multisystem trauma patients, thoracic injuries can further impair both oxygenation and ventilation. Cervical spine fractures occur in about 2% to 5% of patients with TBI and may result in spinal cord injuries that significantly interfere with ventilation.

Adequate oxygen delivery to the injured brain is an essential part of the effort to limit secondary brain injury. Failure to keep the SpO_2 above 90% appears to result in poorer outcomes for brain-injured patients; maintaining SpO_2 above 90% is critical. Assessing for adequate airway and ventilatory effort is crucial in the early stages of managing TBI.

Circulation

As noted previously, maintaining a systolic blood pressure greater than 90 mm Hg is critical for limiting secondary brain injury in the victims of TBI. Therefore, the control of hemorrhage and the prevention and treatment of shock are critical. The prehospital care provider should note and quantify evidence of external bleeding, if possible, and control the hemorrhage rapidly. In the absence of significant external blood loss, a weak, rapid pulse in a victim of blunt trauma suggests life-threatening internal hemorrhage in the pleural spaces, **peritoneum**, **retroperitoneum**, or soft tissues surrounding long-bone fractures. In an infant with open fontanelles, sufficient blood loss can occur inside the cranium to produce hypovolemic shock.

Increased ICP can lead to a recognized series of cardiovascular changes. As ICP rises and cerebral blood flow is affected, the brain and brain stem become hypoxic. This causes stimulation of the sympathetic nervous system in an effort to raise blood pressure. With the increase in blood pressure, the parasympathetic system slows the heart; thus bradycardia becomes manifest. This effect is known as Cushing's reflex. Cushing's triad describes the combination of findings that occur with increased ICP: a slow pulse, increased blood pressure associated with a widened pulse pressure, and irregular respirations, such as Cheyne-Stokes breathing.[32] A slow, forceful pulse may be the result of intracranial hypertension and may indicate impending herniation (Cushing's phenomenon). In a patient with potentially life-threatening injuries, transport should not be delayed to measure blood pressure; it should be performed en route as time permits.

Disability

During the primary assessment and after the initiation of appropriate measures to treat problems identified in the airway, breathing, and circulation assessments, a baseline Glasgow Coma Scale (GCS) score should be calculated to assess the patient's LOC accurately (**Figures 10-10** and **10-11**). As described in the Patient Assessment and Management chapter, the GCS score is calculated by using the best response noted when evaluating the patient's eyes, verbal response, and motor response. Each component of the score should be recorded individually, rather than just providing a total, so that specific changes can be noted over time. If a patient lacks spontaneous eye opening, a verbal command (e.g., "Open your eyes") should be used. If the patient does not respond to a verbal stimulus, a painful stimulus, such as nail bed pressure with a pen or squeezing of anterior axillary tissue, should be applied.

The patient's verbal response can be examined using a question such as, "What happened to you?" If fully oriented, the patient will supply a coherent answer. Otherwise, the patient's verbal response is scored as confused, inappropriate, unintelligible, or absent. If the patient is intubated, the score is calculated from only the eye and motor scales, and a "T" is added to note the inability to assess the verbal response, such as "8T."

The last component of the GCS is the motor score. A simple, unambiguous command should be given to the patient, such as, "Hold up two fingers" or "Show me a hitchhiker's sign." A patient

Figure 10-10 Glasgow Coma Scale

Evaluation	Points
Eye Opening	
Opens eyes spontaneously	4
Opens eyes on command	3
Opens eyes to painful stimulus	2
Does not open eyes	1
Best Verbal Response	
Answers appropriately (oriented)	5
Gives confused answers	4
Gives inappropriate response	3
Makes unintelligible noises	2
Makes no verbal response	1
Best Motor Response	
Follows command	6
Localizes painful stimuli	5
Withdraws from pain (nonlocalizing movement to pain)	4
Responds with abnormal flexion to painful stimuli (decorticate)	3
Responds with abnormal extension to pain (decerebrate)	2
Gives no motor response	1

Note that the lowest possible score is 3 and the highest possible score is 15.

Figure 10-11 Pediatric Glasgow Coma Scale

Activity	Score	Infant	Score	Child
Eye opening	4	Open spontaneously	4	Open spontaneously
	3	Open to speech or sound	3	Open to speech
	2	Open to painful stimuli	2	Open to painful stimuli
	1	No response	1	No response
Verbal	5	Coos, babbles	5	Oriented conversation
	4	Irritable cry	4	Confused conversation
	3	Cries to pain	3	Cries
	2	Moans to pain		Inappropriate words
	1	No response	2	Moans
				Incomprehensible words/sounds
			1	No response
Motor	6	Normal spontaneous movement	6	Obeys verbal commands
	5	Localizes pain	5	Localizes pain
	4	Withdraws to pain	4	Withdraws to pain
	3	Abnormal flexion (decorticate)	3	Abnormal flexion (decorticate)
	2	Abnormal extension (decerebrate)	2	Abnormal extension (decerebrate)
	1	No response (flaccid)	1	No response (flaccid)

who squeezes the finger of a prehospital care provider may simply be demonstrating a grasping reflex as opposed to following a command purposefully. A painful stimulus is used if the patient fails to follow a command, and the patient's best motor response is scored. A patient who attempts to push away a painful stimulus is considered to be "localizing." Other possible responses to pain include withdrawal from the stimulus, abnormal flexion (decorticate) or extension (decerebrate) of the upper extremities, and absence of a motor function.

It is generally accepted that a score of 13 to 15 likely indicates a mild TBI while a score of 9 to 12 is indicative of moderate TBI. A GCS score of 3 to 8 suggests severe TBI. Of course, many other factors can affect the GCS, including the presence of intoxicants or other drugs. In addition, a patient who is dead still has a score of 3. In addition to determining the GCS, the pupils are examined quickly for symmetry and response to light. In adults, the resting pupil diameter is generally between 3 and 5 mm.[33] A difference of greater than 1 mm in pupil size is considered abnormal. A significant portion of the population has **anisocoria**, inequality of pupil size, which is either congenital or acquired as the result of ophthalmic trauma. It is not always possible in the field to distinguish between pupillary inequality caused by trauma and congenital or pre-existing posttraumatic anisocoria. Pupillary inequality should always be treated as secondary to the acute trauma until the appropriate workup has ruled out cerebral edema or motor or ophthalmic nerve injury.[34]

Expose/Environment

Patients who have sustained a TBI frequently have other injuries, which threaten life and limb as well as the brain. All such injuries must be identified. The entire body should be examined for other potentially life-threatening problems.

Secondary Assessment

Once life-threatening injuries have been identified and managed, a thorough secondary assessment should be completed if time permits during transport of the patient to an appropriate receiving facility. The patient's head and face should be palpated carefully for wounds, depressions, and **crepitus**.

Any drainage of clear fluid from the nose or ear canals may be CSF. In most cases, however, the CSF will be mixed with blood, making formal recognition of this finding difficult. One method that is often suggested is to place a drop of the suspected blood–CSF mixture onto a gauze pad. When placed on a gauze pad or white cloth, CSF may diffuse out from blood, producing a characteristic yellowish "halo."[35] If time permits, this test may be attempted during transport; however, there are many false positive results, thus limiting its usefulness.

The pupillary size and response should be rechecked at this time. Because of the incidence of associated cervical spine fractures in patients with TBI, as noted previously, the neck should be examined for tenderness and bony deformities.

The single most important observation is assessment of the patient's mental status and how it is changing in the time you are with the individual. Patients who were initially found with an impaired mental status but are improving are much less concerning than those patients whose mental status deteriorates during your management and transport.

In a cooperative patient, a more thorough neurologic examination may also be performed. This will include assessing the cranial nerves, sensation, and motor function in all extremities. Looking for complete or partial deficits as well as asymmetry in function may reveal important clues to a possible neurologic injury. Findings such as **hemiparesis** (weakness) or **hemiplegia** (paralysis), present on only one side of the body, are considered "lateralizing signs" and usually are indicative of TBI.

History

A SAMPLE history (*s*ymptoms, *a*llergies, *m*edications, *p*ast history, *l*ast meal, *e*vents) can be obtained from the patient, family members, or bystanders if time and circumstances allow. Diabetes mellitus, seizure disorders, and drug or alcohol intoxication can mimic TBI. Any evidence of drug use or overdose should be noted. The patient may have a history of prior head injury and may complain of persistent or recurring headache, visual disturbances, nausea and vomiting, or difficulty speaking.[36]

Serial Examinations

It is important to re-evaluate the GCS and determine what changes are occurring over time. The patient who initially presented with a GCS score that is now decreasing is of much greater concern for serious TBI than a patient who has an improving GCS score. About 3% of patients with apparently mild brain injury (GCS 14 or 15) may experience an unexpected deterioration in their mentation. During transport, both the primary assessment and assessment of the GCS should be repeated at frequent intervals. Patients whose GCS deteriorates by more than two points during transport are at particularly high risk for an ongoing pathologic process.[34,37,38] These patients need rapid transport to an appropriate facility. The receiving facility will use GCS trends during transport in the patient's early management. Trends in the GCS or vital signs should be reported to the receiving facility and documented on the patient care report. Responses to management should also be recorded.[39]

Specific Head and Neck Injuries

Scalp Injuries

As noted in the anatomy section, the scalp is comprised of multiple layers of tissue and is highly vascular; even a small laceration may result in copious hemorrhage. More complex injuries, such as a degloving injury, in which a large area of the scalp is torn back from the skull, can result in hypovolemic shock and even **exsanguination** (**Figure 10-12**). These types of injury often occur in an unrestrained front-seat occupant of a vehicle whose head impacts the windshield, as well as in workers whose long hair becomes caught in machinery. A serious blow to the head may result in the formation of a scalp hematoma, which may be confused with a depressed skull fracture while palpating the scalp.

Skull Fractures

Fractures of the skull can result from either blunt or penetrating trauma. Linear fractures, usually resulting from blunt trauma, account for about 80% of skull fractures; however, a powerful impact may produce a *depressed* skull fracture, in which fragments of bone are driven toward or into the underlying brain tissue (**Figure 10-13**). Although simple linear fractures can be diagnosed only with a radiographic study, depressed skull fractures can often be palpated during a careful physical examination. A closed, nondepressed skull fracture by itself is of little clinical significance, but its presence increases the risk of an intracranial hematoma. Closed, depressed skull fractures may require neurosurgical intervention. Open skull fractures can result from a particularly forceful impact or from a gunshot wound and serve as an entry site for bacteria, predisposing the patient to meningitis. If the dura mater is torn, brain tissue or CSF may leak from an open skull fracture. Because of the risk of meningitis, these wounds require immediate neurosurgical evaluation.

Basilar skull fractures (fractures of the floor of the cranium) should be suspected if CSF is draining from the nostrils or ear canals. **Periorbital ecchymosis** ("raccoon eyes") and Battle's sign, in which ecchymosis is noted over the mastoid area behind the ears, often occur with basilar skull fractures, although they may take several hours after injury to become apparent. If permitted, examination of the tympanic membrane with an otoscope may reveal blood behind the eardrum, indicating a basilar skull fracture.

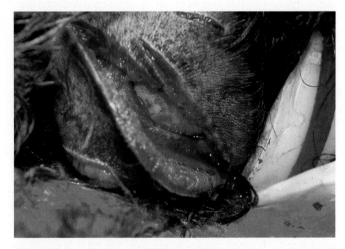

Figure 10-12 Extensive scalp injuries may result in massive external hemorrhage.
Source: Courtesy of Peter T. Pons, MD, FACEP.

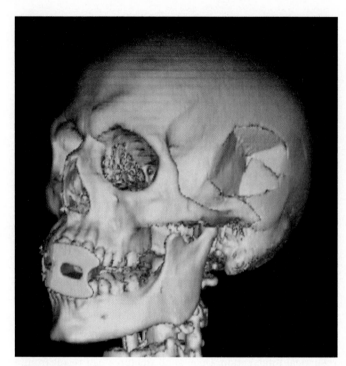

Figure 10-13 A three-dimensional reconstruction of a depressed skull fracture after an assault.
Source: Courtesy of Peter T. Pons, MD, FACEP.

Facial Injuries

Injuries to the face range from minor soft tissue trauma to severe injuries associated with airway compromise or hypovolemic shock. The airway may be compromised by either structural damage or anatomic distortion resulting from the trauma or from fluid or other objects in the airway itself. Structural changes may result from deformities of fractured facial bones or from hematomas that develop in the tissues. Because the head has a high concentration of blood vessels, many injuries to this region result in significant hemorrhage. Blood and blood clots may interfere with the patency of the airway. Facial trauma is often associated with alterations in consciousness and potentially severe trauma to the brain. Trauma to the face may result in fractures or displacement of teeth into the airway lumen. TBIs and swallowed blood from facial injuries may lead to vomiting, which also may lead to airway obstruction.

Trauma to the Eye and Orbit

Injury to the structures of the orbit and eye are common and often result from direct trauma to the face, either from intentional (assault) or unintentional causes. Although injury of the globe (eyeball) itself is not often encountered, it must be considered whenever trauma to the face and orbit is noted, as proper management of a globe injury may result in salvage of the patient's vision.

Eyelid Laceration

In the prehospital setting, laceration of an eyelid must cause consideration of the possibility that the globe itself has been penetrated. Field treatment consists of immediately covering the eye with a protective rigid shield (**NOT** a pressure patch) that is placed over the bony orbit. The primary consideration is to avoid any pressure on the eye that might do further harm by forcing intraocular contents out through a corneal or scleral laceration.

Corneal Abrasion

A corneal abrasion is disruption of the protective **epithelial** covering of the cornea. This abrasion results in intense pain, tearing, light sensitivity (photophobia), and increased susceptibility to infection until the defect has healed (usually in 2 to 3 days). There is typically a history of **antecedent** trauma or contact lens use. Prehospital management for this disorder is to cover the eye with a patch, shield, or sunglasses to reduce the discomfort caused by light sensitivity.

Subconjunctival Hemorrhage

Subconjunctival hemorrhage over the sclera of the eye results from bleeding between the **conjunctiva** and the **sclera** (**Figure 10-14**). It is easily visible without the use of any diagnostic equipment. This injury is innocuous and resolves over a period of several days to several weeks without treatment. In the presence of antecedent trauma, one should be alert for another, more serious injury. In particular, if hemorrhage results in massive swelling of the conjunctiva (**chemosis**), an occult globe rupture should be suspected. Prehospital management of this disorder consists solely of transporting the patient to the hospital so that the diagnosis can be confirmed and other associated disorders ruled out.

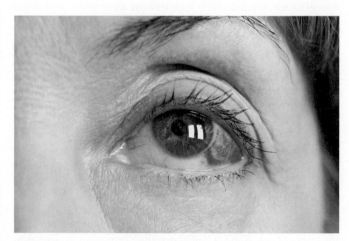

Figure 10-14 Subjunctival hemorrhage.
Source: © Susan Law Cain/ShutterStock, Inc.

Hyphema

The term **hyphema** refers to blood in the anterior chamber of the globe between the **iris** and the **cornea**. This condition is usually seen in the setting of acute trauma from a direct blow to the eye. The eye should be examined with the victim sitting upright. If enough blood is present, it collects at the bottom of the anterior chamber and is visible as a layered hyphema (**Figure 10-15**). This blood may not be appreciated if the victim is examined while in a supine position or if the amount of blood is very small. Hyphema patients should have a protective shield placed over the eye and be transported to the hospital in a sitting position (if there is no other contraindication) so that a complete eye examination can be performed.

Open Globe

If there is a history of trauma and penlight inspection of the eye reveals an obvious **open globe** (wound that goes through the cornea or sclera into the interior of the eyeball), the remainder of the physical examination of the eye should be discontinued and a protective shield immediately placed onto the bony orbit over the eye to protect it from further injury. Do **NOT** apply a pressure patch or instill any topical medication.

There are two primary concerns in the management of this condition. The first is to minimize manipulation of or additional trauma to the eye that might raise intraocular pressure and result in expulsion of intraocular contents through the corneal or scleral defect. The second is to prevent development of **posttraumatic endophthalmitis**, an infection of the **aqueous** humor and the **vitreous humor** of the eye. This typically has devastating visual results, with only 30% of victims in one study retaining visual acuity greater than or equal to 20/400. Expeditious transport to the hospital is warranted for ophthalmologic evaluation and surgical repair.

A penetrating injury to the eye or a ruptured globe may not always be obvious. Clues to occult rupture include large subconjunctival hemorrhage with chemosis, dark uveal tissue (the colored iris) present at or protruding through the limbus (junction

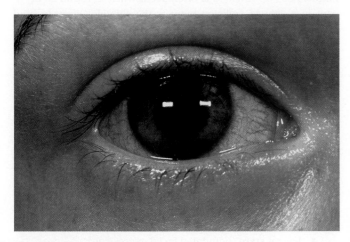

Figure 10-15 Hyphema.
Source: © Dr. Chris Hale/Science Source.

of the cornea and the sclera), distorted pupil (teardrop shaped), leak from a lacerated or punctured wound of the cornea, mechanism of injury (hammering metal on metal, impaling injury, etc.), or decrease in vision. If an occult globe rupture is suspected, the patient should be treated as described previously for an obvious open globe. The relatively less severe appearance of the injury does not eliminate the threat of endophthalmitis, so again rapid transport to the hospital is warranted.

Nasal Fractures

Fracture of the nasal bones is the most common fracture in the face. Indications that a nasal fracture is present include **ecchymosis**, **edema**, nasal deformity, swelling, and epistaxis (nosebleed). On palpation, bony crepitus may be noted.

Fracture of the cribriform plate (the thin, horizontal bone in the skull through which the olfactory [cranial nerve 1] nerve passes) may also present after a high-force midface trauma mechanism of injury in addition to causing nasal bone fracture. Any clear rhinorrhea (CSF leak from the nose) occurring after significant force to the midface is significant for possible cribriform plate fracture.

Midface Fractures

Midfacial fractures can be categorized as follows (**Figure 10-16**):

- *Le Fort I fracture* involves a horizontal detachment of the maxilla from the nasal floor. Although air passage through the nares (nostrils) may not be affected, the oropharynx may be compromised by a blood clot or edema in the soft palate.
- *Le Fort II fracture*, also known as a pyramidal fracture, includes the right and left maxillae, the medial portion of the orbital floor, and the nasal bones. The sinuses are well vascularized, and this fracture may be associated with airway compromise from significant hemorrhage.
- *Le Fort III fracture* involves the facial bones being fractured off the skull (craniofacial disjunction). Because of the forces involved, this injury may be associated with airway compromise, presence of TBI, injuries to the tear ducts, malocclusion (misalignment) of teeth, and CSF leakage from the nares.

Patients with a midface fracture generally have loss of normal facial symmetry. The face may appear flattened, and the patient may be unable to close the jaws or teeth. If conscious, the patient may complain of facial pain and numbness. On palpation, crepitus may be noted over fracture sites.

Mandibular Fractures

Following fractures of the nasal bones, mandibular fractures are the second most common type of facial fracture. In more than 50% of cases, the mandible (jawbone) is broken in more than one location. The most common complaint of a patient with a

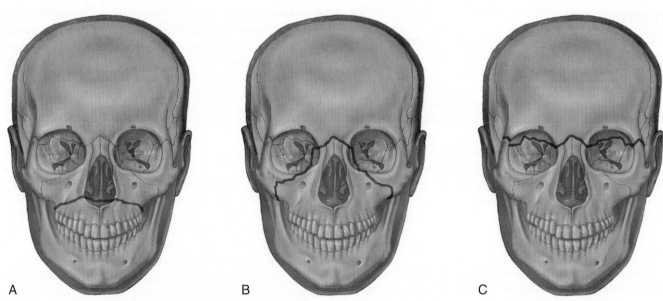

A   B   C

Figure 10-16 Types of Le Fort fractures of the midface. **A.** Le Fort I fracture. **B.** Le Fort II fracture. **C.** Le Fort III fracture.
Source: Modified from Sheehy S. *Emergency Nursing.* 3rd ed. St. Louis, MO: Mosby; 1992.

mandibular fracture, in addition to pain, is malocclusion of the teeth; that is, the upper and lower teeth no longer meet in their usual alignment. Visual examination may reveal a step-off or misalignment of the teeth. On palpation, a step-off type of deformity and crepitance may be noted.

In a supine patient with a mandible fracture, the tongue may occlude the airway as the bony support structure of the tongue is no longer intact.

Laryngeal Injuries

Fractures of the larynx typically result from a blunt blow to the anterior neck, such as when a motorcycle or bicycle rider's anterior neck is struck by an object. The patient may complain of a change in voice (usually lower in tone). On inspection, the prehospital care provider may note a neck contusion or loss of the prominence of the thyroid cartilage (Adam's apple). A fracture of the larynx may result in the patient coughing up blood (hemoptysis) or the development of subcutaneous emphysema in the neck, which may be detected on palpation. Endotracheal intubation is generally contraindicated in the presence of a laryngeal fracture because this procedure may dislodge fracture segments. If a patient with a suspected laryngeal fracture has a compromised airway, a surgical cricothyrotomy may be lifesaving.

Injuries to Cervical Vessels

A carotid artery and internal jugular vein traverse the anterior neck on either side of the trachea. The carotid arteries supply blood to the majority of the brain, and the internal jugular veins drain this region. Open injury to one of these vessels can produce profound hemorrhage. An added danger from internal jugular vein injuries is air embolism. If a patient is sitting up or the head is elevated, venous pressure may fall below atmospheric pressure during inspiration, permitting air to enter the venous system. A large air embolus can be fatal because it can interfere with both cardiac function and cerebral perfusion. An additional concern of trauma to the cervical vasculature is the development of an expanding hematoma that may lead to airway compromise as the hematoma expands and impinges on and distorts the normal anatomy.

Blunt injury to the neck may also result in a tear and dissection of the carotid intima (the innermost layer of the carotid artery) away from the outer layers. This injury can lead to occlusion of the carotid artery and a stroke-like picture. Carotid artery intimal flaps or dissections often occur when a restrained occupant in a vehicle collision impacts the shoulder strap located across the neck.

Brain Injuries
Cerebral Concussion

The diagnosis of a "concussion" is made when an injured patient shows any transient alteration in neurologic function with a subsequent return to normal. Although most people associate a loss of consciousness with the diagnosis of concussion, loss of consciousness is not required to make a diagnosis of concussion; rather, posttraumatic amnesia is the hallmark of concussion. Other neurologic changes include the following:

- Vacant stare (befuddled facial expression)
- Delayed verbal and motor responses (slow to answer questions or follow instructions)

- Confusion and inability to focus attention (easily distracted and unable to follow through with normal activities)
- Disorientation (walking in the wrong direction; unaware of time, date, and place)
- Slurred or incoherent speech (making disjointed or incomprehensible statements)
- Lack of coordination (stumbling, inability to walk tandem/straight line)
- Emotions inappropriate to the circumstances (distraught, crying for no apparent reason)
- Memory deficits (exhibited by patient repeatedly asking the same question that has already been answered)
- Inability to memorize and recall (e.g., three of three words or three of three objects in five minutes)[40]

Severe headache, dizziness, nausea, and vomiting frequently accompany a concussion. Patients exhibiting signs of concussion, especially patients with nausea, vomiting, or neurologic findings on secondary assessment, should be immediately transported for further evaluation. The formal diagnosis of a concussion will be made in the hospital once the patient is evaluated and a head CT scan result shows no observable intracranial pathology.

Although most of these findings last several hours to a couple days, some patients experience a postconcussive syndrome with headaches, dizziness, and difficulty concentrating for weeks, and even months, after a severe concussion. The effects of repetitive concussion on the brain, particularly as relates to sports injuries, have garnered more attention in recent years. While a concussion has often been thought of as a relatively benign injury, it has been recognized that repeated blows to the head resulting in a concussion cause permanent damage that becomes manifest over time. This damage leads to long-term difficulties with concentration and thinking clearly; symptoms such as headache and dizziness; mood disorders including depression, anxiety, and irritability; and sleep disturbances.

It is also important to determine whether the patient has had a recent concussion and, if so, whether the symptoms from that episode have completely resolved. Patients who have sustained a concussion and then have a second concussion before the symptoms from the first one have fully resolved are at risk for sudden deterioration in neurologic status. This phenomenon, which has been termed the **secondary impact syndrome**,[41] has become a particular concern in athletic events where athletes sustain a concussion and are eager to return to the game, often before they have fully recovered from the effects of the initial trauma. In these cases, the brain is compromised as a result of the first impact; when the second trauma occurs, the brain loses its ability to autoregulate and develops sudden and massive edema, leading to herniation and death. This process can occur in as little as 5 minutes. Controversy exists as to whether this is, in fact, a unique and distinct entity or rather a progressive form of cerebral edema.[42] Regardless of whether secondary impact syndrome is a unique disease, the conceptual basis is important. Patients (especially athletes) who have sustained a concussion

should be carefully evaluated to determine the persistence of symptoms. If the patient has not fully recovered from the initial insult, he or she should avoid repeat trauma to the head and brain and, in the case of athletes, not be allowed to return to play.

Intracranial Hematoma

Intracranial hematomas are divided into three general types: epidural, subdural, and intracerebral. Because the signs and symptoms of each of these have significant overlap, specific diagnosis in the prehospital setting (as well as the ED) is almost impossible, although the prehospital care provider may suspect a particular type of hematoma based on the characteristic clinical presentation. Even so, a definitive diagnosis can be made only after a CT scan is performed at the receiving facility. Because these hematomas occupy space inside the rigid skull, they may produce rapid increases in ICP, especially if they are sizable.

Epidural Hematoma

Epidural hematomas account for about 1% to 2% of TBI patients who require hospitalization and about 10% of those who present with traumatic coma. These hematomas often result from a relatively low-velocity blow to the temporal bone, such as the impact from a punch or baseball. A fracture of this thin bone damages the middle meningeal artery, which results in arterial bleeding that collects between the skull and dura mater (**Figure 10-17**). This high-pressure arterial blood can start to dissect or peal the dura off of the inner table of the skull, creating an epidural space full of blood. Such an epidural hematoma has a characteristic lens shape, as seen on the CT scan, created by the dura holding the hematoma against the inner table of the skull. The principal threat to the brain is from the expanding mass of blood displacing the brain and threatening herniation. For this reason, patients whose epidural hematoma is rapidly evacuated often have excellent recoveries.

The classic history for an epidural hematoma is a patient experiencing a brief loss of consciousness, then regaining consciousness, and then experiencing a rapid decline in consciousness. During the period of consciousness, the lucid interval, the patient may be oriented, lethargic, or confused or may complain of a headache. Only about one-third of patients with epidural hematomas actually experience this "lucid interval," however, and it may also occur with other types of intracranial hemorrhages, making it nonspecific for epidural hematoma. Nonetheless, a patient who experiences a "lucid interval," followed by a decline in GCS, is at risk for a progressive intracranial process and needs emergency evaluation.

As a patient's LOC worsens, the physical examination may reveal a dilated and sluggish or nonreactive pupil, most commonly on the same side of the herniation (ipsilateral side). Because motor nerves cross over to the other side above the spinal cord, hemiparesis or hemiplegia typically occurs on the side opposite the impact (contralateral side). The mortality rate for an epidural hematoma is about 20%; however, with rapid recognition and evacuation, the mortality rate can be as low as 2%. This improved rate of outcome is because an epidural hematoma is usually a "pure" space-occupying lesion, with little injury to the brain beneath. If the hematoma is quickly recognized and removed, the pathologic effect is corrected, and the patient can make an excellent recovery. Such rapid removal reduces not only mortality, but also subsequent, significant neurologic morbidity. Epidural hematomas often occur in young people, who are just beginning their careers, emphasizing the societal value as well as the human value of their rapid identification and removal.

Subdural Hematoma

Subdural hematomas account for about 30% of severe brain injuries, with a male to female ratio of 3:1.[43] In young adults, 56% of subdural hematomas are due to motor vehicle crashes and 12% are due to falls, while in the elderly 22% are due to motor vehicle crashes and 56% are due to falls.[44]

In addition to being more common than epidural hematomas, they also differ in etiology, location, and prognosis. Unlike the epidural hematoma, which is caused by arterial hemorrhage, a subdural hematoma generally results from a venous bleed. In this case, bridging veins are torn during a violent blow to the head. Blood collects in the subdural space, between the dura mater and the underlying arachnoid membrane (**Figure 10-18**).

Subdural hematomas present in two different ways. In some patients who have just experienced significant trauma, the disruption of the bridging veins results in relatively rapid accumulation of blood in the subdural space, with rapid onset of mass effect. Adding to this morbidity is associated direct

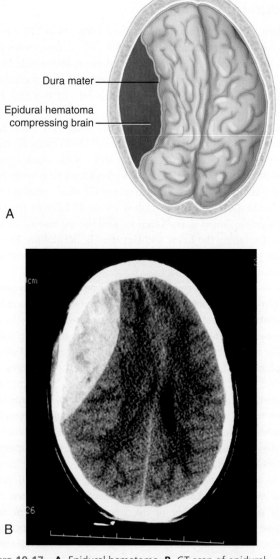

Figure 10-17   A. Epidural hematoma. **B.** CT scan of epidural hematoma.
Source: B. Courtesy of Peter T. Pons, MD, FACEP.

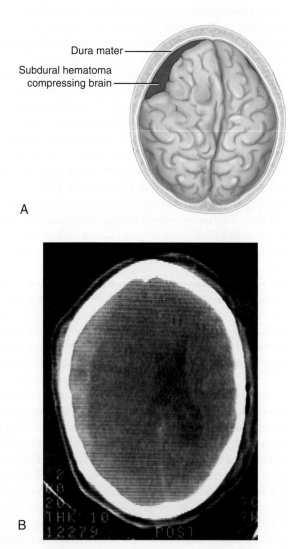

Figure 10-18   A. Subdural hematoma. **B.** CT scan of subdural hematoma.
Source: B. Courtesy of Peter T. Pons, MD, FACEP.

injury to the brain parenchyma itself beneath the subdural hematoma, which occurs as part of the traumatic event leading to the venous disruption. As a result, unlike that of epidural hematomas, the mass effect of subdural hematomas is often caused by both the accumulated blood and the swelling of the injured brain beneath. Patients presenting with such acute mass effect will have an acutely depressed mental status and will need rapid identification of the emergency in the field with emergent transport to an appropriate receiving facility for CT scan, ICP monitoring and management, and possibly surgery.

In some patients, however, clinically occult subdural hematomas can occur. In elderly or debilitated patients, such as those with chronic disease, the subdural space is enlarged secondary to brain atrophy. In such patients, blood may accumulate in the subdural space without exerting mass effect and, thus, may be clinically occult. Such subdural hematomas can occur during falls in elderly persons or during apparently minor trauma. At particular risk are older patients receiving anticoagulants such as warfarin (Coumadin). Because these falls are minor, patients often do not present for evaluation, and the bleeds are not identified. Many patients in whom chronic subdural hematoma is eventually identified do not even recall the traumatic event that caused the bleed because it seemed so minor.

In some patients in whom an occult subdural hematoma is eventually identified, the subdural blood liquefies but is retained within the subdural space. Over time, through a mechanism that includes repeated small bleeds into the liquid hematoma, the now-chronic subdural hematoma can expand and slowly start to exert mass effect on the brain. Because the onset of the mass effect is gradual, the patient will not have the dramatic presentation associated with an acute subdural hematoma, Instead, the patient is more likely to present with headache, visual disturbances, personality changes, difficulty speaking (**dysarthria**), and hemiparesis or hemiplegia of a slowly progressive nature. Only when some of these symptoms become pronounced enough to prompt the patient or caregiver to seek help is the chronic subdural hematoma discovered. On CT scan, a chronic subdural hematoma has a distinct appearance compared with the more emergent, acute subdural hematoma. Often the event precipitating transport for evaluation and care is the most recent of the small, repetitive subdural bleeds that create chronic subdural hematomas, and a small amount of acute blood may be found in a larger collection of chronic blood. The need for and the urgency of surgery are determined by the patient's symptoms, the amount of mass effect, and the patient's overall medical condition.

Prehospital care personnel frequently encounter these patients when called to facilities that care for chronically ill populations. Because the symptoms are nonspecific, diagnosing a chronic subdural hematoma in the field is rarely possible, and the symptoms may be confused with those of a stroke, infection, dementia, or even a generalized decline in the patient.

Although many subdural hematomas in these patients will be chronic, patients taking Coumadin, after an apparently insignificant trauma, may have a subdural hematoma that expands over several hours and progresses to herniation resulting from the patient's inability to clot. These patients can have a benign presentation and then deteriorate several hours after their trauma. Elderly patients, especially patients receiving Coumadin, who have experienced apparently minor falls should be managed with a heightened sense of urgency and care.

Cerebral Contusions

Damage to the brain itself may produce cerebral contusions and, if this damage includes injury to the blood vessels within the brain, actual bleeding into the substance of the brain, or intracerebral hematomas. Cerebral contusions are relatively common, occurring in about 20% to 30% of severe brain injuries and in a significant percentage of moderate head injuries as well. Although typically the result of blunt trauma, these injuries may also occur from penetrating trauma, such as a gunshot wound to the brain. In blunt trauma, cerebral contusions may be multiple. Cerebral contusions result from a complex pattern of transmission and reflection of forces within the skull. As a result, contusions often occur in locations remote from the site of impact, often on the opposite side of the brain, the familiar contrecoup injury.

Cerebral contusions often take 12 to 24 hours to appear on CT scans, and thus, a patient with a cerebral contusion may have an initially normal head CT scan. The only clue to its presence may be a depressed GCS, with many patients showing moderate head injuries (GCS 9 to 13). As the contusion evolves after injury, it not only becomes more apparent on head CT, but it also can cause increased mass effect and create increasing headache. Of particular concern, it may cause moderate head injuries to deteriorate to severe head injuries in about 10% of patients.[45]

Subarachnoid Hemorrhage

Subarachnoid hemorrhage (SAH) is bleeding that occurs beneath the arachnoid membrane, which lies under the subdural space covering the brain. Blood in the subarachnoid space cannot enter the subdural space. Many of the brain's blood vessels are located in the subarachnoid space, so injury to these vessels will cause subarachnoid bleeding, a layering of blood beneath the arachnoid membrane on the surface of the brain. This layering of blood is typically thin and rarely causes mass effect.

SAH is usually thought of as associated with spontaneous rupture of cerebral aneurysms causing the sudden onset of the worst headache of the patient's life. In fact, posttraumatic SAH is the most common cause of subarachnoid bleeding. The trauma patient with SAH will usually complain of headache, which may be severe in nature. Nausea and vomiting are common, as is dizziness. In addition, the presence of blood in the subarachnoid space may cause meningeal signs such as pain and stiffness of the neck, visual complaints, and photophobia (aversion to bright light). These patients may also develop seizures.

Because subarachnoid bleeding rarely causes mass effect, it does not require surgery for decompression. In fact, patients with SAH and a GCS of 13 or greater, generally do extremely well.[46] However, it can be a marker for potentially severe brain injury, and its presence increases the risk for other space-occupying lesions. Patients with traumatic subarachnoid hemorrhage (tSAH) have a 63% to 73% increased risk of a cerebral contusion, and 44% will develop subdural hematomas. Patients with tSAH have an increased risk of elevated ICP and intraventricular hemorrhage. Patients with large amounts of tSAH (greater than 1 cm of blood thickness, blood in the suprasellar or ambient cisterns) have a positive predictive value of 72% to 78% for a poor outcome, and in the Trauma Coma Data Bank, the presence of tSAH doubled the incidence of death in brain-injured patients.[47,48]

Penetrating Cranial Injury

Penetrating trauma of the brain is one of the most devastating neurologic injuries. The penetrating object will cause direct injury to the brain tissue as it passes into and, in some cases, through the brain parenchyma. The nature of the neurologic injury produced depends on the area of the brain injured. Gunshot wounds are particularly destructive because of the energy associated with the missile. As described in the Kinematics of Trauma chapter, not only does a bullet cause direct injury as it passes through tissue, the associated shock wave damages tissue along the cavitation pathway. In particular, gunshot wounds that cross the midline and pass from one side of the brain to the other, thus involving both sides of the brain, are associated with a dismal outcome. In rare instances, such as when the bullet traverses only the frontal lobes, the patient may survive, albeit with significant impairment. The potential for survival is also better if the bullet passes from front to back on one side of the brain. Again, however, the patient will have persistent, significant neurologic deficit.

All penetrating brain injury results in open fracture of the skull. The potential for subsequent infection, if the patient survives, is high. In addition, penetrating injuries of the skull may also damage other important organs such as the eyes, ears, and face, leading to impaired function of the involved organs.

Management

Effective management of a patient with TBI begins with orderly interventions focused on treating any life-threatening problems identified in the primary assessment. Once these problems are addressed, the patient should be rapidly packaged and transported to the nearest facility capable of caring for TBI.

Airway

Patients with a depressed LOC may be unable to protect their airway, and adequate oxygenation of the injured brain is critical to preventing secondary injury. As noted earlier, facial injuries can be associated with hemorrhage and edema that may compromise the airway. Hematomas in the floor of the mouth or in the soft palate may occlude the airway. The manual and simple airway skills are appropriate initial airway interventions (see the Airway and Ventilation chapter). Both oral and nasal airways may become obstructed by edema or blood clots, and intermittent suctioning may be necessary. Patients with facial fractures and laryngeal or other neck injuries will typically assume a position that maintains their airway. Attempts to force a patient to lie supine or wear a cervical collar may be met with extreme combativeness if he or she becomes hypoxic as a result of positional airway impairment. In these situations, airway patency takes precedence over spinal immobilization, and patients may be transported in a sitting or semisitting position, as tolerated.

Cervical collars may be deferred if thought to compromise the airway, while manual stabilization of the spine continues to be performed. Conscious patients can often assist in managing their own airway by suctioning themselves when they feel it is needed; the prehospital care provider can allow them to hold and use the suction device. Facial trauma, including those injuries caused by gunshot wounds, is not a contraindication to endotracheal intubation; however, many of these patients will need to be managed using percutaneous transtracheal ventilation or a needle or surgical cricothyroidotomy.

Definitive airway management of the patient with TBI has historically been focused on endotracheal intubation. However, many of the alternative devices such as supraglottic airways can serve to maintain a patent airway in the prehospital setting.

An early study reported that victims of TBI who were intubated appeared to do better than those who were not intubated.[49] Recent studies, however, have yielded mixed results in TBI casualties intubated in the field.[50-55] The specific explanation for these conflicting data awaits further study and explanation. However, poorly performed intubation appears be more harmful than no intubation at all. Several studies have shown that patients intubated in the field may have unrecognized episodes of hypoxia or hypotension, thus leading to poorer outcomes.[56] In addition, many of these patients undergo unintentional hyperventilation, further complicating their course. The deciding factors on whether or not to intubate a patient may be prehospital care provider skill and length of transport. In urban settings, short transport times allow patients to be managed using alternate techniques and fairly urgently delivered to the ED where the airway can be managed in a more controlled setting. Patients intubated in the field may do worse because of prolonged field times and a less experienced prehospital care provider performing the intubation. Similarly, intubation in a system in which prehospital care providers perform only a few intubations a year may be more detrimental than other means of airway support during transport. Conversely, in systems with longer transport times, intubation may be more beneficial than no intubation at all, even when done by a less experienced prehospital care provider. Future studies should help determine the best practice in the prehospital environment.

With these qualifiers in mind, all patients with a severe TBI (GCS less than 9) should be considered for active airway management. Because this can be extremely challenging due to the patient's combativeness, clenched jaw muscles (trismus), vomiting, and the need to maintain in-line cervical spine stabilization, intubation, if that is the method of airway management chosen, should be performed by the most skilled prehospital care provider who can be available in a timely manner. It is essential that the patient's SpO_2 be monitored throughout the process of managing the airway and that hypoxia (SpO_2 less than 90%) be avoided. The use of neuromuscular blocking agents as part of a rapid-sequence intubation (RSI) protocol may facilitate successful intubation.[57] Blind nasotracheal intubation can serve as an alternative technique, but the presence of midface trauma has been considered a relative contraindication for this procedure. Concern has often been voiced about the possibility of inadvertent cranial and cerebral penetration with the nasotracheal tube in patients who have sustained head trauma. Review of the medical literature reveals that this complication has been reported only twice in head trauma patients.[58,59]

There is no one ideal airway management technique that is preferred over any other. Instead, manual and simple airway skills should be used as the initial interventions and progression to complex airway interventions undertaken if, and only if, the airway cannot be maintained by less invasive means. In many cases, bag-mask ventilation with a nasal or oral airway is sufficient to oxygenate and ventilate the patient. Prolonged attempts at complex airway interventions should be avoided, especially with a short transport time.

Suction equipment should always be readily available. Airway management interventions will often precipitate episodes of vomiting. In addition, the TBI itself will often lead to vomiting.

Breathing

All patients with suspected TBI should receive supplemental oxygen. As mentioned previously in this chapter, the use of pulse oximetry is strongly recommended because hypoxia can worsen neurologic outcome and is often difficult to detect clinically. Oxygen concentration can be titrated when using pulse oximetry; SpO_2 should be at least 90%, with 95% or higher as optimal. If pulse oximetry is not available, oxygen should be provided via a nonrebreather face mask for a spontaneously breathing patient. For intubated patients, an oxygen concentration of 100% (fraction of inspired oxygen [FiO_2] of 1.0) should be maintained with a bag-mask device. If hypoxia persists despite oxygen therapy, the prehospital care provider should attempt to identify and treat all likely etiologies, including aspiration and tension pneumothoraces. Use of positive end-expiratory pressure (PEEP) valves, if available, may be considered to improve oxygenation; however, levels of PEEP greater than 15 centimeters of water ($cm\ H_2O$) may increase ICP.[60,61]

Because both hypocapnia and hypercapnia can aggravate TBI, control of ventilatory rate is important.[62] In the hospital, arterial blood gases (ABGs) are available and $PaCO_2$ is directly measured and maintained in the range of 35 to 40 mm Hg. End-tidal carbon dioxide ($ETCO_2$) can also be used to estimate serum $PaCO_2$ in hemodynamically stable patients. Because the

measured values for $ETCO_2$ and $PaCO_2$ vary widely from patient to patient, each in-hospital patient must have a unique "offset" between $PaCO_2$ and $ETCO_2$ determined by comparison of the $ETCO_2$ value with an ABG to obtain acceptable accuracy from the use of $ETCO_2$. New ABGs are obtained each time the patient's condition changes.

In the prehospital environment, ABGs and $PaCO_2$ are not routinely available to determine the "offset" with $ETCO_2$. In addition, other patient factors, such as changes in pulmonary perfusion, in cardiac output, and in patient temperature, all cause alterations in $ETCO_2$, which cannot be distinguished from $ETCO_2$ changes that result from actual changes in $PaCO_2$. Because physiologic changes occur rapidly in the prehospital phase as patients are resuscitated and warmed as well as ventilated, they are rarely stable enough to allow $ETCO_2$ to be used with any accuracy. Although $ETCO_2$ is an excellent tool for monitoring ventilation, it is not accurate enough to guide hyperventilation therapy meaningfully in the prehospital setting.[63-73]

It is simpler to judge the degree of ventilation by counting breaths per minute. Normal ventilatory rates should be used when assisting ventilation in patients with TBI: 10 breaths/minute for adults, 20 breaths/minute for children, and 25 breaths/minute for infants. Excessively fast ventilatory rates produce cerebral vasoconstriction, which in turn leads to a decrease in cerebral oxygen delivery. Routine prophylactic hyperventilation has been shown to worsen neurologic outcome and should not be used. A subgroup analysis of patients enrolled in the San Diego Paramedic RSI trial showed that both hyperventilation and severe hypoxia in the prehospital setting were associated with an increase in mortality. For adult patients, ventilating with a tidal volume of 350 to 500 ml at a rate of 10 breaths/minute should be sufficient to maintain adequate oxygenation without inducing hypocarbia.[74]

Hyperventilation of a patient in a controlled fashion may be considered in the specific circumstance of signs of herniation. These signs include asymmetric pupils, dilated and nonreactive pupils, extensor posturing or no response on motor examination, or progressive neurologic deterioration defined as a decrease in the GCS of more than 2 points in a patient whose initial GCS was 8 or less. In such cases, mild, controlled hyperventilation in the field may be performed during the prehospital phase of care. Mild hyperventilation is defined as an $ETCO_2$ of 30 to 35 mm Hg as measured by capnography or by careful control of the breathing rate (20 breaths/minute for adults, 25 breaths/minute for children, and 30 breaths/minute for infants less than 1 year of age).[74]

Circulation

Both blood loss and hypotension are important causes of secondary brain injury, so efforts should be taken to prevent or treat these conditions. Hemorrhage control is essential. Direct pressure or pressure dressings should be applied to any external hemorrhage. Complex scalp wounds can produce significant external blood loss. Several gauze pads held in place by an elastic roller bandage create an effective pressure dressing to control bleeding. If this approach fails to control bleeding, the bleeding can often be controlled by applying direct pressure along the wound edges, thereby compressing the scalp vasculature between the skin and soft tissues and the galea. Dramatic bleeding can often be controlled with this maneuver. A pressure dressing should not be applied to a depressed or open skull fracture unless significant hemorrhage is present, because it may aggravate brain injury and lead to an increase in ICP. Direct gentle pressure may also limit the size of extracranial (scalp) hematomas. Gentle handling and immobilization to a long backboard or scoop stretcher in anatomic alignment can minimize interstitial blood loss around fractures.

Hemorrhage from the carotid arteries and internal jugular veins may be massive. In most circumstances, direct pressure will control such external hemorrhage. Injuries to these vessels from penetrating trauma may be associated with internal bleeding, presenting as an expanding hematoma. These hematomas may compromise the airway, and endotracheal intubation may be necessary. However, attempts to intubate a conscious patient with an expanding neck hematoma but no external bleeding may stimulate a cough, which may be sufficient to disrupt a clot that may have formed at a knife or bullet wound, resulting in massive external hemorrhage.

Because hypotension further worsens brain ischemia, standard measures should be employed to combat shock. In patients with TBI, the combination of hypoxia and hypotension is associated with a mortality rate of about 75%. If shock is present and major internal hemorrhage is suspected, prompt transport to a trauma center takes priority over brain injuries.

Hypovolemic and neurogenic shock are aggressively treated by resuscitation with isotonic crystalloid solutions; however, transport should not be delayed to establish intravenous (IV) access. To preserve cerebral perfusion, adequate fluid should be given to maintain a systolic blood pressure of at least 90 to 100 mm Hg. For adult TBI patients with normal vital signs and no other suspected injuries, IV fluid at a rate of no more than 125 ml/hour should be administered and adjusted if signs of shock develop.[74]

A randomized trial of patients with severe TBI showed that those who received prehospital resuscitation with hypertonic saline had almost identical neurologic functioning 6 months after injury compared to those treated with crystalloid.[75] Because of its increased cost and lack of benefit compared to normal saline or lactated Ringer's solution, hypertonic saline is not recommended for routine prehospital volume replacement.

Disability

Assessment of the GCS should be integrated into the primary assessment of all trauma patients after circulation is addressed. Use of the GCS helps evaluate the patient's status and may impact transport and triage decisions, depending on the system in which the prehospital care provider is working.

Prehospital management of TBI patients primarily consists of measures aimed at reversing and preventing factors that cause secondary brain injury. Prolonged or multiple grand mal seizures can be treated with IV administration of a benzodiazepine, such as diazepam, lorazepam, or midazolam. These drugs should be cautiously titrated because hypotension and ventilatory depression may occur.

Because of the significant incidence of cervical spine fractures, patients with suspected TBI as a result of blunt trauma should be placed in spinal immobilization. Some degree of caution must be exercised when applying a cervical collar to a patient with TBI. Some evidence suggests that a tightly fitted cervical collar can impede venous drainage of the head, thereby increasing ICP. *Application of a cervical collar is not mandatory as long as the head and neck are sufficiently immobilized.* Victims of penetrating head wounds generally do not require spine immobilization unless clinical findings clearly demonstrate spinal cord neurologic damage.

Transport

To achieve the best possible outcome, patients with moderate and severe TBI should be transported directly to a trauma center that can perform a CT scan and ICP monitoring and provide prompt neurosurgical consultation and intervention. If such a facility is not available, aeromedical transport from the scene to an appropriate trauma center should be considered.[39]

The patient's pulse rate, blood pressure, SpO_2, and GCS should be reassessed and documented every 5 to 10 minutes during transport. PEEP valves may be used cautiously if persistent hypoxia exists because, as noted, levels of PEEP greater than 15 cm H_2O may increase ICP. The patient's body heat should be preserved during transport.

Controversy exists regarding the optimal position for a patient with TBI. In general, patients with TBI should be transported in a supine position because of the presence of other injuries.[76] Although elevating the head on the ambulance stretcher or long backboard (reverse Trendelenburg position) may decrease ICP, cerebral perfusion pressure may also be jeopardized, especially if the head is elevated higher than 30 degrees.

The receiving facility should be notified as early as possible so that appropriate preparations can be made before the patient's arrival. The radio report should include information regarding the mechanism of injury, initial GCS score and any changes en route, focal signs (e.g., motor exam asymmetry, unilaterally or bilaterally dilated pupils) and vital signs, other serious injuries, and response to management.[39]

Prolonged Transport

As with all patients with suspected TBI, efforts focus on preventing secondary brain injury. A prolonged transport time may lower the threshold for performing airway management. RSI may be used in this setting, especially if aeromedical transport is considered, because a combative patient in the confines of a helicopter threatens the crew, pilot, and himself or herself. Efforts to control the airway should be performed while cervical spine stabilization is being applied. Oxygen should be administered to maintain an appropriate SpO_2 level. Because of the risk of developing pressure ulcers from lying on a hard backboard, the patient may be placed on a padded long backboard, especially if the anticipated transport time is lengthy. Patients should be attached to continuous pulse oximetry, and serial vital signs, including ventilations, pulse, blood pressure, and GCS score, should be measured. Pupils should be periodically checked for response to light and symmetry.

When there is a delay in transport or a prolonged transport time to an appropriate facility, additional management options can be considered. For patients with an abnormal GCS score, the blood glucose level should be checked. If the patient is hypoglycemic, a 50% dextrose solution can be administered intravenously until the blood sugar is restored to a normal level. Benzodiazepines may be titrated intravenously if recurrent or prolonged seizures occur.

External hemorrhage should be controlled, and crystalloid fluids administered if signs of shock are apparent. Fluids should be titrated to maintain the systolic blood pressure greater than 90 mm Hg in the patient with suspected TBI. Associated injuries should be managed while en route to the receiving facility. Fractures should be appropriately splinted to control both internal hemorrhage and pain.

Appropriate management of increased ICP in the prehospital setting is extremely challenging because the ICP is not monitored in the field unless the patient is undergoing interfacility transfer and an ICP monitor or ventriculostomy has been placed at the referring center. Although a declining GCS score may represent increasing ICP, it may also be the result of worsening cerebral perfusion from hypovolemic shock. Warning signs of possible increased ICP and herniation include the following:

- Decline in GCS score of two points or more
- Development of a sluggish or nonreactive pupil
- Development of hemiplegia or hemiparesis
- Cushing's phenomenon

The decision to intervene and manage increased ICP is based on written protocol or made in consultation with medical control at the receiving facility. Possible temporizing management options include sedation, chemical paralysis, osmotherapy (the use of osmotically active agents such as mannitol that may assist in the treatment of intracranial hypertension), and controlled hyperventilation. Small doses of benzodiazepine sedatives should be titrated cautiously because of the potential side effects of hypotension and ventilatory depression. Use of a long-acting neuromuscular blocking agent, such as vecuronium, may be considered if the patient is intubated. If the cervical collar is believed to be too tight, it may be loosened slightly or removed, provided that the head and neck are adequately immobilized with other measures.

Osmotherapy with mannitol (0.25 to 1.0 g/kg) can be given intravenously. However, aggressive diuresis may produce hypovolemia, which can worsen cerebral perfusion. Mannitol should be avoided for patients in whom systemic resuscitation has not been achieved—that is, patients with systolic blood pressure less than 90 mm Hg. If an osmotic agent is used, the patient should be maintained in a euvolemic state. In addition, a Foley catheter should be placed if transport will be extremely prolonged.

An increased rate of ventilation (controlled, mild therapeutic hyperventilation) aimed at maintaining the $ETCO_2$ at 30 to 35 mm Hg may be considered for obvious signs of herniation. The following ventilatory rates should be used: 20 breaths/minute for adults, 25 breaths/minute for children, and 30 breaths/minute for infants. *Prophylactic hyperventilation has no role in TBI, and therapeutic hyperventilation, if instituted, should be stopped if signs of intracranial hypertension resolve.* Steroids have not been shown to improve the outcome of patients with TBI and should not be administered.

The primary focus for the TBI patient during prolonged transport or in austere environments is the best possible maintenance of cerebral oxygenation and perfusion and the best efforts possible to control cerebral edema.

Brain Death and Organ Donation

The diagnosis of brain death is made when there is no clinical evidence of neurologic function in a patient who is warm, whose mental status is not impacted by sedating or paralyzing medications, and who is completely resuscitated with a systolic blood pressure greater than 90 mm Hg and SpO_2 greater than 90% along with a normal blood glucose level.

Assessment for clinical evidence of neurologic function consists of ensuring that there is no evidence of cortical function, followed by an assessment of midbrain and brain stem function down to the respiratory center in the lower medulla. This assessment is performed in the hospital and consists of establishing the absence of response to deep pain, followed by the midbrain and brain stem assessment for nonreactive pupils, absence of a corneal reflex, and absence of response to cold caloric stimulation. In addition, absence of a gag reflex, absence of a cough reflex, and, finally, absence of any effort to breathe, with $PaCO_2$ greater than 60 mm Hg and adequate PO_2, are all determined. In the absence of any activity on these tests, the patient can be declared clinically "brain dead."

Many clinical protocols and some state statutes also require that brain death be confirmed by an ancillary test, such as radionucleotide cerebral blood flow studies or electroencephalography.

The physiologic definition of brain death just described is the definition typically used in the United States. Philosophical, ethical, and legal issues remain about how much of the brain must be dead before "personhood" is lost, and thus, the definition of brain death varies throughout the world. In addition, various hospitals and systems have differing methods for declaring brain death, and in the United States, states have varying legal statutes defining who may declare death and brain death and how it is to be declared. Those interested should inquire within their local system.

The victim of TBI that progresses to brain death provides an important source of organs for transplantation. TBI was the cause of brain death for more than 40% of individuals from whom organs were procured, with the majority of organs coming from those between 18 and 49 years of age. Despite the presence of a fatal brain injury, an individual's heart, lungs, liver, kidneys, pancreas, and corneas may benefit others with chronic illnesses. Enlisting the trust and support of the public in obtaining these organs is critical to ensuring their availability to those who so desperately need them. To gain this trust, the families of TBI victims first need to be sure that the resuscitation of the injured brain has been the first priority of the treating team, and second,

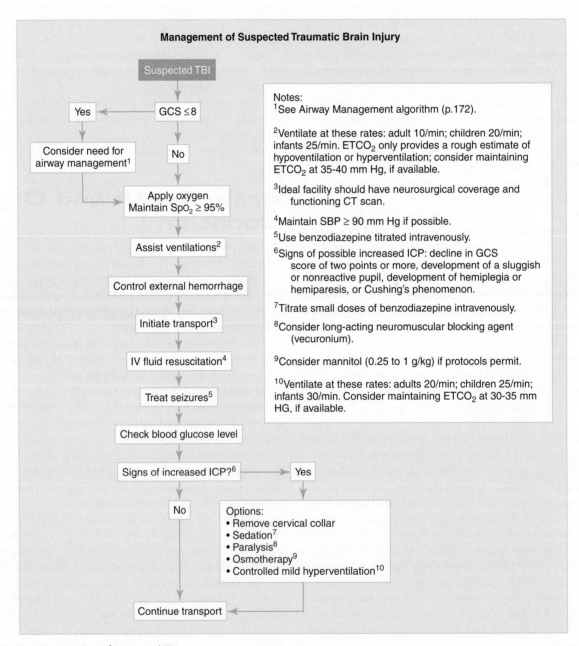

Figure 10-19 Management of suspected TBI.

when that resuscitation has failed, they need to understand the issues surrounding physiologic brain death.

It is essential that health care providers clearly understand the issues surrounding brain death and effectively communicate these issues to the family members of the victims of TBI. In most cases, approaching a family concerning possible organ donation should occur only after all of the medical interventions have been attempted and completed, and the contact should be made by trained representatives of the hospital or organ recovery team (**Figure 10-19**).

Summary

- Preventing the development of or recognizing and treating hypoxia and reduced cerebral blood flow in the field can make the difference between a good and a poor outcome.
- The severity of TBI may not be immediately apparent; therefore, serial neurologic evaluations of the patient, including Glasgow Coma Scale scores and pupillary response, are necessary to recognize changes in the patient's condition.
- TBI is often found in association with multisystem trauma, so all problems are addressed in the appropriate order of priority. Not only are airway, breathing, and circulation always the priorities of patient care, but they are specifically important in the management of TBI in preventing secondary brain injury.
- Prehospital management of the TBI patient involves controlling hemorrhage from other injuries, maintaining a systolic blood pressure of at least 90 to 100 mm Hg, and providing oxygen to maintain oxygen saturation of at least 90%.
- Hyperventilation of patients is performed only when objective signs of herniation are noted.

SCENARIO RECAP

On an 85°F (29°C) summer day, you and your partner are dispatched to the finish line of a marathon race for a 30-year-old man who fell 14 feet (4.3 meters) off a ladder while attempting to secure the finish line banner. Upon your arrival, the patient is supine and unresponsive. A bystander is holding the patient's head and neck in-line. You note an irregular breathing rate that increases and then decreases in depth.

You also note that there is bloody fluid coming from both ears and both nostrils of the patient. The patient's airway is secured with an oropharyngeal airway once absence of the gag reflex is noted. Your partner ventilates the patient with a bag-mask device at a rate of 12 breaths per minute. You notice that the patient's right pupil is dilated. The radial pulse is 54 and regular. Oxygen saturation (Spo_2) is 96%. The patient's skin is cool, dry, and pale. His GCS score is calculated to be 7, with eyes = 2, verbal = 1, and motor = 4 (E2V1M4).

You rapidly prepare the patient for transport and place him into your ambulance to perform the secondary assessment while en route to the hospital. Palpation of the occiput generates a painful moan from the patient. You cover the patient with a warm blanket and measure his blood pressure, which is 184/102. An electrocardiogram reveals sinus bradycardia with infrequent premature ventricular beats noted. The right pupil remains widely dilated.

- What injury is most likely present given the patient's presenting signs?
- What are your management priorities at this point?
- What actions may you need to take to combat increased intracranial pressure and maintain cerebral perfusion during a prolonged transport?

SCENARIO SOLUTION

En route to the hospital, the patient begins to show palmar flexion of both hands. With this sign of impending herniation, you increase the ventilation rate to 16 to 20 breaths/minute. The patient remains unconscious. You consider insertion of a complex airway; however, since the SpO_2 is at 96% and transport time to the trauma center is only a few minutes, you decide to maintain him with the oral airway and bag-mask device with 100% oxygen.

References

1. Centers for Disease Control and Prevention. Traumatic Brain Injury. http://www.cdc.gov/ncipc/tbi/TBI.htm. Accessed November 26, 2013.

2. Bryan-Hancock C, Harrison J. The global burden of traumatic brain injury: preliminary results from the Global Burden of Disease Project. *Inj Prev*. 2010;16(suppl 1):A17.

3. Cipolla MJ. *The Cerebral Circulation*. Morgan & Claypool Life Sciences: San Rafael, CA; 2009.

4. Chestnut RM, Marshall LF, Klauber MR, et al. The role of secondary brain injury in determining outcome from severe head injury. *J Trauma*. 1993;34:216.

5. Fearnside MR, Cook RJ, McDougall P, et al. The Westmead Head Injury Project outcome in severe head injury: a comparative analysis of prehospital, clinical, and CT variables. *Br J Neurosurg*. 1993;7:267.

6. Gentleman D. Causes and effects of systemic complications among severely head-injured patients transferred to a neurosurgical unit. *Int Surg*. 1992;77:297.

7. Marmarou A, Anderson RL, Ward JL, et al. Impact of ICP instability and hypotension on outcome in patients with severe head trauma. *J Neurosurg*. 1991;75:S59.

8. Miller JD, Becker DP. Secondary insults to the injured brain. *J R Coll Surg Edinb*. 1982;27:292.

9. Obrist WD, Gennarelli TA, Segawa H, et al. Relation of cerebral blood flow to neurological status and outcome in head injured patients. *J Neurosurg*. 1979;51:292.

10. Obrist WD, Langfitt TW, Jaggi JL, et al. Cerebral blood flow and metabolism in comatose patients with acute head injury. *J Neurosurg*. 1984;61:241.

11. Marshall LF, Toole BM, Bowers SA. Part 2: patients who talk and deteriorate: implications for treatment. *J Neurosurg*. 1983;59:285.

12. Reilly PL, Adams JH, Graham DI, et al. Patients with head injury who talk and die. *Lancet*. 1975;2:375.

13. Rose J, Valtonen S, Jennett B. Avoidable factors contributing to death after head injury. *BMJ*. 1977;2:615.

14. Miller JD, Sweet RC, Narayan RK, et al. Early insults to the injured brain. *JAMA*. 1978;240:439.

15. Silverston P. Pulse oximetry at the roadside: a study of pulse oximetry in immediate care. *BMJ*. 1989;298:711.

16. Stochetti N, Furlan A, Volta F. Hypoxemia and arterial hypotension at the accident scene in head injury. *J Trauma*. 1996;40:764.

17. Kellie G. An account of the appearances observed in the dissection of two of three individuals presumed to have perished in the storm of the 3rd, and whose bodies were discovered in the vicinity of Leith on the morning of the 4th of November 1821 with some reflections on the pathology of the brain. *Trans Med Chir Sci Edinb*. 1824;1:84.

18. Plum F. The Diagnosis of Stupor and Coma. 3rd ed. New York, NY: Oxford University Press; 1982.

19. Langfitt TW, Weinstein JD, Kassell NF, et al. Transmission of increased intracranial pressure. I. Within the craniospinal axis. *J Neurosurg*. 1964;21:989.

20. Langfitt TW. Increased intracranial pressure. *Clin Neurosurg*. 1969;16:436.

21. Graham DI, Ford I, Adams JH, et al. Ischeaemic brain damage is still common in fatal non-missile head injury. *J Neurol Neurosurg Psychiatry*. 1989;52:346.

22. Marmarou A, Anderson RL, Ward JL, et al. Impact of ICP instability and hypotension on outcome in patients with severe head trauma. *J Neurosurg*. 1991;75:S59.

23. Obrist WD, Wilkinson WE. Regional cerebral blood flow measurement in humans by xenon-133 clearance. *Cerebrovasc Brain Metab Rev*. 1990;2:283.

24. Darby JM, Yonas H, Marion DW, et al. Local "inverse steal" induced by hyperventilation in head injury. *Neurosurgery*. 1988;23:84.

25. Marion DW, Darby J, Yonas H. Acute regional cerebral blood flow changes caused by severe head injuries. *J Neurosurg*. 1991;74:407.

26. Manley GT, Pitts LH, Morabito D, et al. Brain tissue oxygenation during hemorrhagic shock, resuscitation, and alterations in ventilation. *J Trauma Injury Infect Crit Care*. 1999;46:261.

27. Caron MJ, Hovda DA, Mazziotta JC, et al. The structural and metabolic anatomy of traumatic brain injury in humans: a computerized tomography and positron emission tomography analysis. *J Neurotrauma*. 1993;10(suppl 1):S58.

28. Caron MJ, Mazziotta JC, Hovda DA, et al. Quantification of cerebral glucose metabolism in brain-injured humans utilizing positron emission tomography. *J Cereb Blood Flow Metab*. 1993;13(suppl 1):S379.

29. Caron MJ. PET/SPECT imaging in head injury. In: Narayan RK, Wilberger JE, Povlishock JT, eds. *Neurotrauma*. New York, NY: McGraw-Hill; 1996.

30. Lam AM, Winn HR, Cullen BF, et al. Hyperglycemia and neurological outcome in patients with head injury. *J Neurosurg*. 1991;75:545.

31. Young B, Ott L, Dempsey R, et al. Relationship between admission hyperglycemia and neurologic outcome of severely brain-injured patients. *Ann Surg*. 1989;210:466.

32. Ayling J. Managing head injuries. *Emerg Med Serv*. 2002;31(8):42.

33. Jarvis C, ed. *Physical Examination and Health Assessment*. 6th ed. St. Louis, MO: Elsevier Publishers; 2012:71.

34. Brain Trauma Foundation. Glasgow Coma Score. In: Gabriel EJ, Ghajar J, Jagoda A, et al. *Guidelines for Prehospital Management of*

Traumatic Brain Injury. New York, NY: Brain Trauma Foundation; 2000.

35. Dula DJ, Fales W. The "ring sign:" is it a reliable indicator for cerebral spinal fluid? *Ann Emerg Med.* 1993;22:718.

36. American College of Surgeons (ACS). *Advanced Trauma Life Support.* Chicago, IL: ACS; 2004.

37. Servadei F, Nasi MT, Cremonini AM. Importance of a reliable admission Glasgow Coma Scale score for determining the need for evacuation of posttraumatic subdural hematomas: a prospective study of 65 patients. *J Trauma.* 1998;44:868.

38. Winkler JV, Rosen P, Alfrey EJ. Prehospital use of the Glasgow Coma Scale in severe head injury. *J Emerg Med.* 1984;2:1.

39. Brain Trauma Foundation. Hospital transport decisions. In: Gabriel EJ, Ghajar J, Jagoda A, et al. *Guidelines for Prehospital Management of Traumatic Brain Injury.* New York, NY: Brain Trauma Foundation; 2000.

40. American Academy of Neurology. The management of concussion in sports (summary statement). *Neurology.* 1997;48:581.

41. Cantu RC. Second impact syndrome. *Clin Sports Med.* 1998;17:37-44.

42. McCrory P. Does second impact syndrome exist? *Clin J Sport Med.* 2001;11:144-149.

43. Meagher RL, Young WF. Subdural hematoma. eMedicine, Medscape. http://emedicine.medscape.com/article/1137207-overview. Updated March 1, 2013. Accessed November 22, 2013.

44. Coughlin RF, Moser RP. Subdural hematoma. In: Domino FJ, ed. *The 5-Minute Clinical Consult 2013.* 21st ed. Philadelphia, PA: Wolters Kluwer Health/Lippincott Williams & Wilkins; 2013:1246-1247.

45. Rimel RW, Giordani B, Barth JT. Moderate head injury: completing the clinical spectrum of brain trauma. *Neurosurgery.* 11:344, 1982.

46. Quigley MR, Chew BG, Swartz CE, Wilberger JE. The clinical significance of isolated traumatic subarachnoid hemorrhage. *J Trauma Acute Care Surg.* 2013;74:581-584.

47. Brain Trauma Foundation. CT scan features. In: Bullock MR, Chesnut RM, Clifton GL, et al. *Management and Prognosis of Severe Traumatic Brain Injury.* 2nd ed. New York, NY: Brain Trauma Foundation; 2000.

48. Kihtir T, Ivatury RR, Simon RJ, et al. Early management of civilian gunshot wounds to the face. *J Trauma.* 1993;35:569.

49. Winchell RJ, Hoyt DB. Endotracheal intubation in the field improves survival in patients with severe head injury. *Arch Surg.* 1997;132:592.

50. Davis DP, Hoyt DB, Ochs M, et al. The effect of paramedic rapid sequence intubation on outcome in patients with severe traumatic brain injury. *J Trauma Injury Infect Crit Care.* 2003;54:444.

51. Bochicchio GV, Ilahi O, Joshi M, et al. Endotracheal intubation in the field does not improve outcome in trauma patients who present without an acutely lethal traumatic brain injury. *J Trauma Injury Infect Crit Care.* 2003;54:307.

52. Davis DP, Peay J, Sise MJ, et al. The impact of prehospital endotracheal intubation in moderate to severe traumatic brain injury. *J Trauma.* 2005;58:933.

53. Bulger EM, Copass MK, Sabath DR, et al. The use of neuromuscular blocking agents to facilitate prehospital intubation does not impair outcome after traumatic brain injury. *J Trauma.* 2005;58:718.

54. Wang HE, Peitzman AB, Cassidy LD, et al. Out-of-hospital endotracheal intubation and outcome after traumatic brain injury. *Ann Emerg Med.* 2004;44:439.

55. Chi JH, Knudson MM, Vassar MJ, et al. Prehospital hypoxia affects outcome in patients with traumatic brain injury: a prospective multi-center study. *J Trauma.* 2006;61:1134.

56. Dunford JV, Davis DP, Ochs M, et al. Incidence of transient hypoxia and pulse rate reactivity during paramedic rapid sequence intubation. *Ann Emerg Med.* 2003;42:721.

57. Davis DP, Ochs M, Hoyt DB, et al. Paramedic-administered neuromuscular blockade improves prehospital intubation success in severely head-injured patients. *J Trauma Injury Infect Crit Care.* 2003;55:713.

58. Marlow TJ, Goltra DD, Schabel SI. Intracranial placement of a nasotracheal tube after facial fracture: a rare complication. *J Emerg Med.* 1997;15:187.

59. Horellou MD, Mathe D, Feiss P. A hazard of nasotracheal intubation. *Anaesthesia.* 1978;22:78.

60. Cooper KR, Boswell PA, Choi SC. Safe use of PEEP in patients with severe brain injury. *J Neurosurg.* 1985;63:552.

61. McGuire G, Crossley D, Richards J, et al. Effects of varying levels of positive end-expiratory pressure on intracranial pressure and cerebral perfusion pressure. *Crit Care Med.* 1997;25:1059.

62. Warner KJ, Cuschieri J, Copass MK, et al. The impact of prehospital ventilation on outcome after severe traumatic brain injury. *J Trauma.* 2007;62:1330.

63. Christensen MA, Bloom J, Sutton KR. Comparing arterial and end-tidal carbon dioxide values in hyperventilated neurosurgical patients. *Am J Crit Care.* 1995;4:116.

64. Grenier B, Dubreuil M. Noninvasive monitoring of carbon dioxide: end-tidal versus transcutaneous carbon dioxide. *Anesth Analg.* 1998;86:675.

65. Grenier B, Verchere E, Mesli A, et al. Capnography monitoring during neurosurgery: reliability in relation to various intra-operative positions. *Anesth Analg.* 1999;88:43.

66. Isert P. Control of carbon dioxide levels during neuroanaesthesia: current practice and an appraisal of our reliance upon capnography. *Anaesth Intensive Care.* 1994;22:435.

67. Kerr ME, Zempsky J, Sereika S, et al. Relationship between arterial carbon dioxide and end-tidal carbon dioxide in mechanically ventilated adults with severe head trauma. *Crit Care Med.* 1996;24:785.

68. Mackersie RC, Karagianes TG. Use of end-tidal carbon dioxide tension for monitoring induced hypocapnia in head-injured patients. *Crit Care Med.* 1990;18:764.

69. Russell GB, Graybeal JM. Reliability of the arterial to end-tidal carbon dioxide gradient in mechanically ventilated patients with multisystem trauma. *J Trauma Injury Infect Crit Care.* 1994;36:317.

70. Sanders AB. Capnometry in emergency medicine. *Ann Emerg Med.* 1989;18:1287-1290.

71. Sharma SK, McGuire GP, Cruise CJE. Stability of the arterial to end-tidal carbon dioxide difference during anaesthesia for prolonged neurosurgical procedures. *Can J Anaesthesiol.* 1995;42:498.

72. Warner KJ, Cuschieri J, Garland B, et al. The utility of early end-tidal capnography in monitoring ventilation status after severe trauma. *J Trauma.* 2009;66:26-31.

73. Davis DP, Dunford JV, Poste JC, et al. The impact of hypoxia and hyperventilation on outcome after paramedic rapid sequence intubation of severely head injured patients. *J Trauma.* 2004;57:1.

74. Badjatia N, Carney N, Crocco TJ, et al. Treatment: cerebral herniation. In: Gabriel EJ, Ghajar J, Jagoda A, et al. *Guidelines for Prehospital Management of Traumatic Brain Injury.* New York, NY: Brain Trauma Foundation; 2000.

75. Cooper DJ, Myles PS, McDermott FT, et al. Prehospital hypertonic saline resuscitation of patients with hypotension and severe traumatic brain injury: a randomized controlled trial. *JAMA.* 2004;291:1350.

76. Feldman Z, Kanter MJ, Robertson CS. Effect of head elevation on intracranial pressure, cerebral perfusion pressure and cerebral blood flow in head-injured patients. *J Neurosurg.* 1992;76:207.

Suggested Reading

American College of Surgeons (ACS) Committee on Trauma. Head trauma. In: *Advanced Trauma Life Support for Doctors, Student Course Manual.* 9th ed. Chicago, IL: ACS; 2012.

Atkinson JLD. The neglected prehospital phase of head injury: apnea and catecholamine surge. *Mayo Clin Proceed.* 2000;75:37.

Chi JH, Nemani V, Manley GT. Prehospital treatment of traumatic brain injury. *Sem Neurosurg.* 2003;14:71.

Kolb JC, Summer RL, Galli L. Cervical collar–induced changes in intracranial pressure. *Am J Emerg Med.* 1999;17:135.

Rosner MJ, Coley IB. Cerebral perfusion pressure, intracranial pressure and head elevation. *J Neurosurg.* 1986;65:636.

Teasdale G, Jennett B. Assessment of coma and impaired consciousness: a practical scale. *Lancet.* 1974;2:81.

Valadka AB. Injury to the cranium. In: Mattox KL, Feliciano DV, Moore EE. *Trauma.* 4th ed. Norwalk, CN: Appleton & Lange; 2000.

CHAPTER 11

Spinal Trauma

CHAPTER OBJECTIVES

At the completion of this chapter, the reader will be able to do the following:

- Describe the epidemiology of spinal injuries.

- Compare and contrast the most common mechanisms that produce spinal injury in adults with those in children.

- Recognize patients with the potential for spinal trauma.

- Relate the signs and symptoms of spinal injury and neurogenic shock with their underlying pathophysiology.

- Integrate principles of anatomy and pathophysiology with assessment data and

principles of trauma management to formulate a treatment plan for the patient with obvious or potential spinal injury.

- Describe the indications for selective spinal immobilization.

- Discuss factors associated with prehospital findings and interventions that may affect spinal injury morbidity and mortality.

- Understand the principles of selective spinal immobilization and how the application of these principles may change dependent on the patient and the situation.

SCENARIO

You have been dispatched to the scene of a bicyclist who is reported down alongside a roadway. On arrival, you find a 19-year-old woman lying supine on the side of the road away from traffic. The scene is safe, with traffic being controlled by the police. A police officer is kneeling next to the patient trying to talk to her, but she is not responding.

As you begin your primary assessment, you find an unresponsive female patient who fell from her bike while riding along a roadway. You are unable to ascertain the specific cause of the fall, and the police do not know if she was struck by a motor vehicle, as there were no witnesses. She is wearing full cycling gear, including helmet and gloves. She has abrasions on her forehead and an obvious deformity of the right wrist. Her airway is open, and she is breathing regularly. She shows no obvious signs of external blood loss. Her skin appears dry and warm with normal color. As you are performing your primary assessment, she begins to awaken but remains confused as to what happened.

- What pathologic processes explain the patient's presentation?
- What immediate interventions and further assessments are needed?
- What are the management goals for this patient?

Introduction

Spinal trauma, if not recognized and properly managed, can result in irreparable damage to the spinal cord and leave the patient with a lifelong neurologic disability. Some patients sustain immediate spinal cord damage as a result of the trauma event. Others sustain an injury to the spinal column that does not initially damage the spinal cord; spinal cord damage may result later with movement of the spine. Because the central nervous system (CNS) is incapable of regeneration, a severed spinal cord cannot be repaired. Inappropriately moving a patient with a spinal column injury or allowing the patient to move can result in a devastating injury to the spinal cord, if it has not already been damaged. Failure to suspect, properly assess, and immobilize a patient with a potential spine injury may produce a much worse outcome than failure to immobilize a fractured femur properly, for example. Conversely, spinal immobilization of the patient has been shown to have potentially serious consequences and should not be done in patients who have no indications of injury involving the spinal column or cord.

Spinal cord injury can have profound effects on human physiology, lifestyle, and financial circumstances. Human physiology is affected because the use of extremities or other functions is severely limited or completely impaired as a result of spinal cord damage. Lifestyle is affected because spinal cord injury usually results in profound changes to daily activity levels and independence. Spinal cord injury also impacts the financial circumstances of the patient as well as the population in general.[1] A patient with this injury requires both acute and long-term care. The lifetime cost of this care is estimated to be approximately $1.35 million per patient for a permanent spinal cord injury.[2]

About 32 people per 1 million of the population in the United States will sustain some type of spinal cord injury annually.

An estimated 250,000 to 400,000 people live with spinal cord injuries in the United States. Spinal cord injury can occur at any age; however, it usually occurs in those 16 to 35 years of age because this age group is involved in the most violent and high-risk activities. Most trauma patients are 16 to 20 years of age. The second largest group of patients is 21 to 25 years, and the third largest group is 26 to 35 years of age. Males outnumber females. Common causes are motor vehicle crashes (48%), falls (21%), penetrating injuries (15%), sports injuries (14%), and other injuries (2%). Overall, approximately 11,000 people sustain spinal cord injuries annually in the United States.[3]

Sudden violent forces acting on the body can force the spine and its ligaments beyond their normal limits of motion either by impacting directly on the head or neck or by driving the torso out from under the head. The following four concepts help clarify the possible effect of energy on the spine when evaluating the potential for injury:

1. The head is similar to a bowling ball perched on top of the neck, and its mass often moves in a different direction from the torso, resulting in strong forces being applied to the neck (cervical spine, spinal cord).
2. Objects in motion tend to stay in motion, and objects at rest tend to stay at rest (Newton's first law).
3. Sudden or violent movement of the upper legs displaces the pelvis, resulting in forceful movement of the lower spine. Because of the weight and inertia of the head and torso, force in an opposite (contra) direction is applied to the upper spine.
4. Lack of neurologic deficit does not rule out bone or ligament injury to the spinal column or conditions that have stressed the spinal cord to the limit of its tolerance.

Neurologic deficits result from trauma to a number of different central and peripheral nervous system structures. As discussed in the previous chapter, traumatic brain injury is a common cause of neurologic injury. Some trauma patients with neurologic deficit will have a spinal cord injury. Other patients have neurologic deficit caused by either a direct peripheral nerve injury or an extremity injury that is associated with a nerve injury but not a spinal cord injury. In all of these situations, the neurologic damage may be temporary in some instances, but will, most likely, be permanent. It should be assumed that any patient who has been injured as a result of any of the following mechanisms has a potential spinal injury:

- Any blunt mechanism that produced a violent impact on the head, neck, torso, or pelvis
- Incidents that produce sudden acceleration, deceleration, or lateral bending forces to the neck or torso
- Any fall from a height, especially in elderly persons
- Ejection or a fall from any motorized or otherwise powered transportation device
- Any shallow-water diving incident[4,5]

Any such patient should be manually stabilized in a neutral in-line position (unless contraindicated) until the need for spinal immobilization has been assessed.

Anatomy and Physiology

Vertebral Anatomy

The spinal column is composed of 33 bones called vertebrae, which are stacked on top of one another. Except for the first (C1) and second (C2) vertebrae (cervical) at the top of the spine and the fused sacral and coccygeal vertebrae at the lower spine, all the vertebrae are almost alike in form, structure, and motion (**Figure 11-1**). The largest part of each vertebra is the anterior part called the *body*. Each vertebral body bears most of the weight of the vertebral column and torso superior to it. Two curved sides called the **neural arches** are formed by the pedicle and posteriorly by the lamina projecting back from the body. The posterior part of the vertebra is a tail-like structure called the spinous process. In the lower five cervical vertebrae, this **spinous process** points directly posterior; in the thoracic and lumbar vertebrae, it points slightly downward in a caudad direction (toward the feet).

Most vertebrae also have similarly styled protuberances called **transverse processes** at each side near their anterior lateral margins. The transverse and spinous processes serve as points of attachment for muscles and ligaments and are therefore fulcrums for movement. The neural arches and the posterior part of each vertebral body form a near-circular shape with an opening in the center called the **vertebral foramen** (spinal canal). The spinal cord passes through this space. The spinal cord is protected somewhat from injury by the bony vertebrae surrounding it. Each vertebral foramen lines up with that of

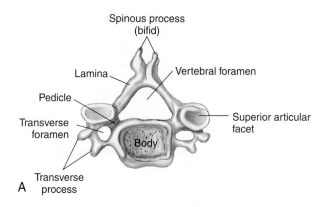

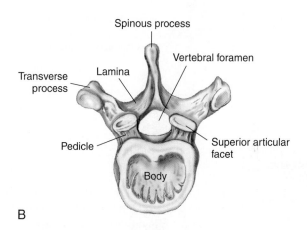

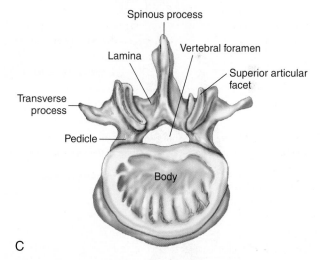

Figure 11-1 Except for the fused sacral and coccygeal vertebrae, each vertebra has the same parts as the other vertebrae. The body (anterior portion) of each vertebra becomes larger and stronger because it must support more weight nearing the pelvis. **A.** Fifth cervical vertebra. **B.** Thoracic vertebra. **C.** Lumbar vertebra.

the vertebrae above and the vertebrae below to form the hollow spinal canal through which the spinal cord passes.

Vertebral Column

The individual vertebrae are stacked in an S-shape column (**Figure 11-2**). This organization allows extensive multidirectional movement while imparting maximum strength. The spinal column is divided into five individual regions for reference. Beginning at the top of the spinal column and descending downward, these regions are the cervical, thoracic, lumbar, sacral, and coccygeal regions. Vertebrae are identified by the first letter of the region in which they are found and their sequence from the top of that region. The first cervical vertebra is called *C1*, the third thoracic vertebra *T3*, the fifth lumbar vertebra *L5*, and so on throughout the entire spinal column. Each vertebra supports increasing body weight as the vertebrae progress down the spinal column. Appropriately, the vertebrae from C3 to L5 become progressively larger to accommodate the increased weight and workload (see Figure 11-1).

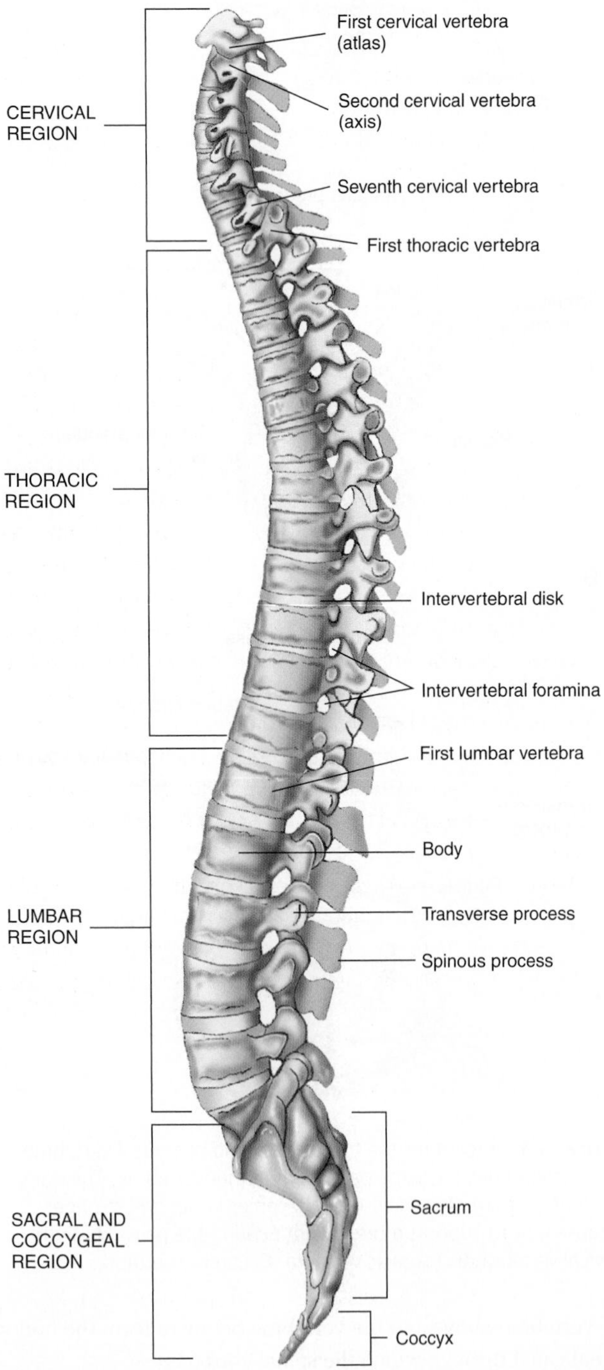

Located at the top end of the spinal column are the seven *cervical* vertebrae that support the head and make up the neck. The cervical region is flexible to allow for total movement of the head. Next are 12 *thoracic* vertebrae. Each pair of ribs connects posteriorly to one of the thoracic vertebrae. Unlike the cervical spine, the thoracic spine is relatively rigid, with less movement. Below the thoracic vertebrae are the five *lumbar* vertebrae. These are the most massive of all the vertebrae. The lumbar area is also flexible, allowing for movement in several directions. The five *sacral* vertebrae are fused, forming a single structure known as the **sacrum**. The four *coccygeal* vertebrae are also fused, forming the *coccyx* (tailbone). Approximately 55% of spinal injuries occur in the cervical region, 15% in the thoracic region, 15% at the thoracolumbar junction, and 15% in the lumbosacral area.

Ligaments and muscles tether the spine from the base of the skull to the pelvis. These ligaments and muscles form a web that sheathes the entire bony part of the spinal column, holding it in normal alignment, providing stability, and allowing for movement. If these ligaments and muscles are torn, excessive movement of one vertebra in relation to another can occur. In the presence of torn spinal ligaments, this excessive movement may result in dislocation of the vertebrae, which can compromise the space inside the spinal canal and, thus, impinge upon and damage the spinal cord.

The anterior and posterior longitudinal ligaments connect the vertebral bodies anteriorly and inside the canal. Ligaments between the spinous processes provide support for flexion–extension (forward and backward) movement, and those between the lamina provide support during lateral flexion (side bending) (**Figure 11-3**).

The head balances on top of the spine, and the spine is supported by the pelvis. The skull perches on the ring-shaped first cervical vertebra (C1), referred to as the **atlas**. The **axis**, C2, is also basically ring shaped but has a spur (the odontoid process) that protrudes upward similar to a tooth, located just behind the anterior arch of the atlas (**Figure 11-4**). The axis allows the head approximately a 180-degree range of rotation.

The human head weighs between 16 and 22 pounds (7 to 10 kilograms [kg]), somewhat more than the average weight of a bowling ball. The weight and position of the head atop the thin and flexible neck, the forces that act on the head, the small size of the supporting muscle, and the lack of ribs or other bones help make the cervical spine particularly susceptible to injury. At the level of C3, the spinal cord occupies approximately 95% of the spinal canal (the spinal cord occupies approximately

Figure 11-2 The vertebral column is not a straight rod, but a series of blocks that are stacked to allow for several bends or curves. At each of the curves, the spine is more vulnerable to fractures; hence the origin of the phrase "breaking the S in a fall."

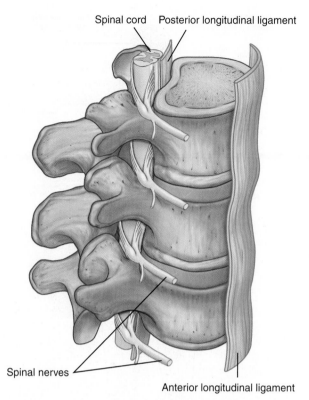

Figure 11-3 Anterior and posterior longitudinal ligaments of vertebral column.

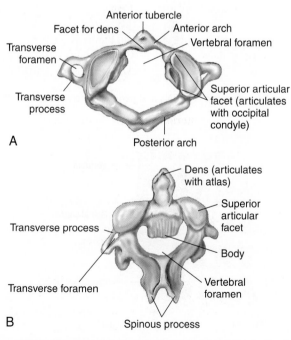

Figure 11-4 The first and second cervical vertebrae are uniquely shaped. **A.** Atlas (C1). **B.** Axis (C2).

point can produce compression of the spinal cord. The posterior neck muscles are strong, permitting up to 60% of the range of flexion and 70% of the range of extension of the head without any stretching of the spinal cord. However, when sudden violent acceleration, deceleration, or lateral force is applied to the body, the significant weight of the head on the narrow cervical spine can amplify the effects of sudden movement. An example of this scenario would be a rear-end collision without the headrest properly adjusted.

The sacrum is the base of the spinal column, the platform on which the spinal column rests. The sacrum supports between 70% and 80% of the body's total weight. The sacrum is a part of both the spinal column and the pelvic girdle, and it is joined to the rest of the pelvis by immovable joints.

Spinal Cord Anatomy

The spinal cord is continuous with the brain and starts from the base of the brain stem, passing through the foramen magnum (the hole at the base of the skull) and through each vertebra via the spinal canal to the level of the second lumbar (L2) vertebra. Blood is supplied to the spinal cord by the vertebral and spinal arteries.

The spinal cord is surrounded by cerebrospinal fluid (CSF) and is encased in a dural sheath. This dural sheath covers the brain and continues down to the second sacral vertebra to a saclike reservoir (the great cistern). CSF produced by the brain passes around the cord and is absorbed in this cistern. CSF performs the same function for the spinal cord as for the brain, acting as a cushion against injury during rapid and severe movement.

The spinal cord itself consists of gray matter and white matter. The gray matter consists of the bodies of the nerve cells. The white matter contains the long axons that make up the anatomic spinal tracts and serve as the communication pathways for nerve impulses. Spinal tracts are divided into two types: ascending and descending (**Figure 11-5**).

Ascending nerve tracts carry sensory impulses from distal body parts through the spinal cord up to the brain. Ascending nerve tracts can be further divided into tracts that carry the different sensations of pain and temperature; touch and pressure;

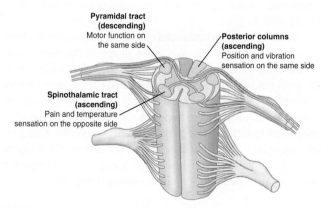

Figure 11-5 Spinal cord tracts.

65% of the spinal canal area at its end in the lumbar region), and only 3 millimeters (mm) of clearance exists between the spinal cord and the canal wall. Even a minor dislocation at this

and sensory impulses of motion, vibration, position, and light touch. The nerve tracts that carry pain and temperature sensation "cross over" in the spinal cord, meaning that the nerve root with the information from the right side of the body crosses over to the left side of the spinal cord and then goes up to the brain. In contrast, the nerve tract that carries the sensory information for position, vibration, and light touch does *not* cross over in the spinal cord. Thus, this sensory information is carried up to the brain on the same side of the spinal cord as the nerve roots.

Descending nerve tracts are responsible for carrying motor impulses from the brain through the spinal cord down to the body, and they control all muscle movement and muscle tone. These descending tracts also do not cross over in the spinal cord. Therefore the motor tract on the right side of the spinal cord controls motor function on the right side of the body. These motor tracts *do* cross over in the brain stem, however, so the left side of the brain controls motor function on the right side of the body, and vice versa.

As the spinal cord continues to descend, pairs of nerves branch off from the spinal cord at each vertebra and extend to the various parts of the body (**Figure 11-6**). The spinal cord has 31 pairs of spinal nerves, named according to the level from which they arise. Each nerve has two roots on each side.

The **dorsal root** is for sensory impulses, and the ventral root is for motor impulses. Neurologic stimuli pass between the brain and each part of the body through the spinal cord and particular pairs of these nerves. As they branch from the spinal cord, these nerves pass through a notch in the inferior lateral side of the vertebra, posterior to the vertebral body, called the **intervertebral foramen**. Cartilage-like intervertebral discs lie between the body of each vertebra and act as shock absorbers (**Figure 11-7**).

These nerve branches have multiple control functions, and their level in the spinal cord is represented by dermatomes on the skin. A **dermatome** is the sensory area on the skin surface of the body for which a nerve root is responsible. Collectively, dermatomes allow the body areas to be mapped out for each spinal level (**Figure 11-8**). Dermatomes help determine the level of a spinal cord injury. Three landmarks to keep in mind are the *clavicles*, which are the C4–C5 dermatome; the *nipple level*, which is the T4 dermatome; and the *umbilicus level*, which is the T10 dermatome. Remembering these three levels can help locate a spinal cord injury.

The process of inhalation and exhalation requires both chest excursion and proper changes in the shape of the diaphragm. The diaphragm is innervated by the phrenic nerves, which originate from the nerves arising from the spinal cord between levels C2 and C5. If the spinal cord above the level of C2 or the phrenic nerves are cut, or the nerve impulses are otherwise disrupted, a patient will lose the ability to breathe spontaneously. A patient with this injury may asphyxiate before the arrival of providers unless bystanders initiate rescue breathing. Positive-pressure ventilation will need to be continued during transport.

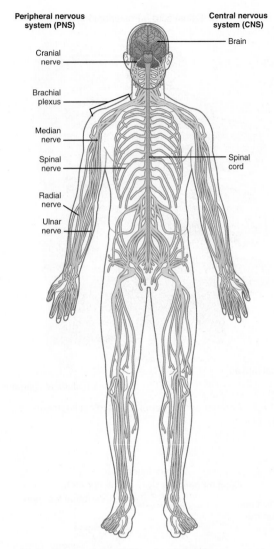

Figure 11-6   Nerves of the CNS and peripheral nervous system (PNS).

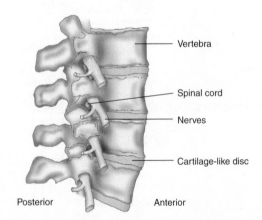

Figure 11-7   The cartilage between each vertebral body is called the intervertebral disc. These discs act as shock absorbers. If damaged, the cartilage may protrude into the spinal canal, compressing the cord or the nerves that come through the intervertebral foramina.

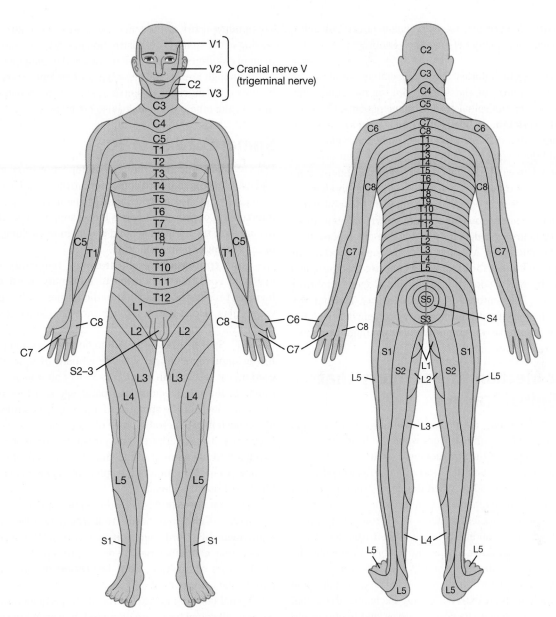

Figure 11-8 Dermatome map shows the relationship between areas of touch sensation on the skin and the spinal nerves that correspond to these areas. Loss of sensation in a specific area may indicate injury to the corresponding spinal nerve.

Pathophysiology

The bony spine can normally withstand forces of up to 1,000 foot-pounds (1,360 joules) of energy. High-speed travel and contact sports can routinely exert forces on the spine well in excess of this amount. Even in a low- to moderate-speed vehicle crash, the body of an unrestrained 150-pound (68-kg) person can easily place 3,000 to 4,000 foot-pounds (4,080 to 5,440 joules) of force against the spine as the head is suddenly stopped by the windshield or roof. Similar force can occur when a motorcyclist is thrown over the front of the motorcycle or when a high-speed skier collides with a tree.

Skeletal Injuries

Various types of injuries can occur to the spine, including the following:

- Compression fractures that produce wedge compression or total flattening of the body of the vertebra
- Fractures that produce small fragments of bone that may lie in the spinal canal near the cord
- **Subluxation**, which is a partial dislocation of a vertebra from its normal alignment in the spinal column

- Overstretching or tearing of the ligaments and muscles, producing instability between the vertebrae[6]

Any of these skeletal injuries may immediately result in the irreversible transection of the spinal cord, or the injury may compress or stretch the spinal cord. In some patients, however, damage to the vertebrae or ligaments results in an *unstable* spinal column injury but does not produce an immediate spinal cord injury. Should the fragments in an unstable spine shift position, they may then damage the spinal cord. In addition, patients who have one spine fracture have a 10% chance of having another spinal fracture. Therefore, the entire spine must be immobilized in patients who have indications for cervical spinal immobilization.

A lack of neurologic deficit does not rule out a bony fracture or an unstable spine. Although the presence of good motor and sensory responses in the extremities indicates that the spinal cord is currently intact, it does not exclude a damaged vertebra or associated bony, ligamentous, or soft-tissue injury. The majority of patients with spine fractures have no neurologic deficit. A full assessment is required to determine the need for immobilization.

Specific Mechanisms of Injury That Cause Spinal Trauma

Axial loading of the spine can occur in several ways. Most often, this compression of the spine occurs when the head strikes an object and the weight of the still-moving body bears against the stopped head, such as when the head of an unrestrained occupant strikes the windshield or when the head strikes an object in a shallow-water diving incident. Compression and axial loading also occur when a patient sustains a fall from a substantial height and lands in a standing position. This drives the weight of the head and thorax down against the lumbar spine while the sacral spine remains stationary. About 20% of falls from a height greater than 15 feet (4.6 m) involve an associated lumbar spine fracture. During such an extreme energy exchange, the spinal column tends to exaggerate its normal curves, and fractures and compressions occur at such areas. The spine is S shaped; therefore, it can be said that the compressive forces tend to "break the patient's S." These forces compress the concave side and open the convex side of the spine.

Excessive flexion (**hyperflexion**), *excessive extension* (**hyperextension**), and *excessive rotation* (**hyper-rotation**) can cause bone damage and tearing of muscles and ligaments, resulting in impingement on or stretching of the spinal cord.

Sudden or excessive lateral bending requires much less movement than flexion or extension before injury occurs because motion in this direction is limited to begin with. During lateral impact, the torso and the thoracic spine are moved laterally. The head tends to remain in place until it is pulled along by the cervical attachments. The center of gravity of the head is above and anterior to its seat and attachment to the cervical spine; therefore, the head will tend to roll sideways. This movement often results in dislocations and bony fractures.

Distraction (*over-elongation of the spine*) occurs when one part of the spine is stable and the rest is in longitudinal motion. This pulling apart of the spine can easily cause stretching and tearing of the spinal cord. Distraction injury is a common mechanism in children's playground injuries and in hangings.

Although any one of these types of violent movements may be the dominant cause of spinal injury in a given patient, one or more of the others will usually also be involved.

Spinal Cord Injuries

Primary injury occurs at the time of impact or force application and may cause spinal cord compression, direct spinal cord injury (usually from sharp unstable bony fragments or projectiles), and interruption of the spinal cord's blood supply. Secondary injury occurs after the initial insult and can include swelling, ischemia, or movement of bony fragments.[7]

Cord concussion results from the temporary disruption of spinal cord functions distal to the injury. **Cord contusion** involves bruising or bleeding into the tissues of the spinal cord, which may also result in a temporary (and sometimes permanent) loss of spinal cord functions distal to the injury (spinal "shock"). **Spinal shock** is a neurologic phenomenon that occurs for an unpredictable and variable amount of time after spinal cord injury, resulting in temporary loss of all sensory and motor function, muscle flaccidity and paralysis, and loss of reflexes below the level of the spinal cord injury. Cord contusion is usually caused by a penetrating type of injury or movement of bony fragments. The severity of injury resulting from the contusion is related to the amount of bleeding into the spinal cord tissue. Damage to or disruption of the spinal blood supply can result in local cord tissue ischemia.

Cord compression is pressure on the spinal cord caused by swelling, but also may occur from traumatic disc rupture and bone fragments. Cord compression may result in tissue ischemia and in some cases may require decompression to prevent a permanent loss of function. **Cord laceration** occurs when spinal cord tissue is torn or cut.

Spinal cord injury usually results in permanent disability if some or all spinal tracts are disrupted; however, neurologic deficits may be reversed if the spinal cord has sustained only slight damage. Spinal cord transection can be categorized as complete or incomplete. In **complete cord transection**, all spinal tracts are interrupted, and all spinal cord functions distal to the site are lost. Because of the additional effects of swelling, determination of the extent of loss of function may not be accurate until 24 hours after the injury. Most complete spinal cord transections result in either paraplegia or quadriplegia, depending on the level of the injury. In **incomplete cord transection**, some tracts and motor/sensory functions remain intact. Prognosis for recovery is greater in these cases than with complete transection.

Types of incomplete cord injuries include the following:

- **Anterior cord syndrome** is typically a result of bony fragments or pressure on spinal arteries (**Figure 11-9**). Symptoms include loss of motor function and pain, temperature, and light touch sensations. However, some light touch, motion, position, and vibration sensations are spared.

- **Central cord syndrome** usually occurs with hyperextension of the cervical area (**Figure 11-10**). Symptoms include weakness or paresthesias in the upper extremities but normal strength and sensation in the lower extremities. This syndrome causes varying degrees of bladder dysfunction.
- **Brown-Séquard syndrome** is caused by penetrating injury and involves hemi-transection of the spinal cord, involving only one side of the spinal cord (**Figure 11-11**). Symptoms include complete spinal cord damage and loss of function on the affected side (motor, vibration, motion, and position) with loss of pain and temperature sensation on the side opposite the injury.[8]

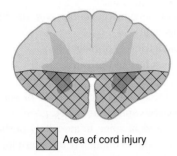

Area of cord injury

Figure 11-9 Anterior cord syndrome.

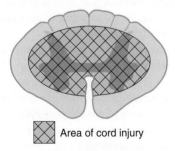

Area of cord injury

Figure 11-10 Central cord syndrome.

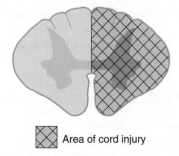

Area of cord injury

Figure 11-11 Brown-Séquard syndrome.

Neurogenic "shock" secondary to spinal cord injury represents a significant additional finding. This condition is different than spinal shock, which was described earlier. Although many people use the terms "neurogenic shock" and "spinal shock" interchangeably, in fact, they represent different entities. When the spinal cord is disrupted, the body's sympathetic control mechanism is interrupted and can no longer maintain constriction of

the muscles in the walls of the blood vessels below the point of disruption. These arteries and arterioles dilate, enlarging the size of the vascular container, which leads to a partial loss of systemic vascular resistance. This causes a relative hypovolemia, and, as a result, the blood pressure will decrease. The skin, however, will be warm and dry, rather than cold and clammy as would be expected with hemorrhagic shock. Instead of the tachycardia usually associated with hypovolemic shock, this type of injury is associated with a normal heart rate or a slight bradycardia.

Although the patient may be hypotensive, neurogenic "shock" often does not cause impairment in oxygen delivery to peripheral tissues (see the Shock chapter). High spinal cord injuries (C5 or above) are more likely to require cardiovascular interventions such as vasopressors and pacemakers.[9] A recent consensus statement recommends prompt correction of hypotension (systolic blood pressure of less than 90 millimeters of mercury [mm Hg]) in the setting of acute spinal cord injury to prevent secondary injury. Ideally, the blood pressure of patients with suspected spinal cord injury should be maintained in a normal range (mean arterial pressure of 85 to 90 mm Hg).[10]

Assessment

Spinal injury, as with other conditions, should be assessed in the context of other injuries and conditions present. The primary assessment is the first priority. However, often the patient first needs to be moved in order to ensure the safety of all individuals at the scene. Therefore, a rapid scene assessment and history of the event should determine if the possibility of a spinal injury exists, in which case the patient's spine must be manually protected. The patient's head is brought into a neutral in-line position, unless contraindicated (see the Manual In-line Stabilization of the Head discussion later in this chapter). The head is maintained in that position until the assessment reveals no indication for immobilization, or the manual stabilization is replaced with a spinal motion restriction device, such as cervical collar with a half-spine board, long backboard, or vest-type device.

Neurologic Examination

In the field, a rapid neurologic examination is performed to identify obvious deficits related to a spinal cord injury. The patient is asked to move the arms, hands, and legs, and any inability to do so is noted. Then the patient is checked for the presence or absence of sensation, beginning at the shoulders and moving down the body to the feet. A complete neurologic examination does not need to be performed in the prehospital setting as it will not provide additional information that will affect the decisions about needed prehospital care and only serves to expend precious time on scene and delay transport.

The rapid neurologic examination should be repeated after the patient has been immobilized, any time the patient is moved, and upon arrival to the receiving facility. This will help identify any changes in patient condition that may have occurred after the primary assessment.

Using Mechanism of Injury to Assess Spinal Cord Injury

Traditionally, prehospital care providers have been taught that suspicion for a spinal injury is based solely on the mechanism of injury and that spinal immobilization is required for any patient with a suggestive mechanism of injury. This generalization has caused a lack of clear clinical guidelines for assessment of spinal cord injuries. However, assessment of the neck and spine for spinal immobilization should also include assessment of the motor and sensory function, presence of pain or tenderness, and patient reliability as predictors of spinal cord injury (**Figure 11-12**). In addition, the patient may not complain of pain in the spinal column because of pain associated with a more distracting painful injury, such as a fractured femur.[9] Alcohol or drugs that the patient may have ingested as well as traumatic brain injury may also blunt the patient's perception of pain and mask serious injury.

Figure 11-12   Indications for Spinal Immobilization

- Tenderness on palpation of the spinal column
- Complaint of pain in the spine
- Altered mental status (e.g., traumatic brain injury, under the influence of alcohol or intoxicating substances)
- Inability to communicate effectively (e.g., extremely young age, language barrier)
- Glasgow Coma Scale (GCS) score of less than 15
- Evidence of distracting injury
- Paralysis or other neurologic deficit or complaint

The primary focus of prehospital care is to recognize the indications for spinal immobilization rather than to attempt to clear the spine.[11-18] Because many patients do not have spinal injury, a selective approach to performing spinal immobilization is appropriate, especially since spinal immobilization has been shown to produce adverse effects in healthy volunteers, including increases in respiratory effort, skin ischemia, and pain.[19] This selective approach to spinal immobilization is even more important with the elderly population, who may be more susceptible to skin breakdown and have underlying pulmonary disease. Prehospital care providers should focus on appropriate indications for performing spinal immobilization.[20]

If no indications are present after a careful and thorough examination, there may be no need for spinal immobilization. The cornerstone to proper spinal care is the same as with all trauma care: superior assessment, with appropriate and timely treatment.

Blunt Trauma

Major causes of spinal injury in adult patients include the following:

1. Motor vehicle crashes
2. Falls
3. Motorcycle crashes
4. Sports injuries
5. Violent trauma
6. Shallow-water incidents

Major causes of spinal injury in pediatric patients include the following:

1. Falls from heights (generally two to three times the patient's height)
2. Falls from a tricycle or bicycle
3. Being struck by a motor vehicle

As a general guideline, the presence of spinal injury and a potentially unstable spine should be presumed, manual stabilization of the cervical spine immediately performed, and an assessment of the spine conducted to determine the need for immobilization with the following situations:

- Any blunt mechanism that produced a violent impact on the head, neck, torso, or pelvis (e.g., assault, entrapment in a structural collapse)
- Incidents that produced sudden acceleration, deceleration, or lateral bending forces to the neck or torso (e.g., moderate- to high-speed motor vehicle crashes, pedestrians struck by vehicle, involvement in explosion)
- Any fall, especially in elderly persons
- Ejection or fall from any motorized or otherwise powered transportation device (e.g., scooters, skateboards, bicycles, motor vehicles, motorcycles, recreational vehicles)
- Any shallow-water incident (e.g., diving, body surfing)

Other situations often associated with spinal damage include the following:

- Head injuries with any alteration   in level of consciousness
- Significant helmet damage
- Significant blunt injury to the torso
- Impacted or other deceleration fractures of the legs or hips
- Significant localized injuries to the area of the spinal column

These mechanisms of injury should mandate a thorough and complete examination of the patient to determine if indications are present that necessitate spinal immobilization. If no indications are found, manual stabilization of the cervical spine can be discontinued.

The wearing of proper seat belt restraints has proven to save lives and reduce head, face, and thoracic injuries. However, the use of proper restraints does not completely rule out the possibility of spinal injury. In significant frontal-impact collisions when sudden severe deceleration occurs, the restrained torso stops suddenly as the seat and shoulder belts engage, but the unrestrained head can continue its forward movement. If the force of deceleration is strong enough, the head will move down until the chin strikes the chest wall, frequently rotating across the diagonal strap of the shoulder restraint. Such rapid, forceful hyperflexion and rotation of the neck can result in compression fractures of the cervical vertebrae, "jumped" facets (dislocation of the articular processes), and stretching of the spinal cord. Different mechanisms can also cause spinal trauma in restrained victims of rear or lateral collisions. The amount of damage to the vehicle and the patient's other injuries are the key factors in determining if a patient needs to be immobilized.

The patient's ability to walk should not be a consideration in determining whether a patient needs to be treated for potential spinal injury. A significant number of patients who require surgical repair of unstable spinal injuries were found "walking around" at the scene or walked into the emergency department (ED) at the hospital.

Penetrating Trauma

Penetrating injury represents a special consideration regarding the potential for spinal trauma.[21] In general, if a patient did not sustain definite neurologic injury at the moment that the penetrating trauma occurred, there is little concern for subsequent development of a spinal cord injury (**Figure 11-13**). This is because of the mechanism of injury and the kinematics associated with the force involved. Penetrating objects generally do not produce unstable spinal fractures because penetrating trauma, unlike blunt injury, produces minimal risk of creating unstable ligamentous or bony injury. A penetrating object causes injury along the path of penetration. If the object did not directly injure the spinal cord as it penetrated, the patient is unlikely to develop a spinal cord injury.

Numerous studies have shown that unstable spinal injuries rarely occur from penetrating trauma to the head, neck, or torso[22-29] and that isolated penetrating injuries by themselves are not indications for spinal immobilization. Because of the very low risk of an unstable spinal injury and because the other injuries created by the penetrating trauma often require a higher priority in management, patients with penetrating trauma need not undergo spinal immobilization. In fact, a retrospective study utilizing the National Trauma Data Bank documented that patients with penetrating trauma who received spinal immobilization in the field had a higher overall mortality rate than those who did not.[30] However, the prehospital care provider must be alert to the fact

Figure 11-13 Penetrating Injuries

Penetrating injuries by themselves are not indications for spinal immobilization.

that there may be blunt trauma involved along with the penetrating trauma. A person who fell down a flight of stairs after being shot or stabbed or was involved in a fight prior to receiving a gunshot wound may well be a candidate for spinal immobilization.

Indications for Spinal Immobilization

The mechanism of injury can be used as an aid to determine indications for spinal immobilization (**Figure 11-14**). The key point always is that a complete physical assessment coupled with good clinical judgment will guide decision making, and *if in doubt, immobilize.*

Patients with a penetrating injury (e.g., gunshot or stab wounds) to the head, neck, or torso should be considered to have a concerning mechanism of injury when they complain of neurologic symptoms or display such findings as numbness, tingling, and loss of motor or sensory function or actual loss of consciousness. However, if patients with penetrating injury have no neurologic complaints, secondary mechanism of injury, or other findings, the spine does not need to be immobilized (although the backboard may still be used for lifting and transport purposes).

In the patient with blunt trauma, the following conditions should mandate spinal immobilization:

1. *Altered level of consciousness*, with Glasgow Coma Scale (GCS) score less than 15. Any factor that alters the patient's perception of pain will hinder the prehospital care provider's assessment for injury; such factors include:
   - Traumatic brain injury
   - Altered mental status other than traumatic brain injury (For example, patients with psychiatric illness, with Alzheimer's disease, or under the influence of intoxicants may have impaired pain perception.)
   - Acute stress reactions, which may cause "pain masking"
2. *Spinal pain or tenderness.* This includes subjective pain or pain on movement, point tenderness, or guarding of the muscles in the spinal area.
3. *Neurologic deficit or complaint.* This includes bilateral paralysis, partial paralysis, paresis (weakness), numbness, prickling or tingling, and neurogenic spinal shock below the level of the injury. In males, a continuing erection of the penis (priapism) may be an additional indication of spinal cord injury.

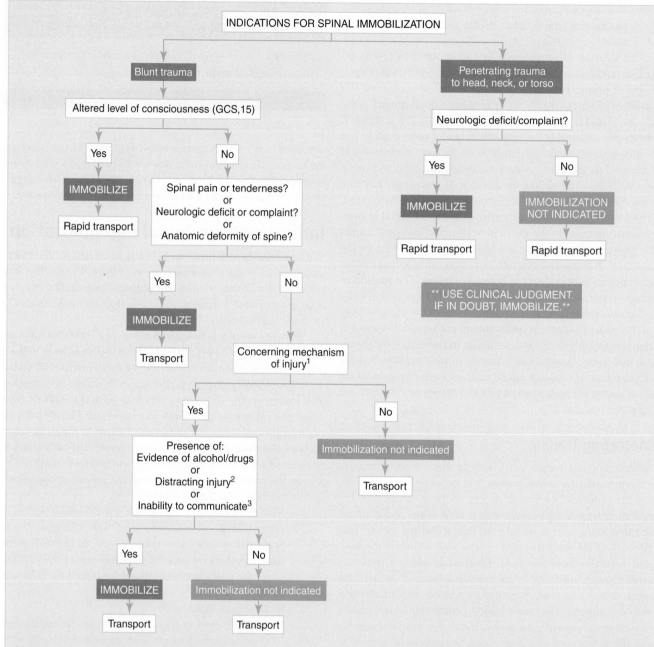

Notes:

[1]Concerning mechanisms of injury
- Any mechanism that produced a violent impact to the head, neck, torso, or pelvis (e.g., assault, entrapment in structural collapse, etc.)
- Incidents producing sudden acceleration, deceleration, or lateral bending forces to the neck or torso (e.g., moderate- to high-speed MVC, pedestrian struck, involvement in an explosion, etc.)
- Any fall, especially in elderly persons
- Ejection or fall from any motorized or otherwise-powered transportation device (e.g., scooters, skateboards, bicycles, motor vehicles, motorcycles, or recreational vehicles)
- Victim of shallow-water diving incident

[2]Distracting injury
Any injury that may have the potential to impair the patient's ability to appreciate other injuries. Examples of distracting injuries include a) long bone fracture, b) a visceral injury requiring surgical consultation, c) a large laceration, degloving injury, or crush injury, d) large burns, or e) any other injury producing acute functional impairment.
(Adapted from Hoffman JR, Wolfson AB, Todd K, Mower WR: Selective cervical spine radiography in blunt trauma: methodology of the National Emergency X-Radiography Utilization Study [NEXUS], *Ann Emerg Med* 461, 1998.)

[3]Inability to communicate.
Any patient who, for reasons not specified above, cannot clearly communicate so as to actively participate in their assessment. Examples: speech or hearing impaired, those who only speak a foreign language, and small children.

Figure 11-14 Indications for spinal immobilization.

4. *Anatomic deformity of the spine.* This includes any deformity of the spine noted on physical examination of the patient.

However, the absence of these signs does not rule out bony spinal injury (**Figure 11-15**).

When a patient has a concerning mechanism of injury in the absence of the conditions just listed, the reliability of the patient must be assessed. A reliable patient is calm and cooperative and has a completely normal mental status. An unreliable patient may exhibit any of the following:

- *Altered mental status.* Patients who have sustained a traumatic brain injury resulting in an alteration in their level of consciousness cannot be adequately evaluated and should be immobilized. Similarly, patients who are under the influence of drugs or alcohol are immobilized and managed as if they had spinal injury until they are calm, cooperative, and sober and physical examination is normal.
- *Distracting painful injuries.* Injuries that are severely painful may distract the patient from other, less painful injuries and interfere with giving reliable responses during the assessment.[9] Examples include a fractured femur or a large burn (see Figure 11-14).
- *Communication barriers.* Communication problems may be encountered in patients who have language barriers, are hearing impaired, are preverbal or very young, or for any reason cannot communicate effectively.

The patient should be continually rechecked for reliability at all phases of an assessment. If at any time the patient exhibits these signs or symptoms or the reliability of the examination is in question, it should be assumed that the patient has a spinal injury, and full immobilization management techniques should be implemented.

Figure 11-15 Signs and Symptoms of Spinal Trauma

- Pain in the neck or back
- Pain on movement of the neck or back
- Pain on palpation of the posterior neck or midline of the back
- Deformity of the spinal column
- Guarding or splinting of the muscles of the neck or back
- Paralysis, paresis, numbness, or tingling in the legs or arms at any time after the incident
- Signs and symptoms of neurogenic shock
- Priapism (in male patients)

In many situations the mechanism of injury is not suggestive of neck injury (e.g., falling on outstretched hand and producing a Colles' fracture [distal radius and ulna fracture]). In these patients, in the presence of a normal examination and proper assessment, spinal immobilization is not indicated.

Management

In the United States, the management for a potentially unstable spine is to immobilize the patient in a supine position, usually on a rigid long backboard in a neutral in-line position. The scoop stretcher is often used as an alternative to a rigid long backboard, as its application often does not require either logrolling or lifting of the patient and it may be more comfortable (**Figure 11-16**). In many countries, a full-body vacuum mattress splint is often used instead of the backboard (**Figure 11-17**). The head, neck, torso, and pelvis should each be immobilized in a neutral in-line position to prevent any further movement of the unstable spine that could result in damage to the spinal cord. Spinal immobilization follows the common principle of fracture management: immobilizing the joint above and the joint below an injury. Because of the anatomy of the spine, this principle of immobilization must be extended beyond just the joint above and below a suspected vertebral injury. The joint above the spine means the head and the joint below means the pelvis.

Moderate anterior flexion or extension of the arms may cause significant movement of the shoulder girdle. Any movement or angulation of the pelvis results in movement of the sacrum and of the vertebrae attached to it. For example, lateral movement of both legs together can result in angulation of the pelvis and lateral bending of the spine.

Fractures of one area of the spine are often associated with fractures of other areas of the spine.[28] Therefore, the entire weight-bearing spine (cervical, thoracic, lumbar, and sacral) should be considered as one entity, and the entire spine immobilized and supported to achieve proper immobilization. The supine position is the most stable position to ensure continued support during handling, carrying, and transporting a patient. It also provides the best access for further examination and additional resuscitation and management of a patient. When the patient is supine, the airway, mouth and nose, eyes, chest, and abdomen can be accessed simultaneously.

Patients usually present in one of four general postures: sitting, semi-prone, supine, or standing. The patient's spine needs to be protected and stabilized immediately and continuously from the time the patient is discovered until the patient is mechanically secured. Techniques and equipment, such as manual stabilization, half-spine boards, immobilization vests, standing take-down, scoop stretchers, proper logroll methods, and rapid extrication with full manual stabilization, are interim techniques used to protect a patient's spine. These techniques allow for a patient's safe movement from the position in which the patient was found until full supine immobilization can be implemented. A recent study suggests that one type of scoop stretcher currently manufactured may be as effective as a standard rigid long backboard.[39]

Figure 11-16 The Scoop Stretcher

The scoop stretcher (also known as clamshell stretcher, Robertson orthopedic stretcher, and scoop) was invented in 1943 by Wallace W. Robinson from Portland, Maine, and was patented in 1947.[31] It utilized just one opening joint at the foot end of the stretcher. The form we know today, with two opening joints, was patented by Ferno® in 1970.

The scoop stretcher has traditionally been made out of metal (aluminum or other lightweight metals), but modern plastics are now used more commonly. It is a two-part device, allowing the separated halves to be placed under each side of the patient without excessive manipulation. After fastening the two halves together, the patient can be lifted and transferred to an ambulance stretcher or vacuum mattress.

In its collapsed state, the scoop stretcher is roughly 5 feet, 5 inches (1.6 m) long and 16 inches (0.4 m) wide, but it can be extended to about 6 feet, 6 inches (2.0 m) to suit the size of the patient. The weight of a scoop is roughly the same as a long backboard. The acceptable patient weight limits vary according to the manufacturer's specifications (generally, 350 to 660 pounds [160 to 300 kg]).

Unlike a long backboard, the scoop stretcher should not be considered a tool for transporting a patient over a long distance. Its primary function is to transfer the patient onto a stretcher or vacuum mattress. If the situation is critical, the scoop stretcher may be used to transport the patient for a short distance, provided the patient is properly secured with belts.

The scoop stretcher has proven to be more comfortable for patients than the long backboard and may result in less spine movement during application of the device.[32]

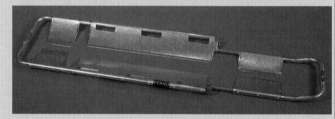

Scoop stretcher.

Source: © Jones and Bartlett Publishers. Courtesy of MIEMSS.

Figure 11-17 The Vacuum Mattress Splint

The vacuum mattress was invented by Loed and Haederlé in France. Other sources give credit to Erik Runereldt, a Swede, who reportedly got the idea for it in the late 1960s after seeing a package of coffee beans being vacuum packed.

The vacuum mattress is a transport and immobilization tool used after the patient has been transferred to it with the scoop stretcher. The splint is an airtight polymer bag filled with small polystyrene balls and a valve. When the air inside the vacuum mattress is removed, the atmospheric pressure outside presses the balls together, forming a rigid "bed" for the patient that molds to the patient's body contours.

The vacuum mattress has evolved considerably in the last decade. It is now wider and longer than the original version and has an improved valve system to more easily remove the air from within the mattress. Removal of the air from the mattress involves using a vacuum pump (either an electric suction unit or a manual hand pump).

The mattress shown here has a V shape, enabling prehospital care providers to package the patient more securely. The belts for fixation and carrying are sewn onto the mattress, which makes it easy to use and handle.

As with all medical tools, there are many different makes of vacuum mattresses; therefore prehospital care providers must be familiar with their particular device and participate in frequent trainings.

Numerous studies have demonstrated that the vacuum mattress provides a much higher degree of comfort to the patient when compared to the long rigid backboard.[33-38] Of particular importance, the vacuum mattress is, similar to most backboards, x-ray penetrable, so the patient does not need to be removed from the immobilizing systems while being evaluated in the ED.

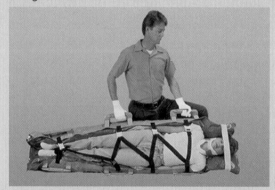

Vacuum mattress splint.

Source: Courtesy of Hartwell Medical.

Often, too much focus is placed on particular immobilization devices without an understanding of the principles of immobilization and how to modify these principles to meet individual patient needs. Specific devices and immobilization methods can be safely used only with an understanding of the anatomic principles that are generic to all methods and equipment. Any inflexible, detailed method for using a device will not meet the varying conditions found in the field. Regardless of the specific equipment or method used, the management of any patient with an unstable spine should follow the general steps described in the next section.

General Method

When the decision is made to immobilize a trauma patient, follow these principles:

1. Move the patient's head into a proper neutral in-line position (unless contraindicated; see next section). Continue manual support and in-line stabilization without interruption.
2. Evaluate the patient by performing the primary assessment, and provide any immediately required intervention.
3. Check the patient's motor ability, sensory response, and circulation in all four extremities, if the patient's condition allows.
4. Examine the patient's neck, and measure and apply a properly fitting, effective cervical collar.
5. Depending on the situation and the criticality of the patient, either position a shortboard or vest-type device on the patient, or use a rapid extrication maneuver if the patient is in a motor vehicle. Place the patient on a long backboard or other appropriate immobilization device if he or she is lying on the ground.
6. Immobilize the patient's torso to the device so that it cannot move up, down, left, or right.
7. Evaluate and pad behind the adult patient's head or pediatric patient's chest as needed.
8. Immobilize the patient's head to the device, maintaining a neutral in-line position.
9. Once the patient is on the immobilization device (if a short device is used), immobilize the legs so that they cannot move anteriorly or laterally.
10. Secure the patients arms if indicated.
11. Re-evaluate the primary assessment and reassess the patient's motor ability, sensory response, and circulation in all four extremities, if the patient's condition allows.

Manual In-line Stabilization of the Head

Once it has been determined from the mechanism of injury that an injured spine may exist, the first step is to provide manual in-line stabilization. The patient's head is grasped and carefully moved into a neutral in-line position unless contraindicated (see below). A proper neutral in-line position is maintained without any

significant traction on the head and neck. Only enough pull should be exerted on a sitting or standing patient to cause axial unloading (taking the weight of the head off the axis and the rest of the cervical spine). The head should be constantly maintained in the manually stabilized, neutral in-line position until mechanical immobilization of the torso and head is completed or the examination reveals no need for spinal immobilization. In this way, the patient's head and neck are immediately immobilized and remain so if indicated until after examination at the hospital. Moving the head into a neutral in-line position presents less risk than if the patient were carried and transported with the head left in an angulated position. In addition, both immobilization and transport of the patient are much simpler with the patient in a neutral position.

Contraindications

Movement of the patient's head into a neutral in-line position is contraindicated in a few cases. If careful movement of the head and neck into a neutral in-line position results in any of the following, the movement must be stopped:

- Resistance to movement
- Neck muscle spasm
- Increased pain
- Commencement or increase of a neurologic deficit, such as numbness, tingling, or loss of motor ability
- Compromise of the airway or ventilation

Neutral in-line movement should not be attempted if a patient's injuries are so severe that the head presents with such misalignment that it no longer appears to extend from the midline of the shoulders. In these situations, the patient's head must be immobilized in the position in which it was initially found. Fortunately, such cases are rare.

Rigid Cervical Collars

Rigid cervical collars alone do not provide adequate immobilization; they simply aid in supporting the neck and promote a lack of movement. Properly sized rigid cervical collars limit flexion by about 90% and limit extension, lateral bending, and rotation by about 50%. A rigid cervical collar is an important adjunct to immobilization but must always be used with manual stabilization or mechanical immobilization provided by a suitable spine-immobilization device. A soft cervical collar is of no use as an adjunct to spinal immobilization in the field.

The unique primary purpose of a cervical collar is to protect the cervical spine from compression. Prehospital methods of immobilization (using a vest, a shortboard, or a long backboard device) still allow some movement of the patient and the spine because these devices only fasten externally to the patient, and the skin and muscle tissue move slightly on the skeletal frame even when the patient is extremely well immobilized. Most rescue situations involve some movement of the patient and spine when extricating, carrying, and loading the patient. This type of movement also occurs when an ambulance accelerates and decelerates in normal driving conditions.

An effective cervical collar sits on the chest, posterior thoracic spine and clavicle, and trapezius muscles, where the tissue movement is at a minimum. It still allows movement at C6, C7, and T1 but prevents compression of these vertebrae. The head is immobilized under the angle of the mandible and at the occiput of the skull. The rigid collar allows the unavoidable loading between the head and the torso to be transferred from the cervical spine to the collar, eliminating or minimizing the cervical compression that could otherwise result.

Even though it does not fully immobilize the spine and head, a cervical collar aids in limiting head movement. The rigid anterior portion of the collar also provides a safe pathway for the lower head strap across the neck as the patient is further immobilized.

The collar must be the correct size for the patient. A collar that is too short will not be effective and will allow significant flexion or compression of the spine from axial loading; a collar that is too large will cause distraction of the spine, hyperextension, or full motion if the chin slips inside of it.[40] Also, a collar must be applied properly. A collar that is too loose will be ineffective in limiting head movement and can accidentally cover the anterior chin, mouth, and nose, obstructing the patient's airway; a collar that is too tight can compress the veins of the neck, causing increased intracranial pressure.

There are many different rigid cervical collars available on the market. The method of determining the correct size and the application of the device should be done according to the manufacturer's recommendations. An ill-fitting, improperly sized cervical collar will not help the patient and may be detrimental if an unstable spinal column is present (**Figure 11-18**).

The collar is applied after bringing the patient's head into a neutral in-line position. If the head cannot be returned to a neutral in-line position, use of any collar is difficult and should not be considered. In this case, the improvised use of a blanket or towel roll may assist in stabilization. A collar that does not allow the mandible to move down and the mouth to open without motion of the spine will produce aspiration of gastric contents into the lungs if the patient vomits and, therefore, should not be used. Alternative methods to immobilize a patient when a collar cannot be used may include use of such items as blankets, towels, and tape. In the prehospital setting, the prehospital care provider may need to be creative when presented with these types of patients. Whatever method is used, the basic concepts of immobilization should be followed (**Figure 11-19**).

There have also been reports of increased intracranial pressure associated with cervical collar use in patients with traumatic brain injury. If a patient with suspected traumatic brain injury shows obvious signs of increasing intracranial pressure, loosening or opening the collar should be considered to provide some relief.[41,42]

Figure 11-18 Proper Cervical Collar Sizing

An ill-fitting, improperly sized cervical collar will not help the patient and may be detrimental if an unstable spinal column is present.

Figure 11-19 Guidelines for Rigid Cervical Collars

Rigid cervical collars:
- Do not adequately immobilize by their use alone
- Must be properly sized for each patient
- Must not inhibit a patient's ability to open the mouth or the prehospital care provider's ability to open the patient's mouth if vomiting occurs
- Should not obstruct or hinder ventilation in any way

Immobilization of Torso to the Board Device

Regardless of the specific device used, the patient must be immobilized so that the torso cannot move up, down, left, or right. The rigid device is strapped to the torso and the torso to the device. The device is secured to the patient's torso so that the head and neck will be supported and immobilized when affixed to it. The patient's torso and pelvis are immobilized to the device so that the thoracic, lumbar, and sacral sections of the spine are supported and cannot move. **The torso should be immobilized to the device before the head is secured.** In this way, any movement of the device that may occur when fastening the torso straps is prevented from angulating the cervical spine.

Many different methods exist for immobilizing the device to the torso. Protection against movement in any direction—up, down, left, or right—should be achieved at both the upper torso (shoulders or chest) and the lower torso (pelvis) to avoid compression and lateral movement of the vertebrae of the torso. Immobilization of the upper torso can be achieved with several specific methods; an understanding of the basic anatomic principles common to each method must be applied. Cephalad movement of the upper torso is prohibited by use of a strap on each side, fastened to the board inferior to the upper margin of each shoulder, which then passes over the shoulder and is fastened at a lower point (**Figure 11-20**). Caudad movement of the torso can be prohibited by use of straps that pass snugly around the pelvis and legs (**Figure 11-21**).

In one method, two straps are used to produce an X. A strap goes from each side of the board over the shoulder, then across the upper chest and through the opposite armpit, to fasten to the board on the armpit side. This approach stops any upward, downward, left, or right movement of the upper torso (**Figure 11-22**).

The same immobilization can be achieved by fastening one strap to the board and passing it through one armpit, then across the upper chest and through the opposite armpit, to fasten to the second side of the board. A strap, or cravat, is then added to each side and passed over the shoulder to fasten it to the armpit strap, similar to a pair of suspenders.

Immobilization of the upper torso of a patient with a fractured clavicle is accomplished by placing backpack-type loops

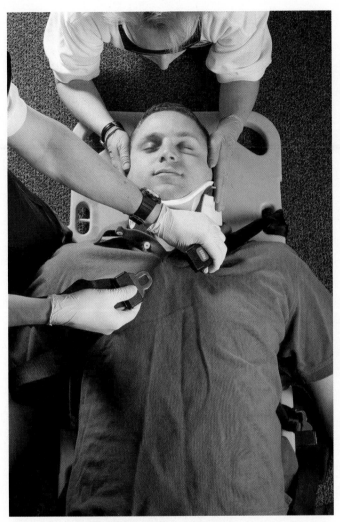

Figure 11-20 Caudad movement of the patient's trunk can be minimized by use of straps that pass snugly around the pelvis and legs.

Source: © Jones & Bartlett Learning. Photographed by Darren Stahlman.

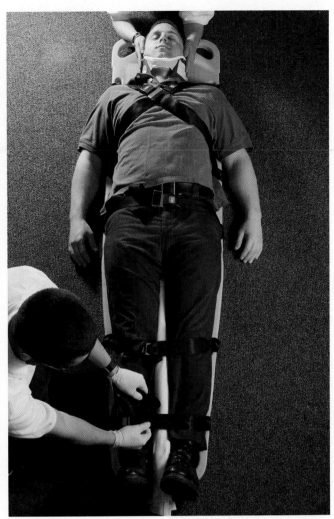

Figure 11-21 Cephalad movement of the patient's trunk is minimized by use of a strap fastened to the board at or below the upper margin of each shoulder, which then passes over the shoulder and is fastened at a lower point.

Source: © Jones & Bartlett Learning. Photographed by Darren Stahlman.

around each shoulder through the armpit and fastening the ends of each loop in the same handhold. The straps remain near the lateral edges of the upper torso and do not cross the clavicles. With any of these methods, the straps are over the upper third of the chest and can be fastened tightly without producing the ventilatory compromise typically produced by tight straps placed lower on the thorax.

Immobilization of the lower torso can be achieved by use of a single strap fastened tightly over the pelvis at the iliac crests. If the long backboard will have to be upended or carried on stairs or over a distance, a pair of groin loops will provide stronger immobilization than the single strap across the iliac crests.

Lateral movement or anterior movement away from the rigid device at the midtorso can be prevented by use of an additional strap around the midtorso. Any strap that surrounds the torso between the upper thorax and the iliac crests should be snug but not so tight that it inhibits chest excursion, impairing ventilatory function, or causes a significant increase in intra-abdominal pressure. Regardless of which strapping device or technique is

used, the principle is to secure the torso and then the head to the backboard. The particular device and technique chosen depend on the judgment of the prehospital care provider and the given situation.

The Backboard Debate

While the backboard provides motion restriction of the entire spine, it is important to understand a number of facts about the backboard itself. Being placed onto a rigid board is an extremely uncomfortable experience for the patient. An unpadded board will lead to complaints of back discomfort after a relatively short time on the board. In addition, being immobilized onto a rigid backboard leads to a significant amount of pressure being placed on bony prominences in contact with the board. Over time, circulation to these areas can become compromised, leading to skin ischemia, necrosis, and decubitus ulcers. All of these factors should prompt the prehospital care provider to place some padding under the patient and to minimize the amount of time a patient spends on the board.

Maintenance of Neutral In-line Position of the Head

In many patients, when the head is placed in a neutral in-line position, the posterior-most portion of the occipital region at the back of the head is between 0.5 and 3.5 inches (1.3 to 8.9 centimeters [cm]) anterior to the posterior thoracic wall (**Figure 11-23A**). Therefore, in most adults, a space exists between the back of the head and the board device when the head is in a neutral in-line position; thus, suitable padding should be added before securing the patient's head to the board device (**Figure 11-23B**). To be effective, this padding must be made of a material that does not readily compress. Firm, semirigid pads designed for this purpose or folded towels can be used. The amount of padding needed must be individualized for each patient; a few individuals require none. If too little padding is inserted or if the padding is of an unsuitable spongy material, the head will be hyperextended when head straps are applied.

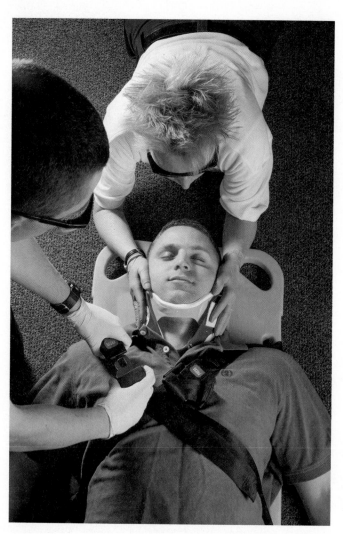

Figure 11-22 Two straps used to produce an X across the upper chest helps to stop any upward, downward, left, or right movement of the upper torso.

Source: © Jones & Bartlett Learning. Photographed by Darren Stahlman.

In addition, some patients, especially bariatric individuals, may experience respiratory compromise from being strapped supine onto a board.

All of these concerns have lead to a growing move to decrease or completely cease the utilization of the backboard or to remove patients from the board once the patient has been placed on the stretcher. While it is clear that too many patients are unnecessarily immobilized based solely on the mechanism of injury, the backboard continues to have an important role in prehospital management of trauma patients. It is useful as an extrication tool as well as for carrying trauma patients from the point of injury to the waiting ambulance stretcher. Critical evaluation of the effect of decreasing backboard use must be in place to determine whether or not this change in practice is in fact beneficial or if inadvertent movement of the spine leading to spinal cord injury results from the decision to not immobilize the trauma patient.

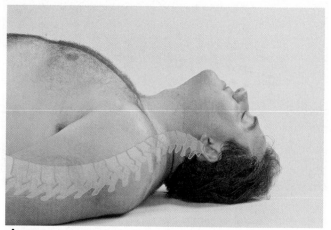

A

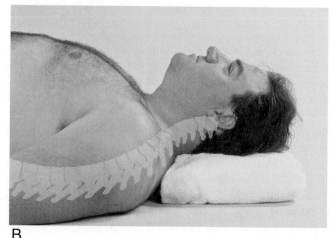

B

Figure 11-23 **A.** In some patients, allowing the skull to fall back to the level of the backboard can produce severe hyperextension of the spine. **B.** Padding is needed between the back of the head and the backboard to prevent such hyperextension.

If too much padding is inserted, the head will be moved into a flexed position. Both hyperextension and flexion of the head can increase spinal cord damage and are contraindicated.

The same anatomic relationship between the head and back applies when most people are supine, whether on the ground or on a backboard. When most adults are supine, the head falls back into a hyperextended position. On arrival, the head should be moved into a neutral in-line position and manually maintained in that position, which in many adults will require holding the head up off the ground. Once the patient is placed on the long backboard and the head is about to be fastened to the board, proper padding (as described) should be inserted between the back of the head and the board to maintain the neutral position. These principles should be used with all patients, including athletes with shoulder pads and patients with abnormal curvature of the spine, such as those with severe kyphosis (**Figure 11-24**).

In small children, generally those with the body size of a 7-year-old or younger, the size of the head is much larger relative to the rest of the body than it is in adults, and the muscles of the back are less developed.[39] When a small child's head is in a neutral in-line position, the back of the head usually extends 1 to 2 inches (2.5 to 5 cm) beyond the posterior plane of the back. Therefore, if a small child is placed directly on a rigid surface, the head will be moved into a position of flexion (**Figure 11-25A**).

The placement of small children on a standard long backboard results in unwanted flexion of the head and neck. The long backboard needs to be modified either by creating a recess in the board for the occiput to fit into or by inserting padding under the torso to maintain the head in a neutral position (**Figure 11-25B**). The padding placed under the torso should be of the appropriate thickness so that the head lies on the board in a neutral position; too much will result in extension, too little in flexion. The padding under the torso must also be firm and evenly shaped. Use of irregularly shaped or insufficient padding, or placing it only under the shoulders, can result in movement and misalignment of the spine.

Completing Immobilization

Head

Once the patient's torso has been immobilized to the rigid device selected and appropriate padding inserted behind the head as needed, the head should be secured to the device. Because of its rounded shape, the head cannot be stabilized on a flat surface with only straps or tape. Use of these alone allows the head to rotate and move laterally. Also, because of the angle of the forehead and the slippery nature of oily and moist skin and hair, a simple strap over the forehead is unreliable and can easily

Figure 11-24 Athletic Equipment Removal

A number of recent publications, including a position paper, have advocated the immobilization of helmeted athletes to a long backboard with the helmet in place.[43-50] A search of the medical literature for supporting evidence reveals that these recommendations are based on, at best, Class III research. Studies criticizing the practice of helmet removal have primarily been done in cadavers. These studies report that extreme hyperextension of the cervical spine occurs when the helmet alone is removed and the shoulder pads are left in place; however, all the studies were done without the placement of appropriate padding under the head to prevent it from falling back onto the backboard. Adherence to proper spinal precautions and application of treatment principles will best accomplish the task of spinal immobilization whether or not the helmet or shoulder pads are removed.

Athletic equipment should be removed by personnel trained and experienced in the removal of sports equipment. Historically, these trained and experienced personnel generally have been those individuals, usually athletic trainers, present at the athletic event site. However, prehospital care providers need to receive training in such

removal, because access to the airway, if needed, can be accomplished only by appropriate access to the patient's face and head, which requires removal of the face mask at a minimum and the helmet in many cases. If the decision is made not to remove the equipment at the scene, someone knowledgeable in sports equipment removal should accompany the patient to the hospital.

While special care for helmeted athletes is needed, the general principles of spinal immobilization taught in Prehospital Trauma Life Support (PHTLS) courses are appropriate and need to be followed. Ideally, the helmet and shoulder pads should be removed as one unit. However, it is still possible to immobilize a player to a long backboard without causing hyperextension of the cervical spine when the helmet alone is removed. This is accomplished by the appropriate use of padding behind the head to maintain the head in neutral alignment with the rest of the spine if the shoulder pads are not removed. Prehospital care providers must determine the specific medical needs for an injured athlete and take appropriate steps to meet those needs, which may often include immediate removal of the athletic equipment.

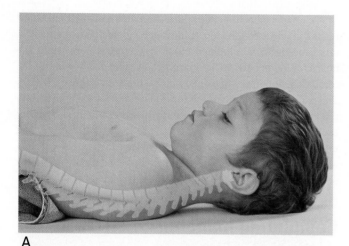

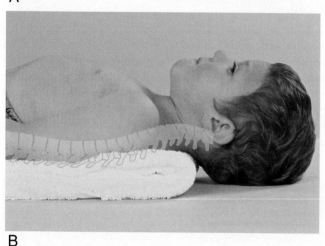

Figure 11-25 **A.** The larger size of a child's head relative to body size, combined with the reduced development of the posterior thoracic muscles, produces hyperflexion of the head when a child is placed on a backboard. **B.** Padding beneath the shoulders and torso will prevent this hyperflexion.

slide off. Although the human head weighs about the same as a bowling ball, it has a significantly different shape. The head is ovoid, longer than it is wide with almost completely flat lateral sides, resembling a bowling ball with about 2 inches (5 cm) cut off to form left and right sides. Adequate external immobilization of the head, regardless of method or device, can be achieved only by placing pads or rolled blankets on these flat sides and securing them with straps or tape. In the case of vest-type devices, this is accomplished with hinged side flaps that are part of the vest.

The side supports, whether they are preshaped foam blocks or rolled blankets, are placed next to both sides of the head. The sidepieces should be at least as wide as the patient's ears, or larger, and be at least as high as the level of the patient's eyes with the patient supine. Two straps or pieces of tape surrounding these headpieces draw the sides together. When it is packaged between the blocks or blankets, the head now has a flat posterior surface that can be realistically fixed to a flat device. The upper forehead strap is placed snugly across the front of the lower

forehead (across the supraorbital ridge) to help prevent anterior movement of the head. If tape is used, avoid placing it directly onto the eyebrows. This strap should be pulled tightly enough to indent the blocks or blankets and rest firmly on the forehead.

The device, regardless of type, that holds the head also requires a lower strap to help keep the sidepieces firmly pressed against the lower sides of the head and to anchor the device further and prevent anterior movement of the lower head and neck. The lower strap passes around the sidepieces and across the anterior rigid portion of the cervical collar. This strap should not place too much pressure on the front of the collar, which could produce airway compression or a venous return problem at the neck.

Sandbags are not recommended for use as side supports because of the weight that may be placed on the head and neck when the immobilized patient is turned on his or her side.[51] The use of sandbags secured to the long backboard on the sides of the head and neck represents a dangerous practice. Regardless of how well they are secured, these heavy objects can shift and move. Should the need arise to rotate the patient and board to the side, such as when the patient needs to vomit, the combined weight of the sandbags can produce localized lateral pressure against the head and cervical spine, forcing them to move. Raising or lowering the head of the board when moving and loading the patient, or any sudden acceleration or deceleration of the ambulance, can also produce shifting of the bags and movement of the head and neck.

The use of chin cups or straps encircling the chin prevents opening of the mouth to vomit, so these devices should not be used.

Legs

Significant outward rotation of the legs may result in anterior movement of the pelvis and movement of the lower spine; tying the feet together eliminates this possibility. Placing a rolled blanket or piece of padding between the legs will increase comfort for the patient.

The patient's legs are immobilized to the board with two or more straps: one strap proximal to the knees at about midthigh and one strap distal to the knees. The average adult measures 14 to 20 inches (35 to 50 cm) from one side to the other at the hips and only 6 to 9 inches (15 to 23 cm) from one side to the other at the ankles. When the feet are placed together, a V shape is formed from the hips to the ankles. Because the ankles are considerably narrower than the board, a strap placed across the lower legs can prevent anterior movement but will not prevent the legs from moving laterally from one edge of the board to the other. If the board is angled or rotated, the legs will fall to the lower edge of the board, which can angulate the pelvis and produce movement of the spinal column.

One way to hold the patient's lower legs effectively in place is to encircle them several times with the strap before attaching it to the board. The legs can be kept in the middle of the board by placing blanket rolls between each leg and the edges of the board before strapping. It is important to ensure that the straps are not so tight as to impair distal circulation.

Arms

For safety, the patient's arms may be secured to the board or across the torso before moving the patient. One way to achieve this is with the arms placed at the sides on the board with the palms in, secured by a strap across the forearms and torso. This strap should be snug but not so tight as to compromise the circulation in the hands.

The patient's arms should not be included in the strap at the iliac crests or in the groin loops. If the straps are tight enough to provide adequate immobilization of the lower torso, they can compromise the circulation in the hands. If the straps are loose, they will not provide adequate immobilization of the torso or arms. Use of an additional strap exclusively to hold the arms allows the strap to be opened for taking a blood pressure measurement or starting an intravenous line once the patient is in the ambulance without compromising the immobilization. If the arm strap is also a torso strap, loosening it to free just an arm has the side effect of loosening the torso immobilization as well.

Rapid Extrication Versus Short Device for the Seated Patient

The decision to use a rapid extrication technique over a short device should be based upon the clinical presentation of the patient, the findings during the primary assessment, and the situation at the scene. If the patient is found to have critical injuries; has airway, breathing, or circulation issues; or is in shock or impending shock, rapid extrication techniques and rapid transport are appropriate. The benefit in rapidly accessing the patient and treating these conditions outweighs the risk of the extrication procedure for these patients. Generally, less than 20% of patients fall into this category. In most stable patients, a short device should be employed. An exception may be when the risk of staying on the scene (e.g., a congested high-speed motorway) may result in vehicle collisions with responders working on the scene of the incident. In this case, the prehospital care provider should weigh the risk versus the benefit of staying on the scene for an extended length of time to apply the short device. Similarly, if the situation at the scene poses a significant hazard to the patient and the prehospital care providers, a rapid extrication of the patient may be warranted.

Most Common Immobilization Mistakes

The following are the most common immobilization errors:

1. *Inadequate immobilization.* The torso can move significantly up or down on the board device or the head can still move excessively.
2. *Improper sizing or improper application of the cervical collar.*
3. *Immobilization with the head hyperextended.* The most common cause is a lack of appropriate padding behind the head.
4. *Immobilizing the head before the torso or readjusting the torso straps after the head has been secured.* This causes movement of the device relative to the torso, which results in movement of the head and cervical spine.
5. *Inadequate padding.* Failure to fill the voids under a patient can allow for inadvertent movement of the spine, resulting in additional injury as well as increased discomfort for the patient.
6. *Placing someone in spinal immobilization who does not meet immobilization criteria.*

Complete spinal immobilization is generally not a comfortable experience for the patient. As the degree and quality of the immobilization increase, the patient's comfort decreases. Spinal immobilization is a balance between the need to protect and immobilize the spine completely and the need to make it tolerable for the patient. This is why proper evaluation of the need for spinal immobilization is indicated (**Figure 11-26**).

Obese Patients

With the increasing size of the current U.S. and world population, care of the *bariatric* (overweight, obese) patient is becoming more common. Transport of a 400-pound (182-kg) patient is becoming an all too common occurrence, and special bariatric transport cots have been developed for this purpose. However, a review of commercially available long backboards shows that most long backboards measure 16 by 72 inches (40 by 183 cm), with a few measuring 18 inches (46 cm) wide. The weight limit for these long backboards varies from 250 pounds (113 kg) to 600 pounds (272 kg). When using backboards on bariatric trauma patients, special care is needed to ensure that the safe operating limits are not exceeded. Also, additional personnel must be present to help lift and extricate bariatric patients, without causing further injury to the patient or prehospital care providers. This subgroup of trauma patients presents the challenge of balancing safe packaging and moving procedures against the short scene times normally recommended for critically injured trauma patients.

Certain obese patients may demonstrate an increased work of breathing to the point of respiratory failure if placed supine on a backboard. This phenomenon occurs secondary to the increased pressure being placed on the diaphragm by the adipose tissue of the abdomen. In these cases the principles of immobilization should still be followed, but the practice may be changed. An obese patient with a potential cervical injury may have his or her cervical spine manually maintained by the prehospital care provider's hands and a cervical collar, while the patient is allowed to remain sitting upright on the stretcher during transport. This approach will provide cervical stabilization without causing increased respiratory distress.

Figure 11-26 Criteria for Evaluating Immobilization Skills

Prehospital care providers must practice their immobilization skills in hands-on sessions using mock patients before use with real patients. At least one study has shown that appropriate immobilization was not performed in a significant number of patients with potential spinal injury.[40] When practicing or when evaluating new methods or equipment, the following criteria will serve as good tools for measuring how effectively the "patient" has been immobilized:

1. Initiate manual in-line stabilization immediately and maintain it until it is replaced mechanically.
2. Check neurologic function distally.
3. Apply an effective, properly sized cervical collar.
4. Secure the torso before the head.
5. Prevent movement of the torso up or down the board device.
6. Prevent movement of the upper and lower torso left or right on the immobilization device.
7. Prevent anterior movement of the torso off the rigid device.
8. Ensure ties crossing the chest do not inhibit chest excursion or result in ventilatory compromise.
9. Effectively immobilize the head so that it cannot move in any direction, including rotationally.
10. Provide padding behind the head, if necessary.
11. Maintain the head in a neutral in-line position.
12. Ensure that nothing inhibits or prevents the mouth from being opened.
13. Immobilize the legs so that they cannot move anteriorly, rotate, or move from side to side, even if the board and patient are rotated to the side.
14. Maintain the pelvis and legs in a neutral in-line position.
15. Ensure that the arms are appropriately secured to the board or torso.
16. Ensure that any ties or straps do not compromise distal circulation in any limb.
17. Re-evaluate the patient if bumped, jostled, or in any way moved in a manner that could compromise an unstable spine while the device was being applied.
18. Complete the procedure within an appropriate time frame.
19. Recheck distal neurologic function.

Many methods and variations can meet these objectives. The selection of a specific method and specific equipment will be based on the situation, the patient's condition, and available resources.

Pregnant Patients

Occasionally a pregnant patient will require spinal immobilization. Depending on the gestational age, placing the patient in a fully supine position may cause compression of the inferior vena cava, leading to a decrease in venous blood return to the heart, thus decreasing the mother's blood pressure. In these circumstances, the patient should be secured to the backboard using standard techniques. Once secured, the backboard is tipped on an angle to place the patient in a left lateral position. This position will move the uterus off of the vena cava, restoring blood pressure (**Figure 11-27**).

Use of Steroids

A series of studies suggested that high doses of the steroid methylprednisolone improve the neurologic outcome of patients with acute spinal cord injuries resulting from blunt trauma, when started within 8 hours of the injury.[52–54] In many centers, it became common for patients with such injuries to receive a bolus of 30 milligrams/kilograms (mg/kg) of methylprednisolone followed by an infusion of 5.4 mg/kg/hour for up to 48 hours, depending upon when the medication was initiated. Spinal cord injuries in children or those resulting from penetrating trauma

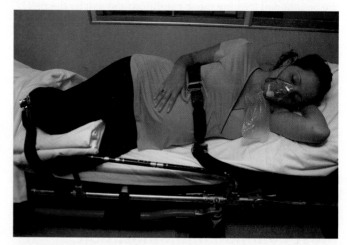

Figure 11-27 Tipping a pregnant female onto her left side helps lift the uterus off of the inferior vena cava and improves blood return to the heart and blood pressure.

Source: © Jones and Bartlett Publishers. Courtesy of MIEMSS.

were not studied, and steroids are not indicated for neurologic deficits resulting from stab or gunshot wounds.

Because steroids have known adverse effects, including suppression of adrenal glands and immune functioning, and because of concerns regarding the scientific validity of these studies, administration of steroids to patients with spinal cord injuries was questioned.[51] In fact, the complications associated with steroid administration may significantly outweigh any benefit, if any, they may confer. Numerous publications no longer recommend steroid use for spinal injury, either in the field or in the hospital.[55-59] Thus, there appears to be no role for the administration of steroids to the spinal cord–injured patient in the prehospital setting.

Prolonged Transport

As with other injuries, the prolonged transport of patients with suspected or confirmed spine and spinal cord injuries presents special considerations. Keeping in mind the goal to move patients with a suspected spinal cord injury only once, care should be taken to pad a long backboard, if that is what is used, prior to securing the patient. Cervical spine stabilization and spinal movement precautions should be utilized as the patient is moved to the padded backboard. Such efforts should help reduce the risk for the development of pressure ulcers in a patient with spinal cord injury. Any areas where there could be pressure on the patient's body, especially over bony prominences, should be sufficiently padded. For transports that will be particularly long, consideration should be given to using a scoop stretcher to carefully lift a patient, removing the long backboard, and then placing the patient down onto the ambulance pram.

Patients who are immobilized to long backboards are at risk for aspiration should they regurgitate. In the event the patient begins to vomit, the backboard and patient should immediately be tipped onto the side. Suction should be kept near the head of the patient so it is readily accessible should vomiting occur. Insertion of a gastric tube (either nasogastric or orogastric), if allowed, and the judicious use of antiemetic medications may help reduce this risk.

Patients with high spinal cord injuries may have involvement of their diaphragm and accessory respiratory muscles (i.e., intercostal muscles) predisposing them to respiratory failure. Impending respiratory failure may be aggravated and hastened by straps placed across the trunk for spinal immobilization that further restrict respiration. Prior to initiating a prolonged transport, double-check that the patient's torso is secured at the shoulder girdle and at the pelvis, and that any straps do not limit chest wall excursion.

As described earlier, patients with high spinal cord injuries may experience hypotension from loss of sympathetic tone (neurogenic "shock"). Although these patients rarely suffer from widespread hypoperfusion of their tissues, crystalloid boluses are generally sufficient to restore their blood pressure to normal. Vasopressors are rarely, if ever, necessary to treat neurogenic shock. Another hallmark of a high cervical spine injury is bradycardia. If associated with significant hypotension, bradycardia may be treated with intermittent doses of atropine, 0.5 to 1.0 mg administered intravenously.

The presence of tachycardia combined with hypotension should raise suspicion for the presence of hypovolemic (hemorrhagic), rather than neurogenic, shock. Careful assessment may pinpoint the source of hemorrhage, although intra-abdominal sources and pelvic fractures are most likely. Insertion of a urinary catheter will allow urine output to be used as another guide to tissue perfusion. In an adult, a urine output of greater than 30 to 50 milliliters per hour (ml/hour) generally indicates satisfactory end-organ perfusion. The loss of sensation that accompanies a spinal cord injury may prevent a conscious patient from perceiving peritonitis or other injuries below the level of the sensory deficit.

Patients with spinal injuries may have significant back pain or pain from associated fractures. As described in the Musculoskeletal Trauma chapter, pain may be managed with small doses of intravenous narcotics titrated until pain is relieved. Narcotics may exaggerate the hypotension associated with neurogenic shock. Padding the backboard as previously described may also provide some comfort for spinal fractures.

Patients with spinal cord injuries lose some ability to regulate body temperature, and this effect is more pronounced with injuries higher in the spinal cord. Thus, these patients are sensitive to the development of hypothermia, especially when they are in a cold environment. Patients should be kept warm (normothermic), but remember that covering them with too many blankets may lead to hyperthermia.

Spine and spinal cord injuries are best managed at facilities that have excellent orthopedic or neurosurgical services and are experienced in the management of these injuries. All level I and II trauma centers should be capable of managing the spinal cord injury and any associated injuries. Some facilities that specialize in the management of spine and spinal cord injuries may directly accept a patient who has suffered only a spinal cord injury (e.g., a shallow-water diving injury with no evidence of aspiration).

Summary

The vertebral column is comprised of 24 separate vertebrae plus the sacrum and coccyx stacked on top of one another.

- The major functions of the spinal column are to support the weight of the body and allow movement.
- The spinal cord is enclosed within the vertebral column and is vulnerable to injury from abnormal movement and positioning. When support for the vertebral column has been lost as a result of injury to the vertebrae or to the muscles and ligaments that help hold the spinal column in place, injury to the spinal cord can occur.

- Because the spinal cord does not regenerate, permanent neurologic injury, often involving paralysis, can result. The presence of spinal trauma and the need to immobilize the patient may be indicated by other injuries that could occur only with sudden, violent forces acting on the body or by specific signs and symptoms of vertebral or spinal cord injury.

- Damage to the bones of the spinal column is not always evident. If an initial injury to the spinal cord has not occurred, neurologic deficit will not be present, even though the spinal column is unstable. Immobilization of spinal fractures, as with other fractures, requires immobilization of the joint above and the joint below the injury. For the spine, the joints above are the head and neck, and the joint below is the pelvis.

- The device selected should immobilize the head, chest, and pelvis areas in a neutral in-line position without causing or allowing movement. Dependent on the patient, the severity of the patient's injuries, and the availability of equipment, the technique chosen should be based on the judgment of the prehospital care provider. Properly fitting and applying equipment are paramount for the successful immobilization of the trauma patient.

SCENARIO RECAP

You have been dispatched to the scene of a bicyclist who is reported down alongside a roadway. On arrival, you find a 19-year-old woman, lying supine on the side of the road away from traffic. The scene is safe, with traffic being controlled by the police. A police officer is kneeling next to the patient trying to talk to her, but she is not responding.

As you begin your primary assessment, you find an unresponsive female patient who fell from her bike while riding along a roadway. You are unable to ascertain the specific cause of the fall, and the police do not know if she was struck by a motor vehicle, as there were no witnesses. She is wearing full cycling gear, including helmet and gloves. She has abrasions on her forehead and an obvious deformity of the right wrist. Her airway is open, and she is breathing regularly. She shows no obvious signs of external blood loss. Her skin appears dry and warm with normal color. As you are performing your primary assessment, she begins to awaken but remains confused as to what happened.

- What pathologic processes explain the patient's presentation?
- What intermediate interventions and further assessments are needed?
- What are the management goals for this patient?

SCENARIO SOLUTION

The patient's vital signs are as follows: pulse 66 beats/minute, ventilatory rate 14 breaths/minute, and blood pressure 96/70 mm Hg. As you continue your examination, you note that the patient is not moving her arms or legs. The physical findings along with the vital signs are suggestive of neurogenic "shock." Interruption of the sympathetic nervous system and unopposed parasympathetic influence on the vascular system below the point of spinal injury result in an increased size of the vascular container and a relative hypovolemia. The patient's response to the spinal cord injury is a low blood pressure and bradycardia.

The first priorities of care are to continue to maintain a patent airway and oxygenation and assist ventilation as necessary to ensure an adequate minute volume while concurrently providing manual stabilization of the cervical spine. You immobilize the patient effectively and efficiently on a long backboard and transport the patient to an appropriate facility 9 minutes away. You manage the hypotension caused by neurogenic shock with a 500-ml bolus of intravenous fluids. You splint the fractured arm while en route.

The goals of prehospital management for this patient are to prevent additional spinal cord trauma, maintain tissue perfusion, care for extremity trauma en route, and transport without delay to an appropriate facility for definitive care.

References

1. DeVivo MJ. Causes and costs of spinal cord injury in the United States. *Spinal Cord*. 1997;35:809.
2. Spinal Cord Injury Information Pages. Spinal cord injury facts and statistics. http://www.sci-info-pages.com/facts.html. Accessed November 26, 2013.
3. Jackson AB, Dijkers M, Devivo MJ, Poczatek RB. A demographic profile of new traumatic spinal cord injuries: change and stability over 30 years. *Arch Phys Med Rehabil*. 2004;85:1740.
4. Meldon SW, Moettus LN. Thoracolumbar spine fractures: clinical presentation and the effect of altered sensorium and major injury. *J Trauma*. 1995;38:1110.
5. Ross SE, O'Malley KF, DeLong WG, et al. Clinical predictors of unstable cervical spine injury in multiply-injured patients. *Injury*. 1992;23:317.
6. Lindsey RW, Gugala Z, Pneumaticos SG. Injury to the vertebrae and spinal cord. In: Feliciano DV, Mattox KL, Moore EE, eds. *Trauma*. New York, NY: McGraw Hill; 2008:479–510.
7. Tator CH, Fehlings MG. Review of the secondary injury theory of acute spinal cord trauma with special emphasis on vascular mechanisms. *J Neurosurg*. 1991;75:15.
8. Tator CH. Spinal cord syndromes: physiologic and anatomic correlations. In: Menezes AH, Sonntag VKH, eds. *Principles of Spinal Surgery*. New York, NY: McGraw-Hill; 1995.
9. Bilello JP, Davis JW, Cunningham MA, et al. Cervical spinal cord injury and the need for cardiovascular intervention. *Arch Surg*. 2003;138:1127.
10. Section on Disorders of the Spine and Peripheral Nerves of the American Association of Neurologic Surgeons/Congress of Neurologic Surgeons. Blood pressure management after acute spinal cord injury. *Neurosurgery*. 2002;50:S58.
11. Ullrich A, Hendey GW, Geiderman J, et al. Distracting painful injuries associated with cervical spinal injuries in blunt trauma. *Acad Emerg Med*. 2001;8:25.
12. Domeier RM, Evans RW, Swor RA, et al. Prospective validation of out-of-hospital spinal clearance criteria: a preliminary report. *Acad Emerg Med*. 1997;4:643.
13. Domeier RM, Swor RA, Evans RW, et al. Multicenter prospective validation of prehospital clinical spinal clearance criteria. *J Trauma*. 2002;53:744.
14. Hankins DG, Rivera-Rivera EJ, Ornato JP, et al. Spinal immobilization in the field: clinical clearance criteria and implementation. *Prehosp Emerg Care*. 2001;5:88.
15. Stroh G, Braude D. Can an out-of-hospital cervical spine clearance protocol identify all patients with injuries? An argument for selective immobilization. *Ann Emerg Med*. 2001;37:609.
16. Dunn TM, Dalton A, Dorfman T, et al. Are emergency medical technician-basics able to use a selective immobilization of the cervical spine protocol? A preliminary report. *Prehosp Emerg Care*. 2004;8:207.
17. Domeier RM, Frederiksen SM, Welch K. Prospective performance assessment of an out-of-hospital protocol for selective spine immobilization using clinical spine clearance criteria. *Ann Emerg Med*. 2005;46:123.
18. Domeier RM, National Association of EMS Physicians Standards and Practice Committee. Indications for prehospital spinal immobilization. *Prehosp Emerg Care*. 1997;3:251.
19. Kwan I, Bunn F. Effects of prehospital spinal immobilization: a systematic review of randomized trials on healthy subjects. *Prehosp Disast Med*. 2005;20:47.
20. National Association of EMS Physicians and American College of Surgeons Committee on Trauma. Position Statement: EMS spinal precautions and the use of the long backboard. *Prehosp Emerg Care*. 2013;17:392–393.
21. Connell RA, Graham CA, Munro PT. Is spinal immobilization necessary for all patients sustaining isolated penetrating trauma? *Injury*. 2003;34:912.
22. Kennedy FR, Gonzales P, Beitler A, et al. Incidence of cervical spine injuries in patients with gunshot wounds to the head. *Southern Med J*. 1994;87:621.
23. Chong CL, Ware DN, Harris JH. Is cervical spine imaging indicated in gunshot wounds to the cranium? *J Trauma*. 1998;44:501.
24. Kaups KL, Davis JW. Patients with gunshot wounds to the head do not require cervical spine immobilization and evaluation. *J Trauma*. 1998;44:865.
25. Lanoix R, Gupta R, Leak L, Pierre J. C-spine injury associated with gunshot wounds to the head: retrospective study and literature review. *J Trauma*. 2000;49:860.
26. Barkana Y, Stein M, Scope A, et al. Prehospital stabilization of the cervical spine for penetrating injuries of the neck: is it necessary? *Injury*. 2003;34:912.
27. Cornwell EE, Chang, DC, Boner JP, et al. Thoracolumbar immobilization for trauma patients with torso gunshot wounds—is it necessary? *Arch Surg*. 2001;136:324.
28. American College of Surgeons (ACS) Committee on Trauma. *Advanced Trauma Life Support for Doctors*. 9th ed. Chicago, IL: ACS; 2012.
29. Stuke LE, Pons PT, Guy JS, Chapleau WP, Butler FK, McSwain NE. Prehospital spine immobilization for penetrating trauma—review and recommendations from the Prehospital Trauma Life Support Executive Committee. *J Trauma*. 2011;71:763.
30. Haut ER, Kalish BT, Efron DT, et al. Spine immobilization in penetrating trauma: more harm than good? *J Trauma*. 2010;68:115–121.
31. Robinson WW, inventor. Scoop Stretcher. US patent 2417378. December 28, 1943
32. Krell JM, McCoy MS, Sparto PJ, Fisher GL, Stoy WA, Hostler DP. Comparison of the Ferno Scoop Stretcher with the long backboard for spinal immobilization. *Prehosp Emerg Care*. 2006;10(1):46-51.
33. Lovell ME, Evans JH. A comparison of the spinal board and the vacuum stretcher, spinal stability and interface pressure. *Injury*. 1994;25(3):179–180.
34. Chan D, Goldberg RM, Mason J, Chan L. Backboard versus mattress splint immobilization: a comparison of symptoms generated. *J Emerg Med*. 1996;14(3):293–298.
35. Johnson DR, Hauswald M, Stockhoff C. Comparison of a vacuum splint device to a rigid backboard for spinal immobilization. *Am J Emerg Med*. 1996;14(4):369–372.
36. Hamilton RS, Pons PT. The efficacy and comfort of full-body vacuum splints for cervical-spine immobilization. *J Emerg Med*. 1996;14(5):553–559.
37. Cross DA, Baskerville J. Comparison of perceived pain with different immobilization techniques. *Prehosp Emerg Care*. 2001;5(3):270–274.
38. Luscombe MD, Williams JL. Comparison of a long spinal board and vacuum mattress for spinal immobilisation. *Emerg Med J*. 2003;20(5):476–478.
39. DeBoer SL, Seaver M. Big head, little body syndrome: what EMS providers need to know. *Emerg Med Serv*. 2004;33:47.
40. Ben-Galim P, Dreiangel N, Mattox KL, Reitman CA, Kalantar SB, MD, Hipp JA. Extrication collars can result in abnormal separation between vertebrae in the presence of a dissociative injury. *J Trauma*. 2010;69(2):447–450.

41. Ho AMH, Fung KY, Joynt GM, Karmakar KM, Peng Z. Rigid cervical collar and intracranial pressure of patients with severe head injury. *J Trauma*. 2002;53:1185–1188.

42. Mobbs RJ, Stoodley MA, Fuller JF. Effect of cervical hard collar on intracranial pressure after head injury. *Anz J Surg*. 2002;72: 389–391.

43. Donaldson WF, Lauerman WC, Heil B, et al. Helmet and shoulder pad removal from a player with suspected cervical spine injury: a cadaveric model. *Spine*. 1998;23:1729.

44. Gastel JA, Palumbo MA, Hulstyn MJ, et al. Emergency removal of football equipment: a cadaveric cervical spine injury model. *Ann Emerg Med*. 1998;32:411.

45. Kleiner DM, Almquist JL, Bailes J, et al. Prehospital care of the spine-injured athlete: a document from the Inter-Association Task Force for Appropriate Care of the Spine-Injured Athlete. Dallas, TX: National Athletic Trainers' Association; 2001.

46. Palumbo MA, Hulstyn MJ. The effect of protective football equipment on the alignment of the injured cervical spine. *Am J Sports Med*. 1996;24:446.

47. Prinsen RKE, Syrotuik DG, Reid DC. Position of the cervical vertebrae during helmet removal and cervical collar application in football and hockey. *Clin J Sport Med*. 1995;5:155.

48. Swenson TM, Lauerman WC, Blanc RO, et al. Cervical spine alignment in the immobilized football player: radiographic analysis before and after helmet removal. *Am J Sports Med*. 1997;25:226.

49. Waninger KN. Management of the helmeted athlete with suspected cervical spine injury. *Am J Sports Med*. 2004;32:1331.

50. Waninger KN. On-field management of potential cervical spine injury in helmeted football players: leave the helmet on! *Clin J Sport Med*. 1998;8:124.

51. Nesathurai S. Steroids and spinal cord injury: revisiting the NASCIS 2 and NASCIS 3 trials. *J Trauma*. 1998;45:1088.

52. Bracken MB, Shepard MJ, Collins, et al. A randomized, controlled trial of methylprednisolone or naloxone in the treatment of acute spinal-cord injury. Results of the Second National Acute Spinal Cord Injury Study. *N Engl J Med*. 1997;322(20):1405–1411.

53. Bracken MB, Shepard MJ, Collins WF Jr, et al. Methylprednisolone or naloxone treatment after acute spinal cord injury: 1-year follow-up data. Results of the Second National Acute Spinal Cord Injury Study. *J Neurosurg*. 1992;76(1):23–31.

54. Otani K, Abe H, Kadoya S, et al. Beneficial effect of methylprednisolone sodium succinate in the treatment of acute spinal cord injury. *Sekitsui Sekizui J*. 1996;7:633–647.

55. Bledsoe BE, Wesley AK, Salomone JP. High-dose steroids for acute spinal cord injury in emergency medical services. *Prehosp Emerg Care*. 2004;8:313.

56. Spine and Spinal Cord Trauma. In: ACS Committee on Trauma. *Advanced Trauma Life Support for Doctors*. Chicago, IL: American College of Surgeons; 2008.

57. Short DJ, El Masry WS, Jones PW. High dose methylprednisolone in the management of acute spinal cord injury—a systematic review from the clinical perspective. *Spinal Cord*. 2000;38:273.

58. Coleman WP, Benzel D. Cahill DW, et al. A critical appraisal of the reporting of the National Acute Spinal Cord Injury Studies (II and III) of methylprednisolone in acute spinal cord injury. *J Spinal Disord*. 2000;13:185.

59. Hurlbert RJ. The role of steroids in acute spinal cord injury: an evidence-based analysis. *Spine*. 2001;26:S39.

Suggested Reading

American College of Surgeons (ACS) Committee on Trauma. *Advanced Trauma Life Support for Doctors, Student Course Manual*. 9th ed. Chicago, IL: ACS; 2012.

Pennardt AM, Zehner WJ. Paramedic documentation of indicators for cervical spine injury. *Prehosp Disaster Med*. 1994;9:40.

SPECIFIC SKILLS

Spine Management

These skills are meant to demonstrate the principles of spinal immobilization. The specific preference as to the particular device used will be determined by each agency, jurisdictional medical oversight, and local protocols.

Cervical Collar Sizing and Application

Principle: To select and apply an appropriate-sized cervical collar to assist in providing neutral alignment and stabilization of the patient's head and neck.

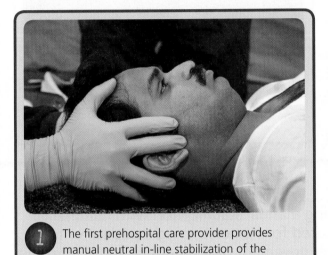

1   The first prehospital care provider provides manual neutral in-line stabilization of the patient's head and neck.

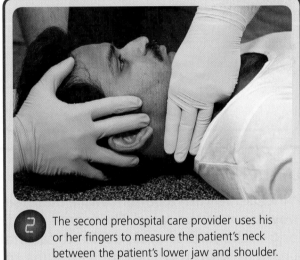

2   The second prehospital care provider uses his or her fingers to measure the patient's neck between the patient's lower jaw and shoulder.

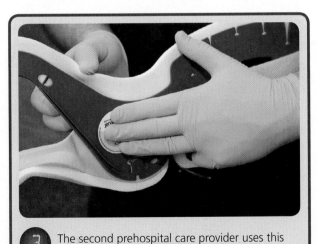

3   The second prehospital care provider uses this measurement to select a properly sized collar or adjust an adjustable collar to the correct size.

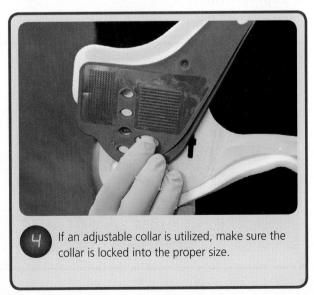

4   If an adjustable collar is utilized, make sure the collar is locked into the proper size.

Spine Management (continued)

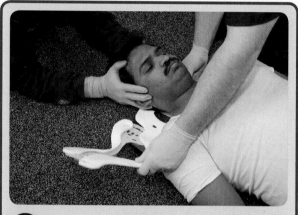

 The second prehospital care provider applies the properly sized collar while the first prehospital care provider continues to maintain the neutral in-line head and neck stabilization.

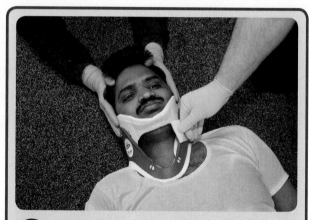

 After applying and securing the cervical collar, manual in-line stabilization of the head and neck is maintained until the patient is secured to an immobilization device.

Logroll

Principle: To turn a patient while maintaining manual stabilization with minimal movement of the spine. The logroll is indicated for (1) positioning a patient onto a long backboard or other device to facilitate movement of the patient and (2) turning a patient with suspected spinal trauma to examine the back.

A. Supine Patient

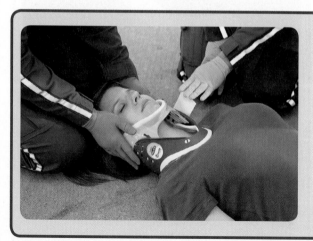

 While one prehospital care provider maintains neutral in-line stabilization at the patient's head, a second prehospital care provider applies a properly sized cervical collar.

Spine Management (continued)

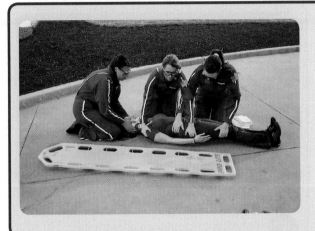

2 While one prehospital care provider maintains neutral in-line stabilization, a second prehospital care provider kneels at the patient's midthorax, and a third prehospital care provider kneels at the level of the patient's knees. The patient's arms are straightened and placed palms-in next to the torso while the patient's legs are brought into neutral alignment. The patient is grasped at the shoulder and hips in such a fashion as to maintain a neutral in-line position of the lower extremities. The patient is "logrolled" slightly onto his or her side.

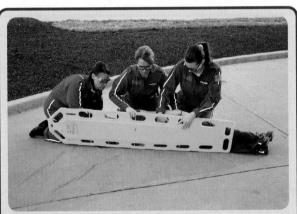

3 The long backboard is placed with the foot end of the board positioned between the patient's knees and ankles (the head of the long backboard will extend beyond the patient's head). The long backboard is held against the patient's back and the patient is logrolled back onto the long backboard, and the board is lowered to the ground with the patient.

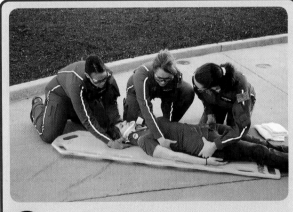

4 Once on the ground, the patient is grasped firmly by the shoulders, the pelvis, and the lower extremities.

Spine Management (continued)

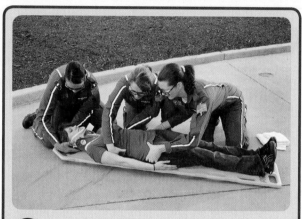

5 The patient is moved upward and laterally onto the long backboard. Neutral in-line stabilization is maintained without pulling on the patient's head and neck.

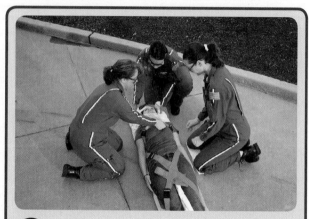

6 The patient is positioned onto the long backboard with the head at the top of the board and the body centered and secured to the device.

B. Prone or Semi-prone Patient

When a patient presents in a prone or semi-prone position, a stabilization method similar to that used for the supine patient can be used. The method incorporates the same initial alignment of the patient's limbs, the same positioning and hand placement of the prehospital care providers, and the same responsibilities for maintaining alignment.

The patient's arms are positioned in anticipation of the full rotation that will occur. When using the semi-prone logroll method, a cervical collar can be safely applied only after the patient is in an in-line position and supine on the long backboard, not before.

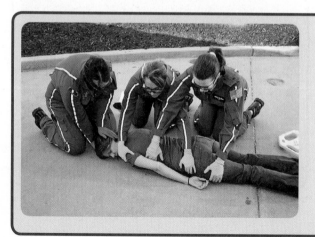

1 Whenever possible, the patient should be rolled away from the direction in which the patient's face initially points. One prehospital care provider establishes in-line manual stabilization of the patient's head and neck. Another prehospital care provider kneels at the patient's thorax and grasps the patient's opposite shoulder and wrist and pelvis area. A third prehospital care provider kneels at the patient's knees and grasps the patient's wrist and pelvis area and lower extremities.

Spine Management (continued)

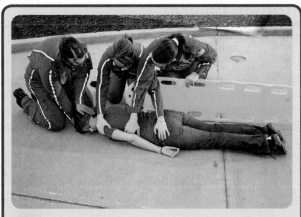

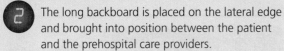

2 The long backboard is placed on the lateral edge and brought into position between the patient and the prehospital care providers.

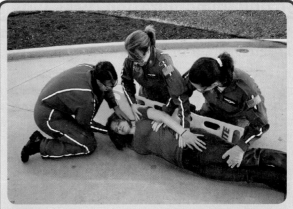

3 The board is placed with the foot of the board between the patient's knees and ankles, and the patient is logrolled onto his or her side. The patient's head rotates less than the torso, so by the time the patient is on his or her side (perpendicular to the ground), the head and torso have come into proper alignment.

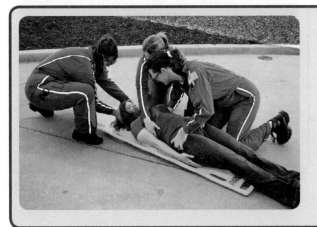

4 Once the patient is supine on the long backboard, the patient is moved upward and toward the center of the board. The prehospital care providers should take care not to pull the patient but to maintain neutral in-line stabilization. Once the patient is positioned properly on the long backboard, a properly sized cervical collar can be applied, and the patient can be secured to the backboard.

Spine Management (continued)

Sitting Immobilization (Vest-Type Extrication Device)

Principle: To immobilize a trauma patient without critical injuries before moving the patient from a sitting position.

This type of immobilization is used when spinal stabilization is indicated for a sitting trauma patient without life-threatening conditions. Several brands of vest-type extrication devices are available. Each model is slightly different in design, but any model can serve as a general example. The **Kendrick Extrication Device (KED)** is used in this demonstration. The details (but not the general sequence) are modified when using a different model or brand of extrication device. Also, during this demonstration, the windshield of the vehicle has been removed for clarification purposes.

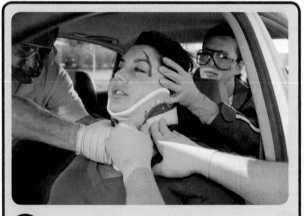

1 Manual in-line stabilization is initiated and a properly sized cervical collar applied.

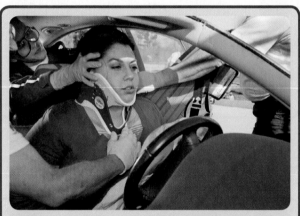

2 The patient is maintained in an upright position slightly forward to provide an adequate amount of space between the patient's back and the vehicle seat for placement of the vest-type device. *Note:* Before placing the vest-type device behind the patient, the two long straps (groin straps) are unfastened and placed behind the vest device.

Spine Management (continued)

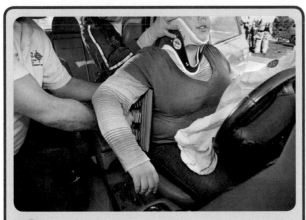

3 After placing the vest device behind the patient, the side flaps are placed around the patient and moved until the side flaps are touching the patient's armpits.

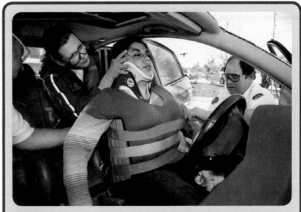

4 The torso straps are positioned and fastened, starting with the middle chest strap and followed by the lower chest strap. Each strap is tightened after attachment. Use of the upper chest strap at this time is optional. If the upper chest strap is used, the prehospital care provider should ensure that it is not so tight that it impedes the patient's ventilations. The upper chest strap should be tightened just before moving the patient.

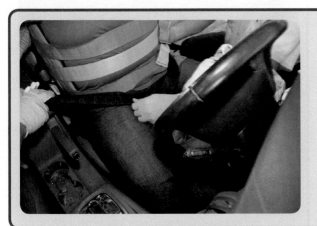

5 Each groin strap is positioned and fastened. Using a back-and-forth motion, each strap is worked under the patient's thigh and buttock until it is in a straight line in the intergluteal fold from front to back. Each groin strap is placed under the patient's leg and attached to the vest on the same side as the strap's origin. Once in place, each groin strap is tightened. The patient's genitalia should not be placed under the straps but to the side of each strap.

Spine Management (continued)

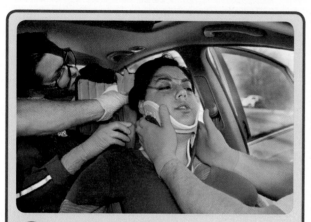

6 Padding is placed between the patient's head and the vest to maintain neutral alignment.

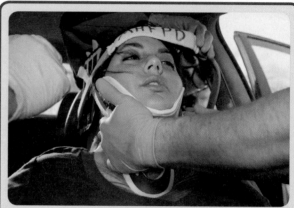

7 The patient's head is secured to the head flaps of the vest device. The prehospital care provider should be careful not to seat the patient's mandible or obstruct the airway. *Note:* The torso straps should be evaluated and readjusted as needed.

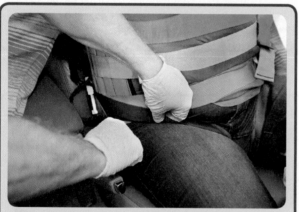

8 All straps should be rechecked before moving the patient. If the upper chest strap has not been secured, it should be attached and tightened.

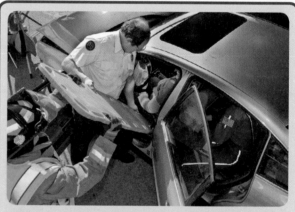

9 If possible, the ambulance cot with a long backboard should be brought to the opening of the vehicle door. The long backboard is placed under the patient's buttocks so that one end is securely supported on the vehicle seat and the other end on the ambulance cot. If the ambulance cot is not available or the terrain will not allow the placement of the cot, other prehospital care providers can hold the long backboard while the patient is rotated and lifted out of the vehicle.

Spine Management (continued)

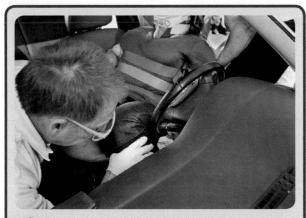

 10 While rotating the patient, the patient's lower extremities must be elevated onto the seat. If the vehicle has a center console, the patient's legs should be moved over the console one at a time.

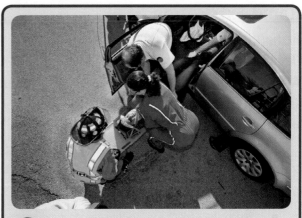

 11 Once the patient is rotated with his or her back to the center of the long backboard, the patient is lowered to the board while keeping the legs elevated. After placing the patient onto the long backboard, the two groin straps are released and the patient's legs are lowered. The patient is positioned by moving him or her up on the board with the vest device in place. The prehospital care provider should consider releasing the upper chest strap at this time.

Once the patient is positioned on the long backboard, the vest device is left secured in place to continue to immobilize the patient's head, neck, and torso. The patient and vest device are secured to the long backboard. The patient's lower extremities are immobilized to the board, and the long backboard is secured to the ambulance cot.

Spine Management (continued)

Rapid Extrication

Principle: To manually stabilize a patient with critical injuries before and during movement from a sitting position.

A. Three or More Prehospital Care Providers

Sitting patients with life-threatening conditions and indications for spinal immobilization (see Figure 11-14) can be rapidly extricated. Immobilization to an interim device before moving the patient provides more stable immobilization than when using only the manual (rapid extrication) method. However, it requires an additional 4 to 8 minutes to complete. The prehospital care provider will use the vest or halfboard methods when (1) the scene and patient's condition are stable and time is not a primary concern or (2) a special rescue situation involving substantial lifting or technical rescue hoisting exists, and significant movement or carrying of the patient is involved before it is practical to complete the supine immobilization to a long backboard.

Rapid extrication is indicated in the following situations:

- When the patient has life-threatening conditions identified during the primary assessment that cannot be corrected where the patient is found
- When the scene is unsafe and clear danger to the prehospital care provider and patient exists, necessitating rapid removal to a safe location
- When the patient needs to be moved quickly to access other, more seriously injured patients

Note: Rapid extrication is selected only when life-threatening conditions are present and not on the basis of personal preference.

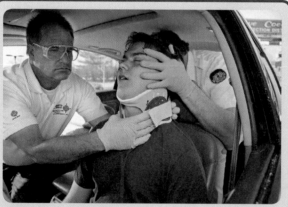

1 Once the decision is made to extricate a patient rapidly, manual in-line stabilization of the patient's head and neck in a neutral position is initiated. This is best accomplished from behind the patient. If a prehospital care provider is unable to get behind the patient, manual stabilization can be accomplished from the side. Whether from behind the patient or the side, the patient's head and neck are brought into a neutral alignment, a rapid assessment of the patient is performed, and a properly sized cervical collar is applied.

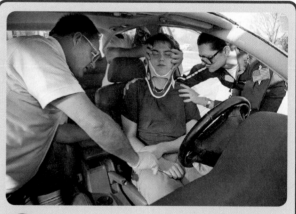

2 While manual stabilization is maintained, the patient's upper torso and lower torso and legs are controlled. The patient is rotated in a series of short, controlled movements.

Spine Management (continued)

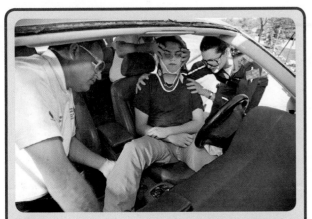

3 If the vehicle has a center console, the patient's legs should be moved one at a time over the console.

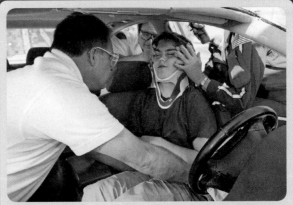

4 The prehospital care provider continues to rotate the patient in short controlled movements until control of manual stabilization can no longer be maintained from behind and inside the vehicle. A second prehospital care provider assumes manual stabilization from the first prehospital care provider while standing outside of the vehicle.

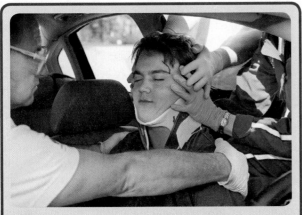

5 The first prehospital care provider can now move outside the vehicle and reassume manual stabilization from the second prehospital care provider.

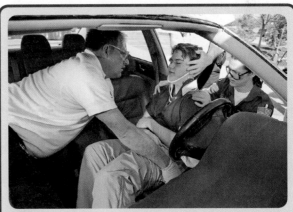

6 The rotation of the patient is continued until the patient can be lowered out of the vehicle door opening and onto the long backboard.

Spine Management (continued)

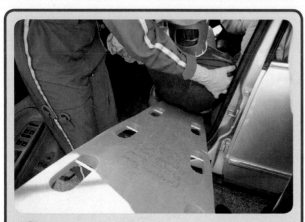

7 The long backboard is placed with the foot end of the board on the vehicle seat and the head end on the ambulance cot. If the cot cannot be placed next to the vehicle, other prehospital care providers can hold the long backboard while the patient is lowered onto it.

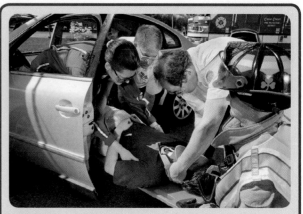

8 Once the patient's torso is down on the board, the weight of the patient's chest is controlled while the patient's pelvis and lower legs are controlled. The patient is moved upward onto the long backboard. The prehospital care provider who is maintaining manual stabilization is careful not to pull the patient but to support the patient's head and neck.

After the patient is positioned onto the long backboard, the prehospital care providers can secure the patient to the board and the board to the ambulance cot. The patient's upper torso is secured first, then the lower torso and pelvis area, then the head. The patient's legs are secured last. If the scene is unsafe, the patient should be moved to a safe area before being secured to the board or cot.

Note: This procedure represents only one example of rapid extrication. Because very few field situations are ideal, prehospital care providers may need to modify the steps for extrication for the particular patient and situation. The principle of rapid extrication should remain the same regardless of the situation: Maintain manual stabilization throughout the extrication process without interruption, and maintain the entire spine in an in-line position without unwarranted movement. Any positioning of the prehospital care providers that works can be successful. However, numerous position changes and hand position takeovers should be avoided because they invite a lapse in manual stabilization.

The rapid extrication technique can effectively provide manual in-line stabilization of the patient's head, neck, and torso throughout a patient's removal from a vehicle. The following are three key points of rapid extrication:

1. One prehospital care provider maintains stabilization of the patient's head and neck at all times, another rotates and stabilizes the patient's upper torso, and a third moves and controls the patient's lower torso, pelvis, and lower extremities.

Spine Management (continued)

2. Maintaining manual in-line stabilization of the patient's head and neck is impossible if attempting to move the patient in one continuous motion. The prehospital care providers need to limit each movement, stopping to reposition and prepare for the next move. Undue haste will cause delay and may result in movement of the spine.

3. Each situation and patient may require adaptation of the principles of rapid extrication. This can only work effectively if the maneuvers are practiced. Each prehospital care provider needs to know the actions and movements of the other prehospital care providers.

B. Two Prehospital Care Providers

In some situations an adequate number of prehospital care providers may not be available to extricate a critical patient rapidly. In these situations a two-provider technique is useful.

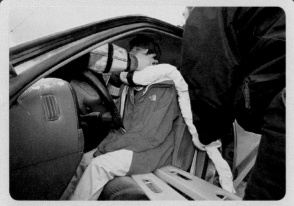

1 One prehospital care provider initiates and maintains manual in-line stabilization of the patient's head and neck. A second prehospital care provider places a properly sized cervical collar on the patient and places a prerolled blanket around the patient. The center of the blanket roll is placed at the patient's midline on the rigid cervical collar. The ends of the blanket roll are wrapped around the cervical collar and placed under the patient's arms.

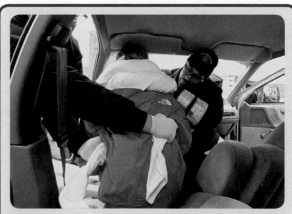

2 The patient is turned using the ends of the blanket roll and until the patient's back is centered on the door opening.

Spine Management (continued)

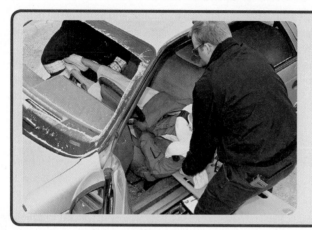

 The first prehospital care provider takes control of the blanket ends, moving them under the patient's shoulders, and moves the patient by the blanket while the second prehospital care provider moves and controls the patient's lower torso, pelvis, and legs.

Child Immobilization Device

Principle: To provide spinal immobilization to a child with a suspected spinal injury.

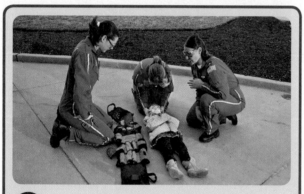

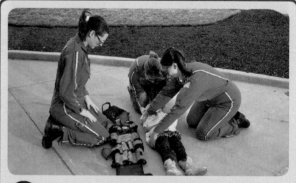

 The first prehospital care provider kneels above the patient's head and provides manual in-line stabilization of the patient's head and neck. The second prehospital care provider sizes and applies a cervical collar while the first prehospital care provider maintains neutral in-line stabilization. The second prehospital care provider straightens the patient's arms and legs, if needed.

The second prehospital care provider now kneels at the patient's side between the shoulders and knees. The second prehospital care provider grasps the patient at the shoulder and hips in such a fashion as to maintain a neutral in-line position of the lower extremities. On command from the first prehospital care provider, the patient is logrolled slightly onto his or her side.

Spine Management (continued)

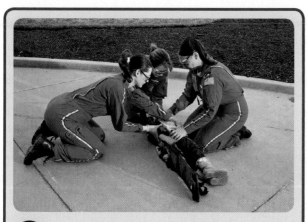

3 A third prehospital care provider positions the immobilization device behind the patient and holds it in place.

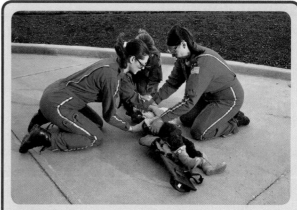

4 The device is held against the patient's back and the patient is logrolled onto the device, and the device is lowered to the ground with the patient.

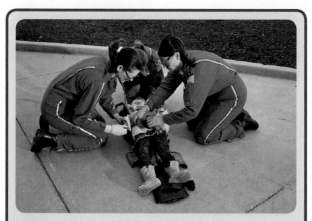

5 The patient is now secured to the immobilization device by the second and third prehospital care provider while the first prehospital care provider maintains head and neck stabilization.

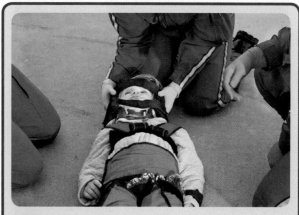

6 After securing the patient's torso and lower extremities to the immobilization device, the patient's head is secured to the immobilization device.

Spine Management (continued)

Helmet Removal

Principle: To remove a safety helmet while minimizing the risk of additional injury.

Patients who are wearing full-face helmets must have the helmet removed early in the assessment process. This provides immediate access for the prehospital care provider to assess and manage a patient's airway and ventilatory status. Helmet removal ensures that hidden bleeding is not occurring into the posterior helmet and allows the prehospital care provider to move the head (from the flexed position caused by large helmets) into neutral alignment. It also permits complete assessment of the head and neck in the secondary assessment and facilitates spinal immobilization when indicated (see Figure 11-14). The prehospital care provider explains to the patient what will occur. If the patient verbalizes that the prehospital care provider should not remove the helmet, the prehospital care provider will explain that properly trained personnel can remove it by protecting the patient's spine. Two prehospital care providers are required for this maneuver.

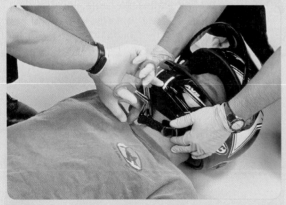

1 One prehospital care provider takes a position above the patient's head. With palms pressed on the sides of the helmet and fingertips curled over the lower margin, the first prehospital care provider stabilizes the helmet, head, and neck in as close to a neutral in-line position as the helmet allows. A second prehospital care provider kneels at the side of the patient, opens or removes the face shield if needed, removes eyeglasses if present, and unfastens or cuts the chin strap.

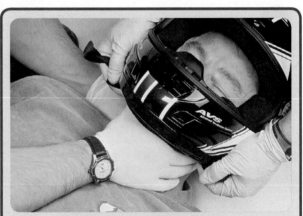

2 The patient's mandible is grasped between the thumb and the first two fingers at the angle of the mandible. The other hand is placed under the patient's neck on the occiput of the skull to take control of manual stabilization. The prehospital care provider's forearms should be resting on the floor or ground or on his or her own thighs for additional support.

Spine Management (continued)

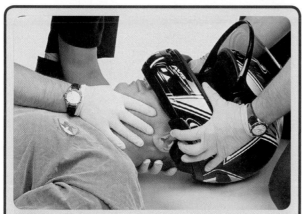

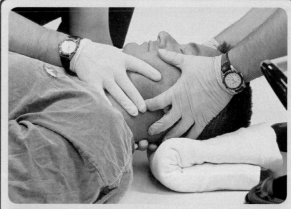

3 The first prehospital care provider pulls the sides of the helmet slightly apart, away from the patient's head, and rotates the helmet with up-and-down rocking motions while pulling it off of the patient's head. Movement of the helmet is slow and deliberate. The prehospital care provider takes care as the helmet clears the patient's nose.

4 Once the helmet is removed, padding should be placed behind the patient's head to maintain a neutral in-line position. Manual stabilization is maintained, and a properly sized cervical collar is placed on the patient.

Note: Two key elements are involved in helmet removal, as follows:

1. While one prehospital care provider maintains manual stabilization of the patient's head and neck, the other prehospital care provider moves. At no time should both prehospital care providers be moving their hands.
2. The prehospital care provider rotates the helmet in different directions, first to clear the patient's nose and then to clear the back of the patient's head.

Vacuum Splint Application

It is important to take proper care when using a vacuum mattress. Any sharp object on the ground or in the patient's clothes may pierce the mattress, rendering it useless.

The steps involved in applying a vacuum splint may vary from the following steps, depending upon the particular vacuum mattress available. Prehospital care providers should become familiar with the steps specific to the particular device used in their agency.

Spine Management (continued)

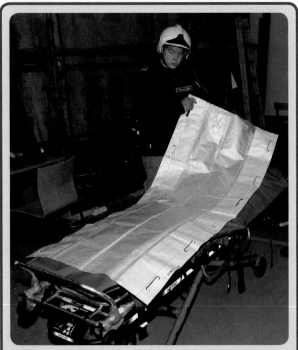

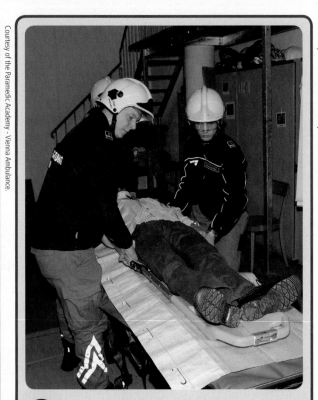

1 A prehospital care provider places a vacuum mattress on a lowered stretcher. The mattress should be deflated partially with the valve of the mattress at the head. The plastic balls inside the mattress should be spread out evenly and form a relatively flat surface. A prehospital care provider then places a sheet on the vacuum mattress.

2 A scoop stretcher is used to transfer the patient onto the vacuum mattress.

Spine Management (continued)

Courtesy of the Paramedic Academy - Vienna Ambulance.

3 The scoop stretcher is removed carefully from beneath the patient.

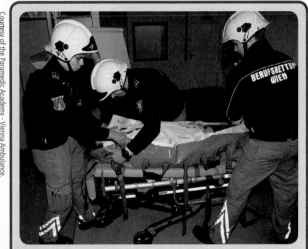

Courtesy of the Paramedic Academy - Vienna Ambulance.

4 The vacuum mattress is molded to the body contours of the patient while one prehospital care provider maintains manual in-line stabilization of the patient's head. Once the mattress is molded to the patient, the valve of the vacuum mattress is opened and suction is applied to deflate the mattress.

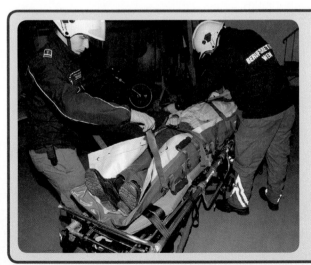

Courtesy of the Paramedic Academy - Vienna Ambulance.

5 Then the valve is closed and the patient secured with belts. A sheet or blanket should be placed over the patient.

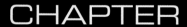
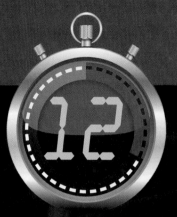

CHAPTER 12

Thoracic Trauma

CHAPTER OBJECTIVES

At the completion of this chapter, the reader will be able to do the following:

- Discuss the normal anatomy and physiology of the thoracic organs.

- Explain the alterations in anatomy and physiology that result from thoracic injury.

- Discuss the relationships among the kinematics of trauma, thoracic anatomy and physiology, and various assessment findings, leading to an index of suspicion for various injuries.

- Differentiate between patients in need of rapid stabilization and transport and patients in whom further on-scene assessment and management is warranted or appropriate.

- Discuss the impact of an urban or suburban and rural or austere setting on assessment and management of thoracic injury.

- Relate the signs, symptoms, pathophysiology, and management of the following specific thoracic injuries:

  - Rib fractures
  - Flail chest
  - Pulmonary contusion
  - Pneumothorax (simple, open, and closed)
  - Tension pneumothorax
  - Hemothorax
  - Blunt cardiac injury
  - Cardiac tamponade
  - Commotio cordis
  - Traumatic aortic disruption
  - Tracheobronchial disruption
  - Traumatic asphyxia
  - Diaphragmatic rupture

SCENARIO

You and your partner are dispatched to an industrial construction area for a worker who was struck by a piece of metal. Upon arrival, you are met at the gate by the site safety officer, who leads you to an interior work area. En route to the work area, the safety officer states the patient was helping to install metal studs. When he turned to grab another stud, he ran into the end of a stud his partner had just trimmed, cutting through his shirt and puncturing his chest.

In the work area, you find an approximately 35-year-old man sitting upright on a pile of lumber, leaning forward and holding a rag to the right side of his chest. You ask the patient what happened, and he tries to tell you but has to stop after every five to six words to catch his breath. As you move the rag, you notice an open laceration approximately 2 inches (5 centimeters) long with a small amount of blood-tinged, "bubbling" fluid. The patient is diaphoretic and has a rapid radial pulse. Decreased breath sounds are noted on the right side with auscultation. No other abnormal physical findings are noted.

- Is this patient in respiratory distress?
- Does he have life-threatening injuries?
- What interventions should you undertake in the field?
- What modality should be used to transport this patient?
- How would a different location (e.g., rural) impact your management and plans during prolonged transport?
- What other injuries do you suspect?

Introduction

As with other forms of injury, thoracic trauma can result from blunt or penetrating mechanisms. Blunt force applied to the thoracic cage in motor vehicle crashes, high falls, beatings, or crush injuries can cause disruption of the normal anatomy and physiology of the thoracic organs. Similarly, penetrating wounds from gunshots, knives, or impalement on objects such as rebar can injure the thorax. Definitive management of most thoracic injuries does not require *thoracotomy* (opening the chest cavity operatively). In fact, only 15% to 20% of all chest injuries require thoracotomy. The remaining 85% are well managed with relatively simple interventions, such as supplemental oxygen, ventilatory support, analgesia, and tube *thoracostomy* (chest tube placement) when necessary.[1-3]

Nevertheless, thoracic injuries can be quite significant. The thoracic organs are intimately involved in the maintenance of oxygenation, ventilation, and perfusion and oxygen delivery. Injury to the chest, especially if not promptly recognized and appropriately managed, can lead to significant morbidity. *Hypoxia* (insufficient oxygen in the blood), **hypercarbia** (excessive carbon dioxide in the blood), *acidosis* (excessive acid in the blood), and *shock* (insufficient oxygen reaching the body's organs and tissues) can result from inadequate management of

chest injury in the short term and thereby contribute to late complications, such as multisystem organ failure which accounts for the 25% of trauma deaths that result from thoracic injury.[1-3]

Anatomy

The chest is roughly a hollow cylinder formed by its bony and muscular structures. There are 12 paired ribs. The upper 10 pairs attach to the spinal column in the back and either the sternum or the rib above in the front. The lower two pairs of ribs attach only in back to the spine. In the front they are free and thus referred to as "floating ribs." This bony cage provides a great deal of protection to the internal organs of the chest cavity and, thanks to the lower ribs, even shields the organs of the upper abdomen (most notably the spleen and liver). This framework of ribs is reinforced with muscle. The **intercostal muscles** lie between and connect the ribs to one another.

A number of muscle groups move the upper extremity and are part of the chest wall, including the major and minor *pectoral muscles*, anterior and posterior *serratus muscles*, and *latissimus dorsi muscles*, along with the various muscles of the back (**Figure 12-1**). All this "padding" means it takes a considerable amount of force to injure the internal organs.

Also found in the thorax are muscles involved in the process of breathing (ventilation), including the intercostal muscles; the

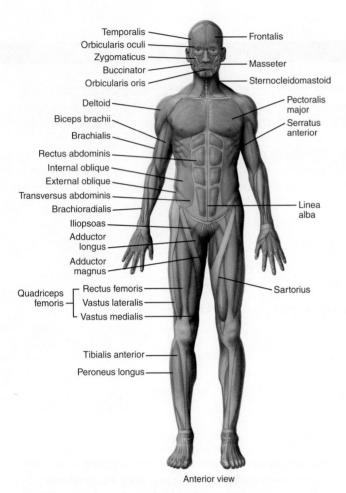

Figure 12-1 The muscular system.

Source: Background image © Carol and Mike Werner/Science Source.

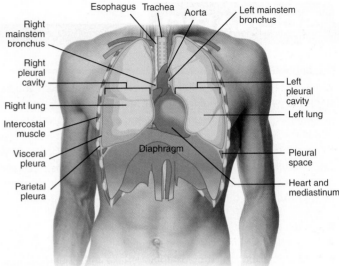

Figure 12-2 The thoracic cavity, including the ribs, intercostal muscles, diaphragm, mediastinum, lungs, heart, great vessels, bronchi, trachea, and esophagus.

Source: Background image © Mariya L/ShutterStock.

Physiology

The two components of chest physiology that are most likely to be impacted by injury are *breathing* and *circulation*.[1-3] Both processes need to be working properly and in conjunction with one another for oxygen to reach the body's organs, tissues, and ultimately cells and to expel carbon dioxide. To best understand what happens to patients when their chests are injured and how to manage their injuries, it is important to understand the physiology of these two processes.

Ventilation

The lay terms "breathing" and "respiration" actually refer to the physiologic process of ventilation. *Ventilation* is the mechanical act of drawing air through the mouth and nose into the trachea and bronchi and then into the lungs, where it arrives in small air sacs known as *alveoli*. **Respiration** is ventilation plus the delivery of oxygen to the cells. The process of drawing air in is called **inhalation**. Oxygen in that inhaled air is transported across the lining membrane of the alveoli, into adjacent small blood vessels known as **capillaries**, where it attaches to hemoglobin in the red blood cells for transport to the rest of the body. This process is known as **oxygenation**. Simultaneously, carbon dioxide, which is dissolved in the blood, diffuses out into the air within the alveoli for expulsion when that air is blown out again in the process of exhalation (**Figure 12-3**). **Cellular respiration** is the use of oxygen by the cells to produce energy (see the Physiology of Life and Death and the Airway and Ventilation chapters).

diaphragm, which is a dome-shaped muscle attached around the lower aspect of the chest; and muscles in the neck that attach to upper ribs. An artery, vein, and nerve course along the lower edge of each rib and provide blood and stimulation to the intercostal muscles.

Lining the cavity formed by these structures is a thin membrane called the **parietal pleura**. A matching thin membrane covers the two lungs within the chest cavity, called the **visceral pleura**. There is normally no space between these two membranes. In fact, a small amount of fluid between the two membranes holds them together, much as a thin layer of water will hold two sheets of glass together. This pleural fluid creates a surface tension, which opposes the elastic nature of the lungs, preventing their otherwise natural tendency to collapse.

The lungs occupy the right and left sides of the chest cavity (**Figure 12-2**). Between them and enveloped by them is a space called the **mediastinum**, which contains the trachea, the main bronchi, the heart, the major arteries and veins to and from the heart, and the esophagus.

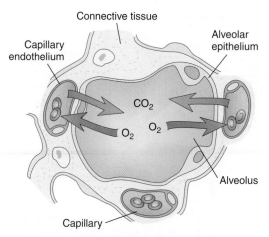

Figure 12-3 The capillaries and alveoli lie in close proximity; therefore, oxygen (O_2) can easily diffuse through the capillary, alveolar walls, capillary walls, and red blood cells. Carbon dioxide (CO_2) can diffuse back in the opposite direction.

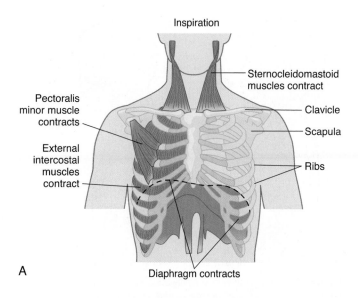

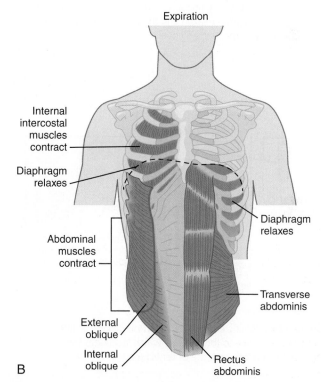

Inhalation is brought about by contraction of the muscles of respiration (primarily the intercostal muscles and the diaphragm), which results in a lifting and separating of the ribs and downward motion of the diaphragm. This action increases the size of the thoracic cavity and creates a negative pressure within the chest compared with the air pressure outside the body. As a result, air flows into the lungs (**Figures 12-4** and **12-5**). *Expiration* is achieved by relaxing the intercostal muscles and diaphragm, resulting in the return of the ribs and diaphragm to their resting positions. This return causes the pressure within the chest to exceed the pressure outside the body, and air from the lungs is emptied through the bronchi, trachea, mouth, and nose to the outside.

Ventilation is under the control of the respiratory center of the brain stem. The brain stem controls ventilation through monitoring of the partial pressure of arterial carbon dioxide ($PaCO_2$) and partial pressure of arterial oxygen (PaO_2) by specialized cells known as **chemoreceptors**. Chemoreceptors are located in the brain stem and in the aorta and carotid arteries. If the chemoreceptors detect increased $PaCO_2$, they stimulate the respiratory center to increase the depth and frequency of breaths, eliminating more carbon dioxide and returning $PaCO_2$ to normal (**Figure 12-6**). This process is very efficient and can increase the volume of air moved in and out of the lungs per minute by a factor of 10. Mechanoreceptors, found in the airways, lungs, and chest wall, measure the degree of stretch in these structures and provide feedback to the brain stem about lung volume.

In certain lung diseases, such as emphysema, or chronic obstructive pulmonary disease (COPD), the lungs are not able to eliminate carbon dioxide as effectively. This results in a chronic elevation of the carbon dioxide level in the blood. The

Figure 12-4 **A.** During inspiration, the diaphragm contracts and flattens. Accessory muscles of inspiration—such as the external intercostal, pectoralis minor, and sternocleidomastoid muscles—lift the ribs and sternum, which increases the diameter and volume of the thoracic cavity. **B.** In expiration during quiet breathing, the elasticity of the thoracic cavity causes the diaphragm and ribs to assume their resting positions, which decreases the volume of the thoracic cavity. In expiration during labored breathing, muscles of expiration—such as the internal intercostal and abdominal muscles—contract, causing the volume of the thoracic cavity to decrease more rapidly.

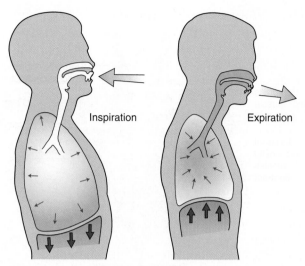

Figure 12-5 When the chest cavity expands during inspiration, the intrathoracic pressure decreases and air goes in the lungs. When the diaphragm relaxes and the chest returns to its resting position, the intrathoracic pressure increases and air is expelled. When the diaphragm is relaxed and the glottis is open, the pressure inside and outside the lungs is equal.

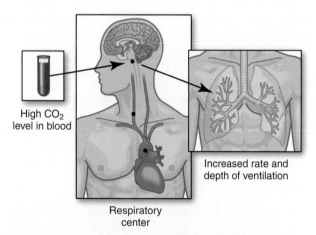

Figure 12-6 An increased level of carbon dioxide is detected by nerve cells sensitive to this change, which stimulates the lung to increase both depth and rate of ventilation.

chemoreceptors become insensitive to changes in $PaCO_2$. As a result, the chemoreceptors in the aorta and carotid arteries stimulate breathing when the PaO_2 falls. Similar to when the brain stem chemoreceptors detect an increase in $PaCO_2$ and stimulate increased respirations to lower the carbon dioxide level, the oxygen chemoreceptors send feedback to the respiratory center that stimulate the respiratory muscles to be more active, increasing the ventilatory rate and depth to raise the PaO_2 to more normal

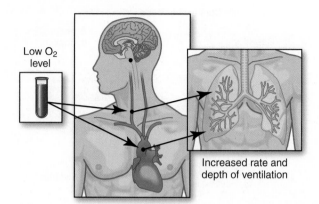

Figure 12-7 Receptors located in the aorta and carotid arteries are sensitive to the oxygen level and will stimulate the lungs to increase air movement into and out of the alveolar sacs.

values (**Figure 12-7**). This mechanism is often referred to as "hypoxic drive," as it is related to falling levels of oxygen in the blood.

The concept of the hypoxic drive has led to recommendations to limit the amount of oxygen given to trauma patients with pre-existing COPD for fear of suppressing their impetus to breathe. Trauma patients who are hypoxic should never be deprived of supplemental oxygen in the prehospital setting.[4] The true existence of the hypoxic drive remains controversial. If it truly exists, it will not manifest itself in the acute setting.

Figure 12-8 defines several terms that are important in discussing and understanding the physiology of ventilation.[5]

Circulation

The other major physiologic process that may be affected following thoracic injury is circulation. The Shock chapter covers this topic more extensively, but the following discussion sets the stage for the pathophysiology of chest injury.

The heart, which lies in the center of the chest within the mediastinum, functions as a biologic pump. For a pump to work, it must be primed with fluid and the fluid level maintained. For the heart, this priming function is provided by the return of blood through two large veins, the **superior vena cava** and the **inferior vena cava**. The heart then normally contracts 70 to 80 times per minute on average (normal range 60 to 100 beats per minute), ejecting approximately 70 milliliters (ml) of blood with each beat out to the body through the aorta.

Processes that interfere with the return of blood to the heart through the superior and inferior venae cavae (e.g., loss of blood through hemorrhage, increased pressure in the chest cavity from tension pneumothorax) cause the output of the heart and thus the blood pressure to decrease. Similarly, processes

Figure 12-8 Pulmonary Volumes and Relationships

- *Dead space*. Amount of air brought into the lungs that does not have the opportunity to exchange oxygen and carbon dioxide with the blood in the alveolar capillaries (e.g., air in trachea and bronchi).
- **Minute ventilation** $(\dot{V})$. Total volume of air moved into and out of the lungs in 1 minute.
- **Tidal volume** (VT). Amount of air that is inhaled then exhaled during a normal breath (0.4 to 0.5 liters).
- **Total lung capacity** (TLC). Total volume the lungs contain when maximally inflated. This volume declines with age from 6.0 liters in young adults to approximately 4.0 liters in elderly persons.
- **Work of breathing**. Physical work or effort performed in moving the chest wall and diaphragm to breathe. This work increases with rapid breathing, increasing minute ventilation, and when the lungs are abnormally stiff.

that injure the heart itself (e.g., blunt cardiac injury) may make the heart a less efficient pump, causing the same physiologic abnormalities. Just as chemoreceptors recognize changes in carbon dioxide or oxygen levels, **baroreceptors** located in the arch of the aorta and the carotid sinuses of the carotid arteries recognize changes in blood pressure and direct the heart to change the rate and forcefulness of its beating to return the blood pressure to normal.

Pathophysiology

As mentioned earlier, both blunt and penetrating mechanisms may disrupt the physiologic processes just described. There are common elements in the disturbances created by these mechanisms.

Penetrating Injury

In penetrating injuries, objects of varying size and type traverse the chest wall, enter the thoracic cavity, and possibly injure the organs within the thorax. Normally, no space exists between the pleural membranes. However, when a penetrating wound creates a communication between the chest cavity and the outside world, air can enter into the pleural space through the wound during inspiration when the pressure inside the chest is lower than the pressure outside the chest. Air may be further encouraged to enter a wound if the resistance to

airflow through the wound is less than that through the airways. Air in the pleural space (**pneumothorax**) disrupts the adherence between the pleural membranes created by the thin film of pleural fluid. All these processes together allow the lung to collapse, preventing effective ventilation. Penetrating wounds result in an open pneumothorax only when the size of the chest wall defect is large enough that the surrounding tissues do not close the wound at least partially during inspiration and/or expiration.

Wounds of the lung caused by a penetrating object allow air to escape from the lung into the pleural space and result in collapse of the lung. In either case, the patient becomes short of breath. To make up for the lost ventilation capacity, the respiratory center will stimulate more rapid breathing. This increases the work of breathing. The patient may be able to tolerate the increased workload for a time, but if not recognized and treated, the patient is at risk for ventilatory failure, which will be manifested by increasing respiratory distress as the carbon dioxide levels in the blood rise and the oxygen levels fall.

If there is continued entry of air into the chest cavity without any exit, pressure will begin to build within the pleural space, leading to **tension pneumothorax**. This will further impede the patient's ability to properly ventilate. It also will begin to impact circulation negatively as venous return to the heart is reduced by the increasing intrathoracic pressure, and shock may ensue. In extreme cases with displacement of the *mediastinal structures* (organs and vessels located in the middle of the chest between the two lungs) into the opposite side of the chest, venous return is highly compromised, leading to decreased blood pressure and jugular venous distension, and the classic, but late, finding of **tracheal shift** away from the midline toward the uninvolved side of the chest may be detected.

Lacerated tissues and torn blood vessels bleed. Penetrating wounds to the chest may result in bleeding into the pleural space (**hemothorax**) from the chest wall muscles, the intercostal vessels, and the lungs. Penetrating wounds to the major vessels in the chest result in catastrophic bleeding. Each pleural space can accommodate approximately 3,000 ml of fluid. Thoracic bleeding into the pleural space may not be readily apparent externally, but it may be of sufficient magnitude to create a shock state. The presence of large volumes of blood in the pleural space will also impede the patient's ability to breathe; the blood in the pleural space prevents expansion of the lung on that side. It is not uncommon for an injury to the lung to result in both a hemothorax and a pneumothorax, termed a *hemopneumothorax*. A hemopneumothorax results in collapse of the lung and impaired ventilation from both the air in the pleural space and the accumulation of blood in the thoracic cavity.

Wounds of the lung may also result in bleeding into the lung tissue itself. This blood floods the alveoli, preventing them from filling with air. Alveoli filled with blood cannot participate in gas exchange. The more alveoli that are flooded, the more the patient's ventilation and oxygenation may be compromised.

Blunt Force Injury

Blunt force applied to the chest wall is transmitted through the chest wall to the thoracic organs, especially the lungs. This wave of energy can tear lung tissue, which may result in bleeding into the alveoli. In this setting the injury is called a **pulmonary contusion**. A pulmonary contusion is essentially a bruise of the lung. It can be made worse by overaggressive fluid resuscitation. The impact on oxygenation and ventilation is the same as with penetrating injury.

If the force applied to the lung tissue also tears the visceral pleura, air may escape from the lung into the pleural space, creating a pneumothorax and the potential for a tension pneumothorax, as previously described. Blunt force trauma to the chest can also break ribs, which can then lacerate the lung, resulting in pneumothorax as well as hemothorax (both caused by bleeding from the broken ribs and from the torn lung and intercostal muscles). Blunt force injury typically associated with sudden deceleration incidents may cause shearing or rupture of the major blood vessels in the chest, particularly the aorta, leading to catastrophic hemorrhage. Finally, in some cases, blunt force can disrupt the chest wall, leading to instability of the chest wall and compromise of the changes in intrathoracic pressure, leading to impaired ventilation.

Assessment

As in all aspects of medical care, assessment involves taking a history and performing a physical examination. In trauma situations, we speak of a **SAMPLE history**, in which the patient's symptoms, age and allergies, medications, past history, time of the last meal, and the events surrounding the injury are elucidated (see the Patient Assessment and Management chapter).[6]

Besides the overall mechanism that resulted in injury, patients are asked about any symptoms they may be experiencing if they are conscious and able to communicate. Victims of chest trauma will likely be experiencing chest pain, which may be sharp, stabbing, or constricting. Frequently, the pain is worse with respiratory efforts or movement. The patient may report a sense of being short of breath or being unable to take in an adequate breath. The patient may feel apprehensive or lightheaded if shock is developing. It is important to remember that the absence of symptoms does not equate to the absence of injury.

The next step in assessment is the performance of a physical examination. There are four components to the physical examination: observation, palpation, percussion, and auscultation.

The assessment should also include a determination of vital signs. Placement of a pulse oximeter to assess arterial oxygen saturation is a useful adjunct in the assessment of the injured patient.[6,7]

- **Observation**. The patient is observed for pallor of the skin and sweating, which may indicate the presence of shock. The patient may also appear apprehensive. The presence of **cyanosis** (bluish discoloration of skin, especially around mouth and lips) may be evident in advanced hypoxia. The frequency of respirations and whether the patient appears to be having trouble breathing (gasping, contractions of the accessory muscles of respiration in the neck, nasal flaring) should be noted. Is the trachea in the midline, or deviated to one side or the other? Are the jugular veins distended? The chest is examined for contusions, abrasions, lacerations, and whether the chest wall expands symmetrically with breathing. Does any portion of the chest wall move paradoxically with respiration? (That is, instead of moving out during inspiration, does it collapse inward, and vice versa during exhalation?) If any wounds are identified, they are carefully examined to see if they are bubbling air as the patient breathes in and out.
- **Auscultation**. The entire chest is evaluated. Decreased breath sounds on one side compared to the other may indicate pneumothorax or hemothorax on the examined side. Pulmonary contusions may result in abnormal breath sounds (crackles). Although often difficult to discern in the field, muffled heart sounds from blood collecting around the heart and murmurs from valvular damage may also be noted on auscultation of the heart.
- **Palpation**. By gently pressing the chest wall with hands and fingers, assessment for the presence of tenderness, crepitus (either bony or **subcutaneous emphysema**), and bony instability of the chest wall is performed.
- **Percussion**. This examination technique is difficult to perform in the field because the environment is often noisy, making evaluation of the percussion note difficult. In addition, there is little additional information to be obtained from percussion that will change the prehospital management.
- **Pulse oximetry**. This should be performed to assess the level of oxygen bound to hemoglobin and followed to indicate changes in the patient's condition and responses to therapy. The oxygen saturation should be maintained at 95% or greater.
- **Waveform capnography**. Whether by sidestream assessment with a nasal probe, by mask, or by in-line assessment in an intubated patient, capnography (end-tidal carbon dioxide) is used to assess the level of carbon dioxide in expired air and is followed to indicate

changes in the patient's condition and responses to therapy. In-line sampling measures the end-tidal carbon dioxide directly at the point of sampling, whereas sidestream assessment takes a sample of expired air and performs the carbon dioxide determination at the monitor location, which is remote from the sampling site.

Repeat determinations of the ventilatory rate during patient reassessment may be the most important assessment tool in recognizing that a patient is deteriorating. As patients become hypoxic and compromised, an early clue to this change is a gradual increase in the ventilatory rate.

Assessment and Management of Specific Injuries

Rib Fractures

Rib fractures are commonly encountered by prehospital care providers and are present in approximately 10% of all trauma patients. Several factors have been shown to contribute to the morbidity and mortality of patients with multiple rib fractures, including total number of ribs fractured, the presence of bilateral fractures, and increased age (65 years or older).[8] The elderly are especially susceptible to rib fractures, likely due to loss of cortical bone mass (osteoporosis), which allows the ribs to fracture after sustaining less kinetic force. Regardless of age, mortality increases as more ribs are fractured. The mortality rate for a single rib fracture is 5.8%, increasing to 10% in those with five fractured ribs. The mortality rate is 34% in those with eight rib fractures.[9,10]

Despite the ribs being fairly well protected by overlying musculature, rib fractures are a common occurrence in thoracic trauma. The upper ribs are broad, thick, and particularly well protected by the shoulder girdle and muscles.[1-3] Because it requires great energy to fracture the upper ribs, patients with upper rib fractures are at risk for harboring other significant injuries, such as traumatic disruption of the aorta. Rib fractures occur most often in ribs 4 to 8 laterally, where they are thin and have less overlying musculature. The broken ends of the ribs may tear muscle, lung, and blood vessels, with the possibility of an associated pulmonary contusion, pneumothorax, or hemothorax.[1,3,11] Underlying pulmonary contusion is the most commonly associated injury seen with multiple rib fractures. Compression of the lung may rupture the alveoli and lead to pneumothorax, as discussed previously. Fracture of the lower ribs[11-13] may be associated with injuries of the spleen and liver and may indicate the potential for other intra-abdominal injuries. These injuries may present with signs of blood loss or shock.[1,3,11]

Assessment

Patients with simple rib fractures will most often complain of chest pain with breathing or movement and difficulty breathing. They may have labored respirations. Careful palpation of the chest wall will usually reveal point tenderness directly over the site of the rib fracture, and crepitus may be felt as the broken ends of the rib grind against each other. The prehospital care provider assesses vital signs, paying particular attention to the ventilatory rate and depth of breathing. Pulse oximetry also should be performed, as well as capnography if available.[1,14,15]

Management

Pain relief is a primary goal in the initial management of patients with rib fractures. This may involve reassurance and positioning of the patient's arms using a sling and swath. It is important to reassure and continuously reassess the patient, keeping in mind the potential for deterioration in ventilation and the development of shock. Establishing intravenous (IV) access should be considered, depending on the patient's condition and anticipated transport time. Administration of IV narcotic analgesics may be appropriate in some situations for advanced units with appropriate protocols and medical control. The patient is encouraged to take deep breaths and cough to prevent the collapse of the alveoli (**atelectasis**) and the potential for pneumonia and other complications. Rigid immobilization of the rib cage with tape or straps should be avoided because these interventions predispose to the development of atelectasis and pneumonia.[1,3] Administration of supplemental oxygen and assisting ventilations may be necessary to ensure adequate oxygenation.

Flail Chest

Flail chest occurs when two or more adjacent ribs are fractured in more than one place along their length. The result is a segment of chest wall that is no longer in continuity with the remainder of the chest. When the respiratory muscles contract to raise the ribs up and out and lower the diaphragm, the flail segment paradoxically moves inward in response to the negative pressure being created within the thoracic cavity (**Figure 12-9**). Similarly, when these muscles relax, the segment may move outward as pressure inside the chest increases. This paradoxical motion of the flail segment makes ventilation less efficient. The degree of inefficiency is directly related to the size of the flail segment.

The significant force necessary to produce such a lesion is generally transmitted to the underlying lung, resulting in a pulmonary contusion. The patient thus may have two mechanisms to compromise ventilation and gas exchange, the flail segment and the underlying pulmonary contusion (which is the bigger problem when it comes to compromising ventilation). As described earlier, the pulmonary contusion does not allow for gas exchange in the contused portion of the lung because of alveolar flooding with blood.

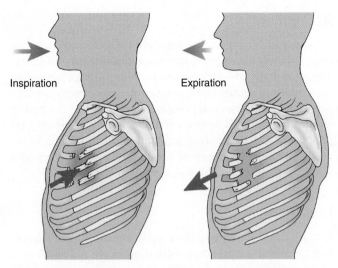

Inspiration   Expiration

Figure 12-9 Paradoxical motion. If stability of the chest wall has been lost by ribs fractured in two or more places, as intrathoracic pressure decreases during inspiration, the external air pressure forces the chest wall inward. When intrathoracic pressure increases during expiration, the chest wall is forced outward.

Assessment

As with a simple rib fracture, assessment of flail chest will reveal a patient in pain. The pain is typically more severe, however, and the patient usually appears to be in distress. The ventilatory rate is elevated, and the patient does not take deep breaths because of the pain. Hypoxia may be present, as demonstrated by pulse oximetry or cyanosis. Paradoxical motion may or may not be evident or easily recognized. Initially, the intercostal muscles will be in spasm and tend to stabilize the flail segment. As these muscles fatigue over time, the paradoxical motion becomes increasingly evident. The patient will have tenderness and potentially bony crepitus over the injured segment. The instability of the segment may also be appreciated on palpation.

Management

Management of flail chest is directed toward pain relief, ventilatory support, and monitoring for deterioration. The ventilatory rate may be the most important parameter to follow and carefully measure. Patients who are developing underlying pulmonary contusion and respiratory compromise will demonstrate an increase in their ventilatory rate over time. Pulse oximetry, if available, is also useful to detect hypoxia.[7] Oxygen should be administered to ensure an oxygen saturation of at least 95%.

Intravenous access may be obtained, except in cases of extremely short transport times. Narcotic analgesics may be carefully titrated to provide pain relief.

Support of ventilation with bag-mask device assistance, continuous positive airway pressure (CPAP), or endotracheal intubation and positive-pressure ventilation may be necessary (particularly with prolonged transport times) for those patients who are having difficulty maintaining adequate oxygenation.[14]

Efforts to stabilize the flail segment with sandbags or other means are contraindicated as they may further compromise chest wall motion and, thus, impair ventilations.[1]

Pulmonary Contusion

When lung tissue is lacerated or torn by blunt or penetrating mechanisms, bleeding into the alveolar air spaces can result in *pulmonary contusion*. As the alveoli fill with blood, gas exchange is impaired because air cannot enter these alveoli from the terminal airways. In addition, blood and edema fluid in the tissue between the alveoli further impede gas exchange in the alveoli that are ventilated. Pulmonary contusion is almost always present in the patient with a flail segment and is a common—and potentially lethal—complication of thoracic injury.[3,11] Deterioration to the point of respiratory failure may occur over the first 24 hours after injury.

Assessment

Assessment findings of the patient are variable depending on the severity of the contusion (percentage of involved lung). Early assessment typically may reveal no respiratory compromise. As the contusion progresses, the ventilatory rate will increase and rales may be heard on auscultation. In fact, a rising ventilatory rate is often the earliest clue that a patient is deteriorating from a pulmonary contusion. A high index of suspicion is necessary, particularly in the presence of a flail segment.

Management

Management is directed toward support of ventilation. The prehospital care provider should repeatedly reassess the ventilatory rate and any signs of respiratory distress. Continuous pulse oximetry and capnography, if available, should be utilized. Supplemental oxygen should be provided to all patients with suspected pulmonary contusion with a goal of maintaining oxygen saturation in the normal range. CPAP can be used to improve oxygenation in patients in whom supplemental oxygen alone proves to be inadequate for maintaining acceptable oxygen saturation levels.[16] Support of ventilation with bag-mask device or endotracheal intubation may be necessary.[15]

In the absence of hypotension (systolic blood pressure less than 90 millimeters of mercury [mm Hg]), aggressive IV fluid administration may further increase edema and compromise ventilation and oxygenation. Instead, IV fluids should be administered to maintain normal pulse and blood pressure. Pulmonary contusion is another example in which fluid resuscitation must be balanced with the patient's other needs. (See the Shock chapter.)

Pneumothorax

Pneumothorax is present in up to 20% of severe chest injuries.[9] The three types of pneumothorax represent increasing levels of severity: simple, open, and tension.

Simple pneumothorax is the presence of air within the pleural space. As the amount of air in the pleural space increases, the lung on that side collapses (**Figure 12-10**). **Open pneumothorax** ("sucking chest wound") involves a pneumothorax associated with a defect in the chest wall that allows air to enter and exit the pleural space from the outside with ventilatory effort. *Tension pneumothorax* occurs when air continues to enter and is trapped in the pleural space with gradual increase in intrathoracic pressure. This leads to shift of the mediastinum and results in decreased venous blood return to the heart and compromised circulatory function.

Simple Pneumothorax

Assessment

Assessment in simple pneumothorax is likely to demonstrate findings similar to those in rib fracture. The patient frequently complains of pleuritic chest pain (pain while breathing) and shortness of breath that may vary from mild to severe, and may exhibit varying symptoms and signs of respiratory dysfunction. The classic findings are decreased breath sounds on the side of injury. Any patient with respiratory distress and diminished breath sounds should be assumed to have a pneumothorax.

Management

The prehospital care provider administers supplemental oxygen, obtains IV access, and prepares to treat shock if it develops. Monitoring of pulse oximetry and waveform capnography, if available, is essential to expectant management of the patient in order to detect early signs of respiratory deterioration.[9-13,17,18] If spinal immobilization is not necessary, the patient may be more comfortable in a semi-recumbent position. Rapid transport is essential.[13,15,17] If the prehospital care provider is functioning at the basic level and transport time will be prolonged, rendezvous with an advanced life support (ALS) unit should be considered.

A key point in management is the recognition that a simple pneumothorax may quickly evolve into a tension pneumothorax. The patient needs to be continuously monitored for development of tension pneumothorax so that timely intervention can occur before there is a serious compromise of circulation.

Open Pneumothorax

Open pneumothorax, as with simple pneumothorax, involves air entering the pleural space, causing the lung to collapse. A defect in the chest wall that results in a communication between the outside air and the pleural space is the hallmark of an open pneumothorax. Mechanisms leading to open pneumothorax include gunshot wounds, shotgun blasts, stabbings, impalements, and rarely blunt trauma. When the patient attempts to inhale, air crosses the open wound and enters the pleural space because of the negative pressure created in the thoracic cavity as the muscles of respiration contract. In larger wounds, there may be free flow of air in and out of the pleural space with the different phases of respiration (**Figure 12-11**). Audible noise is often created as air travels in and out of the hole in the chest wall; thus, this wound has been referred to as a "sucking chest wound."

Because airflow follows the path of least resistance, this abnormal airflow through the chest wall may occur preferentially to the normal flow through the upper airway and trachea into the lung, especially if the open defect is similar or larger in size than the glottic opening to the lower airway. Resistance to the flow of air through a wound decreases as the defect size increases. Effective ventilation is then inhibited both by the collapse of the lung on the injured side and with the preferential flow of air into the pleural space through the wound rather than via the trachea into the alveoli of the lung. Though the patient is breathing, oxygen is prevented from entering the circulatory system.

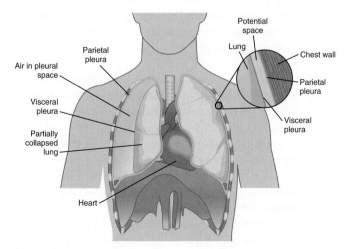

Figure 12-10 Air in the pleural space forces the lung in, decreasing the amount that can be ventilated and, therefore, decreasing oxygenation of the blood leaving the lung.

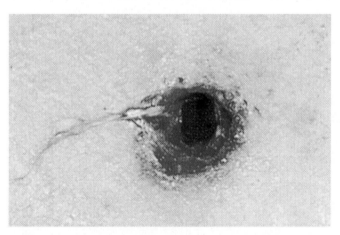

Figure 12-11 A gunshot or stab wound to the chest produces a hole in the chest wall through which air can flow both into and out of the pleural cavity.

Source: Courtesy Norman McSwain, MD, FACS, NREMT-P.

Assessment

Assessment of the patient with open pneumothorax generally reveals obvious respiratory distress. The patient will typically be anxious and tachypneic (breathing rapidly). The pulse rate will be elevated and potentially thready. Examination of the chest wall will reveal the wound, which may make audible sucking sounds during inspiration, with bubbling during expiration.

Management

Initial management of an open pneumothorax involves sealing the defect in the chest wall and administering supplemental oxygen. Airflow through the wound into the pleural cavity is prevented by applying an occlusive dressing using commercial products such as the Halo, Asherman, or Bolin chest seals or improvised methods such as application of aluminum foil or plastic wrap; unlike plain gauze, these materials do not allow airflow through them.

A patient with an open pneumothorax virtually always has an injury to the underlying lung, allowing for two sources of air leak, the first being the hole in the chest wall and the second being the hole in the lung. Even if an injury to the chest wall is sealed with an occlusive dressing, air leakage into the pleural space can continue from the injured lung, setting the stage for the development of a tension pneumothorax (**Figure 12-12**).

The traditional teaching has been that for an open pneumothorax, the occlusive dressing is secured on three sides.[1] This prevents airflow into the chest cavity during inspiration while allowing air to escape through the loose side of the dressing during exhalation and hopefully preventing the development of a tension pneumothorax (**Figure 12-13**). In contrast, taping the occlusive dressing on all four sides has been advocated as preferable to taping only on three sides; however, no definitive answer to this issue has been determined.

A recent study in animals compared the physiologic response of an open pneumothorax that has been completely sealed with a commercial unvented occlusive dressing to the response in

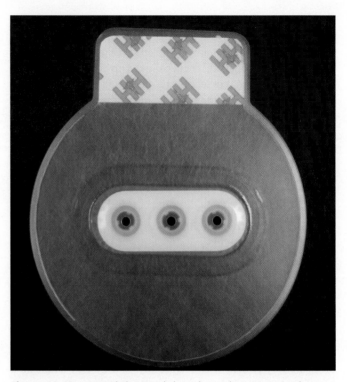

Figure 12-13 Vented chest seals have been shown in animal studies to prevent the development of tension pneumothorax after sealing of an open chest wound.
Source: Courtesy of H & H Medical Corporation.

those cases sealed with a vented dressing.[19] This study showed that both seals improved the respiratory physiology associated with an open pneumothorax; however, the vented seal prevented the development of tension pneumothorax, which the unvented seal did not. This finding has led the military's Committee on Tactical Combat Casualty Care to recommend that, if available, a vented chest seal is preferred over an unvented chest seal.[20] An unvented chest seal is an acceptable alternative if the vented type is not available; however, the patient must be carefully observed for the subsequent development of a tension pneumothorax.

In view of the research, Prehospital Trauma Life Support now recommends the following approach to the management of an open pneumothorax:

- Place a vented chest seal over the open chest wound.
- If a vented seal is not available, place a plastic or foil square over the wound and tape on three sides.
- If none of the above are available, an unvented chest seal or a material such as petroleum gauze that prevents ingress and egress of air may be used; however, this approach may allow the development of tension pneumothorax, so the patient must be observed carefully for signs of deterioration.
- If the patient develops tachycardia, tachypnea, or other indications of respiratory distress, remove the dressing for a few seconds and assist ventilations as necessary.
- If respiratory distress continues, assume the development of a tension pneumothorax and perform a needle thoracostomy using a large-bore (10- to 16-gauge) needle

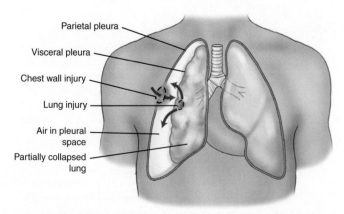

Figure 12-12 Because of the proximity of the chest wall to the lung, it would be extremely difficult for the chest wall to be injured by penetrating trauma and the lung not to be injured. Stopping the hole in the chest wall does not necessarily decrease air leakage into the pleural space; leakage can come from the lung just as easily.

that is 3.5 inches (8 cm) in length in the second intercostal space in the midclavicular line or at the nipple line in the midaxillary line.

If these measures fail to support the patient adequately, endotracheal intubation and positive-pressure ventilation may be necessary.[14] If positive pressure is utilized and a dressing has been applied to seal the open wound, the prehospital care provider needs to monitor the patient carefully for the development of tension pneumothorax. If signs of increasing respiratory distress develop, the dressing over the wound should be removed to allow for decompression of any accumulating tension. If this is ineffective, needle decompression and positive-pressure ventilation should be considered, if not already employed.[21]

In those cases in which positive-pressure ventilation is being performed, the wound does not need to be sealed. The positive-pressure ventilation effectively manages the pathophysiology usually associated with the open pneumothorax by ventilating the lung directly.

Tension Pneumothorax

Tension pneumothorax is a life-threatening emergency. As air continues to enter the pleural space without any exit or release, intrathoracic pressure builds up. As intrathoracic pressure rises, ventilatory compromise increases and venous return to the heart decreases. The decreasing cardiac output coupled with worsening gas exchange results in profound shock. The increasing pressure on the injured side of the chest may eventually push the structures in the mediastinum toward the other side of the chest (**Figure 12-14**). This distortion of anatomy may further impede

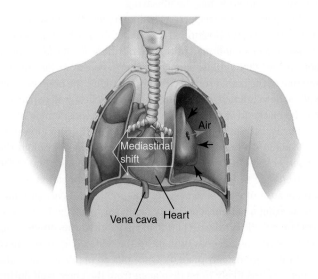

Figure 12-14 Tension pneumothorax. If the amount of air trapped in the pleural space continues to increase, not only is the lung on the affected side collapsed, but the mediastinum is shifted to the opposite side. The lung on the opposite side is then compressed and intrathoracic pressure increases, which kinks the vena cava and decreases blood return to the heart.

venous return to the heart through the kinking of the inferior vena cava as it passes through the diaphragm. Additionally, inflation of the lung on the uninjured side is increasingly restricted, and further respiratory compromise results.

Any patient with thoracic injury is at risk for development of tension pneumothorax. Patients at particular risk are those who likely have a pneumothorax (e.g., patient with signs of rib fracture), those who have a known pneumothorax (e.g., patient with a penetrating wound to the chest), and those with chest injury who are undergoing positive-pressure ventilation. Such patients must be continuously monitored for signs of increasing respiratory distress associated with circulatory impairment and rapidly transported to an appropriate facility.

Assessment

The findings during assessment depend on how much pressure has accumulated in the pleural space (**Figure 12-15**). Initially, patients will exhibit apprehension and discomfort. They will generally complain of chest pain and difficulty breathing. As the tension pneumothorax worsens, they will exhibit increasing agitation, tachypnea, and respiratory distress. In severe cases, cyanosis and apnea may occur.

The classic findings are tracheal deviation away from the side of injury, diminished breath sounds on the side of injury, and a tympanitic percussion note. It is difficult to detect diminished breath sounds in the field environment. Constant practice with auscultation of all patients will hone the prehospital care provider's skill and make detection of this important finding more likely. Detection of a tympanitic percussion note in the field is basically impossible, but the finding is mentioned for the sake of completeness. Transport and treatment should never be delayed for purposes of performing percussion of the chest.

Other physical findings that may be evident are jugular venous distension, chest wall crepitus, and cyanosis. Tachycardia and tachypnea become increasingly prominent as the intrathoracic pressure builds and the pulse pressure narrows, culminating in hypotension and uncompensated shock.

Management

The priority in management involves decompressing the tension pneumothorax.[14] Decompression should be performed when the following three findings are present:

1. Worsening respiratory distress or difficulty ventilating with a bag-mask device
2. Unilateral decreased or absent breath sounds
3. Decompensated shock (systolic blood pressure less than 90 mm Hg with a narrowed pulse pressure)[14-18,21]

Depending upon the clinical setting and the training level of the prehospital care provider, several options (discussed below) for pleural decompression exist. If decompression is not an option (i.e., only basic life support [BLS] available and no occlusive dressing to remove), rapid transport to an appropriate facility while administering high-concentration oxygen (fraction of inspired oxygen [FiO_2] ≥ 85%) is imperative. Positive-pressure

Figure 12-15   Signs of Tension Pneumothorax

Although the following signs are frequently discussed with a tension pneumothorax, many may not be present or are difficult to identify in the field.

Observation

- *Cyanosis* may be difficult to see in the field. Poor lighting, variation in skin color, and dirt and blood associated with trauma often render this sign unreliable.
- *Distended neck veins* are described as a classic sign of tension pneumothorax. However, since a patient with a tension pneumothorax may also have lost a considerable amount of blood, distended neck veins may not be prominent.

Palpation

- *Subcutaneous emphysema* is a common finding. As the pressure builds up within the chest cavity, air will begin to dissect through the tissues of the chest wall. Because tension pneumothorax involves significantly elevated intrathoracic pressure, the subcutaneous emphysema can often be palpated across the entire chest wall and neck

and sometimes can involve the abdominal wall and face as well.

- *Tracheal deviation* is usually a late sign. Even when it is present, it can be difficult to diagnose by physical examination. In the neck, the trachea is bound to the cervical spine by fascial and other supporting structures; thus, the deviation of the trachea is more of an intrathoracic phenomenon, although deviation may be palpated in the jugular notch if it is severe. Tracheal deviation is not often noted in the prehospital environment.

Auscultation

- *Decreased breath sounds on the injured side*. The most helpful part of the physical examination is checking for decreased breath sounds on the side of the injury. However, to use this sign, the prehospital care provider must be able to distinguish between normal and decreased sounds. Such differentiation requires a great deal of practice. Listening to breath sounds during every patient contact will help.

---

ventilatory assistance should be used only if the patient is hypoxic and fails to respond to supplemental oxygen, as this situation may rapidly worsen the tension pneumothorax. Assisting ventilations may result in air accumulating more rapidly in the pleural space. If ALS intercept is an option, it should be accomplished if the intercept will be faster than delivery to an appropriate facility.

Removal of an Occlusive Dressing

In the patient with an open pneumothorax, if an occluding dressing has been applied, it should be briefly opened or removed. This should allow the tension pneumothorax to decompress through the wound with a rush of air. This procedure may need to be repeated periodically during transport if symptoms of tension pneumothorax recur. If removing the dressing for several seconds is ineffective or if there is no open wound, an ALS provider may proceed with a needle thoracostomy.

Needle Decompression (Needle Thoracostomy)

Insertion of a needle into the pleural space of the affected side permits accumulated air, under pressure, to escape. While studies in human patients have primarily been anecdotal reports, needle decompression has been shown to be effective in an

animal model.[22] The immediate improvement in oxygenation and in ease of ventilation may be lifesaving.

If a patient with suspected tension pneumothorax was previously intubated, the position of the endotracheal (ET) tube should be assessed and confirmed prior to performing needle decompression. If the ET tube has slipped farther down from the trachea into one of the main bronchi (usually the right), the opposite lung will not be ventilated and breath sounds and chest wall expansion may be markedly diminished. In these cases, repositioning of the ET tube is warranted prior to considering needle decompression.

Needle decompression is typically performed through the second or third intercostal space in the midclavicular line of the involved side of the chest (**Figure 12-16**). This location is chosen because of ease of access for the prehospital care provider transporting a patient who likely has been "packaged for transport" on a backboard with cervical collar, with arms down along the sides (making access difficult to the midaxillary line, where chest tubes are usually placed). Once placed in this location, the catheter is less likely to be displaced from the chest wall during patient movement. The lung on the affected side is collapsed and shifted toward the contralateral side; therefore, it is unlikely to be injured during the procedure. The needle and catheter should be advanced until the return of a rush of air is achieved and advanced no farther. Once the decompression is achieved, the

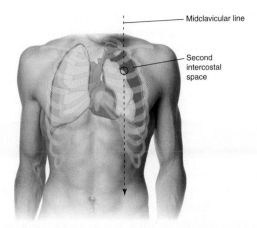

Midclavicular line

Second intercostal space

Figure 12-16 Needle decompression of the thoracic cavity is most easily accomplished and produces the least chance for complication if it is done at the midclavicular line through the second intercostal space.

Source: Background image © Mariya L/ShutterStock.

catheter is taped to the chest to prevent dislodgement. Improper placement (location or depth) may result in injuries to the lungs, heart, or great vessels.[23]

Several recent studies have questioned this location for placement, noting that chest wall thickness in the midclavicular line is often greater than the length of the catheter commonly used for decompression. Recent evidence suggests that placement of the catheter in the fifth intercostal space of the anterior or middle axillary line could provide greater success. A study using computed tomography (CT) scan to review chest wall thickness of trauma patients noted an average chest wall thickness in the midclavicular line to be 46 mm (right) and 45 mm (left). In the same patients, the average chest wall thickness was 33 mm (right) and 32 mm (left) in the anterior axillary line. The study's authors noted that needle decompression using a standard 5-cm needle would fail in 42.5% of cases in the midclavicular line versus only 16.7% in the anterior axillary line.[24] The authors also noted in a cadaveric study that needle decompression in the fifth intercostal space, midaxillary line resulted in 100% successful placement into the thoracic cavity compared to only 57.5% in the midclavicular line.[25]

Each location has clear advantages and disadvantages. Decompression in the midclavicular line has the advantage of ease of access for the prehospital care provider and lower chance of dislodgement or kinking during patient movement. However, there is a risk of inducing major hemorrhage from inadvertent placement of the catheter into the subclavian vessels (superiorly) or internal mammary artery, heart, or pulmonary vessels (medially).[26,27] Additionally as noted earlier, chest wall thickness often results in the catheter never actually entering the thoracic cavity. Advantages of the midaxillary placement of the catheter include its relative safety and efficacy. Recent data from the military does suggest a higher rate of catheter kinking and failure when placed in the midaxillary line, primarily due to movement of the patient.[28]

Regardless of the method chosen, decompression should be performed with a large-bore (10- to 16-gauge) IV needle that is at least 8 cm (3.5 inches) in length. Careful monitoring of the patient following the procedure is mandatory. A recent review noted a 26% mechanical failure rate due to kinking, obstruction, or dislodgement, with 43% of attempts ultimately failing to relieve the tension pneumothorax.[29]

This procedure, when successfully performed, converts the tension pneumothorax into a negligible open pneumothorax. The relief to respiratory effort far outweighs the negative effect of the open pneumothorax. Because the diameter of the decompression catheter is significantly smaller than the patient's airway, it is unlikely that any air movement through the catheter will significantly compromise ventilatory effort. Thus, creation of a one-way valve (Heimlich valve) is probably unnecessary from a clinical standpoint. Using a manufactured valve is costly, and fashioning a valve from a glove is time consuming. Continued provision of supplemental oxygen, as well as ventilatory support as needed, is appropriate.

As a general rule, bilateral tension pneumothorax is exceedingly rare in patients who are not intubated and ventilated with positive pressure. The first step in reassessing the patient is to confirm the location of the ET tube, ensure that it has no kinks or bends causing compression of the tube, and ensure that the tube has not inadvertently moved down into a main bronchus. Extreme caution should be exercised with bilateral needle decompression in patients who are not being ventilated with positive-pressure ventilation. If the prehospital care provider's assessment is in error, the creation of bilateral pneumothoraces can cause severe respiratory distress.

The patient should be rapidly transported to an appropriate facility. Intravenous access should be obtained unless transport time is particularly short. The patient must be closely observed for deterioration. Repeat decompression and endotracheal intubation may become necessary.

Tube Thoracostomy (Chest Tube Insertion)

In general, insertion of a chest tube (tube thoracostomy) is not performed in the prehospital setting because of concerns of time, procedural complications, infection, and training issues. Needle decompression can be accomplished in a fraction of the time required to perform a tube thoracostomy because fewer steps are necessary and less equipment is used. Published complication rates with tube thoracostomy range from 2.8% to 21%,[30,31] and include damage to the heart or lungs and malposition in the subcutaneous tissues of the chest wall or in the peritoneal cavity. This procedure requires a sterile field, which is challenging to create in the field. A break in sterile technique, such as contamination of the chest tube or instruments may result in the development of an empyema (collection of pus in the pleural space), requiring surgical intervention and drainage. Significant training is required to develop this skill, and ongoing practice is required to maintain skill proficiency.

Patients being transported with a chest tube in place are still at risk for the development of a tension pneumothorax, particularly if they are undergoing positive-pressure ventilatory assistance. If signs of a tension pneumothorax begin to manifest, first ensure that there are no kinks in the chest tube or connecting tubing. Next, ensure that the connecting tubing is correctly connected to a water seal and drainage device. Even with no identified problems, the patient with signs of an increasing tension pneumothorax may require needle decompression. Do not delay just because there is already a chest tube in place (**Figure 12-17**).

Figure 12-17 Troubleshooting Tube Thoracostomy

Three Basic Components of Chest Tube Drainage Systems

1. *Seal*. Allows air to escape pleural space but not return. The seal is generally a water seal that bubbles as air escapes the pleural space and rises with inspiratory negative pressure.
2. *Collecting system*. Collects and measures output. Observe for changes in volume of output and nature.
3. *Suction*. Provides negative pressure to assist drainage and expansion. Ensure that suction is appropriately attached and functioning. Review the basic operation of any drainage system with the patient's health care team prior to transfer of the patient.

Changes in Respiratory Status in Patients with Chest Tubes

- Assess vital signs, including pulse oximetry. If the chest tube is not working properly, the patient may become tachycardic, tachypneic, and hypoxic. If tension pneumothorax is developing, subcutaneous emphysema, increasing respiratory distress, narrowing pulse pressure, and hypotension may result.
- Assess lung sounds. The lung sounds may become diminished in the involved side if the chest is no longer functioning and instead is allowing air to reaccumulate within the chest.
- Assess ventilatory effort. Ventilatory effort will increase when the chest tube is not functioning.
- Assess circulation. If the chest tube is not working properly and is allowing air to accumulate within the chest, the patient may become tachycardic. If tension pneumothorax is developing, narrowing pulse pressure and hypotension may result.
- Assess level of consciousness. If hypoxia or signs of shock develop, the patient may become agitated and anxious. As these complications progress, the patient's level of consciousness will decrease.

Troubleshooting Steps

- Assess the dressing and tube site to ensure that the chest tube has not been dislodged during transfers.
- Check that the chest tubing is all tightly connected and unobstructed, with no kinks or clamps.
- Check that the chest seal is intact and functioning. Is there any bubbling and/or variation with ventilations?
- Assess whether the chest tube is fogging and/or drainage is continuing.
- Ensure that the suction is functioning. Is there continuous bubbling or a negative pressure indicator throughout the ventilation cycle?
- If the patient's ventilatory status continues to deteriorate, assess closely for signs of developing tension pneumothorax. If indicated, disconnect the chest tube from the drainage system, which should allow release of tension if the chest tube is properly placed and unobstructed. If this step does not relieve the condition, consider needle decompression and contact online medical control.

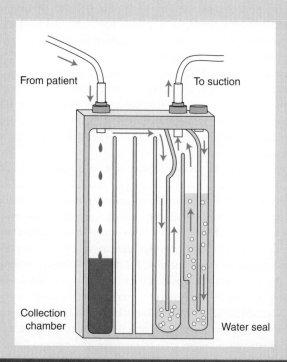

Hemothorax

Hemothorax occurs when blood enters the pleural space. Because this space can accommodate a large volume of blood (2,500 to 3,000 ml), hemothorax can represent a source of significant blood loss. In fact, the loss of circulating blood volume from bleeding into the pleural space represents a greater physiologic insult to the patient with chest injury than the collapse of the lung that the hemothorax produces (**Figure 12-18**). It is rare that enough blood accumulates to create a "tension hemothorax." The mechanisms resulting in hemothorax are the same as those causing the various types of pneumothorax. The bleeding may come from the chest wall musculature, intercostal vessels, lung parenchyma, pulmonary vessels, or great vessels of the chest.

Assessment

Assessment reveals a patient in some distress, depending upon the degree of blood lost into the chest and compression of the lung on the involved side. Chest pain and shortness of breath are again prominent features, generally with signs of significant shock. The prehospital care provider monitors the patient for signs of shock: tachycardia, tachypnea, confusion, pallor, and hypotension. Breath sounds on the side of the injury are diminished or absent, but the percussion note is dull (compared to tympanitic for a pneumothorax). Pneumothorax may be present in conjunction with hemothorax, increasing the likelihood for cardiorespiratory compromise. Because of loss of circulating blood volume, distended neck veins often are not present.

Management

Management includes constant observation to detect physiologic deterioration while providing appropriate support. High-concentration oxygen should be administered and ventilation supported if necessary with bag-mask device or endotracheal intubation if available and indicated. Hemodynamic status is closely monitored. Intravenous access should be obtained and appropriate fluid therapy provided with a goal of maintaining adequate perfusion without large volumes indiscriminately administered. Rapid transport to an appropriate facility capable of immediate blood transfusion and surgical intervention completes the management algorithm for hemothorax.

Blunt Cardiac Injury

Cardiac injury most often results from application of force to the anterior chest, especially in a deceleration event such as a motor vehicle crash with violent frontal impact.[1,2,32] The heart is then compressed between the sternum anteriorly and the spinal column posteriorly (**Figure 12-19**). This compression of the heart causes an abrupt increase in the pressure within the ventricles to several times normal, which results in cardiac contusion, sometimes valvular injury, and rarely cardiac rupture, as follows:

- *Cardiac contusion*. The most common result of cardiac compression is cardiac contusion. The heart muscle is bruised, with varying amounts of injury to the myocardial cells. This injury most often results in abnormal heart rhythms, such as sinus tachycardia.[32] Of greater concern, but less common, are premature ventricular contractions or nonperfusing rhythms such as ventricular tachycardia and ventricular fibrillation. If the septal region of the heart is injured, the electrocardiogram (ECG) may demonstrate intraventricular conduction abnormalities, such as right bundle branch

Figure 12-18 Hemothorax. The amount of blood that can accumulate in the thoracic cavity (leading to hypovolemia) is a much more severe condition than the amount of lung compressed by this blood loss.

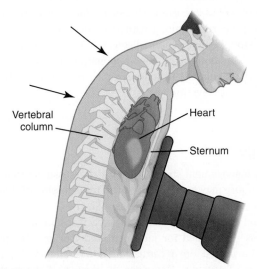

Figure 12-19 The heart can be compressed between the sternum (as the sternum stops against the steering column or dashboard) and the posterior thoracic wall (as the wall continues its forward motion). This compression can contuse the myocardium.

block. If a sufficient volume of myocardium is injured, the contractility of the heart may be impaired, and cardiac output falls, resulting in cardiogenic shock. Unlike the other forms of shock usually encountered in the trauma setting, this shock does not improve with fluid administration and may actually worsen.

- *Valvular rupture.* Rupture of the supporting structures of the heart valves or the valves themselves typically renders the valves incompetent. The patient will present in varying degrees of shock with symptoms and signs of congestive heart failure (CHF), such as *tachypnea*, rales, and new-onset heart murmur.
- *Blunt cardiac rupture.* A rare event, blunt cardiac rupture occurs in less than 1% of patients with blunt chest trauma.[32-34] Most of these patients will die at the scene from *exsanguination* into the chest or fatal cardiac tamponade. The surviving patients will typically present with cardiac tamponade.

Assessment

Assessment of the patient with the potential for blunt cardiac injury reveals a mechanism that imparted a frontal impact to the center of the patient's chest. A bent steering column accompanied by bruising over the sternum implies such a mechanism. As with other chest injuries, the patient is likely to complain of chest pain and/or shortness of breath. If a dysrhythmia is present, the patient may complain of palpitations. Physical findings of concern are bruising over the sternum, crepitus over the sternum, and sternal instability. With a floating sternum (**flail sternum**), the ribs on either side of the sternum are broken, allowing it to move paradoxically with respirations, similar to flail chest, as described earlier. If valvular disruption has occurred, a harsh murmur may be detectable over the precordium along with signs of acute CHF, such as hypotension, jugular venous distension, and abnormal breath sounds. ECG monitoring may demonstrate tachycardia, premature ventricular contractions, other rhythm disturbances, or ST-segment elevation.

Management

The key management strategy is correct assessment that blunt cardiac injury may have occurred and transmission of that concern along with the clinical findings to the receiving hospital. In the meantime, high-concentration oxygen is administered and IV access established for judicious fluid therapy. The patient should be placed on a cardiac monitor to detect dysrhythmias and ST-segment elevations, if present. If dysrhythmias are present and ALS providers are present, standard antidysrhythmic pharmacotherapy should be instituted. There are no data to support prophylactic antidysrhythmic therapy in blunt cardiac injury. As always, ventilatory support measures should be implemented as indicated.

Cardiac Tamponade

Cardiac tamponade occurs when a wound of the heart allows fluid (usually blood) to acutely accumulate between the pericardial sac and the heart.[1,32] The pericardial sac is comprised of a fibrous, inelastic tissue. Normally, there is a small amount of fluid in the pericardial sac, similar to the pleural space, as described earlier. Because the pericardium is inelastic, pressure begins to rise rapidly within the pericardial sac as fluid accumulates within it. This rising pericardial pressure impedes venous return to the heart. This, in turn, leads to diminished cardiac output and blood pressure. With each contraction of the heart, additional blood may enter the pericardial sac, further impeding the heart's ability to fill in preparation for the next contraction (**Figure 12-20**). This condition can become profound enough to precipitate **pulseless electrical activity**, a life-threatening injury requiring coordinated response by prehospital care providers in all phases of care to achieve an optimal outcome. The normal adult pericardium may be able to accommodate as much as 300 ml of fluid before pulselessness occurs, but as little as 50 ml is usually enough to impede cardiac return and, thus, cardiac output.[1]

Most often, cardiac tamponade is caused by a stab wound to the heart. This mechanism of injury may result in penetration into one of the cardiac chambers or just a laceration of the myocardium. The right ventricle is the most anterior chamber in the heart and is therefore the most commonly injured chamber in penetrating trauma. Regardless of the anatomic location of injury, bleeding into the pericardial sac occurs. The rising pressure within the pericardium results in the cardiac tamponade physiology. At the same time, the increased pressure within the pericardium may also temporarily impede further bleeding from the cardiac wound, allowing the patient to survive long enough to reach definitive medical care. In the case of gunshot wounds to the heart, the damage to the heart and

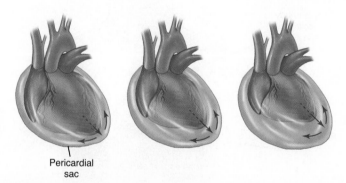

Pericardial sac

Figure 12-20 Cardiac tamponade. As blood courses from the cardiac lumen into the pericardial space, it limits expansion of the ventricle. Therefore, the ventricle cannot fill completely. As more blood accumulates in the pericardial space, less ventricular space is available to accumulate blood, and cardiac output is reduced.

pericardium is usually so severe that the pericardium cannot contain the hemorrhage, resulting in rapid exsanguination into the chest cavity. The same is true in the case of impalements. Blunt rupture of a cardiac chamber can result in cardiac tamponade but more often causes exsanguinating hemorrhage.

Cardiac tamponade should be kept in mind as a possibility when evaluating any patient with a thoracic penetration. This index of suspicion should be raised to the level of "present until proven otherwise" when the penetrating injury is within a rectangle (the cardiac box) formed by drawing a horizontal line along the clavicles, vertical lines from the nipples to the costal margins, and a second horizontal line connecting the points of intersection between the vertical lines and the costal margin (**Figure 12-21**). The presence of such a wound should be communicated to the receiving institution as soon as it is recognized to allow for appropriate preparation to manage the patient.

Assessment

Assessment involves quickly recognizing the presence of at-risk wounds, as previously described, in combination with an appreciation for the physical findings of pericardial tamponade. Beck's triad is a constellation of findings indicative of cardiac tamponade: (1) distant or muffled heart sounds (the fluid around the heart makes it difficult to hear the sounds of the valves closing); (2) jugular venous distension (caused by the increasing pressure in the pericardial sac backing blood up into the neck veins); and (3) low blood pressure. Another physical finding described in cardiac tamponade is paradoxical pulse (**Figure 12-22**).

Detection of some of these signs is difficult in the field, especially muffled heart tones and paradoxical pulse. Additionally, the components of Beck's triad are present in only 22% to 77% of cases of tamponade.[35,36] Thus, the prehospital care provider needs to maintain a high index of suspicion, based on the

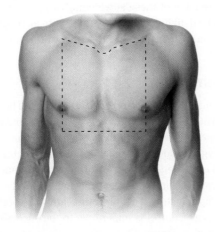

Figure 12-21 In a series of 46 patients with penetrating cardiac injuries, 40 had a wound within the "cardiac box."
Source: Background image © Mariya L/ShutterStock.

> ### Figure 12-22   Paradoxical Pulse
>
> The **paradoxical pulse**, also known as pulsus paradoxus, is actually an accentuation of the normal, slight drop in systolic blood pressure (SBP) that occurs during inspiration. As the lungs expand, there is preferential filling and ejection of blood from the right side of the heart at the expense of the left side. Thus, peripheral blood pressure falls. This decrease in SBP is usually less than 10 to 15 mm Hg. A greater decrease in SBP constitutes the so-called paradoxical pulse.

location of the wounds and hypotension, and implement therapy accordingly.

Management

Management requires rapid, monitored transport to a facility that can perform immediate surgical repair.[13,16,37-41] The prehospital care provider first needs to recognize that cardiac tamponade likely exists and to inform the receiving facility so that preparations can be made for emergent surgical intervention. Oxygen in high concentration should be administered. Intravenous access should be obtained and judicious fluid therapy initiated, because this can augment central venous pressure and, thus, improve cardiac filling for a time. The prehospital care provider should strongly consider endotracheal intubation and positive-pressure ventilation if the patient is hypotensive.[18,39,40]

Definitive therapy requires release of the tamponade and repair of the cardiac injury. A patient with a suspected cardiac tamponade should be transported directly to a facility capable of immediate surgical intervention, if available. Draining some of the pericardial fluid by **pericardiocentesis** (insertion of a needle into the pericardial space) is often an effective temporizing maneuver. Risks of pericardiocentesis include injury to the heart and coronary arteries, resulting in increased tamponade and injury to the lung, great vessels, and liver. In very rare cases, resuscitative thoracotomy (opening the chest to control bleeding and repair internal wounds) has been performed in the field by physicians in systems in which they respond to field emergencies.[42,43]

Commotio Cordis

The term **commotio cordis** refers to the clinical situation in which an apparently innocuous blow to the anterior chest results in sudden cardiac arrest.[44,45] Commotio cordis is believed to account for about 20 deaths per year in the United States, predominantly in children and adolescents (mean age about 13 years). Most experts theorize that commotio cordis results from a relatively minor, nonpenetrating blow to the precordium (area over the heart), occurring at an electrically vulnerable portion of the cardiac cycle, whereas some believe that coronary artery vasospasm may play a role in its development. Regardless of the mechanism, the terminal result is a cardiac dysrhythmia resulting in ventricular fibrillation and sudden cardiac arrest.

This condition most frequently occurs during amateur sporting events in which the victim is struck in the midanterior chest by a projectile or object, such as a baseball (most common), ice hockey puck, lacrosse ball, or softball. However, commotio cordis has also been reported after bodily impacts (e.g., karate blows), a low-velocity motor vehicle crash, and the collision of two outfielders trying to catch a baseball. After the impact, victims have been known to walk a step or two and then suddenly drop to the ground in cardiac arrest. Typically, no injury is noted to the ribs, sternum, or heart at autopsy. Most victims have no known history of heart disease. The condition may be prevented through the use of equipment such as safety baseballs.[46]

Assessment

Patients who have sustained commotio cordis are found in cardiopulmonary arrest. In some victims, a minor bruise is noted over the sternum. Ventricular fibrillation is the most common rhythm, although complete heart block and left bundle branch block with ST-segment elevations have also been seen.

Management

Once cardiac arrest is confirmed, cardiopulmonary resuscitation (CPR) is initiated. Commotio cordis is managed in a manner similar to cardiac arrests resulting from myocardial infarction rather than those resulting from trauma and blood loss. The cardiac rhythm should be determined as expeditiously as possible, with rapid defibrillation administered if ventricular fibrillation is identified. Prognosis is poor, with the chance of survival at 15% or less.[45] Virtually all survivors of this condition received both rapid, bystander-initiated CPR and immediate defibrillation, often with an automated external defibrillator. Precordial thumps have not been shown to consistently terminate ventricular fibrillation; however, they may be attempted if a defibrillator is not immediately available. The initiation of CPR and electrical defibrillation should not be delayed to perform a precordial thump.[47] If immediate attempts at defibrillation are unsuccessful, the airway is secured and IV access initiated. Epinephrine and antidysrhythmic pharmacologic agents may be administered as outlined in medical cardiac arrest protocols.

Traumatic Aortic Disruption

Traumatic aortic disruption results from a deceleration/acceleration mechanism of significant force.[48] Examples include high-speed frontal-impact motor vehicle crashes and high falls in which the patient lands flat.

The aorta arises from the upper portion of the heart in the mediastinum. The heart, ascending aorta, and aortic arch are relatively mobile within the chest cavity. As the arch of the aorta transitions to the descending aorta, it is "wrapped" with an investing layer of tissue and becomes adherent to the vertebral column. Thus, the descending aorta is relatively immobile. When there is a sudden deceleration of the body, such as occurs in a high-speed frontal impact, the heart and the aortic arch continue to move forward relative to the fixed (immobile) descending aorta. This contrast in velocity produces shear forces in the aortic wall at the junction between these two segments of the aorta.[40] Thus, the typical location for a traumatic aortic injury is just distal to the takeoff of the left subclavian artery. This shear force can disrupt the wall of the aorta in varying degrees (**Figure 12-23**). When the tear extends through the full thickness of the aortic wall, the patient rapidly exsanguinates into the pleural cavity. However, if the tear is only partially through the wall, leaving the outer layer (adventitia) intact, the patient may survive for a variable length of time, making rapid identification and treatment essential for a successful outcome.[48]

Assessment

Assessment of aortic disruption hinges on index of suspicion. A high index should be maintained in situations involving high-energy deceleration/acceleration mechanisms. For such a devastating injury, there may be little external evidence of chest injury. The prehospital care provider needs to assess the adequacy of the airway and breathing and should perform careful auscultation and palpation. Careful examination may demonstrate that the pulse quality may be different between the two upper extremities (pulse stronger in the right arm than the left) or between the upper (brachial artery) and lower extremities (femoral artery). Blood pressures, if measured, may be higher in the upper extremities than the lower extremities, comprising the signs of a pseudo-coarctation (narrowing) of the aorta.

Definitive diagnosis of aortic disruption requires radiographic imaging in the hospital. Plain chest radiographs may demonstrate a variety of signs suggesting the injury is present. The most reliable of these is widening of the mediastinum. The injury can be definitively demonstrated with **aortography**, CT of the chest, and **transesophageal echocardiography**.[48]

Management

Management of traumatic aortic disruption in the field is supportive. A high index of suspicion for its presence is maintained when the appropriate mechanism exists. High-concentration supplemental oxygen is administered and IV access is obtained, except in cases of extremely short transport times. Communication with the receiving facility about the mechanism and suspicion for aortic disruption should occur at the earliest opportunity. Strict blood pressure control is imperative to the successful outcome of these injuries (**Figure 12-24**). Traumatic aortic disruption represents another situation in which balanced resuscitation is clinically useful. Fluid resuscitation that results in normal or elevated blood pressure may result in rupture of the remaining tissue of

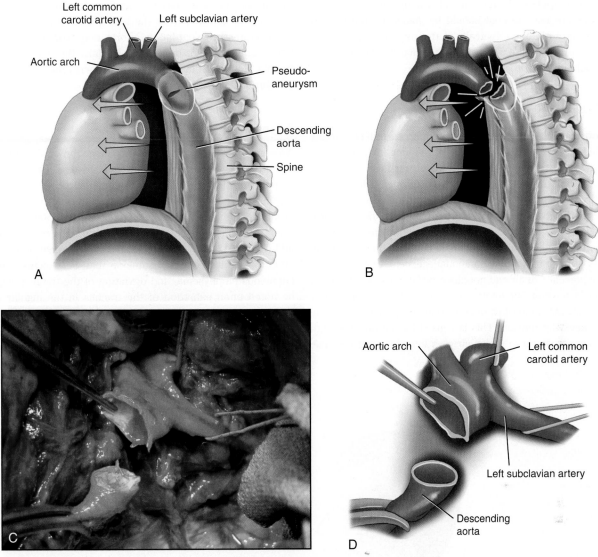

Figure 12-23 **A.** The descending aorta is a fixed structure that moves with the thoracic spine. The arch, aorta, and heart are freely movable. Acceleration of the torso in a lateral-impact collision or rapid deceleration of the torso in a frontal-impact collision produces a different rate of motion between the arch-heart complex and the descending aorta. This motion may result in a tear of the inner lining of the aorta that is contained within the outermost layer, producing a pseudoaneurysm. **B.** Tears at the junction of the arch and descending aorta may also result in a complete rupture, leading to immediate exsanguination in the chest. **C** and **D.** Operative photograph and drawing of a traumatic aortic tear.

Source: C., D. Courtesy Norman McSwain, MD, FACS, NREMT-P.

Figure 12-24 Blood Pressure Maintenance

Caution: When performing interhospital transfer of patients with suspected aortic disruption, it is important not to raise the patient's blood pressure aggressively because this may lead to exsanguinating hemorrhage (see the Shock chapter). Many of these patients may be given infusions of medications, such as beta blockers (e.g., esmolol, metoprolol), to maintain the blood pressure at a lower level, typically a mean arterial pressure of 70 mm Hg or less. Such therapy typically requires invasive monitoring, such as insertion of an arterial line, so that blood pressure can be monitored much more carefully.

the aorta and rapid exsanguination. If transport times are longer, blood pressure management should be guided by the highest blood pressure obtained, typically in the right arm. Control of both blood pressure and contractile force may be accomplished with the administration of beta blockers.[49]

Tracheobronchial Disruption

Tracheobronchial disruption is an uncommon, but potentially highly lethal, entity.[49] All lacerations of the lung involve disruption of airways to some degree; however, in these cases, the intrathoracic portion of the trachea itself or one of the main or secondary bronchi is disrupted. This disruption results in high flow of air through the injury into the mediastinum or pleural space (**Figure 12-25**). Pressure rapidly accumulates, resulting in tension pneumothorax or even tension pneumomediastinum, which is similar to cardiac tamponade except that it results from the presence of air and not blood or fluid. Unlike the usual situation in tension pneumothorax, needle thoracostomy may result in the continuous flow of air through the catheter and may fail to relieve the tension. This is caused by the ongoing high flow of air across these major airways into the pleural space.

Respiratory function may be significantly impaired because of preferential airflow across the lesion as well as the pressure. Positive-pressure ventilation efforts may worsen the tension. Penetrating trauma is more likely to cause this injury than blunt trauma. However, blunt injury of high energy may also cause tracheobronchial disruption.[50]

Assessment

Assessment of the patient with tracheobronchial disruption demonstrates an individual in obvious distress. The patient may be pale and diaphoretic and will demonstrate signs of respiratory distress, such as use of accessory muscles of respiration, grunting, and nasal flaring. Extensive subcutaneous emphysema, especially in the upper chest and neck, may be identified (**Figure 12-26**). Although traditionally taught as important findings, jugular venous distension may be obscured by subcutaneous emphysema, and deviation of the trachea may only be noted upon palpation of the trachea in the jugular notch. Ventilatory rate will be elevated, and oxygen saturation may be diminished. The patient may or may not be hypotensive and may cough up blood (hemoptysis). The hemorrhage associated

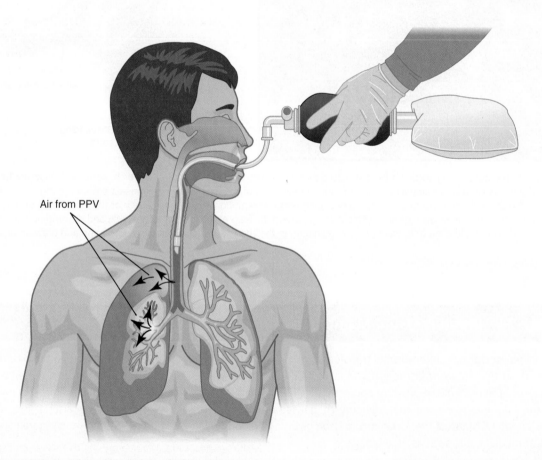

Figure 12-25   Tracheal or bronchial rupture. Positive-pressure ventilation (PPV) can directly force large amounts of air through the trachea or bronchus, rapidly producing a tension pneumothorax.

asphyxia, upper chest) as patients who have been strangled. Unlike strangled patients, however, traumatic asphyxia patients do not suffer from true asphyxia (cessation of air and gas exchange). The similarity in appearance to strangulation patients results from the impaired venous return from the head and neck that is present in both groups of patients.

The mechanism for traumatic asphyxia is an abrupt, significant increase in thoracic pressure resulting from a crush to the torso (e.g., car falling off a jack onto the patient's chest). This pressure results in blood being forced back out of the heart and into the veins in a retrograde direction. Because the veins of the arms and lower extremities contain valves, backward flow into the extremities is limited. However, the veins of the neck and head lack such valves, and blood is preferentially forced into these areas. Subcutaneous venules and small capillaries rupture and blood leaks out, resulting in the purplish discoloration of the skin. Rupture of small vessels in the brain and retina may result in brain and eye dysfunction. Traumatic asphyxia is reported to be a marker for blunt cardiac rupture.[51]

Assessment

The hallmark of traumatic asphyxia is plethora, a bodily condition characterized by an excess of blood and turgescence (i.e., swelling and distension of blood vessels), with a reddish coloration of the skin. This appearance is most prominent above the level of the crush (**Figure 12-27**). The skin below the level of injury is normal. Because of the force applied to the chest necessary to cause this injury, many of the injuries already discussed in this chapter may be present, as well as injuries to the spine and spinal cord.

Management

Management is supportive. High-concentration oxygen is administered, IV access obtained, and judicious ventilatory support provided, if indicated. The reddish-purple discoloration typically fades within 1 to 2 weeks in survivors.

Diaphragmatic Rupture

Small lacerations of the diaphragm may occur in penetrating injuries to the thoracoabdominal region.[1] Because the diaphragm rises and falls with respiration, any penetration that is below the level of the nipples anteriorly or the level of the scapular tip posteriorly is at risk for having traversed the diaphragm. Generally, these lesions do not present any acute problems on their own, but they usually require surgical repair because of the risk in the future for herniation and strangulation of abdominal contents through the defect. Significant injuries to thoracic or abdominal organs may accompany these otherwise apparently innocuous injuries.

Blunt diaphragmatic rupture results from the application of sufficient force to the abdomen to increase abdominal pressure acutely, abruptly, and sufficiently to disrupt the diaphragm. Unlike the small tears that usually accompany penetrating injury, the tears resulting from blunt mechanisms are frequently large

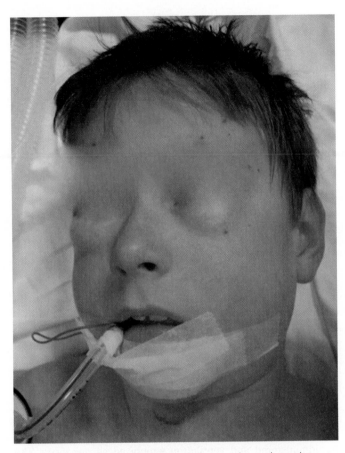

Figure 12-26 Patient with trauma to the anterior neck causing a tracheal disruption and subcutaneous emphysema of the face (eyelids) and neck.
Source: Photograph provided courtesy of J.C. Pitteloud M.D., Switzerland.

with penetrating trauma may not be present in the blunt cases, but hemothorax is a possibility in both penetrating and blunt trauma.

Management

Successful management of tracheobronchial disruption requires administration of supplemental oxygen and judicious use of ventilatory assistance. If assisted ventilation makes the patient more uncomfortable, only oxygen is administered and the patient is transported as quickly as possible to an appropriate facility. Continuous monitoring for signs of progression toward a tension pneumothorax is imperative, and rapid needle decompression should be attempted if these signs present. Complex advanced airway management, such as selective main bronchus intubation, is difficult to accomplish in the field and has the potential for worsening a major bronchial injury.

Traumatic Asphyxia

Traumatic asphyxia is so named because the victims physically resemble strangulation patients. They exhibit the same bluish discoloration of the face and neck (and in the case of traumatic

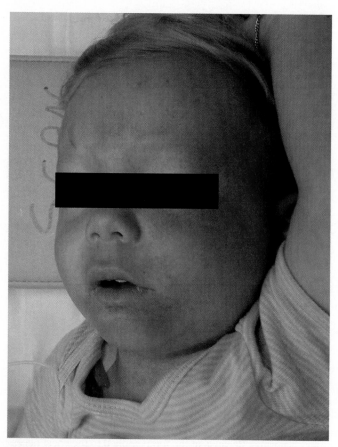

Figure 12-27 Child with traumatic asphyxia. Note the purple discoloration, particularly on the chin, and the multiple petecchiae on the face and forehead.

Source: Photograph provided courtesy of J.C. Pitteloud M.D., Switzerland.

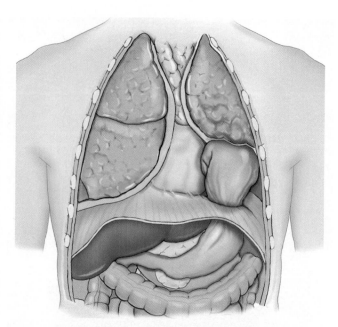

Figure 12-28 Diaphragmatic rupture may cause the bowel or other structures to herniate through the tear, causing partial compression of the lung and respiratory distress.

Management

Prompt recognition that diaphragmatic rupture may be present is necessary. Supplemental oxygen in high concentration should be administered and ventilation supported as necessary. The patient should be rapidly transported to an appropriate facility.

Prolonged Transport

Priorities for managing patients with known or suspected thoracic injuries during prolonged transport remain fundamental, including managing the airway, supporting ventilation and oxygenation, controlling hemorrhage, and providing appropriate volume resuscitation. When faced with a prolonged transport, prehospital care providers may have a lower threshold for securing the airway with endotracheal intubation. Indications for performing endotracheal intubation include increasing respiratory distress or impending respiratory failure (after exclusion or treatment of a tension pneumothorax), a flail chest, open pneumothorax, or multiple rib fractures. Oxygen should be provided to maintain oxygen saturation at 95% or greater.

Ventilations should be assisted as necessary. Pulmonary contusions worsen over time, and the use of CPAP, positive end-expiratory pressure (PEEP) with a transport ventilator, or PEEP valves with bag-mask device may facilitate oxygenation. Any patient with significant thoracic trauma may have or develop a tension pneumothorax, and ongoing assessment should look for the hallmark signs. In the presence of decreased or absent breath sounds, worsening respiratory distress, difficulty squeezing the bag-mask device, increasing peak inspiratory pressures in patients on a ventilator, and hypotension, pleural decompression should be performed. A tube thoracostomy (insertion of a

and allow acute herniation of the abdominal viscera into the chest cavity[1] (**Figure 12-28**). Respiratory distress results from the pressure of the herniated organs on the lungs, preventing effective ventilation, as well as from contusion of the lungs. This impairment of ventilation may be life threatening. In addition to the ventilatory dysfunction, rib fractures, hemothorax, and pneumothorax may occur. Injury of intra-abdominal organs may also accompany the injury to the diaphragm, including injuries to the liver, spleen, stomach, or intestines, as these organs are forced through the tear in the diaphragm into the pleural cavity. These patients are frequently in acute distress and require rapid intervention to recover.

Assessment

Assessment frequently reveals a patient in acute respiratory distress who appears anxious, tachypneic, and pale. The patient may have contusions of the chest wall, bony crepitus, or subcutaneous emphysema. Breath sounds on the affected side may be diminished, or bowel sounds may be auscultated over the chest. The abdomen may be scaphoid if enough of the abdominal contents have herniated into the chest.

chest tube) may be performed by authorized personnel, typically air medical flight crews, if the patient requires needle decompression or is found to have an open pneumothorax. Intravenous access should be secured and IV fluids administered judiciously.

Patients with suspected intrathoracic, intra-abdominal, or retroperitoneal hemorrhage should be maintained with systolic blood pressure in the range of 80 to 90 mm Hg. Overaggressive volume resuscitation may significantly worsen pulmonary contusions, as well as lead to recurrent internal hemorrhage (see the Shock chapter).

Patients with severe pain from multiple rib fractures may benefit from small doses of narcotics titrated intravenously. If narcotic administration results in hypotension and respiratory failure, volume resuscitation and ventilatory support should be provided.

Patients with cardiac dysrhythmias associated with blunt cardiac injury may benefit from the use of antidysrhythmic medications. Any interventions performed should be carefully documented on the patient care report (PCR), and the receiving facility must be made aware of the procedures.

Summary

- Thoracic injuries are particularly significant because of the potential for compromise of respiratory and circulatory function and because thoracic injuries are frequently associated with multisystem trauma.
- Patients with chest injury need to be managed aggressively and transported quickly to definitive care.
- Particular attention should be paid to the administration of supplemental high-concentration oxygen and the need for ventilatory support in any patient suspected of having chest trauma.
- Pulse oximetry and sidestream or in-line waveform capnography are useful adjuncts for assessing ventilatory status and responses to therapy.
- Signs of tension pneumothorax should be carefully sought because treatment in the field with needle decompression may correct this possible, rapidly fatal problem.
- Because of the high risk of multisystem trauma in patients with blunt thoracic trauma, spinal immobilization is considered and hemorrhage is controlled.
- Intravenous access should be obtained en route to the medical facility and fluid therapy administered with appropriate goals in mind.
- Electrocardiographic monitoring may suggest blunt cardiac injury.
- Although many thoracic injuries can be managed without surgical intervention, the patient with a chest injury must still be evaluated and managed at an appropriate medical facility.

SCENARIO RECAP

You and your partner are dispatched to an industrial construction area for a worker who was struck by a piece of metal. Upon arrival you are met at the gate by the site safety officer, who leads you to an interior work area. En route to the work area, the safety officer states the patient was helping to install metal studs. When he turned to grab another stud, he ran into the end of a stud his partner had just trimmed, cutting through his shirt and puncturing his chest.

In the work area you find an approximately 35-year-old man sitting upright on a pile of lumber, leaning forward and holding a rag to the right side of his chest. You ask the patient what happened, and he tries to tell you but has to stop after every five to six words to catch his breath. As you move the rag, you notice an open laceration approximately 2 inches (5 centimeters) long with a small amount of blood-tinged, "bubbling" fluid. The patient is diaphoretic and has a rapid radial pulse. Decreased breath sounds are noted on the right side with auscultation. No other abnormal physical findings are noted.

- Is this patient in respiratory distress?
- Does he have life-threatening injuries?
- What interventions should you undertake in the field?
- What modality should be used to transport this patient?
- How would a different location (e.g., rural) impact your management and plans during prolonged transport?
- What other injuries do you suspect?

SCENARIO SOLUTION

The scene report, patient complaints, and physical examination lead you to suspect that this patient may have serious and potentially life-threatening injuries. He is awake and speaking coherently, indicating that he has a stable airway. He is experiencing severe respiratory distress. The location of the wound, bubbling fluid, and decreased breath sounds indicate an open pneumothorax.

You move quickly to apply an occlusive dressing, provide the patient with supplemental oxygen, and consider ventilatory assistance with a bag-mask device as necessary. The first priorities in this scenario are to recognize the seriousness of the injuries, stabilize the patient, and initiate transfer to an appropriate facility. Given this patient's respiratory distress and findings, he is at significant risk for complications. Transport to the closest trauma center is appropriate. Intravenous access should be obtained en route.

There is risk for respiratory deterioration, and the patient's ventilatory status needs to be monitored closely. Signs of progressing circulatory compromise and respiratory distress would prompt you to first remove the occlusive dressing and, if there is no improvement, to perform needle decompression. If transport time will be extended, air transport should be considered.

References

1. American College of Surgeons (ACS). Thoracic trauma. In: ACS Committee on Trauma. *Advanced Trauma Life Support for Doctors, Student Course Manual.* 9th ed. Chicago, IL: ACS; 2012.

2. Wall MJ, Huh J, Mattox KL. Thoracotomy. In Mattox KL, Feliciano DV, Moore EE. *Trauma.* 5th ed. New York, NY: McGraw-Hill; 2004.

3. Livingston DH, Hauser CJ. Trauma to the chest wall and lung. In: Mattox KL, Feliciano DV, Moore EE. *Trauma.* 5th ed. New York, NY: McGraw-Hill; 2004.

4. Howes DS, Bellazzini MA. Chronic obstructive pulmonary disease. In: Wolfson AB, Hendey GW, Ling LJ, et al., eds. *Harwood-Nuss' Clinical Practice of Emergency Medicine.* 5th ed. Philadelphia, PA: Wolters Kluwer/Lippincott, Williams & Wilkins; 2010.

5. Wilson RF. Pulmonary physiology. In: Wilson RF. *Critical Care Manual: Applied Physiology and Principles of Therapy.* 2nd ed. Philadelphia, PA: Davis; 1992.

6. American College of Surgeons (ACS). Initial assessment. In: ACS Committee on Trauma. *Advanced Trauma Life Support for Doctors.* 9th ed. Chicago, IL: ACS; 2012.

7. Silverston P. Pulse oximetry at the roadside: a study of pulse oximetry in immediate care. *BMJ.* 1989;298:711.

8. Pressley CM, Fry WR, Philip AS, et al. Predicting outcome of patients with chest wall injury. *Am J Surg.* 2012;204(6):900–904.

9. Flagel BT, Luchette FA, Reed RL, et al. Half-a-dozen ribs: the break-point for mortality. *Surgery.* 2005;138:717–725.

10. Jones KM, Reed RL, Luchette FA. The ribs or not the ribs: which influences mortality? *Am J Surg.* 2011;202(5):598–604.

11. Richardson JD, Adams L, Flint LM. Selective management of flail chest and pulmonary contusion. *Ann Surg.* 1982;196:481.

12. Di Bartolomeo S, Sanson G, Nardi G, et al. A population-based study on pneumothorax in severely traumatized patients. *J Trauma.* 2001;51(4):677.

13. Regel G, Stalp M, Lehmann U, et al. Prehospital care: importance of early intervention outcome. *Acta Anaesthesiol Scand Suppl.* 1997;110:71.

14. Barone JE, Pizzi WF, Nealon TF, et al. Indications for intubation in blunt chest trauma. *J Trauma.* 1986;26:334.

15. Mattox KL. Prehospital care of the patient with an injured chest. *Surg Clin North Am.* 1989;69(1):21.

16. Simon B, Ebert J, Bokhari F, Capella J, Emhoff T, Hayward T 3rd, Rodriguez A, Smith L, Eastern Association for the Surgery of Trauma. Management of pulmonary contusion and flail chest: an Eastern Association for the Surgery of Trauma practice management guideline. *J Trauma Acute Care Surg.* 2012 Nov;73(5 Suppl 4):S351–61.

17. Cooper C, Militello P. The multi-injured patient: the Maryland Shock Trauma Protocol approach. *Semin Thorac Cardiovasc Surg.* 1992;4(3):163.

18. Barton ED, Epperson M, Hoyt DB, et al. Prehospital needle aspiration and tube thoracostomy in trauma victims: a six-year experience with aeromedical crews. *J Emerg Med.* 1995;13:155.

19. Kheirabadi BS, Terrazas IB, Koller A, et al. Vented vs. unvented chest seals for treatment of pneumothorax (PTx) and prevention of tension PTx in a swine model. *J Trauma Acute Care Surg.* 2013;75:150–156.

20. Butler FK, Dubose JJ, Otten EJ, et al. Management of open pneumothorax in tactical combat casualty care: TCCC guidelines change 13-02. *J Special Ops Med.* 2013;13(3):81–86.

21. Eckstein M, Suyehara DL. Needle thoracostomy in the pre-hospital setting. *Prehosp Emerg Care.* 1998;2:132.

22. Holcomb JB, McManus JG, Kerr ST, Pusateri AE. Needle versus tube thoracostomy in a swine model of traumatic tension hemopneumothorax. *Prehosp Emerg Care.* 2009;13(1):18–27.

23. Butler KL, Best IM, Weaver WL, et al. Pulmonary artery injury and cardiac tamponade after needle decompression of a suspected tension pneumothorax. *J Trauma.* 2003;54:610.

24. Inaba K, Ives C, McClure K, et al. Radiologic evaluation of alternative sites for needle decompression of tension pneumothorax. *Arch Surg.* 2012;147(9):813–818.

25. Inaba K, Branco BC Exkstein M, et al. Optimal positioning for emergent needle thoracostomy: a cadaver-based study. *J Trauma.* 2011;71:1099–1103.

26. Netto FA, Shulman H, Rizoli SB, et al. Are needle decompressions for tension pneumothoraces being performed appropriately for appropriate indications? *Am J Em Med.* 2008;26:597–602.

27. Riwoe D, Poncia H. Subclavian artery laceration: a serious complication of needle decompression. *Em Med Aust.* 2011;23:651–653.

28. Beckett A, Savage E, Pannell D, et al. Needle decompression for tension pneumothorax in tactical combat casualty care: do catheters placed in the midaxillary line kink more often than those in the midclavicular line? *J Trauma.* 2011;71:S408–S412.

29. Martin M, Satterly S, Inaba K, Blair K. Does needle thoracostomy provide adequate and effective decompression of tension pneumothorax? *J Trauma.* 2012;73(6):1410–1415.

30. Davis DP, Pettit K, Rum CD, et al. The safety and efficacy of prehospital needle and tube thoracostomy by aeromedical personnel. *Prehosp Emerg Care.* 2005;9:191.

31. Etoch SW, Bar-Natan MF, Miller FB, et al. Tube thoracostomy: factors related to complications. *Arch Surg.* 1995;130:521.

32. Newman PG, Feliciano DV. Blunt cardiac injury. *New Horizons.* 1999;7(1):26.

33. Ivatury RR. The injured heart. In: Mattox KL, Feliciano DV, Moore EE. *Trauma.* 5th ed. New York, NY: McGraw-Hill; 2004:555.

34. Symbas NP, Bongiorno PF, Symbas PN. Blunt cardiac rupture: the utility of emergency department ultrasound. *Ann Thorac Surg.* 1999;67(5):1274.

35. Demetriades D. Cardiac Wounds. *Ann Surg.* 1986;203(3): 315–317.

36. Jacob S, Sebastian JC, Cherian PK, et al. Pericardial effusion impending tamponade: a look beyond Beck's triad. *Am J Em Med.* 2009;27:216–219,

37. Ivatury RR, Nallathambi MN, Roberge RJ, et al. Penetrating thoracic injuries: in-field stabilization versus prompt transport. *J Trauma.* 1987;27:1066.

38. Bleetman A, Kasem H, Crawford R. Review of emergency thoracotomy for chest injuries in patients attending a UK accident and emergency department. *Injury.* 1996;27(2):129.

39. Durham LA III, Richardson RJ, Wall MJ Jr, et al. Emergency center thoracotomy: impact of prehospital resuscitation. *J Trauma.* 1992;32(6):775.

40. Honigman B, Rohweder K, Moore EE, et al. Prehospital advanced trauma life support for penetrating cardiac wounds. *Ann Emerg Med.* 1990;19(2):145.

41. Lerer LB, Knottenbelt JD. Preventable mortality following sharp penetrating chest trauma. *J Trauma.* 1994;37(1):9.

42. Wall MJ Jr, Pepe PE, Mattox KL. Successful roadside resuscitative thoracotomy: case report and literature review. *J Trauma.* 1994;36(1):131.

43. Coats TJ, Keogh S, Clark H, et al. Prehospital resuscitative thoracotomy for cardiac arrest after penetrating trauma: rationale and case series. *J Trauma.* 2001;50(4):670.

44. Zangwill SD, Strasburger JF. Commotio cordis. *Pediatr Clin North Am.* 2004;51(5):1347–1354.

45. Perron AD, Brady WJ, Erling BF. Commodio cordis: an underappreciated cause of sudden cardiac death in young patients: assessment and management in the ED. *Am J Emerg Med.* 2001;19(5):406–409.

46. Madias C, Maron BJ, Weinstock J, et al. Commotio cordis—sudden cardiac death with chest wall impact. *J Cardiovasc Electrophysiol.* 2007;18(1):115–122.

47. 2010 American Heart Association Guidelines for Cardiopulmonary Resuscitation and Emergency Cardiovascular Care Science. *Circulation.* 2010;122;S745–S746.

48. Mattox KL, Wall MJ, Lemaire SA. Injury to the thoracic great vessels. In: Mattox KL, Feliciano DV, Moore EE. *Trauma.* 5th ed. New York, NY: McGraw-Hill; 2004.

49. Fabian TC. Roger T. Sherman Lecture: advances in the management of blunt thoracic aortic injury: Parmley to the present. *Am Surg.* 2009;75(4):273–278.

50. Riley RD, Miller PR, Meredith JW. Injury to the esophagus, trachea, and bronchus. In: Mattox KL, Feliciano DV, Moore EE. *Trauma.* 5th ed. New York, NY: McGraw-Hill; 2004.

51. Rogers FB, Leavitt BJ. Upper torso cyanosis: a marker for blunt cardiac rupture. *Am J Emerg Med.* 1997;15(3):275.

Suggested Reading

Bowley DM, Boffard KD. Penetrating trauma of the trunk. *Unfallchirurg.* 2001;104(11):1032.

Brathwaite CE, Rodriguez A, Turney SZ, et al. Blunt traumatic cardiac rupture: a 5-year experience. *Ann Surg.* 1990;212(6):701.

Helm M, Schuster R, Hauke J. Tight control of prehospital ventilation by capnography in major trauma victims. *Br J Anaesth.* 2003;90(3):327.

Lateef F. Commotio cordis: an underappreciated cause of sudden death in athletes. *Sports Med.* 2000;30:301.

Papadopoulos IN, Bukis D, Karalas E, et al. Preventable prehospital trauma deaths in a Hellenic urban health region: an audit of prehospital trauma care. *J Trauma.* 1996;41(5):864.

Rozycki GS, Feliciano DV, Oschner MG, et al. The role of ultrasound in patients with possible penetrating cardiac wounds: a prospective multicenter study. *J Trauma.* 1999;46:542.

Ruchholtz S, Waydhas C, Ose C, et al. Prehospital intubation in severe thoracic trauma without respiratory insufficiency: a matched-pair analysis based on the Trauma Registry of the German Trauma Society. *J Trauma.* 2002;52(5):879.

Streng M, Tikka S, Leppaniemi A. Assessing the severity of truncal gunshot wounds: a nation-wide analysis from Finland. *Ann Chir Gynaecol.* 2001;90(4):246.

SPECIFIC SKILLS

Thoracic Trauma Skills

Needle Decompression

Principle: To decease intrathoracic pressure from a tension pneumothorax affecting the patient's breathing, ventilation, and circulation.

In patients with increasing intrathoracic pressure from a developing tension pneumothorax, the side of the thoracic cavity that has the increased pressure should be decompressed. If this pressure is not relieved, it will progressively limit the patient's ventilatory capacity and cause inadequate venous return, producing inadequate cardiac output and death.

In patients in whom an open pneumothorax has been treated by the use of an occlusive dressing and a tension pneumothorax develops, decompression can usually be achieved through the wound, which provides an existing opening into the thorax. Opening the occlusive dressing over the wound for a few seconds should initiate a rush of air out of the wound as increased pressure in the thorax is relieved.

Once this pressure has been released, the wound is resealed with the occlusive dressing to allow for proper alveolar ventilation and to stop air from "sucking" into the wound. The patient should be monitored carefully and, if any signs of tension recur, the dressing should be "burped" again to release the intrathoracic pressure.

Decompression in a closed-tension pneumothorax is achieved by providing an opening—a thoracostomy—in the affected side of the chest. Different methods for performing a thoracostomy exist. Because needle thoracostomy is the most rapid method and does not require special equipment, it is the preferred method for use in the field.

Needle decompression carries minimal risk and can greatly benefit the patient by improving oxygenation and circulation. Needle decompression should be performed only when the following three criteria are met:

1. Evidence of worsening respiratory distress or difficulty with a bag-mask device
2. Decreased or absent breath sounds
3. Decompensated shock (systolic blood pressure less than 90 mm Hg)

Necessary equipment for needle chest decompression includes a needle, a syringe, 1/2-inch adhesive tape, and alcohol swabs. The needles should be large-bore, over-the-needle IV catheters between 10 and 14 gauge, at least 3.5 inches (8 cm) in length. A 16-gauge catheter can be used if a larger bore is not available.

One prehospital care provider attaches the needle to the syringe while a second prehospital care provider auscultates the patient's chest to confirm which side has the tension pneumothorax, which is indicated by absent or diminished breath sounds.

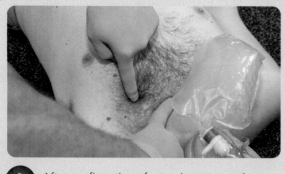

 After confirmation of a tension pneumothorax, the anatomic landmarks are located on the affected side (midclavicular line, second or third intercostal space).

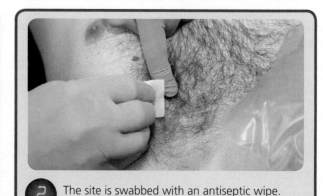

2 The site is swabbed with an antiseptic wipe.

Thoracic Trauma Skills (continued)

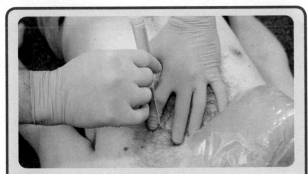

3 The skin over the site is stretched between the fingers of the nondominant hand. The needle and syringe are positioned over the top of the rib.

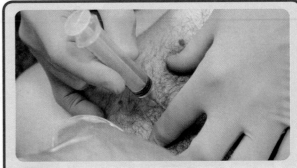

4 Once the needle enters into the thoracic cavity, air will escape into the syringe, and the needle should not be advanced further.

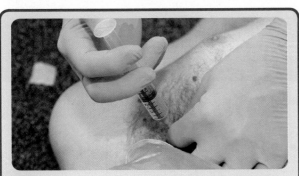

5 The catheter should be left in place and the needle removed, with care not to kink the catheter. As the needle is removed, a rush of air from the hub of the catheter should be heard. If no air escapes, the catheter should be left in place to indicate that needle decompression of the chest was attempted.

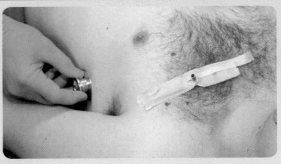

6 After the needle is removed, the catheter is taped in place with adhesive tape. After securing the catheter, the chest is auscultated to check for increased breath sounds. The patient is monitored and transported to an appropriate facility. The prehospital care provider need not waste time applying a one-way valve. Needle decompression may need to be repeated if the catheter becomes occluded with a blood clot and tension pneumothorax reoccurs.

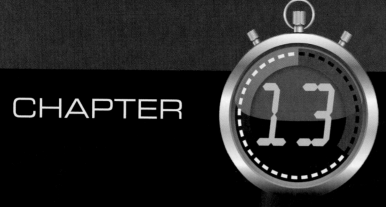

CHAPTER 13

Abdominal Trauma

CHAPTER OBJECTIVES

At the completion of this chapter, the reader will be able to do the following:

- Analyze scene assessment data to determine the level of suspicion for abdominal trauma.

- Recognize the physical examination findings indicative of intra-abdominal bleeding.

- Correlate external signs of abdominal injury to the potential for specific abdominal organ injuries.

- Anticipate the pathophysiologic effects of a blunt or penetrating injury to the abdomen.

- Identify the indications for rapid intervention and transport in the context of abdominal trauma.

- Understand appropriate field management decisions for patients with suspected abdominal trauma, including those with impaled objects, evisceration, and external genital trauma.

- Correlate the anatomic and physiologic changes associated with pregnancy to the pathophysiology and management of trauma.

- Discuss the effects of maternal trauma on the fetus and the priorities of management.

SCENARIO

You are called to a construction site for a male patient in his mid-20s who fell 3 hours earlier and is now complaining of increasing abdominal pain. He states that he tripped on a piece of wood at the site and fell, striking his left lower chest and abdomen on some stacked wood. The patient notes moderate pain over his lower left rib cage when he takes deep breaths and complains of mild difficulty breathing. His coworkers wanted to call for assistance when he fell, but he said the symptoms weren't so bad and told them to hold off. He states that the discomfort has been increasing in intensity and that he is now feeling lightheaded and weak.

You find the patient sitting on the ground in visible discomfort. He is holding the left side of his lower chest and upper abdomen. He has a patent airway, a ventilatory rate of 28 breaths/minute, a heart rate of 124 beats/minute, and a blood pressure of 94/58 millimeters of mercury (mm Hg). The patient's skin is pale and diaphoretic. You lay him down, and on physical examination, he has tenderness on palpation of the left lower ribs without obvious bony crepitus. His abdomen is nondistended and soft to palpation, but he has tenderness and voluntary guarding in the left upper quadrant. No external ecchymosis or subcutaneous emphysema is present.

- What are the patient's possible injuries?
- What are the priorities in the care of this patient?
- Are signs of peritonitis present?

Introduction

Unrecognized abdominal injury is one of the major causes of preventable death in the trauma patient. Because of the limitations of prehospital assessment, patients with suspected abdominal injuries are best managed by prompt transport to the closest appropriate facility.

Early death from severe abdominal trauma typically results from massive blood loss caused by either penetrating or blunt injuries. Any patient with unexplained shock after sustaining a traumatic injury to the trunk of the body should be assumed to have an intra-abdominal hemorrhage until proven otherwise, which can only be accomplished by appropriate diagnostic studies in the hospital. Complications and death may occur from liver, spleen, colon, small intestine, stomach, or pancreatic injuries that were not initially detected. The absence of local signs and symptoms does not rule out the possibility of abdominal trauma, as they often take time to develop and are especially difficult to identify in the patient whose level of consciousness is altered by alcohol, drugs, or traumatic brain injury (TBI). Consideration of the kinematics will raise the index of suspicion of the alert prehospital care provider to possible abdominal trauma and intra-abdominal hemorrhage. It is not necessary to be concerned with pinpointing the exact extent of abdominal trauma, but rather to recognize the likelihood of injury and to treat the clinical findings.

Anatomy

The abdomen contains the major organs of the digestive, endocrine, and urogenital systems and major vessels of the circulatory system. The abdominal cavity is located below the diaphragm; its boundaries include the anterior abdominal wall, the pelvic bones, the vertebral column, and the muscles of the abdomen and flanks. The abdominal cavity is divided into two regions based upon the relationship to the *peritoneum*, which covers many of the organs of the abdomen. The **peritoneal cavity** (the "true" abdominal cavity) contains the spleen, liver, gallbladder, stomach, portions of the large intestine (transverse and sigmoid colon), most of the small intestines (primarily the jejunum and ileum), and female reproductive organs (uterus and ovaries) (**Figure 13-1**). The **retroperitoneal space** is the area in the abdominal cavity that is located behind the peritoneum and contains the kidneys, ureters, inferior vena cava, abdominal aorta, pancreas, much of the duodenum, ascending and descending colon, and rectum (**Figure 13-2**). The urinary bladder and male reproductive organs (penis, testes, and prostate) lie inferior to the peritoneal cavity.

A portion of the abdomen lies in the lower thorax. This is because the dome shape of the diaphragm allows the upper abdominal organs to rise up into the lower chest. This superior portion of the abdomen, sometimes referred to as the thoracoabdomen, is protected in front and along the flanks by the ribs and in back by the vertebral column. The thoracoabdomen contains the liver, gallbladder, spleen, and parts of the stomach anteriorly and the lower lobes of the lungs posteriorly, separated by the diaphragm. Because of their location, the same forces that fracture ribs may injure the underlying lungs, liver, or spleen.

The relationship of these abdominal organs to the lower portion of the thoracic cavity changes with the respiratory cycle. At peak expiration, the dome of the relaxed diaphragm rises to the level of the fourth intercostal space (nipple level in the male), providing greater protection to abdominal organs from the rib cage. Conversely, at peak inspiration, the dome of the contracted

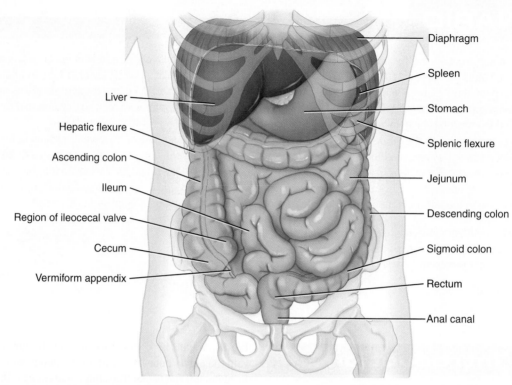

Figure 13-1   The organs inside the peritoneal cavity frequently produce peritonitis when injured. Organs in the peritoneal cavity include solid organs (spleen and liver), hollow organs of the gastrointestinal tract (stomach, small intestine, and colon), and the reproductive organs.

diaphragm lies at the level of the sixth intercostal space; the inflated lungs almost fill the thorax and largely push these abdominal organs out from under the rib cage. Thus, the organs injured by penetrating trauma to the thoracoabdomen may differ depending upon which phase of respiration the patient is in when injured (**Figure 13-3**).

The most inferior portion of the abdomen is protected on all sides by the pelvis. This area contains the rectum, a portion of the small intestine (especially when the patient is upright), the urinary bladder, and, in the female, the reproductive organs. Retroperitoneal hemorrhage associated with a fractured pelvis is a major concern in this portion of the abdominal cavity.

The abdomen between the rib cage and the pelvis is protected only by the abdominal muscles and other soft tissues anteriorly and laterally. Posteriorly, the lumbar vertebrae and the thick, strong *paraspinal* and *psoas* muscles located along the length of the spine provide more protection (**Figure 13-4**).

For purposes of patient assessment, the surface of the abdomen is divided into four quadrants. These quadrants are formed by drawing two lines: one in the middle from the tip of the xiphoid to the symphysis pubis and one perpendicular to this midline at the level of the umbilicus (**Figure 13-5**). Knowledge of anatomic landmarks is important because of the

high correlation of organ location to pain response. The right upper quadrant includes the liver and gallbladder, the left upper quadrant contains the spleen and stomach, and the right lower quadrant and left lower quadrant contain primarily the intestines, the distal ureters, and, in women, the ovaries. A portion of the intestinal tract exists in all four quadrants. The urinary bladder and the uterus in women are midline between the lower quadrants.

Pathophysiology

Dividing the abdominal organs into hollow, solid, and vascular (blood vessel) groups helps explain manifestations of injury to these structures. When injured, solid organs (liver, spleen) and blood vessels (aorta, vena cava) bleed, whereas hollow organs (intestine, gallbladder, urinary bladder) primarily spill their contents into the peritoneal cavity or retroperitoneal space, although they too bleed but often not as briskly as do solid organs. Loss of blood into the abdominal cavity, regardless of its source, can contribute to or can be the primary cause of the development of hemorrhagic shock. The release of acids, digestive enzymes, and/or bacteria from the gastrointestinal tract into the peritoneal cavity results in **peritonitis** (inflammation of the peritoneum or the lining of the abdominal cavity) and **sepsis** (systemic infection)

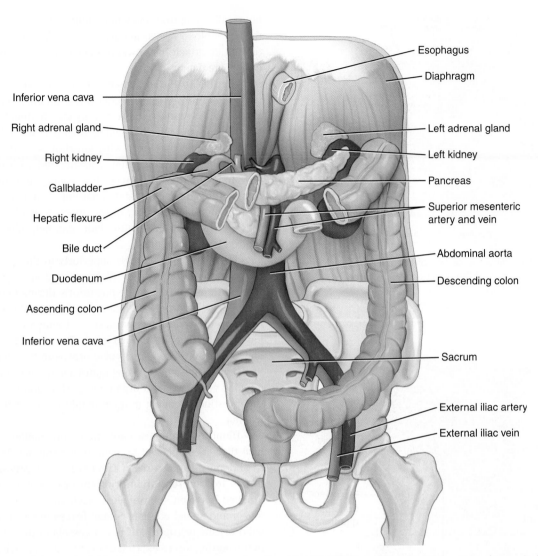

Figure 13-2 The abdomen is divided into two spaces: peritoneal cavity and retroperitoneal space. The retroperitoneal space includes the portion of the abdomen behind the peritoneum. Because the retroperitoneal organs are not within the peritoneal cavity, injury to these structures generally does not produce peritonitis; however, injury to the large blood vessels and solid organs may produce rapid and massive hemorrhage.

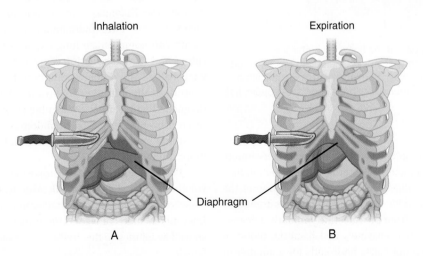

Figure 13-3 Relationship of abdominal organs to the thorax in different phases of respiration in a patient with a stab wound. **A.** Expiration. **B.** Inhalation.

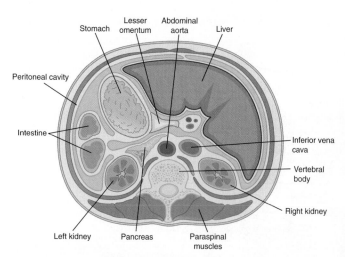

Figure 13-4 This transverse section of the abdominal cavity provides an appreciation of the organ's positions in the anteroposterior direction.

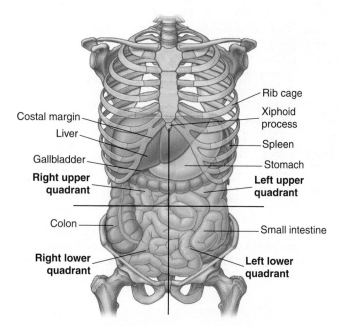

Figure 13-5 As with any part of the body, the better the description of pain, tenderness, guarding, and other signs, the more accurate the diagnosis. The most common system of identification divides the abdomen into four quadrants: left upper, right upper, left lower, and right lower.

if not recognized and promptly treated by surgical intervention. Because urine and bile are generally sterile (do not contain bacteria) and do not contain digestive enzymes, perforation of the gallbladder or urinary bladder does not produce peritonitis as quickly as material spilled from the intestine. Similarly, because it also lacks acids, digestive enzymes, and bacteria, blood in the peritoneal cavity does not cause peritonitis for a number of

hours. Bleeding from intestinal injury is typically minor, unless the larger blood vessels in the *mesentery* (the folds of peritoneal tissue that attach the bowel to posterior wall of the abdominal cavity) are damaged.

Injuries to the abdomen can be caused by either penetrating or blunt trauma. Penetrating trauma, such as a gunshot or stab wound, is more readily visible than blunt trauma. Multiple organs may be damaged as a result of penetrating trauma, more commonly with gunshot wounds versus stab wounds given the high energy associated with the "missile" type injury and the relatively low energy and limited length of most objects used to stab a patient. A mental visualization of the potential trajectory of the penetrating object, such as a bullet or the path of a knife blade, can help identify possible injured internal organs.

The diaphragm extends superiorly to the fourth intercostal space anteriorly, the sixth intercostal space laterally, and the eighth intercostal space posteriorly during maximum expiration (see Figure 13-3). Patients who sustain a penetrating injury to the thorax below these anatomic locations may also have sustained an abdominal injury. Penetrating wounds of the flanks and buttocks may involve organs in the abdominal cavity as well. These penetrating injuries may cause bleeding from a major vessel or solid organ and perforation of a segment of the intestine, the most frequently injured organ in penetrating trauma.

Blunt trauma injuries are often more challenging to recognize than those caused by penetrating trauma. These injuries to abdominal organs result from either compression or shear forces. In **compression injuries**, the organs of the abdomen are crushed between solid objects, such as between the steering wheel and spinal column. **Shear forces** create rupture of the solid organs or rupture of blood vessels in the cavity because of the tearing forces exerted against their supporting ligaments. The liver and spleen can shear and bleed easily, and blood loss can occur at a rapid rate. Increased intra-abdominal pressure produced by compression can rupture the diaphragm, causing the abdominal organs to move upward into the pleural cavity (see the Kinematics of Trauma and the Thoracic Trauma chapters). The intra-abdominal contents forced into the chest cavity can compromise lung expansion and affect both respiratory and cardiac function (**Figure 13-6**). Although rupture of each half of the diaphragm is now believed to occur equally, rupture of the left *hemidiaphragm* (half of the diaphragm) is diagnosed more often, as the underlying liver on the right side often prevents herniation of abdominal contents into the right chest and makes the diagnosis of a right-side diaphragm injury more difficult.

Pelvic fractures may be associated with the loss of large volumes of blood caused by damage to the many smaller blood vessels adjacent to the pelvis. Other injuries associated with pelvic fractures include damage to the urinary bladder and the rectum, as well as injuries to the urethra in the male and the vagina in the female.

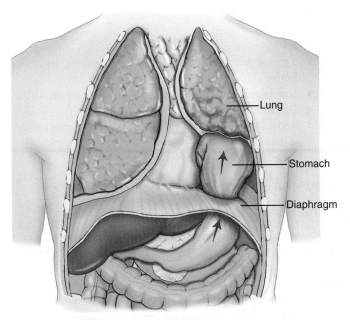

Figure 13-6 With increased pressure inside the abdomen, the diaphragm can rupture, allowing intra-abdominal organs such as the stomach or small intestine to herniate into the chest.

Assessment

The assessment of abdominal injury can be difficult, especially with the limited diagnostic capabilities available in the prehospital setting. A high index of suspicion for abdominal injury should develop from a variety of sources of information, including kinematics, the findings from the physical examination, and input from the patient or bystanders.

Kinematics

As with other types of trauma, knowledge of the mechanism of injury, whether blunt or penetrating, plays an important role in shaping the prehospital care provider's index of suspicion for abdominal trauma.

Penetrating Trauma

Most penetrating trauma in the civilian setting results from stab wounds and gunshot wounds from handguns. Occasionally, impalement with or onto an object occurs when, for example, someone falls onto a projecting piece of wood or metal. These low to moderate kinetic energy forces lacerate or cut abdominal organs along the pathway of the knife, projectile, or penetrating object. High-velocity injuries, such as those created by high-powered rifles and assault weapons, tend to create more serious injuries because of the larger temporary cavities created as the projectile moves through the peritoneal cavity. Projectiles may strike bones (ribs, spine, or pelvis), resulting in fragments that may perforate internal organs. Stab wounds are less likely to penetrate the peritoneal cavity than projectiles fired from a handgun, rifle, or shotgun.

When the peritoneum is penetrated, stab wounds are most likely to injure the liver (40%), small bowel (30%), diaphragm (20%), and colon (15%), whereas gunshot wounds most commonly damage the small bowel (50%), colon (40%), liver (30%), and abdominal vessels (25%).[1] Because of the thicker musculature of the back, penetrating trauma to the back is less likely to result in injuries of intraperitoneal structures than wounds to the anterior abdominal wall. Overall, only about 15% of patients with stab wounds to the abdomen will require surgical intervention, whereas about 85% of patients with gunshot wounds will need surgery for definitive management of their abdominal injuries. Tangential gunshot wounds may pass through subcutaneous tissues but never enter the peritoneal cavity. Explosive devices may also propel fragments that penetrate the peritoneum and injure internal organs.

Blunt Trauma

Numerous mechanisms lead to the compression and shear forces that may damage abdominal organs. A patient may experience considerable deceleration or compression forces when involved in motor vehicle and motorcycle crashes, when struck or run over by a vehicle, or after falling from a significant height. Although abdominal organs are most often injured in events associated with significant kinetic injury, such as those with rapid deceleration or severe compression, abdominal injuries may result from more innocuous-appearing mechanisms, such as assaults, falls down a flight of stairs, and sporting activities (e.g., being tackled in football). Any protective devices or gear used by the patient should be noted, including seat belts, air bags, or sports padding.

Compression of a solid organ may result in splitting of its structure (e.g., hepatic laceration); whereas such forces applied to a hollow structure, such as a loop of bowel or the bladder, may cause the structure to burst open ("rupture"), spilling its contents into the abdomen. Shearing forces may result in tears of structures at sites of tethering to other structures, such as where the more mobile small bowel joins the ascending colon, which is fixed in the retroperitoneum. The organs most commonly injured following blunt trauma to the abdomen include the spleen (40–55%), liver (35–45%), and small bowel (5–10%). Not all injuries to solid organs require surgical intervention (**Figure 13-7**). Many of these types of solid organ injuries are now observed carefully in the hospital, as they will often stop bleeding on their own.

History

History may be obtained from the patient, family, or bystanders and should be documented on the patient care report and relayed to the receiving facility. In addition to the components of the SAMPLE history (**s**ymptoms, **a**llergies and **a**ge, **m**edications,

Figure 13-7 Nonoperative Management of Solid Organ Injuries

Suspected injuries of the spleen, liver, or kidney no longer mandate surgical exploration in the modern trauma center. Experience has shown that many of these injuries will stop bleeding prior to the development of shock and then heal without surgical repair. Research in the last 20 years has shown that even significant solid organ injuries may be safely observed, provided the patient is not experiencing hypovolemic shock or peritonitis. Patients are admitted to the hospital for close monitoring of their vital signs, blood count, and abdominal exam, initially in the intensive care unit. The advantage of this approach is that it prevents the patient from undergoing a potentially unnecessary operation. Since the spleen performs an important role in fighting infections, removal of the spleen (splenectomy) predisposes patients (especially children) to certain bacterial infections.

Successful nonoperative management of these injuries was first reported for splenic injuries in children, but this approach is now often applied to adult patients, as well as to patients suffering injuries to the liver and kidney. Following blunt trauma, recent data indicate that about 50% of splenic injuries and about 67% of liver injuries can be managed in this manner, with reported success rates ranging from 70% to over 90%.[2]

The risk of failure of this technique (rebleeding, with the development of shock requiring surgical intervention) is greatest in the first 7 to 10 days following injury. Prehospital care providers should be aware of this approach, as they may respond to patients who have experienced rebleeding after discharge from the hospital.

past medical/surgical history, last meal, events preceding injury), questions should be tailored to the type of injury and the presence of comorbid conditions that will potentially increase mortality or morbidity. For example, in the case of a motor vehicle crash, questions may be asked to determine the following:

- Type of collision, position of patient in the vehicle, or ejection from the vehicle
- Estimated vehicle speed at time of crash
- Extent of vehicle damage, including intrusion into the passenger compartment, steering wheel deformity, windshield damage, and requirement for prolonged extrication
- Use of safety devices, including seat belts, deployment of air bags, and presence of child safety seats

In the case of penetrating injury, questions may be asked to determine the following:

- Type of weapon (handgun vs. rifle, caliber, length of knife)
- Number of times the patient was shot or stabbed
- Distance from which the patient was shot
- Amount of blood at the scene (although accurate estimation is often difficult)

Physical Examination

Primary Assessment

Most severe abdominal injuries will present as abnormalities identified in the primary assessment, primarily in the evaluation of breathing and circulation. Unless there are associated injuries, patients with abdominal trauma generally present with a patent airway. The alterations found in the breathing, circulation, and disability assessments generally correspond to the degree of shock present. Patients with early, compensated shock may have a mild increase in their ventilatory rate, whereas those with severe hemorrhagic shock demonstrate marked tachypnea. Rupture of a hemidiaphragm often compromises respiratory function when abdominal contents herniate into the chest on the affected side, and bowel sounds may be heard over the thorax when breath sounds are auscultated. Similarly, shock from intra-abdominal hemorrhage may range from mild tachycardia, with few other findings, to severe tachycardia, marked hypotension, and pale, cool, clammy skin.

The most reliable indicator of intra-abdominal bleeding is the presence of hypovolemic shock from an unexplained source.[1] When assessing disability, the prehospital care provider may note only subtle signs, such as mild anxiety or agitation, in the patient with compensated shock from abdominal trauma, whereas patients with life-threatening hemorrhage may have serious depression in their mental status. When abnormalities are found in the assessment of these systems and while preparing for immediate transport, the abdomen should be exposed and examined for evidence of trauma, such as bruising or penetrating wounds.

Secondary Assessment

During the secondary assessment, the abdomen is examined in greater detail. This examination primarily involves inspection and palpation of the abdomen and should be approached systematically.

Inspection

The abdomen is examined for soft-tissue injuries and distension. Intra-abdominal injury may be suspected when soft-tissue trauma is noted over the abdomen, flanks, or back. Such injuries may include contusions, abrasions, stab or gunshot wounds, obvious bleeding, and unusual findings such as evisceration, impaled objects, or tire marks. The "seat belt sign" (ecchymosis or abrasion across the abdomen resulting from compression of the abdominal wall against the shoulder harness or lap belt) indicates that significant force was applied to the abdomen as a result of sudden deceleration (**Figure 13-8**). Although the incidence of intra-abdominal injuries in adult patients with seat belt signs is about 20%, the incidence may approach 50% in children. The injuries associated with restraints are typically to the bowel and its supporting mesentery, as they are compressed and crushed between the seat belt and anterior abdominal wall and the spinal column posteriorly, and often present in a delayed fashion. *Grey-Turner's sign* (ecchymosis involving the flanks) and *Cullen's sign* (ecchymosis around the umbilicus) indicate retroperitoneal bleeding; however, these signs are often delayed and may not be seen in the first few hours after injury.

The contour of the abdomen should be noted, assessing if it is flat or distended. Distension of the abdomen may indicate significant internal hemorrhage; however, the adult peritoneal cavity can hold up to 1.5 liters of fluid before showing any obvious signs of distension. Abdominal distension may also be the result of a stomach filled with air, as can occur during artificial ventilation with a bag-mask device. Although these signs may indicate intra-abdominal injury, some patients with substantial internal injury may lack these findings.

Palpation

Palpation of the abdomen is undertaken to identify areas of tenderness. Ideally, palpation is begun in an area in which

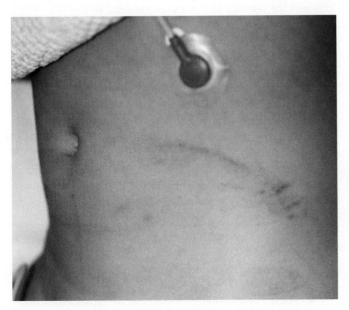

Figure 13-8 An abdominal "seat belt sign" resulting from the patient decelerating against a lap belt.
Source: Courtesy of Peter T. Pons, MD, FACEP.

the patient does not complain of pain. Then, each of the abdominal quadrants is palpated. While palpating a tender area, the prehospital care provider may note that the patient "tenses up" the abdominal muscles in that area. This reaction, called **voluntary guarding**, protects the patient from the pain resulting from palpation. **Involuntary guarding** represents rigidity or spasm of the abdominal wall muscles in response to peritonitis. **Figure 13-9** lists physical findings consistent with the presence of peritonitis. Unlike voluntary guarding, involuntary guarding remains when the patient is distracted (e.g., with conversation) or the abdomen is surreptitiously palpated (e.g., with pressure on the stethoscope while appearing to auscultate bowel sounds). Although the presence of **rebound tenderness** has long been considered an important finding indicating peritonitis, many surgeons now believe that this maneuver—pressing deeply on the abdomen and then quickly releasing the pressure—causes excessive pain. If rebound tenderness is present, the patient will note more severe pain when the abdominal pressure is released.

Deep or aggressive palpation of an obviously injured abdomen should be avoided because, in addition to the pain it causes, palpation may dislodge blood clots and restart hemorrhage and may spill contents from the gastrointestinal tract if perforations are present. Great care during palpation should also be exercised if there is an impaled object in the abdomen. In fact, there is little additional useful information to be gained by palpating the abdomen in a patient with an impaled object.

Although tenderness is an important indicator of intra-abdominal injury, several factors may confound the assessment of tenderness. Patients with altered mental status, such as those with a TBI or those under the influence of drugs or alcohol, may have an *unreliable* examination; that is, the patient may not report tenderness or respond to palpation even when significant internal injuries are present. Pediatric and geriatric patients are more likely to have unreliable abdominal examinations because of impaired pain responses. Conversely, patients with lower rib fractures or a pelvic fracture may have an *equivocal* (ambiguous) examination, with

Figure 13-9	**Findings from the Physical Examination that Support a Diagnosis of Peritonitis**

- Significant abdominal tenderness on palpation or with coughing (either localized or generalized)
- Involuntary guarding
- Percussion tenderness
- Diminished or absent bowel sounds

tenderness resulting from either the fractures or associated internal injuries. If the patient has distracting pain from injuries, such as extremity or spinal fractures, abdominal pain may not be elicited on palpation.

Palpation of the pelvis in the prehospital setting provides little information that will alter the management of the patient. If time is taken to perform this examination, it is performed only once, as any clot that has formed at the site of an unstable fracture may be disrupted, thus exacerbating hemorrhage. During this examination, the pelvis is palpated gently for instability and tenderness. This evaluation involves three steps:

1. Pressing inward on the iliac crests
2. Pulling outward on the iliac crests
3. Pressing posteriorly on the symphysis pubis

If instability is noted during any step of the examination, no further palpation of the pelvis should take place.

Auscultation

Hemorrhage and spillage of intestinal contents in the peritoneal cavity may result in an *ileus*, a condition in which the peristalsis of the bowel ceases. This results in a "quiet" abdomen, as bowel sounds are diminished or absent. Auscultation of bowel sounds is generally not a helpful prehospital assessment tool. Time should not be wasted trying to determine their presence or absence because this diagnostic sign will not alter the prehospital management of the patient. If bowel sounds are heard over the thorax during auscultation of breath sounds, however, the presence of a diaphragmatic rupture may be considered.

Percussion

Although percussion of the abdomen may reveal tympanitic or dull sounds, this information does not alter prehospital management of the trauma patient and only expends valuable time; therefore it is not recommended as a prehospital assessment tool. Significant tenderness on percussion or pain when the patient is asked to cough represents a key finding of peritonitis. Peritoneal signs are summarized in Figure 13-9.

Special Examinations and Key Indicators

Surgical evaluation and, in many cases, intervention remain key needs for most patients who have sustained abdominal injuries; time should not be wasted in attempts to determine the exact details of injury. In many patients, identification of specific organ injury will not be revealed until the abdomen is further evaluated by computed tomography (CT) scanning or surgical exploration.

In the emergency department, ultrasound has become the primary bedside modality used to assess a trauma patient for intra-abdominal hemorrhage.[1,3-6] The focused assessment with sonography for trauma (FAST) examination involves three views of the peritoneal cavity and a fourth view of the pericardium to assess for the presence of fluid, presumably blood, around the heart (**Figure 13-10**). Because fluid does not reflect the ultrasound waves back to the device, fluid appears anechoic (sonographically black). Presence of fluid in one or more areas is worrisome; however, ultrasonography cannot differentiate blood from other types of fluids (ascites, urine from a ruptured bladder, etc.). Compared to other techniques used to evaluate the peritoneal cavity, FAST can be rapidly performed at the patient's bedside, does not interfere with resuscitation, is noninvasive, and is much less costly than CT scanning. The primary disadvantage of FAST is that it does not definitively diagnose injury, but only indicates the presence of fluid that may represent blood. Other disadvantages of the FAST exam are that imaging is dependent upon the operator's skill and experience and its utility is compromised in patients who are obese, have subcutaneous air, and have had previous surgery. Perhaps most importantly, a negative FAST exam does not rule out the presence of an injury, including one that might require surgical intervention. A negative FAST exam means only that, at the moment when the exam was performed, fluid was not visualized in the abdomen. This result could be because no injury exists or because not enough blood has accumulated in the abdomen to be seen (which is a real possibility given a rapid response by emergency medical services [EMS] to the trauma incident scene).

Because of ease of use and improved ultrasound technology, some ground and air EMS systems and military teams have explored the use of FAST in the prehospital setting. The FAST exam has been shown to be feasible in the field, but no published data have demonstrated that use of this technology results in improved outcomes for patients with abdominal trauma.[7-13] FAST may have utility in the austere environment or a mass-casualty situation. However, use of FAST is not recommended by Prehospital Trauma Life Support for routine prehospital care, especially in that it may delay transport to the receiving facility or may provide false reassurance about the actual condition of the patient.

Despite all these different components, the assessment of abdominal injury can be difficult. The following are key indicators for establishing the index of suspicion for abdominal injury:

- Obvious signs of trauma (e.g., soft-tissue injuries, gunshot wounds)
- Presence of hypovolemic shock without another obvious cause
- Degree of shock greater than can be explained by other injuries (e.g., fractures, external hemorrhage)
- Presence of peritoneal signs

Figure 13-10   Focused Assessment with Sonography for Trauma (FAST)*

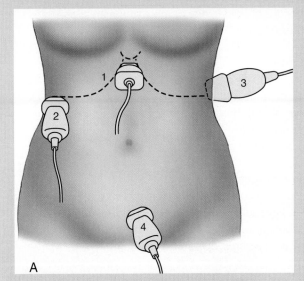

A. Four views constituting the FAST examination.

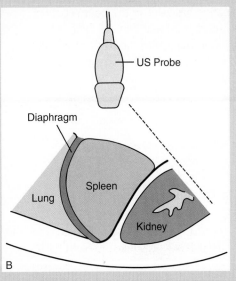

B. Normal splenorenal view identifying organs.

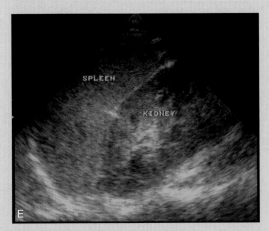

C. Normal view of the right upper quadrant.

Source: Photo courtesy of John Kendall, MD.

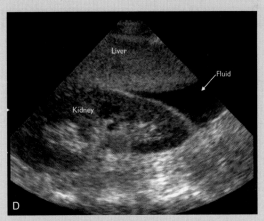

D. Abnormal view of the right upper quadrant demonstrating the presence of fluid (blood).

Source: Photo courtesy of John Kendall, MD.

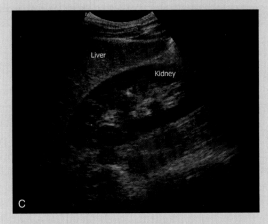

E. Normal view of the left upper quadrant.

Source: Photo courtesy of John Kendall, MD.

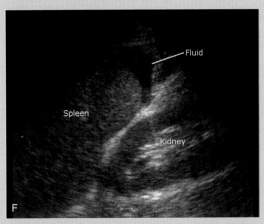

F. Abnormal view of the left upper quadrant demonstrating the presence of fluid (blood).

Source: Photo courtesy of John Kendall, MD.

(Continues on next page)

Figure 13-10   Focused Assessment with Sonography for Trauma (FAST)* (Continued)

The FAST examination has value in the trauma patient because most significant intra-abdominal injuries are associated with hemorrhage into the peritoneal cavity. Although ultrasound cannot differentiate the type of fluid present, any fluid in the trauma patient is presumed to be blood.

Technique
- Four acoustic windows (views) are imaged, three of which evaluate the peritoneal cavity:
  1. Pericardial
  2. Perihepatic (Morrison's pouch)
  3. Perisplenic
  4. Pelvic
- Accumulated fluid appears anechoic (sonographically black).

- Presence of fluid in one or more of the areas indicates a positive scan.

Advantages
- Can be rapidly performed
- Can be done at the bedside
- Does not interfere with resuscitation
- Is noninvasive
- Is less costly than CT

Disadvantages
- Results are compromised in patients who are obese, who have subcutaneous air, or who have had previous abdominal surgery.
- Skill at imaging is operator dependent.

*FAST has been studied in several prehospital systems.[9-12]

Management

The key aspects of prehospital management of patients with abdominal trauma are to recognize the presence of potential injury and initiate rapid transport, as appropriate, to the closest appropriate facility that is capable of managing the patient.

Abnormalities in vital functions identified in the primary assessment are supported during transport. Supplemental oxygen is administered to maintain saturation at 95% or greater, and ventilations are assisted as needed. External hemorrhage is controlled with direct pressure or a pressure dressing. If the patient has sustained blunt trauma that could have also produced spinal injury, immobilization of the spine is performed as appropriate (see the Spinal Trauma chapter). Victims of penetrating trauma to the torso do not need spinal immobilization.

The patient is rapidly packaged and transport is initiated. Patients with abdominal trauma often require transfusion and surgical intervention to control internal hemorrhage and repair injuries; therefore, patients should be transported to facilities that have immediate surgical capability, such as a trauma center, if available, when the following findings are noted: evidence of abdominal trauma associated with hypotension or peritoneal signs, or the presence of an evisceration or impaled object. Taking a patient with intra-abdominal injuries to a facility that does not have an available operating room and a surgical team defeats the purpose of rapid transport. In a rural setting where there is no hospital with general surgeons on staff, consideration should be given to direct transfer to a trauma center, either by ground or air. Early surgical intervention is the key to survival of the unstable patient with abdominal trauma.

During transport, intravenous (IV) access is obtained. The decision to administer crystalloid fluid replacement en route depends on the patient's clinical presentation. Abdominal trauma represents one of the key situations in which balanced resuscitation is indicated. As discussed in the Shock chapter, aggressive administration of IV fluid may elevate the patient's blood pressure to levels that will disrupt any clot that has formed and result in recurrence of bleeding that had ceased because of blood clotting and hypotension. Thus, prehospital care providers must achieve a delicate balance: maintenance of a blood pressure that provides perfusion to vital organs without restoring blood pressure to normal (which may reinitiate bleeding sites in the abdomen). In the absence of TBI, the target systolic blood pressure is 80 to 90 mm Hg (mean arterial pressure of 60 to 65 mm Hg). For patients with suspected intra-abdominal bleeding and a TBI, the systolic blood pressure is maintained at a minimum of 90 mm Hg.

Special Considerations
Impaled Objects

Because removal of an impaled object may cause additional trauma and because the object's distal end may be actively controlling (*tamponading*) the bleeding, removal of an impaled object in the prehospital environment is contraindicated (**Figure 13-11**). The prehospital care provider should neither move nor remove an object impaled in a patient's abdomen. In the hospital, these objects are not removed until their shape and location have been identified by radiographic evaluation

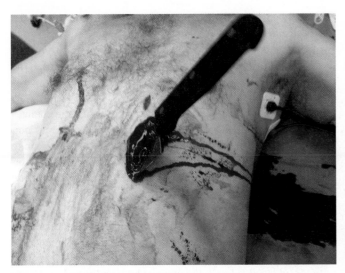

Figure 13-11 Knife impaled in the abdomen.
Source: Courtesy of Lance Stuke, MD, MPH.

and until blood replacement and a surgical team are present and ready. Often these objects are removed in the operating room.

A prehospital care provider may stabilize the impaled object, either manually or mechanically, to prevent any further movement in the field and during transport. In some circumstances the impaled object may need to be cut in order to free that patient and permit transport to the trauma center. If bleeding occurs around it, direct pressure should be applied around the object to the wound with the palm of the hand. Psychological support of the patient is important, especially if the impaled object is visible to the patient.

The abdomen should not be palpated or percussed in these patients because these actions may produce additional organ injury from the distal end of the object. Further examination is unnecessary because the presence of impaled objects indicates the need for management by a surgeon.

Evisceration

In an abdominal **evisceration**, a section of intestine or other abdominal organ is displaced through an open wound and protrudes externally outside the abdominal cavity (**Figure 13-12**). The tissue most often visualized is the fatty **omentum** that lies over the intestines. Attempts should not be made to replace the protruding tissue in the abdominal cavity. The **viscera** should be left on the surface of the abdomen or protruding as found.

Treatment efforts should focus on protecting the protruding segment of intestine or other organ from further damage. Most of the abdominal contents require a moist environment. If the intestine or some of the other abdominal organs become dry, cell death will occur. Therefore, the eviscerated abdominal contents should be covered with a clean or sterile dressing that has been moistened with saline (normal saline IV fluid can be used). These dressings should be periodically remoistened with saline to prevent them from drying out. Wet dressings may be covered with a large, dry or occlusive dressing to keep the patient warm.

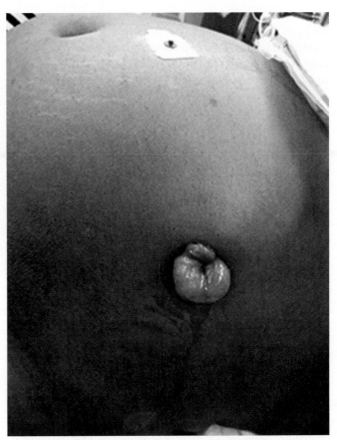

Figure 13-12 Bowel eviscerated through a wound in the abdominal wall.
Source: Courtesy of Lance Stuke, MD, MPH.

Psychological support is extremely important for patients with an abdominal evisceration, and care should be taken to keep the patient calm. Any action that increases pressure within the abdomen, such as crying, screaming, or coughing, can force more of the organs outward. These patients should be expeditiously transported to a facility that has surgical capability.

Trauma in the Obstetrical Patient
Anatomic and Physiologic Changes

Pregnancy causes both anatomic and physiologic changes to the body's systems. These changes can affect the patterns of injuries seen and make the assessment of an injured pregnant patient especially challenging. The prehospital care provider is dealing with two or more patients and must be aware of the changes that have occurred to the woman's anatomy and physiology throughout the pregnancy.

A human pregnancy typically lasts about 40 weeks from conception to birth, and this gestational period is divided into three sections, or trimesters. The first trimester ends at about the 12th week of gestation, and the second trimester is slightly longer than the other two, ending at about week 28.

Following conception and implantation of the fetus, the uterus continues to enlarge through the 38th week of pregnancy. Until about the 12th week, the growing uterus remains protected by the bony pelvis. By the 20th week of gestation, the top of the uterus (fundus) is at the umbilicus, and the fundus approaches the xiphoid process by the 38th week. This anatomic change makes the uterus and its contents more susceptible to both blunt and penetrating injury (**Figure 13-13**). Injury to the uterus can include rupture, penetration, *abruptio placentae* (when a portion of the placenta is pulled away from the uterine wall), and premature rupture of the membranes (**Figure 13-14**). The placenta and gravid uterus are highly vascular; injuries to these structures can result in profound hemorrhage. Because the hemorrhage can also be concealed inside the uterus or peritoneal cavity, it may not be externally visible.

Although a marked protuberance of the abdomen is obvious in late pregnancy, the rest of the abdominal organs remain essentially unchanged, with the exception of the uterus. Intestine that is displaced superiorly is shielded by the uterus in the last two trimesters of pregnancy. The increased size and weight of the uterus alter the patient's center of gravity and increase the risk of falls. Because of its prominence, the gravid abdomen is often injured in a fall.

In addition to these anatomic changes, physiologic changes also occur throughout pregnancy. The woman's heart rate normally increases throughout pregnancy by 15 to 20 beats/minute above normal by the third trimester.[14] This makes the interpretation of tachycardia more difficult. Systolic and diastolic blood pressures normally drop 5 to 15 mm Hg during the second trimester but often return to normal at term.[14] By the 10th week of pregnancy, the woman's cardiac output increases by 1 to 1.5 liters/minute. By term, the woman's blood volume has increased by about 50%. *Because of these increases in cardiac output and blood volume, the pregnant patient may lose 30% to 35% of her blood volume before signs and symptoms of hypovolemia become apparent.*[14] Hypovolemic shock may induce premature labor in patients in the third trimester. Oxytocin, which is released along with antidiuretic hormone in response to loss of circulating blood volume, stimulates uterine contractions.

Some women may have significant hypotension when supine. This supine hypotension of pregnancy typically occurs in the third trimester and is caused by the compression of the vena cava by the enlarged uterus.[14] This dramatically decreases venous return to the heart, and because there is less filling, cardiac output and blood pressure fall (**Figure 13-15**).

The following maneuvers may be used to relieve supine hypotension:

1. The woman may be placed on her left side (left lateral decubitus position), or if spinal immobilization is indicated, 4 to 6 inches (10 to 15 cm) of padding should be placed under the right side of the long backboard (**Figure 13-16**).

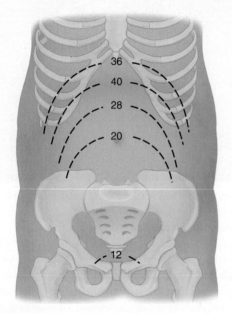

Figure 13-13   Fundal height.

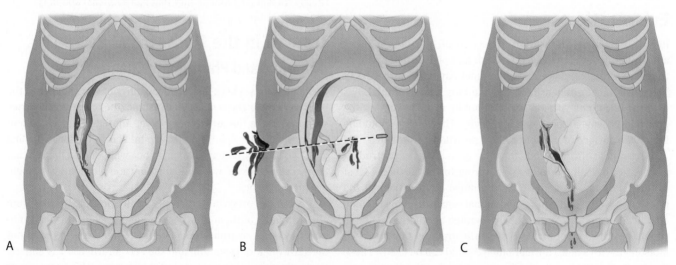

Figure 13-14   Diagram of uterine trauma. **A.** Abruptio placentae. **B.** Gunshot to the uterus. **C.** Ruptured uterus.

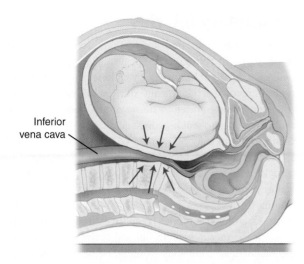

Inferior
vena cava

Figure 13-15 Full-term uterus compressing the vena cava.

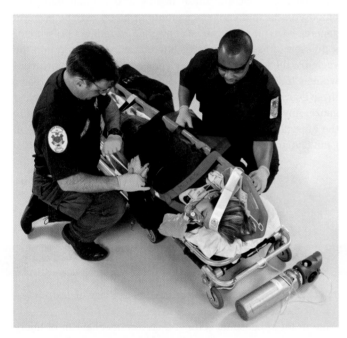

Figure 13-16 Photo of immobilized pregnant patient tilted to side.

2. If the patient cannot be rotated, her right leg should be elevated to displace the uterus to the left.
3. The uterus may be manually displaced toward the patient's left side.

These three maneuvers reduce compression on the vena cava, increasing venous return to the heart and improving cardiac output.

During the third trimester, the diaphragm is elevated and may be associated with mild dyspnea, especially when the

patient is supine. Peristalsis (propulsive, muscular movements of intestines) is slower during pregnancy, so food may remain in the stomach many hours after eating. Therefore, the pregnant patient is at greater risk for vomiting and subsequent aspiration.

Toxemia of pregnancy (also known as eclampsia) is a late complication of pregnancy. Whereas *pre-eclampsia* is characterized by edema and hypertension, **eclampsia** is characterized by mental status changes and seizures, thus mimicking TBI. A careful neurologic assessment and asking about potential complications of pregnancy and other medical conditions such as known diabetes, hypertension, or seizure history are important.[11,12]

Assessment

Pregnancy typically does not alter the woman's airway, but significant respiratory distress may occur when a patient in her third trimester is placed supine on a long backboard. The decrease in peristalsis of the gastrointestinal tract makes vomiting and aspiration more likely. Airway patency and pulmonary function are assessed, including auscultation of breath sounds and monitoring of pulse oximetry.

As with hemoperitoneum from other sources, intra-abdominal bleeding associated with uterine injury may not produce peritonitis for hours. More likely, blood loss from an injury may be masked by the pregnant female's increased cardiac output and blood volume. Therefore, a high index of suspicion and assessment for subtle changes (e.g., skin color) may provide important clues.

In general, the condition of the fetus often depends on the condition of the woman; however, the fetus may be in jeopardy while the woman's condition and vital signs appear hemodynamically normal. This occurs because the body shunts blood away from the uterus (and fetus) to the vital organs. Neurologic changes should be noted and documented, although the exact etiology may not be identifiable in the prehospital setting.

As with the nonpregnant patient, auscultation of bowel sounds is generally not helpful in the prehospital setting. Similarly, spending valuable minutes searching for fetal heart tones at the scene is also not useful; their presence or absence will not alter prehospital management. The external genitalia should be checked for evidence of vaginal bleeding, and the patient should be asked about the presence of contractions and fetal movement. Contractions may indicate that premature labor has begun, whereas a decrease in fetal movement may be an ominous sign of profound fetal distress.

Palpation of the abdomen may reveal tenderness. A firm, hard, tender uterus is suggestive of abruptio placentae, which is associated with visible vaginal bleeding in approximately 70% of cases.[14]

Management

With an injured pregnant patient, the survival of the fetus is best ensured by focusing on the woman's condition. In essence, for the fetus to survive, usually the woman needs to survive. Priority is given to ensuring an adequate patent airway and supporting ventilatory function. Sufficient oxygen should be administered to maintain a pulse oximetry reading of 95% or higher. Ventilations may need to be assisted, especially in the later stages of pregnancy. It is wise to anticipate vomiting and have suction nearby.

The goals of shock management are essentially the same as for any patient and include judicious IV fluid administration, especially if evidence of decompensated shock is present. Any evidence of vaginal bleeding or a rigid, boardlike abdomen with external bleeding in the last trimester of pregnancy may indicate abruptio placentae or a ruptured uterus. These conditions threaten not only the life of the fetus, but also that of the woman because exsanguination can occur rapidly. No good data exist to define the best target blood pressure for an injured pregnant patient. However, restoration of normal systolic and mean blood pressures will most likely result in better fetal perfusion, despite the risk of promoting additional internal hemorrhage in the woman.

Transport of the pregnant trauma patient should not be delayed. Every pregnant trauma patient should be rapidly transported—even those who appear to have only minor injuries—to the closest appropriate facility. An ideal facility is one that has both surgical and obstetric capabilities immediately available. Adequate resuscitation of the woman is the key to survival of the woman and fetus.

Genitourinary Injuries

Injuries to the kidneys, ureters, and bladder are most often present with *hematuria* (blood in the urine). This sign will not be noted unless the patient has a urinary catheter inserted. Because the kidneys receive a significant portion of cardiac output, blunt or penetrating injuries to these organs may result in life-threatening retroperitoneal hemorrhage.

Pelvic fractures may be associated with lacerations of the urinary bladder and the walls of the vagina or the rectum. Open pelvic fractures, such as those with deep groin or perineal lacerations, may result in severe external hemorrhage.

Trauma to the external genitalia may occur from multiple mechanisms, although injuries resulting from ejection from a motorcycle or motor vehicle, an industrial accident, straddle-type mechanisms, gunshot wounds, or sexual assault predominate. Because of the numerous nerve endings in these organs, such injuries are associated with significant pain and psychological concern. These organs also contain numerous blood vessels, and copious amounts of blood may be seen. In general, such bleeding can be controlled with direct pressure or a pressure dressing. Dressings should not be inserted into the vagina or the urethra to control bleeding, particularly in pregnant women. If direct pressure is not required to control hemorrhage, these injuries should be covered with moist, clean, saline-soaked gauze. Any amputated parts should be managed as described in the Musculoskeletal Trauma chapter. Further evaluation of all genital injuries should occur at the hospital.

Summary

- Intra-abdominal injuries are often life threatening because of internal hemorrhage and spillage of gastrointestinal contents into the peritoneal cavity.
- The extent of internal injuries is not identifiable in the prehospital setting; therefore mechanism of injury in combination with signs of abdominal trauma should increase the prehospital care provider's index of suspicion.
- Management of the patient with abdominal trauma includes oxygenation, hemorrhage control, and rapid packaging for transport. Spinal immobilization is not necessary for penetrating torso trauma.
- Balanced resuscitation with crystalloid solutions permits perfusion of vital organs while potentially minimizing the risk of aggravating internal hemorrhage.
- As emergent surgical intervention may be lifesaving, a patient with abdominal trauma should be transported to a facility with immediate surgical capability.
- The anatomic and physiologic changes of pregnancy have implications for the pattern of injury, presentation of signs and symptoms of trauma, and management of the pregnant trauma patient.
- Management of potential fetal compromise caused by trauma is accomplished through effective resuscitation of the woman.

SCENARIO RECAP

You are called to a construction site for a male patient in his mid-20s who fell 3 hours earlier and is now complaining of increasing abdominal pain. He states that he tripped on a piece of wood at the site and fell, striking his left lower chest and abdomen on some stacked wood. The patient notes moderate pain over his lower left rib cage when he takes deep breaths and complains of mild difficulty breathing. His coworkers wanted to call for assistance when he fell, but he said the symptoms weren't so bad and told them to hold off. He states that the discomfort has been increasing in intensity and that he is now feeling lightheaded and weak.

You find the patient sitting on the ground in visible discomfort. He is holding the left side of his lower chest and upper abdomen. He has a patent airway, a ventilatory rate of 28 breaths/minute, a heart rate of 124 beats/minute, and a blood pressure of 94/58 mm Hg. The patient's skin is pale and diaphoretic. You lay him down, and on physical examination, he has tenderness on palpation of the left lower ribs without obvious bony crepitus. His abdomen is nondistended and soft to palpation, but he has tenderness and voluntary guarding in the left upper quadrant. No external ecchymosis or subcutaneous emphysema is present.

- What are the patient's possible injuries?
- What are the priorities in the care of this patient?
- Are signs of peritonitis present?

SCENARIO SOLUTION

The patient is tender over his left lower ribs and left upper quadrant. These findings can represent injuries to the thorax, intra-abdominal organs, or both. His vital signs are consistent with compensated hypovolemic shock, and a hemothorax or intra-abdominal bleeding must be considered. More likely, the tenderness over the lower ribs may indicate fractured ribs with an associated laceration of the spleen, resulting in intraperitoneal hemorrhage.

Oxygen is administered, and the patient is packaged for transport. En route to the trauma center, intravenous access is obtained; however given the patient's blood pressure, crystalloid fluid is administered prudently, as aggressive fluid infusion may raise his blood pressure and lead to increased bleeding.

References

1. American College of Surgeons (ACS) Committee on Trauma. Abdominal trauma. In: ACS Committee on Trauma. *Advanced Trauma Life Support for Doctors, Student Course Manual.* 8th ed. Chicago, IL: ACS; 2008:111-126.

2. Roberts I, Blackhall K, Dickinson KJ. Medical anti-shock trousers (pneumatic anti-shock garments) for circulatory support in patients with trauma. *Cochrane Database Syst Rev.* 1999;(4):CD001856.

3. Rozycki GS, Ochsner MG, Jaffin JH, et al. Prospective evaluation of surgeons' use of ultrasound in the evaluation of trauma patients. *J Trauma Injury Infect Crit Care.* 1993;34(4):516.

4. Rozycki GS, Ochsner MG, Schmidt JA, et al. A prospective study of surgeon-performed ultrasound as the primary adjuvant modality for injured patient assessment. *J Trauma Injury Infect Crit Care.* 1995;39(3):492.

5. Rozycki GS, Ochsner MG, Feliciano DV, et al. Early detection of hemoperitoneum by ultrasound examination of the right upper quadrant: a multicenter study. *J Trauma Injury Infect Crit Care.* 1998;45(5):878.

6. Rozycki GS, Ballard RB, Feliciano DV, et al. Surgeon-performed ultrasound for the assessment of truncal injuries: lessons learned from 1540 patients. *Ann Surg.* 1998;228(4):557.

7. Polk JD, Fallon WF Jr. The use of focused assessment with sonography for trauma (FAST) by a prehospital air medical team in the trauma arrest patient. *Prehosp Emerg Care.* 2000;4(1):82.

8. Melanson SW, McCarthy J, Stromski CJ, et al. Aeromedical trauma sonography by flight crews with a miniature ultrasound unit. *Prehosp Emerg Care.* 2001;5(4):399.

9. Walcher F, Kortum S, Kirschning T, et al. Optimized management of polytraumatized patients by prehospital ultrasound. *Unfall-chirurg.* 2002;105(11):986.

10. Strode CA, Rubal BJ, Gerhardt RT, et al. Wireless and satellite transmission of prehospital focused abdominal sonography for trauma. *Prehosp Emerg Care.* 2003;7(3):375.

11. Heegaard WG, Ho J, Hildebrandt DA. The prehospital ultrasound study: results of the first six months (abstract). *Prehosp Emerg Care.* 2009;13(1):139.

12. Heegard WG, Hildebrandt D, Spear D, et al. Prehospital ultrasound by paramedics: results of field trial. *Acad Em Med.* 2010;17(6):624-630.

13. Jorgensen H, Jensen CH, Dirks J. Does prehospital ultrasound improve treatment of the trauma patient? A systematic review. *Eur J Emerg Med.* 2010;17(5):249-253.

14. American College of Surgeons (ACS) Committee on Trauma. Trauma in pregnancy and intimate partner violence. In: ACS Committee

on Trauma. *Advanced Trauma Life Support for Doctors, Student Course Manual.* 9th ed. Chicago, IL: ACS; 2012:288-297.

Suggested Reading

Berry MJ, McMurray RG, Katz VL. Pulmonary and ventilatory responses to pregnancy, immersion and exercise. *J Appl Physiol.* 1989:66(2):857.

Coburn M. Genitourinary trauma. In: Moore EE, Feliciano DV, Mattox KL, eds. *Trauma.* 5th ed. New York, NY: McGraw-Hill; 2004:809.

Knudson MM, Rozycki GS, Paquin MM. Reproductive system trauma. In: Moore EE, Feliciano DV, Mattox KL, eds. *Trauma.* 5th ed. New York, NY: McGraw-Hill; 2004.

Raja AS, Zabbo CP. Trauma in pregnancy. *Emerg Med Clin North Am.* 2012;30:937-948.

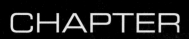
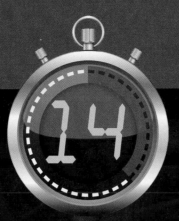

CHAPTER 14

Musculoskeletal Trauma

CHAPTER OBJECTIVES

At the completion of this chapter, the reader will be able to do the following:

- List the three categories used to classify patients with extremity injuries, and relate this classification to priority of care.

- Describe the primary and secondary assessments as related to extremity trauma.

- Discuss the significance of hemorrhage in both open and closed fractures of the long bones, pelvis, and ribs.

- List the five major pathophysiologic problems associated with extremity injuries that may require management in the prehospital setting.

- Explain the management of extremity trauma as an isolated injury and in the presence of multisystem trauma.

- Given a scenario involving an extremity injury, select an appropriate splint and splinting method.

- Describe the special considerations involved in femur fracture management.

- Discuss the management of amputations.

SCENARIO

It is a beautiful Saturday afternoon in June. You have been dispatched to a local motorcycle racetrack for a rider who has been injured. Upon arrival, you are escorted by track officials to an area on the track just in front of the grandstand where the track's medical crew (two-person, emergency medical responders, nontransport) is attending to a single patient lying supine on the track.

One of the emergency medical responders tells you that the patient was a rider in a 350-cc class race with 14 other motorcycles when 3 of them collided in front of the grandstands. The other two riders were not injured, but the patient was unable to stand or move without significant pain in his right leg and pelvis. There was no loss of consciousness and no other complaints besides his leg pain. The medical crew has maintained the patient in a supine position with manual stabilization of the right lower extremity.

As you assess the patient, you find that he is a 19-year-old man, conscious and alert without past medical or trauma history. The patient's initial vital signs are as follows: Blood pressure is 104/68 millimeters of mercury (mm Hg), pulse rate is 112 beats/minute, ventilatory rate is 24 breaths/minute, and skin is pale and diaphoretic. The patient states that he collided with another rider when he came out of a corner and fell down. He states his right leg was run over by at least one other bike. Visual inspection of his right leg reveals shortening of the leg when compared to the left side with tenderness and bruising of the mid-anterior thigh area.

- What do the kinematics of this event tell you about the potential injuries for this patient?
- What type of injury does this patient have and what would your management priorities be?

Introduction

Musculoskeletal injury, although common in trauma patients, rarely poses an immediate life-threatening condition. Skeletal trauma can be life threatening, however, when it produces significant blood loss (hemorrhage), either externally or from internal bleeding into the extremity or the retroperitoneum (in the case of the pelvis).

When caring for a critical trauma patient, the prehospital care provider has three primary considerations with regard to extremity injuries:

1. Maintain assessment priorities. Do not be distracted by dramatic, non-life-threatening musculoskeletal injuries (**Figure 14-1**).
2. Recognize potentially life-threatening musculoskeletal injuries.
3. Recognize the kinematics that created the musculoskeletal injuries and the potential for other life-threatening injuries caused by that energy transfer.

If a life-threatening or potentially life-threatening condition is discovered during the primary assessment, the secondary assessment should not be started. Any problems found during the primary assessment should be corrected before moving to the secondary assessment (see later discussion). This may mean delaying the secondary assessment until the patient is en route to the hospital or even, in some cases, waiting until arrival at the emergency department (ED).

Critical trauma patients may be secured to and transported on longboards to facilitate moving the patient and to allow for resuscitation and treatment of both critical and noncritical injuries. Use of a longboard allows for immobilization of the entire patient and all of his or her injuries, when appropriate, on a single platform that makes it possible to move the victim without disturbing the splinting. Although some injuries are more obvious than others, the prehospital care provider should treat every painful musculoskeletal injury as a possible fracture or dislocation and immobilize it to limit the potential for further injury and to provide some comfort and reduction of pain.

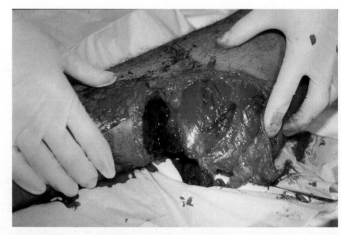

Figure 14-1 Some extremity injuries, although dramatic in appearance, are not life threatening.
Source: Courtesy of Peter T. Pons, MD, FACEP.

Anatomy and Physiology

Understanding the gross anatomy and physiology of the human body is an important piece of the prehospital care provider's fund of knowledge. Anatomy and physiology are the foundations on which assessment and management are based. Without a good grasp of the structures of the bones and muscles, the prehospital care provider will not be able to relate kinematics and superficial injuries to injuries that are internal. Although this textbook does not discuss all of the anatomy and physiology of the musculoskeletal system, it reviews some of the basics.

The mature human body has approximately 206 bones separated into categories by shape: long, short, flat, sutural, irregular, and sesamoid. **Long bones** include the femur, humerus, ulna, radius, tibia, and fibula. **Short bones** include metacarpals, metatarsals, and phalanges. **Flat bones** are usually thin and compact, such as the sternum, ribs, and scapulae. **Sutural bones** are part of the skull and are located between the joints of certain cranial bones. Irregular bones include the vertebrae, mandible, and bones of the pelvis. **Sesamoid bones** are bones located within tendons; the patella is the largest sesamoid bone (**Figure 14-2**).

The skeleton is divided into two primary divisions: the axial skeleton and the **appendicular skeleton**. The axial skeleton is comprised of the bones of the central part of the body, including the skull, spine, sternum, and ribs. The appendicular skeleton is made up of the bones of the upper and lower extremities, shoulder girdle, and pelvis (excluding the sacrum).

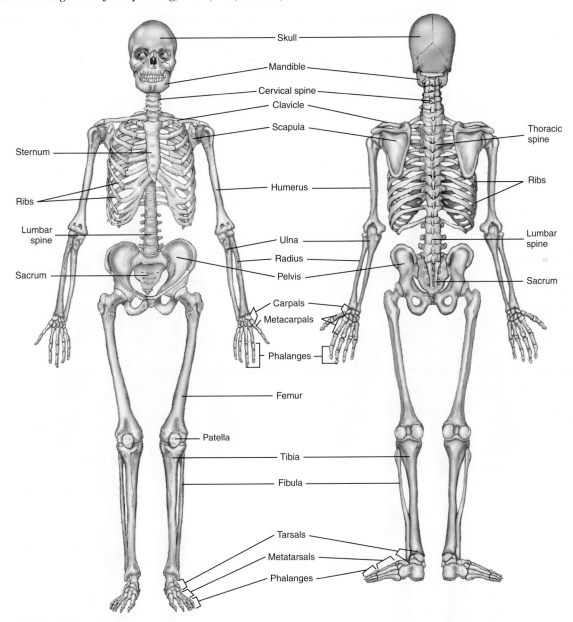

Figure 14-2 The human skeleton.

The human body has almost 650 individual muscles, which are categorized by their function. The muscles that are specific to this chapter are the voluntary, or skeletal, muscles. These muscles are categorized as *skeletal* because they move the skeletal system. Muscles in this category voluntarily move the structures of the body (**Figure 14-3**).

Other important structures discussed in this chapter are tendons and ligaments. A **tendon** is a band of tough, inelastic, fibrous tissue that connects a muscle to bone. It is the white part at the end of a muscle that directly attaches a muscle to the bone that it will move. A **ligament** is a band of tough, fibrous tissue connecting bone to bone; its function is to hold joints together.

Assessment

Musculoskeletal trauma can be categorized into the following three main types:

1. Life-threatening injuries resulting from musculoskeletal trauma, such as external hemorrhage, or internal hemorrhage associated with pelvic or femur fractures with life-threatening blood loss

2. Non-life-threatening musculoskeletal trauma associated with multisystem life-threatening trauma (life-threatening injuries plus limb fractures)

3. Isolated non-life-threatening musculoskeletal trauma (isolated limb fractures)

The purpose of the primary assessment is to identify and treat life-threatening conditions. The presence of a non-life-threatening musculoskeletal injury can be an indicator of possible multisystem trauma and should not distract the prehospital care provider from performing a complete primary assessment. Although the presence of musculoskeletal trauma should not distract the prehospital care provider from the care of more life-threatening conditions, the injuries should be looked at as possible indicators for potential life-threatening conditions. Evaluating the kinematics that created the obvious injuries may point to occult serious injuries.

Kinematics

Understanding the kinematics involved in an injury is one of the most important functions of the assessment and management

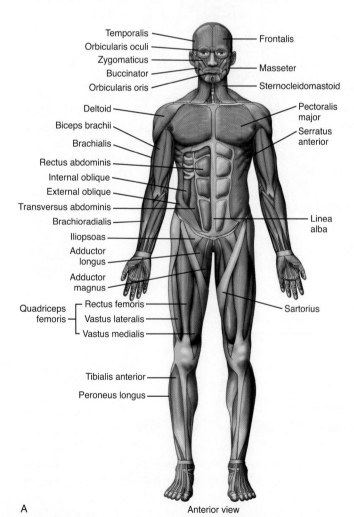

A   Anterior view

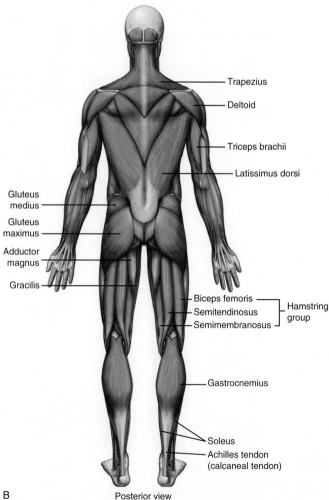

B   Posterior view

Figure 14-3 Major muscles of the human body.

of a trauma patient. Rapidly determining the kinematics and whether it involved low-energy versus high-energy transference (e.g., falling from a bicycle vs. being thrown from a motorcycle) will lead the prehospital care provider to the recognition of most critical injuries or conditions. The best source for determining the kinematics is directly from the patient. If the patient is unresponsive, details of the mechanism of injury can be obtained from witnesses. Rarely, a "best guess" to the events that caused the patient's trauma may be hazarded based on what was observed at the scene and the pattern of injuries found on physical examination if no one was present at the time of the incident. This information should be reported to the receiving facility and documented on the patient care report (PCR).

Based on the kinematics, the prehospital care provider may develop a high index of suspicion for the injuries that a patient might have sustained. Consideration of the kinematics may bring to mind additional injuries for which the prehospital care provider should assess, given knowledge of various injury patterns. For example:

- If a patient jumps out of a window feet first, the primary injury suspicion would be fractures of the calcaneus (heel bone), tibia, fibula, femur, pelvis, and spine and aortic **shear** injuries. However, secondary injuries might include abdominal injury or head injury from tumbling forward after hitting the ground.
- If a patient is involved in a motorcycle collision with a telephone pole and hits his or her head on the pole, primary injuries will include head, cervical spine, and thoracic injury. A secondary injury might include a femur fracture from "striking" the femur on the handlebars of the motorcycle.

Another example involves a patient riding in the passenger side of a vehicle that sustains a side-impact collision. As discussed in the Kinematics of Trauma chapter, Newton's first law of motion states that a body in motion will stay in motion until acted on by an equal but opposite force. The vehicle is the moving object until acted on by the other vehicle. The door of the target vehicle is pushed against the upper arm, which can then be pushed into the chest wall, producing rib fractures, lung contusion, and possibly a fractured humerus. Given the kinematics of this motor vehicle crash, suspicion for musculoskeletal injury would include humerus, pelvis, and femur fractures. Further injury suspicion would include rib fractures, chest wall muscle injury, and liver, lung, and heart injuries. Another secondary injury to consider is abrasion from a deployed air bag.

Another possible injury from a side-impact collision results from an unrestrained passenger becoming a missile (moving object) inside the vehicle. The other vehicle striking the passenger side sets the passenger in motion until he or she is stopped by another object, such as the driver. However, near-side injuries are more severe than far-side injuries. In this case, the kinematics to consider for the driver is the energy delivered by the unrestrained passenger's body.

A basic understanding of kinematics guides the prehospital care provider's assessment for the less obvious injuries.

Primary and Secondary Assessment

Primary Assessment

The first steps of any patient assessment are to ensure scene safety and evaluate the situation. Once the scene is as safe as possible, the patient can be assessed. The primary assessment identifies and addresses the immediate life-threatening conditions. Although angulated fractures or partial amputations may draw the prehospital care provider's attention because of their visual impact, life-threatening conditions must take priority. Airway, breathing, circulation, disability, and expose (ABCDE) remain the most important parts of the primary assessment. For a patient with life-threatening conditions identified in the primary assessment, management of musculoskeletal trauma is delayed until those problems are corrected. However, external hemorrhage is included in the primary assessment and must be controlled when deemed life threatening. If the patient has no life-threatening injuries, the prehospital care provider can proceed to the secondary assessment.

Secondary Assessment

Assessment of the extremities occurs during the secondary assessment. To facilitate the physical examination, the prehospital care provider considers removing any clothing that was not removed during the primary assessment, as allowed by the environment. If the mechanism of injury is not obvious, the patient or bystanders can be questioned about how the injuries occurred. The patient should also be queried about the presence of pain in the extremities. Most patients with significant musculoskeletal injuries have pain, unless a spinal cord or peripheral nerve injury is present.

Assessment of the extremities also includes evaluating any pain, weakness, or abnormal sensations in the extremities. Specific attention is paid to the following:

- *Bones and joints.* This evaluation is accomplished by inspecting for deformities that may represent fractures or dislocations (**Figure 14-4**) and palpating the extremity for tenderness and crepitus. Crepitus is the grinding feeling that bones make when the fractured ends rub against one another. Crepitus can be elicited by palpating the site of injury and by movement of the extremity. Crepitus sounds like a "snap, crackle, and pop" or the popping of plastic "bubble wrap" used for packing. This feeling of bones grating against one another during the assessment of a patient can produce further injury; therefore, once the crepitus is noted, no additional or repetitive steps should be taken to produce it. Crepitus is a distinct feeling that is not easily forgotten.
- *Soft-tissue injuries.* The prehospital care provider visually inspects for swelling, lacerations, abrasions, hematomas, skin color, and wounds. Any wound adjacent to a fracture suggests the presence of an open fracture. Firmness and tenseness of the soft tissues along with pain that appears out of proportion to the general findings may indicate presence of a **compartment syndrome**.
- *Perfusion.* Perfusion is evaluated by palpating distal pulses (radial or ulnar in the upper extremity and dorsalis

pedis or posterior tibial in the lower extremity) and noting capillary refill time in the fingers or toes. Absence of distal pulses in the extremities can indicate disruption of an artery, compression of the vessel by a hematoma or bone fragment, or a compartment syndrome. Large or expanding hematomas may indicate the presence of an injury to a large vessel.

- *Neurologic function.* The prehospital care provider assesses both motor and sensory function in the extremities. If a long-bone fracture is suspected, do not ask the patient to move the extremity, as such movement can induce significant pain and possibly convert a closed fracture to an open fracture. For most situations in the prehospital setting, evaluating gross neurologic functioning is sufficient.

- *Motor function.* Motor function can be assessed by first asking the patient if any weakness is noted. Motor function in the upper extremity is evaluated by having the patient open and close a fist and by testing the patient's grip strength (the patient squeezes the prehospital care provider's fingers), while lower extremity motor function is tested by having the patient wiggle his or her toes and push and pull against the examiner's hands.

- *Sensory function.* Sensory function is evaluated by asking about the presence of any abnormal sensations or numbness and testing to see if the patient feels the prehospital care provider touching various locations on the extremities, including the fingers and toes. **Figures 14-5** and **14-6** provide information on performing more detailed evaluations of motor and sensory function of the extremities.

Repeat evaluation of extremity perfusion and neurologic functioning should be performed after any splinting procedure.

Figure 14-4   Common Joint Dislocation Deformities

Joint	Direction	Deformity
Shoulder	Anterior	Squared off, abducted, externally rotated
	Posterior	Locked in internal rotation
Elbow	Posterior	Olecranon prominent posteriorly
Hip	Anterior	Flexed, abducted, externally rotated
	Posterior	Flexed, adducted, internally rotated
Knee	Anteroposterior	Loss of normal contour, extended
Ankle	Lateral is most common	Externally rotated, prominent medial malleolus
Subtalar joint	Lateral is most common	Laterally displaced os calcis

Source: Adapted From: American College of Surgeons Committee on Trauma: Advanced Trauma Life Support, ed 9, page 211, Chicago, 2012, ACS.

Figure 14-5   Peripheral Nerve Assessment of Upper Extremities

Nerve	Motor	Sensation	Injury
Ulnar	Index finger abduction	Little finger	Elbow injury
Median distal	Thenar contraction with opposition	Index finger	Wrist dislocation
Median, anterior interosseous	Index tip flexion	—	Supracondylar fracture of humerus (children)
Musculocutaneous	Elbow tip flexion	Lateral forearm	Anterior shoulder dislocation
Radial	Thumb, finger metacarpophalangeal extension	First dorsal web space	Distal humeral shaft, anterior shoulder dislocation
Axillary	Deltoid	Lateral shoulder	Anterior shoulder dislocation, proximal humerus fracture

Source: From: American College of Surgeons Committee on Trauma, Advanced Trauma Life Support, ed 9, page 217, Chicago, 2012, ACS.

Associated Injuries

While performing the secondary assessment, clues to the kinematics may be uncovered and an injury pattern may be suspected. Such injury patterns can prompt the prehospital care provider to assess for occult injuries associated with specific fractures. An example would be a thoracic injury associated with a shoulder injury. Thorough examination of the entire body will ensure injuries are not missed. **Figure 14-7** provides some examples of associated injuries.

Figure 14-6 Peripheral Nerve Assessment of Lower Extremities

Nerve	Motor	Sensation	Injury
Femoral	Knee extension	Anterior knee	Pubic rami fractures
Obturator	Hip adduction	Medial thigh	Obturator ring fractures
Posterior tibial	Toe flexion	Sole of foot	Knee dislocation
Superficial peroneal	Ankle eversion	Lateral dorsum of foot	Fibular neck fracture, knee dislocation
Deep peroneal	Ankle/toe dorsiflexion	Dorsal first to second web space	Fibular neck fracture, compartment syndrome
Sciatic nerve	Plantar dorsiflexion	Foot	Posterior hip dislocation
Superior gluteal	Hip abduction	—	Acetabular fracture
Inferior gluteal	Gluteus maximus hip extension	—	Acetabular fracture

Source: From: American College of Surgeons Committee on Trauma, Advanced Trauma Life Support, ed 9, page 217, Chicago, 2012, ACS.

Figure 14-7 Injuries Associated with Musculoskeletal Injuries

Injury	Missed/Associated Injury
Clavicle fracture Scapular fracture Fracture and/or dislocation of shoulder	Major thoracic injury, especially pulmonary contusion and rib fractures
Displaced thoracic spine fracture	Thoracic aortic rupture
Spine fracture	Intra-abdominal injury
Fracture/dislocation of elbow	Brachial artery injury Median, ulnar, and radial nerve injury
Major pelvic disruption (motor vehicle occupant)	Abdominal, thoracic, or head injury
Major pelvic disruption (motorcyclist or pedestrian)	Pelvic vascular hemorrhage
Femur fracture	Femoral neck fracture Posterior hip dislocation
Posterior knee dislocation	Femoral fracture Posterior hip dislocation
Knee dislocation or displaced tibial plateau fracture	Popliteal artery and nerve injuries
Calcaneal fracture	Spine injury or fracture Fracture–dislocation of hindfoot Tibial plateau fracture
Open fracture	70% incidence of associated nonskeletal injury

Source: From: American College of Surgeons Committee on Trauma, Advanced Trauma Life Support, ed 9, page 221, Chicago, 2012, ACS.

Specific Musculoskeletal Injuries

Injuries to the extremities result in two primary problems that require management in the prehospital setting: hemorrhage and instability from fractures and dislocations.

Hemorrhage

Bleeding can be dramatic or subtle. Regardless of the wound's appearance—the capillary ooze of a large abrasion, the dark red blood flowing from a superficial laceration, or the bright red spurting of an open artery—it is the amount of blood lost and the rate of its loss that will determine whether the patient will be able to compensate for the loss of blood volume or whether he or she will descend into shock. A good rule to remember is, "No bleeding is minor; every red blood cell counts." Even a small trickle of blood can add up to substantial blood loss if it is ignored for a long period.

External Hemorrhage

External arterial bleeding should be identified during the primary assessment. Generally, this type of bleeding is easily recognized, but assessment can be difficult when blood is hidden underneath a patient or in heavy or dark clothing. Ideally, obvious hemorrhage is controlled while the patient's airway and breathing are being managed, if sufficient assistance is present; otherwise, it is controlled when identified during assessment of circulation or when the patient's clothing is removed.

Estimation of external blood loss is extremely difficult. Although less experienced individuals tend to overestimate the amount of external hemorrhage, underestimation is also possible, as overt signs of external blood loss are not always apparent. One study suggested that prehospital estimates of blood loss were inaccurate and not clinically beneficial.[1] The reasons for these inaccurate blood loss estimates are many and include that the patient may have been moved from the site of injury or that lost blood may have been absorbed by clothing or soil or washed away in water or by rain.

Internal Hemorrhage

Internal hemorrhage is also common with musculoskeletal trauma. It may result from damage to major blood vessels (many of which are located in close proximity to the long bones of the body), from disrupted muscle, and from the marrow of fractured bones. Continued swelling of an extremity or a cold, pale, pulseless extremity could indicate internal hemorrhage from major arteries or veins. Significant internal blood loss can be associated with fractures (**Figure 14-8**).

Both the potential internal and the external blood loss associated with extremity trauma must be considered when evaluating the patient. This will help the prehospital care provider

Figure 14-8	Approximate Internal Blood Loss Associated with Fractures
Bone fractured	**Internal blood loss (milliliters [ml]) per fracture (Average total blood volume in an adult = 5000 to 6000 ml)**
Rib	125
Radius or ulna	250–500
Humerus	500–750
Tibia or fibula	500–1000
Femur	1000–2000
Pelvis	1000–massive

Note: This table describes the average blood loss from an isolated bone fracture. Injury to underlying organs and tissues can significantly increase these numbers. For example, a rib fracture that also lacerates an intercostal artery or damages the spleen could lead to major hemorrhage in the chest or abdomen, respectively.

anticipate the potential for development of shock, prepare for the possibility of systemic deterioration, and intervene appropriately to minimize its occurrence.

Management

The initial management of external hemorrhage involves the application of direct pressure to the wound. As discussed in the Shock chapter, elevation of an extremity has not been shown to slow hemorrhage, and in musculoskeletal trauma, it may aggravate injuries that are present. If hemorrhage is not controlled with direct pressure or a pressure dressing, a tourniquet should be applied, following the principles described in the Shock chapter. A second tourniquet should be applied next to the first if hemorrhage control is not achieved with initial placement of the first tourniquet. A recommended topical hemostatic agent can be considered for hemorrhage that is not amenable to use of a tourniquet, such as in the groin or axilla. Such agents may also be considered for prolonged-transport situations.

Tourniquet use, once considered taboo, is now the standard of care in the prehospital management of exsanguinating extremity injuries. This paradigm shift in extremity trauma management is due primarily to the experience of the U.S. military in the Iraq and Afghanistan conflicts. Military data document that a leading cause of preventable battlefield death has been uncontrolled hemorrhage from extremity trauma.[2] Since the implementation of widespread training and application of tourniquets, the preventable death rate from isolated extremity trauma has decreased significantly. Similar results are noted in a U.S.

civilian study, which found that 86% of patients who died from an isolated exsanguinating penetrating limb injury had signs of life at the scene but had no discernible pulse or blood pressure upon arrival to the hospital.[3] No patient in this series had a prehospital tourniquet placed.

Previous concerns over potential complications of tourniquet use, such as *nerve palsy* (impairment of nerve function), blood clot, and limb ischemia led to unfounded fear of their use. Tourniquets are routinely used by trauma, vascular, and orthopedic surgeons in the operating room for up to several hours with no long-term *sequelae* (after-effects). The U.S. military reviewed their data and found no major complications from tourniquet use. Minor complications occurred in less than 1% of cases and all resolved over time.[4]

A clear survival advantage has been noted with early tourniquet placement. The patient must have a tourniquet in place before the onset of shock. Patients with a tourniquet placed in the absence of shock had a survival rate greater than 90% versus a less than 10% survival rate in those whose tourniquet was placed after development of shock.[5] Delaying tourniquet placement until arrival at the hospital also increases mortality.[6] The tourniquet should be placed prior to extrication (if required) and prior to departure from the scene. The time of placement should be noted and relayed to the trauma team at the receiving hospital. If possible, the patient should be transported to a hospital with immediate surgical capabilities.

After controlling bleeding in patients with life-threatening hemorrhage from an extremity, prehospital care providers can reassess the primary assessment and focus on resuscitation and rapid transport to the facility that can best treat the patient's condition. During transport, administration of oxygen and initiation of intravenous (IV) fluid resuscitation for patients with shock can begin, keeping in mind that when internal hemorrhage is suspected, the target systolic blood pressure is 80 to 90 mm Hg (mean blood pressure is 60 to 65 mm Hg) and 90 to 100 mm Hg for patients with suspected traumatic brain injury. For patients with more minor bleeding and no signs of shock or other life-threatening problems, bleeding can be controlled with direct pressure and the secondary assessment performed.

Instability (Fractures and Dislocations)

Tears of the supporting structures of a joint, fracture of a bone, and major muscle or tendon injury affect the ability of an extremity to support itself. The two injuries that cause instability of bones or joints are fractures and dislocations.

Fractures

If a bone is fractured, immobilizing it will reduce the potential for further injury and pain. Movement of the sharp ends of the fractured bone may damage blood vessels, resulting in internal and external hemorrhage. Additionally, fractures can damage muscle tissue and nerves.

In general, fractures are classified as either closed or open. In a **closed fracture**, the skin is not punctured by the bone ends, whereas in an **open fracture**, the integrity of the skin has been interrupted (**Figure 14-9A**). Orthopedic surgeons may classify fractures by their pattern (e.g., greenstick, comminuted), but these types cannot be differentiated without an x-ray, and knowledge of the fracture pattern does not alter field management.

Closed Fractures

Closed fractures are fractures in which the bone has been broken but the patient has no loss of skin integrity (i.e., the skin is not broken) (**Figure 14-9B**). Signs of a closed fracture include pain, tenderness, deformity, hematomas, swelling, and crepitus, although in some patients, pain and tenderness may be the only findings. Pulses, skin color, and motor and sensory function should be assessed distal to the suspected fracture site. Asking a patient to move the fractured extremity could result in conversion of a closed fracture into an open fracture. It is not always true that an extremity is not fractured because the patient can voluntarily move it or, in the case of a lower extremity, even walk on it; adrenalin from a traumatic event may motivate patients to endure pain they would not tolerate normally. Additionally, some patients have a remarkably high pain tolerance.

Open Fractures

Open fractures usually occur when a sharp bone end penetrates the skin from the inside or an injury lacerates the skin and muscle down to a fracture site (**Figure 14-9C**). When a fracture is open to the outside environment, the ends of the fracture bone can be contaminated with bacteria from the overlying skin or from contamination from the environment. This can lead to the serious complication of a bone infection (*osteomyelitis*), which can interfere with healing of the fracture. Although the skin wound associated with an open fracture often is not associated with significant hemorrhage, persistent bleeding may come from the marrow cavity of the bone or from the decompressing of a hematoma deep inside the tissue.

Any open wound near a possible fracture needs to be considered an open fracture and treated as such. A protruding bone or bone end should generally not be intentionally replaced; however, the bones occasionally return to a near-normal position when realigned or by the muscle spasms that usually occur with fractures. Inadequate splinting or rough handling of a fractured extremity may convert a closed fracture into an open one.

Open fractures may not always be easy to identify in a trauma patient. Although bone protruding from a wound is obvious, soft-tissue injuries in proximity to a fracture/deformity may have resulted from a bone end that broke through the surface of the skin only to recede back into the tissue.

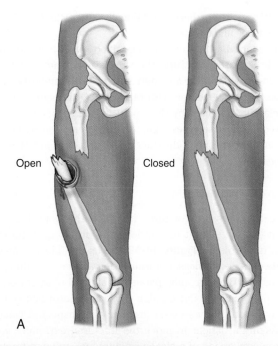

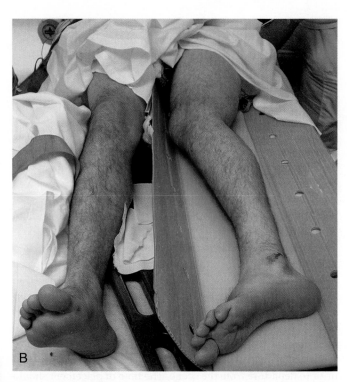

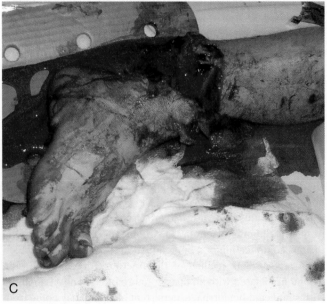

Figure 14-9 **A.** Open versus closed fracture. **B.** Closed fracture of the femur. Note the internal rotation and shortening of the left leg. **C.** Open fracture of the tibia. *Source:* B. Courtesy of Norman McSwain, MD, FACD, NREMT-P; C. Courtesy of Peter T. Pons, MD FACEP.

Internal Hemorrhage

As noted earlier, fractures may result in significant internal hemorrhage into the tissue planes surrounding the fracture. The two most common fractures associated with the greatest hemorrhage are femur and pelvic fractures. An adult can lose 1,000 to 2,000 ml of blood into each thigh. Thus, internal hemorrhage associated with bilateral femur fractures may be sufficient to result in death from hypovolemic shock.

Pelvic fractures also are a common cause of significant hemorrhage (**Figure 14-10**). Multiple small blood vessels lie adjacent to the pelvis and may be torn by bone ends or as the sacroiliac joints of the pelvis fracture or open up. Overaggressive palpation or manipulation of the pelvis (pelvic rock) can significantly increase blood loss when an unstable pelvic fracture is present. In most cases, physical examination of the pelvis does not affect how the patient will be managed.

To assess the pelvis, gentle palpation is acceptable but should be performed only once. Gentle manual pressure anterior to posterior and from the sides may identify crepitus or instability. The area around the pelvis is a "potential space" because it can expand and accommodate a huge amount of blood. Because of the amount of space in the pelvic cavity, hemorrhage may occur with few, if any, external signs of compromise.

Open fractures of the pelvis, often resulting when a pedestrian is struck by a car or when an occupant is ejected from a motor vehicle, are particularly deadly. Falls can also result in pelvic fracture, so it is important to consider pelvic fracture with any mechanism that involves energy absorbed by the pelvis or complaints of pain around the pelvis. Often, massive external—rather than internal—hemorrhage results, and bone ends may lacerate the rectum or vagina, resulting in severe pelvic infection.

Pelvic Fractures

Pelvic fractures can range from minor, relatively insignificant fractures to complex injuries associated with massive internal and external hemorrhage. Fractures of the **pelvic ring** are associated with overall mortality of 6%, whereas mortality from open fractures may exceed 50%. Blood loss is the leading cause of death in patients with pelvic fractures; the remaining deaths are from traumatic brain injury and multiple organ failure.

Because the pelvis is a strong bone and difficult to fracture, patients with pelvic fractures frequently have associated injuries, including traumatic brain injuries (51%), long-bone fractures (48%), thoracic injuries (20%), urethral disruption in men (15%), splenic trauma (10%), and liver and kidney trauma (7% each). Examples of pelvic fractures include the following:

- *Rami fractures.* Isolated fractures of the inferior or superior rami are generally minor and do not require surgical stabilization. Individuals who fall forcibly on their perineum may fracture all four rami ("straddle" injury). These fractures typically are not associated with significant internal hemorrhage.
- *Acetabular fractures.* These fractures occur when the head of the femur is driven into the acetabulum of the pelvis. Surgical intervention is generally needed to optimize normal hip function. These injuries may be associated with significant internal hemorrhage.

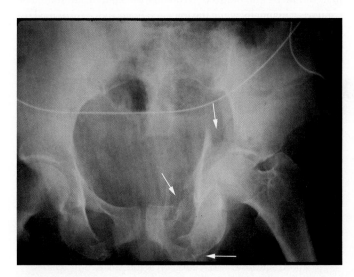

Figure 14-10 Fracture of the pelvis. The arrows show multiple fractures involving the pubic rami and the acetabulum.
Source: Courtesy of Peter T. Pons, MD, FACEP.

- *Pelvic ring fractures.* Fractures of the pelvic ring are typically classified into three categories. Life-threatening hemorrhage is probably most common with vertical shear fractures, but it may be associated with each type of pelvic ring fracture. The prehospital care provider may palpate crepitus and note bony instability with each of these pelvic ring fractures.

1. Lateral compression fractures account for the majority of pelvic ring fractures (**Figure 14-11A**). These injuries may occur when forces are applied to the lateral aspects of the pelvis (e.g., pedestrian is struck by a car). The volume of the pelvis is decreased in these fractures.
2. Anterior–posterior compression fractures account for about 15% of pelvic ring fractures (**Figure 14-11B**). These injuries occur when forces are applied in an anteroposterior direction (e.g., person pinned between a vehicle and wall). These injuries are also known as "open book" pelvic fractures because usually the symphysis pubis is separated and the volume of the pelvis greatly increased.
3. Vertical shear fractures account for the smallest proportion of pelvic ring fractures but tend to cause the highest mortality (**Figure 14-11C**). They occur when a vertical force is applied to the hemi-pelvis (e.g., fall from a height, landing on one leg first). Because one half of the pelvis is sheared off the remaining portion, blood vessels are often torn, resulting in severe internal hemorrhage.

Management
Open and Closed Fracture

The first consideration in managing fractures is to control hemorrhage and treat for shock. Direct pressure and pressure dressings will control virtually all external hemorrhage encountered

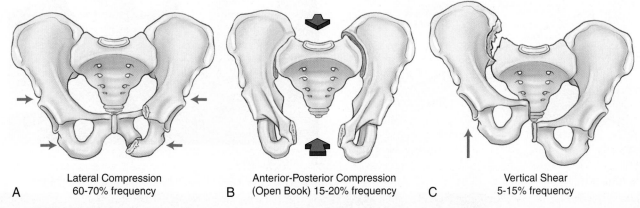

Figure 14-11 Pelvic fractures. **A.** Lateral compression. **B.** Anterior–posterior compression. **C.** Vertical shear.

in the field. Open wounds or exposed bone ends should be covered with a sterile dressing moistened with sterile normal saline or water. Internal hemorrhage is primarily controlled by immobilization, which has the added benefit of providing pain relief. If the bone ends of an open fracture retract into the wound during splinting, this information must be documented on the PCR and reported to ED personnel. There is usually little to be gained from administering IV antibiotics to patients with open fractures in the field, especially in the urban or suburban setting, but doing so may be important with prolonged transport times.

An injured extremity should be moved as little as possible, both during the secondary assessment and during application of a splint. Prior to splinting, an injured extremity should generally be returned to its normal anatomic position, including the use of gentle traction if necessary to restore an extremity to its normal length. The two primary contraindications to this procedure are significant pain and resistance to movement experienced during an attempt to restore a normal anatomic position. Traditional teaching was to splint a suspected fracture "in the position found"; however, there is good rationale for restoring normal anatomic position. First, a "reduced fracture," one that is returned to normal anatomic alignment, is easier to splint. Secondly, reducing a fracture may alleviate compression of arteries or nerves

and result in improved perfusion and neurologic functioning. Reduction of fractures also decreases hemorrhage.

If the fracture is open and bone is exposed, the bone end should be gently rinsed with sterile water or normal saline to remove obvious contamination prior to an attempt to restore normal anatomic position. It is not of major concern if the bone ends retract back into the skin during this manipulation, as open fractures require irrigation and **debridement** in the operating room regardless. However, the fact that the bone was exposed prior to reduction is key information that should be passed on during the patient report at the receiving facility. No more than two attempts should be made to restore an extremity to normal position, and, if unsuccessful, the extremity should be splinted "as is."

The primary objective of splinting is to prevent movement of the fractured body part. Doing so will help decrease the patient's pain and prevent further soft-tissue damage and hemorrhage. To immobilize any long bone in an extremity effectively, the entire limb should be immobilized. To do this, the injured site should be supported manually while the joint and bone above (proximal to) and the joint and bone below (distal to) the injury site are immobilized. Numerous types of splints are available, and most can be used with both open and closed fractures (**Figure 14-12**).

Figure 14-12 Types of Splints

Various splints and splinting materials are available, including the following:

- *Rigid splints* cannot be changed in shape. They require that the body part be positioned to fit the splint's shape. Examples of rigid splints include board splints (wood, plastic, or metal), fracture packs, and inflatable "air splints." This group of splints also includes the long backboard. Rigid splints are best used for long-bone injuries.

- *Formable splints* can be molded into various shapes and combinations to accommodate the shape of the injured extremity. Examples of formable splints include vacuum splints, pillows, blankets, cardboard splints, wire-ladder splints, and foam-covered moldable metal splints. Formable splints are best used for ankle, wrist, and long-bone injuries.
- *Traction splints* are designed to maintain mechanical in-line traction to help realign fractures. Traction splints are most often used to stabilize femur fractures.

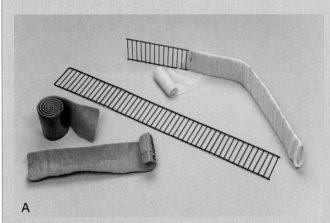

A

A. Formable splint.

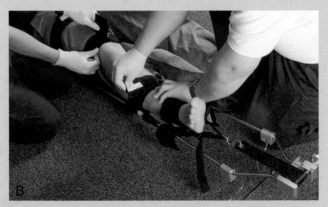

B

B. Traction splint.

Source: © Jones & Bartlett Learning. Photographed by Darren Stahlman.

(Continues on next page)

Figure 14-12   Types of Splints (*Continued*)

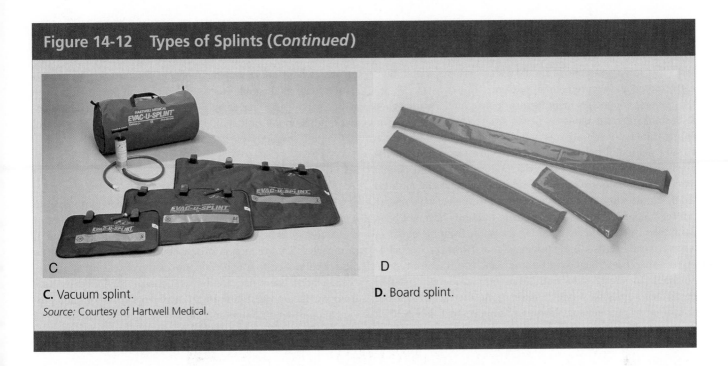

C. Vacuum splint.
Source: Courtesy of Hartwell Medical.

D. Board splint.

With virtually all splinting techniques, further inspection of the extremity is limited, and a thorough assessment should be performed before splinting.

Four additional points are important to remember when applying any type of splint:

1. Pad splints to prevent movement of the extremity inside the splint, to help increase the patient's comfort, and to prevent pressure sores.
2. Remove jewelry and watches so that these objects will not inhibit circulation as additional swelling occurs. Lubrication with soap, lotion, or a water-soluble jelly may facilitate removal of tight rings.
3. Assess neurovascular functions distal to the injury site before and after applying any splint and periodically thereafter. A pulseless extremity indicates either a vascular injury or a compartment syndrome, and rapid transport to an appropriate facility becomes even more of a priority.
4. After splinting, consider elevating the extremity, if possible, to decrease edema and throbbing. Ice or cold packs can also be used to decrease pain and swelling and may be placed on the splinted extremity near the suspected fracture site.

Femur Fractures

Femur fractures represent a unique splinting situation because of the musculature of the thigh. In addition to providing key structural support for the lower extremity, the femur provides resistance to the powerful thigh muscles, keeping the leg extended to its proper length. When the femur is fractured in the midshaft area, this resistance to contraction is removed. As these muscles contract, the sharp bone ends tear through muscle tissue, producing additional internal hemorrhage and pain and predisposing the patient to an open fracture.

In the absence of life-threatening conditions, a traction splint should be applied to stabilize suspected midshaft femoral fractures. The application of traction, both manually and by use of a mechanical device, will help decrease internal bleeding as well as decrease the patient's pain.

One study of prehospital use of traction splints documented that almost 40% of the patients had an injury that either complicated or contraindicated use of a traction splint.[7] Contraindications to the use of a traction splint include the following:

- Suspected pelvic fracture
- Suspected femoral neck (hip) fracture
- Avulsion or amputation of the ankle and foot
- Suspected fractures adjacent to the knee (A traction splint may be used as a rigid splint in this situation, but traction should not be applied.)

When midshaft femoral fractures are encountered in a patient with additional injuries that are life threatening, time should not be taken to apply a traction splint. Instead, attention should be focused on the critical problems, and the suspect lower extremity fractures will be sufficiently stabilized when the patient is immobilized to a long backboard.

Pelvic Fractures

Severe pelvic fractures present a number of challenging problems for prehospital care providers. The first is identification of an unstable pelvis fracture. In many, if not most, cases, this requires x-ray evaluation of the pelvis in order to accurately diagnose the problem. The greatest concern is internal hemorrhage, which can be very difficult to manage. Management of some types of unstable pelvic fractures involves wrapping a bed sheet tightly around the lower aspect of the pelvis and tying it as a sling. The lower extremities should also be adducted and internally rotated and secured in that position.

Several companies manufacture "pelvic binders," designed to stabilize certain types of pelvic fractures. When used on appropriate types of fractures in the hospital, these devices can close a disrupted pelvic ring and decrease the volume of the pelvis. The specific type of pelvis fracture that would benefit from these sorts of treatments cannot be identified by physical examination alone. For numerous reasons, pelvic binders are not recommended for use when pelvic fractures have not been confirmed by x-ray, such as during transport from the scene of a motor vehicle crash to the trauma center. However, if a pelvic fracture has been diagnosed by x-ray and the fracture type is amenable to management with a binder, consideration should be given to applying a binder prior to an interfacility transfer (i.e., from a nontrauma center to a trauma center), especially if the patient is in shock (**Figure 14-13**). At present, there are no published studies of prehospital use of pelvic binders.

Another related concern is that patients with grossly unstable pelvic fractures may be difficult to move, and even turning the patient using a modified logroll procedure can shift bone fragments, causing additional hemorrhage. The best way to move a patient with an unstable fracture identified on palpation may be with a scoop stretcher or by a direct patient lift while maintaining spine immobilization and placement onto a long backboard. This action should be carried out expeditiously.

Dislocations

Joints are held together by ligaments. The bones that make up a joint are attached to their muscles by tendons. Movement of an extremity is accomplished by the contraction (shortening) of muscles. This reduction of muscle length pulls the tendons that are attached to a bone and moves the extremity at a joint. A dislocation is a separation of two bones at the joint, resulting from significant disruption to the ligaments that normally provide supporting structure and stability at a joint (**Figures 14-14** and **14-15**). A dislocation, similar to a fracture, produces an area of instability that the prehospital care provider needs to secure.

Figure 14-13   Pelvic Binders

At least three pelvic binders are commercially available: Pelvic Binder (Pelvic Binder, Inc.), Sam Sling (Sam Products), and Trauma Pelvic Orthotic Device (TPOD; BioCybernetics International).

Rationale
Some pelvic ring fractures are associated with an increase in the pelvic volume (e.g., anteroposterior compression fracture), permitting large amounts of intra-abdominal hemorrhage. Because the volume is increased, there is less tissue surrounding the pelvis to **tamponade** bleeding. Before the development of pelvic binders, patients with these injuries and hemodynamic instability (shock) would undergo external fixation of the pelvis to decrease the pelvic volume and increase the likelihood of tamponade of hemorrhage. Although external fixation seemed to decrease blood requirements, minimal published data exist to suggest that external fixation lowered mortality from these fractures.

Problems
Several potential problems exist with the use of pelvic binders in the prehospital setting:

1. Pelvic fractures are difficult to diagnose in the absence of an x-ray film. No published data show that

prehospital care providers can reliably diagnose a pelvic fracture based on clinical examination. Furthermore, not all pelvic fractures benefit from compression. Although anteroposterior compression fractures may benefit, lateral compression fractures already have a decreased pelvic volume.

2. Limited data exist on efficacy. Only a few retrospective case series have reported on patients with in-hospital use of pelvic binders. Although some demonstrate that the pelvic volume is significantly decreased, few address transfusion requirements, and none has shown a decrease in mortality in those treated with a pelvic binder.

3. No published research exists on the use of pelvic binders in the prehospital setting, and therefore no data show improved outcome.

4. There is significant cost for this single-use device.

Potential Use
One conceivable use for the pelvic binder in the out-of-hospital setting would be the interfacility transfer of a patient with an anteroposterior compression fracture, confirmed by x-ray film, and associated Class II, III, or IV shock. In these patients, the pelvic binder could be applied before transfer, especially to those in decompensated shock. The decision to use the pelvic binder should be made in conjunction with medical control.

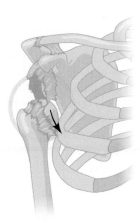

Figure 14-14 A dislocation is a separation of a bone from a joint.

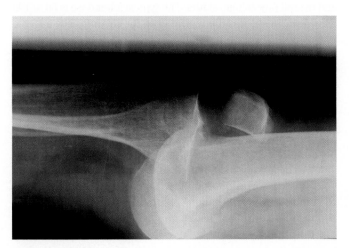

Figure 14-15 Right anterior knee dislocation with overriding tibia on the femur.
Source: © Wellcome Image Library/Custom Medical Stock Photo.

Dislocations can produce great pain. A dislocation can be difficult to distinguish clinically from a fracture and may be associated with fractures as well (fracture–dislocation). Deformity of a joint provides a clue to the type of dislocation.

Individuals who have had prior dislocations have ligaments that are more lax than normal and may be prone to more frequent dislocations unless the problem is corrected surgically. Unlike those sustaining a dislocation for the first time, these patients are often familiar with their injury and can help in assessment and stabilization.

Management

As a general rule, suspected dislocations should be splinted in the position found. Gentle manipulation of the joint can be done to try to return blood flow when the pulse is absent or weak. When faced with a brief transport time to the hospital, however, the better decision is to initiate transport rather than attempt manipulation. This manipulation will cause the patient great pain, so the patient should be prepared before moving the extremity. A splint should be used to immobilize most dislocations, while a sling is used for shoulder injuries. Documentation of how the injury was found and of the presence of pulses, movement, sensation, and color before and after splinting is important. During transport, ice or cold packs can be used to decrease pain and swelling. Analgesia should also be provided to reduce pain.

Attempted reduction of a dislocation should be undertaken only when permitted by written protocols or online medical control, and when the prehospital care provider has been properly trained in the appropriate techniques. All attempts at reduction of a dislocation should be properly documented.

Special Considerations
Critical Multisystem Trauma Patient

Adherence to the primary assessment priorities in patients with multisystem trauma that includes injured extremities does not imply that extremity injuries should be ignored or that injured extremities should not be protected from further harm. Rather, it means that *life takes precedence over limb* when faced with a critically injured trauma patient with extremity injuries that are not bleeding. The focus should be on maintaining vital functions through resuscitation, and only limited measures should be taken to address the extremity injuries, regardless of how dramatic the injuries appear. By properly immobilizing a patient to a long backboard, all extremities and the entire skeleton are essentially splinted in an anatomic position and the patient is easily moved. A secondary assessment need not be completed if the life-threatening problems identified in the primary assessment require ongoing interventions and if transport time is short. If a secondary assessment is deferred for this reason, the prehospital care provider can simply document the findings that precluded performing the secondary assessment.

Pain Management

Analgesia should be considered in patients with isolated extremity trauma and hip fractures.[8] Basic interventions that provide effective pain relief should be attempted first (i.e., immobilization of suspected fractures and use of ice packs), as well as good communication skills with the patient to decrease anxiety. Protocols for analgesic use should be in place with clear indications and contraindications. Examples of acceptable pharmaceutical intervention include morphine sulfate, fentanyl, nitrous oxide, and nonsteroidal anti-inflammatory drugs (NSAIDs).

The patient must be monitored with proper documentation before and after administration of the analgesic. Appropriate monitoring includes continuous pulse oximetry and serial vital signs, including pulse, ventilatory rate, and blood pressure. Continuous capnography may provide early warning signs that a patient is becoming overmedicated ("narcotized").[9] Any pain management protocol should include ensuring that naloxone is immediately available if reversal of the side effects of narcotic analgesics is needed.

Analgesics are recommended for isolated joint and limb injuries but are generally not advocated in multisystem trauma patients. Once the fracture or dislocation is stabilized and splinted, the patient should experience a marked reduction in pain. Stabilizing the affected extremity decreases the amount of movement of the area, thus decreasing the amount of discomfort. The patient should be observed for signs of alcohol or drug use if he or she does not appear to be in much pain despite significant injuries.

Pain medications should be used judiciously and as tolerated by the patient. Analgesics should not be administered when:

1. The patient presents with or develops signs and symptoms of shock
2. Pain is significantly relieved with stabilization and splinting
3. The patient appears under the influence of drugs or alcohol

Medication should not be administered without understanding the potential complications.

Moderate to severe pain may be treated with an NSAID, such as ketorolac, administered IV, while severe pain is typically treated with narcotics (opiates). Morphine and fentanyl are the most commonly used narcotics. Respiratory depression, even apnea, is the greatest concern of the possible detrimental effects of narcotics. Another worrisome adverse effect is that narcotics are vasodilators. This is of particular concern for trauma patients because patients who are in a compensated state of shock (Class II) may have their hypovolemia "unmasked" by the narcotic, and profound hypotension may occur. In patients with potential compensated shock, the lowest possible dose should be administered IV and slowly titrated upward until satisfactory pain relief is noted. Narcotics are best given IV in trauma patients because intramuscular doses may be absorbed erratically if hypoperfusion is present. Other possible adverse reactions for all narcotics include nausea and emesis, dizziness, sedation, and euphoria. For this reason, these agents should be used with caution in patients with head injuries because intracranial hypertension may be exaggerated. Data suggest that the analgesic and adverse effects of morphine and fentanyl are comparable.[10]

Morphine

Morphine is for use in patients with moderate to severe pain. Dosage should be titrated to the patient's response to the pain and physiologic status. It can be given IV, intramuscularly, or subcutaneously. Adult IV dosage is typically 2.5 to 15 mg (or 0.05 to 0.1 mg/kg), administered slowly over several minutes while monitoring the patient for relief and complications. For intramuscular or subcutaneous administration, the adult dose is 10 mg per 70 kg body weight.

Fentanyl

Fentanyl has properties that make it attractive for prehospital trauma patients. Fentanyl has rapid onset and does not cause an increase in the release of histamine (as morphine does), which can exacerbate hypotension in hypovolemic patients. As with all narcotics, the dose should be titrated to patient relief and overall physiologic status. The typical adult dose is 50 to 100 mcg; 1 to 2 mcg/kg is the typical dose for children. The adverse effects are similar to morphine, but specific contraindications include allergy to fentanyl, traumatic brain injury with possible increased intracranial pressure, respiratory depression, and loss of airway control.

Ketamine

Ketamine, a dissociative agent in higher doses and an analgesic in lower doses, has a limited effect on the respiratory drive and does not cause hypotension.[11] Ketamine has commonly been used in Europe and is gaining acceptance in the United States, although its administration as an analgesic is an off-label use. The Committee on Tactical Combat Casualty Care has recently recommended ketamine as an option for pain control on the battlefield, and it has been incorporated into the Tactical Combat Casualty Care (TCCC) course. It can be administered via many routes, including IV, intramuscular, intraosseous, intranasal, oral, and rectal. The standard initial dose is 15 to 30 mg IV, 50 mg intranasally (via nasal atomizer), or 50 to 75 mg intramuscularly for pain control, although higher doses may be required for procedural sedation in situations such as intubation. Because it does not cause hypotension and, in fact, increases both heart rate and blood pressure, ketamine can be used to provide analgesia in patients with decreased blood pressure when narcotic analgesics would be inappropriate. Limited evidence suggests ketamine may increase intracranial pressure and intraocular pressure. Therefore, the use of ketamine is currently not recommended in patients with suspected traumatic brain injury or penetrating eye trauma; however, both of these concerns have recently been questioned.[12-14] Prehospital use of ketamine for analgesia and procedural sedation has proven to be safe and effective.[15,16]

Relief of Anxiety (Anxiolysis)

Treating pain in trauma patients involves managing both the physical pain and the anxiety about the pain and the situation in which patients find themselves. Analgesics manage the pain, and sedatives address the anxiety. Benzodiazepines such as diazepam (Valium), midazolam (Versed), lorazepam (Ativan), and alprazolam (Xanax) are the best known and have the added benefit of antegrade amnesia. The patients often will not remember details of what happened for a period of time after the drug is administered. The use of a narcotic and benzodiazepine together can have a synergistic effect that can be of added benefit in relieving pain and anxiety; however, extreme caution must be used when administering simultaneous doses of both a benzodiazepine and a narcotic as the combined effect on the respiratory and circulatory systems can lead to respiratory depression and hypotension.

Amputations

When tissue has been totally separated from an extremity, the tissue is completely without nutrition and oxygenation. This type of injury is termed an amputation or avulsion. An amputation is the loss of part or all of a limb, and an avulsion involves the tearing away of skin and the underlying soft tissue. Initially, bleeding may be severe with these injuries; however, vessels at the injured site may constrict and retract, and clotting may combine to diminish the blood loss. Movement may disrupt the blood clot, and bleeding can recur. All amputations may be accompanied by significant bleeding but more so with partial amputations. When vessels are completely transected, they retract and constrict, and blood clots may form, decreasing or stopping hemorrhage; however, when a vessel is only partially transected, the two ends cannot retract, and blood continues to pour out of the hole.

Amputations are often evident on the scene (**Figure 14-16**). This type of injury receives great attention from bystanders, and the patient may or may not know that the extremity is missing. Psychologically, the prehospital care provider needs to deal with this injury cautiously (**Figure 14-17**). The patient may not be ready to confront the loss of a limb and should be told after being assessed and treated.

The missing extremity should be located for possible reattachment. Even if it is not possible to regain complete function of the extremity, the patient may regain partial function. The primary assessment should be performed before looking for a missing extremity, unless adequate numbers of emergency response personnel are present to assist. The appearance of an amputation may be horrifying, but if the patient does not have a patent airway or is not breathing, the loss of the limb is secondary to the life-threatening priorities.

Amputations are very painful. Pain management should be employed once life-threatening problems have been excluded in the primary assessment (**Figure 14-18**).

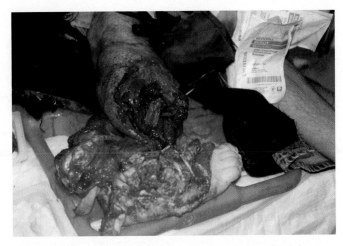

Figure 14-16 Complete amputation of the right leg after it became entangled in machinery.
Source: Courtesy of Peter T. Pons, MD, FACEP.

Figure 14-17 Phantom Pain

In some circumstances, the patient may complain of pain distal to the amputation. This phantom pain is the sensation that pain exists in a missing extremity. The reason for phantom pain is not understood completely, but the brain may not realize that the extremity is not present. This sensation is usually not present at the time of the initial injury.

Management

Principles of managing an amputated part include the following:

1. Clean the amputated part by gentle rinsing with lactated Ringer's (LR) solution.
2. Wrap the part in sterile gauze moistened with LR solution and place it in a plastic bag or container.
3. After labeling the bag or container, place it in an outer container filled with crushed ice.
4. Do not freeze the part by placing it directly on the ice or by adding another coolant such as dry ice.
5. Transport the part along with the patient to the closest appropriate facility.[17]

The longer the amputated portion is without oxygen, the less likely that it can be replaced successfully. Cooling the

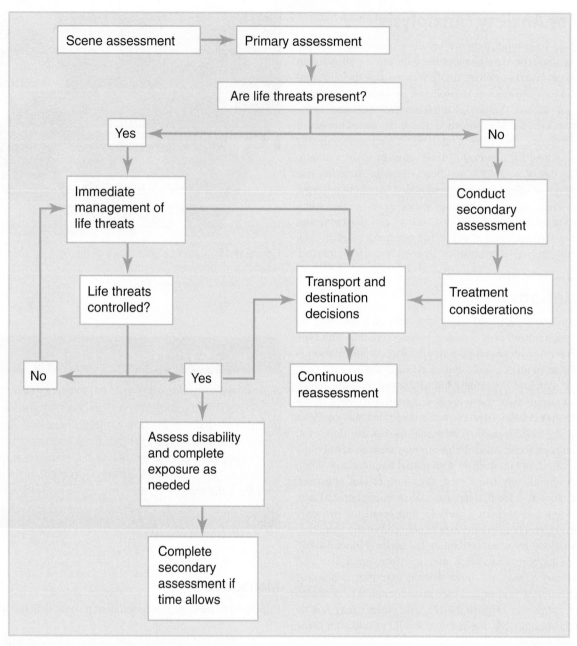

Figure 14-18 Primary assessment algorithm.

amputated body part, without freezing it, will reduce the metabolic rate and prolong this critical time. However, replantation is not a guarantee of successful attachment or ultimate function. Because lower extremity prostheses generally allow the patient to resume a near-normal life, lower extremities are rarely considered for replantation. Furthermore, only cleanly separated amputations in otherwise healthy, younger individuals are usually considered for replantation. Smokers are less likely to have successful replantation because the nicotine in tobacco is a potent vasoconstrictor and may compromise blood flow to the replanted segment. Patients who are candidates for replantation of fingers (particularly the thumb) or a hand/forearm should be transported to a level I trauma center because level II and III facilities often lack replantation capability.

Transport of a patient should not be delayed to locate a missing amputated part. If the amputated part is not readily found, law enforcement officials or other emergency responders should remain at the scene to search for it. When the amputated part is transported in a separate vehicle from the patient, the prehospital care provider ensures that the transporters of the amputated part understand clearly where the patient is being transported and how to handle the part once it is located. The receiving facility should be notified as soon as the part is located, and transport of the part should be initiated as soon as possible.

Field Amputation

In general, many extremities that appear hopelessly entrapped can be released with additional extrication expertise. If the patient has the extremity entangled in a machine, an often-overlooked expert is the maintenance person who repairs the machine. This person usually has the technical knowledge for expeditiously disassembling and removing parts from a machine, thereby facilitating extrication. But, on rare occasions, a patient may have an entrapped extremity for which a field amputation may be the only reasonable option. A regional trauma system should consider development of an appropriately equipped field amputation team (**Figure 14-19**). While rarely utilized, such a team has been shown to save lives.[18] Although formal field amputation is not considered part of the scope of practice of prehospital care providers in the United States, some entrapped extremities may be connected by only a small strand of tissue. The decision to cut this tissue or wait for a physician to arrive at the scene must be made in consultation with medical oversight. If a substantial amputation is necessary, it should ideally be performed by a trained physician because of the anatomic knowledge and technical expertise required. Significant sedation may need to be administered for the procedure, including intubation.

Compartment Syndrome

Compartment syndrome refers to a limb-threatening condition in which the blood supply to an extremity is compromised by increased pressure in that limb. The muscles of extremities are enveloped by dense connective tissue called **fascia**. This fascia forms numerous compartments in the extremities in which the muscles are contained. The forearm has three compartments, and the lower leg (calf) has four. Muscle fascia has

Figure 14-19   Field Amputation Set

An amputation set can be assembled and maintained in a medical director's or supervisor's vehicle in case a field amputation is ever necessary. The following lists provide an example of the various components of an amputation kit.

Medical instruments:

▪ Curved Mayo scissors	1 each
▪ Curved hemostats	4 each
▪ Kelly clamps, regular	2 each
▪ Needle holder, regular	2 each
▪ Towel clamps	4 each
▪ Forceps with teeth, regular	1 each
▪ Rake retractor, six prong, sharp	2 each
▪ Gigli saw handles	2 each
▪ Gigli saw wire	3 each
▪ Amputation knife	1 each
▪ Bone cutter	1 each

Disposable materials:
- Surgical gowns, sterile
- Surgical gloves, sterile
- Scalpel, #10 blade
- Sterile towels (4 pack)
- Lap pads (10 pack)

- Drapes
- Bone wax

Suturing supplies:
- 2–0 silk ties
- 0 silk ties
- 0 silk on atraumatic needle
- 2–0 silk on gastrointestinal (GI) needle, multipack
- 3–0 silk on GI needle, multipack

Dressing supplies:
- Roller gauze
- Army Battle Dressing (**ABD**) pads, large
- Elastic bandages, 4 inch
- Elastic bandages, 6 inch

Medications:
- Neuromuscular blocking agents (succinylcholine, vecuronium, etc.)
- Ketamine
- Fentanyl

Airway management (if not on EMS units):
- Intubation tray
- Endotracheal tubes

minimal stretch, and anything that increases the pressure inside the compartments may result in a compartment syndrome.

The two most common causes of compartment syndrome are hemorrhage within a compartment from a fracture or vascular injury and third-space edema that forms when ischemic muscle tissue is reperfused after a period of diminished or absent blood flow. However, a splint or cast that is applied too tightly may also produce a compartment syndrome. As the pressure in the compartment increases beyond that of capillary pressure (about 30 mm Hg), flow is impaired to the capillaries. The tissue served by these vessels then becomes ischemic. The pressure may continue to build to the point that even arterial flow is compromised by compression in the arteries.

The two earliest signs of a developing compartment syndrome are pain and *paresthesias* (abnormal sensations such as burning, pricking, pins and needles, or tingling) of the involved extremity. Pain is often described as out of proportion to the injury. This pain may be dramatically increased on passive movement of a finger or toe in that extremity. Nerves are extremely sensitive to their blood supply, and any compromised blood flow soon manifests as paresthesia. The fact that these symptoms are normally associated with a fracture underscores the need for baseline circulatory, motor, and sensory examinations and repeated serial examinations so that the prehospital care provider can identify changes.

The other three "classic" signs of compartment syndrome—pulselessness, pallor, and paralysis—are late findings and indicate a clear compartment syndrome and a limb in jeopardy of muscle death (necrosis). Pulselessness is a relatively uncommon finding because it indicates either the presence of a vascular injury, which is less common than a fracture, or that pressure in the compartment that contains the blood vessel in question has exceeded systolic pressure, which is a very late complication. Compartments may also be extremely tense and firm to palpation, although it is difficult to judge the compartment pressures by physical examination alone.

Management

In the hospital, compartment pressures are measured in extremities in which compartment syndrome is suspected. Compartment syndrome can be definitively managed only in the hospital. In the hospital, compartment syndrome is managed with surgical intervention (*fasciotomy*), with an incision through the skin and fascia into the affected compartments to decompress the compartment syndrome.

Only basic maneuvers can be attempted in the field. Any tightly applied splint or dressings should be removed and distal perfusion reassessed. Because compartment syndrome may develop during a long-distance transfer, serial examinations are essential for early identification of this problem.

Crush Syndrome

Crush syndrome, also known as **traumatic rhabdomyolysis**, is a clinical entity characterized by renal failure and death after severe muscle trauma. Crush syndrome was first described in World War I in German soldiers rescued from collapsed trenches, then again in World War II in patients rescued from collapsed buildings during the London Blitz. In World War II, crush syndrome had a mortality rate in excess of 90%. During the Korean War, mortality was 84%, but after the advent of hemodialysis, mortality decreased to 53%. In the Vietnam War, the mortality rate was approximately the same at 50%.

The importance of crush syndrome, however, should not be limited to historical or military interest. Approximately 3% to 20% of the survivors of earthquakes have sustained a crush injury, and approximately 40% of survivors from collapsed buildings will have crush injuries.[19,20] In 1978, an earthquake near Beijing, China, injured more than 350,000 persons, with 242,769 deaths. More than 48,000 of these people died from crush syndrome. More commonly, mechanisms of crush syndrome include entrapment from a trench collapse, construction collapse, or motor vehicle collision.

Crush syndrome arises from a crushing-type injury to large muscle masses, commonly involving the thigh or calf. It occurs when destruction of muscle releases the molecule known as myoglobin. **Myoglobin** is a protein found in muscle cells that is responsible for giving meat its characteristic red color. The function of myoglobin in muscle tissue is to serve as an intracellular storage site for oxygen. When myoglobin is released from damaged muscle, however, it is capable of causing damage to the kidneys, leading to acute renal failure.

Patients with crush syndrome are identified by the following:

- Prolonged entrapment
- Traumatic injury to muscle mass
- Compromised circulation to the injured area

Traumatic injury to the muscle causes release of not only myoglobin but also potassium. Once the patient has been extricated, the affected limb suddenly becomes reperfused with new blood; at the same time, the old blood with elevated levels of myoglobin and potassium is washed out of the injured area and into the rest of the body. Elevated potassium can result in life-threatening cardiac dysrhythmias, and free myoglobin will produce tea- or cola-colored urine and will eventually result in renal failure.

Of note, traumatic rhabdomyolysis can also occur in patients, often the elderly, who fall, perhaps fracture a hip, and are unable to get up or patients who fall in a bathroom and become wedged next to the bathtub and toilet. They are found hours or days later, having lain in the same position, often on a hard surface. The weight of their body on the muscles for a prolonged period of time leads to muscle breakdown and the findings of traumatic rhabdomyolysis.

Management

The key in improving outcomes in crush syndrome is early and aggressive fluid resuscitation. It is important for the prehospital care provider to remember that toxins are accumulating within the entrapped limb during the extrication process. Once the entrapped limb is freed, the accumulated toxins wash into the central circulation, similar to a bolus of poison. Therefore, success will depend on minimizing the toxic effects of accumulated myoglobin and potassium before release of the limb. Resuscitation needs to occur before extrication.[21] A delay in fluid resuscitation will result in renal failure in 50% of the patients, and a delay of 12 hours or more produces renal failure in almost 100% of the patients. Some authors have advocated that final extrication be delayed until the patient has been adequately resuscitated.[22] A poorly resuscitated patient may go into cardiac arrest during extrication because of the sudden release of metabolic acid and potassium into the bloodstream when the compression on the extremity is released.[23]

Fluid resuscitation should proceed with normal saline at a rate of up to 1,500 ml per hour to ensure adequate renal output of 150 to 200 ml per hour. LR solution is avoided until urine output is adequate because of the presence of potassium in the IV fluid. The addition of 50 milliequivalents (mEq) of sodium bicarbonate and 10 grams of mannitol to each liter of fluid used during the extrication period may help decrease the incidence of renal failure. Once the patient has been extricated, the normal saline fluids can be slowed to 500 ml per hour, alternating with 5% dextrose in water (D_5W), with one ampule of sodium bicarbonate per liter.[24]

Once the blood pressure is stabilized and volume status restored, attention is turned toward prophylaxis against **hyperkalemia** and the toxic effects of serum myoglobin. Hyperkalemia in the field will be recognized by the development of peaked T waves on the cardiac monitor. Treatment of the increased potassium follows standard protocols for hyperkalemia, including IV sodium bicarbonate administration, inhaled beta-agonists (albuterol), administration of dextrose and insulin (if available), and, if life-threatening cardiac dysrhythmias occur, IV calcium chloride. Alkalinization of the urine will provide some degree of protection to the kidneys; however, the key is to maintain increased urine output (typically in the range of 50 to 100 ml/hr).

Mangled Extremity

A "mangled extremity" refers to a complex injury resulting from high-energy transfer in which significant injury occurs to two or more of the following: (1) skin and muscle, (2) tendons, (3) bone, (4) blood vessels, and (5) nerves (**Figure 14-20**). Common mechanisms producing mangled extremities include motorcycle crash, ejection from a motor vehicle crash, and a pedestrian being struck by an automobile. When encountered, patients may be in shock from either external blood loss or hemorrhage from associated injuries, which are common because

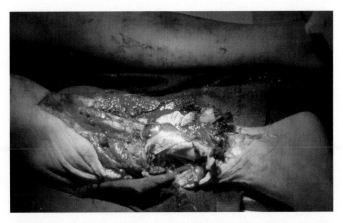

Figure 14-20 Mangled extremity resulting from crushing injury between two vehicles. The patient has fractures and extensive soft-tissue injury.
Source: Courtesy of Peter T. Pons, MD, FACEP.

of the high-energy mechanism. Most mangled extremities involve severe open fractures, and amputation may be necessary in 50% to 75% of patients. Limb salvage is possible in some patients, typically involving six to eight procedures, and success often depends on the experience of the trauma and orthopedic surgeons.

Management

Even with a mangled extremity, the focus is still on the primary assessment to rule out or address life-threatening conditions. Hemorrhage control, including the use of a tourniquet, may be required. The mangled extremity should be splinted, if the patient's condition allows. These patients are probably best cared for at high-volume, level I trauma centers.

Sprains

A **sprain** is an injury in which ligaments are stretched or torn. Sprains are caused by a sudden twisting of the joint beyond its normal range of motion. They are characterized by significant pain, swelling, and possible hematoma. Externally, sprains may resemble a fracture or dislocation. Definitive differentiation between a sprain and a fracture is accomplished only through a radiographic study. In the prehospital setting, it is reasonable to splint a suspected sprain in case it turns out to be a fracture or dislocation. An ice or cold pack may help relieve pain, as well as use of narcotic pain medication.

Management

The general management for suspected extremity injury includes the following steps:

1. Identify and treat any and all life-threatening injuries found in the primary assessment.

2. Stop any external bleeding and treat the patient for shock.
3. Evaluate for distal neurovascular function.
4. Support the area of injury.
5. Immobilize the injured extremity, including the joint above and the joint below the injury site.
6. Re-evaluate the injured extremity after immobilization for changes in distal neurovascular function.
7. Provide pain management as appropriate.

Prolonged Transport

Patients with extremity trauma often have coexisting injuries. Ongoing internal blood loss may be from abdominal or thoracic injuries, and during a prolonged transport, the primary assessment will need to be reassessed frequently to ensure that all life-threatening conditions are identified and no new ones have emerged. Vital signs should be obtained at regular intervals. Intravenous crystalloid solutions should be administered at a rate to maintain adequate perfusion, unless significant internal hemorrhage is suspected in the pelvis, abdomen, or thorax.

During long transports, the prehospital care provider needs to focus greater attention on extremity perfusion. In limbs with compromised vascular supply, the prehospital care provider can attempt to restore normal anatomic positioning to optimize the chance for improved blood flow.

Similarly, dislocation with impaired distal circulation should be considered for reduction in the field. Distal perfusion, including pulses, color, and temperature, as well as motor and sensory function, should be examined in a serial manner. Compartments should be palpated for the development of potential compartment syndromes.

Measures to ensure patient comfort should be taken. Splinting devices should be comfortable and well padded. The limbs should be assessed for any potential points inside the splint where pressure could contribute to the creation of an ulcer, especially in an extremity with compromised perfusion. Parenteral narcotic analgesia should be given at regular intervals, with monitoring of ventilatory rate, blood pressure, pulse oximetry, and capnography, if available. If properly trained personnel are present, nerve blocks may be particularly comforting to the patient, such as a femoral nerve block for a midshaft femoral fracture.

Contaminated wounds should be flushed with normal saline irrigation so that gross particulate matter (e.g., soil, grass) is removed. If the transport will take longer than 120 minutes, and if protocols allow and appropriate personnel are present, antibiotics may be administered for patients with open fractures. A first-generation cephalosporin, cefazolin, is sufficient for minor open fractures, whereas a broader-spectrum agent, such as cefoxitin, might be administered for a more serious open fracture. If a body part has been amputated, it should also be periodically assessed so that it remains cool but does not freeze or become macerated (softened) by soaking in water.

Summary

- In patients with multisystem trauma, attention is directed toward the primary assessment and the identification and management of all life-threatening injuries, including internal or external hemorrhage in the extremities.
- Prehospital care providers must be careful not to be distracted from addressing life-threatening conditions by the gross, dramatic appearance of any noncritical injuries or by the patient's request for their management.
- Once the patient has been fully assessed and found to have only isolated injuries without systemic implication, those noncritical injuries should be addressed.
- Musculoskeletal injuries, in the order of their threat to life, should be immobilized in order to prevent further injury and provide comfort as well as some relief from pain.
- When the mechanism of injury indicates sudden, violent changes in motion, multisystem trauma, or spinal trauma, potential systemic decline needs to be anticipated and the patient's age, physical condition, and medical history included in the evaluation.

SCENARIO RECAP

It is a beautiful Saturday afternoon in June. You have been dispatched to a local motorcycle racetrack for a rider who has been injured. Upon arrival, you are escorted by track officials to an area on the track just in front of the grandstand where the track's medical crew (two-person, emergency medical responders, nontransport) is attending to a single patient lying supine on the track.

One of the emergency medical responders tells you that the patient was a rider in a 350-cc class race with 14 other motorcycles when 3 of them collided in front of the grandstand. The other two riders were not injured, but the patient was unable to stand or move without significant pain in his right leg and pelvis. There was no loss of consciousness and no other complaints besides his leg pain. The medical crew has maintained the patient in a supine position with manual stabilization of the right lower extremity.

As you assess the patient, you find that he is a 19-year-old man, conscious and alert without past medical or trauma history. The patient's initial vital signs are as follows: Blood pressure is 104/68 mm Hg, pulse is 112 beats/minute, respirations are 24 breaths/minute, and skin is pale and diaphoretic. The patient states that he collided with another rider when he came out of a corner and fell down. He states his right leg was run over by at least one other bike. Visual inspection of his right leg reveals shortening of the leg when compared to the left side, with tenderness and bruising of the mid-anterior thigh area.

- What do the kinematics of this event tell you about the potential injuries for this patient?
- What type of injury does this patient have and what would your management priorities be?

SCENARIO SOLUTION

With your partner's help, you were able to apply a traction splint to the midshaft femur fracture of the right leg. After securing your patient to the backboard, you were able to move the patient to the ambulance for transport to the hospital. Once in the ambulance, oxygen via mask was administered and an IV was established. The patient stated that after the splint was applied, his pain improved significantly and that he did not need any analgesic at the moment. The patient's vital signs remained unchanged throughout the transport.

References

1. Williams B, Boyle M. Estimation of external blood loss by paramedics: is there any point? *Prehosp Disaster Med.* 2007;22(6):502–506.
2. Beekley AC, Sebesta JA, Blackbourne LH, et al. Prehospital tourniquet use in Operation Iraqi Freedom: effect on hemorrhage control and outcomes. *J Trauma.* 2008;64:S28–S37.
3. Dorlac WC, DeBakey ME, Holcomb JB, et al. Mortality from isolated civilian penetrating extremity injury. *J Trauma.* 2005;59:217–222.
4. Kragh JF, Walters TJ, Baer DG, et al. Practical use of emergency tourniquets to stop bleeding in major limb trauma. *J Trauma.* 2008;64:S38–S50.
5. Kragh JF, Walters TF, Baer DG, et al. Survival with emergency tourniquet use to stop bleeding in major limb trauma. *Ann Surg.* 2009;249:1–7.
6. Kragh JF, Littrel ML, Jones JA, et al. Battle casualty survival with emergency tourniquet use to stop limb bleeding. *J Emerg Med.* 2011;41(6):590–597.
7. Wood SP, Vrahas M, Wedel S. Femur fracture immobilization with traction splints in multisystem trauma patients. *Prehosp Emerg Care.* 2003;7:241.
8. Alonso-Serra HM, Wesley K. Prehospital pain management. *Prehosp Emerg Care.* 2003;7:842.
9. Hatlestad D. Capnography in sedation and pain management. *J Emerg Med Serv.* 2005;34:65.
10. Galinski M, Dolveck F, Borron SW, et al. A randomized, double-blind study comparing morphine with fentanyl in prehospital analgesia. *Am J Emerg Med.* 2005;23:114.
11. Schmid RL, Sandler AN, Katz J. Use and efficacy of low-dose ketamine in the management of acute postoperative pain: a review of current techniques and outcomes. *Pain.* 1999;82:111–125.
12. Green SM, Roback MG, Kennedy RM, Krauss B. Clinical practice guideline for emergency department dissociative sedation: 2011 update. *Ann Emerg Med.* 2011;57:449–461.
13. Drayna PC, Estrada C, Wang W, Saville BR, Arnold DH. Ketamine sedation is not associated with clinically meaningful elevation of intraocular pressure. *Am J Emerg Med.* 2012;30:1215–1218.
14. Halstead S, Deakyne S, Bajaj L, et al. The effect of ketamine on intraocular pressure in pediatric patients during procedural sedation. *Acad Emerg Med.* 2012;19:1145–1150.
15. Bredmose PP, Lockey DJ, Grier G, et al. Pre-hospital use of ketamine for analgesia and procedural sedation. *Emerg Med J.* 2009;26:62–64.
16. Sibley A, Mackenzie M, Bawden J, et al. A prospective review of the use of ketamine to facilitate endotracheal intubation in the helicopter emergency medical services (HEMS) setting. *Emerg Med J.* 2011;28:521–525.

17. Seyfer AE, American College of Surgeons (ACS) Committee on Trauma. *Guidelines for Management of Amputated Parts.* Chicago, IL: ACS; 1996.

18. Sharp CF, Mangram AJ, Lorenzo M, Dunn EL. A major metropolitan "field amputation" team: a call to arms... and legs. *J Trauma.* 2009;67(6):1158–1161.

19. Pepe E, Mosesso VN, Falk JL. Prehospital fluid resuscitation of the patient with major trauma. *Prehosp Emerg Care.* 2002;6:81.

20. Better OS. Management of shock and acute renal failure in casualties suffering from crush syndrome. *Ren Fail.* 1997;19:647.

21. Michaelson M, Taitelman U, Bshouty Z, et al. Crush syndrome: experience from the Lebanon war, 1982. *Isr J Med Sci.* 1984;20:305.

22. Pretto EA, Angus D, Abrams J, et al. An analysis of prehospital mortality in an earthquake. *Prehosp Disaster Med.* 1994;9:107.

23. Collins AJ, Burzstein S. Renal failure in disasters. *Crit Care Clin.* 1991;7:421.

24. Sever MS, Vanholder R, Lameire N. Management of crush-related injuries after disasters. *N Engl J Med.* 2006;354:1052.

Suggested Reading

American College of Surgeons (ACS) Committee on Trauma. Musculoskeletal trauma. In: ACS Committee on Trauma. *Advanced Trauma Life Support.* 9th ed. Chicago, IL: ACS; 2012:206-229.

Ashkenazi I, Isakovich B, Kluger Y, et al. Prehospital management of earthquake casualties buried under rubble. *Prehosp Disast Med.* 2005;20:122.

Coppola PT, Coppola M. Emergency department evaluation and treatment of pelvic fractures. *Emerg Med Clin North Am.* 2003;18(1):1.

SPECIFIC SKILLS

Traction Splint for Femur Fractures

Principle: To immobilize femur fractures to minimize ongoing internal thigh hemorrhage.

This type of immobilization is used for fractures of the shaft of the femur. The application of traction and immobilization helps to reduce muscle spasm and pain while, at the same time, decreasing the potential for the fractured ends of the bone to produce additional damage and increased bleeding. Traction splints should be applied only if the patient's condition is stable and time permits. Traction splints should not be used if there are associated fractures or injuries to the knee or tibia. The Hare traction splint is shown for illustrative purposes. Other traction splints, such as the Sager traction splint, may be used in accordance with local protocol and policy.

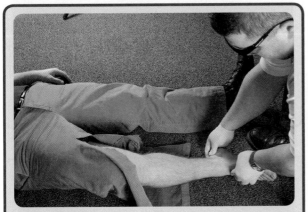

1 The prehospital care provider exposes the leg and assesses the patient's neurovascular status both before and after any manipulation. The prehospital care provider explains to the patient what is going to happen and then performs the action..

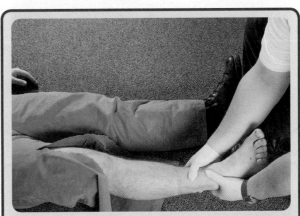

2 If the fractured extremity has marked deformity, the second prehospital care provider grasps the ankle and foot and applies gentle traction to straighten out the fracture and restore the patient's leg to length.

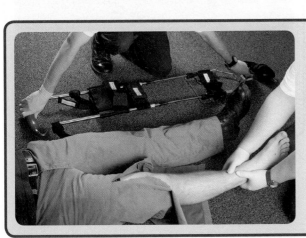

3 The splint is measured against the uninjured leg and adjusted to the appropriate length (approximately 8 to 10 inches [20 to 25 cm] beyond the heel of the leg).

Traction Splint for Femur Fractures (continued)

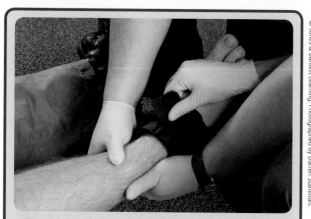

4 The ankle strap is applied to the injured leg. The strap may be used to maintain traction as necessary.

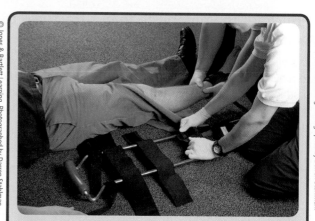

5 All Velcro securing straps are opened.

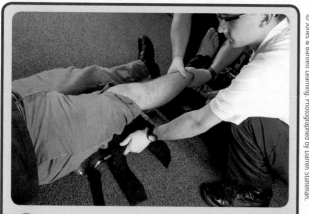

6 The patient's leg is elevated and the proximal end of the traction splint is seated against the ischial tuberosity of the pelvis.

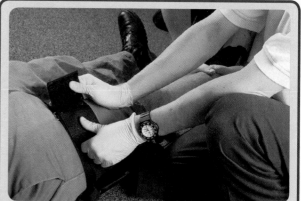

7 The prehospital care provider applies the proximal (pubic) strap around the proximal thigh to secure it in place.

Traction Splint for Femur Fractures (continued)

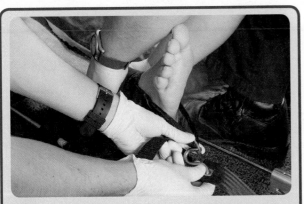

8 The ankle strap is attached to the traction hitch at the distal end of the splint.

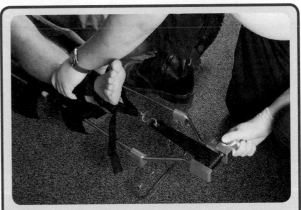

9 While maintaining manual traction, the prehospital care provider slowly turns the traction hitch mechanism to take over the traction function. Once the patient's leg has been restored to the same length as the uninjured leg, the prehospital care provider stops turning the traction hitch mechanism.

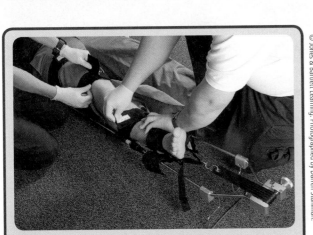

10 The prehospital care provider applies all remaining Velcro straps to secure the leg to the traction splint.

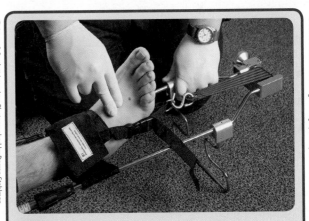

11 The prehospital care provider reassesses the patient's neurovascular status.

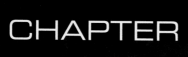

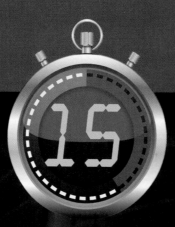

CHAPTER 15

Burn Injuries

CHAPTER OBJECTIVES

At the completion of this chapter, the reader will be able to do the following:

- Define various depths of burns.

- Describe the zones of burn injuries.

- Explain how ice can deepen the depth of burns.

- Estimate burn size using the rule of nines.

- Calculate fluid resuscitation using the Parkland formula

- Calculate fluid resuscitation using the Rule of Ten.

- Describe the additional fluid needs in pediatric patients with burns.

- Describe appropriate burn dressings for prehospital care.

- Explain the unique concerns of electrical injuries.

- Relate the management concerns in patients with circumferential burns.

- Describe the three elements of smoke inhalation.

- Apply the principles of zones of control for scene management in hazardous materials scenes.

- Discuss the criteria for the transfer of patients to burn centers.

SCENARIO

You are called to a residential structure fire. When your unit arrives, you witness a two-story house that is fully involved with fire and thick black smoke pouring out of the roof and windows. You are directed to a victim who is being cared for by emergency medical responders (EMRs). They tell you that the patient re-entered the burning building in an attempt to rescue his dog, and he was carried out unconscious by fire fighters.

Your patient is a man who appears to be in his thirties. The majority of his clothes have been burned off. He has obvious burns to his face, and his hair has been singed. He is unconscious; he is breathing spontaneously, but with snoring respirations. The EMRs have placed the patient on high-flow oxygen with a nonrebreather mask. On physical examination, his airway is patent with manual assistance (jaw thrust); he ventilates easily. The sleeves of his shirt have been burned off. His arms have circumferential burns, but his radial pulse is easily palpable. His heart rate is 118 beats/minute, blood pressure is 148/94 mm Hg, ventilatory rate is 22 breaths/minute, and oxygen saturation (Spo$_2$), taken by pulse oximeter, is 92%. On physical examination, you determine that the patient is burned on his entire head and has blistering of the anterior chest and abdomen, along with full-thickness burns of his entire right and left arm and hand.

- What is the extent of burns for this patient?
- What are the initial steps for managing this patient?
- How does the prehospital care provider recognize an inhalation injury?

Introduction

Many people consider burns to be the most frightening and dreaded of all injuries. In the course of our daily lives, we have all sustained a burn of some degree and have experienced the intense pain and anxiety associated with even a small burn. Burns are common in industrialized and agricultural societies and in civilian and military settings. Burns can range from small to catastrophic injuries covering large regions of the body. Regardless of size, all burns are serious. Even minor burns can result in serious disability.

Burns result from a variety of sources. While the most common etiology of burn injury is thermal, from fire or scald, other causes include chemical, electrical, and radiation exposure. Consideration of the etiology of burns will prevent the rescuer from exposing himself or herself to the burn source and sustaining unnecessary injury, as well as provide optimal care for the victim.

A common misconception is that burns are injuries isolated to the skin only. On the contrary, large burns can be extensive, multisystem injuries capable of life-threatening effects involving the heart, lungs, kidneys, gastrointestinal (GI) tract, and immune system. The most common cause of death in a fire victim is not from the direct complications of the burn wound, but from complications of respiratory failure.

Although considered a form of trauma, burns have some significant differences from other types of trauma that merit consideration. After a trauma, such as a motor vehicle crash or a fall, the victim's physiologic response is to initiate several adaptive mechanisms to preserve life. These responses can include the shunting of blood from the periphery of the body to vital organs,

increase in cardiac output, and increase in production of various protective serum proteins. In contrast, after a burn, the patient's body essentially attempts to shut down, go into shock, and die. A substantial portion of initial burn care is directed at reversal of this initial shock. In patients who have traumatic injuries as well as burns, actual mortality of these combined injuries is much greater than the combined predicted mortality of each injury individually.

Smoke inhalation is a life-threatening injury that is often more dangerous to the patient than the burn injury itself. Inhalation of toxic fumes from smoke is a greater predictor of burn mortality than the age of the patient or the size of the burn.[1] A victim does not need to inhale a large quantity of smoke to experience a severe injury. Often, life-threatening complications from smoke inhalation may not manifest for several days.

The circumstances in which the burn occurred should be considered, because a large percentage of burns in both children and adults result from an intentional injury. Approximately 20% of all burn victims are children, and 20% of these children are the victims of intentional injury or child abuse.[2,3] Most health care providers are surprised to learn that, of the forms of physical violence inflicted on children, intentional burn injury is second only to beating. Burns as a form of abuse are not limited to children. It is common to see women burned in cases of domestic violence, as well as elderly persons in cases of elder abuse.

Anatomy of Skin

Skin serves several complex functions, including protection from the external environment, regulation of fluids, thermoregulation, sensation, and metabolic adaptation (**Figure 15-1**).

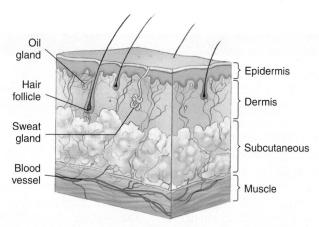

Figure 15-1 Normal skin. The skin in composed of three tissue layers—epidermis, dermis, and subcutaneous layer—and associated muscle. Some layers contain structures such as glands, hair follicles, blood vessels, and nerves. All these structures are interrelated to the maintenance, loss, and gain or body temperature.

The skin covers about 1.5 to 2.0 square meters in the average adult. It is made up of three layers—the **epidermis**, the **dermis**, and the **subcutaneous (or hypodermis) layer**. The outer *epidermis* is about 0.05 millimeters (mm) thick in areas such as the eyelids and can be as thick as 1 mm on the sole of the foot. The deeper *dermis* is on average 10 times thicker than the epidermis. The subcutaneous layer, or hypodermis, is made up of adipose (fat) and connective tissue that helps keep the outer layers of the skin attached to the underlying structures. The subcutaneous layer also contains some of the larger blood vessels and nerves.

The skin of males is thicker than the skin of females, and the skin of children and elderly persons is thinner than that of the average adult. These facts explain why one individual can sustain burns of varying depths from exposure to a singular burning agent, why a child might experience a deep burn while an adult with the same exposure has only a superficial injury, or why an elderly person will sustain a deeper burn than a younger adult.

Burn Characteristics

The creation of a burn is similar to frying an egg. When you break an egg into a hot skillet, the egg is initially liquid and transparent. As the egg is exposed to the high temperatures, it rapidly becomes opaque and solidifies. A virtually identical process occurs when a patient is burned. In the case of the egg, the proteins of the egg break down and change shape and are destroyed in a process known as *denaturation*. When a patient is injured by burning, the elevated or freezing temperature, radiation, or chemical agent causes the proteins in the skin to be severely damaged, resulting in protein denaturation.

Injury to the skin can occur in two phases: immediate and delayed. The damage that occurs at the moment of exposure to the burning source is immediate, whereas delayed injury results from inadequate resuscitation, inappropriate treatment

such as application of ice, and progression of the burn. Skin is capable of tolerating temperatures of 40°C (104°F) for brief periods. However, once temperatures exceed this point, there is a *logarithmic* increase in the magnitude of tissue destruction.[4]

A full-thickness burn, also known as a third-degree burn, has three zones of tissue injury that form essentially concentric circles[5] (**Figure 15-2**). The central zone is known as the **zone of coagulation**, and this is the region of greatest tissue destruction. The tissue in this zone is *necrotic* (dead) and is not capable of tissue repair.

Adjacent to the zone of necrosis is a region of lesser injury. This zone is referred to as the **zone of stasis** because immediately after injury, the blood flow to this region is stagnant. The cells in this zone are injured, but not irreversibly. If they are subsequently deprived of the delivery of oxygen or blood flow, these viable cells will die and become necrotic. Timely and appropriate burn care will preserve blood flow and oxygen delivery to these injured cells. Resuscitation of the patient will eliminate this stasis and re-establish delivery of oxygen to the injured and susceptible cells. Failure to resuscitate the patient appropriately results in death of the cells in the injured tissue, and a partial-thickness burn then converts to a full-thickness burn.

Consider for a moment a patient who is suffering from myocardial ischemia or a cerebrovascular accident. A decrease in blood flow deprives the tissues of the heart or brain of the oxygen necessary for cellular survival. In the model of a burn injury, the tissues of the zone of stasis are also afflicted with inadequate oxygen delivery. Deprived of blood flow and oxygen delivery for too long, the tissue will die; if blood flow is preserved or re-established, the vulnerable tissue in the zone of stasis will remain viable.

A common error that results in damage to the zone of stasis is the application of ice by a well-meaning bystander or prehospital care provider. When ice is applied to the skin in an effort to stop the burning process, the ice causes vasoconstriction, preventing re-establishment of blood flow that is needed to minimize the resulting burn injury. It is argued that when ice is applied to a burn the patient will experience some reduction in pain; however, the *analgesia* (pain relief) will be at the expense of additional tissue destruction. For these reasons, ice should be withheld and any ongoing burning should be arrested with the use of ambient

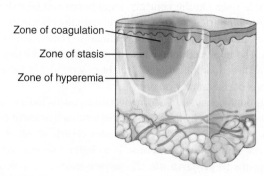

Figure 15-2 Three zones of burn injury.

or room-temperature water, and analgesia should be provided with oral or *parenteral* (all other routes) medications.

The outermost zone is known as the **zone of hyperemia**. This zone has minimal cellular injury and is characterized by increased blood flow secondary to an inflammatory reaction initiated by the burn injury.

Burn Depth

Estimation of burn depth can be deceptively difficult to even the most experienced prehospital care provider. Often, a burn that appears to be **partial thickness** (second degree) will prove to be **full thickness** (third degree) in 24 to 48 hours. The surface of a burn may appear to be partial thickness at first glance, but later, on **debridement** in the hospital, the superficial epidermis separates, revealing a white, full-thickness burn **eschar** underneath. Because the burn may evolve over time, it is often wise to withhold final judgment of burn depth for up to 48 hours after injury. Often it is best simply to tell patients that the injury is either superficial or deep and that time is required to determine ultimate burn depth. Furthermore, the prehospital care provider should never attempt to estimate burn depth until attempts have been made to initially debride the wound in the hospital.

Superficial Burns

Superficial burns, historically referred to as *first-degree* burns, involve only the epidermis and are characterized as red and painful (**Figure 15-3**). These burns are rarely clinically significant, with the exception of large areas of sunburn, which expose the patient to significant pain and risk of dehydration without attention to appropriate oral hydration, especially in young children or the elderly. These wounds heal typically within a week, and the patients will not scar. Burns of this depth are not included when calculating the percentage of total body surface area that is burned or used for fluid administration.

Partial-Thickness Burns

Partial-thickness burns, once referred to as *second-degree burns*, are those that involve the epidermis and varying portions of the underlying dermis (**Figure 15-4**). They can be further classified as

either *superficial* or *deep*. Partial-thickness burns will appear as blisters (**Figure 15-5**) or as **denuded** burned areas with a glistening or wet-appearing base. These wounds are painful. Because remnants of the dermis survive, these burns can often heal in 2 to 3 weeks.

In partial-thickness burns, the zone of necrosis involves the entire epidermis and varying depths of the superficial dermis. If not well cared for, the zone of stasis in these injuries can progress to necrosis, making these burns

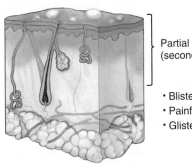

Partial thickness (second degree)

• Blistering
• Painful
• Glistening wound bed

Figure 15-4 Partial-thickness burn.

Figure 15-5 Blisters

Much discussion has been generated about blisters, including whether or not to open and debride them and how to approach the blister associated with partial-thickness burns. A blister occurs when the epidermis separates from the underlying dermis and fluid that is leaking from nearby vessels fills the space between the layers. The presence of *osmotically active* proteins in the blister fluid draws additional fluid into the blister space, causing the blister to continue to enlarge. As the blister enlarges, it creates pressure on the injured tissue of the wound bed, which increases the patient's pain.

Many think that the skin of the blister acts as a dressing and prevents contamination of the wound. However, the skin of the blister is not normal and, therefore, cannot serve as a protective barrier. Additionally, maintaining the blister intact prevents application of topical antibiotics directly on the injury. For these reasons, most burn specialists open and debride blisters after arrival of the patient to the hospital.[6]

In the prehospital setting, blisters are generally best left alone during the relatively short transport time—in most cases, to the hospital where the burn injury can be managed in a cleaner environment. Blisters that have already ruptured should be covered with a clean, dry dressing.

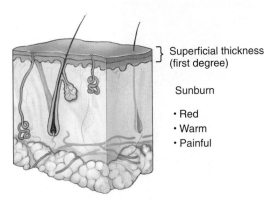

Superficial thickness (first degree)

Sunburn

• Red
• Warm
• Painful

Figure 15-3 Superficial burn.

larger and perhaps converting the wound to a full-thickness burn. A superficial partial-thickness burn will heal with vigilant wound care. Deep partial-thickness burns often require surgery in order to minimize scarring and prevent functional deformities of high-function areas such as the hands.

Full-Thickness Burns

Full-thickness burns may have several appearances (**Figure 15-6**). Most often these wounds will appear as thick, dry, white, leathery burns, regardless of race or skin color (**Figure 15-7**). This thick leathery damaged skin is referred to as eschar. In severe cases, the skin will have a charred appearance with visible *thrombosis* (clotting) of blood vessels (**Figure 15-8**). This burn injury has, in the past, also been called third degree.

There is a common misconception that full-thickness burns are pain free, owing to the fact that the injury destroys the nerve endings in the burned tissue. Patients with these burns have varying degrees of pain. Full-thickness burns are typically surrounded by areas of partial- and superficial-thickness burns. The nerves in these areas are intact and continue to transmit pain sensations from the damaged tissues. Burns of this depth can be disabling and life threatening. Prompt surgical excision and intensive rehabilitation at a specialized center are required.

Fourth-Degree Burns

Fourth-degree burns are those that not only burn all layers of the skin, but also burn underlying fat, muscles, bone, or internal organs (**Figures 15-9** and **15-10**). Although the descriptive terminology used for classifying burns does not include a formal name for these burns and the "fourth-degree" burn terminology persists, these burns are, in fact, full-thickness burns with deep tissue damage. These burns can be extremely debilitating and disfiguring as a result of the damage done to the skin and underlying tissues and structures. Significant debridement of dead and **devitalized** tissue may result in extensive soft-tissue defects.

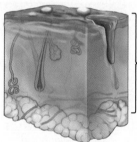

Full thickness
(third degree)

- Leathery
- White to charred
- Dead tissue
- Victims will have pain from burned areas adjacent to the full-thickness burn.

Figure 15-6   Full-thickness burn.

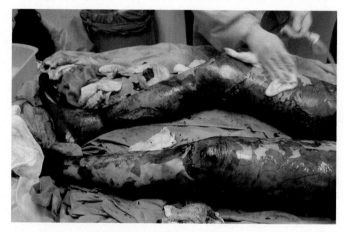

Figure 15-8   Example of deep, full-thickness burn with charring of the skin and visible thrombosis of blood vessels.
Source: Courtesy of Jeffrey Guy, MD.

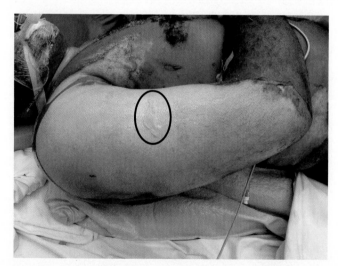

Figure 15-7   This patient has suffered from partial-thickness and a full-thickness burn, characterized as white and leathery in appearance.
Source: Courtesy of Jeffrey Guy, MD.

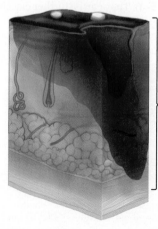

Fourth Degree
(full-thickness with deep tissue damage)

Figure 15-9   Fourth-degree burn.

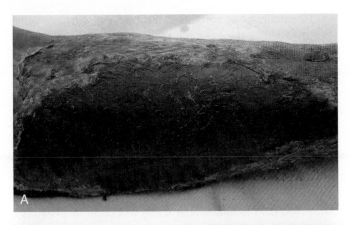

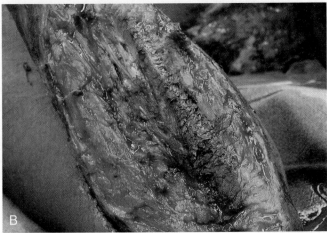

Figure 15-10 Fourth-degree burns to the arm, with burns not only to the skin but also to the subcutaneous fat, muscle, and bone.
Source: Courtesy of Jeffrey Guy, MD.

Burn Assessment
Primary Assessment and Resuscitation

The goal of the primary assessment is to systematically evaluate and treat life-threatening disorders in order of importance to preserve life. The ABCDE (airway, breathing, circulation, disability, and expose) method of trauma care applies to the management of the burn patient, although burn patients provide unique challenges in every step of the resuscitation.

Major burns are often a very lethal injury. However, aside from burn-related compromise of the airway or breathing, burns by themselves are not typically an immediately life-threatening injury. The overall appearance of the burns can be dramatic and even grotesque. The sophisticated prehospital care provider will be mindful that the patient may also have suffered from a mechanical trauma and have less apparent, internal injuries that pose a more immediate life threat.

Airway

Preserving the airway's patency is the highest priority in caring for a burn victim. The heat from the fire can cause edema of the airway above the level of the vocal cords and can occlude the airway. Therefore, careful initial, as well as continuous, evaluation is required. It is a mistake to believe that once the prehospital care provider has completed the assessment of the ABCs that step in the patient assessment process is complete and all is well with the patient's airway. Prehospital care providers who are likely to experience prolonged transport times need to be particularly vigilant about airway assessment. For example, a burned patient may have a patent airway on the initial airway evaluation. In the time that follows, the face, as well as the airway, will likely swell. As a result, an airway that was satisfactory initially may become critically narrowed or obstructed by edema 30 to 60 minutes later. The airway can narrow to such a degree that it becomes obstructed and air cannot pass.

A more likely scenario is related to the physiologic effect of a narrowed, but not obstructed, airway. Narrowing of the trachea from swelling of the mucosa increases resistance to the inflow of air during inhalation. An increase in airway resistance produces an increase in the work of breathing for the patient. An increase in the work of breathing from a swollen airway can contribute to or produce respiratory arrest even when the patient has a patent airway.

To avoid catastrophic airway narrowing or occlusion, early control of the airway is prudent. Intubation of these patients is often difficult and hazardous because of the distorted anatomy. Repeated, unsuccessful attempts to intubate a patient will lead to further increase in the amount of swelling present and distortion of the anatomy.

Another method of intubation often considered in these cases is rapid sequence induction or rapid sequence intubation. This procedure uses pharmacologic agents to sedate and paralyze the patient for airway management. If the prehospital care provider feels that the injury is significant enough, he or she can utilize this procedure to secure the airway, or the provider can request a team that is capable of this procedure for an assessment and implementation. However, pharmacologic interventions will suppress or completely obliterate the patient's ability to manage the airway, and if intubation is unsuccessful, alternate methods of securing a patent airway must be prepared in advance.

Often, patients with burns are the individuals best suited to manage their own airway by assuming a position that maintains an open airway and allows for comfortable respiration. In those instances in which intervention is required, the airway should be managed by the most experienced prehospital care provider available.

If the patient is intubated, special precautions must be taken when securing the endotracheal (ET) tube and preventing inadvertent dislodgement or extubation. Following facial burns, the skin of the face will often peel or weep fluid, rendering adhesive tapes not suitable for securing the ET tube (**Figure 15-11**). The ET tube can be secured using two umbilical tapes or pieces of intravenous (IV) tubing wrapped around the head. One piece should be draped over the ear and the second under the ear (Figure 15-11). Commercially available cloth and Velcro devices are also suitable.

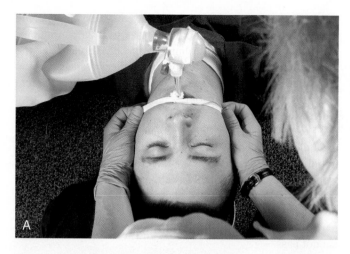

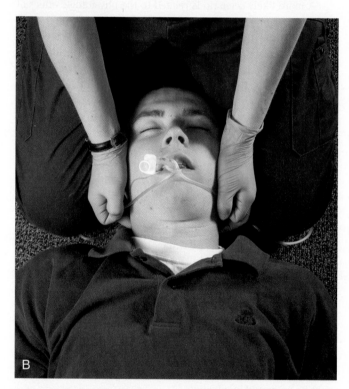

Figure 15-11 Prehospital care providers can use umbilical tape or IV tubing to secure an ET tube if the patient has burns to the face. **A.** Umbilical tape. **B.** IV tubing.

Source: © Jones & Bartlett Learning. Photographed by Darren Stahlman.

Breathing

As with any trauma patient, breathing can be adversely affected by such problems as fractured ribs, pneumothoraces, and other closed or open chest wounds. In the event of a circumferential chest wall burn, the chest wall compliance progressively decreases to such an extent that it inhibits the patient's ability to inhale. Following a burn injury, the burned skin will start to harden and contract while the deeper, soft tissues will simultaneously swell. The net result is that the burns constrict the chest wall similarly to having several leather belts progressively tightening around the patient's chest. As time progresses, the patient cannot move the chest wall to breathe.

When attempting to ventilate patients with circumferential chest wall burns, the bag-mask device may become difficult or impossible to compress. In such cases, prompt escharotomies of the chest wall will allow re-establishment of ventilation. An **escharotomy** is a surgical procedure that involves making an incision through the hardened burn eschar, allowing the burn and chest to expand and move with the patient's respiratory movements.

Circulation

Evaluation and management of circulation includes the measurement of blood pressure, evaluation of circumferential burns (see the Circumferential Burns section in this chapter), and establishment of IV catheters. Accurate measurement of blood pressure becomes difficult or impossible with burns to the extremities, and if a blood pressure can be obtained, it may not correctly reflect systemic arterial blood pressure because of full-thickness burns and edema of the extremities. Even if the patient has adequate arterial blood pressure, distal limb perfusion may be critically reduced because of circumferential injuries. Burned extremities should be elevated during transport to reduce the degree of swelling in the affected limb.

Establishment of two large-bore IV catheters capable of the rapid flow rate needed for large-volume resuscitation is a requirement for burns that involve more than 20% of the total body surface area. Ideally, the IV catheters should not be placed through or adjacent to burned tissue; however, placement through the burn is appropriate if no alternative sites are available. When the catheter is placed in or near a burn, special measures must be taken to ensure that the catheter is not inadvertently dislodged. Adhesive tapes and dressings typically used to secure IV catheters will be ineffective when applied on or adjacent to burned tissue. Alternative means to secure the lines include wrapping the site with Kerlix or Coban rolls. In some patients, the prehospital care provider may not be able to obtain venous access. Intraosseous (IO) access is an alternative and reliable method to administer IV fluids as well as narcotics.

Burn patients are trauma patients and may have sustained injuries other than the thermal injuries. Burns are obvious and sometimes intimidating injuries, but it is vital to assess for other, less obvious internal injuries that may be more immediately life threatening than the burns. For example, in attempts to escape being burned, patients may leap from the windows of buildings; elements of the burning structure may collapse and fall on the patient; or the patient may be trapped in the burning wreckage of a motor vehicle crash. In all of these cases, the patient will have sustained both burns and associated trauma. The immediate life threat is hemorrhage from the traumatic injury and not the burn.

Disability

A source of life-threatening neurologic disability that is unique to burn victims is the effect of inhaled toxins such as carbon monoxide and hydrogen cyanide gas. These toxins can produce asphyxiation (see the section on Smoke Inhalation Injuries).

Evaluate the patient for neurologic and motor deficits as one would do for any other trauma patient. Identify and splint fractures of long bones after applying a clean sheet or dressing if the extremity is burned. Perform spinal immobilization if you suspect a potential spinal injury.

Expose/Environment

The next priority is to expose the patient completely. Every square inch of the patient should be exposed and inspected. All jewelry should be promptly removed because the gradually developing swelling of burned areas will cause jewelry to act as a constricting band and compromise distal circulation. In the event of mechanical trauma, all of the patient's clothes are removed in order to identify injuries that might be concealed by the clothing. In a burn victim, removal of the clothing can potentially have a therapeutic benefit. Clothing and jewelry can retain residual heat, which may continue to injure the patient. Following chemical burns, the clothing may be soaked with the agent that burned the patient. In the case of chemical burns, improper handling of the victim's clothing that has been saturated with a potentially hazardous material can result in injury to both the patient and the prehospital care provider.

Controlling the environmental temperature is critical when caring for patients with large burns. Patients with burns are not able to retain their own body heat and are extremely susceptible to hypothermia. The burn leads to vasodilation in the skin, which, in turn, allows for increased heat loss. In addition, as open burn wounds weep and leak fluid, evaporation further exacerbates the patient's body heat loss. Make every effort to preserve the patient's body temperature. Apply several layers of blankets. Keep the passenger compartment of the transporting ambulance or aircraft warm, regardless of the time of year. As a general rule, if the prehospital care providers are comfortable, then ambient temperature is not warm enough for the patient.

Secondary Assessment

After completing the primary assessment, the next objective is completion of the secondary assessment. The secondary assessment of a patient with a burn injury is no different than that of any other trauma patient. The prehospital care provider should complete a head-to-toe evaluation, attempting to identify additional injuries or medical conditions. The appearance of the burns can be dramatic; however, these wounds are not typically immediately life threatening. A thorough and systematic evaluation needs to be performed the same as would be done for any other trauma patient.

Burn Size Estimation (Assessment)

Estimation of burn size is necessary to resuscitate the patient appropriately and prevent the complications associated with hypovolemic shock from burn injury. Burn size determination is also used as a tool for stratifying injury severity and triage. The most widely applied method is the rule of nines. This method applies the principle that major regions of the body in adults are considered to be 9% of the total body surface area (**Figure 15-12**). The perineum, or genital area, represents 1%.

Children have different proportions than adults. Children's heads are proportionally larger than adults' heads, and children's

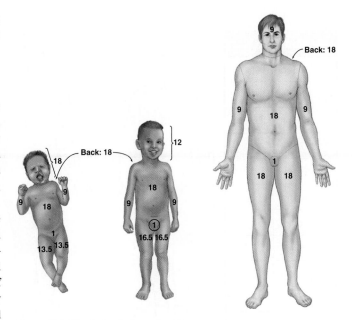

Figure 15-12 Rule of nines.
Source: © Jones & Bartlett Learning.

legs are shorter in proportion than adults' legs. Because these proportions vary with differing age groups, it is not appropriate to apply the rule of nines to pediatric patients. Charts and diagrams are available to assist in estimating burn size in children.

The *Lund-Browder chart* is a diagram that takes into account age-related changes in children. Using these charts, a prehospital care provider maps the burn and then determines burn size based on an accompanying reference table (**Figure 15-13**). This method requires drawing a map of the burns and then converting the map to a calculated burned surface area. The complexity of this method makes it difficult to use in a prehospital situation.

Small burns can be assessed using the rule of palms (**Figure 15-14**) . The use of the patient's palm has been a widely accepted and long-standing practice for estimating the size of smaller burns. However, there has not been uniform acceptance of what defines a palm and how large it is.[7] The average area of the palm alone (not including the extended fingers) is 0.5% total body surface area (TBSA) in males and 0.4% in females. Including the palmar aspect of all five extended digits along with the palm, the area increases to 0.8% total body surface area (TBSA) for males and 0.7% TBSA for females.[7] Aside from gender differences of palm size, the size of the palm also varies with body weight of the patient. As the patient's body mass index (BMI) increases, the total skin surface area of the body increases and the TBSA percentage of the palm decreases.[8] Therefore, in most cases, the palm plus the fingers of the patient can be considered to be approximately 1% of the patient's TBSA.

Dressings

Before transport, the wounds should be dressed. The goal of the dressings is to prevent ongoing contamination and prevent airflow over the wounds, which will help with pain control.

Region	%
Head	
Neck	
Ant. Trunk	
Post. Trunk	
Right arm	
Left arm	
Buttocks	
Genitalia	
Right leg	
Left leg	
Total burn	

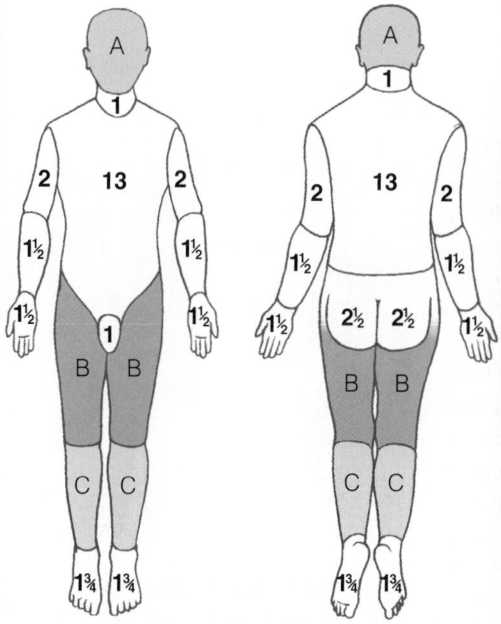

Relative percentages of body surface area affected by growth

Age (years)	A (½ of head)	B (½ of one thigh)	C (½ of one leg)
0	9½	2¾	2½
1	8½	3¼	2½
5	6½	4	2¾
10	5½	4¼	3
15	4½	4½	3¼
Adult	3½	4¾	3

Figure 15-13 Lund-Browder chart.

Source: Adapted from Lund, C. C., and Brower, N. C. *Surg Gynecol Obstet.* 1944. 79: 352–358.

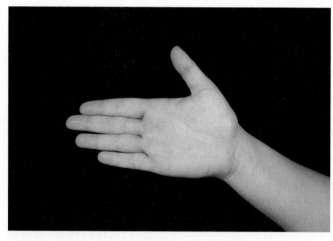

Figure 15-14 The rule of palms uses the patient's palm plus the fingers to estimate the size of smaller burns.

Source: © Jones & Bartlett Learning. Photographed by Kimberly Potvin.

Dressings in the form of a dry sterile sheet or towel are sufficient before transporting the patient. Several layers of blankets are then placed over the sterile burn sheets to help the patient maintain body heat. Topical antibiotic ointments and creams should not be applied until the patient has been evaluated by the burn center.

Transport

Patients who have multiple injuries in addition to their burns should first be transported to a trauma center, where immediately life-threatening injuries can be identified and surgically treated, if necessary. Once stabilized at a trauma center, the patient with

burns can then be transported to a burn center for definitive burn care and rehabilitation. The American Burn Association and the American College of Surgeons have identified criteria for transport or transfer of burn patients to a burn center, as outlined in **Figure 15-15**. In those geographic areas without easy access to a burn center, local medical direction will determine the preferred destination for such cases.

Management

Initial Burn Care

The initial step in the care of a burn patient is to stop the burning process. The most effective and appropriate method of terminating the burning is irrigation with copious volumes of room-temperature water. Use of cold water or ice is contraindicated. The application of ice will stop the burning and provide analgesia, but it also will increase the extent of tissue damage in the zone of stasis (**Figure 15-16**). Remove all clothing and jewelry; these items maintain residual heat and will continue to burn the patient. In addition, jewelry may constrict digits or extremities as the tissues begin to swell.

To effectively dress a recent burn, sterile, non-adherent dressings are applied and the area is covered with a clean, dry sheet. If a sheet is not readily available, substitute a sterile surgical gown, drapes, towels, or Mylar rescue blanket. The dressing will prevent ongoing environmental contamination while helping to prevent the patient from experiencing pain from air flowing over the exposed nerve endings (**Figure 15-17**).

Prehospital care providers have often been unsatisfied and frustrated with the simple application of sterile sheets to a burn. However, topical ointments and conventional topical antibiotics

Figure 15-15 Injuries Requiring Burn Unit Care

Patients with serious burns should receive care at centers that have special expertise and resources. Initial transport or early transfer to a burn unit results in a lower mortality rate and fewer complications. A burn unit may treat adults, children, or both.

The Committee on Trauma of the American College of Surgeons recommends referral to a burn unit for patients with burn injuries who meet the following criteria:

1. Inhalation injury
2. Partial-thickness burns over greater than 10% of the TBSA
3. Full-thickness (third-degree) burns in any age group
4. Burns that involve the face, hands, feet, genitalia, perineum, or major joints
5. Electrical burns, including lightning injury
6. Chemical burns
7. Burn injury in patients with pre-existing medical disorders that could complicate management, prolong recovery, or affect mortality
8. Any patients with burns and concomitant trauma (e.g., fractures) in which the burn injury poses the greatest risk of morbidity or mortality; if trauma poses the greater immediate risk, the patient may be initially stabilized in a trauma center before transfer to a burn unit
9. Children with burns in hospitals without qualified personnel or equipment for the care of children
10. Burn injury in patients who will require special social, emotional, or long-term rehabilitative intervention

Source: Data from the American College of Surgeons (ACS) Committee on Trauma: *Resources for Optimal Care of the Injured Patient:* 2006, Chicago, ACS.

Figure 15-16 Burn Cooling

A potentially controversial topic is the practice of burn cooling. Several investigators have evaluated the effect of various cooling methods on the microscopic appearance of the burned tissue, as well as the impact on wound healing. In one study, the researchers concluded that burn cooling had a beneficial effect on the experimental burn wound.[9] Burns treated with cooling had less cellular damage than those that were not cooled.

Investigators have been able to directly measure the impact of cooling on the temperature of the burned dermis, the microscopic structure of the tissue, and wound healing. A study evaluated the outcomes of various cooling methods. These investigators compared burns cooled with tap water (15°C [59°F]) to application of a commercially available gel. Each of these methods was applied immediately after the burns as well as after a 30-minute delay. Immediate tap water cooling was almost twice as effective in reducing the temperature within the burned tissue. In this trial, wounds that were cooled had better microscopic appearance and wound healing at 3 weeks after injury.[10]

Overaggressive cooling with ice is harmful and will increase the injury to the tissue already damaged by the burn. This finding was demonstrated in an animal model; cooling the burn immediately by the application of ice was more harmful than application of tap water or no treatment at all.[11] The application of ice water at a temperature of 1–8°C (34–46°F) resulted in more tissue destruction than was seen in burns that received no cooling treatment at all. In contrast, cooling with tap water at a temperature of 12–18°C (54–64°F) showed less tissue necrosis and a faster rate of healing than was observed in wounds not cooled.[12]

An important consideration is that the research on cooling was performed on experimental animals, and the burns were very limited in size. Ten percent TBSA was the largest burn size evaluated.

In summary, not all methods of burn cooling are equivalent. Cooling that is too aggressive will lead to tissue damage. If delayed, it is not likely to be beneficial. In patients with large burns, burn wound cooling is likely to induce hypothermia. Another potential hazard of cooling a burn is that in the patient with both burns and mechanical trauma, systemic hypothermia has predictable and detrimental effects on the ability of blood to form clot.

Figure 15-17 Prevent Airflow Over Patient's Burn

Most adults have experienced the pain associated with a dental cavity. The pain is intensified when air is inhaled over the exposed nerve. With a partial-thickness burn, thousands of nerves are exposed, and the air currents in the environment produce pain in the patient when they come into contact with the exposed nerves of the wound. By keeping burns covered, the patient will experience less pain.

---

should not be applied because they prevent a direct inspection of the burn. Such topical ointments and antibiotics are removed on admission to the burn center to allow direct visualization of the burn and determination of burn severity. Also, some topical medications may complicate the application of tissue-engineered products used to aid wound healing.

High-concentration antimicrobial-coated dressings have become the mainstay of wound care in burn centers (**Figure 15-18**). These dressings are coated with a form of silver, which is time-released over several days when applied to an open burn wound. The released silver provides rapid antimicrobial coverage of the common organisms contaminating and infecting wounds. Recently, these dressings have been adapted from burn center use to prehospital applications. These large antimicrobial sheets can be rapidly applied to the burn and can eradicate any contaminating organisms. This method of wound care allows prehospital care providers to apply a non-pharmaceutical device that greatly reduces burn wound contamination within 30 minutes of application.[13-15] An advantage of these dressings in wilderness and military applications is their compact size and light weight. An entire adult can be covered with antibiotic dressings that can be stored in a container the size of a manila envelope with minimal weight.

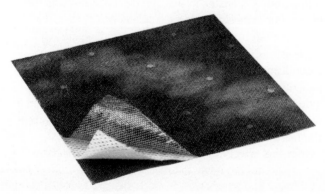

Figure 15-18 Acticoat dressing.
Source: Courtesy of Smith & Nephew.

Fluid Resuscitation

Administration of large amounts of IV fluids is needed over the course of the first day postburn to prevent a patient with burns from going into hypovolemic shock. After sustaining a burn, the patient loses a substantial amount of intravascular fluid in the form of obligatory whole-body edema, as well as evaporative losses at the site of the burn. Massive fluid shifts will occur, even though total body water may remain unchanged. Evaporative losses can be enormous. However, excessive fluid administration is harmful. Therefore, although large fluid requirements are needed to treat burn shock, too much fluid will complicate the patient's management and even worsen the patient's wounds.

The resuscitation of a patient with a burn injury is aimed not only at the restoration of the loss of intravascular volume but also at the replacement of anticipated intravascular losses at a rate that mimics those losses as they occur (**Figure 15-19**). In trauma patients, the prehospital care provider is replacing the volume that the patient has already lost from hemorrhage from an open fracture or bleeding viscera. In contrast, when treating the patient with a burn injury, the objective is to calculate and replace the fluids that the patient has already lost as well as replace the volume that the prehospital care provider anticipates the patient will lose over the first 24 hours after the burn injury.

Figure 15-19 Resuscitating a Patient with a Burn Injury

Resuscitating a patient with a burn injury can be compared to filling a leaking bucket. The bucket is leaking water at a constant rate. The bucket has a line drawn inside near the top of the bucket. The objective is to keep the water level with the line. Initially the water depth will be very low. The longer the bucket has been unattended, the lower the water level and the greater the amount of fluid that will need to be replaced. The container will continue to leak, so once the bucket has been filled to an appropriate level, water will need to be continuously added at a constant rate to maintain the desired level.

The longer the patient with a burn injury is not resuscitated or is under-resuscitated, the more hypovolemic the patient becomes. Therefore, greater amounts of fluids are required to establish a "level" of homeostasis. Once the patient has been resuscitated, the vascular space continues to leak in the same manner as the bucket. To maintain equilibrium with this homeostatic point, additional fluids need to be provided to replace the ongoing losses.

Intravenous access should be considered for those situations involving long transport time to the hospital. In urban settings with short transport times, the need for obtaining IV access is based not upon the burn but upon other conditions, such as associated trauma.

Adult Patient

The use of IV fluids, especially lactated Ringer's solution, is the best way initially to manage a burn patient. The amount of fluids administered in the first 24 hours after injury is typically 2 to 4 milliliters (ml) multiplied by the patient's body weight in kilograms (kg) multiplied by the percentage of TBSA burned (using only the total of second- and third-degree burn). There are several formulas that guide fluid resuscitation in the burn patient. The most notable is the *Parkland formula*, which delivers 4 ml × body weight in kg × percentage of area burned. Half of this fluid needs to be administered within the first 8 hours of injury, and the remaining half of the volume from hours 8 to 24.

Note, the first half of the fluid is administered within 8 hours from the time the patient was injured, not from the time the prehospital care provider started to resuscitate the patient. This detail is especially important in wilderness or military settings, in which there may be an initial delay in treatment. For example, if the patient presents for emergency care 3 hours after the injury with no or little fluid administration, the first half of the calculated total needs to be administered over the next 5 hours. Thus, the patient will have received the target volume by hour 8 after the injury.

Lactated Ringer's is preferred to 0.9% normal saline for burn resuscitation. Burn patients typically require large volumes of IV fluids. Patients who receive large amounts of normal saline in the course of burn resuscitation will often develop a condition known as **hyperchloremic acidosis** because of the large amounts of chloride in the normal saline solution.

Calculation of Fluid Resuscitation Measures

For example, consider an 80-kg (176-pound) man who has sustained third-degree burns to 30% of his TBSA and who is managed on scene shortly after the injury. The fluid resuscitation volume would be calculated as follows:

24-hour fluid total = 4 ml/kg × weight in kg × % TBSA burned
= 4 ml/kg × 80 kg × 30% TBSA burned
= 9,600 ml

Note that in this formula, the units of kilograms and percent cancel out so that only ml is left, thus making the calculation 4 ml × 80 × 30 = 9,600 ml.

Once the 24-hour total is calculated, divide that number by 2:

Amount of fluid to be given from time of injury to hour 8 = 9,600 ml/2 = 4,800 ml

To determine the hourly rate for the first 8 hours, divide this total by 8:

Fluid rate for the first 8 hours = 4,800 ml/8 hours = 600 ml/hour

The fluid requirement for the next period (hours 8 to 24) is calculated as follows:

Amount of fluid to be given from hours 8 to 24 = 9,600 ml/2 = 4,800 ml

To determine the hourly rate for the final 16 hours, divide this total by 16:

Fluid rate for final 16 hours = 4,800 ml/16 hours = 300 ml/hour

The Rule of Ten for Burn Resuscitation

In an effort to simplify the process of calculating fluid requirements for burn patients in the prehospital setting, researchers from the U.S. Army Institute of Surgical Research developed the Rule of Ten to help guide initial fluid resuscitation.[16] The percentage of BSA burned is calculated and rounded to the nearest 10. For example, a burn of 37% would be rounded to 40%. The percentage is then multiplied by 10 to get the number of ml per hour of crystalloid. Thus, in the previous example, the calculation would be 40 × 10 = 400 ml per hour. This formula is used for adults weighing 40 to 70 kg (88 to 154 pounds). If the patient exceeds this weight range, for each 10 kg in body weight over 70 kg, an additional 100 ml per hour is given.

If the Rule of Ten is compared to the Parkland formula, it will immediately become apparent that the fluid volumes calculated differ to a small extent. Regardless of which method is used to calculate fluid requirements, the calculated volume is an estimate of the fluid needs, and the actual volume given to the patient must be adjusted based upon the clinical response of the patient.

Pediatric Patient

Children require relatively larger volumes of IV fluids than adults with similar-sized burns. Also, children have less metabolic reserves of the molecule glycogen in their livers to maintain adequate blood glucose during the periods of burn resuscitation. For these reasons, children should receive 5% dextrose containing IV fluids (D_5LR) at a standard maintenance rate in addition to burn resuscitation fluids.

Smoke Inhalation—Fluid Management Considerations

The patient with both thermal burns and smoke inhalation will require significantly more fluid than the burn patient without smoke inhalation.[17] In an attempt to "protect the lungs," prehospital care providers will often administer less fluid than calculated. Withholding fluids actually increases the severity of the pulmonary injury.

Analgesia

Burns are extremely painful and, as such, require appropriate attention to pain relief beginning in the prehospital setting. Narcotic analgesics such as fentanyl (1 mcg per kg body weight) or morphine (0.1 mg per kg body weight) in adequate dosages will be required to control pain.

Special Considerations
Electrical Burns

Electrical injuries are devastating injuries that can easily be underappreciated. In many cases the extent of apparent tissue damage does not accurately reflect the magnitude of the actual injury. Tissue destruction and necrosis are much greater than the visually apparent trauma because most of the destruction occurs internally as the electricity is conducted through the patient. The patient will have external burns at the points of contact with the electrical source as well as grounding points (**Figure 15-20**). As the electricity courses through the patient's body, deep layers of tissue are destroyed despite seemingly minor injuries on the surface.

Electrical and crush injuries share many similarities. In both injuries, there is massive destruction of large muscle groups with resultant release of both potassium and myoglobin (see the Musculoskeletal Trauma chapter). The release of muscle potassium causes a significant increase in the serum level, which can result in cardiac dysrhythmias. Elevated potassium levels can make administration of the depolarizing muscle relaxant succinylcholine prohibitively dangerous.[18] If chemical paralysis of the patient is required, such as for rapid sequence intubation, nondepolarizing agents such as vecuronium or rocuronium may be used. **Myoglobin** is a molecule found in the muscle that assists the muscle tissue in transportation of oxygen. When released into the bloodstream in considerable amounts, the myoglobin is toxic to the kidneys and can cause kidney failure. This condition, **myoglobinuria**, is evidenced by tea- or cola-colored urine (**Figure 15-21**).

Prehospital care providers are commonly called upon to provide interhospital transfers of patients after electrical injuries.

Patients with electrical burns should ideally be transported with a urinary catheter in place. Patients with myoglobinuria require aggressive fluid administration to maintain a urine output of greater than 100 ml/hour in adults or 1 mL/kg/hour in children to avoid acute kidney injury. Sodium bicarbonate is administered in some cases to make the myoglobin more soluble in urine and reduce the likelihood of renal injury; however, its actual benefit in preventing acute kidney injury remains a topic of debate.

The electrical burn patient may have associated mechanical injuries as well. Approximately 15% of patients with electrical injuries will also have traumatic injuries. This rate is twice that seen in patients burned by other mechanisms.[19] Tympanic membranes may rupture, resulting in hearing difficulties. Intense and sustained muscle contraction (*tetany*) can result in shoulder dislocations and compression fractures of multiple levels of the spine as well as long bones, and for this reason patients with electrical injury should have their spine immobilized. Long-bone fractures should be splinted when detected or suspected. Intracranial bleeds and cardiac dysrhythmias may also occur.

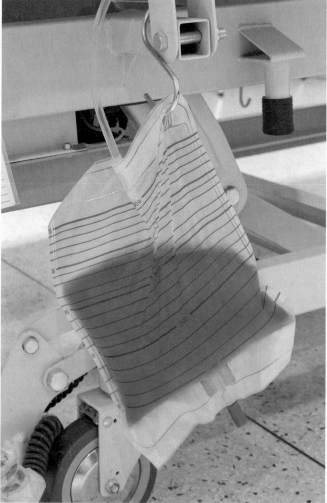

Figure 15-21 Urine of patient after electrical injury from high-tension wires. The patient has myoglobinuria after extensive muscle destruction.
Source: © Suphatthra China/ShutterStock, Inc.

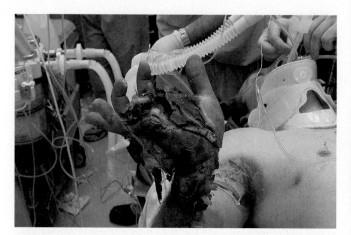

Figure 15-20 Patient after electrical injury from high-tension wires.
Source: Courtesy of Jeffrey Guy, MD.

Electrical flash burns are the result of superheated air. Nevertheless, because of the catastrophic and occult nature of conduction injuries, it is imperative that providers maintain a high index of suspicion for the presence of a transmission type of injury.

Circumferential Burns

Circumferential burns of the trunk or limbs are capable of producing a life- or limb-threatening condition as a result of the thick, inelastic eschar that is formed. Circumferential burns of the chest can constrict the chest wall to such a degree that the patient suffocates from the inability to inhale. Circumferential burns of the extremities create a tourniquet-like effect that can render an arm or leg pulseless. Therefore, all circumferential burns should be handled as an emergency and patients transported to a burn center or to the local trauma center, if a burn center is not available. As discussed previously, escharotomies are surgical incisions made through the burn eschar to allow expansion of the deeper tissues and decompression of previously compressed and often occluded vascular structures (**Figure 15-22**).

Smoke Inhalation Injuries

The leading cause of death in fires is not thermal injury but the inhalation of toxic smoke. Any patient with a history of exposure to smoke in an enclosed space should be considered to be at risk of having an inhalation injury. Victims with burns to the face or

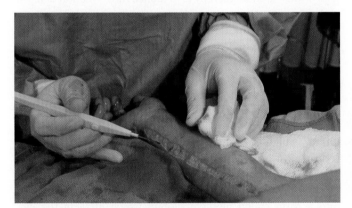

Figure 15-22 Escharotomies are performed to release the constricting effect of circumferential burns.
Source: Courtesy of Jeffrey Guy, MD.

Figure 15-23 Conditions Suggesting Smoke Inhalation

- Burn in a confined space
- Confusion or agitation
- Burns to face or chest
- Singeing of eyebrows or nasal hair
- Soot in the sputum
- Hoarseness, loss of voice, or stridor

soot in the sputum are at risk for a smoke-inhalation injury; however, the absence of these signs does not exclude the diagnosis of a toxic inhalation (**Figure 15-23**). Maintaining a high index of suspicion is vitally important because signs and symptoms may not manifest for days after the exposure.

There are three elements of smoke inhalation: thermal injury, asphyxiation, and delayed toxin-induced lung injury. Dry air is a poor conductor of heat; the inhalation of heated air associated with a structure fire rarely induces thermal injury to the airways below the level of the vocal cords. The large surface area of the nasopharynx acts effectively as a heat exchanger and cools the inhaled, heated air to about body temperature by the time the air reaches the level of the vocal cords. When heated dry air at 300°C (572°F) is inhaled, the air is cooled to 50°C (122°F) by the time it is at the level of the trachea.[20] The vocal cords provide additional protection by reflexively moving into an adducted or closed position.[21] The exception to this is the inhalation of steam. Steam has 4,000 times the heat-carrying capacity of dry air and is capable of burning the distal airways and bronchioles when inhaled.[20]

Asphyxiants

Two gaseous products that are clinically important as asphyxiants are *carbon monoxide* and *cyanide gas*. Both molecules are classified as asphyxiants and, thus, cause cell death by cellular hypoxia or asphyxia. Patients with asphyxia from smoke containing one or both of these compounds will have inadequate delivery of oxygen to tissues despite an adequate blood pressure or pulse oximeter reading.

Carbon monoxide binds to hemoglobin with much greater affinity than oxygen does. The symptoms of carbon monoxide inhalation depend on the duration or severity of exposure and the resultant serum levels. Symptoms can range from mild headache to coma and death (**Figure 15-24**). Traditional teaching is

Figure 15-24 Symptoms of Carbon Monoxide Poisoning

- **Mild**
  - Headache
  - Fatigue
  - Nausea
- **Moderate**
  - Severe headache
  - Vomiting
  - Confusion
  - Drowsiness/sleepiness
  - Increased heart rate and ventilatory rate
- **Severe**
  - Seizures
  - Coma
  - Cardiorespiratory arrest
  - Death

that patients poisoned with carbon monoxide develop "classic" cherry-red skin coloration. Unfortunately, this is often a late sign and should not be relied upon when considering the diagnosis.

Portable pulse carbon monoxide monitors that noninvasively measure the amount of carbon monoxide in the bloodstream are available for use in the prehospital settings (**Figure 15-25**). These monitors look and work similar to pulse oximeters. Patients will generally complain of mild symptoms with levels of 10–20% carboxyhemoglobin. As the level of carbon monoxide in the blood further increases, symptoms progressively get worse. As levels exceed 50–60%, seizures, coma, and death result.

Pulse oximeters cannot be used to guide recognition or treatment. Pulse oximetry will give a falsely normal or elevated reading because the detection of oxyhemoglobin depends on the colorimetric analysis performed by the oximeter and that analysis is fooled by the similar color of carboxyhemoglobim.

Treatment of carbon monoxide toxicity is removal of the patient from the source and administration of oxygen. When breathing room air (21% oxygen), the body will eliminate half the carbon monoxide in 250 minutes.[22] When the patient is placed on 100% oxygen, the half-life of the carbon monoxide–hemoglobin complex is reduced to 40 to 60 minutes.[23] For many years, hyperbaric oxygen has been considered the treatment of choice for moderate or severe carbon monoxide poisoning. The use of hyperbaric oxygen reduces the half-life of carbon monoxide to 20 to 30 minutes and has been thought to decrease the incidence of long-term sequelae from the carbon monoxide exposure. Recently, the benefit of hyperbaric oxygen treatment over standard 100% oxygen therapy has been questioned.[24] In addition, if the patient has significant burn injuries or other traumatic injuries, providing needed care in a hyperbaric chamber is

extremely difficult. Therefore, in the majority of cases, bypassing a burn or trauma center in favor of a facility with a hyperbaric chamber is not warranted.

Cyanide gas is produced from the burning of plastics or polyurethane. Cyanide poisons the cellular processes of energy production, preventing the body's cells from using oxygen. The patient can die from asphyxia despite having adequate amounts of oxygen available in the blood. Symptoms of cyanide toxicity include altered level of consciousness, dizziness, headache, and tachycardia or tachypnea. Patients with carbon monoxide toxicity from a structure fire should also be considered to be at risk for cyanide poisoning. The treatment of cyanide poisoning is the rapid administration of antidote. The preferred antidote for cyanide poisoning is a medication that directly binds to the cyanide molecule, rendering it harmless. *Hydroxocobalamin* (Cyanokit) detoxifies the cyanide by directly binding to it and forming cyanocobalamin (vitamin B$_{12}$), which is nontoxic. Hydroxocobalamin is available for prehospital use in Europe and in the United States. A second chelating agent that has been used in Europe for cyanide poisoning is *dicobalt edetate*; however, if this medication is administered in the absence of cyanide poisoning, cobalt toxicity is a risk.

The "Lilly kit" or "Pasadena kit" has been the traditional cyanide antidote kit used in the United States and may still be utilized in some settings. This method of treating cyanide poisoning was developed in the 1930s and found to be effective in detoxifying animals poisoned with 21 times the lethal dose of cyanide.[25] The goal of this antidote therapy is to induce the formation of a second poison (methemoglobin) in the patient's blood. This therapeutically induced poison binds with the cyanide and allows the body to slowly detoxify and excrete the cyanide.

The Lilly kit contains three medications. The first medication to be administered for victims of cyanide poisoning is a nitrate, either amyl nitrate or sodium nitrate, both of which are provided in the kit. Amyl nitrate comes in an ampule that is broken open, releasing fumes that the patient inhales; sodium nitrate, which is given IV, is the preferred method of administration as it is a more efficient delivery modality and avoids exposure of healthcare providers to amyl nitrate fumes. The nitrate medications change some of the patient's hemoglobin into a form called methemoglobin, which attracts the cyanide away from the site of toxic action in the mitochondria of the cell. Once the cyanide binds with the methemoglobin, the mitochondria can once again begin to produce energy for the cell. Unfortunately, methemoglobin is toxic because it does not carry oxygen to cells as well as hemoglobin does. This decrease in oxygen delivery can exacerbate the tissue hypoxia associated with increased carbon monoxide levels that the victim may also have as a result of smoke inhalation.[26,27]

The third medication in the kit is sodium thiosulfate, which is given IV after the nitrate. The thiosulfate and cyanide from the methemoglobin are metabolized to thiocyanate, which is safely excreted in the patient's urine.

Because of the toxicity of methemoglobin and the time needed to administer the full Lilly kit, hydroxocobalamin has become the preferred antidote for the treatment of cyanide poisoning.

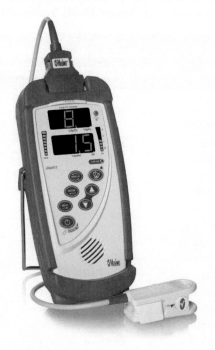

Figure 15-25 Masimo prehospital carbon monoxide monitor, Rad-57.
Source: Courtesy of Masimo Corporation.

Toxin-Induced Lung Injury

The thermal and asphyxiant components of an inhalation injury are usually apparent at the time of the rescue. In contrast, the signs and symptoms of toxin-induced lung injury typically do not manifest themselves for several days. The first several days after a smoke inhalation injury are often described as the "honeymoon period." During this period, the patient may appear deceptively stable with little or no pulmonary dysfunction. The severity of this lung injury is largely dependent on two factors: the composition of the smoke and the duration of exposure.[28]

In simplified terms, smoke is the product of incomplete combustion—that is, chemical dust. The chemicals in the smoke react with the lining of the trachea and lungs and damage the cells lining the airways and lungs.[29-31] Compounds such as ammonia, hydrogen chloride, and sulfur dioxide form corrosive acids and alkalis when they are inhaled and react with water.[32] These poisons cause necrosis of the cells lining the trachea and bronchioles. Normally, these cells have tiny hairlike structures called *cilia*. On these cilia is a blanket of mucus that captures and transports normally inhaled debris to the oropharynx, where the debris is swallowed into the GI tract. Several days after an inhalation injury, these cells die. The debris from these necrotic cells and the debris these cells typically capture accumulate instead of being removed. The result is an increase in secretions, plugging of the airways with mucus and cellular debris, and an increased rate of life-threatening pneumonia.

Prehospital Management

The initial and most important element of caring for a patient with smoke exposure is determining the need for orotracheal intubation. Continuous re-evaluation of airway patency is required in order to recognize developing signs of airway obstruction. Change in the character of the voice, difficulty handling secretions, or drooling are signs of impending airway occlusion. Whenever patency of the patient's airway is in doubt, the prehospital care provider can proceed with securing the airway using orotracheal intubation.[33,34] In some cases, rapid sequence intubation may be necessary, if allowed, to manage the airway. In the event of long transport times, rendezvous with an agency capable of providing definitive airway management should be considered.

Patients with smoke inhalation should be transported to burn centers even in the absence of surface burns. Burn centers treat a greater volume of patients with smoke inhalation and offer unique modes of mechanical ventilation.

Child Abuse

Approximately 20% of all child abuse is the result of intentional burning. The majority of the children intentionally burned are 1 to 2 years of age.[35] Many jurisdictions require health care providers to report cases of suspected child abuse.

The most common form of burn child abuse is forcible immersion. These injuries typically occur when an adult places a child in hot water, often as a punishment related to toilet training.[36] Factors that determine the severity of injury include age of the patient, temperature of the water, and duration of exposure. The child may sustain deep second- or third-degree burns of the hands or feet in a glove-like or stocking-like pattern. Such findings are especially suspicious when the burns are symmetric and lack splash patterns[37] (**Figures 15-26** and **15-27**). In cases of intentional scalding, the child will tightly flex the arms and legs into a defensive posture because of fear or pain. The resultant burn pattern will spare the flexion creases of the popliteal fossa (knees), the antecubital fossa (elbows), and the groin. Sharp lines of demarcation will also be seen between burned and unburned tissue, essentially indicating a dip[38,39] (**Figure 15-28**).

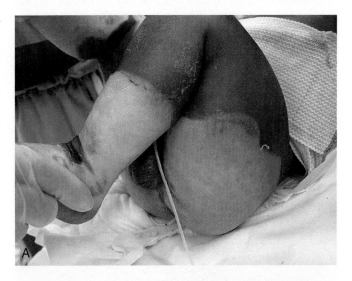

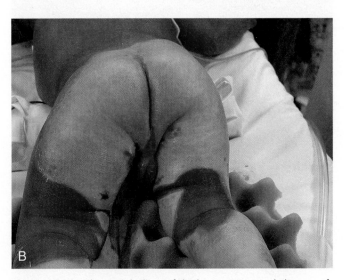

Figure 15-26 The straight lines of the burn pattern and absence of splash marks indicate that this burn is the result of abuse.
Source: Courtesy of Jeffrey Guy, MD.

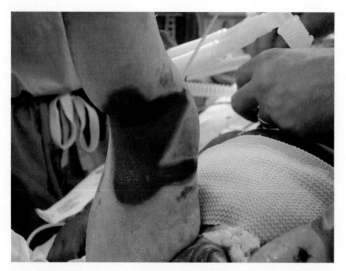

Figure 15-27 The sparing of the areas of flexion and the sharp lines of demarcation between burned and unburned skin indicate that this child was in a tightly flexed, defensive position before injury. Such a posture indicates that the scald is not accidental.

Source: Courtesy of Jeffrey Guy, MD.

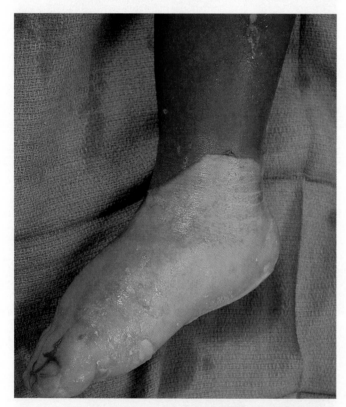

Figure 15-28 The stocking-type scald of the child's foot indicates intentional immersion burn injury consistent with child abuse.

Source: Courtesy of Jeffrey Guy, MD.

In accidental scald injuries, the burns will have variable burn depth, irregular margins, and smaller burns remote from the large burns, indicating splash.[40]

Contact Burns

Contact burns are the second most common mechanism of burn injury in children, whether accidental or intentional. All body surfaces have some degree of curvature. When an accidental contact burn occurs, the burning agent makes contact with the curved body surface area. The burning instrument is deflected off the curved surface, or the victim withdraws from the hot object. The resultant injury has an irregular burn edge and depth. When a child receives an intentional contact burn, the inflicting implement is pressed onto the child's skin. The resultant injury has sharp lines of demarcation between burned and unburned tissue and uniform depth.[39] Common objects involved in contact burns include curling irons, steam irons, radiators, and hot pots and pans.

Radiation Burns

The severity of burns produced from various forms of radiation is a product of the amount of energy absorbed by the target tissue. The various forms of radiation include electromagnetic radiation, x-rays, gamma rays, and particulate radiation. The different forms of radiation are able to transfer varying degrees of energy to tissue. Additionally, some forms of radiation (e.g., electromagnetic) can pass through tissue or an individual, resulting in no damage. In contrast, other forms of radiation (e.g., neutron exposure) are absorbed by the target tissue and result in significant injury. It is the absorption of the radiation that results in damage to the absorbing tissue. The absorption capacity of the radiation is more damaging than the actual dose of radiation. Equivalent doses of different forms of radiation will have dramatically different effects on an individual.

The typical exposure to radiation occurs in the setting of an industrial or occupational incident. However, with the increasing threat of global terrorism, the detonation of a "dirty bomb" or radiation dispersal device (conventional explosive with radioactive material added) or a small, improvised nuclear device (i.e., "dirty nuke") is a possibility. (See the Explosions and Weapons of Mass Destruction chapter for more detail.)

The detonation of a dirty bomb is designed to spread radioactive material over a large area. While the explosion itself would likely injure or kill individuals in close proximity to the blast, the risk from the radioactive material is, in reality, relatively small. There is little likelihood of absorbing a large enough dose of radiation to produce clinical illness.

The detonation of a nuclear weapon in a metropolitan area, on the other hand, would injure and kill many people by three mechanisms: thermal burns from the initial firestorm, supersonic destructive blast causing blunt and penetrating trauma, and production of radiation. Mortality from a combination of thermal and radiation burns is greater than that from either thermal or radiation burns alone of equal magnitude. The combination of thermal and radiation burns has a synergistic effect on mortality.[41]

Radiation is a hazardous material, and many of the initial priorities are the same as for any patient exposed to a hazardous material. The initial priorities are to utilize appropriate personal protective equipment, remove the patient from the source of contamination, remove contaminated clothing, and irrigate the patient with water. Remember that any removed clothing should be considered contaminated and should be handled with caution. Irrigation is done carefully to remove any radioactive debris or particles from contaminated areas without spreading the injury to uncontaminated body surfaces. Irrigation should continue until contamination has been minimized to a steady state, as determined by a full-body survey with a Geiger counter.[42]

The exception to this approach is the patient who has sustained major trauma in addition to their radiation injury. In these cases, clothing should be removed immediately, then the traumatic injury is dealt with and the patient stabilized. Patients with burns should undergo fluid resuscitation similar to any other patient with burn injury. Irradiated patients may experience vomiting and diarrhea, which will necessitate an increase in resuscitation fluids.

The physiologic consequences of whole-body radiation are termed **acute radiation syndrome** (ARS). The initial symptoms of ARS typically appear within hours of exposure. The cells of the body that are most sensitive to the effects of radiation are those that typically undergo rapid division. These rapidly dividing cells are found in the skin, GI tract, and bone marrow; therefore, these tissues manifest the first signs of ARS. Within a few hours after significant radiation exposure, the patient will experience nausea, vomiting, and cramping abdominal pain. Aggressive fluid management is required to prevent the development of renal failure. Over the following days, the patient may develop bloody diarrhea, ischemia of the bowel, and overwhelming infection, and may die. Bone marrow is extremely sensitive to the effects of radiation and will stop production of white blood cells needed to fight infections and platelets needed to make blood clots. The resultant infections and bleeding complications are often fatal.

After a nuclear event, IV supplies, infusion pumps, and receiving medical facilities may be in short supply. If the prehospital care provider is unable to provide the patient with IV resuscitation, the patient can be resuscitated with oral fluids. A cooperative patient should be encouraged to drink a balanced salt solution to maintain a large urine output; alternatively, fluids can be delivered by nasogastric or nasoenteric tubes. Oral balanced salt solutions include Moyer's solution (4 grams sodium chloride [0.5 teaspoon of salt] and 1.5 grams sodium bicarbonate [0.5 teaspoon baking soda] in 1 liter water) and World Health Organization oral rehydration solution (WHO ORS). Animal research has shown encouraging results with such resuscitation strategies in patients with burns as large as 40% TBSA. Administration of balanced salt solution to the GI tract at a rate of 20 ml/kg provided resuscitation equivalent to standard IV fluid resuscitation.[43]

Chemical Burns

All prehospital care providers need to be familiar with the basics of treating chemical injuries. Prehospital care providers in urban settings may be called to a chemical incident at an industrial setting, whereas a rural prehospital care provider may be summoned to an incident involving agents used in agriculture. Tons of hazardous materials are transported through urban and rural settings daily by both highways and rail systems. Military prehospital care providers may treat casualties of chemical burns caused by weapons or incendiary devices, chemicals used to fuel or maintain equipment, or chemical spills after damage to civilian installations.

Injuries from chemicals are often the result of prolonged exposure to the offending agent, in contrast to thermal injuries, which usually involve a very brief exposure duration. The severity of chemical injury is determined by four factors: nature of the chemical, concentration of the chemical, duration of contact, and mechanism of action of the chemical.

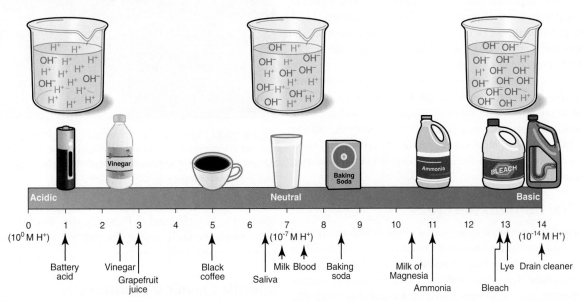

Figure 15-29 Chemical agents are classified as acid, neutral, or base, depending upon the amount of hydrogen or hydroxide ions. Many household items will be acid or base and require care in handling.

Source: © Jones & Bartlett Learning.

Chemical agents are classified as acid, base, organic, or inorganic. **Acids** are chemicals with a pH between 7 (neutral) and 0 (strong acid). **Bases** are agents with a pH between 7 and 14 (strong base) (**Figure 15-29**). Acids damage tissue by a process called **coagulative necrosis**; the damaged tissue coagulates and transforms into a barrier that prevents deeper penetration of the acid. In contrast, alkali burns destroy the tissue by **liquefaction necrosis**; the base liquefies the tissue, allowing the chemical to penetrate more deeply and cause increasingly deeper tissue damage.

Prehospital Management

The greatest priority in the care of a patient exposed to chemical agents is personal and scene safety. As in an emergency, the prehospital care provider should always be protected first. If there is any possibility of exposure to a chemical hazard, ensure scene safety and determine if any special garment or breathing apparatus is required. Avoid contamination of equipment and emergency vehicles; a contaminated vehicle creates an exposure risk to all others in its path. Attempt to obtain identification of the chemical agent as soon as possible.

Remove all clothing from the patient, as it may be contaminated with the chemical agent in either liquid or powder form. The contaminated clothing needs to be discarded with care. If any particulate substance is on the skin, it should be brushed away. Next, wash (*lavage*) the patient with copious amounts of water. Lavage will dilute the concentration of the injurious agent and wash away any remaining reagent. The key to lavage is to use large amounts of the water. A common error is to rinse 1 or 2 liters of water across the patient, then stop the lavage process once the water starts to pool and accumulate on the floor. When lavaged with only small amounts of fluid, the offending agent is spread across the patient's body surface area and not flushed away.[44,45]

Failure to provide adequate runoff and drainage of lavage fluid may cause injury to previously unexposed and uninjured areas of the patient's body as the contaminated lavage accumulates beneath the patient. One simple way of promoting runoff in a prehospital setting is to place the patient on a backboard and then tilt it with cribbing or other means to elevate the head. At the lower end of the board, tuck a large plastic garbage bag to capture the contaminated runoff.

Neutralizing agents for chemical burns are typically avoided. Often in the neutralizing process the neutralizing agents give off heat in an exothermic reaction. Therefore, a well-meaning prehospital care provider may create a thermal burn in addition to the chemical burn. Most commercially available decontamination solutions are made for the purpose of decontaminating equipment, not people.

Chemical Burns to the Eye

Injuries to the eye caused by exposure to alkali may be encountered. A small exposure to the eye can result in a vision-threatening injury. The eyes should be immediately irrigated with large amounts of irrigation fluid. If possible, ocular decontamination with continuous irrigation using a Morgan lens is performed (**Figure 15-30**). If a Morgan lens is not available, continuous irrigation may be accomplished manually with handheld IV tubing or, if both eyes are involved, a nasal cannula placed on the bridge of the nose and

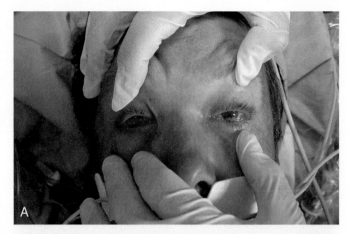
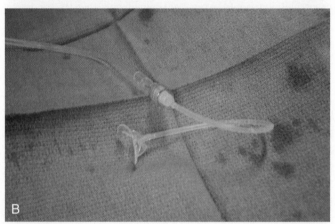
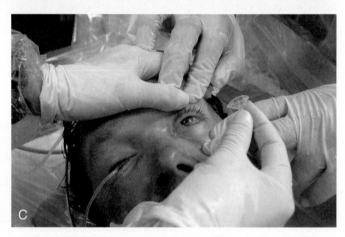

Figure 15-30 Eyes that have sustained a chemical injury require prompt irrigation with copious amounts of saline. A Morgan lens can be placed on the eye to provide appropriate ocular irrigation.
Source: Courtesy of Jeffrey Guy, MD.

attached to IV tubing and an IV bag. Application of an ophthalmic local anesthetic such as proparacaine will simplify the patient's care for the prehospital care provider.

Specific Chemical Exposures

Cement is an alkali that may be retained on the clothing or in the footwear of individuals. The powdered cement will react with the victim's sweat in a reaction that gives off heat and excessively dries, or *desiccates*, the skin.[46] This exposure typically presents with a burn injury hours or the day after contact with the cement. The initial treatment includes brushing the cement powder away followed by copious irrigation.

Fuels such as gasoline and kerosene can cause contact burns after prolonged exposure. These organic hydrocarbons can dissolve cell membranes, resulting in skin necrosis.[47] Decontamination of the patient covered with fuel is accomplished by irrigation with large volumes of water. Gasoline contact exposure can lead to full-thickness tissue injury. An exposure of sufficient duration or severity also may result in systemic toxicity. Severe cardiovascular, renal, pulmonary, neurologic, and hepatic complications may follow absorption through the topical wounds. In cases of suspected systemic toxicity, prompt surgical debridement may be warranted if there is concern for ongoing absorption of toxins from the wound.

Hydrofluoric acid is a dangerous substance widely used in domestic, industrial, and military settings. It is primarily found in the manufacturing of refrigerants but is also used when making herbicides, pharmaceuticals, high-octane gasoline, aluminum, plastics, electrical components, and fluorescent light bulbs. In addition, it is used to etch glass and metal and is found in rust removers and automobile wheel cleaners. The real danger of this chemical is the fluoride ion, which produces profound alterations of electrolytes, especially calcium and magnesium.[48] Even small amounts of hydrofluoric acid can lead to profound, and potentially lethal, *hypocalcemia* (low serum calcium level). Left untreated, hydrofluoric acid will liquefy tissues and leach calcium from the patient's bones. Initial treatment for hydrofluoric acid exposure is irrigation with water, followed by application of calcium gluconate gel at an emergency department. Patients with hydrofluoric acid burns should be promptly transferred to a burn center for additional treatment.

Injuries from phosphorus are often seen in military settings. **White phosphorus** (WP) is a powerful incendiary agent used in the production of munitions. It burns violently when exposed to air, producing brilliant flames and dense smoke. It will continue to burn until all of the agent has been consumed or is deprived of oxygen. When in contact with skin, WP will produce deep chemical and thermal burns.

The initial treatment is to deprive the WP of access to oxygen. All clothing needs to be rapidly removed because it may contain some retained phosphorus particles that could ignite the clothing. Keep the affected areas immersed in water or saline-soaked dressings, and remoisten the dressings during transport. If the dressings dry out, any retained WP will reignite and could ignite the dressings and burn the patient.

Hypochlorite solutions are often used to produce household bleaches and industrial cleaners. These solutions are strong alkalis; the commonly available solutions are 4% to 6% and are not usually lethal unless large areas of the body are exposed to the chemical. In greater concentrations, however, small volumes are potentially lethal. About 30 ml of a 15% solution is considered a life-threatening exposure.

Sulfur and **nitrogen mustards** are compounds that are classified as **vesicants** or **blister agents**. These agents have been used as chemical weapons and are recognized as a threat in chemical terrorism. These chemicals will burn and blister skin on exposure. They are irritants to the skin and cause irritation to the lungs and the eyes. After exposure, patients will complain of a burning sensation in the throat and eyes. The skin involvement develops several hours later as redness is followed by blistering in the exposed or contaminated areas. After intense exposure, victims will develop full-thickness necrosis and respiratory failure.[49-51] The principal treatment in the field is decontamination to prevent inadvertent cross-contamination.

In caring for victims of vesicant exposure, prehospital care providers must wear appropriate gloves, garments, and breathing equipment (**Figure 15-31**). The patients must be decontaminated and irrigated with water or saline. Other agents used to decontaminate victims, used by specially trained personnel, include dilute hypochlorite solution and Fuller's earth powder, which is available commercially and functions as an absorbent agent. Additional specialized treatment is required when the patient arrives at a burn center.

Figure 15-31 Hazardous Materials Scene Control Zones

To limit the spread of a hazardous material, the National Institute of Occupational Safety and Health (NIOSH), the Occupational Safety and Health Administration (OSHA), the U.S. Coast Guard, and the Environmental Protection Agency (EPA) have developed and advocated the use of control zones.[52] The objective of this concept is to perform specific activities in specific zones. By adherence to such principles, the likelihood of spread of contamination and injury to emergency response personnel and bystanders is reduced.

The zones are three concentric circles. The innermost zone is the **hot zone**. This is the region immediately involved with and adjacent to the hazardous materials incident. Personnel entering this area must be fully protected, in most cases using Level A personal protective equipment (PPE), against the potential hazard (see the Explosions and Weapons of Mass Destruction chapter). The task of rescuers in the hot zone is to evacuate injured patients before decontamination or patient care. The next zone is the **warm zone**, where decontamination of patients, personnel, and equipment occurs, again by personnel using appropriate protective equipment. In this zone, the only patient care administered is a primary assessment and spine immobilization, as indicated. The outermost zone is the **cold zone**, where equipment and personnel are staged. Once the patient is evacuated to the cold zone, providers can then deliver definitive care without the need for chemical PPE.

If a patient arrives to your hospital or aid station from a hazardous materials scene and has not been decontaminated, you should follow the concepts of these hazardous materials zones.

Tear gas and similar chemicals are known as **riot control agents**. A riot control agent will rapidly and briefly disable those exposed to it by causing irritation to the skin, mucous membranes, lungs, and eyes. The extent of the injury is determined by the magnitude of exposure to the agent. The duration of the irritation typically lasts 30 to 60 minutes. Treatment consists of removing those exposed to the riot control agent from the source of the exposure, removing contaminated clothing, and irrigating the patients' skin and eyes.

Summary

- All burns are serious, regardless of their size.
- Potentially life-threatening burns include large thermal burns, electrical injuries, and chemical burns.
- Unlike in mechanical trauma (e.g., penetrating, blunt), the body has little to no adaptive mechanisms to survive a burn injury.
- Burn injuries are not isolated to the skin; these are systemic injuries of unparalleled magnitude. Patients with major burn injury will experience dysfunction of the cardiovascular, pulmonary, gastrointestinal, renal, and immune systems.
- Failure to provide appropriate fluid resuscitation will lead to refractory shock, multiorgan dysfunction, and even deepening of the burns. The role of the prehospital care provider is, therefore, crucial in optimizing survival after a burn injury.
- Although complicated and dangerous, burns are rarely rapidly fatal. A patient with severe smoke inhalation and large thermal burns may take several hours or days to die. Patients with burns also are likely to have other mechanical trauma.
- Dramatic burns may focus the prehospital care provider's attention away from other, potentially life-threatening injuries. Performing primary and secondary assessments will reduce the likelihood of missing these injuries (e.g., pneumothorax, pericardial tamponade, splenic rupture).
- Constant vigilance is required to avoid becoming a victim. Often the injuring agent still poses a risk for injuring the prehospital care providers.
- Even small burns in areas of high function (hands, face, joints, perineum) may result in long-term impairment from scar formation.
- Familiarity with burn center transport criteria will help ensure that all patients can achieve maximal function recovery after burn injury.
- The leading cause of death in patients with burns is complications from smoke inhalation: asphyxiation, thermal injury, and delayed toxic-induced lung injury. Frequently, patients do not develop symptoms of respiratory failure for 48 hours or longer. Even without burns to the skin, victims of smoke inhalation should be transported to burn centers.
- Victims of burn injury from hazardous materials, such as chemicals or radioactive agents, should undergo decontamination to avoid inadvertent spread of the material to prehospital and health care providers.

SCENARIO RECAP

You are called to a residential structure fire. When your unit arrives, you witness a two-story house that is fully involved with fire and thick, black smoke pouring out of the roof and windows. You are directed to a victim who is being cared for by EMRs. They tell you that the patient re-entered the burning building in an attempt to rescue his dog, and he was carried out unconscious by fire fighters.

Your patient is a man who appears to be in his thirties. The majority of his clothes have been burned off. He has obvious burns to his face, and his hair has been singed. He is unconscious; he is breathing spontaneously, but with snoring respirations. The EMRs have placed the patient on high-flow oxygen with a nonrebreather mask. On physical examination, his airway is patent with manual assistance (jaw thrust); he ventilates easily. The sleeves of his shirt have been burned off. His arms have circumferential burns, but his radial pulse is easily palpable. His heart rate is 118 beats/minute, blood pressure is 148/94 mm Hg, ventilatory rate is 22 breaths/minute, and oxygen saturation (Spo_2), taken by pulse oximeter, is 92%. On physical examination, you determine that the patient is burned on his entire head and has blistering of the anterior chest and abdomen, along with full-thickness burns of his entire right and left arm and hand.

- What is the extent of burns for this patient?
- What are the initial steps for managing this patient?
- How does the prehospital care provider recognize an inhalation injury?

SCENARIO SOLUTION

The patient has sustained critical injuries. Given that the patient was found collapsed in a burned building with burns to the face and labored respirations, you must be concerned that the patient has inhaled a large amount of smoke.

Evaluate and re-evaluate for airway edema and an inhalation injury. Airway patency needs to be a concern; however, the patient currently is managing his own airway. Keeping in mind that often the best person to manage an airway is the patient, you need to balance the time required to transport the patient with the difficulties of airway management in a patient with an edematous airway. If transport will be prolonged or delayed, secure the airway by tracheal intubation. The patient clearly needs 100% oxygen given the exposure to smoke and concerns about asphyxiants. If you elect to intubate this patient, be careful to secure the ET tube. Anchor the tube securely. A portable carbon monoxide monitor placed on the patient reports a carboxyhemoglobin level of 16%, which is already being treated since the patient is on 100% oxygen. You consult the local protocol regarding management of smoke inhalation with potential cyanide poisoning.

Both upper extremities have deep, full-thickness burns. You are not able to identify any veins to establish an IV line. Neither leg is burned, nor is there evidence of any fractures. An IO line is started in the left tibia, and an infusion of lactated Ringer's is begun.

The patient is burned on the entire head, both upper extremities, and the anterior trunk. Each limb is approximately 9% of TBSA, the anterior trunk is 18%, and the head is approximately 9%. Therefore, the estimated TBSA burned is approximately 45%. The patient weighs approximately 175 pounds, or 80 kg. Estimate the patient's fluid needs using the Parkland formula, as follows:

45% TBSA burned × 80 kg × 4 ml/kg/TBSA burned = 14,400 ml to be administered in first 24 hours

Half this fluid total is administered in the first 8 hours after injury. Therefore, the hourly rate for the first 8 hours is:

14,400 ml/2 = 7,200 ml to be administered in first 8 hours

Calculate the hourly fluid rate:

7,200 ml/8 = 900 ml per hour for hours 0 to 8

References

1. Tredget EE, Shankowsky HA, Taerum TV, et al. The role of inhalation injury in burn trauma: a Canadian experience. *Ann Surg.* 1990;212:720.

2. Herndon D, Rutan R, Rutan T. Management of the pediatric patient with burns. *J Burn Care Rehabil.* 1993;14(1):3.

3. Rossignal A, Locke J, Burke J. Pediatric burn injuries in New England, USA. *Burns.* 1990;16(1):41.

4. Mortiz AR, Henrique FC Jr. Studies of thermal injury: the relative importance of time and surface temperature in the causation of cutaneous burn injury. *Am J Pathol.* 1947;23:695.

5. Robinson MC, Del Becaro EJ. Increasing dermal perfusion after burning by decreasing thromboxane production. *J Trauma.* 1980;20:722.

6. Heggers JP, Ko F, Robson MC, et al. Evaluation of burn blister fluid. *Plast Reconstr Surg.* 1980;65:798.

7. Rossiter ND, Chapman P, Haywood IA. How big is a hand? *Burns.* 1996;22(3):230–231.

8. Berry MG, Evison D, Roberts AH. The influence of body mass index on burn surface area estimated from the area of the hand. *Burns.* 2001;27(6):591–594.

9. de Camara DL, Robinson MC. Ultrastructure aspects of cooled thermal injury. *J Trauma.* 1981;21:911–919.

10. Jandera V, Hudson DA, de Wet PM, Innes PM, Rode H. Cooling the burn wound: evaluation of different modalities. *Burns.* 2000;26:265–270.

11. Sawada Y, Urushidate S, Yotsuyanagi T, Ishita K. Is prolonged and excessive cooling of a scalded wound effective? *Burns.* 1977;23(1):5558.

12. Venter TH, Karpelowsky JS, Rode H. Cooling of the burn wound: the ideal temperature of the coolant. *Burns.* 2007;33:917–922.

13. Dunn K, Edwards-Jones VT. The role of Acticoat with nanocrystal-line silver in the management of burns. *Burns.* 2004;30(suppl):S1.

14. Wright JB, Lam K, Burrell RE. Wound management in an era of increasing bacterial antibiotic resistance: a role for topical silver treatments. *Am J Infect Control.* 1998;26:572.

15. Yin HQ, Langford R, Burrell RE. Comparative evaluation of the antimicrobial activity of Acticoat antimicrobial dressing. *J Burn Care Rehabil.* 1999;20:195.

16. Chung KK, Salinas J, Renz EM, et al. Simple derivation of the initial fluid rate for the resuscitation of severely burned adult combat casualties: in silico validation of the rule of 10. *J Trauma.* 2010;69:S49–S54.

17. Navar PD, Saffle JR, Warden GD. Effect of inhalation injury on fluid resuscitation requirements after thermal injury. *Am J Surg.* 1985;150:716.

18. RxList. Anectine: warnings. http://www.rxlist.com/anectine-drug/warnings-precautions.htm Reviewed January 31, 2011. Accessed September 1, 2013.

19. Layton TR, McMurty JM, McClain EJ, Kraus DR, Reimer BL. Multiple spine fractures from electrical injuries. *J Burn Care Rehabil.* 1984;5:373–375.

20. Moritz AR, Henriques FC, McClean R. The effects of inhaled heat on the air passages and lungs. *Am J Pathol.* 1945;21:311.

21. Peters WJ. Inhalation injury caused by the products of combustion. *Can Med Assoc J.* 1981;125:249.

22. Forbes WH, Sargent F, Roughton FJW. The rate of carbon monoxide uptake by normal men. *Am J Physiol.* 1945;143:594.

23. Mellins RB, Park S. Respiratory complications of smoke inhalation in victims of fires. *J Pediatr.* 1975;87:1.

24. Buckley NA, Juurlink DN, Isbister G, Bennett MH, Lavonas EJ. Cochrane Summaries. There is insufficient evidence to support the use of hyperbaric oxygen for treatment of patients with carbon monoxide poisoning. http://summaries.cochrane.org/CD002041/. Published April 13, 2011. Accessed September 1, 2013

25. Chen KK, Rose CL, Clowes GH. Comparative values of several antidotes in cyanide poisoning. *Am J Med Sci.* 1934;188:767.

26. Feldstein M, Klendshoj NJ. The determination of cyanide in biological fluids by microdiffusion analysis. *J Lab Clin Med.* 1954;44:166.

27. Vogel SN, Sultan TR. Cyanide poisoning. *Clin Toxicol.* 1981;18:367.

28. Crapo R. Smoke inhalation injuries. *JAMA.* 1981;246:1694.

29. Herndon DN, Traber DL, Niehaus GD, et al. The pathophysiology of smoke inhalation in a sheep model. *J Trauma.* 1984;24:1044.

30. Till GO, Johnson KJ, Kunkel R, et al. Intravascular activation of complement and acute lung injury. *J Clin Invest.* 1982;69:1126.

31. Thommasen HV, Martin BA, Wiggs BR, et al. Effect of pulmonary blood flow on leukocyte uptake and release by dog lung. *J Appl Physiol Respir Environ Exerc Physiol.* 1984;56:966.

32. Trunkey DD. Inhalation injury. *Surg Clin North Am.* 1978;58:1133.

33. Haponik E, Summer W. Respiratory complications in the burned patient: diagnosis and management of inhalation injury. *J Crit Care.* 1987;2:121.

34. Cahalane M, Demling R. Early respiratory abnormalities from smoke inhalation. *JAMA.* 1984;251:771.

35. Hight DW, Bakalar HR, Lloyd JR. Inflicted burns in children: recognition and treatment. *JAMA.* 1979;242:517.

36. U.S. Department of Justice, Office of Justice Programs, Office of Juvenile Justice and Delinquency Prevention. *Burn Injuries in Child Abuse.* 2001. https://www.ncjrs.gov/pdffiles/91190-6.pdf. Accessed December 17, 2013.

37. Chadwick DL. The diagnosis of inflicted injury in infants and young children. *Pediatr Ann.* 1992;21:477.

38. Adronicus M, Oates RK, Peat J, et al. Nonaccidental burns in children. *Burns.* 1998;24:552.

39. Purdue GF, Hunt JL, Prescott PR. Child abuse by burning: an index of suspicion. *J Trauma.* 1988;28:221.

40. Lenoski EF, Hunter KA. Specific patterns of inflicted burn injuries. *J Trauma.* 1977;17:842.

41. Brooks JW, Evans EI, Ham WT, Reid JD. The influence of external body radiation on mortality from thermal burns. *Ann Surg.* 1953;136:533.

42. American Burn Association (ABA). Radiation injury. In: *Advanced Burn Life Support Course.* Chicago, IL: ABA; 1999:66.

43. Michell MW, Oliveira HM, Vaid SU, et al. Enteral resuscitation of burn shock using intestinal infusion of World Health Organization oral rehydration solution (WHO ORS): a potential treatment for mass casualty care. *J Burn Care Rehabil.* 2004;25:S48.

44. Bromberg BF, Song IC, Walden RH. Hydrotherapy of chemical burns. *Plast Reconstr Surg.* 1965;35:85.

45. Leonard LG, Scheulen JJ, Munster AM. Chemical burns: effect of prompt first aid. *J Trauma.* 1982;22:420.

46. Alam M, Moynagh M, Orr DS, Lawlor C. Cement burns—the Dublin national burns experience. *J Burns Wounds.* 2007;7:33–38.

47. Mozingo DW, Smith AD, McManus WF, et al. Chemical burns. *J Trauma.* 1998;28:64.

48. Mistry D, Wainwright D. Hydrofluoric acid burns. *Am Fam Physician.* 1992;45:1748.

49. Willems JL. Clinical management of mustard gas casualties. *Ann Med Milit Belg.* 1989;3S:1.

50. Papirmeister B, Feister AJ, Robinson SI, et al. The sulfur mustard injury: description of lesions and resulting incapacitation. In: Papirmeister B, Feister A, Robinson S, Ford R. *Medical Defense Against Mustard Gas.* Boca Raton, FL: CRC Press; 1990:13.

51. Sidell FR, Takafuji ET, Franz DR. *Medical Aspects of Chemical and Biological Warfare.* Washington, DC: Office of the Surgeon General; 1997.

52. Centers for Disease Control and Prevention. NIOSH/OSHA/USCG/EPA recommended zones. http://wonder.cdc.gov/wonder/prevguid/p0000018/p0000018.asp#Figure_5 Accessed September 2, 2013.

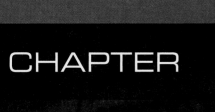

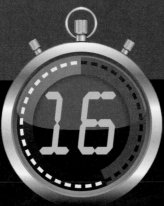

CHAPTER 16

Pediatric Trauma

CHAPTER OBJECTIVES

At the completion of this chapter, the reader will be able to do the following:

- Identify the anatomic and physiologic differences in children that account for unique pediatric injury patterns.

- Demonstrate an understanding of the special importance of managing the airway and restoring adequate tissue oxygenation in pediatric patients.

- Identify the quantitative vital signs for pediatric patients.

- Demonstrate an understanding of management techniques for the various injuries found in pediatric patients.

- Calculate the Pediatric Trauma Score.

- Describe the signs of pediatric trauma suggestive of nonaccidental trauma.

SCENARIO

You are called to the scene of a motor vehicle crash on a heavily traveled highway. Two vehicles have been involved in a frontal offset collision. One of the vehicle's occupants is a child improperly restrained in a child booster seat. No weather-related factors are involved on this spring afternoon.

On arrival at the scene, you see that the police have secured and blocked traffic from the area around the crash. As your partner and the other arriving crew are assessing the other patients, you approach the child. You see a young boy, approximately 2 years of age, sitting in the booster seat, which is slightly turned at an angle; there is blood on the back of the headrest of the seat in front of him. Despite numerous abrasions and minor bleeding from the head, face, and neck, the child appears very calm.

Your primary and secondary assessments reveal a 2-year-old boy who weakly repeats "ma-ma, ma-ma." His pulse rate is 180 beats/minute, with the radial pulses weaker than the carotid; his blood pressure is 50 millimeters of mercury (mm Hg) by palpation. His ventilatory rate is 18 breaths/minute, slightly irregular, but without abnormal sounds. As you continue to assess him, you note that he has stopped saying "ma-ma" and seems to just stare into space. You also note that his pupils are slightly dilated, and his skin is pale and sweaty. A woman who identifies herself as the family's nanny tells you that the mother is en route and that you should wait for her.

- What are the management priorities for this patient?
- What are the most likely injuries in this child?
- Where is the most appropriate destination for this child?

Introduction

Annual data reporting from the Centers for Disease Control and Prevention (CDC) continues to show that, although the leading cause of death continues to vary by age group, injury is the most common cause of death for children in the United States. More than 8.5 million children are injured annually, with approximately one child death from injuries every 30 minutes.[1,2] Tragically, as many as 80% of these deaths may be avoidable, either by effective injury-prevention strategies or by ensuring proper care in the acute injury phase.[3]

As with all aspects of pediatric care, proper assessment and management of an injured child require a thorough understanding of not only the unique characteristics of childhood growth and development (including their immature anatomy and developing physiology) but also their unique mechanisms of injury.

The adage holds true that "children are not just little adults." Children have distinct, reproducible patterns of injury, different physiologic responses, and special treatment needs, based on their physical and psychosocial development at the time of injury.

This chapter first describes the special characteristics of the pediatric trauma patient, then reviews optimal trauma management and its rationale. Although the unique characteristics of pediatric injury are important for the prehospital care provider to understand, the fundamental basic and advanced life support treatment approach using the primary and secondary assessments is the same for every patient, regardless of age or size.

The Child as Trauma Patient

Demographics of Pediatric Trauma

The unique needs and characteristics of pediatric patients require special attention when assessing the acutely injured child. The incidence of blunt (versus penetrating) trauma is highest in the pediatric population. The National Pediatric Trauma Registry (NPTR), the National Trauma Data Bank (NTDB) of the American College of Surgeons (ACS), continues to identify blunt trauma as the most common mechanism of injury, with penetrating injury accounting for only 10% of pediatric cases. While penetrating trauma will often result in injury to one body system, blunt trauma mechanisms have a greater propensity for multisystem injury.

Falls, pedestrians struck by automobiles, and occupant injury as a result of motor vehicle crashes are the most common causes of pediatric injury in the United States, with falls alone accounting for more than 2.5 million injuries a year.[2] Worldwide, the World Health Organization estimates that approximately 950,000 children die from trauma and tens of millions are hospitalized with nonfatal injuries.[4] As in the United States, traffic-related accidents are the most common cause of death, with burns, homicide, and falls the next most common.

For a variety of reasons, to be discussed throughout this chapter, multisystem involvement is the rule rather than the exception in major pediatric trauma. Although there may only be minimal external evidence of injury present, potentially life-threatening internal injury may still exist and must be evaluated for at an appropriate trauma center.

Kinematics of Pediatric Trauma

A child's size produces a smaller target to which forces from fenders, bumpers, and falls are applied. Minimal cushioning from body fat, increased elasticity of connective tissues, and proximity of the viscera to the surface of the body limit children's ability to dissipate these forces as in the adult; therefore, energy is more readily transmitted to underlying organs. Additionally, the skeleton of a child is incompletely calcified, contains multiple active growth centers, and is more resilient than that of an adult. As a result, there may be significant internal injuries without obvious evidence of external trauma.

Common Patterns of Injury

The unique anatomic and physiologic characteristics of the pediatric patient, combined with the age-specific common mechanisms of injury, produce distinct, but predictable, patterns of injury (Figure 16-1). Improper seat belt usage or front seat placement in the vehicle with resulting air bag impact can lead to significant injury in the pediatric patient (**Figure 16-2**). Trauma is frequently a time-critical illness, and familiarity with these patterns will assist the prehospital care provider in optimizing management decisions for the injured child in an expeditious manner. For example, blunt pediatric trauma involving closed head injury results in apnea, hypoventilation, and hypoxia much more commonly than hypovolemia and hypotension. Therefore, clinical care guidelines for pediatric trauma patients should include greater emphasis on focused management of the airway and breathing.

Thermal Homeostasis

The ratio between a child's body surface area and body mass is highest at birth and diminishes throughout infancy and childhood. Consequently, more surface area exists through which heat can quickly be lost, not only providing additional stress to the child but also altering the child's physiologic responses to metabolic derangements and shock. Profound hypothermia can result in severe *coagulopathy* and potentially irreversible cardiovascular collapse. In addition, many of the clinical signs of hypothermia are similar to those of impending decompensated shock, thereby potentially muddying the prehospital care provider's clinical assessment.

Psychosocial Issues

The psychological ramifications for an injured child can also present a major challenge. Particularly with a very young child, regressive psychological behavior may result when stress, pain, or other perceived threats impair the child's ability to process frightening events. Unfamiliar individuals in strange

Figure 16-1 Common Patterns of Injury Associated with Pediatric Trauma	
Type of Trauma	**Patterns of Injury**
Motor vehicle crash (child is passenger)	Unrestrained: Multisystem trauma (including chest and abdomen), head and neck injuries, scalp and facial lacerations Restrained: Chest and abdomen injuries, lower spine fractures Side impact: Head, neck, and chest injuries; extremity fracture Deployed air bag: Head, face, chest injuries; upper extremity fractures
Motor vehicle crash (child is pedestrian)	Low speed: Lower extremity fractures High speed: Multisystem trauma (including chest and abdomen), head and neck injuries, lower extremity fractures
Fall from a height	Low: Upper extremity fractures Medium: Head and neck injuries, upper and lower extremity fractures High: Multisystem trauma (including chest and abdomen), head and neck injuries, upper and lower extremity fractures
Fall from bicycle	Without helmet: Head and neck lacerations, scalp and facial lacerations, upper extremity fractures With helmet: Upper extremity fractures Striking handlebar: Internal abdominal injuries

Source: Modified from American College of Surgeons Committee on Trauma: Pediatric trauma. In ACS Committee on Trauma: *Advanced trauma life support for doctors, student course manual*, ed 9, Chicago, 2012, ACS.

Figure 16-2 Pediatric Injuries Associated with Seat Belts and Air Bags

Despite laws in all 50 states requiring the use of car safety seats or child restraint devices for young children, in almost half of motor vehicle crashes, the child is not restrained or is improperly restrained.[5] Furthermore, if a child is the front-seat occupant in a vehicle with a passenger-side air bag, the child is just as likely to sustain serious injury whether appropriately restrained or not.[6] A child exposed to a passenger-side air bag is twice as likely to sustain significant injury as a front-seat passenger without an air bag.[7]

Children with lap belt or inappropriate seat belt placement are thought to be at increased risk for bowel injury in motor vehicle crashes. The incidence is difficult to determine. In one study, 20% of injured children had a visible seat belt bruise, and 50% of these children had significant intra-abdominal injuries; almost 25% of these children had intestinal perforation.[8] Others have shown an increased risk, but not to this extent, with only 5%

of injured children having an abdominal wall bruise from the seat belt, and only 13% of those with bruising having intestinal injury.[9] It is reasonable to assume that any child found restrained by a lap belt with abdominal wall bruising after a motor vehicle crash has an intra-abdominal injury until proved otherwise.

Approximately 1% of all motor vehicle crashes involving children also resulted in exposure of the child to a deployed passenger air bag. Of these children, 14% suffered serious injury, compared with 7.5% of restrained front-seat passengers not exposed to an air bag. Overall risk of any injury was 86% versus 55% in the control group of patients (those not exposed to an air bag).[7] Minor air bag injury included minor upper torso and facial burns and lacerations. Major air bag injury consisted of significant chest, neck, face, and upper extremity injury.[10] There has been a documented decapitation of a child by a passenger air bag.[2]

---

surroundings can limit a child's ability to fully cooperate with history taking, physical examination, and treatment. An understanding of these characteristics and a willingness to soothe and comfort an injured child are frequently the most effective means of achieving good rapport and obtaining a comprehensive assessment of the child's physiologic state.

The child's parents, or caregivers, also frequently have unique needs and issues, such as information about the child's injuries and planned treatment or reassurance about the child's condition, that, if addressed, may assist the prehospital care provider in caring for the child successfully; however, if ignored, these needs and issues can cause parents to become angry or aggressive and present significant obstacles to effective care. Whenever a child is sick or injured, the caregivers are also affected and should be considered to be patients as well. The treatment of all patients begins with effective communication, but communication becomes even more important when dealing with these "parent patients." It may only consist of simple words of compassion, or great lengths of patience, but you cannot be an effective prehospital care provider for the pediatric patient if you are ignorant of the parents'/caregivers' needs. When you include the parents/caregivers in the process, they can often act as functional members of their child's emergency care team. Furthermore, parental engagement will be a signal to the child that you are endorsed as a "safe" person, increasing the likelihood of the child's cooperation.

Recovery and Rehabilitation

Also unique to the pediatric trauma patient is the effect that even minor injury may have on subsequent growth and development. Unlike an anatomically mature adult, a child must not only

recover from the injury but also continue normal growth. The effect of injury on this process, especially in terms of permanent disability, growth deformity, or subsequent abnormal development, cannot be overestimated. Children sustaining even minor traumatic brain injury (TBI) may have prolonged disability in cerebral function, psychological adjustment, or other regulated organ systems. As many as 60% of children who have sustained severe multiple trauma have personality changes, with 50% having subtle cognitive or physical handicaps. These disabilities can have a substantial effect on siblings and parents, resulting in a high incidence of family dysfunction, including divorce.

The effects of inadequate or suboptimal care in the acute injury phase may have far-reaching consequences not only on the child's immediate survival but also, perhaps more importantly, on the long-term quality of the child's life. Therefore, it is extremely important to maintain a high index of suspicion for injury and to use clinical "common sense" when caring and making transport decisions for the acutely injured child.

Pathophysiology

The final outcome for the injured child may be determined by the quality of care rendered in the first moments following an injury. During this critical period, a coordinated, systematic primary assessment is the best strategy to avoid unnecessary morbidity and prevent overlooking a potentially fatal injury. As in the adult patient, the three most common causes of immediate death in the child are hypoxia, massive hemorrhage, and overwhelming central nervous system (CNS) trauma. Expedient triage, stabilizing emergency medical treatment, and transport to the most appropriate center for treatment can optimize the potential for a meaningful recovery.

Hypoxia

The first priority in prehospital care is always to maintain a patent airway, whether by basic supportive measures or through advanced techniques. Confirming that a child has an open and functioning airway does not preclude the need for supplemental oxygen and assisted ventilation, especially when CNS injury, hypoventilation, or hypoperfusion is present. Well-appearing, injured children can rapidly deteriorate from mild tachypnea to a state of total exhaustion and apnea. Once an airway is established, the rate and depth of ventilation should be carefully evaluated to confirm adequate ventilation. If ventilation is inadequate, merely providing an excessive concentration of oxygen will not prevent ongoing or worsening hypoxia.

The effects of even *transient* (brief) hypoxia on the traumatically injured brain deserve special attention. A child may have significant alteration in level of consciousness (LOC), yet retain an excellent potential for a complete functional recovery if cerebral hypoxia is avoided.

Pediatric patients who require aggressive airway management should be preoxygenated before attempting to place an advanced airway device. This simple maneuver may not only begin the reversal of existing hypoxia but also provide sufficient reserves to improve the margin of safety when placement of an advanced airway is performed. A period of hypoxia during multiple or prolonged attempts at placing an advanced airway may be more detrimental to the child than simply ventilating the child with a bag-mask and rapidly transporting.[11-13] In light of recent data, attempting advanced airway management is unnecessary and potentially harmful if the child is adequately ventilated and oxygenated using good basic life support skills, such as bag-mask ventilation.

Hemorrhage

Most pediatric injuries do not cause immediate exsanguination. However, children who sustain injuries that result in major blood loss frequently die within moments of the injury or shortly after arrival at a receiving facility. These fatalities frequently result from multiple injured internal organs, with at least one significant injury causing acute blood loss. This bleeding may be minor, such as a simple laceration or contusion, or may be a life-threatening hemorrhage, such as a ruptured spleen, lacerated liver, or avulsed kidney.

As in adults, the injured child compensates for hemorrhage by increasing systemic vascular resistance; however, this is at the expense of peripheral perfusion. Children are physiologically more adept at this response because pediatric vasoconstriction is not limited by pre-existing peripheral vascular disease. Utilizing blood pressure measurements alone is an inadequate strategy to identify the early signs of shock. Tachycardia, although it may be the result of fear or pain, should be considered to be secondary to hemorrhage or hypovolemia until proven otherwise.

A narrowing pulse pressure and increasing tachycardia may be the first subtle signs of impending shock.

Furthermore, the prehospital care provider must pay close attention to signs of ineffective organ perfusion as evidenced by alterations in respiratory efforts, decreased LOC, and diminished skin perfusion (decreased temperature, poor color, and prolonged capillary refill). Unlike in the adult, these early signs of hemorrhage in the child may be subtle and difficult to identify, leading to a delayed recognition of shock. If the prehospital care provider misses these early signs, a child may lose enough circulating blood volume that compensatory mechanisms fail. When this happens, cardiac output plummets, organ perfusion decreases, and the child can rapidly decompensate, often leading to irreversible, fatal hypotension and shock. Therefore, every child who sustains blunt trauma should be carefully monitored to detect these subtle signs that might signal that there is ongoing hemorrhage, long before frank vital sign abnormalities.

A major reason for the rapid transition to decompensated shock is the loss of red blood cells (RBCs) and their corresponding oxygen-carrying capacity. Restoration of lost intravascular volume with crystalloid solutions will provide a transient increase in blood pressure, but circulating volume will dissipate quickly as the fluid shifts across capillary membranes. It is generally thought that when replacing the intravascular volume with isotonic crystalloid solutions, a 3:1 ratio of crystalloid to the suspected blood loss is needed to compensate for this fluid shift. As blood is lost and intravascular volume is replaced with crystalloids, the remaining RBCs are diluted in the bloodstream, reducing the blood's ability to carry oxygen to the tissues. Therefore, it should be assumed that any child who requires more than one 20 milliliter per kilogram (ml/kg) bolus of crystalloid solution may be rapidly deteriorating and not only needs intravascular volume resuscitation with crystalloid solution but will likely also require a transfusion of RBCs so that oxygen-delivery capacity is restored in parallel to the intravascular volume.

However, once vascular access has been secured, there is a tendency to inadvertently over-resuscitate an injured child who is not in frank shock. In the child with moderate bleeding, no evidence of end-organ hypoperfusion, and normal vital signs, fluid resuscitation should be limited to no more than one or two normal saline boluses of 20 ml/kg. The intravascular component of one bolus represents approximately 25% of a child's blood volume. Therefore, if more than two boluses are required, the prehospital care provider must take care to reassess the child for sources of previously undetected ongoing bleeding.

In the child with TBI, fluid resuscitation should be given to prevent hypotension, a known and preventable secondary insult to head injury.[14,15] The cerebral perfusion pressure is the difference between the intracranial pressure (the pressure inside the skull) and the mean arterial pressure (the pressure driving blood into the skull). Traumatic brain injury can cause an increase in intracranial pressure, therefore even though blood may be adequately oxygenated, if the systemic blood pressure is low, oxygenated blood may not perfuse the brain; thus, hypoxic brain injury can still occur. Although over-resuscitation should be avoided to prevent an **iatrogenic** cerebral edema, hypotension must be prevented or quickly treated with fluid resuscitation, as a single episode of hypotension can increase mortality by as much as 150%.[16] Careful assessments of the child's vital signs and frequent re-evaluation after therapeutic interventions should guide ongoing management decisions.

Isotonic crystalloid solutions should be the fluid of choice for resuscitation of the child with TBI, because hypotonic crystalloid solutions (e.g., dextrose in water) are known to increase cerebral edema. Furthermore, although hypertonic crystalloid solutions (e.g., hypertonic saline) may be useful for treatment of cerebral edema in the pediatric intensive care unit where there is extensive monitoring, evidence to date has not demonstrated improved outcomes of pediatric trauma patients when administered in the field.

Central Nervous System Injury

The pathophysiologic changes after CNS trauma begin within minutes. Early and adequate resuscitation is the key to increased survival of children with CNS trauma. Although some CNS injuries are overwhelmingly fatal, many children with the appearance of a devastating neurologic injury go on to a complete and functional recovery after deliberate coordinated efforts to prevent secondary injury. These recoveries are achieved through the prevention of subsequent episodes of hypoperfusion, hypoventilation, hyperventilation, and ischemia. Adequate ventilation and oxygenation (while avoiding hyperventilation) are as critical in the management of TBIs as the avoidance of hypotension.[15]

For given degrees of CNS injury severity, children have lower mortality and a higher potential for survival than their adult counterparts. However, the addition of injuries outside the brain lessens the child's chances of favorable outcome, illustrating the potentially negative effect of shock from associated injuries.

Children with TBI frequently present with an alteration in consciousness, possibly sustaining a period of unconsciousness not witnessed during the initial evaluation. A history of loss of consciousness is one of the most important prognostic indicators of potential CNS injury and should be recorded for every case. In the event that the injury was not witnessed, amnesia to the event is commonly used as a surrogate for a loss of consciousness. Further, complete documentation of baseline neurologic status is important, including the following:

1. Glasgow Coma Scale score (modified for pediatrics)
2. Pupillary reaction
3. Response to sensory stimulation
4. Motor function

These are essential steps in the initial pediatric trauma assessment for neurologic injury. The absence of an adequate baseline assessment makes ongoing follow-up and evaluation of interventions extremely difficult.

Attention to detail in history taking is especially important in pediatric patients with possible cervical spine injury. A child's skeleton is incompletely calcified with multiple active growth centers, often preventing radiographic diagnosis of injury from a mechanism causing a stretching, contusion, or blunt injury to the spinal cord. This condition is called spinal cord injury without radiographic abnormality, or SCIWORA. A transient neurologic deficit that resolves prior to facility arrival may be the only indicator of a significant spinal cord injury. Despite quick symptom resolution, children with SCIWORA can develop spinal cord edema up to 4 days after the initial injury, with devastating neurologic disabilities if left untreated.

Assessment
Primary Assessment

The small and variable size of the pediatric patient (Figure 16-3), the diminished caliber and size of the blood vessels and circulating volume, and the unique anatomic characteristics of the airway frequently make the standard procedures used in basic life

Figure 16-3 Height and Weight Range for Pediatric Patients

Group	Age	Range of Mean Norms Average Height (cm [inches])	Average Weight (kg [lb])
Newborn	Birth to 6 weeks	51 to 63 (20 to 25)	4 to 5 (8 to 11)
Infant	6 weeks to 1 year	56 to 80 (22 to 31)	4 to 11 (8 to 24)
Toddler	1 to 2 years	77 to 91 (30 to 36)	11 to 14 (24 to 31)
Preschooler	2 to 6 years	91 to 122 (36 to 48)	14 to 25 (31 to 55)
School-age child	6 to 13 years	122 to 165 (48 to 65)	25 to 63 (55 to 139)
Adolescent	13 to 16 years	165 to 182 (65 to 72)	62 to 80 (139 to 176)

support extremely challenging and technically difficult. Effective pediatric trauma resuscitation mandates the availability of appropriately sized airways, laryngoscope blades, endotracheal (ET) tubes, nasogastric tubes, blood pressure cuffs, oxygen masks, bag-mask devices, and associated equipment. Attempting to place an overly large intravenous (IV) catheter or an inappropriately sized airway can do more harm than good, not only because of the potential physical damage to the patient, but also because it may delay transport to the appropriate facility. Color-coded, length-based resuscitation guides (discussed later in the chapter) provide practical medication and equipment references.[17]

Airway

As in the injured adult, the immediate priority and focus in the acutely injured child are on airway management. However, there are several anatomic differences that complicate the care of the injured child. Children have a relatively large occiput and tongue and have an anteriorly positioned airway. Additionally, the smaller the child, the greater the size discrepancy between the cranium and the midface. Therefore, the relatively large occiput forces passive flexion of the cervical spine (Figure 16-4). These factors all predispose children to a higher risk of anatomic airway obstruction than adults. In the absence of trauma, the pediatric patient's airway is best protected by a slightly superior–anterior position of the midface, known as the **sniffing position** (Figure 16-5). In the presence of trauma, however, the **neutral position** best protects the cervical spine by keeping it immobilized to prevent the flexion at the fifth and sixth cervical vertebrae (C5 to C6) and the extension at C1 to C2 that occurs with the sniffing position. In this position, a jaw-thrust maneuver can be used to facilitate airway opening if needed.

Manual stabilization of the cervical spine is done during airway management and maintained until the child is immobilized with an appropriate cervical immobilization device, whether it is commercially purchased or a simple solution such as towel rolls. Additionally, placing a pad or blanket of 2 to 3 centimeters (cm; about 1 inch) in thickness under an infant's torso can lessen the acute flexion of the neck and help keep the airway patent.

Bag-mask ventilation with high-flow (at least 15 liters per minute) 100% oxygen probably represents the best choice when the injured child requires assisted ventilation.[11] If the child is unconscious, an oropharyngeal airway may be considered, but due to risk of vomiting, it should not be used in the child with an intact gag reflex. This is also true of the laryngeal mask and King LT airways, both of which are supraglottic airways; when sized appropriately, these devices can be considered for airway management in pediatric trauma patients who cannot be ventilated by simple bag-mask device. In very young children, especially those weighing less than 20 kg, these devices can cause iatrogenic upper airway obstruction by causing the relatively larger pediatric epiglottis to fold into the airway.

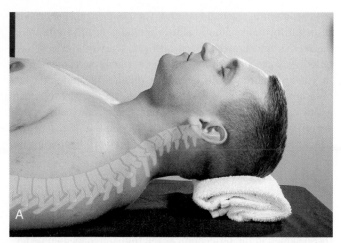

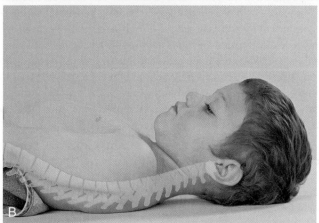

Figure 16-4 Compared to an adult (A), a child has a larger occiput and less shoulder musculature. When placed on a flat surface, these factors result in flexion of the neck (B).

Source: A. © Jones & Bartlett Learning. Photographed by Darren Stahlman.

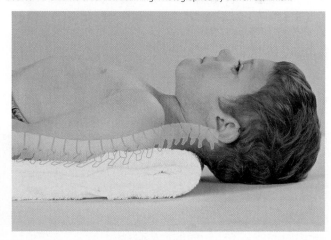

Figure 16-5 Sniffing position.

In comparison to that of the adult, the child's larynx is smaller in size and is slightly more anterior and *cephalad* (forward and toward the head), making it more difficult to visualize the vocal cords during intubation attempts (**Figure 16-6**). Endotracheal intubation, despite being the most reliable means of ventilation in the child with airway compromise, should be reserved for those situations in which bag-mask ventilation is ineffective and nonvisualized advanced airway devices have failed. Nasotracheal intubation is generally not recommended in young children. This technique requires a spontaneously breathing patient, involves blind passage around the relatively acute posterior nasopharyngeal angle, and can cause more severe bleeding in children. Additionally, in the patient with a basilar skull fracture, it can even inadvertently penetrate the cranial vault.

If unable to receive effective bag-mask ventilation, a child with craniofacial injuries causing upper airway obstruction may be considered for percutaneous transtracheal jet ventilation with a large angiocatheter. This should be performed only by those skilled in the procedure, as the thin and malleable pediatric trachea can be easily damaged, resulting in permanent iatrogenic airway loss. This procedure is only a temporary measure to improve oxygenation and does not provide adequate ventilation. Increasing hypercarbia dictates that a more definitive airway be established as soon as safely possible. Surgical cricothyroidotomy is usually not indicated in the care of the pediatric trauma patient, though it may be considered in the larger child (usually at the age of 12 years).[18]

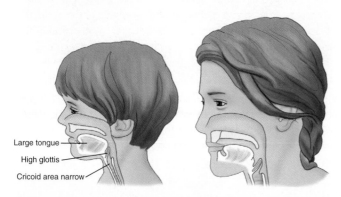

Large tongue
High glottis
Cricoid area narrow

Figure 16-6 Comparison of the adult and child airways.

Breathing

As in all trauma patients, a significantly traumatized child typically needs an oxygen concentration of 85% to 100% (fraction of inspired oxygen [FiO_2] of 0.85 to 1.0). This concentration is maintained by the use of supplemental oxygen and an appropriately sized clear plastic pediatric mask. When hypoxia occurs in the small child, the body compensates by increasing the ventilatory rate (tachypnea) and by a strenuous increase in ventilatory effort, including increased thoracic excursion efforts and the use of accessory muscles in the neck and abdomen. This increased metabolic demand can produce severe fatigue and result in ventilatory failure, as an increasing percentage of the patient's cardiac output becomes devoted to maintaining this respiratory effort. Ventilatory distress can rapidly progress from a compensated ventilatory effort to ventilatory failure, then respiratory arrest, and ultimately a hypoxic cardiac arrest. Central (rather than peripheral) cyanosis is a fairly late and often inconsistent sign of respiratory failure and should not be depended on to recognize impending respiratory failure.

Evaluation of the child's ventilatory status with early recognition of the signs of distress and the provision of ventilatory assistance are key elements in the management of the pediatric trauma patient. The normal ventilatory rate of infants and children younger than 4 years is typically two to three times that of adults (**Figure 16-7**).

Tachypnea with signs of increased effort or difficulty may be the first manifestations of respiratory distress and shock. As distress increases, additional signs and symptoms include shallow breathing or minimal chest movement. Breath sounds may be weak or infrequent, and air exchange at the nose or mouth may be reduced or minimal. Ventilatory effort becomes more labored and may include the following:

- Head bobbing with each breath
- Gasping or grunting
- Flared nostrils

Figure 16-7	Ventilatory Rates for Pediatric Patients		
Group	**Age**	**Ventilatory Rate (breaths/minute)**	**Ventilatory Rate (breaths/minute) That Indicates Possible Need for Ventilatory Assistance with Bag-Mask Device**
Newborn	Birth to 6 weeks	30 to 50	< 30 or > 50
Infant	6 weeks to 1 year	20 to 30	< 20 or > 30
Toddler	1 to 2 years	20 to 30	< 20 or > 30
Preschooler	2 to 6 years	20 to 30	< 20 or > 30
School-age child	6 to 13 years	12 to 25	< 12 or > 25
Adolescent	13 to 16 years	12 to 20	< 12 or > 20

- Stridor or snoring respirations
- Suprasternal, supraclavicular, subcostal, or intercostal retractions
- Use of accessory muscles, such as neck and abdominal wall muscles
- Distension of the abdomen when the chest falls (seesaw effect between the chest and abdomen)

The effectiveness of a child's ventilation should be evaluated using the following indicators:

- Rate and depth (minute volume) and effort indicate adequacy of ventilation.
- Pink skin may indicate adequate ventilation.
- Dusky, gray, cyanotic, or mottled skin indicates insufficient oxygenation and perfusion.
- Anxiety, restlessness, and combativeness can be early signs of hypoxia.
- Lethargy, depressed LOC, and unconsciousness are probably advanced signs of hypoxia.
- Breath sounds indicate the depth of exchange.
- Wheezing, rales, or rhonchi may indicate inefficient oxygenation.
- Declining pulse oximetry and/or declining capnography indicate respiratory failure.

A rapid evaluation of ventilation includes assessment of the patient's ventilatory rate (particularly tachypnea), ventilatory effort (degree of labor, nostril flaring, accessory muscle use, retraction, and seesaw movement), auscultation (air exchange, bilateral symmetry, and pathologic sounds), skin color, and mental status.

In the child initially presenting with tachypnea and increased ventilatory effort, normalization of the ventilatory rate and apparent lessening of the respiratory effort should not be immediately interpreted as a sign of improvement as it may indicate exhaustion or impending respiratory failure. As with any change in the patient's clinical status, frequent reassessment is necessary to determine if this is an improvement or deterioration in physiologic status.

Ventilatory assistance should be given to those children in acute ventilatory distress. Because the main problem is one of inspired volume rather than concentration of oxygen, assisted ventilation is best given by use of a bag-mask device, supplemented with an oxygen reservoir attached to high-concentration oxygen (FiO_2 of 0.85 to 1.0). Because a child's airway is so small, it is prone to obstruction from increased secretions, blood, body fluids, and foreign materials; therefore, early and periodic suctioning may be necessary. In infants, who are obligate nose breathers, the nostrils should also be suctioned.

When obtaining a mask seal in infants, caution should be exercised to avoid compressing the soft tissues underneath the chin because doing so pushes the tongue against the soft palate and increases the risk of occluding the airway. Pressure on the uncalcified, soft trachea should also be avoided. One or two hands can be used to obtain a mask seal, depending on the size and age of the child.

Use of the correct-sized bag-mask is essential for obtaining a proper mask seal, providing the proper tidal volume, and ensuring that the risks of hyperinflation and barotrauma are minimized. Ventilating a child too forcefully or with too large of a tidal volume can lead to gastric distension. In turn, gastric distension can result in regurgitation, aspiration, or prevention of adequate ventilation by limiting diaphragmatic excursion. Hyperinflation can lead to a tension pneumothorax that can result in both severe respiratory distress and sudden cardiovascular collapse, as the mediastinum is more mobile in the child. This mobility protects the child from traumatic aortic injuries but increases the susceptibility to tension pneumothorax. The more mobile mediastinum compresses easily, allowing for earlier respiratory compromise and cardiovascular collapse than occurs in an adult.

Changes in a child's ventilatory status can be subtle, but ventilatory effort can rapidly deteriorate until ventilation is inadequate and hypoxia ensues. The patient's breathing should be evaluated as part of the primary assessment and carefully and periodically reassessed to ensure its continued adequacy. Pulse oximetry should also be monitored, and efforts should be made to keep oxygen saturation (SpO_2) at greater than 95% (at sea level).

Whenever a child is manually ventilated, it is important to carefully control the rate at which ventilations are being administered. It is relatively easy to inadvertently hyperventilate the patient, which will decrease the carbon dioxide level in the blood and cause cerebral vasoconstriction. This can lead to poorer outcomes in patients with TBI. Furthermore, excessive ventilation pressures can lead to gastric insufflation. The distended stomach can subsequently push up into the more pliable pediatric thorax and limit tidal volume capacity.

Circulation

The survival rate from immediate exsanguinating injury is low in the pediatric population. Fortunately, the incidence of this type of injury is also low. External hemorrhage should be quickly identified and controlled by direct manual pressure during the primary assessment. Injured children usually present with at least some circulating blood volume and should respond appropriately to volume replacement.

As in the assessment of the airway, a single measurement of heart rate or blood pressure does not equate with physiologic stability. Serial measurements and changing trends of vital signs are critical in gauging a child's evolving hemodynamic state in the acute injury phase. Close monitoring of vital signs is absolutely essential to recognizing the signs of impending shock, enabling the appropriate interventions to be performed to prevent clinical deterioration. Figures 16-8 and 16-9 provide the normal ranges for pulse rate and blood pressure by pediatric age groups.

If the primary assessment suggests hypotension, the most likely cause is blood loss through a major external wound that is readily observable (e.g., large scalp laceration, open femur fracture), an intrathoracic injury (identifiable by diminished

Figure 16-8   Pulse Rate for Pediatric Patients

Group	Age	Pulse Rate (beats/minute)	Pulse Rate (beats/minute) That Indicates a Possible Serious Problem*
Newborn	Birth to 6 weeks	120 to 160	< 100 or > 160
Infant	6 weeks to 1 year	80 to 140	< 80 or > 150
Toddler	1 to 2 years	80 to 130	< 60 or > 140
Preschooler	2 to 6 years	80 to 120	< 60 or > 130
School-age child	6 to 13 years	60 to 110	< 60 or > 120
Adolescent	13 to 16 years	60 to 100	< 60 or > 100

*Bradycardia or tachycardia.

Figure 16-9   Blood Pressure (BP) for Pediatric Patients

Group	Age	Expected BP Range (mm Hg)*	Lower Limit of Systolic BP (mm Hg)
Newborn	Birth to 6 weeks	74 to 100 50 to 68	> 60
Infant	6 weeks to 1 year	84 to 106 56 to 70	> 70
Toddler	1 to 2 years	98 to 106 50 to 70	> 70
Preschooler	2 to 6 years	98 to 112 64 to 70	> 75
School-age child	6 to 13 years	104 to 124 64 to 80	> 80
Adolescent	13 to 16 years	118 to 132 70 to 82	> 90

*Top numbers represent systolic range; bottom numbers represent diastolic range.

ventilatory mechanics and auscultatory findings), or a major intra-abdominal injury. Because blood is not a compressible medium, blood loss from a major intra-abdominal injury can produce abdominal distension and increasing abdominal girth. However, increased abdominal girth in the young pediatric trauma patient can also commonly be caused by gastric distension from crying and air swallowing. Gastric decompression through a nasogastric or orogastric tube can help to distinguish between these causes of distension, although it is best to assume that a distended abdomen is a sign of potentially significant abdominal injury.

A major consideration in the assessment of a pediatric patient is compensated shock. Because of their increased physiologic reserve, children with hemorrhagic injury frequently present with only slightly abnormal vital signs. Although initial tachycardia may be from hypovolemia, psychological stress, pain, or fear can also increase the heart rate. All injured children should have their heart rate, ventilatory rate, and overall CNS status monitored closely. An accurate blood pressure reading may be difficult to obtain in the prehospital setting, and focus should be placed on other signs of perfusion. A pediatric patient's systolic blood pressure, if measured, may seem alarmingly low when compared to that of an adult, but may be within the normal range for a healthy child.

A child with hemorrhagic injury can maintain adequate circulating volume by increasing peripheral vascular resistance to maintain mean arterial pressure. Clinical evidence of this compensatory mechanism includes prolonged capillary refill, peripheral pallor or mottling, cool peripheral skin temperature, and decreased intensity of the peripheral pulses. In the child, signs of significant hypotension develop with the loss of approximately 30% of the circulating volume. If initial resuscitation is inadequate, increased peripheral vascular resistance will not be able to compensate for loss of circulating volume and the blood pressure will fall. The concept of evolving shock must be of paramount concern in the initial management of an injured child and is a major indication for transport to an appropriate trauma facility for expeditious evaluation and treatment.

Disability

After assessment of airway, breathing, and circulation, the primary assessment must include an assessment of neurologic status. Although the AVPU scale (**A**lert, responds to **V**erbal stimulus, responds to **P**ainful stimulus, **U**nresponsive) remains a simple, rapid assessment tool for the child's neurologic status, it remains less informative than the Glasgow Coma Scale (GCS). It should be combined with a careful examination of the pupils to determine whether they are equal, round, and reactive to light. As in adults, the GCS provides a more thorough assessment of neurologic status and should be calculated for each pediatric trauma patient. The scoring for the verbal section for children younger than 4 years of age must be modified because of developing communication skills in this age group, and the child's behavior should be observed carefully (Figure 16-10).

The GCS score should be repeated frequently and used to document progression or improvement of neurologic status during the postinjury period (refer to the Scene Assessment and the Shock chapters for a review of the GCS). A more thorough assessment of motor and sensory function should be performed in the secondary assessment if time permits.

Expose/Environment

Children should be examined for other potentially life-threatening injuries; however, they may be frightened at attempts to remove their clothes. In addition, because of children's high body surface area, they are more prone to developing hypothermia. Once the examination to identify other injuries is complete, the pediatric patient should be covered to preserve body heat and prevent further heat loss.

Pediatric Trauma Score

The decision as to which child requires what level of care must proceed from a careful and rapid evaluation of the entire child. Overlooking potential organ system injury and inadequately managing the pediatric patient are two common problems, both in the field and in the hospital. For this reason, the **Pediatric Trauma Score** (PTS) was developed to provide a reliable and simple protocol for assessment that is predictive of outcome; however, the PTS is not used in the CDC's field triage algorithm as the physiologic, anatomic, and mechanistic considerations in the field triage algorithm have been considered adequate for the initial field assessment (Figure 16-11).

To calculate the PTS, six components of pediatric injury are graded and then added together to produce a score predictive of injury severity and potential for mortality. The six components are the pediatric patient's size, airway, LOC, systolic blood pressure, presence of fractures, and skin condition. The system is based on an analysis of pediatric injury patterns and is designed to provide a protocol checklist to ensure that all the major injury factors related to injury outcome are considered in the initial evaluation of the child. The PTS is different than the Revised Trauma Score (RTS), which considers only the blood pressure, ventilatory rate, and GCS score.

Size is the first component because it is readily observed and is a major consideration in the infant/toddler group. The airway is assessed next, because the functional status and the level of care required to provide adequate ventilation and oxygenation must be considered.

The most important historical factor in primary assessment of the CNS is loss of consciousness (LOC). Because children frequently sustain transient LOC during an injury, the obtunded grade (+1) is applied to any child with loss of consciousness, no matter how fleeting. This grade identifies children at higher risk of developing potentially fatal, yet frequently treatable, intracranial injuries that may lead to secondary brain injury.

Systolic blood pressure (SBP) is used to identify children in whom evolving preventable shock may occur (SBP 51 to 90 mm Hg; +1). Regardless of size, a child whose SBP is less than 50 mm Hg (−1) is in obvious jeopardy (**Figure 16-12**). A child whose SBP exceeds 90 mm Hg (+2) falls into a better outcome category. If the appropriately sized blood pressure cuff is not available, SBP is assessed as +2 if the radial or pedal pulse is palpable, +1 if only the carotid or femoral pulse is palpable, and −1 if no pulse is palpable.

Because of the high incidence of skeletal injury in the pediatric population and its potential contribution to mortality and disability, the presence of a long-bone fracture is included in the PTS as a component. Finally, the skin is assessed for open wounds and penetrating injury.

Figure 16-10 Pediatric Verbal Score

Verbal Response	Verbal Score
Appropriate words or social smile; fixes and follows	5
Crying but consolable	4
Persistently irritable	3
Restless, agitated	2
No response	1

Figure 16-11 Pediatric Trauma Score

Component	+2	+1	−1
Size	Child/adolescent >20 kg	Toddler 11–20 kg	Infant <10 kg
Airway	Normal	Assisted: O₂ mask, cannula	Intubated: ETT, cricothyroidotomy
Consciousness	Awake	Obtunded, lost consciousness	Coma, unresponsive
Systolic blood pressure	90 mm Hg Good peripheral pulses, perfusion	51–90 mm Hg Carotid, femoral pulse palpable	<50 mm Hg Weak or no pulses
Fracture	None seen or suspected	Single closed fracture anywhere	Open or multiple fractures
Cutaneous	No visible injury	Contusion, abrasion, laceration <7 cm not through fascia	Tissue loss, any gun shot wound or stab through fascia

Note: The Pediatric Trauma Score (PTS) is primarily designed to function as a checklist. Each component can be assessed by basic physical examination. Airway evaluation is designed to reflect intervention required for effective care. An open fracture is graded −1 for fracture and −1 for cutaneous injury. As clinical observation and diagnostic evaluation continue, further definition and reassessment will establish a trend that predicts severity of injury and potential outcome.

Figure 16-12 Pediatric Vital Signs and Quantitative Norms

The term pediatric or child includes a vast range of physical development, emotional maturity, and body sizes. The approach to the patient and the implications of many injuries vary greatly between an infant and an adolescent.

In most anatomic and therapeutic dosage considerations, a child's weight (or specific height or length) serves as a more accurate indicator than exact chronologic age.[17] Figure 16-3 lists the average height and weight for healthy children of varying ages.

The acceptable ranges of vital signs vary for the different ages within the pediatric population. Adult norms cannot be used as guidelines in smaller children. An adult ventilatory rate of 30 breaths/minute is tachypneic, and an adult heart rate of 120 beats/minute is tachycardic. Both are considered alarmingly high in an adult and are significant pathologic findings. However, the same findings in an infant may be within the normal ranges.

Normal ranges of vital signs for different age groups may not be consistent across all pediatric references. In an injured child without a previous history of normal vital signs, borderline vital signs may be viewed as pathologic, even though the signs may be physiologically acceptable in that specific child. The guidelines in Figures 16-8, 16-8, and 16-9 can aid in evaluating vital signs in pediatric patients. These tables present statistically common ranges into which most children in these age groups will fall.

Several commercially available items serve as rapid reference guides for pediatric vital signs and equipment size. These include the length-based resuscitation tape and several slide-rule-type plastic scales.

The following guideline formulas can also be used to estimate the expected finding for ages 1 to 10 years:

$$\text{Weight (kg)} = 8 + (2 \times \text{Child's age [years]})$$

$$\text{Lowest acceptable SBP (mm Hg)} = 70 + (2 \times \text{Child's age [years]})$$

$$\text{Total vascular blood volume (ml)} = 80 \text{ ml} \times \text{Child's weight (kg)}$$

Quantitative vital signs in children, although important, are only one piece of information used in making an assessment. A child with a normal set of vital signs can rapidly deteriorate into either critical ventilatory difficulty or decompensated shock. Vital signs should be considered along with mechanism of injury and other clinical findings.

By nature of its design, the PTS serves as a straightforward checklist that ensures that all of the components necessary to identify a critically injured pediatric patient are considered. As a predictor of injury, the PTS has a statistically significant, direct linear relationship with the Injury Severity Score (ISS) and an inverse linear relationship with patient mortality. There is a threshold score of 8, below which injured pediatric patients should be taken to an appropriate pediatric trauma center because they have the greatest potential for preventable mortality and morbidity. Although research has shown that other scores, such as the RTS, the unresponsive element (U) of the AVPU score, and a best motor response of 1 from the GCS, predict mortality at least as well as the PTS, the PTS remains the only score that includes size, skeletal injury, and open wounds. Although the PTS is a readily available assessment and triage tool, it has not been universally accepted. Other methods of triage are used, and it is the prehospital care provider's responsibility to be well versed in local protocols and procedures.

Secondary Assessment (Detailed Physical Examination)

The secondary assessment of the pediatric patient should follow the primary assessment only after life-threatening conditions have been identified and managed. The head and neck should be examined for obvious deformities, contusions, abrasions, punctures, burns, tenderness, lacerations, or swellings. The thorax should be re-examined. Potential pulmonary contusions may become evident after volume resuscitation, manifested by respiratory distress or abnormal lung sounds. Trauma patients are infrequently *nil per os* (NPO [fasting]) at the time of their injuries, so insertion of a nasogastric or orogastric tube may be indicated, if local protocols allow. This protocol is especially important for children who are **obtunded** or who have post-traumatic seizure activity.

Examination of the abdomen should focus on distension, tenderness, discoloration, ecchymoses, and presence of a mass. Careful palpation of the iliac crests may suggest an unstable pelvic fracture and increase the suspicion for possible retroperitoneal or urogenital injury as well as increased risk for hidden blood loss. An unstable pelvis should be noted, but repeated examinations of the pelvis should not be performed, as this may result in further injury and increased blood loss. The pediatric patient should be appropriately immobilized on a longboard and prepared for transfer to a pediatric trauma facility.

Each extremity should be inspected and palpated to rule out tenderness, deformity, diminished vascular supply, and neurologic deficit. A child's incompletely calcified skeleton, with its multiple growth centers, increases the possibility of epiphyseal (growth plate) disruption. Accordingly, any area of edema, pain, tenderness, or diminished range of motion should be treated as if it were fractured until evaluated by radiographic examination. In children, as in adults, a missed orthopedic injury in an extremity may have little effect on mortality but may lead to long-term deformity and disability.

Management

The keys to pediatric patient survival from a traumatic injury are rapid cardiopulmonary assessment, age-appropriate aggressive management, and transport to a facility capable of managing pediatric trauma. A color-coded, length-based resuscitation tape was devised to serve as a guide that allows for rapid identification of a patient's height with a correlated estimation of weight, the size of equipment to be used, and appropriate dosages of potential resuscitative drugs. In addition, most prehospital systems have a guideline for selecting appropriate destination facilities for pediatric trauma patients.

Airway

Ventilation, oxygenation, and perfusion are as essential to an injured child as to an adult. Thus, the primary goal of the initial resuscitation of an injured child is restoration of adequate tissue oxygenation as quickly as possible. The first priority of assessment and resuscitation is the establishment of a patent airway.

A patent airway should be ensured and maintained with suctioning, manual maneuvers, and airway adjuncts. As in the adult, initial management in the pediatric patient includes in-line cervical spine stabilization. Unless a specialized pediatric spine board that has a depression at the head is used, adequate padding (2 to 3 cm [about 1 inch]) should be placed under the torso of the small child so that the cervical spine is maintained in a straight line rather than forced into slight flexion because of the disproportionately large occiput (**Figure 16-13**). When adjusting and maintaining airway positioning, compressing the soft tissues of the neck and trachea should be avoided.

Once manual control of the airway is achieved, an oropharyngeal airway can be placed if no gag reflex is present. The device should be inserted carefully and gently, parallel to the course of the tongue rather than turned 90 or 180 degrees in the posterior oropharynx as in the adult. Use of a tongue blade to depress the tongue can be helpful in pediatric patients.

Endotracheal intubation under direct visualization of the trachea may be indicated for long transports (**Figure 16-14**). However, this should only be initiated by experienced personnel and when adequate oxygenation cannot be maintained by a bag-mask device. Importantly, there are no data to show improved survival or neurologic outcome in pediatric trauma patients intubated early in the field versus those who underwent bag-mask ventilation. In fact, there is some evidence suggesting worse outcomes.[16] A more recent study in a rural setting found that multiple prehospital intubation attempts were associated with significant complications (**Figure 16-15**).[19,20]

Although the Combitube has been a proven rescue airway device for adult trauma victims,[21,22] its large size and the lack of smaller sizes make it inadequate as a rescue device for small children (under 4 feet [1.2 m] in height). The laryngeal mask airway and now the smaller sizes of the King LT airways provide an alternate airway device choice in older children (> 8 years of age, when the airway is more similar to that of adults) and are reasonable alternatives to endotracheal intubation in certain situations.[23]

For pediatric patients, the risks may outweigh the benefits of endotracheal intubation and must be carefully considered before attempting the procedure, especially in the pediatric patient in whom bag-mask ventilation is providing adequate ventilation and oxygenation. Consideration of the risks associated with endotracheal intubation is increasingly important as additional nonvisualized advanced airway devices become available and added into the prehospital care provider's practice.

Breathing

The pediatric patient's minute volume and ventilatory effort should be evaluated carefully. Because of the potential for rapid deterioration from mild hypoxia to ventilatory arrest, ventilation should be assisted if dyspnea and increased ventilatory effort are observed. A properly sized bag-mask device with a reservoir and high-flow oxygen to provide an oxygen concentration of between 85% and 100% (FiO_2 of 0.85 to 1.0) should be used. Continuous pulse oximetry serves as an adjunct for ongoing assessment of airway and breathing. The SpO_2 should be kept at greater than 95% (at sea level).

In the intubated pediatric patient with a closed head injury, ET tube placement should be confirmed in multiple fashions, including directly visualizing the ET tube pass through the vocal folds, listening for the presence of equal bilateral breath sounds, and listening for the absence of sounds over the epigastrium

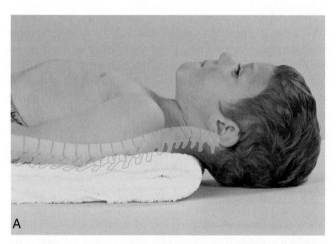
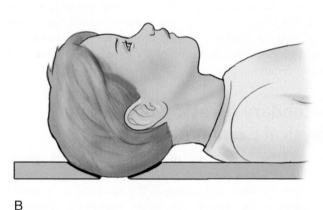

A   B

Figure 16-13 Provide adequate padding under the child's torso or use a spine board with a cutout for the child's occiput.

Figure 16-14   Pediatric Endotracheal Intubation

Endotracheal intubation of a pediatric patient should include careful attention to cervical spine immobilization. One prehospital care provider should maintain the pediatric patient's spine in a neutral position while another prehospital care provider intubates.

The narrowest portion of the pediatric airway is the cricoid ring, creating a "physiologic cuff." Although uncuffed ET tubes were previously used in pediatric patients due to this difference, newer recommendations endorse the use of cuffed tubes in all ages. The cuffed tube allows prehospital care providers to inflate the cuff fully, partially, or not at all, depending on the strength of the seal. To prevent iatrogenic tracheal injury, cuff pressures should not exceed 25 centimeters of water (cm H_2O). The appropriate size for a cuffed ET tube can be estimated by using the diameter of the child's fifth finger or the external nares, or by using the formula age/4 + 3.5.

A slight amount of cricoid pressure frequently brings the anterior structures of the child's larynx into better view. However, pediatric tracheal rings are relatively soft and pliable, and overzealous cricoid pressure may completely occlude the airway.

A common error that occurs during the intubation of pediatric patients under emergency circumstances is aggressive advancement of the ET tube resulting in its placement into the right main bronchus. The ET tube should never be advanced more than three times the ET tube size (in centimeters). For example, a 3.0-cm ET tube should rest at a depth no greater than 9 cm.

The chest and epigastrium should always be auscultated after the ET tube is placed and end-tidal carbon dioxide ($ETCO_2$) capnometry used when available. ET tube placement should be frequently reassessed, especially after any movement of the patient. In addition to confirming ET tube placement, auscultation may rule out the possibility of other pulmonary injury. The pediatric patient with a compromised airway and a pulmonary injury who has been successfully intubated may be in greater jeopardy for the development of a tension pneumothorax as a result of positive-pressure ventilation.

Figure 16-15 Prehospital Pediatric Intubation: The Great Debate

It would almost seem intuitive that providing an ET tube as early as possible in the management of the pediatric patient with TBI would be of benefit. A retrospective review showed improved survival in adult patients with TBI who were intubated prior to arrival at the receiving hospital.[24] Subsequent studies evaluated rapid-sequence intubation (RSI), demonstrating its improved efficiency and success rate in intubation of adults and children.[25,26] However, many retrospective and prospective case-control studies found that prehospital intubation compared with bag-mask ventilation did not improve survival or neurologic outcome and even might have been detrimental.[12,27,28] A prospective randomized trial in children comparing endotracheal intubation to bag-mask ventilation in an urban area with short transport times demonstrated no difference in survival or neurologic outcome between the two groups but an increased incidence of complications in the intubated group.[11]

Prolonged periods of hypoxia are often associated with the intubation process, as well as periods of overaggressive ventilation following intubation in patients transported to the trauma center.[13]

Data supporting prehospital pediatric endotracheal intubation are limited and ambiguous. In the spontaneously breathing child, endotracheal intubation with or without pharmacologic assistance is not recommended. Emergency medical services programs that perform pediatric prehospital intubation should include at least the following:[29]

1. Close medical direction and supervision
2. Training and continuing education, including hands-on operating room experience
3. Resources for patient monitoring, drug storage, and ET tube placement confirmation
4. Standardized RSI protocols
5. Availability of an alternate airway such as a laryngeal mask airway or King LT airway
6. Intensive continuing quality assurance/quality control and performance review program

when ventilated. Continuous end-tidal carbon dioxide ($ETCO_2$) monitoring should be used to document continuing appropriate ET tube placement and avoid extremes of hypercarbia and hypocarbia, both of which can be just as detrimental to recovery from a closed head injury as hypoxia. $ETCO_2$ should be targeted at 30 to 40 mm Hg.[13]

Tension Pneumothorax

Children are more susceptible than adults to acute cardiovascular collapse from a tension pneumothorax. Most children with tension pneumothoraces will present with acute cardiac decompensation secondary to decreased venous return before any detectable changes in oxygenation and ventilation have occurred. Any child who acutely decompensates, especially after initiation of positive-pressure ventilation by bag-mask device or advanced airway placement, should be emergently assessed for tension pneumothorax.

Jugular venous distension may be difficult to determine because an extrication collar has been applied or because of the presence of hypovolemia from hemorrhage. Tracheal shift is a late sign of tension pneumothorax and may only be determined by palpating the trachea in the jugular notch. In these pediatric patients, unilateral absent breath sounds, in association with cardiovascular compromise, represent an indication for emergency needle decompression. In the intubated pediatric patient, diminished sounds on the left may indicate a right main bronchus intubation, but when associated with acute cardiac decompensation, these sounds may represent tension pneumothorax.

Careful reassessment of the patient's airway and respiratory status is needed to distinguish these subtle differences in the presentation.

Needle decompression is performed using the same landmarks as in the adult, but it is often more immediately effective in the child because the mediastinum rapidly shifts back to its normal position and venous return is quickly restored.

Circulation

Once the pediatric patient's external hemorrhage is controlled, perfusion should be evaluated. Controlling external hemorrhage involves applying direct manual pressure on the bleeding point, the use of advanced hemostatic dressings, and the selective use of tourniquets in extreme cases in which other measures have failed. Managing an external hemorrhage is not just a matter of covering the bleeding site with layer after layer of absorbent dressing. If the initial dressing becomes saturated in blood, it is best to add an additional dressing rather than to replace it, as the removal may dislodge any clot that has begun to form, while at the same time performing additional interventions to stop the ongoing hemorrhage.

The pediatric vascular system is usually able to maintain a normal blood pressure until severe collapse occurs, at which point it is often unresponsive to resuscitation. Fluid resuscitation should be started whenever signs of compensated hypovolemic shock are present and must be started immediately in pediatric patients who present with decompensated shock. Lactated Ringer's (LR) or normal saline (NS) solution in 20-ml/kg boluses should be used.

For pediatric trauma patients who display any signs of hemorrhagic shock or hypovolemia, key factors to survival are appropriate volume resuscitation and rapid initiation of transport to a suitable facility. Transport should not be delayed to obtain vascular access or administer IV fluid.

Vascular Access

Fluid replacement in a pediatric patient with severe hypotension or signs of shock must deliver adequate fluid volume to the right atrium to avoid further reduction in cardiac preload. The most appropriate initial sites for IV access are the *antecubital fossa* (anterior aspect of the forearm at the elbow) and the saphenous vein at the ankle. Access through the external jugular vein is another possibility, but airway management takes priority in such a small space and spinal immobilization makes the neck poorly accessible.

In the unstable or potentially unstable pediatric patient, attempts at peripheral access should be limited to two in 90 seconds. If peripheral access is unsuccessful, intraosseous access should be established (**Figure 16-16**).

Placement of a subclavian or internal jugular catheter in a pediatric patient should be performed only under the most controlled circumstances within the hospital; this should not be attempted in the prehospital environment.

The determination of which pediatric patients should have intravascular access depends on the severity of injury, the experience of the involved prehospital care providers, and transport times, among other factors. If uncertainty exists as to which pediatric patients need intravascular access, or if fluid replacement is needed during transport, online medical direction should be obtained.

Fluid Therapy

Lactated Ringer's solution, or NS solution if LR solution is unavailable, is the initial resuscitation fluid of choice for a hypovolemic pediatric patient. As discussed in the Shock chapter, the time that a crystalloid fluid remains in the intravascular space is relatively short, which is why a 3:1 ratio of crystalloid fluid to blood lost has been recommended.

An initial fluid bolus for a pediatric patient is 20 ml/kg, which is approximately 25% of the normal circulating blood volume of the child. As much as 40 to 60 ml/kg may be required to achieve adequate and rapid initial replacement in response to significant blood loss. Any pediatric patient who does not show at least a minor improvement in hemodynamic status with the first 20-ml/kg fluid bolus and stabilization after the second 20-ml/kg bolus should receive a blood transfusion. The crystalloid bolus may temporarily restore cardiovascular stability as it transiently

Figure 16-16   Pediatric Intraosseous Infusion

Intraosseous (IO) infusion can provide an excellent alternative site for resuscitative volume replacement in injured children of all ages. This is an effective route for infusion of medications, blood, or high-volume fluid administration.

The most accessible site for IO infusion is the anterior tibia just inferior and medial to the tibial tuberosity. After preparing the skin antiseptically and securing the leg adequately, a site is chosen on the anterior portion of the tibia, 1 to 2 cm (0.4 to 0.8 inches) below and medial to the tibial tuberosity. Specially manufactured IO infusion needles are optimal for the procedure, but spinal or bone marrow needles may also be used. Spinal needles that are 18- to 20-gauge work well because they have a trocar to prevent the needle from being obstructed as it passes through the bony cortex into the marrow. Any 14- to 20-gauge needle can be used in an emergency.

There are a variety of commercially available devices that ease the difficulty of placing an IO needle, using various mechanical devices. For example, one device uses a high-speed drill to insert a specially designed IO needle, and another uses a spring-loaded mechanism. The needle is placed at a 90-degree angle to the bone and advanced firmly through the cortex into the marrow.

Evidence that the needle is adequately within the marrow includes the following:
1. A soft "pop" is heard and no resistance is felt after the needle has passed through the cortex.
2. Bone marrow aspirates into the needle.
3. Fluid flows freely into the marrow without evidence of subcutaneous infiltration.
4. The needle is secure and does not appear loose or wobbly.

IO infusion should be considered during initial resuscitation if percutaneous venous cannulation (venous IV insertion) has been unsuccessful. Because the flow rate is limited by the bone marrow cavity, the administration of fluids and medications should normally be done under pressure, and the IO route alone will seldom be sufficient after initial resuscitation.

Proper location of the insertion site is extremely important in the pediatric patient. Failure to properly identify landmarks could lead to misplacement of the IO device and damage of the epiphyseal plate (growth center) of the bone, which, in turn, can result in growth problems of the bone and unequal extremity lengths.

fills and then leaks from the circulatory system. However, until circulating RBCs are replaced and oxygen transport is restored, hypoxic injury can continue.

Pain Management

As with adults, pain management should be considered for children in the prehospital setting. Indications for analgesia include isolated limb injury and suspected spinal fracture. Small doses of a narcotic analgesia that are appropriately titrated will not compromise the neurologic or abdominal examination. Both morphine and fentanyl are acceptable choices, but they should be administered only according to written prehospital care guidelines or with orders from online medical control. Because of the side effects of hypotension and hypoventilation, all pediatric patients receiving IV narcotics should be monitored with pulse oximetry and serial vital signs. In general, benzodiazepines should not be administered in combination with narcotics because of their synergistic effects on respiratory depression or even respiratory arrest.

Unfortunately, the trend to undertreat pediatric pain remains an issue in emergency medical services (EMS). In one study of children with long-bone fractures, only 10% received any analgesia while en route to the hospital.[30]

Transport

Because timely arrival at the most appropriate facility may be the key element in the pediatric patient's survival, triage is an important consideration in the management of a pediatric patient.

The tragedy of preventable pediatric traumatic death has been documented in multiple studies reported over the past three decades. It is estimated that as many as 80% of pediatric trauma deaths can be classified as preventable or potentially preventable. These statistics have been one of the primary motivations for the development of regionalized pediatric trauma centers, where continuous, coordinated, high-quality, sophisticated care can be provided.

Many urban areas have both pediatric trauma centers and adult trauma centers. Ideally, the pediatric multisystem trauma patient will benefit from the initial resuscitation capability and definitive care available at a pediatric trauma center because of its specialization in treating traumatized children. It may be appropriate to bypass an adult trauma center in favor of transport to a pediatric-capable trauma center. For many communities, however, the nearest specialized pediatric trauma center may be hours away. In these cases, the seriously traumatized child should be transported to the nearest adult trauma center because early resuscitation and evaluation before transport to a pediatric facility may improve the pediatric patient's chances of survival.[31]

In areas where no specialized pediatric trauma center is nearby, personnel working in adult trauma centers should be experienced in the resuscitation and treatment of both adult and pediatric trauma patients. In areas where neither facility is readily close, the seriously injured child should be transported to the nearest appropriate hospital capable of caring for trauma victims, according to local prehospital triage guidelines.

Aeromedical transport may be considered in rural areas to expedite transport. There is little evidence that aeromedical transport provides any benefit in urban areas in which ground transport to a pediatric trauma center is almost as quick.[32] It is becoming increasingly evident that utilizing aeromedical transport exposes both the patient and the crew to a significant amount of risk. These concerns must be carefully weighed when deciding whether to utilize this resource.

Review of more than 15,000 records in the NPTR indicates that 25% of the pediatric patients were injured severely enough to require triage to a designated pediatric trauma center. Use of the PTS can help with appropriate triage. Many EMS and trauma systems use other pediatric triage criteria, which may be dictated by state, regional, or local guidelines. All prehospital care providers need to be familiar with the triage protocols in place within their own systems.

Specific Injuries
Traumatic Brain Injury

Traumatic brain injury (TBI) is the most common cause of death in the pediatric population. Of the fatalities included in the first 40,000 patients in the NPTR, 89% had a CNS injury as either the primary or the secondary contributor to mortality. Although many of the most severe injuries are treatable only by prevention, initial resuscitative measures may minimize secondary brain injury and, consequently, the severity of the pediatric patient's injury. Adequate ventilation, oxygenation, and perfusion are needed to prevent secondary morbidity. While the recovery of pediatric patients sustaining severe TBI is typically considered to be better than in adults, growing evidence indicates that a wide variety of impairments persist, including functional, cognitive, and behavioral abnormalities.

The results of the initial neurologic assessment are useful for prognosis. Even with a normal initial neurologic evaluation, however, any child who sustains a significant head injury may be susceptible to cerebral edema, hypoperfusion, and secondary insults (**Figure 16-17**). Furthermore, victims of nonaccidental trauma may have very little external evidence of trauma, yet may have sustained considerable intracranial injury. A baseline GCS score should be assessed and frequently repeated during transport. Supplemental oxygen should be administered, and if possible, pulse oximetry should be monitored. Although vomiting is common after a concussion, persistent or forceful projectile vomiting is of concern and requires further evaluation.

As with hypoxia, hypovolemia may dramatically worsen the original TBI. External hemorrhage must be controlled and the pediatric patient's fractured extremities immobilized to limit internal blood loss associated with these injuries. An attempt should be made to keep these pediatric patients in a *euvolemic* (normal volume) state with IV volume resuscitation. On rare occasions, infants younger than about 6 months of age may

Figure 16-17   Pediatric Concussion

The issue of concussion in pediatric patients, particularly those engaged in sports activities, has become a topic of great importance.[33] In the past, when a pediatric athlete sustained a concussion, the child was kept out of the game for a short time and was allowed to return to play as soon as he or she felt able to play again. More recently, it has been recognized that repeated blows to the head and brain lead to long-term difficulties with cognition, behavior, and function. It is now recommended that any pediatric athlete who has sustained a concussion be removed from play and not be permitted to participate for the duration of the event.

The recognition of concussion is of key importance. Where it was once thought that concussion involved a brief loss of consciousness with a return to normal function, it is now understood that loss of consciousness is not necessary to make the diagnosis. Concussion may involve a variety of symptoms and complaints, including headache, nausea, balance problems, feeling dazed or stunned, confusion, and asking questions slowly or repetitively. It is recommended that medical personnel present at a sporting event have a formal method for assessing pediatric athletes for concussion using a standard sideline assessment tool as well as a neurologic examination.

Full recovery from a concussion may take a week or longer—in some cases, months. Until the pediatric athlete has fully recovered from the concussion and is asymptomatic, the child should not be allowed to return to play. Once the pediatric athlete is asymptomatic, he or she may be returned to activity and play in a graded, structured format with repeat evaluations to assess for relapse of symptoms. Return of symptoms indicates incomplete recovery, and the pediatric athlete should refrain from participation in sports until improvement has occurred.

---

become hypovolemic as a result of intracranial bleeding because they have open cranial sutures and fontanelles. An infant with an open fontanelle may better tolerate an expanding intracranial hematoma and thus not become symptomatic until rapid expansion occurs. An infant with a bulging fontanelle should be considered to have a more severe TBI.

For pediatric patients with a GCS score of eight or less, adequate oxygenation and ventilation should be the goal at all times, not the placement of an ET tube. Prolonged attempts at securing an endotracheal airway may increase periods of hypoxia and delay transport to an appropriate facility. The best airway for a pediatric patient is the one that is both safest and most effective. Ventilation with a bag-mask device while being prepared to suction emesis, should it occur, is often the best airway for the pediatric patient with TBI.[11-13]

A pediatric patient with signs and symptoms of intracranial hypertension or increased intracranial pressure, such as a sluggishly reactive or nonreactive pupil, systemic hypertension, bradycardia, and abnormal breathing patterns, may benefit from temporary mild hyperventilation to lower intracranial pressure. However, this effect of hyperventilation is transient and also decreases overall oxygen delivery to the CNS, actually causing additional secondary brain injury.[34] It is strongly recommended that this strategy not be used unless the pediatric patient is exhibiting signs of active herniation or *lateralizing* signs (distal neurologic abnormalities such as weakness on one side from injury to an area of the brain). $ETCO_2$ monitoring should guide management in the intubated pediatric patient, with the target range about 35 mm Hg. Hyperventilation to an $ETCO_2$ of less than 25 mm Hg has been associated with worse neurologic outcome.[13] If capnography is not available, a ventilation rate of 25 breaths/minute for children and 30 breaths/minute for infants should be used.[35]

During prolonged transports, small doses of mannitol (0.5 to 1 g/kg body weight) may benefit pediatric patients with evidence of intracranial hypertension, if local protocols permit. However, use of mannitol in the setting of insufficient volume resuscitation may result in hypovolemia and worsening shock. Mannitol should not be given in the field without discussing this option with online medical control, unless permitted by standing orders or protocol.

Brief seizures may occur soon after TBI and, aside from ensuring patient safety, oxygenation, and ventilation, often do not require specific treatment by prehospital care providers. However, recurrent seizure activity is worrisome and may require IV boluses of a benzodiazepine, such as diazepam (0.1 to 0.2 mg/kg/dose). Depending on local protocols, midazolam or lorazepam may also be used, but all benzodiazepines should be used with extreme caution because of the potential side effects of ventilatory depression and hypotension, as well as their ability to cloud the neurologic examination.

Spinal Trauma

The indication for spinal immobilization in a pediatric patient is based on the mechanism of injury and physical findings; the presence of other injuries that suggest violent or sudden movement of the head, neck, or torso; or the presence of specific signs of spine injury, such as deformity, pain, or a neurologic deficit. As with adult patients, the correct prehospital management of a suspected spine injury is in-line manual stabilization followed by the use of a properly fitting cervical collar and immobilization of the pediatric patient to an appropriate device so that the head, neck, torso, pelvis, and legs are maintained in a neutral in-line position. This should be achieved without impairing the pediatric patient's ventilation or ability to open the mouth or disrupting any other resuscitative efforts.

The threshold for performing spinal immobilization is lower in young children because of their inability to communicate or otherwise participate in their own assessment. No studies have validated the safety of clinically clearing a pediatric patient's spine in the field. The same immaturity previously discussed also contributes to children's fear and lack of cooperation with immobilization. A child who strongly fights attempts at immobilization may be at increased risk of worsening any existing spinal injuries. It may be valid to decide not to restrain such a pediatric patient if the child can be persuaded to lie quietly without restraints. However, any decision to stop immobilization attempts in the interest of patient safety must be supported by careful and thorough documented reasoning as well as serial assessment of neurologic status during and immediately after transport. Ideally, this decision would be made in concert with online medical control.

When most small children are placed on a rigid surface, the relatively larger size of the child's occiput will result in passive neck flexion. Unless using a specialized pediatric spine board that has a depression at the head to accommodate the occiput, sufficient padding (2 to 3 cm [about 1 inch]) should be placed under the pediatric patient's torso to elevate it and allow the head to be in a neutral position. The padding should be continuous and flat from the shoulders to the pelvis and extend to the lateral margins of the torso to ensure that the thoracic, lumbar, and sacral spine are on a flat, stable platform without the possibility of anterior–posterior movement. Padding should also be placed between the lateral sides of the pediatric patient and the edges of the board to ensure that no lateral movement occurs when the board is moved or if the pediatric patient and board need to be rotated to the side to avoid aspiration during vomiting episodes.

Various new pediatric immobilization devices are available. The prehospital care provider needs to regularly practice and be familiar with any specialized equipment used in the prehospital care provider's system as well as the required adjustments necessary when immobilizing a pediatric patient using adult-sized equipment. If a vest-type device is used on a pediatric patient, adequate immobilization while at the same time preventing respiratory compromise must be ensured. In the past, it was recommended that an infant or young child be immobilized in a car safety seat if that is where they were found.[36,37] The National Highway Traffic Safety Administration now recommends that it is better to transport the pediatric patient immobilized in an appropriately sized pediatric immobilization device instead of the car seat. Keeping the injured child in an upright position in the car seat increases the axial load placed on the spine by the patient's head; therefore, standard immobilization techniques are preferred to the car seat.[38]

Thoracic Injuries

The extremely resilient rib cage of a child often results in less injury to the bony structure of the thorax, but there is still risk for pulmonary injury, such as pulmonary contusion, pneumothorax,

or hemothorax. Although rib fractures are rare in childhood, they are associated with a high risk of intrathoracic injury when present. Crepitus may be appreciated on examination and may be a sign of pneumothorax. The risk of mortality increases with the number of ribs fractured. A high index of suspicion is the key to identifying these injuries. Every pediatric patient who sustains trauma to the chest and torso should be carefully monitored for signs of respiratory distress and shock. Abrasions or contusions over the pediatric patient's torso after blunt force trauma may be the only clues to the prehospital care provider that the child has suffered thoracic trauma.

Additionally, when transporting a pediatric patient who has sustained a high-impact blunt thoracic injury, the pediatric patient's cardiac rhythm should be monitored once en route to a medical facility. In all cases, the key items in managing thoracic trauma involve careful attention to ventilation, oxygenation, and timely transport to an appropriate facility.

Abdominal Injuries

The presence of blunt trauma to the abdomen, an unstable pelvis, post-traumatic abdominal distension, rigidity or tenderness, or otherwise unexplained shock can be associated with possible intra-abdominal hemorrhage. A "seat belt sign" (or mark) across the abdomen of a pediatric patient is often an indicator of serious internal injuries (Figure 16-18).

The key prehospital elements in management of abdominal injuries include fluid resuscitation, supplemental high-concentration oxygen, and rapid transport to an appropriate facility with continued careful monitoring en route. There are really no definitive interventions that prehospital care providers can offer to pediatric patients with intra-abdominal injuries, and, as such, there should be every effort to transport pediatric patients rapidly to the closest, most appropriate facility.

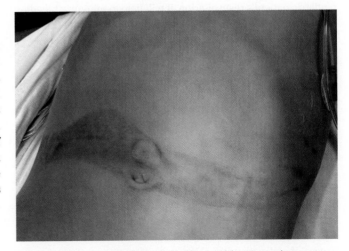

Figure 16-18 "Seat belt sign" in a 6-year-old patient who was found to have a ruptured spleen. Seat belt signs are often associated with serious intra-abdominal injuries.
Source: Courtesy of Jeffrey Guy, MD.

Extremity Trauma

Compared with the adult skeleton, the child's skeleton is actively growing and consists of a large proportion of cartilaginous tissue and metabolically active growth plates. The ligamentous structures that hold the skeleton together are frequently stronger and better able to withstand mechanical disruption than the bones to which they are attached. As a result, children with skeletal trauma frequently sustain major traumatic forces before developing long-bone fractures, dislocations, or deformities. Incomplete ("greenstick") fractures are common and may be indicated only by bony tenderness and pain on use of the affected extremity.

Primary joint disruption from injury other than penetrating injury is uncommon compared with disruption of the *diaphyseal* (shaft) or *epiphyseal* (end) segments of bone. Fractures that involve the growth plate are unique in that they must be carefully identified and managed in the acute injury phase to not only ensure adequate healing, but also prevent subsequent displacement or deformity as the child continues to develop. The association of neurovascular injuries with orthopedic injuries in children should always be considered, and the distal vascular and neurologic examination should be carefully evaluated. Often, the presence of a potentially debilitating injury can be determined only by radiologic study or, when the slightest suggestion of a decrease in distal perfusion exists, by *arteriography* (x-ray study of a blood vessel that has been injected with radioopaque contrast material).

The apparent gross deformity sometimes associated with extremity injury should not distract focus from potentially life-threatening injuries. Uncontrolled hemorrhage represents the most life-threatening consequence of extremity trauma. In multisystem pediatric and adult trauma patients alike, the initiation of transport to an appropriate facility without delay after completion of the primary assessment, resuscitation, and rapid packaging remains paramount in reducing mortality. If basic splinting can be provided en route without detracting from the pediatric patient's resuscitation, it will help to minimize bleeding and pain from long-bone fractures, but attention to life-threatening injuries should always remain the primary focus.

Thermal Injuries

Following motor vehicle crashes and drowning, burns rate third as a cause of pediatric trauma deaths.[1] Caring for an injured child always poses significant physical and emotional challenges to the prehospital care provider, and these difficulties are only amplified when caring for the pediatric patient with burns. The pediatric patient with burns may have an *edematous (swollen) airway*, IV access may be complicated by burns of the extremity, and the pediatric patient may be hysterical from pain.

The primary assessment should be followed as in other causes of pediatric trauma, but every step of the primary assessment may be more complicated than in a pediatric patient without thermal injuries. Most deaths related to structure fires are not directly related to soft-tissue burns but are secondary to smoke inhalation. When children are trapped in a structure fire, they often hide from the fire under beds or in closets. These children frequently die, and their recovered bodies often have no burns; they die from carbon monoxide or hydrogen cyanide toxicity and hypoxia. More than 50% of children younger than 9 years old in structure fires have some degree of smoke-inhalation injury.

Thermally induced edema of the airway is always a concern in patients with burns, but especially in pediatric patients. The smaller diameter of the pediatric trachea means that 1 mm of edema will produce a greater magnitude of airway obstruction than in an adult with a larger-diameter airway. A pediatric patient with an edematous airway may be sitting forward and drooling, or complaining of hoarseness or voice changes. These symptoms should prompt rapid preparations for and initiation of transport to the hospital. While en route, supplemental oxygen is administered and preparations made for airway intervention should the symptoms progress or the pediatric patient develop respiratory or cardiac arrest.

If an ET tube is placed, it needs to be protected against inadvertent dislodgement or removal. If the pediatric patient accidentally becomes extubated, the prehospital care provider may not be able to intubate the pediatric patient again due to progressive edema, and the results could be disastrous. Securing an ET tube in a pediatric patient who has peeling facial skin and moist wounds is difficult. Securing the ET tube to the face with adhesive tape should not be attempted in a pediatric patient with facial burns. The ET tube should be secured with two pieces of umbilical tape, with one piece draped above the ear and the second piece placed below the ear. An effective alternative to umbilical tape is IV tubing. If these supplies are not available but extra hands are, designate a prehospital care provider to be solely responsible for holding the airway in place.

Fluid Resuscitation

Rapid establishment of intravascular access is vital to prevent the development of shock. Delayed fluid resuscitation in pediatric patients has been associated with significantly worse clinical outcomes and an increased mortality rate, especially in burned infants.

After securing an airway, providing adequate ventilation and oxygenation, it is critical that venous access be obtained quickly. Children have a relatively small intravascular volume, and a delay in fluid resuscitation may lead to the rapid development of hypovolemic shock. To provide the large volumes of IV fluids required in critical burns, such pediatric patients usually require two peripheral IV catheters to achieve the required IV flow rates. The insertion of a single large-bore IV catheter is often challenging, so two IV catheters is all the more so. Burns on the extremities may make it difficult to impossible to establish enough access for an appropriate fluid resuscitation.

In pediatric patients with burns, as in adult patients with burns, fluid needs are calculated from the time of the injury, so even a delay of 30 minutes to the beginning of fluid resuscitation can result in hypovolemic shock. Excessive fluids can result in respiratory complications as well as excessive edema, which can complicate burn care.

The amount of fluids typically given to a patient with burns is calculated based on the estimated percentage of body surface area burned using the "rule of nines," a rapid and imprecise method of estimating resuscitative fluid needs based on adult battlefield burn casualties. The premise of this method of burn size estimation is that major regions of the adult body (e.g., head, arm, anterior torso) each comprise 9% of the total body surface area. Children's anatomic regions are proportionally different than those in adults; children have larger heads and smaller limbs. Therefore, estimation of pediatric burn size should use diagrams that are age specific, such as the Lund-Browder chart, and not the rule of nines. If charts and diagrams are not available, the "rule of palms" may be utilized. Using this method, the size of the pediatric patient's palm plus fingers represents approximately 1% of the body surface area. (See the Burn Injuries chapter for further discussion of these burn estimation methods.)

Based on the percentage of body surface area burned, the volume of IV fluids needed for resuscitation is determined (see the Burn Injuries chapter). Two important pediatric considerations merit mention. First, small children have a limited reserve of glycogen. Glycogen is essentially glucose molecules strung together and is used for carbohydrate storage purposes. These glycogen molecules can then be mobilized in times of stress. If these limited glycogen stores become depleted, the child may rapidly develop hypoglycemia. Second, children have a large volume-to-surface area ratio; the general shape of an adult is a cylinder, whereas children resemble a sphere. The clinical implication is that a child will require more IV fluids. To address both of these issues, in addition to the calculated resuscitative fluids, maintenance fluids containing 5% dextrose are administered. In prolonged transports of a pediatric patient with a Foley catheter, the fluids should be titrated to ensure a urine output of 1 ml/kg/hour. If the urine output is not adequate, a fluid bolus of 20 ml/kg is administered, and the rate of administration of the resuscitative fluids is increased to achieve the desired urine output.

Once peripheral IV access has been obtained, provisions must be made to ensure that the IV line is not inadvertently removed or dislodged. The usual techniques used to secure IV lines are often ineffective when a line is placed in or adjacent to a burn because adhesive tape and dressings may not adhere to burned tissue. If possible, the IV line is secured with a Kerlix dressing, though circumferential dressings must be frequently monitored as edema develops, to prevent tissue damage from the dressing becoming a constricting band.

When peripheral venous access cannot be obtained, intraosseous catheters should be used for the unstable and/or unconscious pediatric patient. Although previously advocated only for pediatric patients younger than 3 years of age, intraosseous infusions are now used in older children as well as adults.

Abuse

Each year approximately 1.5 million children are abused by burning, accounting for 20% of all incidents of child abuse.[21,39] Approximately 20% to 25% of children admitted to a pediatric burn center are victims of child abuse.[40,41] An increased awareness of this problem among prehospital care providers can improve detection of this cause of pediatric trauma. Careful documentation of the situation surrounding the injury, as well as of the injury patterns themselves, can aid officials in the prosecution of the offenders.[42]

The two most common mechanisms by which these children receive burns are scalds and contact burns. Scalds are the most common source of nonaccidental burns. Scalding injuries typically are inflicted on children of toilet-training age. The usual scenario is that children soil themselves and are subsequently immersed in a tub of scalding water. These scald burns are characterized by a pattern of sharp demarcation between burned and unburned tissue and sparing of flexion creases, as the child will frequently draw his or her legs up to avoid the scalding water (see the Burn Injuries chapter).

Contact burns are the second most common mechanism of abuse burns. Common items used to inflict contact burns are curling irons, clothing irons, and cigarettes. Cigarette burns appear as round wounds measuring slightly over 1 cm in diameter (typically 1.3 cm). To conceal these injuries, the abuser may place the burns in areas usually covered by clothing, above the hairline in the scalp, or even in the axillae.

All the surfaces of the human body have some degree of curvature; a hot item that falls onto the body surface will have an initial point of contact and will then deflect from the point of contact. The resultant accidental contact burns will have irregular borders and uneven depths. In contrast, when a hot item is deliberately used to burn someone, the item is pressed onto the region of the body. The burn will have a pattern with a sharp regular outline and uniform burn depth (see the Burn Injuries chapter).

A high index of suspicion for abuse is important, and all cases of suspected abuse should be reported. Make meticulous observations of the surroundings, such as the position of various pieces of furniture, presence of curling irons, and depth of bath water. Record the names of the individuals present at the scene. Any pediatric patient suspected of being abused by burns, regardless of the size of the burns, needs to be cared for at a center experienced in pediatric burn care.

Child abuse and neglect are further discussed later in this chapter.

Motor Vehicle Injury Prevention

The American Academy of Pediatrics (AAP) has defined optimal restraint for children in motor vehicles. The AAP recommends that children should always ride in the rear seat and face the rear of the seat until 2 years of age. Children should be in child safety seats until 4 years of age, and then graduate into a belt-positioning booster seat until they are 8 to 10 years old. At that time, the standard three-point (seat belt–shoulder harness combination) adult restraint can be used. The lap belt alone should never be used.

Suboptimal restraint is defined as the lack of use of a child safety seat or booster seat for anyone younger than 8 years of age, and lack of a three-point restraint for a child older than 8 years (see **Figure 16-2**).[43] In a recent review, when these guidelines were observed, the risk of abdominal injury in children appropriately restrained was 3.5 times less than in the suboptimally restrained pediatric population.[44] The protective benefit of the rear-seat position is such that risk of death is decreased by at least 30%, even if restrained with a lap belt only in the rear seat versus three-point restraint in the front seat.[45]

Child Abuse and Neglect

Child abuse (maltreatment or nonaccidental trauma) is a significant cause of childhood injury. As mentioned previously, almost 20% of all burns in pediatric patients involve either child abuse or child neglect.[42] Prehospital care providers must always consider the possibility of child abuse when circumstances warrant.

Prehospital care providers should suspect abuse or neglect if they note any of the following scenarios:

- Discrepancy between the history and the degree of physical injury, or frequent changes in the reported history.
- Inappropriate response from the family.
- Prolonged interval between time of injury and call for medical care.
- History of the injury inconsistent with the developmental level of the child. For example, a history indicating that a newborn rolled off a bed would be suspect because newborns are developmentally unable to roll over.

Certain types of injury also suggest abuse, such as the following (**Figure 16-19**):

- Multiple bruises in varying stages of resolution (excluding the palms, forearms, tibial areas, and the forehead in ambulatory children, who are frequently injured in normal falls). Accidental bruises usually occur over bony prominences.
- Bizarre injuries such as bites, cigarette burns, rope marks, or any pattern injury.
- Sharply demarcated burns or scald injuries in unusual areas (see the Burn Injuries chapter).

In many jurisdictions, prehospital care providers are legally mandated reporters if they identify potential child abuse. Generally, prehospital care providers who act in good faith and in the best interests of the child are protected from legal action. Reporting procedures vary, so prehospital care providers should be familiar with

the appropriate agencies that handle child abuse cases in their location. The need to report abuse is emphasized by data suggesting that up to 50% of maltreated children are released back to their abusers because abuse was not suspected or reported (**Figure 16-20**).

Prolonged Transport

Occasionally a situation arises as a result of patient location, triage decisions, or environmental considerations in which transport will be prolonged or delayed and prehospital personnel need to manage the ongoing resuscitation of a pediatric patient. Even though this may be suboptimal because of the lack of field resources (e.g., blood) and the inability to perform diagnostic and therapeutic interventions, by applying the principles discussed in this chapter in an organized fashion, the pediatric patient can be safely managed until arrival at a trauma center. If radio or cell phone contact with the receiving facility is possible, constant communication and feedback are crucial for both prehospital and hospital-based members of the trauma team.

Management consists of continued serial evaluation of the components of the primary assessment. The pediatric patient should be securely stabilized on a backboard with spinal precautions. The board should be padded as well as possible to prevent pressure sores. If the airway is tenuous and the crew is well trained in pediatric airway management, including endotracheal intubation, then airway management should be performed. Otherwise, conscientious bag-mask ventilation is still an acceptable management strategy, assuming it provides adequate oxygenation and ventilation.

Pulse oximetry should be monitored and preferably $ETCO_2$ as well, especially in the pediatric patient with a head injury. If signs of shock exist, 20-ml/kg boluses of LR or NS solution are administered until the pediatric patient improves or is transferred to definitive care.

The GCS score should be calculated early and followed serially. Assessment for other injuries should continue, and all efforts to keep the pediatric patient normothermic should be standard practice. Fractures should be splinted and stabilized with serial neurovascular assessments. This cycle of continued assessment of the primary assessment should be repeated until the pediatric patient can be safely transported or transferred to definitive care.

Any change or decompensation in the pediatric patient's condition requires immediate reassessment of the primary assessment. For example, if SpO_2 begins to decline, is the ET tube still secure and in the airway? If so, has the pediatric patient developed a tension pneumothorax? Is the ET tube now in the right main bronchus? If the pediatric patient has received what was thought to be sufficient fluid and is still in shock, is there now cardiac tamponade, severe cardiac contusion, or perhaps an occult source of bleeding, such as intra-abdominal injury or missed scalp laceration? Has the GCS score changed? Are there now lateralizing signs suggesting progressive head injury and requiring more aggressive treatments? Is the circulation and

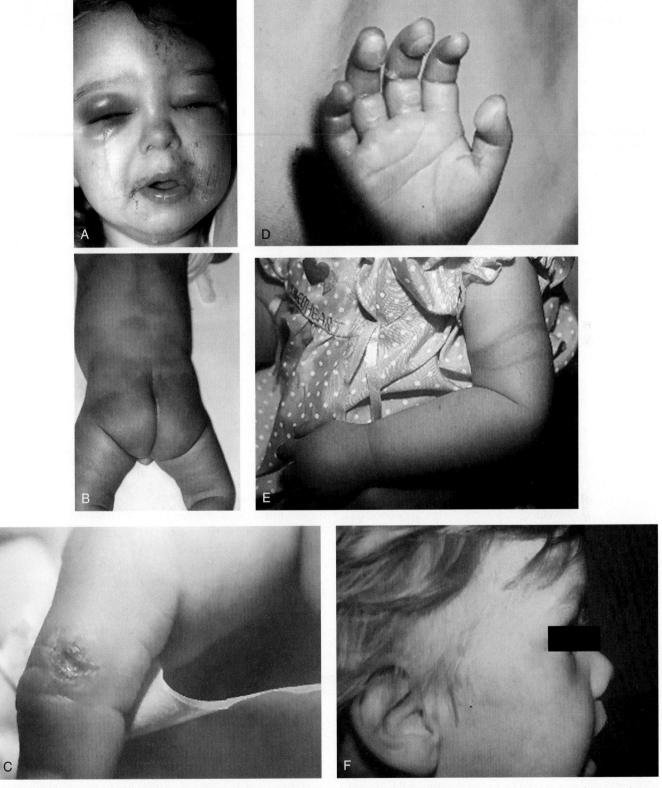

Figure 16-19   Indicators of possible nonaccidental trauma. **A.** "Raccoon eyes," or periorbital bruising, a possible indication of anterior fossa skull fracture. **B.** Mongolian blue spots, shown here on the trunk and buttocks of a newborn Asian infant, which can be easily confused with bruising. **C.** Well-circumscribed lesions with blistering, seen here as a result of a cigarette burn. **D.** Fingertip burns caused by having the hand held forcibly against an electric stove burner. The burns are confined to the tips because the child tried to prevent her hand from being flattened against the burner. **E.** Abrasion caused by a ligature. **F.** Facial bruising from a slap to the face. The handprint can just be identified.

Source: Taylor S, Raffles A: Diagnosis in color: Pediatrics, London, 1997, Mosby-Wolfe.

Figure 16-20 Documenting Nonaccidental Trauma in Children

Prehospital care providers may be the only medical responders to a potential crime scene involving nonaccidental (abuse) trauma. Although prehospital care providers are under intense pressure at an emergency scene, they are in a unique position to collect items of evidentiary importance that may assist in determining the mechanism of injury and identifying the abuser.

The prehospital care provider's response to a "child in need of assistance" call should ideally involve 10 fundamental actions:

1. Document all adults and children present.
2. Document all statements and the demeanors of all persons present. As recorders of "scene" statements, prehospital care providers must be familiar with the general requirements that allow certain statements to be used in court.
   a. Identify and document the maker of the statement.
   b. Record all statements in the official report.
   c. Record verbatim content, using quotation marks when appropriate.
   d. Document the time when the statement was made.
   e. Record the speaker's demeanor.
   f. Explain the prehospital care provider's responsibilities as necessary.
   g. Ask open-ended, nonleading follow-up questions, but do not become exposed to risk if aggression occurs during further questioning.
   h. Record the question. The content of an answer can often be understood only by knowing the question that was asked.
   i. List all persons present who heard the statement.
3. Document the environment. Prehospital care providers may arrive before caregivers clean up, modify, or destroy evidence.

4. Collect significant items. Preserving the potential mechanism of injury is vital to verifying a suspect's history.
5. Identify and record the child's age and developmental stage.
6. Recognize and document the signs of abuse and neglect.
   a. Signs of physical abuse: unexplained fractures, bruises, black eyes, cuts, burns, and welts; pattern injuries and bite marks; antisocial behavior; fear of adults; signs of apathy, depression, hostility, or stress; eating disorders
   b. Signs of sexual abuse: difficulty walking or sitting, overcompliance, excessive aggressiveness, nightmares, bed-wetting, drastic change in appetite, inappropriate interest or knowledge of sexual acts, fear of a particular person
   c. Signs of neglect: unsuitable clothing; unbathed/dirty; severe body odor; severe diaper rash; underweight; lack of food, formula, or toys; parent or child use of drugs or alcohol; apparent lack of supervision; unsuitable living conditions
7. Assess other children present.
8. Evaluate children and adults with disabilities.
9. Adhere to mandatory reporting requirements and procedures.
10. Interact with the multidisciplinary team (MDT).

Nonaccidental pediatric trauma and neglect cases are fraught with difficult issues. Holding abusers responsible for their acts requires meticulous documentation; thorough, coordinated investigations; and teamwork. Prehospital care providers are uniquely positioned to observe and document vital information when assessing the possibility of child abuse.

Source: Modified from Rogers LL: Emergency medical professionals: assisting in identifying and documenting child abuse and neglect. *NCPCA Update Newslett* 17(7):1, 2004.

neurologic function of the extremities still intact? Is the pediatric patient normothermic? If radio contact is available, continued advice and guidance should be sought throughout the resuscitation and transport.

By paying attention to the basics and continually reassessing your pediatric patient, adequate resuscitation can be performed until the pediatric patient can be transferred to definitive care.

Summary

- The primary assessment and management of the pediatric patient in the prehospital setting require application of standard trauma life support principles modified to account for the unique characteristics of pediatric patients.
- Traumatic brain injury is the leading cause of death from trauma, as well as the most common injury for which pediatric patients require airway management.
- Children have the ability to compensate for volume loss longer than adults, but when they decompensate, they deteriorate suddenly and severely.
- Significant underlying organ and vascular injury can occur with few or no obvious signs of external injury.
- Pediatric patients with the following signs are unstable and should be transported without delay to an appropriate facility, ideally a pediatric trauma center:
    - Respiratory compromise
    - Signs of shock or circulatory instability
    - Any period of postinjury unconsciousness
    - Significant blunt trauma to the head, thorax, or abdomen
    - Fractured ribs
    - Pelvic fracture
- Always consider the possibility of abuse or nonaccidental trauma when the history of the injury does not match the presentation of the patient.

SCENARIO RECAP

You are called to the scene of a motor vehicle crash on a heavily traveled highway. Two vehicles have been involved in a frontal offset collision. One of the vehicle's occupants is a child improperly restrained in a child booster seat. No weather-related factors are involved on this spring afternoon.

On arrival at the scene, you see that the police have secured and blocked traffic from the area around the crash. As your partner and the other arriving crew are assessing the other patients, you approach the child. You see a young boy, approximately 2 years of age, sitting in the booster seat, which is slightly turned at an angle; there is blood on the back of the headrest of the seat in front of him. Despite numerous abrasions and minor bleeding from the head, face, and neck, the child appears very calm.

Your primary and secondary assessments reveal a 2-year-old boy who weakly repeats "ma-ma, ma-ma." His pulse rate is 180 beats/minute, with the radial pulses weaker than the carotid; his blood pressure is 50 mm Hg by palpation. His ventilatory rate is 18 breaths/minute, slightly irregular, but without abnormal sounds. As you continue to assess him, you note that he has stopped saying "ma-ma" and seems to just stare into space. You also note that his pupils are slightly dilated, and his skin is pale and sweaty. A woman who identifies herself as the family's nanny tells you that the mother is en route and that you should wait for her.

- What are the management priorities for this patient?
- What are the most likely injuries in this child?
- Where is the most appropriate destination for this child?

SCENARIO SOLUTION

You correctly identify this child as a victim of multisystem trauma who is in shock and critically injured. Because of the probable traumatic brain injury combined with the change in mentation, you have to determine the greatest threat to his survival—the brain injury and other injuries not yet identified. You correctly identify hypotension and tachycardia, which you assume are related to hypovolemic shock, probably the result of an unrecognized intra-abdominal injury.

Initially, the patient's breathing is supported with high-concentration oxygen through a nonrebreathing mask. You realize that his ventilatory rate is low for a child of his age and are prepared to provide more aggressive airway control with a bag-mask if his condition deteriorates. As you consider options for airway management, you ask your partner to hold manual stabilization of the head and neck.

Because of the nature of the child's injuries, you consult with online medical control, who agrees that helicopter transport to the closest pediatric trauma center is more appropriate than ground transport to a nearby community hospital that has no pediatric critical care, neurosurgical, or orthopedic resources. Brief efforts at peripheral venous access are successful. You begin crystalloid infusion through the IV line. The pediatric patient's mother arrives just as you are transferring care to the helicopter crew.

References

1. Centers for Disease Control and Prevention, National Center for Injury Prevention and Control, Web-Based Injury Statistics Query and Reporting System (WISQARS). Leading causes of death reports, 2010. http://webappa.cdc.gov/sasweb/ncipc/leadcaus10_us.html. Accessed January 5, 2014.
2. Centers for Disease Control and Prevention, Web-Based Injury Statistics Query and Reporting System (WISQARS). Leading causes of nonfatal injury reports, 2012. http://webappa.cdc.gov/sasweb/ncipc/nfilead2001.html. Accessed January 5, 2014.
3. Gaines BA, Ford HR. Abdominal and pelvic trauma in children. *Crit Care Med*. 2002;30(11 suppl):S416.
4. World Health Organization. *World Report on Child Injury Prevention*. http://whqlibdoc.who.int/publications/2008/9789241563574_eng.pdf. Accessed September 4, 2013.
5. Winston FK, Durbin DR, Kallan MJ, Moll EK. The danger of premature graduation to seat belts for young children. *Pediatrics*. 2000;105(6):1179.
6. Grisoni ER, Pillai SB, Volsko TA, et al. Pediatric airbag injuries: the Ohio experience. *J Pediatr Surg*. 2000;35(2):160.
7. Durbin DR, Kallan M, Elliott M, et al. Risk of injury to restrained children from passenger air bags. *Traffic Injury Prev*. 2003;4(1):58.
8. Bensard DD, Beaver BL, Besner GE, Cooney DR. Small bowel injury in children after blunt abdominal trauma: is diagnostic delay important? *J Trauma Injury Infect Crit Care*. 1996;41(3):476.
9. Allen GS, Moore FA, Cox CS Jr, et al. Hollow visceral injury and blunt trauma. *J Trauma Injury Infect Crit Care*. 1998;45(1):69.
10. Durbin DR, Kallan M, Elliott M, et al. Risk of injury to restrained children from passenger air bags. *Annu Proc Assoc Adv Auto Med*. 2002;46:15.
11. Gausche M, Lewis RJ, Stratton SJ, et al. Effect of out-of-hospital pediatric endotracheal intubation on survival and neurological outcome: a controlled clinical trial. *JAMA*. 2000;283(6):783.
12. Davis DP, Hoyt DB, Ochs M, et al. The effect of paramedic rapid sequence intubation on outcome in patients with severe traumatic brain injury. *J Trauma Injury Infec Crit Care*. 2003;54(3):444.
13. Davis DP, Dunford JV, Poste JC, et al. The impact of hypoxia and hyperventilation on outcome after paramedic rapid sequence intubation of severely head-injured patients. *J Trauma Injury Infect Crit Care*. 2004;57(1):1.
14. York J, Arrillaga A, Graham R, Miller R. Fluid resuscitation of patients with multiple injuries and severe closed-head injury: experience with an aggressive fluid resuscitation strategy. *J Trauma Injury Infect Crit Care*. 2000;48(3):376.
15. Manley G, Knudson MM, Morabito D, et al. Hypotension, hypoxia, and head injury: frequency, duration, and consequences. *Arch Surg*. 2001;136(10):1118.
16. Chesnut RM, Marshall LF, Klauber MR, et al. The role of secondary brain injury in determining outcome from severe head injury. *J Trauma*. 1993;34(2):216–222.
17. Luten R. Error and time delay in pediatric trauma resuscitation: addressing the problem with color-coded resuscitation aids. *Surg Clin North Am*. 2002;82(2):303.
18. American College of Surgeons (ACS) Committee on Trauma. Pediatric trauma. In: ACS Committee on Trauma. *Advanced Trauma Life Support for Doctors, Student Course Manual*. 8th ed. Chicago, IL: ACS; 2008:225–245.
19. National Vital Statistics System, Centers for Disease Control and Prevention. Deaths: final data for 1997. *MMWR*. 1999;47(19):1.
20. Ehrlich PF, Seidman PS, Atallah D, et al. Endotracheal intubation in rural pediatric trauma patients. *J Pediatr Surg*. 2004;39:1376.
21. Heins M. The "battered child" revisited. *JAMA*. 1984;251:3295.
22. Davis DP, Valentine C, Ochs M, et al. The Combitube as a salvage airway device for paramedic rapid sequence intubation. *Ann Emerg Med*. 2003;42(5):697.
23. Martin SE, Ochsner MG, Jarman RH, et al. Use of the laryngeal mask airway in air transport when intubation fails. *J Trauma Injury Infect Crit Care*. 1999;47(2):352.
24. Winchell RJ, Hoyt DB. Endotracheal intubation in the field improves survival in patients with severe head injury. *Arch Surg*. 1997;132(6):592.
25. Davis DP, Ochs M, Hoyt DB, et al. Paramedic-administered neuromuscular blockade improves prehospital intubation success in

severely head-injured patients. *J Trauma Injury Infect Crit Care.* 2003;55(4):713.

26. Pearson S. Comparison of intubation attempts and completion times before and after the initiation of a rapid sequence intubation protocol in an air medical transport program. *Air Med J.* 2003;22(6):28.

27. Stockinger ZT, McSwain NE Jr. Prehospital endotracheal intubation for trauma does not improve survival over bag-valve-mask ventilation. *J Trauma Injury Infect Crit Care.* 2004;56(3):531.

28. Murray JA, Demetriades D, Berne TV, et al. Prehospital intubation in patients with severe head injury. *J Trauma Injury Infect Crit Care.* 2000;49(6):1065.

29. Davis BD, Fowler R, Kupas DF, Roppolo LP. Role of rapid sequence induction for intubation in the prehospital setting: helpful or harmful? *Curr Opin Crit Care.* 2002;8(6):571.

30. Dong L, Donaldson A, Metzger R, Keenan H. Analgesic administration in the emergency department for children requiring hospitalization for long-bone fracture. *Pediatr Emerg Care.* 2012;28:109.

31. Larson JT, Dietrich AM, Abdessalam SF, Werman HA. Effective use of the air ambulance for pediatric trauma. *J Trauma Injury Infect Crit Care.* 2004;56(1):89.

32. Eckstein M, Jantos T, Kelly N, Cardillo A. Helicopter transport of pediatric trauma patients in an urban emergency medical services system: a critical analysis. *J Trauma Injury Infect Crit Care.* 2002;53(2):340.

33. Halstead ME, Walter KD, Council on Sports Medicine and Fitness. Clinical report—sport-related concussion in children and adolescents. *Pediatrics.* 2010;126;597.

34. Carmona Suazo JA, Maas AI, van den Brink WA, et al. CO_2 reactivity and brain oxygen pressure monitoring in severe head injury. *Crit Care Med.* 2000;28(9):3268.

35. Adelson PD, Bratton SL, Carney NA, et al. Guidelines for the acute medical management of severe traumatic brain injury in infants, children, and adolescents. Chapter 4. Resuscitation of blood pressure and oxygenation and prehospital brain-specific therapies for the severe pediatric traumatic brain injury patient. *Pediatr Crit Care Med.* 2003;4(3 suppl):S12.

36. De Lorenzo RA. A review of spinal immobilization techniques. *J Emerg Med.* 1996;14(5):603.

37. Valadie LL. Child safety seats and the emergency responder. *Emerg Med Serv.* 2004;33(7):68.

38. U.S. Department of Transportation, National Highway Traffic Safety Administration. Working group best-practice recommendations for the safe transportation of children in emergency ground ambulances. DOT HS 811 677. September 2012.

39. Weimer CL, Goldfarb IW, Slater H. Multidisciplinary approach to working with burn victims of child abuse. *J Burn Care Rehabil.* 1988;9:79.

40. Feldman KW, Schaller RT, Feldman JA, McMillon M. Tap water scald burns in children. *Pediatrics.* 1978;62:1.

41. Montrey JS, Barcia PJ. Nonaccidental burns in child abuse. *South Med J.* 1985;78:1324.

42. Hight DW, Bakalar HR, Lloyd JR. Inflicted burns in children: recognition and treatment. *JAMA.* 1979;242:517.

43. American Academy of Pediatrics Committee on Injury and Poison Prevention. Selecting and using the most appropriate car safety seats for growing children: guidelines for counseling parents. *Pediatrics.* 2002;109(3):550.

44. Nance ML, Lutz N, Arbogast KB, et al. Optimal restraint reduces the risk of abdominal injury in children involved in motor vehicle crashes. *Ann Surg.* 2004;239(1):127.

45. Braver ER, Whitfield R, Ferguson SA. Seating positions and children's risk of dying in motor vehicle crashes. *Injury Prev.* 1998;4(3):181.

Suggested Reading

EMSC Partnership for Children/National Association of EMS Physicians model pediatric protocols: 2003 revision [no authors listed]. *Prehosp Emerg Care.* 2004;8(4):343.

CHAPTER 17

Geriatric Trauma

CHAPTER OBJECTIVES

At the completion of this chapter, the reader will be able to do the following:

- Discuss the epidemiology of trauma in the elderly population.

- Describe the anatomic and physiologic effects of aging as a factor in causes of geriatric trauma and as a factor in the pathophysiology of trauma.

- Explain the interaction of various pre-existing medical problems with traumatic injuries in geriatric patients and how these interactions produce differences in the pathophysiology and manifestations of trauma.

- Discuss the physiologic effects of specific common classes of medications on the pathophysiology and manifestations of geriatric trauma.

- Compare and contrast the assessment techniques and considerations used in the elderly population with those used in younger populations.

- Demonstrate modifications in spinal immobilization techniques for safe and effective spinal immobilization of the elderly patient with the highest degree of comfort possible.

- Compare and contrast the management of the elderly trauma patient with that of the younger trauma patient.

- Assess the scene and elderly patients for signs and symptoms of abuse and neglect.

SCENARIO

Your unit is dispatched to the home of a 78-year-old woman who has fallen down a flight of stairs. Her daughter states that they had spoken on the telephone just 15 minutes earlier and that she was coming to her mother's house to do some shopping. When she got to the house, she found her mother on the floor and called for an ambulance.

Upon initial contact, you find the patient lying at the bottom of a flight of stairs. You note that the patient is an elderly woman whose appearance matches her reported age. While maintaining in-line stabilization of the spine, you note that the patient is unresponsive to your commands. She has a visible laceration of the forehead and an obvious deformity of the left wrist. She is wearing a Medic Alert bracelet that indicates that she is diabetic.

- Did the fall cause the change in mental status, or was there an antecedent event?
- How do the patient's age, medical history, and medications interact with the injuries received to make the pathophysiology and manifestations different from those in younger patients?
- Should advanced age alone be used as an additional criterion for transport to a trauma center?

Introduction

The elderly population represents the fastest-growing age group in the United States. Gerontologists (medical specialists who study and care for elderly patients) divide the term elderly into three specific categories, as follows:

- *Middle age*: 50 to 64 years of age
- *Late age*: 65 to 79 years of age
- *Older age*: 80 years of age and older

Although such definitions are important for epidemiologic data, it is also important to recognize that the physiologic changes of aging occur along the entire age spectrum and vary among individuals. Recovery from closed head injury starts to decline beginning in the mid-20s age group, and overall survival from trauma starts to decline in the late 30s. In addition, increasing age is often associated with multiple pre-existing medical conditions, which further complicate the recovery from trauma. The approach to the elderly patient includes recognition of this fact, although younger patients with comorbidities may share similar attributes.

Over 41 million Americans (13.3% of the U.S. population) are 65 years of age or older, and the size of this group has risen dramatically during the last 100 years.[1] At the same time, fertility rates have dropped, meaning that there will be fewer people under 65 years of age to support the costs of health care and living expenses of those over 65 years of age. By the year 2050, nearly 25% of Americans will be eligible for Medicare, and the population over 85 years of age will have grown from 5.5 million to 19 million people.[2] The United Nations Population Division estimates the worldwide number of those older than 60 years of age to be just under 800 million today (representing 11% of the world population) and projects that it will increase to just over 2 billion in 2050 (representing 22% of the world population).[3]

The injured elderly present unique challenges in prehospital (and hospital) care management, second only to those encountered with infants. Sudden illness and trauma in elderly patients present a different prehospital care dimension than in younger patients. Some of the earliest data looking at the effect of age on outcome are from the Major Trauma Outcome Study by the American College of Surgeons Committee on Trauma.[4] Data from more than 3,800 patients aged 65 years and older were compared to almost 43,000 patients younger than 65 years of age. Mortality increased in ages 45 to 55 years and doubled by age 75 years. The age-adjusted risk of death occurs across the spectrum of injury severity, suggesting that injuries that could be easily tolerated by younger patients may result in mortality in those of advanced age.

Because older persons are more susceptible to critical illness and trauma than the rest of the population, a wider range of difficulties in patient assessment and management needs to be considered. Because elderly patients often access medical care through emergency systems (e.g., 9-1-1), rendering care is different than for younger patients. The range of disabilities experienced by elderly patients is enormous, and field assessment may take longer than with younger patients. Difficulties in assessment can be expected as a result of age-related sensory impairments in hearing and vision, senility, and physiologic changes.

Advances in medicine and an increasing awareness of healthier lifestyles during the last several decades have resulted in a significant increase in the percentage of the population over 65 years of age. Although trauma occurs most frequently in young people, and geriatric emergencies are most often medical problems, a growing number of geriatric calls result from or include trauma. Trauma is the fourth leading cause of death in persons aged 55 to 64 years and is the ninth highest cause of death in those aged 65 years and older.[5] Approximately 15% of injury-related deaths in elderly patients are classified as homicide. Trauma deaths in this age group account for 25% of all trauma deaths nationwide.[6]

Specific patterns of injury are also unique to the geriatric population.[7] Although motor vehicle crashes are the leading cause of death from trauma overall, falls are the predominant cause of traumatic death in patients over 75 years of age. As with small children (age younger than 5 years), scald injuries account for a greater percentage of burns in those over 65 years.

Progress in recent years has not only increased adult life expectancy but has also affected the quality of life and, therefore, the range of physical activities performed at older ages. As more people live longer and enjoy better health in their older years, more of them travel, drive, and continue active physical pursuits that can result in an associated increase in geriatric trauma. Many who could retire now continue to work despite a health problem or advancing age.

Recent social changes have increased the number of older people living in independent housing, retirement communities, and other assisted-living facilities compared with those in nursing homes or other, more guarded and limited environments. This shift in home environment suggests a probable increase in the incidence of simple household trauma, such as falls, in elderly persons. The past few years have also seen an increase in geriatric victims of crime in the home and on the streets. Older people are often singled out as "easy marks" and can sustain substantial trauma from crimes of seemingly limited violence, such as purse snatching, when they are struck, knocked down, or fall.

With the growing awareness of this expanding population at risk, the prehospital care provider must understand the unique needs of an elderly trauma patient. Specifically, the aging process and the effects of coexisting medical problems on an elderly patient's response to trauma and trauma management must be understood. The special considerations outlined in this chapter should be included in the assessment and management of any trauma patient who is 65 years of age or older, physically appears elderly, or is middle-aged and has any of the significant medical problems typically associated with the elderly population.

Anatomy and Physiology of Aging

The aging process causes changes in physical structure, body composition, and organ function, and it can create unique problems during prehospital care. The aging process influences mortality and morbidity rates.

Aging, or **senescence**, is a natural biologic process and is sometimes referred to as a process of "biologic reversal" that begins during the years of early adulthood. At this time,

organ systems have achieved maturation, and a turning point in physiologic growth has been reached. The body gradually loses its ability to maintain **homeostasis** (the state of relative constancy of the body's internal environment), and viability declines over a period of years until death occurs.

The fundamental process of aging occurs at the cellular level and is reflected in both anatomic structure and physiologic function. The period of "old age" is generally characterized by frailty, slower cognitive processes, impairment of psychological functions, diminished energy, the appearance of chronic and degenerative diseases, and a decline in sensory acuity. Functional abilities are lessened, and the well-known external signs and symptoms of older age appear, such as skin wrinkling, changes in hair color and quantity, osteoarthritis, and slowness in reaction time and reflexes (**Figure 17-1**).

Influence of Chronic Medical Problems

As people age, they experience the normal physiologic changes of advancing years and can also experience more medical problems. Although some individuals can reach an advanced age without any serious medical problems, statistically an older person is more likely to have one or more significant medical conditions (**Figure 17-2**). Seniors presently consume more than one-third of health care resources in the United States.[8] Usually, proper medical care can control these conditions, helping to avoid or minimize exacerbations from becoming repeated acute and often life-threatening episodes.

Some older individuals have reached advanced age with minimal medical problems, whereas others may live with chronic

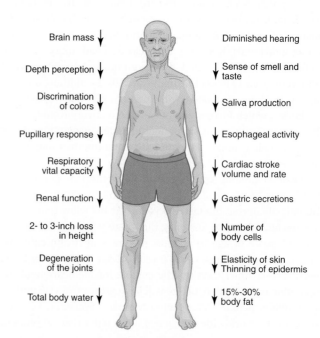

Brain mass ↓
Depth perception ↓
Discrimination of colors ↓
Pupillary response ↓
Respiratory vital capacity ↓
Renal function ↓
2- to 3-inch loss in height
Degeneration of the joints
Total body water ↓

Diminished hearing
↓ Sense of smell and taste
↓ Saliva production
↓ Esophageal activity
↓ Cardiac stroke volume and rate
↓ Gastric secretions
↓ Number of body cells
↓ Elasticity of skin Thinning of epidermis
↓ 15%-30% body fat

Figure 17-1 Changes caused by aging.

Figure 17-2   Percentage of Patients with Pre-existing Disease (PED)

Age (years)	PED (%)
13–39	3.5
40–64	11.6
65–74	29.4
75–84	34.7
85+	37.3

illnesses and depend on modern medical means to survive. This latter group can deteriorate more rapidly in an emergency situation.

Repeated acute episodes of a medical problem or even the single occurrence of a significant episode can result in chronic residual effects on the body. A patient who has previously had an acute myocardial infarction sustains permanent heart damage. The resultant reduced cardiac capacity continues for the rest of the patient's life, affecting the heart and, because of the ensuing chronic impairment of circulation, other organs as well.

As a person's age advances, additional medical problems can occur. None is truly isolated because the effect on the body is cumulative. The total influence on the body usually is greater than the sum of each individual effect. As each condition progresses and reduces the quality of the body's vital functions, the individual's ability to withstand even modest anatomic or physiologic insults is greatly diminished.

Regardless of whether the patient is pediatric, middle-aged, or elderly, the priorities, intervention needs, and life-threatening conditions that usually result from serious trauma are the same. However, because of these pre-existing physical conditions, elderly patients often die from less severe injuries and die sooner than younger patients. Data support that pre-existing conditions play a role in the mortality of an elderly trauma patient and that the more conditions a trauma patient has, the higher his or her mortality rate (**Figure 17-3**). Certain conditions are associated with a higher

Figure 17-3   Number of Pre-existing Diseases (PEDs) and Patient Outcome After Trauma

Number of PEDs	Survived	Died	Mortality Rate (%)
0	6341	211	3.2
1	868	56	6.1
2	197	36	15.5
3 or more	67	22	24.7

Figure 17-4   Prevalence of Pre-existing Diseases (PEDs) and Associated Mortality Rates After Trauma

PED	Number of Patients	PED Present (%)	Total (%)	Mortality Rate (%)
Hypertension	597	47.9	7.7	10.2
Pulmonary disease	286	23	3.7	8.4
Cardiac disease	223	17.9	2.9	18.4
Diabetes	198	15.9	2.5	12.1
Obesity	167	13.4	2.1	4.8
Malignancy	80	6.4	1	20
Neurologic disorder	45	3.6	0.6	13.3
Renal disease	40	3.2	0.5	37.5
Hepatic disease	41	3.3	0.5	12.2

mortality rate because of the way in which they interfere with an elderly patient's ability to respond to trauma (**Figure 17-4**).[9]

Ears, Nose, and Throat

Tooth decay, gum disease, and injury to teeth result in the need for various dental prostheses. The brittle nature of capped teeth, fixed bridges, or loose, removable bridges and dentures poses a special problem; these foreign bodies can be easily broken and aspirated and can subsequently obstruct the airway.

Changes in the contours of the face result from resorption of the mandible, in part because of the absence of teeth (**edentulism**). This resorption causes a characteristic look of an infolding and shrinking mouth. These changes can adversely affect the ability to create an effective seal with a bag-mask device and to sufficiently visualize the airway during endotracheal intubation.

The nasopharyngeal tissues become increasingly fragile with age. In addition to the risk this change poses during the initial trauma, interventions such as insertion of nasopharyngeal tubes may induce profuse bleeding if not performed with care.

Respiratory System

Ventilatory function declines in the elderly person partly as a result of the decreased ability of the chest wall to expand and contract and partly from stiffening of the airway. The increased stiffness in the chest wall is associated with a reduction in expansion of the chest wall and a stiffening of cartilaginous connections of the ribs. As a result of these changes, the chest cage is less pliable. With declines in the efficiency of the respiratory system, the elderly person requires more work to breathe and greater exertion to carry out daily activities.

The alveolar surface area in the lungs decreases with age; it is estimated to decrease by 4% for each decade after 30 years of age. A 70-year-old person, for example, would have a 16% reduction in alveolar surface area. Any alteration of the already-reduced alveolar surface decreases oxygen uptake. Additionally, as the body ages, its ability to saturate hemoglobin with oxygen decreases, leading to lower baseline oxygen saturation as a normal finding and less oxygen reserve available.[10] Because of impaired mechanical ventilation and diminished surface for gas exchange, the elderly trauma patient is less capable of compensating for physiologic losses associated with trauma.

Changes in the airway and lungs of elderly persons may not always be related to senescence alone. Cumulative chronic exposure to environmental toxins over the course of their lives may be caused by occupational hazards or tobacco smoke. Impaired cough and gag reflexes, along with poor cough strength and diminished esophageal sphincter tone, result in an increased risk of **aspiration pneumonitis**. A reduction in the number of **cilia** (hair-like projections of the cells in the respiratory tract that propel foreign particles and mucus from the bronchi) predisposes the elderly person to problems caused by inhaled particulate matter.

Another factor that affects the respiratory system is a change in the spinal curvature. Curvature changes, primarily increasing **kyphosis**, accompanied by an anteroposterior hump (as seen in osteoporosis patients) often lead to additional ventilatory difficulty (**Figure 17-5**).

Changes that affect the diaphragm can also contribute to ventilatory problems. Stiffening of the rib cage can cause more reliance on diaphragmatic activity to breathe. This increased reliance on the diaphragm makes an older person especially sensitive to changes in intra-abdominal pressure. Thus, a supine position or a full stomach from a large meal can provoke ventilatory insufficiency. Obesity can also play a part in diaphragm movement restriction, especially when fat distribution tends to be central.

Cardiovascular System

Diseases of the cardiovascular system are the primary cause of death in the elderly population. Cardiovascular disease accounts for more than 3,000 deaths per 100,000 persons over 65 years of age. In 2010, myocardial infarction accounted for 27% of deaths in the United States, with an additional 6% caused by stroke.[5]

Age-related decreases in arterial elasticity lead to increased peripheral vascular resistance. The myocardium and blood vessels rely on their elastic, contractile, and *distensible* (stretchable) properties to function properly. With aging, these properties decline, and the cardiovascular system becomes less efficient at moving circulatory fluids around the body. The cardiac output diminishes by approximately 50% from 20 to 80 years of age. Among patients over 75 years of age, as many as 10% will have some degree of overt congestive heart failure.

Atherosclerosis is a narrowing of the blood vessels, a condition in which the inner layer of the artery wall thickens as fatty deposits build up within the artery. These deposits, called plaque, protrude above the surface of the inner layer and decrease the diameter of the internal channel of the vessel. The same luminal narrowing occurs in the coronary vessels. Almost 50% of the U.S. population has coronary artery stenosis by age 65 years.[5]

One result of this narrowing is **hypertension**, a condition that affects one of six adults in the United States. Calcification of the arterial wall reduces the ability of the vessels to change size in response to endocrine and central nervous system stimuli. The decrease in circulation can adversely affect any of the vital organs and is a common cause of heart disease. Of particular concern is that the baseline normal blood pressure of the elderly trauma patient may be higher than in younger patients. What would otherwise be accepted as normotension may indicate profound hypovolemic shock in the patient with pre-existing hypertension.

With age, the heart itself shows an increase in fibrous tissue and size (**myocardial hypertrophy**). Atrophy of the cells of the conduction system results in the increased incidence of cardiac dysrhythmias. In particular, the normal reflexes in the heart that respond to hypotension diminish with age, resulting in the inability of elderly patients to increase their heart rate appropriately to compensate adequately for a low blood pressure. Maximal heart rate also begins to decrease starting at age 40 years, estimated by the formula 220 minus the age in years. Patients with a permanent pacemaker have a fixed heart rate and cardiac output that cannot meet the demands of increased myocardial oxygen consumption accompanying the stress of trauma. Patients with hypertension taking beta blocker medications may also not have an increase in heart rate to compensate for hypovolemia.

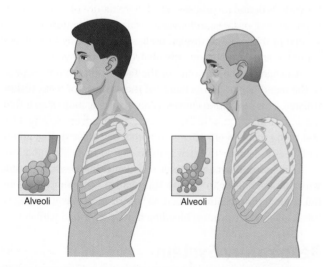

Figure 17-5 Spinal curvature can lead to an anteroposterior hump, which can cause ventilatory difficulties. Reduction in the alveolar surface area can also reduce the amount of oxygen that is exchanged in the lungs.

In the elderly trauma patient, this reduced circulation contributes to cellular hypoxia. The result is cardiac dysrhythmia, acute heart failure, and even sudden death. The body's ability to compensate for blood loss or other causes of shock is significantly lowered in the elderly person because of a diminished *inotropic* (cardiac contraction) response to **catecholamines**. In addition, total circulating blood volume decreases, creating less physiologic reserve for blood loss from trauma. Diastolic dysfunction makes the patient more dependent on atrial filling to augment cardiac output, which is diminished in hypovolemic states.

The reduced circulation and circulatory-defense responses, coupled with increasing cardiac failure, produce a significant problem in managing shock in the elderly trauma patient. Fluid resuscitation needs to be carefully monitored because of the reduced compliance of the cardiovascular system and the often "stiff" right ventricle. As the patient ages, cardiac muscle loses its elastic properties and becomes "stiffer." As a result, its ability to compensate for a sudden increase in circulating volume is limited. Care must be taken when treating hypotension and shock to avoid causing volume overloading with aggressive fluid resuscitation.[11]

Nervous System

As individuals age, brain weight and the number of neurons (nerve cells) decrease. The weight of the brain reaches its peak (1.4 kilogram, or 3 pounds) at approximately 20 years of age. By 80 years of age, the brain has lost about 10% of its weight, with progressive cerebral atrophy.[12] The body compensates for the loss of size with increased cerebrospinal fluid. Although this additional space around the brain can protect it from contusion, it also allows for more brain movement in response to acceleration/deceleration injuries. The increased space in the cranial vault also explains why the elderly patient may have significant volumes of blood accumulate around the brain with minimal or no symptoms.

The speed with which nerve impulses are conducted along certain nerves also decreases. These decreases result in only small effects on behavior and thinking. Reflexes are slower, but not to a significant degree. Compensatory functions can be impaired, particularly in patients with diseases such as Parkinson's disease, resulting in an increased incidence of falls. The peripheral nervous system is also affected by the slowing of nerve impulses, resulting in tremors and an unsteady gait.

General information and vocabulary abilities increase or are maintained, whereas skills requiring mental and muscular activity (psychomotor ability) may decline. The intellectual functions that involve verbal comprehension, arithmetic ability, fluency of ideas, experiential evaluation, and general knowledge tend to increase after 60 years of age in those who continue learning activities. Exceptions are those who develop senile dementia and other disorders such as Alzheimer's disease.

The normal biologic aging of the brain is not a predictor for diseases of the brain. However, decreases in the cortical structure of the brain may be involved in mental impairment. As changes occur in the brain, memory can be affected, and personality changes and other reductions in brain function can occur. These changes may involve the need for some form of mental health service. About 10% to 15% of elderly persons require professional mental health services. However, when assessing an elderly trauma patient, any impairment in mentation should be assumed to be the result of an acute traumatic insult, such as shock, hypoxia, or brain injury.

Sensory Changes
Vision and Hearing

Overall, approximately 28% of elderly persons have hearing impairment, and approximately 13% have visual impairment. Men tend to be more likely to have hearing difficulties, whereas both genders have a similar incidence of eye-related impairment.

Loss of vision is challenging at any age, and it may be even more problematic for the elderly person. The inability to read directions (e.g., on a prescription label) can lead to a disastrous effect. In addition, elderly persons experience decreases in visual acuity, ability to differentiate colors, and night vision.

The cells of the lens of the eye are incapable of restoration to their original molecular structure. One of the destructive agents over years of exposure is ultraviolet radiation. Eventually, the lens loses its capability to increase in thickness and curvature. The result is almost universal farsightedness (*presbyopia*) in persons over 40 years of age, requiring glasses for reading.

As a result of changes to the various structures of the eye, elderly persons have more difficulty seeing in dimly lit environments. Decreased tear production leads to dry eyes—itching and burning—and the inability to keep the eyes open for long periods.

With age, the lens of the eye begins to become cloudy and impenetrable to light. This gradual process results in a **cataract**, or a milky lens that blocks and distorts light that enters the eye and blurs vision. Some degree of cataract formation is present in 95% of elderly persons. This deterioration of vision increases the risk of a motor vehicle crash, particularly when driving at night.[13]

A gradual decline in hearing (*presbycusis*) is also characteristic of aging. **Presbycusis** is usually caused by loss of conduction of sound into the inner ear; the use of hearing aids can compensate for this loss to some degree. This hearing loss is most pronounced when the person attempts to discriminate complex sounds, such as when many people are speaking at once, or with loud, ambient noise present, such as the wailing of sirens.

Pain Perception

Because of the aging process and the presence of diseases such as diabetes, elderly persons may not perceive pain normally, placing them at increased risk of injury from excesses in heat and cold exposure. Many elderly persons have conditions such as arthritis that result in chronic pain. Living with daily pain can cause an increased tolerance to pain, which may result in a patient's failure to identify areas of injury. In evaluating patients, especially those who usually "hurt all over" or who appear to have a high tolerance to pain, areas in which the pain has increased or in which the painful area has enlarged should be located. It is also important to note whether the pain's characteristics or exacerbating factors have changed since the trauma occurred.

Renal System

Changes common with aging include reduced levels of filtration by the kidneys and a reduced excretory capacity. These changes should be considered when administering drugs normally cleared by the kidneys. Chronic renal inhibition typically affects elderly persons and contributes to a reduction in a patient's over-all health status and ability to withstand trauma. For example, renal dysfunction may be one cause of chronic anemia, which would lower a patient's **physiologic reserve**.

Musculoskeletal System

Bone loses mineral as it ages. The loss of bone (**osteoporosis**) is unequal among the genders. During young adulthood, bone mass is greater in women than in men. However, bone loss is more rapid in women and accelerates after menopause. With this higher incidence of osteoporosis, older women have a greater probability of fractures, particularly of the neck of the femur (hip). Causes of osteoporosis include loss of estrogen levels, increased periods of inactivity, and inadequate intake and inefficient use of calcium.

Osteoporosis contributes significantly to hip fractures and spontaneous compression fractures of the vertebral bodies. The incidence approaches 1% per year for men and 2% for women over age 85 years.[14]

Older persons are sometimes shorter than they were in young adulthood because of dehydration of the vertebral discs. As the discs flatten, a loss of approximately 2 inches (5 centimeters) in height occurs between 20 and 70 years of age. *Kyphosis* (curvature of the spine) in the thoracic region can also contribute to height loss and is often caused by osteoporosis (**Figure 17-6**). As the bones become more porous and fragile, erosion occurs anteriorly, and compression fractures of the vertebrae may develop. As the thoracic spine becomes more curved, the head and shoulders appear to be pushed forward. If chronic obstructive pulmonary disease (COPD), particularly emphysema, is present, the kyphosis may be more pronounced because of the increased development of the accessory muscles of breathing.

Absolute levels of growth hormones decrease with aging, in conjunction with a decline in responsiveness to anabolic hormones. The combined effect is a reduction in muscle mass of about 4% per decade after age 25 years until age 50 years, when the process accelerates to between 10% and 35% per decade. Muscle loss is measured microscopically by both absolute number of muscle cells and reduction in cell size.

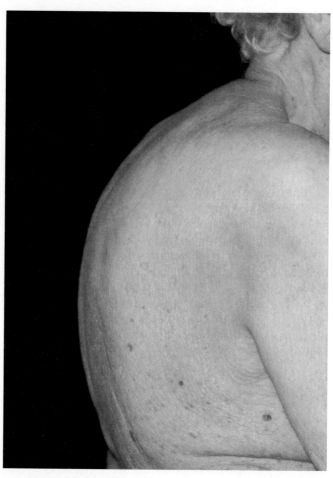

Figure 17-6 Kyphosis, typically caused by osteoporosis. Because of the elderly person's tendency to flex the legs, the arms appear longer.
Source: © Dr. P. Marazzi/Science Source.

Deficits that relate to the musculoskeletal system (e.g., inability to flex the hip or knee adequately with changes in terrain) predispose the elderly person to falls. Muscle fatigue can cause many problems that affect movement, especially falls. Changes in the body's normal posture are common, and changes in the spine make the curvature become more acute with aging. Some degree of osteoporosis is universal with aging. Because of this progressive bone resorption, the bones become less pliant, more brittle, and more easily broken. The decrease in bone strength, coupled with reduced muscle strength caused by less active exercise, can result in multiple fractures with only mild or moderate force. The most common sites of long-bone fracture in elderly persons include the proximal femur, hip, humerus, and wrist. The increased incidence of falls as a mechanism of injury results in Colles' fractures of the distal radius, as the dorsiflexed hand is outstretched in an effort to break the fall.

The entire vertebral column changes with age, primarily because of the effects of osteoporosis, **osteophytosis** (bone spurs), and calcification of the supporting ligaments. This calcification results in decreased range of motion and narrowing of the spinal canal. The narrowed canal and progressive osteophytic disease put these patients at high risk for spinal cord injury with even minor trauma. The narrowing of the spinal canal is called **spinal stenosis** and increases the likelihood of cord compression without any actual break in the bony cervical spine. The thoracic and lumbar spine degenerate progressively as well, and the combined forces of osteoporosis and posture changes lead to increased falls. A high level of suspicion for spinal injury is needed during patient assessment because more than 50% of vertebral compression fractures are asymptomatic.[15]

Skin

Significant changes in the skin and connective tissues are associated with aging and result in difficulties with response to trauma as well as direct wound healing. Cell numbers decrease, tissue strength is lost, and the skin has impaired functional status. As the skin ages, sweat and sebaceous glands are lost. Loss of sweat glands reduces the body's ability to regulate temperature. Loss of sebaceous glands, which produce oil, makes the skin dry and flaky. Production of melanin, the pigment that gives color to skin and hair, declines, causing an aging pallor. The skin thins and appears translucent, primarily because of changes in underlying connective tissue, and therefore is more prone to sustaining damage from relatively minor trauma. The thinning and drying of the skin also reduce its resistance to minor injury and microorganisms, resulting in an increased infection rate from open wounds. As elasticity is lost, the skin stretches and falls into wrinkles and folds, especially in areas of heavy use, such as those overlying the facial muscles of expression. Thinning of the skin also results in the potential for significant tissue loss and injury in response to relatively low-energy transfers.

Loss of fatty tissue can predispose the elderly person to hypothermia. The loss of up to 20% of dermal thickness with advanced age and an associated loss in vascularity are also responsible for impaired thermoregulatory dysfunction. However, hypothermia should also suggest the possibility of occult sepsis, hypothyroidism, or phenothiazine overdose in the elderly population. This loss of fatty tissue also leads to less padding over bony prominences, such as the head, shoulders, spine, buttocks, hips, and heels. Prolonged immobilization without additional padding can result in tissue necrosis and ulceration as well as increased pain and discomfort during treatment and transport.

Nutrition and the Immune System

With aging, a reduction in lean body mass and decreases in metabolic rate cause a reduction in caloric needs. However, because of inefficient utilization mechanisms, protein needs may actually increase. These competing changes often result in pre-existing malnutrition in the elderly trauma patient. The financial status of retired individuals may also affect their choices of and access to quality nutrition.

The ability of the immune system to function decreases as it ages. Grossly, organs associated with the immune response (thymus, liver, and spleen) all decrease in size. A decrease in

cell-mediated and humoral responses to infection also results. Coupled with any pre-existing nutritional problems common in the elderly population, there is an increased susceptibility to infection. *Sepsis* is a common cause of late death after severe or even insignificant trauma in the elderly patient.

Assessment

Prehospital assessment of the elderly patient is based on the same method used for all trauma patients. Although the methodology is unchanged, the process may be altered in elderly patients. As with all trauma patients, however, the mechanism of injury should be considered first. This section discusses some special considerations in assessing an elderly trauma patient.

Kinematics

Falls

Falls are the leading cause of trauma death and disability in those over 75 years of age. Approximately one-third of community-dwelling people over 65 years of age fall each year, increasing to 50% by 80 years of age. Men and women fall with equal frequency, but women are more than twice as likely to sustain a serious injury because of more pronounced osteoporosis. Falls in the elderly, even those that occur from a standing position, can result in serious injury and life-threatening trauma.

Most falls result from the inherent nature of aging, with the changes in posture and gait.[16] Declining visual acuity from cataracts, glaucoma, and loss of night vision contributes to the loss of visual clues used by elderly persons to navigate safely. Diseases of the central and peripheral nervous systems and the vascular instability of cardiovascular disease further precipitate falls. Not only do pre-existing conditions predispose the geriatric patients to more serious complications, but also the use of medications to treat these conditions, such as anticoagulants and beta blockers, interferes with the normal physiologic and compensatory responses to trauma. However, the most important variables contributing to falls in elderly persons are physical barriers in their environment, such as slippery floors, throw rugs, stairs, poorly fitting shoes, and poor lighting.

Long-bone fractures account for the majority of injuries, with fractures of the hip resulting in the greatest mortality and morbidity rates. The mortality rate from hip fractures is 20% at 1 year after the injury and rises to 33% at 2 years. Mortality is most often secondary to pulmonary embolus and the effects of decreased mobility.

Vehicular Trauma

Motor vehicle crashes are the leading cause of trauma death in the geriatric population between 65 and 74 years of age. An elderly patient is five times more likely to be fatally injured in a motor vehicle crash than a younger driver, even though excessive speed is rarely a causative factor in the older age group.[17] For many reasons, elderly persons are often involved in collisions during daylight hours, during good weather, and close to their domicile (**Figure 17-7**).

These high fatality rates have been attributed to certain physiologic changes. In particular, subtle changes in memory and judgment together with impaired visual and auditory acuity can result in delayed reaction time. A common finding at crash investigations is that the elderly driver failed to yield to oncoming traffic.

Figure 17-7   Older Drivers

The National Highway Traffic Safety Administration has produced a CD-ROM program to assist physicians in assessing and counseling older drivers.

Alcohol is rarely involved, unlike with motor vehicle crashes in younger persons. Only 5% of fatally injured elderly persons are intoxicated, compared with 25% for all other age categories.[17]

Elderly pedestrians represent more than 20% of all pedestrian fatalities. Because of slower walking speeds, the time allowed by traffic signals may be too short for the elderly person to traverse the crosswalk safely. This may explain the observation that more than 45% of all elderly pedestrian fatalities occur near a crosswalk.

Assault and Domestic Abuse

Abuse is defined as willful infliction of injury, unreasonable confinement, intimidation, or cruel punishment resulting in physical or psychological harm or pain, or the withholding of services that would prevent these conditions. The elderly are highly vulnerable to this crime. Violent assaults have been estimated to account for more than 10% of trauma admissions in elderly patients. The need for chronic care because of debilitation may predispose an elderly person to abuse or neglect from his or her caregivers. It is estimated that only about 15% of cases of geriatric abuse are reported to the proper authorities[18,19] (see the later discussion on Elder Maltreatment).

Burns

Elderly patients represent 20% of burn unit admissions, with an estimated 1,500 fire-related deaths per year. Burn fatalities in elderly patients occur from burns of smaller size and severity compared with other age groups. Fatality rates are seven times those of younger burn victims.

Because of impairments in visual and auditory acuity, elderly persons may have delayed recognition of house fires. Decreased pain perception can result in more significant burns. Thinning of dermal elements may result in a deeper thickness of burns.

The presence of pre-existing medical conditions, such as cardiovascular disease and diabetes, results in poor tolerance to the resuscitative care of burns. Vascular collapse and infection are the most common causes of death from burns in elderly patients.

Traumatic Brain Injury

The brain has undergone a 10% reduction in mass by 70 years of age. The dura mater adheres more closely to the skull, resulting in a loss of some brain volume. The dural bridging veins become more stretched and, thus, susceptible to tearing. This results in a lower frequency of epidural hemorrhage and a higher frequency of subdural hemorrhage. Because of brain atrophy, a fairly large subdural hemorrhage can exist with minimal clinical findings. The combination of head trauma and hypovolemic shock yields a greater fatality rate. Pre-existing medical conditions or their treatment may be a cause of altered mentation in elderly patients. When in doubt as to whether confusion represents an acute or a chronic process, the injured patient should be assumed to have sustained a traumatic brain injury and preferentially transported to a trauma center for evaluation when possible.

Primary Assessment

Airway

Evaluation of the elderly patient begins with assessment of the airway. Changes in mentation may be associated with the tongue blocking the airway. The oral cavity should be examined for foreign bodies, such as dentures or fractured teeth that have become dislodged.

Breathing

Elderly patients who breathe at a rate of less than 10 or greater than 30 breaths/minute, similar to any other adult, will not have adequate minute volume and will require positive-pressure assisted ventilations. In most adults, a ventilatory rate between 12 and 20 breaths/minute is normal and confirms that an adequate minute volume is present. However, in an elderly patient, reduced tidal volume capacity and pulmonary function may result in an inadequate minute volume, even at rates of 12 to 20 breaths/minute. Breath sounds should be immediately assessed if the ventilatory rate is abnormal; however, these sounds may be harder to hear because of smaller tidal volumes.

An elderly patient's vital capacity is diminished by 50%. Kyphotic changes of the spine (anteroposterior) result in a ventilation–perfusion mismatch at rest. Hypoxia is much more likely to be a consequence of shock than in younger patients. Elderly patients also have a decreased ability for chest excursions. Lower tidal volumes and lower minute volumes are typical. Reductions in capillary oxygen and carbon dioxide exchange are significant. Hypoxemia tends to be progressive.

Circulation

Some findings can only be interpreted properly by knowing the individual patient's pre-event, or "baseline," status. Expected ranges of vital signs and other findings usually accepted as normal are not "normal" in every individual, and deviation is much more common in the elderly patient. Although the typical ranges are broad enough to include most individual adult differences, an individual of any age may vary beyond these norms; therefore, such variation in elderly patients should be expected.

Medication may contribute to these changes. For example, in the average adult, a systolic blood pressure of 120 millimeters of mercury (mm Hg) is considered normal and generally unimpressive. However, in the chronically hypertensive patient who normally has a systolic blood pressure of 150 mm Hg or higher, a pressure of 120 mm Hg would be a concern, suggestive of hidden bleeding (or some other mechanism causing hypotension) of such a degree that decompensation has occurred. Likewise, heart rate is a poor indicator of trauma in elderly patients because of the effects of medications such as beta blockers and the heart's poor response to circulating catecholamines (epinephrine). Quantitative information or signs should not be used in isolation from other findings. However, failing to recognize that such a change occurred or that it is a serious pathologic finding in a particular patient can produce a poor outcome for the patient.

Delayed capillary refilling time is common in the elderly because of less efficient circulation (peripheral arterial disease); therefore, it is a poor indicator of acute circulatory changes in these patients. Some degree of decreased distal motor, sensory, and circulatory ability in the extremities represents a common normal finding in elderly patients.

Disability

All findings should be viewed collectively to maintain an increased level of suspicion for neurologic injury in the elderly patient. Wide differences in mentation, memory, and orientation (to the past and present) can exist in elderly persons. Significant neurologic trauma should be identified in light of the individual's preinjury, normal status. Unless someone on the scene can describe this status, it should be assumed that the patient has a neurologic injury, hypoxia, or both. The ability to distinguish between a patient's chronic status and acute changes is an essential factor to prevent underreaction or overreaction to the patient's present neurologic status when evaluating his or her overall condition. However, unconsciousness remains a serious sign in all cases.

The elderly patient's orientation to time and place should be assessed by careful and complete questioning. People who work 5 days a week with weekends off usually know the day of the week. If they do not, it can be assumed that they have some level of disorientation. For those who no longer work a traditional job and who are often surrounded by others who do not, a lack of distinction between days of the week or even months of the year may not indicate disorientation but only a lack of "calendar" importance in the structure of their lives.

Similarly, people who no longer drive pay less attention to roads, town borders, locations, and maps. Although normally oriented, they may not be able to identify their present location. Confusion or the inability to recall events and details long past may be more indicative of how long ago the events occurred rather than how forgetful the individual is. Likewise, the repeated retelling of events long past and more attention paid to the far past than the immediate past often simply represent a nostalgic lingering on years and events. Such social and psychological compensations should not be considered as signs of senility or a diminished mental capacity.

Expose/Environment

Elderly persons are more susceptible to ambient environmental changes. They have a decreased ability to respond to temperature changes, decreased heat production, and a decreased ability to rid the body of excessive heat. Thermoregulatory problems are related to an imbalance of electrolytes (e.g., potassium depletion, hypothyroidism, diabetes mellitus). Other factors include a decreased basal metabolic rate, decreased ability to shiver, arteriosclerosis, and effects of drugs and alcohol. Hyperthermia may result from cerebrovascular accidents (strokes) and administration of diuretics, antihistamines, and antiparkinsonian drugs. Hypothermia is often associated with decreased metabolism, less fat, less efficient peripheral vasoconstriction, and poor nutrition.

Secondary Assessment (Detailed History and Physical Examination)

The secondary assessment of the elderly trauma victim is performed in the same manner as for younger patients and after urgent life-threatening conditions have been addressed. However, a number of factors may complicate assessment of the geriatric patient, meaning prehospital care providers may need to take more than the average amount of time when assessing elderly patients.

Communication Challenges

Many factors come into play when communicating with geriatric patients, from the normal biologic effects of the aging process to generational expectations of the provider–patient relationship. Understanding how best to communicate with individuals in this age group will help the prehospital care provider deliver prompt, efficient care.

- *Additional patience may be needed because of the elderly patient's hearing or visual impairments.* Empathy and compassion are essential. A patient's intelligence should not be underestimated merely because communication may be difficult or absent. If the patient has close associates or relatives, they may participate in giving information or may stay nearby to help validate information. However, not all elderly patients have significant deficits. Speaking in a louder tone or slower cadence to the elderly patient may be unnecessary and insulting.

- *Assessment of the elderly patient requires different questioning tactics.* The patient should be asked for specific versus general information because elderly persons often respond "yes" to all questions during the assessment process. Asking open-ended questions is a useful tool in evaluating most patients, including the elderly. When dealing with a problem, however, providing specific details from which to choose can be helpful. For example, instead of saying, "Describe the pain in your hip," the prehospital care provider can ask, "Is the pain in your hip sharp, stabbing, or dull?" or "On a scale of 1 to 10, with 10 being the most intense pain, how would you rate the pain?"

- *A significant other may need to be involved.* With the patient's permission, involving the caregiver or spouse may be necessary to gather valid information. It is important, however, to not approach elderly patients as if they are small children. A common mistake by health care providers in both prehospital and emergency department settings is to treat the elderly in this way. Often, well-meaning relatives are so aggressive in reporting the events for an elderly loved one that they take over as the respondent to all inquiries. In such a situation, the prehospital care provider can easily overlook that the clinical impression and history are from someone other than the patient and may not be correct. Not only does this increase the danger of obtaining incomplete or inaccurate information through a third party's impressions and interpretation of what is transpiring, but it also discounts the patient as a mature adult.

  Some elderly patients may be reluctant to give information without the assistance of a relative or support person. However, the elderly patient may not want any other person present for many reasons, including abuse problems. The elderly patient may fear punishment for telling someone, in the presence of the abuser, why he or she has multiple bruise marks. Also, some problems may embarrass the elderly patient, and the person may not want any family members to know about them.

- *Pay attention to impaired hearing, sight, comprehension, and mobility capabilities.* Eye contact should be made with the patient. The patient may be hearing impaired and depend on watching your lips and other facial movements. Noise, distractions, and interruptions should be minimized. Fluency in speech, an involuntary movement, cranial nerve dysfunction, or difficulty breathing should be noted. Is the patient's movement easy, unsteady, or unbalanced?

- *Be respectful and avoid language that may be interpreted as condescending.* The patient should be addressed by his or her last name, unless otherwise instructed by the patient. Use of a patient's first name without his or her permission or use of pet names such as "honey" may insult the patient and make him or her a less willing participant. Phrases such as, "Now, now, you'll be fine," which may be considered patronizing or dismissive, should be avoided.

Physiologic Changes

The prehospital care provider must be prepared for the physiologic distinctions often encountered in the geriatric age group.

- *The body may not respond the same as in younger patients.* Typical findings of serious illness, such as fever, pain, or tenderness, may take longer to develop and, thus, make it more difficult to evaluate the elderly patient. In addition, many medications will alter the body's response. Often a prehospital care provider will have to depend on the patient's history alone.

- *Altered comprehension or neurologic disorders are a significant problem for many elderly patients.* These impairments can range from confusion to senile dementia of the type associated with Alzheimer's disease. Not only may these patients have difficulty in communicating, but they may also be unable to comprehend or help in the assessment. They may be restless and sometimes combative.

- *Elderly patients may not be properly nourished or hydrated.* Shake the patient's hand to feel for grip strength, skin turgor, and body temperature. Look at the patient's state of nourishment. Does the patient appear to be well, thin, or emaciated? Elderly patients have a decreased thirst response, and they also have a decreased amount of body fat (15% to 30%) and total body water.

- *Elderly patients have a decrease in skeletal muscle weight, widening and weakening of bones, degeneration of joints, and osteoporosis.* They have an increased probability of fractures with minor injuries and a greatly increased risk of fractures to the vertebrae, hip, and ribs. The ease of rising or sitting should be observed as it provides clues as to muscle strength.

- *Elderly patients have degeneration of heart muscle cells and fewer pacemaker cells.* Elderly persons are prone to dysrhythmia as a result of a loss of elasticity of the heart and major arteries. Widespread use of beta blockers, calcium channel blockers, and diuretics further complicates this problem. Often after injury, elderly patients present with low cardiac output with hypoxia and have no lung injury. Cardiac stroke volume and rate decrease, as does cardiac reserve, all leading to morbidity and mortality in the elderly trauma patient. An elderly patient with a systolic blood pressure of 120 mm Hg or lower should be considered to be in hypovolemic shock until proved otherwise.

Environmental Factors

The environment in which the patient is found can tell you a lot about the patient's well-being.

- *Look for behavioral problems or manifestations that do not fit the scene.* Look at the patient's physical appearance and grooming. Are the patient's attire and grooming appropriate for where and how the patient was found? Is the patient able to care for him- or herself? Is the living environment clean and well-kept? Is there the potential for elder abuse or neglect?

Detailed History

Medications

Knowledge of a patient's medications can provide key information in determining prehospital care. Pre-existing disease in the elderly trauma patient is a significant finding. The following classes of drugs are of particular interest because of their frequent use by elderly persons and their potential to affect the assessment and care of the trauma patient:

- Beta blockers (e.g., propranolol, metoprolol) may account for a patient's absolute or relative bradycardia. In this situation, an increasing tachycardia as a sign of developing shock may not occur. The drug's inhibition of the body's normal sympathetic compensatory mechanisms can mask the true level of the patient's circulatory deterioration. Such patients can rapidly decompensate, seemingly without warning.
- Calcium channel blockers (e.g., verapamil) may prevent peripheral vasoconstriction and accelerate hypovolemic shock.
- Nonsteroidal anti-inflammatory agents (e.g., ibuprofen) may contribute to platelet dysfunction and increase bleeding.
- Anticoagulants (e.g., clopidogrel, aspirin, warfarin) may increase blood loss. Data suggest that use of warfarin increases the risk of isolated head injury and adverse outcome. Any bleeding from trauma will be more brisk and difficult to control when a patient is taking an anticoagulant. More importantly, internal bleeding can progress rapidly, leading to shock and death.
- Hypoglycemic agents (e.g., insulin, metformin, rosiglitazone) may be causally related to the events that caused

injury, affect mentation, and may make blood glucose therapy difficult if their use is unrecognized.

- Over-the-counter medications, including herbal preparations and supplements, are frequently used by elderly persons. Their inclusion in the list of medications is often omitted by patients, who should be specifically questioned about their use. These preparations are unregulated and, thus, have unpredictable dose effects and possible drug interactions. Complications of these agents include bleeding (garlic) and myocardial infarction (ephedrine/ma huang).

Assessing the elderly trauma patient's medication list can prove challenging if, for example, the patient has lost consciousness or is struggling to recount an extensive list of medications with difficult names. In some communities, emergency medical services (EMS) agencies have promoted programs such as the File of Life Project (www.folife.org). In this program, the patient's detailed medical history is placed in a common location in any house: the refrigerator door. The patient completes a medical history form that is then placed into a magnetic holder that is applied to the refrigerator, alerting prehospital care providers to the File of Life (**Figure 17-8**).

Because geriatric patients are often taking numerous medications, the possibility of drug interactions or inadvertent overdose must be considered as a possible cause of the patient's trauma, altered mental status, or changes in vital signs.

Medical Conditions

Numerous medical conditions may predispose individuals to traumatic events, especially those that result in an alteration in the level of consciousness or other neurologic deficit. Common examples include seizure disorders, insulin shock from diabetes mellitus, syncopal episodes from antihypertensive medication, cardiac dysrhythmia from an acute coronary syndrome, and cerebrovascular accidents. Because the incidence of chronic medical conditions increases with age, geriatric patients are more prone to suffering trauma as the result of such a medical problem than are younger victims. The astute prehospital care provider always keeps this concept in mind during the assessment and notes clues from the primary and secondary assessments that may point to a medical problem that precipitated the injury, such as the following:

- Observations made by bystanders that a victim appeared unconscious prior to a crash
- A Medic Alert bracelet that indicates the patient has an underlying condition such as diabetes
- An irregular heartbeat or cardiac dysrhythmia seen during electrocardiogram monitoring

This key information is passed on to the receiving facility.

A

FILE OF LIFE

KEEP INFORMATION UP TO DATE !!
Review At Least Every Six Months !
MEDICAL DATA REVIEWED AS OF___MO.___YR.

Name: Sex: M F
Address:
Doctor: Phone #:
Doctor: Phone #:

EMERGENCY CONTACTS

Name: Phone #:
Address:
Name: Phone #:
Address:

B

KEEP INFORMATION UP TO DATE !!
Review At Least Every Six Months !
MEDICAL DATA REVIEWED AS OF MO. YR.

Name: Sex: M F
Address:
Doctor: Phone #:
Preferred Hospital:

EMERGENCY CONTACTS

Name: Phone #:
Address:
Name: Phone #:
Address:

MEDICAL DATA

Use pencil for ease in making changes.

Special Conditions/Remarks:

Medication	Dosage	Frequency

Pharmacy: Phone:
Date of Birth:
Blood Type: Religion:
Health Care Proxy on file at:
Living Will on file at:

® FILE OF LIFE **SEE BACK OF CARD FOR ADDITIONAL INFORMATION**

C

Use Pencil for ease in making changes

Recent Surgery: **Date:**

Do you have an EMS-NO CPR Directive or a DNR form ?
YES ☐ **NO** ☐ **Where is it located ?**

MEDICAL CONDITIONS

Check all that exi st

- ☐ No known medical conditions
- ☐ Abnormal EKG
- ☐ Adrenal Insufficiency
- ☐ Angina
- ☐ Asthma
- ☐ Bleeding Disorder
- ☐ Cancer
- ☐ Cardiac Dysrhythmia
- ☐ Cataracts
- ☐ Clotting Disorder
- ☐ Coronary Bypass Graft
- ☐ Dementia ☐ Alzheimer's ☐
- ☐ Diabetes/Insulin Dependent
- ☐ Eye Surgery
- ☐ Glaucoma
- ☐ Hearing Impaired
- ☐ Heart Valve Prosthesis
- ☐ Other:
- ☐ Hemodialysis
- ☐ Hemolytic Anemia
- ☐ Hepatitis-Type [ ]
- ☐ Hypertension
- ☐ Hypoglycemia
- ☐ Laryngectomy
- ☐ Leukemia
- ☐ Lymphomas
- ☐ Memory Impaired
- ☐ Myasthenia Gravis
- ☐ Pacemaker
- ☐ Renal Failure
- ☐ Seizure Disorder
- ☐ Sickle Cell Anemia
- ☐ Stroke
- ☐ Tuberculosis
- ☐ Vision Impaired

ALLERGIES

- ☐ Aspirin
- ☐ Barbiturate
- ☐ Codeine
- ☐ Demerol
- ☐ Horse Serum
- ☐ Environmental:
- ☐ Other:
- ☐ Insect Stings
- ☐ Latex
- ☐ Lidocaine
- ☐ Morphine
- ☐ Novocaine
- ☐ Penicillin
- ☐ Sulfa
- ☐ Tetracycline
- ☐ X-Rays Dyes
- ☐ No Known Allergies

MEDICAL INSURANCE

Med Ins Co:
Policy #:
Other Med Ins Co:
Policy #:
Medicaid #: Medicare #:

Figure 17-8 File of Life.

Source: Courtesy of the File of Life Foundation.

Management

Airway

The presence of dentures, common in the elderly population, may affect airway management. Ordinarily, dentures should be left in place to maintain a better seal around the mouth with a mask. However, partial dentures (plates) may become dislodged during an emergency and may completely or partially block the airway; these should be removed.

Fragile nasopharyngeal mucosal tissues and the possible use of anticoagulants put the elderly trauma patient at increased risk of bleeding from placement of a nasopharyngeal airway. This hemorrhage may further compromise the patient's airway and result in aspiration.

Arthritis may affect the temporomandibular joints and cervical spine. The decreased flexibility of these areas may make endotracheal intubation more difficult.

The objective of airway management is primarily to ensure a patent airway for the delivery of adequate tissue oxygenation. Early mechanical ventilation by either bag-mask device or advanced airway interventions should be considered in elderly trauma patients because of their greatly limited physiologic reserve.[19]

Breathing

In all trauma patients, supplemental oxygen should be administered as soon as possible. Oxygen saturation should generally be kept at greater than 95%. The elderly population has a high prevalence of COPD. Even if a patient has severe COPD, it is unlikely that high-flow oxygen administration will be detrimental to the respiratory drive during routine urban or suburban transports. However, if the prehospital care provider notes *somnolence* (a state of drowsiness) or a slowing of ventilatory rate, ventilations can be assisted with a bag-mask device with consideration for advanced airway management.

Elderly persons experience increased stiffness of the chest wall. In addition, reduced chest-wall muscle power and stiffening of the cartilage make the chest cage less flexible. These and other changes are responsible for reductions in lung volumes. The elderly patient may need ventilatory support by assisted ventilations with a bag-mask device earlier than younger trauma patients. The mechanical force applied to the resuscitation bag may need to be increased to overcome the increased chest wall resistance.

Circulation

Elderly persons may have poor cardiovascular reserve. Vital signs are a poor indicator of shock in the elderly patient because the patient who is normally hypertensive may be in shock with a blood pressure that is considered "normal" for a younger patient. Reduced circulating blood volume, possible chronic anemia, and pre-existing myocardial and coronary disease leave the patient with very little tolerance for even modest amounts of blood loss.

Because of the laxity of skin or use of anticoagulant agents, geriatric patients are prone to the development of larger hematomas and potentially more significant internal hemorrhage. Early control of hemorrhage through direct pressure on open wounds, stabilization or immobilization of fractures, and rapid transport to a trauma center are essential. Fluid resuscitation should be guided by the index of suspicion for serious bleeding based on the mechanism of injury and an overall appearance of shock. At the same time, over-administration of IV fluids is to be avoided, as the elderly patient often poorly tolerates an excessive fluid load. The kidney's ability to concentrate urine is decreased, leading to dehydration even before an injury occurs. Urine output is a poor measure of perfusion in elderly persons.

Immobilization

Protection of the cervical spine, particularly in trauma patients who have sustained multisystem blunt injury, is an expected standard of care. In the elderly population, this standard of care must apply not only in trauma situations but also during acute medical problems in which attempts to maintain airway patency are a priority. Degenerative arthritis of the cervical spine may subject the elderly patient to spinal cord injury from positioning and manipulating the neck to manage the airway, even if the patient has no injury to the bony spine. Another consideration with improper movement of the cervical spine is the possibility of occlusion of the arteries to the brain, which can result in unconsciousness and even stroke.

A cervical collar applied to an elderly patient with severe kyphosis should not compress the airway or carotid arteries. Less traditional means of immobilization, such as a rolled towel and head block, can be considered if standard collars are inappropriate.

Padding may need to be placed under the patient's head and between the shoulders when immobilizing the kyphotic supine elderly patient (**Figure 17-9**). In those systems that have access to vacuum mattresses, the vacuum mattress can mold to the patient's anatomy and provide appropriate support and greater comfort. Because of the thin skin and lack of *adipose tissue* (fat) in the frail, elderly patient, geriatric patients are more likely to develop pressure (*decubitus*) ulcers from lying on their back; therefore, additional padding will be required when the patient is immobilized to a long backboard. It is always a good idea to check for pressure points when the patient is resting on the board and pad appropriately. When applying the straps to secure the patient, the elderly patient may not be able to straighten his or her legs fully because of decreased range of motion of the hips and knees. This may require the placement of padding under the legs for comfort and security of the patient during transport.[20]

Temperature Control

The elderly patient should be monitored closely for hypothermia and hyperthermia during treatment and transport. Although it is appropriate to expose the patient to facilitate a thorough

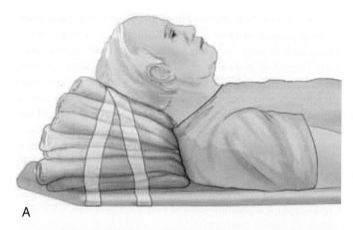

A

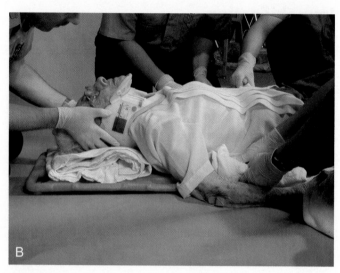

B

Figure 17-9 Immobilization of a kyphotic patient. (Note: Other straps and the cervical collar are not shown for clarity of illustration purposes.)

Source: B. © Jones & Bartlett Learning.

examination, elderly persons are especially prone to heat loss. Once the physical examination is complete, the patient should be covered with a blanket or other available covering to preserve body heat.

The effects of various medications such as those used to treat Parkinson's disease, depression, psychosis, and nausea and vomiting may mean that a patient is more prone to overheating; therefore, some means of cooling the patient should be considered if the patient is unable to be moved quickly to a controlled environment. (See the chapter titled Environmental Trauma I: Heat and Cold for a detailed discussion of management of hyperthermia.)

Prolonged extrication in the extremes of heat and cold may place the elderly patient at risk and should be rapidly addressed. External methods of heating or cooling the elderly trauma patient should be balanced by the possibility of direct thermal injury to the site of application with the patient's attenuated skin structure. Therefore, a sheet or some of the patient's clothing should be placed between the heat or cooling source and the patient's skin.

Legal Considerations

Several legal considerations can become issues when providing care to the elderly trauma patient. Recent evidence demonstrates that although mortality increases with age, 80% of discharged geriatric trauma patients return to a high functional level. Under certain circumstances, the patient or family member may choose to forego potentially lifesaving interventions and provide comfort measures only (e.g., elderly patient with extensive burns). The most appropriate care plan for the patient can be determined by identifying a living will, advance directives, or other legal documents, if available to the prehospital care providers at the scene.

In most of the United States, spouses, siblings, children, spouses of children, and parents have no legal standing in making medical decisions for an adult. Persons with power of attorney or court-appointed conservators may have authority over an individual's financial affairs, but they do not necessarily have control over that individual's personal medical decisions. Court-appointed custodians or guardians may or may not have the power to make medical decisions, depending on the local laws and the specific charge of their appointment. Such powers are considered to exist only when a guardianship of person or a durable power of attorney for health care is specified and clear documentation of such third-party powers is present.

In the midst of a trauma scene, it may be difficult to make such a fine legal distinction. Because the ambulance was summoned and a "call for help" was made, the concept of "implied consent" to care for the patient applies in cases of patients who are unconscious or have reduced mental capacity. If relatives object to the actions of the prehospital providers or attempt to interfere with care of the patient, law enforcement should be summoned to the scene to assist in dealing with the relatives. In addition, the prehospital providers can contact their medical direction and have their online supervising physician speak directly with the relatives.

Reporting Elder Abuse

In many states, health care workers, including prehospital care providers, are required by law to report cases of suspected elder maltreatment to authorities. Should further clarification be necessary or should anyone attempt to interfere with the prehospital care, law enforcement should be called to the scene (if not already present) and the problem presented to the police officer in charge. The law generally provides a protocol for a law enforcement officer to make a timely decision at the scene, with clarification to occur later at the hospital when time allows. Such events should be documented carefully and completely as a part of the run report.

Elder Maltreatment

Elder abuse is defined as any action by an elderly person's family member (any relative), associated persons who have daily household contact (housekeeper, roommate), anyone the elderly person relies on for daily needs of food, clothing, and shelter, or a professional caregiver who takes advantage of the elderly person's property or emotional state.

Reports and complaints of abuse, neglect, sexual assault, and other related problems among the elderly population are increasing. The exact extent of elder abuse is not known for the following reasons:

1. Elder abuse has been largely hidden from society.
2. Abuse and neglect of elderly persons have varying definitions.
3. Elders are uneasy or fearful of reporting the problem to law enforcement agencies or human and social welfare personnel. A typical victim of elder abuse may be a parent who feels ashamed or guilty because he or she raised the abuser. The abused may also feel traumatized by the situation or fear continued reprisal by the abuser.
4. Some jurisdictions lack formal reporting mechanisms. Some areas do not even have a statutory provision requiring the reporting of elder abuse.

The physical and emotional signs of abuse, such as rape, beating, or nutritional deprivation, are often overlooked or perhaps are not accurately identified. Older women in particular are not likely to report incidents of sexual assault to law enforcement agencies. Sensory deficits, senility, and other forms of altered mental status (e.g., drug-induced depression) may make it impossible or extremely difficult for the elderly patient to report the maltreatment.

Profile of the Abused

The elderly adult most likely to be abused fits into the following profile:

- Over 65 years of age, especially women over 75 years of age
- Frail
- Multiple chronic medical conditions
- Demented
- Impaired sleep cycle, sleepwalking, or loud shouting at night
- Incontinent of feces, urine, or both
- Dependent on others for activities of daily living or incapable of independent living

Profile of the Abuser

Because many elderly people live in a family environment and are typically women older than 75 years of age, that environment may provide clues. The abuser is frequently the spouse of the patient or the middle-aged child or in-law of the patient who is caring for dependent children and dependent parents while perhaps holding full-time or part-time employment. Most of these abusers are untrained in the particular care required

by the elderly and have little relief time from the constant care demands of their family.

Abuse is not restricted to the home. Other environments such as nursing, convalescent, and continuing care centers are sites where the elderly may sustain physical, chemical, or pharmacologic harm. Care providers in these environments may consider elderly persons to represent management problems or categorize them as obstinate or undesirable patients.

The usual profile of the abuser includes the following signs:

- Existence of household conflict
- Marked fatigue
- Unemployment
- Financial difficulties
- Substance abuse
- Previous history of abuse

Categories of Maltreatment

Abuse can be categorized in the following ways:

1. *Physical abuse* includes assault, neglect, malnutrition, poor maintenance of the living environment, and poor personal care. The signs of physical abuse or neglect may be obvious, such as the imprint left by an item (e.g., fireplace poker) or may be subtle (e.g., malnutrition). The signs of elder abuse are similar to those of child abuse (**Figure 17-10**) (see the Pediatric Trauma chapter).
2. *Psychological abuse* can take the forms of neglect, verbal abuse, infantilization, or deprivation of sensory stimulation.

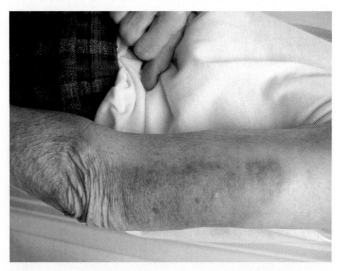

Figure 17-10 Bruises in varying stages of healing are highly suggestive of physical abuse. For example, if a 70-year-old man were brought from his caregiver's home to the emergency department with bruises such as the ones depicted here, providers would need to consider the possibility of abuse.
Source: © Libby Welch/Photofusion/Getty Images.

3. *Financial abuse* can include theft of valuables or embezzlement.
4. *Sexual assault and/or abuse.*
5. *Self-abuse.*

Important Points

Many abused patients are terrorized into making false statements for fear of retribution. In the case of elder abuse by family members, fear of removal from the home environment can cause the elderly patient to lie about the origin of the abuse. In other cases of elder abuse, sensory deprivation or dementia may deter adequate explanation. The prehospital care provider should identify abuse and uncover any pathology reported by the patient. Any history of maltreatment or findings consistent with it should be documented on the patient care report.

Further trauma to a patient may be reduced by identifying an abusive situation. Reporting a high index of suspicion for abuse can allow for referral to and protective services from human, social, and public safety agencies (**Figure 17-11**).

Disposition

One of the greatest challenges with prehospital care of the injured patient is defining which patients are most likely to benefit from the surgeons and advanced treatment options available at a trauma center. For many of the reasons mentioned previously, triage criteria may be less reliable in the elderly patient because of physiologic or pharmacologic effects. A major recommendation in the *Guidelines for Geriatric Trauma* of the Eastern Association for the Surgery of Trauma is that prehospital care providers treating trauma patients of advanced age should have a lower threshold to triage these victims directly to a trauma center.[21] The Centers for Disease Control and Prevention's Guidelines for Field Triage of Injured Patients recommends that patients over the age of 55 years be transported to a trauma center.[22] Furthermore, potentially preventable mortality in the geriatric trauma population is lower at trauma centers.

Prolonged Transport

The majority of care of the elderly trauma patient follows the general guidelines for prehospital care of the injured patient. However, several special circumstances exist in prolonged transport scenarios. For example, geriatric patients with less significant anatomic injuries should be triaged directly to trauma centers.

Treatment of shock in the prehospital environment over an extended period requires careful reassessment of vital signs during transport. After control of hemorrhage with local measures, fluid resuscitation should be titrated to physiologic response to optimize resuscitation of intravascular volume status while avoiding potential volume overload in a patient with impaired cardiac function.

Figure 17-11 Reporting Elder Abuse and Neglect

In many states, EMS personnel are legally considered to be mandated reporters of suspected elder (or adult) abuse, neglect, and exploitation. Abuse is considered the deliberate infliction of pain, injury, mental anguish, unreasonable confinement, or nonconsensual sexual contact. Neglect involves living in conditions in which the adult or responsible caretaker is not providing care required to maintain the elderly person's physical and mental health and well-being. Exploitation is the illegal use of an adult's resources for another's gain or advantage. In recent years, elder abuse has been increasingly recognized. However, younger adults who have incapacitating conditions such as mental illness, mental retardation, and physical disability are also at risk for abuse and neglect.

Signs of abuse and neglect include unexplained or unusual injuries; conflicting accounts of how an injury occurred; a caregiver who prevents the adult from speaking with others; dehydration or malnutrition; depression; lack of access to medications, eyeglasses, dentures, or other aids; lack of personal hygiene; unkempt environment; and lack of adequate heating and cooling.

Mandated reporters must report directly to the social services agency responsible for investigating adult abuse, rather than relying on intermediaries such as hospital personnel. If the individual is in immediate danger or has been sexually assaulted, law enforcement must be notified as well. In the event that a death appears to have been caused by abuse or neglect, mandatory reporters generally must notify the office of the medical examiner or coroner and law enforcement.

Mandatory reporters are liable for failing to report suspected abuse, neglect, and exploitation. However, they are protected against civil and criminal liability associated with reporting, they may be able to keep their identity confidential, and they are allowed to share medical information that is related to the case, although this information would be protected under the Health Insurance Portability and Accountability Act (HIPAA) in normal circumstances. Laws governing the mandatory reporting of elder abuse are enacted at the state level. All prehospital care providers must be aware of the laws in the state in which they work.

Immobilization on a long backboard places the geriatric patient at increased risk for pressure-related skin breakdown over extended transports. Weakened skin structure and impaired vascular supply may lead to earlier complications than expected in younger trauma patients. Prior to a long transport, consideration should be given to clearing the spine or logrolling a patient onto an appropriately padded long backboard to protect the patient's skin. Agencies in remote regions should consider purchasing a specially designed, low-pressure backboard that immobilizes the patient while limiting the potential for skin breakdown.

Environmental control is essential in geriatric patients with a lengthy transport. Limiting body exposure and controlling the ambient temperature of the vehicle may limit hypothermia. The hypothermic patient may shiver, producing anaerobic metabolism, leading to lactic acidosis, and accelerating shock.

Finally, transport of the geriatric trauma patient from remote regions may be a valid use of aeromedical transport. Transport via helicopter may limit the duration of environmental exposure, reduce the duration of shock, and ensure earlier access to trauma center care, including early surgery and blood transfusion.

Summary

- Elderly persons are living healthier, more active, and longer lives than ever before.
- Although general guidelines for care of the injured patient remain the same, several specific approaches are unique to care of the injured geriatric patient.
- Anatomic and physiologic changes associated with aging, chronic disease, and medications can make certain types of trauma more likely, complicate traumatic injuries, and cause a decreased ability to compensate for shock. Older patients have less physiologic reserve and tolerate physical insult poorly.
- Knowledge of the elderly trauma patient's medical history and medications is an essential component of care.
- Many factors in elderly trauma patients can mask early signs of deterioration, increasing the possibility of sudden, rapid decompensation without apparent warning.
- With an elderly trauma patient, more serious injury may have occurred than indicated by the initial presentation.
- A lower threshold for direct triage of these patients to trauma centers is important.

SCENARIO RECAP

Your unit is dispatched to the home of a 78-year-old woman who has fallen down a flight of stairs. Her daughter states that they had spoken on the telephone just 15 minutes earlier and that she was coming to her mother's house to do some shopping. When she got to the house, she found her mother on the floor and called for an ambulance.

Upon initial contact, you find the patient lying at the bottom of a flight of stairs. You note that the patient is an elderly woman whose appearance matches her reported age. While maintaining in-line stabilization of the spine, you note that the patient is unresponsive to your commands. She has a visible laceration of the forehead and an obvious deformity of the left wrist. She is wearing a Medic Alert bracelet that indicates that she is diabetic.

- Did the fall cause the change in mental status, or was there an antecedent event?
- How do the patient's age, medical history, and medications interact with the injuries received to make the pathophysiology and manifestations different from those in younger patients?
- Should advanced age alone be used as an additional criterion for transport to a trauma center?

SCENARIO SOLUTION

When dealing with trauma in the elderly patient, you cannot always determine immediately whether the trauma was the primary event or whether it was secondary to a medical event, such as a stroke, myocardial infarction, or syncopal episode. However, you always need to consider the possibility that a significant medical event preceded the trauma. Your primary assessment reveals that the patient is maintaining a patent airway and is breathing at 16 times per minute. There is no major external hemorrhage and the bleeding from the forehead laceration is easily controlled with pressure.

The patient's heart rate is 84 beats/minute and blood pressure is 154/82 mm Hg. You manually control the head and spine and immobilize the patient to a longboard with appropriate padding underneath. Because the patient is a known diabetic, you check her blood sugar to see if there is a correctable cause for her altered mentation. Given her age, the apparent head trauma, and the magnitude of the fall, you transport her emergently to the closest trauma center.

References

1. U.S. Census Bureau. State and county quickfacts. http://quickfacts.census.gov/qfd/states/00000.html. Accessed February 24, 2013.
2. Scommegna P. United States growing bigger, older, and more diverse. Population Reference Bureau. http://www.prb.org/Publications/Articles/2004/USGrowingBiggerOlderandMoreDiverse.aspx. Accessed December 26, 2013.
3. United Nations, Department of Economic and Social Affairs, Population Division. World population prospects: the 2012 revision. http://esa.un.org/unpd/wpp/Excel-Data/population.htm. Accessed September 3, 2013.
4. Champion H, Copes WS, Sacco WJ, et al. The Major Trauma Outcome Study: establishing national norms for trauma care. *J Trauma*. 1990;30(11):1356.
5. National Center for Injury Prevention and Control, Centers for Disease Control and Prevention, Web-Based Injury Statistics Query and Reporting System (WISQARS). Ten leading causes of death by age group, United States - 2010, http://www.cdc.gov/injury/wisqars/pdf/10LCID_All_Deaths_By_Age_Group_2010-a.pdf. Accessed January 5, 2014.
6. American College of Surgeons (ACS) Committee on Trauma. *Advanced Trauma Life Support for Doctors, Student Course Manual*. 9th ed. Chicago, IL: ACS; 2012:272–284.
7. Jacobs D. Special considerations in geriatric injury. *Curr Opin Crit Care*. 2003;9(6):535.
8. Cohen RA, Bloom B, Simpson G, Parsons PE. Access to health care. Part 3: Older adults. *Vital Health Stat 10*. 1997;(198):1–32.
9. Milzman DP, Boulanger BR, Rodriguez A, et al. Pre-existing disease in trauma patients: a predictor of fate independent of age and injury severity score. *J Trauma*. 1992;32:236.
10. Smith T. Respiratory system: aging, adversity, and anesthesia. In: McCleskey CH, ed. *Geriatric Anesthesiology*. Baltimore, MD: Williams & Wilkins; 1997.
11. Deiner S, Silverstein JH, Abrams K. Management of trauma in the geriatric patient. *Curr Opin Anaesthesiol*. 2004;17(2):165.
12. Carey J. Brain facts: a primer on the brain and nervous system. Washington, DC: Society for Neuroscience; 2002.
13. U.S. Department of Health and Human Services, National Institutes of Health, National Eye Institute. Facts about cataracts. http://www.nei.nih.gov/health/cataract/cataract_facts.asp. Accessed January 5, 2014.
14. EPOS Group. Incidence of vertebral fracture in Europe: Results from the European Prospective Osteoporosis Study (EPOS). *J Bone Miner Res*. 2002;17:716–24
15. Blackmore C. Cervical spine injury in patients 65 years old and older: epidemiologic analysis regarding the effects of age and injury mechanism on distribution, type, and stability of injuries. *Am J Roentgenol*. 2002;178:573.
16. Tinetti M. Preventing falls in elderly persons. *N Engl J Med*. 2003;348:42.
17. Centers for Disease Control and Prevention,. Older adult drivers: Get the facts. 2013 http://www.cdc.gov/motorvehiclesafety/older_adult_drivers/adult-drivers_factsheet.html. Accessed January 5, 2014
18. U.S. Department of Health and Human Services, U.S. Administration on Aging, National Center on Elder Abuse, Elder Abuse: The Size of the Problem. http://www.ncea.aoa.gov/Library/Data/index.aspx. Accessed January 5, 2014
19. Heffner J, Reynolds S. Airway management of the critically ill patient. *Chest*. 2005;127:1397.
20. American Geriatric Society. *Geriatric Education for Emergency Medical Services (GEMS)*. Sudbury, MA: Jones & Bartlett Publishers; 2003.
21. Eastern Association for the Surgery of Trauma. Geriatric trauma, triage of. http://www.east.org/tpg/geriatric.pdf. Published 2001. Accessed December 26, 2013.
22. Sasser SM, Hunt RC, Faul M. Guidelines for field triage of injured patients: recommendations of the National Expert Panel on Field Triage 2011. *MMWR*. 2012;61(1):1–20.

Suggested Reading

American College of Surgeons (ACS) Committee on Trauma. Extremes of age: Geriatric trauma. In: ACS Committee on Trauma. *Advanced Trauma Life Support for Doctors, Student Course Manual*. 9th ed. Chicago, IL: ACS; 2012:272–284.

Callaway D, Wolfe R. Geriatric trauma. *Emer Med Clin North Am*. 2007;25(3):837–860.

Lavoie A, Ratte S, Clas D, et al. Pre-injury warfarin use among elderly patients with closed head injuries in a trauma center. *J Trauma*. 2004;56:802.

Tepas JJ III, Veldenz HC, Lottenberg L, et al. Elderly trauma: a profile of trauma experience in the sunshine (retirement) state. *J Trauma*. 2000;48:581.

Victorino GP, Chong TJ, Pal JD. Trauma in the elderly patient. *Arch Surg*. 2003;138:1093–1097.

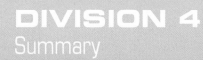
CHAPTER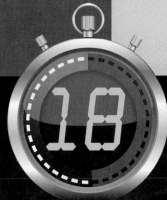

Golden Principles of Prehospital Trauma Care

CHAPTER OBJECTIVES

At the completion of this chapter, the reader will be able to do the following:

- Relate the importance of the "Golden Period."

- Discuss why trauma patients die.

- Discuss the 15 "Golden Principles" of prehospital trauma care.

Introduction

In the late 1960s, R Adams Cowley, MD, conceived the idea of a crucial time period during which it is important to begin definitive patient care for a critically injured trauma patient. In an interview he said:

> There is a "golden hour" between life and death. If you are critically injured, you have less than 60 minutes to survive. You might not die right then—it may be three days or two weeks later—but something has happened in your body that is irreparable.[1]

Is there a basis for this concept? The answer is definitely yes. However, it is important to realize that a patient does not always have the luxury of a "Golden Hour." A patient with a penetrating wound to the heart may have only a few minutes to reach definitive care before the shock caused by the injury becomes irreversible. At the other end of the spectrum is a patient with slow, ongoing internal hemorrhage from an isolated femur fracture. Such a patient may have several hours or longer to reach definitive care and resuscitation.

Because the Golden *Hour* is not a strict 60-minute time frame and varies from patient to patient based on the injuries, the more appropriate term is Golden *Period*. If a critically injured patient is able to obtain definitive care—that is, hemorrhage control and resuscitation—within that particular patient's Golden Period, the chance of survival is improved greatly.[2] The American College of Surgeons (ACS) Committee on Trauma has used this concept of a Golden Period to emphasize the importance of transporting a patient to a facility where expert trauma care is immediately available.

No call, scene, or patient is the same. Each requires flexibility of the health care providers to act and react to situations as they develop. The management of prehospital trauma must reflect these contingencies. The goals, however, do not change:

1. Gain access to the patient.
2. Identify and treat life-threatening injuries.
3. Package and transport the patient to the closest appropriate facility in the least amount of time.

The majority of the techniques and principles discussed are not new, and most are taught in initial training programs. Prehospital Trauma Life Support (PHTLS) is different in the following ways:

1. It provides current, evidence-based management practices for the trauma patient.
2. It provides a systematic approach for establishing priorities of patient care for trauma patients who have sustained injury to multiple body systems.
3. It provides an organizational scheme for interventions.

The PHTLS program teaches that the prehospital care provider can make correct judgments leading toward a good outcome only if the prehospital care provider is supplied with a good base of knowledge. The foundation of the PHTLS program is that patient care should be *judgment* driven, not *protocol* driven—hence the medical detail provided in this course. This chapter addresses the key aspects of prehospital trauma care and "brings it all together."

Why Trauma Patients Die

Studies that analyze the causes of death in trauma patients reveal several common themes. A study from Russia of more than 700 trauma deaths found that most patients who rapidly succumbed to their injuries fall into one of three categories: massive acute blood loss (36%), severe injury to vital organs such as the brain (30%), and airway obstruction and acute ventilatory failure (25%).[3] A study published in 2010 documented that 76% of patients who died rapidly did so from nonsurvivable injuries to the head, aorta, and heart.[4] In an analysis of 753 trauma patients who died of their injuries at a level I trauma center, Dr. Ronald Stewart and coworkers found that 51% of trauma patients died from severe trauma to the central nervous system (CNS) (e.g., traumatic brain injury), 21% from irreversible shock, 25% from both severe CNS trauma and irreversible shock, and 3% from multiple organ failure.[5]

But what is happening to these patients on a cellular level? As discussed in the Physiology of Life and Death chapter, the metabolic processes of the human body are driven by energy, similar to any other machine. Shock is viewed as a failure of energy production in the body. As with machines, the human body generates its own energy but must have fuel to do so. Fuel for the body is oxygen and glucose. The body can store glucose as complex carbohydrates (glycogen) and fat to use at a later time. However, oxygen cannot be stored. It must be constantly supplied to the cells of the body. Atmospheric air, containing oxygen, is drawn into the lungs by the action of the diaphragm and intercostal muscles. Oxygen diffuses across the alveolar and capillary walls, where it binds to the hemoglobin in the red blood cells (RBCs) and is then transported to the body's tissues by the circulatory system. In the presence of oxygen, the cells of the tissues then "burn" glucose through a complex series of metabolic processes (glycolysis, Krebs cycle, and electron transport) to produce the energy needed for all body functions. This energy is stored as adenosine triphosphate (ATP). Without sufficient energy (ATP), essential metabolic activities cannot function normally, and cells begin to die and organs to fail.

The sensitivity of the cells to oxygen deprivation varies from organ to organ (**Figure 18-1**). The cells within an organ can be fatally damaged but can continue to function for a period of time (see the Physiology of Life and Death and the Shock chapters for complications of prolonged shock). This delayed death of cells, leading to organ failure, is what Dr. Cowley was referring to in

Figure 18-1   Shock

When the heart is deprived of oxygen, the myocardial cells cannot produce enough energy to pump blood to the other tissues. For example, a patient has lost a significant number of red blood cells and blood volume following a gunshot wound to the aorta. The heart continues to beat for several minutes before failing. Refilling the vascular system after the heart has been without oxygen for several minutes will not restore the function of the injured cells of the heart. This process is called irreversible shock.

Although ischemia, as seen in severe shock, may damage virtually all tissues, the damage to the organs does not become apparent at the same time. In the lungs, acute respiratory distress syndrome often develops within 48 hours of an ischemic insult, whereas acute renal failure and hepatic failure typically occur several days later. Although all body tissues are affected by insufficient oxygen, some tissues are more sensitive to ischemia. For example, a patient who has sustained a traumatic brain injury may develop cerebral edema (swelling) that results in permanent brain damage. Although the higher level brain cells cease to function and die, the rest of the body survives and may live for years.

---

his earlier quote. Shock results in death if a patient is not treated promptly, which is why Dr. Cowley advocated the rapid transport of the patient to the operating room for control of internal hemorrhage.

The Golden Period represents a time interval during which the cascade of events in shock is worsening and long-term survival and outcome are jeopardized, but this condition is almost always *reversible* if proper care is received rapidly. Failure to initiate appropriate interventions aimed at improving oxygenation and controlling hemorrhage allows shock to progress, becoming *irreversible*. For trauma patients to have the best chance of survival, interventions should start with a solid emergency communications system that is easy for citizens to access. Trained dispatchers can begin the process of providing care in the field by offering pre-arrival instructions such as hemorrhage control. Care in the field continues with the arrival of prehospital care providers and proceeds to the emergency department (ED), the operating room (OR), and the intensive care unit (ICU). Trauma is a "team sport." The patient "wins" when all members of the trauma team—from those in the field to those in the trauma center—work together to care for the individual patient.

The Golden Principles of Prehospital Trauma Care

The preceding chapters discussed the assessment and management of patients who have sustained injury to specific body systems. Although this text presents the body systems individually, most severely injured patients have injury to more than one body system—hence the term multisystem trauma patient (also known as *polytrauma*). A prehospital care provider needs to recognize and prioritize the treatment of patients with multiple injuries, following the "Golden Principles of Prehospital Trauma Care."

1. Ensure the Safety of the Prehospital Care Providers and the Patient

Scene safety remains the highest priority on arrival to all calls for medical assistance. Prehospital providers must develop and practice situational awareness of all scene types (**Figure 18-2**). This awareness includes not only the safety of the patient but also the safety of all emergency responders. Based on information provided by dispatch, potential threats can often be anticipated before arrival at the scene. For a motor vehicle crash, threatening situations may include traffic, hazardous materials, fires, fuel spills, and downed power lines. In an incident involving a victim with a gunshot wound, the perpetrator may still be in the area.

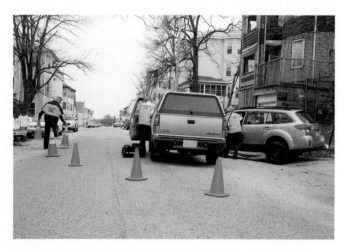

Figure 18-2 Ensure the safety of the prehospital care providers and the patient.
Source: © Jones & Bartlett Learning. Photographed by Darren Stahlman.

When a violent crime is involved, law enforcement personnel must partner with EMS to enter the scene in order to secure the area and expedite care of injured patients. A prehospital care provider who takes needless risk may also become a victim. By becoming a victim, the prehospital care provider is no longer of help to the original trauma patient and instead adds to the scene management difficulties. The same concerns also apply to natural disasters, such as earthquakes and tornadoes, and disasters caused by humans, such as explosions or mass shootings. Only those with proper training should attempt to enter these scenes to perform rescue activities.

Another fundamental aspect of safety involves the use of standard precautions. Blood and other body fluids can transmit infections, such as human immunodeficiency virus (HIV) and hepatitis B virus (HBV). Protective gear, such as gloves, should always be worn, especially when caring for trauma patients in the presence of blood and body fluids.

The safety of the patient and possible hazardous situations should also be identified. Even if a patient involved in a motor vehicle crash has no life-threatening conditions identified in the primary assessment, rapid extrication is appropriate if threatening conditions to the patient's safety are noted, such as a significant potential for fire or a precarious vehicle position.

2. Assess the Scene Situation to Determine the Need for Additional Resources

During the response to the scene and immediately upon arrival, a quick assessment is performed to determine the need for additional or specialized resources. Examples include additional emergency medical services (EMS) units to accommodate the number of patients, fire suppression equipment, special rescue teams, power company personnel, medical helicopters, and physicians to aid in the triage of a large number of patients. The need for these resources should be anticipated and requested as soon as possible, and a designated communications channel should be secured.

3. Recognize the Kinematics That Produced the Injuries

The Kinematics of Trauma chapter provides the reader with a foundation of how kinetic energy can translate into injury to the trauma patient. As the scene and the patient are approached, the kinematics of the situation are noted (**Figure 18-3**). Understanding the principles of kinematics leads to better patient assessment. Knowledge of specific injury patterns aids in predicting injuries and knowing where to examine. Consideration of the kinematics should not delay the initiation of patient assessment and care but can be included in the global scene assessment and in the questions directed to the patient and bystanders.

The kinematics may also play a key role in determining the destination facility for a given trauma patient. The Centers for Disease Control and Prevention have described the mechanism of injury criteria for triage to trauma centers (**Figure 18-4**).

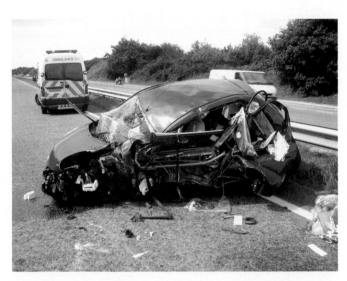

Figure 18-3 Recognize the kinematics that produced the injuries.
Source: Courtesy of Mark Woolcock.

Figure 18-4 Mechanism of Injury Criteria for Triage to Trauma Centers

- Falls
  - Adults: Greater than 20 feet (6.1 meters [m]) (one story is equal to 10 feet)
  - Children: Greater than 10 feet (3 m), or two or three times the child's height
- High-risk auto crash
  - Intrusion, including roof: Greater than 12 inches (0.3 m) occupant site; greater than 18 inches (0.5 m) any site

- Ejection (partial or complete) from automobile
- Death in same passenger compartment
- Vehicle telemetry data consistent with a high risk of injury
- Vehicle versus pedestrian or bicyclist who is thrown, run over, or significantly impacted (at greater than 20 miles per hour [mph])
- Motorcycle crash at greater than 20 mph

Source: Adapted from the Field Triage Decision Scheme: The National Trauma Triage Protocol, US Department of Health and Human Services, Centers for Disease Control and Prevention.

The key aspects of the kinematics noted at the scene should also be documented and described to the staff at the receiving trauma facility.

4. Use the Primary Assessment to Identify Life-Threatening Conditions

The central concept in the PHTLS program is the emphasis on the primary assessment (primary survey) adopted from the Advanced Trauma Life Support (ATLS) Program for Doctors, taught by the ACS Committee on Trauma. This brief survey allows vital functions to be rapidly assessed and life-threatening conditions to be identified through systematic evaluation of the ABCDEs: **a**irway, **b**reathing, **c**irculation, **d**isability, and **e**xpose/**e**nvironment (**Figure 18-5**). On initial approach to the scene and as field care is provided, input is received from several senses (sight, hearing, smell, touch) that must be sorted—placed in a priority scheme of life-threatening or limb-threatening injuries—and used to develop a plan for correct management.

The primary assessment involves a "treat as you go" philosophy. As life-threatening problems are identified, care is initiated at the earliest possible time. Although taught in a stepwise fashion, many aspects of the primary assessment can be performed simultaneously. During transport, the primary assessment should be reassessed at reasonable intervals so that the effectiveness of the interventions can be evaluated and new concerns addressed.

In children, pregnant patients, and elderly persons, injuries should be considered:

1. To be more serious than their outward appearance
2. To have a more profound systemic influence
3. To have a greater potential for producing rapid decompensation

In pregnant patients, there are at least two patients to care for—the woman and the fetus—both of whom may have sustained injury. Addressing the needs of the woman improves the chances of survival for both mother and fetus. Compensatory mechanisms differ in the pregnant female and may not reveal abnormalities until the patient is profoundly compromised (see the Abdominal Trauma chapter, under Trauma in the Obstetrical Patient).

The primary assessment also provides a framework to establish management priorities when faced with numerous patients. At a multiple-casualty incident, for example, patients who have serious problems identified with their airway, ventilation, or perfusion are managed before patients with only altered levels of consciousness. The Disaster Management chapter discusses triage in greater detail.

Figure 18-5 Critical or Potentially Critical Trauma Patient: Scene Time of 10 Minutes or Less

Presence of any of the following life-threatening conditions:

1. Inadequate or threatened airway
2. Impaired ventilation as demonstrated by any of the following:
   - Abnormally fast or slow ventilatory rate
   - Hypoxia (oxygen saturation [SpO_2] less than 95% even with supplemental oxygen)
   - Dyspnea
   - Open pneumothorax or flail chest
   - Suspected pneumothorax
   - Suspected tension pneumothorax
3. Significant external hemorrhage or suspected internal hemorrhage
4. Shock, even if compensated
5. Abnormal neurologic status
   - Glasgow Coma Scale (GCS) score of 13 or less
   - Seizure activity
   - Sensory or motor deficit

6. Penetrating trauma to the head, neck, or torso, or proximal to the elbow and knee in the extremities
7. Amputation or near-amputation proximal to the fingers or toes
8. Any trauma in the presence of the following:
   - History of serious medical conditions (e.g., coronary artery disease, chronic obstructive pulmonary disease, bleeding disorder)
   - Age greater than 55 years
   - Children
   - Hypothermia
   - Burns
   - Pregnancy greater than 20 weeks
   - Prehospital care provider judgment of high-risk condition

5. Provide Appropriate Airway Management While Maintaining Cervical Spine Stabilization as Indicated

Management of the airway remains the highest priority in the treatment of critically injured patients. This should be accomplished while maintaining the head and neck in a neutral in-line position, if indicated by the mechanism of injury. All prehospital care providers must be able to perform the "essential skills" of airway management with ease: manual clearing of the airway, manual maneuvers to open the airway (trauma jaw thrust and trauma chin lift), suctioning, and the use of oropharyngeal and nasopharyngeal airways.

The need for advanced or complex airway management and choice of technique and device for securing the airway depend on the critical-thinking capabilities of the prehospital care provider as well as factors such as the training level and skill of the prehospital care provider, the ease of management, anatomic considerations, and the time needed to reach the receiving facility.

For many years, endotracheal intubation has been the preferred technique for controlling the airway of a critically injured trauma patient in the prehospital setting. This recommendation, although based upon ATLS standards, has become increasingly controversial as more prehospital data on airway management have emerged (see the Airway and Ventilation chapter). As previously discussed, concerns related to prehospital endotracheal intubation include unrecognized malpositioning, insufficient performance of the procedure to maintain proficiency, and conflicting data on outcome of patients who have received endotracheal intubation. One study has shown that prehospital patients with significant injuries who are managed by endotracheal intubation versus those managed by bag-mask ventilation prior to arrival at a trauma center have the same outcome.[6] *In some circumstances, such as given the close proximity of an appropriate receiving facility, the most prudent decision may be to focus on the essential skills of airway management and rapidly transport the patient to that facility.* Bag-mask ventilation must be performed correctly and with the same attention to the details of adequate ventilation as when an endotracheal intubation is performed.

Endotracheal intubation may be considered for patients with the following:

- A Glasgow Coma Scale (GCS) score of 8 or less
- Requirement for high concentrations of oxygen to maintain oxygen saturation (SpO_2) greater than 95%
- Requirement for assisted ventilations because of a decreased ventilatory rate or decreased minute volume
- An expanding hematoma in the neck
- Airway or pulmonary burns
- Altered mental status that affects positioning of the tongue

Although performing endotracheal intubation in the field seems to make sense, there is no conclusive evidence that endotracheal intubation results in lower morbidity or mortality rates in the trauma patient. Several studies performed in San Diego, California, demonstrated that hyperventilation was common after endotracheal intubation and was associated with worse outcome and reduced survival.[7,8] The authors noted that the device itself was not the problem; rather it was the postinsertion maintenance and attention to ventilation details that produced complications.

After an endotracheal tube has been placed, its proper position must be ascertained and confirmed using a combination of clinical assessments and adjunct devices, particularly continuous capnometry (see the Airway and Ventilation chapter). Endotracheal tube placement should always be reconfirmed when there is a sudden change in capnography or oxygen saturation readings, after moving an intubated patient onto or off the gurney at the scene, after moving the patient into or out of the ambulance, after encountering sharp or jolting turns or when transporting on rough roadways, and after transferring the patient onto the gurney in the ED.

There are many devices other than the endotracheal tube that may be used to manage the airway. In addition, when endotracheal intubation is indicated but cannot be performed, these devices provide good alternative options (see the airway management algorithm provided in the Airway and Ventilation chapter). Ventilation can be attempted using the essential skills alone or with such devices as a dual-lumen airway or a laryngeal mask airway. If adequate ventilation can be achieved, additional attempts at intubation using retrograde or digital techniques may be considered. If ventilation cannot be accomplished, cricothyroidotomy is an acceptable option.

6. Support Ventilation and Deliver Oxygen to Maintain an SpO_2 Greater Than 95%

Assessment and management of ventilation is another key aspect in the management of the critically injured patient. The normal ventilatory rate in the adult patient is 12 to 20 ventilations per minute. A rate slower than this often significantly interferes with the body's ability to oxygenate the RBCs passing through the pulmonary capillaries and to remove the carbon dioxide produced by the tissues. These patients with bradypnea require assisted or total ventilatory support with a bag-mask device connected to supplemental oxygen (fraction of inspired oxygen [FiO_2] greater than 0.85).

When patients are tachypneic (adult rate greater than 20 breaths/minute), their minute ventilation (tidal volume multiplied by their ventilatory rate) should be estimated. For a patient with a significant decrease in minute volume (rapid, shallow ventilations), ventilation should be assisted with a bag-mask device connected to supplemental oxygen (FiO_2 greater than 0.85).

If available, end-tidal carbon dioxide monitoring ($ETCO_2$) can prove useful to ensure sufficient ventilatory support. A sudden decrease in the $ETCO_2$ may indicate dislodgment of the endotracheal tube, if placed, or a sudden decrease in perfusion (profound hypotension or cardiopulmonary arrest).

Supplemental oxygen should be administered to any trauma patient with obvious or suspected life-threatening conditions. If available, pulse oximetry can be used to maintain the SpO_2 greater than 95% (at sea level). If concern exists about the accuracy of a pulse oximetry reading or if this technology is not available, oxygen can be administered through a nonrebreathing mask to the spontaneously breathing patient or with a bag-mask device connected to supplemental oxygen (FiO_2 greater than 0.85) for those patients receiving assisted or total ventilatory support.

If providing assisted ventilations, care must be taken to avoid inadvertent hyperventilation. Hyperventilation of the traumatic brain injury patient in the absence of signs of increased intracranial pressure and herniation can compromise cerebral blood flow by causing vasoconstriction and lead to worse outcomes for the patient.

7. Control Any Significant External Hemorrhage

In the trauma patient, significant external hemorrhage is a finding that requires immediate attention. Because blood is not available for administration in the prehospital setting, hemorrhage control becomes a paramount concern for prehospital care providers in order to maintain a sufficient number of circulating RBCs; *every red blood cell counts*. Extremity injuries and scalp wounds, such as lacerations and partial avulsions, may be associated with life-threatening blood loss.

Most external hemorrhage is readily controlled by the application of direct pressure at the bleeding site or, if resources are limited, by the use of a pressure dressing created with gauze 4×4 pads and an elastic bandage. To properly apply pressure, the gauze must be packed tightly into the wound so that the gauze is in direct contact with the bleeding surface, not just lying over the top of it. The goal of properly packing a wound is to put pressure directly on the cut or torn blood vessels; the gauze is not merely a catchment device used to keep the blood from running down the patient. After the gauze has been packed tightly into the wound, pressure must be put on the packing to keep it tightly against the bleeding site. This is accomplished by the application of hand pressure onto the dressing for 5 to 6 minutes or more to ensure that the bleeding has stopped. However, if the patient is on some type of anticoagulant medication (including aspirin), more time is required.

If direct pressure or a properly packed pressure dressing fails to control external hemorrhage from an extremity, the next step is to restrict the blood flow into the extremity by using a properly applied tourniquet. The military use of this important device in the conflicts in Iraq and Afghanistan has demonstrated its effectiveness and revealed minimal complications. On occasion, the application of a single tourniquet may not completely occlude the artery and stop the hemorrhage. In these cases, a second tourniquet applied just proximal to the first may be required (see the Shock chapter).

For external hemorrhage from locations where a tourniquet cannot be applied to compress a bleeding blood vessel (torso, neck, high extremity, or groin), a hemostatic agent may be used. Similar to packing a wound, the gauze-impregnated agent must be inserted and packed into the wound and pressure applied for a minimum of 3 minutes.

For a patient in obvious shock from external hemorrhage, measures aimed at resuscitation (e.g., administration of intravenous [IV] fluids) should be avoided before adequately controlling the bleeding. *Attempted resuscitation will never be successful in the presence of ongoing external hemorrhage.*

Control of external hemorrhage and recognition of suspected internal hemorrhage, combined with prompt transport to the closest appropriate facility, represent opportunities for the prehospital care provider to make significant impact and save many lives.

8. Provide Basic Shock Therapy, Including Appropriately Splinting Musculoskeletal Injuries and Restoring and Maintaining Normal Body Temperature

At the end of the primary assessment, the patient's body is exposed so that the prehospital care provider can quickly scan for additional life-threatening injuries. Once this is completed, the patient should be covered again because hypothermia can be fatal to a critically injured trauma patient. The patient in shock is already handicapped by a marked decrease in energy production resulting from widespread inadequate tissue perfusion. Allowing the loss of heat by unnecessary exposure provides a negative effect on the critical trauma patient. The triad of death (hypothermia, acidosis, and *coagulopathy* [decreased ability for blood clotting to occur]) are all symptoms of reduced energy production and anaerobic metabolism. A cold, shivering patient has already started down the path of death. If the temperature in the ambulance is comfortable for you, fully clothed, then it is likely too cold for the patient.

Severe hypothermia can ensue if the patient's body temperature is not maintained. Hypothermia drastically impairs the ability of the body's blood clotting system to achieve hemostasis. Blood coagulates (clots) as the result of a complex series of enzymatic reactions leading to the formation of a fibrin matrix that traps RBCs and stems bleeding. These enzymes function within a very narrow temperature range. A drop in body temperature below 95°F (35°C) may significantly contribute to the development of a coagulopathy. Therefore, it is important to maintain body heat through the use of blankets and restore it with resuscitation and a warmed environment inside the ambulance.

When fracture of a long bone occurs, surrounding muscle and connective tissue are often torn. This tissue damage, along with bleeding from the ends of the broken bones, can result in significant internal hemorrhage. This blood loss can range from about 500 ml from a humerus fracture up to 1 to 2 liters from a single femur fracture. Rough handling of a fractured extremity can worsen the tissue damage and aggravate bleeding. Splinting assists in reducing the loss of additional blood into surrounding tissues, helping to preserve circulating RBCs for oxygen transport. For this reason, as well as for pain management, fractured extremities are splinted.

With a critically injured trauma patient, there may be no time to splint each individual fracture. Instead, immobilizing the patient to a long backboard will splint virtually all fractures in an anatomic position and diminish internal hemorrhage. The one possible exception to this is a midshaft fracture of the femur. Because of the spasm of the very strong muscles in the thigh, the muscles contract, causing the bone ends to override one another, thereby damaging additional tissue. These types of fractures are best managed by use of a traction splint if time allows its application during transport. For the vast majority of trauma calls, when no life-threatening conditions are identified in the primary assessment, each suspected extremity injury can be appropriately splinted.

9. Maintain Manual Spinal Stabilization Until the Patient Is Immobilized

When contact with the trauma patient is made, manual stabilization of the cervical spine should be initiated and maintained until the patient is either (1) immobilized on an appropriate device or (2) deemed not to meet indications for spinal immobilization (**Figure 18-6**). Satisfactory spinal immobilization involves immobilization from the head to the pelvis. Immobilization should not interfere with the patient's ability to open the mouth and should not impair ventilatory function.

Spinal immobilization after blunt trauma is indicated if the patient has an altered level of consciousness (GCS score less than 15), neck pain, a neurologic complaint, spinal tenderness, an anatomic abnormality, or a motor or sensory deficit identified on physical examination. If the patient has sustained a mechanism of injury that causes concern, spinal immobilization is indicated if the patient has evidence of alcohol or drug intoxication, a significant distracting injury, or an inability to communicate because of age or a language barrier (see the Spinal Trauma chapter, under Indications for Spinal Immobilization).

For the victim of penetrating trauma, spinal immobilization is performed only if the patient has spine-related neurologic complaints or if a motor or sensory deficit is noted on physical examination. One study found that the outcome is worse for patients with penetrating trauma who undergo unneeded prehospital spinal immobilization.[9]

10. For Critically Injured Trauma Patients, Initiate Transport to the Closest Appropriate Facility as Soon as Possible After EMS Arrival on Scene

Numerous studies have demonstrated that delays in transporting trauma patients to appropriate receiving facilities lead to increases in mortality rates (**Figure 18-7**). Although prehospital care providers have become proficient at airway management, ventilatory support, and administration of IV fluid therapy, most critically injured trauma patients are in hemorrhagic shock

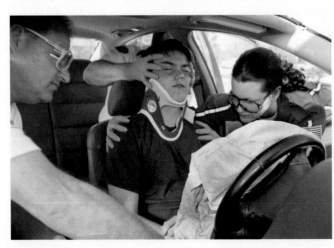

Figure 18-6   Maintain manual spinal immobilization until the patient is immobilized.
Source: Courtesy of Rick Brady.

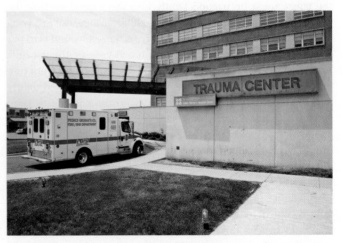

Figure 18-7   For critically injured trauma patients, initiate transport to the closest appropriate facility within 10 minutes of arrival on scene.
Source: Courtesy of Rick Brady.

and are in need of two things that cannot be provided in the prehospital setting: (1) Blood (specifically RBCs) to carry oxygen and plasma to provide internal clotting and (2) control of internal hemorrhage. Because human blood is a perishable product, it is impractical for administration in the field in most circumstances. Crystalloid solution temporarily restores intravascular volume but does not replace the oxygen-carrying capacity of the lost RBCs and the lost clotting factors of plasma, and it rapidly leaks into the interstitial space, creating oxygen exchange problems. Some EMS units now carry liquid plasma for long transport times. This plasma does not require thawing and can last up to 30 days with refrigeration. In Europe, EMS units are now carrying *lyophilized* (freeze-dried) plasma, which does not require refrigeration and has a long shelf life. It is reconstituted by dilution with crystalloid.

Similarly, control of internal hemorrhage almost always requires emergent surgical intervention best performed in an OR. Resuscitation can never be achieved in the patient with ongoing internal hemorrhage. Therefore, the goal of the prehospital care provider is to spend as little time on scene as possible.

This concern for limiting scene time should not be construed as a "scoop-and-run" mentality in which no attempts are made to address key problems before initiating transport. Instead, PHTLS advocates a philosophy of "limited scene intervention," focusing on a rapid assessment aimed at identifying threats to life and performing interventions that are *believed* to improve outcome. Examples include airway and ventilatory management, control of external hemorrhage, and spinal immobilization. Precious time should not be wasted on procedures that can be instituted en route to the receiving facility. Patients who are critically injured (see Figure 18-5) should be transported as soon as possible after EMS arrival on scene, ideally within 10 minutes, whenever possible—the "Platinum 10 Minutes" of the Golden Period. Reasonable exceptions to the Platinum 10 Minutes include situations that require extensive extrication or time needed to secure an unsafe scene, such as law enforcement ensuring that a perpetrator is no longer present.

The *closest* hospital may not be the *most appropriate* receiving facility for many trauma patients. Those patients who meet certain physiologic, anatomic, or mechanism of injury criteria benefit from being taken to a trauma center—a facility that has special expertise and resources for managing trauma. Ideally, patients who meet physiologic, anatomic, or mechanism of injury criteria, and those with special circumstances, should be transported directly to a trauma center if one is within a reasonable distance (i.e., 30 minutes driving time). Air medical helicopters can also be utilized to transport patients from the scene directly to trauma centers, provided the delay in transport related to awaiting arrival of the helicopter does not exceed the time of ground transport to the closest hospital when a trauma center is not readily available.

Each community, through a consensus of surgeons, emergency physicians, and prehospital care providers, must decide where these types of trauma patients should be transported. These decisions should be incorporated into protocols that designate the best destination facility—the closest *appropriate*

facility. In most situations, it is appropriate to bypass nontrauma centers to reach a trauma center. Even if this causes a moderate increase in the transport time, the overall time to definitive care will be shorter. Ideally, in the urban setting, a critically injured patient arrives at a trauma center within 25 to 30 minutes of being injured.

The hospital must work as efficiently as the prehospital care providers to continue resuscitation and, if necessary, transport the patient quickly to the OR (all within the Golden Period) to control hemorrhage and keep shock from becoming irreversible.

11. Initiate Warmed Intravenous Fluid Replacement En Route to the Receiving Facility

Initiation of transport of a critically injured trauma patient should never be delayed simply to insert IV catheters and administer fluid therapy. Although crystalloid solutions do restore lost blood volume and improve perfusion, they do not transport oxygen. Additionally, restoring normal blood pressure may result in additional hemorrhage from clot disruption in damaged blood vessels that initially clotted off, thereby increasing patient mortality.

While en route to the receiving facility, two large-bore IV catheters can be inserted and an infusion of warmed (102°F [39°C]) crystalloid solution started, preferably lactated Ringer's. Warmed solution is given to aid in the prevention of hypothermia. Volume resuscitation is individualized to the clinical situation and involves balancing the need for perfusion of vital organs with the risk of rebleeding as the blood pressure increases (see the Shock chapter, under Managing Volume Resuscitation).

For adult patients with suspected uncontrolled hemorrhage in the chest, abdomen, or retroperitoneum, IV fluid therapy is titrated to maintain a mean arterial pressure of 60 to 65 millimeters of mercury (mm Hg) (systolic blood pressure of 80 to 90 mm Hg) unless a CNS injury (traumatic brain injury or spinal cord injury) is suspected, in which case a target systolic blood pressure of at least 90 mm Hg is appropriate. If an isolated external hemorrhage has been controlled (e.g., via application of a tourniquet to an amputated extremity), warmed IV fluid is provided in order to return vitals to normal levels unless the patient develops evidence of recurrent Class III or IV shock, in which case fluid is titrated to a mean arterial pressure of 60 to 65 mm Hg. IV lines and fluid therapy may be initiated during extrication or while awaiting the arrival of an air medical helicopter. These situations do not result in a delay in transport to initiate volume resuscitation.

Basic life support (BLS) providers should consider a rendezvous with an advanced life support (ALS) service (by air or ground units) when faced with a critical patient and prolonged transport time to provide interventions and monitoring that are not available from the basic-level prehospital providers.

12. Ascertain the Patient's Medical History and Perform a Secondary Assessment When Life-Threatening Problems Have Been Satisfactorily Managed or Have Been Ruled Out

If life-threatening conditions are found in the primary assessment, key interventions should be performed and the patient transported within the Platinum 10 Minutes. Conversely, if life-threatening conditions are not identified, a secondary assessment is performed. The secondary assessment is a systematic, head-to-toe physical examination that serves to identify all injuries. A SAMPLE history (**s**ymptoms, **a**llergies, **m**edications, **p**ast medical history, **l**ast meal, **e**vents preceding the injury) is also obtained during the secondary assessment.

For critically injured trauma patients, a secondary assessment is performed only if time permits and once life-threatening conditions have been managed appropriately. In some situations in which the patient is located close to an appropriate receiving facility, a secondary assessment may never be completed. This approach ensures that the prehospital care provider's attention is focused on the most serious problems—those that may result in death if not properly managed—and not on lower-priority injuries.

The patient's airway, respiratory, and circulatory status along with vital signs should be reassessed frequently because patients who initially present without life-threatening injuries may subsequently develop them.

13. Provide Adequate Pain Relief

Patients who have sustained serious injury will experience significant amounts of pain. It is appropriate to provide analgesics to relieve that pain as long as no other contraindications to the administration of analgesics are present, such as hypotension, which can be made worse by the medication.

It was once thought that providing pain relief would mask the patient's symptoms and impair the ability of the trauma team to adequately assess the patient after arrival to the hospital. Numerous studies have shown that this is, in fact, not the case. Patients should not be allowed to suffer from pain during their transport. Prehospital care providers should administer analgesics to provide adequate pain relief.

14. Provide Thorough and Accurate Communication Regarding the Patient and the Circumstances of the Injury to the Receiving Facility

Communication about a trauma patient with the receiving hospital involves three components:

- Pre-arrival warning
- Verbal report upon arrival

- Written documentation of the encounter in the patient care report (PCR)

Care of the trauma patient is a team effort. The response to a critical trauma patient begins with the prehospital care provider and continues in the hospital. Delivering information from the prehospital setting to the receiving hospital allows for notification and mobilization of appropriate hospital resources to ensure an optimal reception of the patient. Upon arrival at the receiving facility, ideally a trauma center for the most critically injured, the prehospital care provider relates a verbal report to those who are assuming the care of the trauma patient. This report should be succinct and accurate and should serve to inform receiving personnel of:

- The patient's presenting condition
- Kinematics of the injury
- Assessment findings
- Interventions performed
- The patient's response to those interventions

Because of the prehospital care provider's ability to interview family members and bystanders and because a patient's mental status may deteriorate during transport, prehospital care providers may have key information essential to assessment and management of the patient that the hospital personnel may not be able to ascertain. Direct communication from prehospital provider to hospital provider during the patient hand-off in the receiving facility ensures continuity of care.

Upon completion of patient care duties, the prehospital care provider carefully and accurately completes a PCR. Like other medical records, this document serves as an organized record of the encounter with the patient. A PCR includes all important information provided by the patient and family or bystanders, as well as findings identified in the physical examination. Additionally, interventions performed are listed as well as any changes that were noted in the patient's condition during the ongoing assessment and reassessment.

Although several different options exist for documentation, all PCRs should "paint a picture" to the reader of the patient's appearance and provide a chronology of interventions. PCRs should be accurate because they are a medicolegal document. They provide crucial information that is included in hospital trauma registries and may be utilized for research.

15. Above All, Do No Further Harm

The medical principle that states "Above all, do no further harm" dates back to the ancient Greek physician Hippocrates. Applied to the prehospital care of the trauma patient, this principle can take many forms: developing a backup plan for airway management before initiating rapid sequence intubation, protecting a patient from flying debris during extrication from a damaged vehicle, or controlling significant external hemorrhage before initiating volume resuscitation. Recent experience has shown that prehospital care providers can safely perform many of the lifesaving skills that can be delivered in a trauma center. However, the issue in the prehospital setting is not, "What *can* prehospital care providers do for critically injured trauma patients?" but rather, "What *should* prehospital care providers do for critically injured trauma patients?"

When caring for a critically injured patient, prehospital care providers need to ask themselves if their actions at the scene and during transport will reasonably benefit the patient. If the answer to this question is no or is uncertain, those actions should be withheld and emphasis placed on transporting the trauma patient to the closest appropriate facility. Interventions should be limited to those that prevent or treat physiologic deterioration.

Trauma care must follow a given set of priorities that establish an efficient and effective plan of action, based on available time frames and any dangers present at the scene, if the patient is to survive (**Figure 18-8**). Appropriate intervention and stabilization should be integrated and coordinated between the field, the ED, and the OR. It is essential that every health care provider at

every level of care and at every stage of treatment be in harmony with the rest of the team.

Another important component to the principle of "Above all, do no further harm" relates to the issue of secondary injury. It has become clear that injury occurs, not only from the initial traumatic event, but also from the physiologic consequences that result from the direct trauma. Specifically, hypoxia, hypotension, and hypothermia all produce additional injury, over and above the primary injury. Failure to recognize that these problems are present, allowing them to develop during the course of treatment, or failure to correct them in a timely fashion, offers an opportunity for added complications and greater morbidity and mortality.

In discussing the issue of doing no further harm, the concept of "financial harm" should be considered in addition to the common thought of physical harm. Specifically, on a regular basis, manufacturers introduce new medications and devices designed to replace or improve existing modalities of treatment. It is important to consider a number of issues prior to implementing new treatments, including:

- What is the medical evidence supporting the efficacy of the new treatment?
- Is the new intervention as good as or better than existing interventions?
- How does the cost of providing the new intervention compare to the existing intervention?

As a general principle, there should be convincing medical evidence demonstrating that a new intervention is at least as good as, and preferably better than, existing treatments before it is formally accepted and implemented. The cost of a new intervention often exceeds that of an existing intervention. In the absence of evidence indicating superiority of the new intervention, the added charges to the patient are not justified and therefore constitute financial harm.

Finally, doing no further harm sometimes means doing less. As discussed in the chapter titled PHTLS: Past, Present, and Future, critically injured trauma patients arriving at a trauma center can have a worse outcome when transported by EMS rather than private vehicle. A significant factor that probably accounts for the increased mortality rate is the actions of well-intentioned prehospital care providers who fail to understand that trauma is a surgical disease; most critically injured patients require immediate surgery to save their lives. Anything that delays surgical intervention translates into more hemorrhage, more shock, and ultimately death.

Even with the best-planned and executed resuscitation, not all trauma patients can be saved. However, with attention focused on the reasons for early traumatic death, a much larger percentage of patients may survive, with a lower residual morbidity rate than would otherwise result without the benefit of correct and expedient field management. *The fundamental principles taught in PHTLS—rapid assessment, key field interventions, and rapid transport to the closest appropriate facility—have been shown to improve outcomes in critically injured trauma patients.*

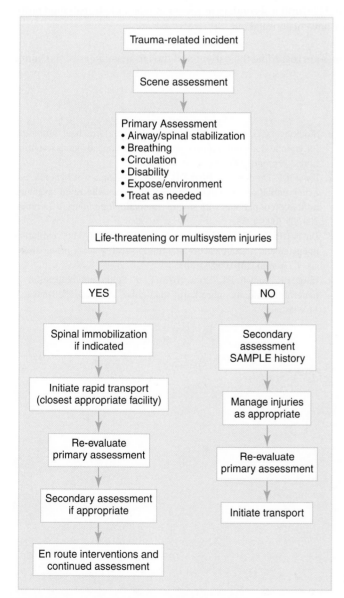

Figure 18-8 Trauma response algorithm.

Summary

The following are the Golden Principles of Prehospital Trauma Care:

1. Ensure the safety of the prehospital care providers and the patient.
2. Assess the scene situation to determine the need for additional resources.
3. Recognize the kinematics that produced the injuries.
4. Use the primary assessment approach to identify life-threatening conditions.
5. Provide appropriate airway management while maintaining cervical spine stabilization as indicated.
6. Support ventilation and deliver oxygen to maintain an SpO_2 greater than 95%.
7. Control any significant external hemorrhage.
8. Provide basic shock therapy, including appropriately splinting musculoskeletal injuries and restoring and maintaining normal body temperature.
9. Maintain manual spinal stabilization until the patient is immobilized.
10. For critically injured trauma patients, initiate transport to the closest appropriate facility as soon as possible after EMS arrival on scene.
11. Initiate warmed intravenous fluid replacement en route to the receiving facility.
12. Ascertain the patient's medical history and perform a secondary assessment when life-threatening problems have been satisfactorily managed or have been ruled out.
13. Provide adequate pain relief.
14. Provide thorough and accurate communication regarding the patient and the circumstances of the injury to the receiving facility.
15. Above all, do no further harm.

References

1. University of Maryland Medical Center. History of the Shock Trauma Center: tribute to R Adams Cowley, MD. http://umm.edu/programs/shock-trauma/about/history Updated December 16, 2013. Accessed January 2, 2014.
2. Lerner EB, Moscati RM. The Golden Hour: scientific fact or medical "urban legend"? *Acad Emerg Med.* 2001;8:758.
3. Tsybuliak GN, Pavlenko EP. Cause of death in the early post-traumatic period. *Vestn Khir Im I I Grek.* 1975;114(5):75.
4. Gunst M, Ghaemmaghami V, Gruszecki A, Urban J, Frankel H, Shafi S. Changing epidemiology of trauma deaths leads to a bimodal distribution. *Proc (Bayl Univ Med Cent).* 2010;23(4):349–354.
5. Stewart RM, Myers JG, Dent DL, et al. 753 Consecutive deaths in a level 1 trauma center: the argument for injury prevention. *J Trauma.* 2003;54:66.
6. Stockinger ZT, McSwain NE Jr. Prehospital endotracheal intubation for trauma does not improve survival over bag-valve-mask ventilation. *J Trauma.* 2004;56(3):531–536.
7. Davis DP, Dunford JV, Hoyt DB, et al. The impact of hypoxia and hyperventilation on outcome following paramedic rapid sequence intubation of patients with severe traumatic brain injury. *J Trauma.* 2007;62:1330–1338.
8. Davis DP, Peay J, Sise MJ, et al. Prehospital airway and ventilation management: a trauma score and injury severity score-based analysis. *J Trauma.* 2010;69:294–301.
9. Haut ER, Kalish BT, Efron DT, et al. Spine immobilization in penetrating trauma: more harm than good? *J Trauma.* 2010;68(1):115–120.

CHAPTER

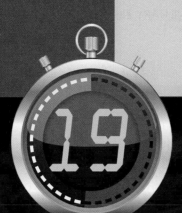

Disaster Management

CHAPTER OBJECTIVES

At the completion of this chapter, the reader will be able to do the following:

- Identify the five phases of the disaster cycle.

- Explain the comprehensive emergency management process.

- Discuss common pitfalls encountered during disaster response.

- Understand and discuss the components that comprise the medical response to a disaster.

- Recognize how disaster response may affect the psychological well-being of prehospital care providers.

SCENARIO

You are dispatched to a local high school that has been placed into service as a shelter following community-wide flooding from a large weather event. Your community's mayor and other dignitaries are in attendance at the school to address the community's concerns about closed roads and the lack of electrical power.

While en route to the scene, dispatch updates you that there are multiple reports of many casualties following the structural collapse of elevated bleachers in the gym that were being used as seating during a storm update. Police and fire resources are also en route to the scene but have limited available resources due to other ongoing, storm-related public safety incidents.

- What safety and security concerns would you expect to encounter?
- What triage system should be utilized?
- How should the response to this incident be organized?

Introduction

Unlike the trauma patient who has a finite period of time for presentation, treatment, and recovery, the response to and recovery from a disaster are time consuming, encompass multiple agencies, and include not only medical and psychosocial issues but also the rebuilding of public health, physical safety, and sociologic resources and infrastructures.

The World Health Organization (WHO) has defined a disaster as:

A serious disruption of the functioning of a community or a society causing widespread human, material, economic, or environmental losses which exceed the ability of the affected community or society to cope using its own resources.[1]

This broad definition does not provide specific reference to any medical issues or the emergency medical response, but is inclusive of the overall community response and sociopolitical response to any disaster of significant magnitude.

From a medical perspective, the definition can be more focused. A disaster is defined as a situation in which the number of patients presenting for medical assistance within a given time and at a given place is such that the health care providers cannot provide care for them with the usual resources at hand and require additional, and sometimes external, assistance.[2] This concept applies to all medical care settings, including hospitals and prehospital services. This situation is commonly referred to as a **mass-casualty incident (MCI)**. The abbreviation MCI has also been used to refer to "multiple-casualty incidents," which are events that involve more than one casualty but that can be handled with the community's standard resources. In this text, MCI will be used to refer to mass-casualty incidents that overwhelm the community's available resources.

It is important to understand that these definitions identify two key concepts: (1) A disaster is independent of a specific number of victims, and (2) the impact of the disaster exceeds the available resources of the medical response. Simply stated, all MCIs are a component of a disaster, but not all disasters are MCIs.

Disasters are often thought to follow no rules because no one can predict the time, location, or complexity of the next disaster. Traditionally, health care providers have thought that all disasters are different, especially those involving terrorism. However, all disasters, regardless of etiology, have similar medical and public health consequences. Disasters differ in the degree to which these consequences occur and the degree to which they disrupt the medical and public health infrastructure of the disaster locale.

The key principle of disaster medical care is to do the greatest good for the greatest number of patients with the resources available. This objective is different from that of "conventional" non-disaster-related medical care, which is to do the greatest good for the individual patient.

Natural disasters, man-made disasters, and terrorism encompass the spectrum of possible disaster threats. **Weapons of mass destruction (WMDs)**, creating huge numbers of casualties and contaminated environments, may be the greatest challenge of all (see the Explosions and Weapons of Mass Destruction chapter).

A consistent approach to the management of disasters, based on an understanding of their common features and the response expertise required to deal with the incident, is becoming the accepted practice throughout the world. This strategy forms the framework for **mass-casualty incident (MCI) response**. The primary objective of the MCI response is to reduce the morbidity (injury and disease) and mortality (death) caused by the disaster. All prehospital care providers need to incorporate the key principles of the MCI response into their training, given the complexity of current disasters (**Figure 19-1**).

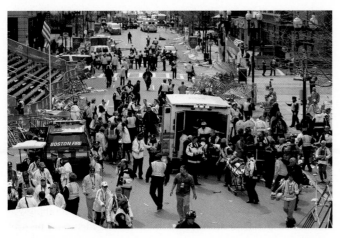

Figure 19-1 Mass casualty management at the scene of the Boston Marathon bombings.
Source: © Charles Krupa/AP Images.

The Disaster Cycle

Eric Noji, MD,[3] and others have defined a theoretic framework by which the sequence of events in a disaster can be broken down and analyzed. This conceptual description not only provides an overview of the natural history of a disaster but also provides the basis for the development of the response process.[3,4] Five phases have been identified:

1. The **quiescence or interdisaster period** represents the time in between disasters or MCIs during which risk assessment and mitigation activities should be undertaken and plans for the response to likely events are developed, tested, and implemented.

2. The next phase is the **prodrome (predisaster) phase**, or **warning phase**. At this point, a specific event has been identified as inevitable. This could reflect a natural weather condition (e.g., impending landfall of a hurricane) or the active unfolding of a hostile and potentially violent situation. During this period, specific steps may be taken to mitigate the effects of the ensuing events. These defensive maneuvers may include such actions as fortifying physical structures, initiating evacuation plans, and mobilizing public health resources to mount a postevent response. It must be noted, however, that not all incidents will have a warning phase. For example, an earthquake may occur without warning.

3. The third phase is the **impact phase**, or the occurrence of the actual event. During this period, there is often little that can be done to alter the impact or outcome of what is occurring.

4. The fourth phase is the **rescue, emergency, or relief phase**, which is the period immediately following the impact during which response occurs and appropriate management and intervention can save lives. The skills of emergency medical responders, prehospital care

providers, rescue teams, and medical support services will be brought to bear to maximize the number of survivors of the event.

5. The fifth phase is the **recovery or reconstruction phase**, during which community resources are called upon to endure, emerge from, and rebuild after the effects of the disaster through the coordinated efforts of the medical, public health, and community infrastructure (physical and political). This period is by far the longest, lasting months, and perhaps years, before a community fully recovers.

Understanding the disaster cycle (**Figure 19-2**) allows prehospital care providers to evaluate the preparations that have been made in anticipation of the likely hazards and events that may be encountered in their community. After an incident has occurred, there follows an opportunity for critical evaluation of the after-action report and assessment of the prehospital care provider's individual area of responsibility and response, as well as the response of others, to determine the efficiency and efficacy of the response process and identify areas for future improvement. These concepts apply to all disasters, regardless of size.

The duration of each phase of the disaster life cycle will vary depending upon the frequency with which incidents occur in a given community, the nature of the incident, and the degree to which the community is prepared. For example, the quiescent period in some locations can be extremely long (measured in years), whereas in other communities it may be measured in months. A specific example is that of hurricanes. The southeastern states of the United States prepare for hurricanes annually with a quiescent period between events of approximately 6 to 8 months. In contrast, although the New England states have

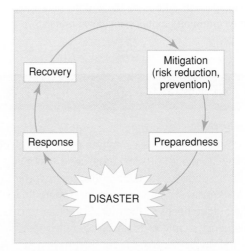

Figure 19-2 The life cycle of a disaster. The quiescence phase is represented by the mitigation and preparedness arrows. The warning phase comes just before the impact of the event. It is followed by the rescue and recovery phases.

been the victims of hurricanes, it is a rare event with a quiescent period of years in between hurricane strikes. Similarly, the rescue and recovery phases can vary significantly depending on the particular incident. The rescue and recovery from something like a plane crash will be measured in hours or at most days, whereas the rescue and recovery from a major flood may take weeks to months or longer.

Comprehensive Emergency Management

Knowledge of the life cycle of disasters can be used to implement the steps involved in **comprehensive emergency management**. Comprehensive emergency management defines the specific steps needed to manage an incident and consists of four components: mitigation, preparation, response, and recovery.

- **Mitigation**: This component of emergency management generally occurs during the quiescence phase of the disaster cycle. Potential hazards or likely etiologies of MCIs in the community are identified and assessed. Steps are then taken to prevent these hazards from causing an incident or to minimize their effect should something unexpected occur.
- **Preparedness**: This step of comprehensive emergency management involves identification in advance of an incident of the specific supplies, equipment, and personnel that would be needed to manage an incident, as well as the specific action plan that would be taken if an incident occurred.
- **Response**: This phase involves the activation and deployment of the various resources identified in the preparedness phase in order to manage an incident that has now occurred.
- **Recovery**: This component of comprehensive emergency management addresses the actions necessary to return the community to its preincident status.

While this process is typically applied to the management of a disaster, these same steps may also be utilized for the individual emergency preparedness of each emergency responder.

Personal Preparedness

Just as it is vital that each community and each agency undertake a comprehensive planning process in order to be prepared to meet the challenges of dealing with a disaster, each prehospital care provider must be ready to face the many issues that a disaster may present.

Prehospital care providers must have a complete understanding of the many potential hazards that may accompany a disaster response in advance of the actual incident and be prepared to take the necessary steps to protect themselves from these dangers. Gaps in knowledge about such issues as building collapse, hazardous materials incidents, WMDs and their effects on treatment, personal protection equipment, and overall incident management should be identified in advance and addressed.

Many disasters will go on for a long period of time and prehospital care providers must discuss their roles, responsibilities, and potentially prolonged absence with their families. This includes preparing their families for what they should do and where they should go during such an event to ensure their safety. Just as the local emergency medical service (EMS) procures supplies and equipment before a disaster, prehospital care providers should ensure that adequate supplies are available at home to meet their families' needs (**Figures 19-3, 19-4,** and **19-5**). An additional resource that provides information about personal and family preparation in the event of a disaster is the Ready Campaign sponsored by the Federal Emergency Management Agency (FEMA), available online at www.ready.gov.

Taking these actions will help reassure prehospital care providers that their families are safely dealing with their own needs during the incident, will provide comfort to the providers' families, who will know that the prehospital care provider is as prepared as possible for his or her role in disaster response, and

---

Figure 19-3 Emergency Supply List

All homes should have some basic supplies on hand in order to survive for at least 3 days if an emergency occurs. The following is a list of some basic items that every emergency supply kit should include. It is important that individuals review this list and consider where they live and the unique needs of their family in order to create an emergency supply kit that will meet their specific needs. Individuals should also consider having at least two emergency supply kits, one full kit at home and smaller portable kits in their workplace, vehicle, or other places where they spend time.

- Water—1 gallon per person and pet, per day (3-day supply for evacuation, 2-week supply for home)
- Food—nonperishable, easy to prepare items (3-day supply for evacuation, 2 week supply for home) (see Figure 19-4)
- Cell phone with chargers
- Battery-powered or hand-cranked radio and a National Oceanic and Atmospheric Administration (NOAA) Weather Radio with tone alert and extra batteries for both
- Flashlight and extra batteries
- First aid kit (see Figure 19-5)

(Continues on next page)

Figure 19-3 Emergency Supply List (*Continued*)

- Whistle to signal for help
- Dust mask, to help filter contaminated air, and plastic sheeting and duct tape to shelter in place
- Moist towelettes, garbage bags, and plastic ties for personal sanitation
- Wrench or pliers to turn off utilities
- Can opener for food (if kit contains canned food)
- Local maps

Additional items to consider adding to an emergency supply kit:

- *Items for infants*, including formula, diapers, bottles, pacifiers, powdered milk, and medications not requiring refrigeration
- *Items for seniors, disabled persons, or anyone with serious allergies*, including special foods, denture items, extra eyeglasses, hearing aid batteries, prescription and nonprescription medications that are regularly used, inhalers, and other essential equipment
- Prescription medications and glasses
- Pet food and extra water for your pet
- Important family documents such as copies of insurance policies, identification, and bank account records in a waterproof, portable container
- Cash or traveler's checks and change
- Emergency reference material such as a first aid book or information from www.ready.gov
- Sleeping bag or warm blanket for each person (Consider additional bedding if you live in a cold-weather climate.)
- Complete change of clothing, including a long-sleeved shirt, long pants, and sturdy shoes (Consider additional clothing if you live in a cold-weather climate.)
- Household chlorine bleach and medicine dropper (When diluted 9 parts water to 1 part bleach, bleach can be used as a disinfectant. In an emergency, you can use it to treat water by using 16 drops of regular household liquid bleach per gallon of water. Do not use bleaches that are scented or color safe or that have added cleaners.)
- Fire extinguisher (A-B-C type)
- Matches in a waterproof container
- Paper and pencil
- Entertainment—including games and books, favorite dolls, and stuffed animals for small children
- Kitchen accessories—a manual can opener; mess kits or disposable cups, plates, and utensils; utility knife; sugar and salt; aluminum foil and plastic wrap; resealable plastic bags; paper towels
- Sanitation and hygiene items—shampoo, deodorant, toothpaste, toothbrushes, comb and brush, lip balm, sunscreen, contact lenses and supplies, any medications regularly used, toilet paper, moist towelettes, soap, hand sanitizer, liquid detergent, feminine supplies, plastic garbage bags (heavy-duty) and ties (for personal sanitation uses), medium-sized plastic bucket with tight lid, disinfectant, household chlorine bleach
- Needles and thread
- A map of the area marked with places you could go and their telephone numbers
- An extra set of keys and IDs—including keys for cars and any properties owned and copies of driver's licenses, passports, and work identification badges
- Cash and coins and copies of credit cards
- Copies of medical prescriptions
- A small tent, compass, and shovel

Pack the items in easy-to-carry containers, label the containers clearly, and store them where they would be easily accessible. Duffle bags, backpacks, and covered trash receptacles are good candidates for containers. In a disaster situation, a family may need access to the disaster supplies kit quickly—whether sheltering at home or evacuating. Ensuring that family vehicles are filled with gasoline will allow for immediate evacuation to a safe location. Following a disaster, having the right supplies can help a household endure home confinement or evacuation.

Make sure the needs of everyone who would use the kit are covered, including infants, seniors, and pets. It is a good idea to involve whoever is going to use the kit, including children, in assembling it.

Source: Adapted from FEMA: Ready America (www.ready.gov) and the Centers for Disease Control and Prevention: Emergency Preparedness and Response (www.bt.cdc.gov/planning/).

Figure 19-4   Food Kit

- Store at least a 3-day supply of nonperishable food.
- Select foods that require no refrigeration, preparation, or cooking and little or no water.
- Pack a manual can opener and eating utensils.
- Avoid salty foods, as they will make you thirsty.
- Choose foods your family will eat.
- Suggested foods include the following:
  - Ready-to-eat canned meats, fruits, and vegetables
  - Protein or fruit bars
  - Dry cereal or granola
  - Peanut butter

- Dried fruit
- Nuts
- Crackers
- Canned juices
- Nonperishable pasteurized milk
- High-energy foods
- Vitamins
- Food for infants
- Comfort/stress foods
- Bring a propane stove or grill for cooking (with extra propane tank).

Source: Data from FEMA: Ready America (www.ready.gov) and the Centers for Disease Control and Prevention: Emergency Preparedness and Response (www.bt.cdc.gov/planning/).

Figure 19-5   First Aid Kit

In any emergency, a family member may be cut or burned or may suffer other injuries. An emergency kit should include the following:

- Two pairs of latex gloves or other sterile gloves (if anyone has latex allergies)
- Sterile dressings to stop bleeding
- Cleansing agent/soap and antibiotic towelettes to disinfect
- Antibiotic ointment to prevent infection
- Burn ointment to prevent infection
- Adhesive bandages in a variety of sizes
- Eye wash solution to flush the eyes or to use as a general decontaminant
- Thermometer
- Daily prescription medications such as insulin, heart medicine, and asthma inhalers (Periodically rotate medicines to account for expiration dates.)

- Prescribed medical supplies such as glucose and blood pressure monitoring equipment and supplies

Other things it may be useful to include:

- Cell phone with charger
- Scissors
- Tweezers
- Tube of petroleum jelly or other lubricant
- Nonprescription drugs:
  - Aspirin or nonaspirin pain reliever
  - Antidiarrhea medication
  - Antacid (for upset stomach)
  - Laxative

Source: Data from FEMA: Ready America (www.ready.gov) and the Centers for Disease Control and Prevention: Emergency Preparedness and Response (www.bt.cdc.gov/planning/).

will allow prehospital care providers to continue to provide care to those requiring emergency medical assistance.

Mass-Casualty Incident Management

The severity and diversity of injuries and illness in a disaster or MCI, in addition to the number of victims, will be major factors in determining whether an MCI requires resources and assistance from outside the impacted community.

Today's complex disasters, especially those involving terrorism and WMDs (chemical, biologic, radiologic, or nuclear), may result in an austere environment. An **austere environment** is a setting in which resources, supplies, equipment, personnel, transportation, and other aspects of the physical, political, social, and economic environments are limited. As a result of these limitations, severe constraints on the availability and adequacy of immediate care for the population in need will be imposed. Prehospital care providers must anticipate the reality that, in such situations, the level of care provided to the sick and injured will be altered and interventions normally offered to all patients may be provided only to those individuals who meet specific criteria and who are likely to survive.[5]

Emergency medical concerns related to MCIs include the following five elements:

■ *Search and rescue.* This activity involves the process of systematically looking for those individuals who have been impacted by an event and rescuing them from hazardous situations. Depending on the situation, this often requires the use of specially trained teams, particularly when extrication issues are involved.
■ *Triage and initial stabilization.* This is the process of systematically evaluating and categorizing each victim according to the seriousness of the injury or illness and providing initial medical care to address immediate life- or limb-threatening problems.
■ *Patient tracking.* This is a system by which patients are uniquely identified and followed through their initial contact with search and rescue, evacuation, transport, and ultimately discharge from definitive care.
■ *Definitive medical care.* This component is the provision of the specific medical care needed to treat the patient's specific injuries. This care will usually be provided at hospitals; however, alternate care facilities may be used in major events when hospitals are overwhelmed with casualties or when hospitals have been directly impacted and damaged by the incident.
■ *Evacuation.* This is the process of transporting disaster victims and injured patients away from the disaster site, either to a safe location or to a definitive care facility.

Public health concerns related to MCIs include the following:

■ Water (ensuring a supply of safe, potable water)
■ Food (ideally nonperishable and needing no refrigeration or cooking)
■ Shelter (a place for cover, protection, and refuge)
■ Sanitation (protection from contact with human and animal feces, solid waste, and wastewater)
■ Security and safety
■ Transportation
■ Communication (dissemination of information to the affected population, including information about communicable diseases)
■ Endemic and epidemic diseases (Endemic diseases are ones that are always present in a given area or population but that usually occur with low frequency, whereas an epidemic disease is one that develops and spreads rapidly to the population at risk.)

Both medical and public health disaster-response activities are coordinated through one organizational structure: the incident command system.

The National Incident Management System

The National Incident Management System (NIMS) was developed to provide a template for a comprehensive, nationwide, systematic approach to managing an incident, regardless of cause, size, location, or complexity. NIMS offers a set of preparedness concepts and principles for all hazards and events. It outlines the essential principles for a common operating structure and interoperability of communications and information management systems. It also provides standardized resource management procedures. NIMS uses the incident command system to oversee the direct response to an incident.

Incident Command System

Many different organizations participate in the response to a disaster. The **incident command system (ICS)** was created to allow different types of agencies and multiple jurisdictions of similar agencies (fire, police, EMS) to work together effectively, using a common organizational structure and language to better manage the response to a disaster or other major incident (**Figure 19-6**) (see the Scene Assessment chapter). Representatives from the various responding agencies will usually come together in an incident command post to facilitate interagency communications and decision making and work together to unify the command process.

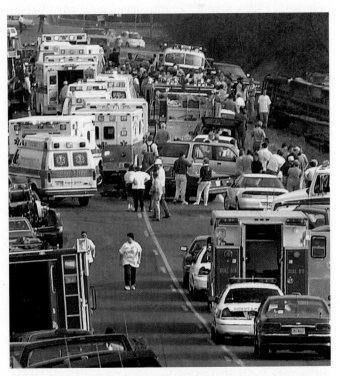

Figure 19-6 The incident command system (ICS) allows integration of fire, police, and EMS assets at a disaster scene.
Source: © David Crigger, Bristol Herald Courier/AP Images.

The ICS recognizes that, regardless of the specific nature of the incident (police, fire, or medical), there are a number of functions that must always happen. The ICS is organized around these necessary functions. Its components are:

- Command
    - Safety officer
    - Information officer
    - Liaison officer
- Planning
- Logistics
- Operations
- Finance

These functions apply to all incidents and are now used in medical settings of all types, from prehospital to in-hospital, to organize the response to a disaster.

From a medical perspective, several important ICS principles will help during an MCI response:

1. ICS must be started early, preferably upon arrival of the emergency responder to the scene, before the incident management gets out of control.
2. Medical and public health responders, often used to working independently, need to implement the ICS management structure and coordinate their response assets to better respond to an MCI.
3. Using ICS will allow for the integration of the medical response into the overall response to the incident.

Detailed information and training about the ICS is available on the FEMA website (http://training.fema.gov/EMIWeb/IS/ICSResource/index.htm [accessed January 7, 2014]).

Characteristics of the Incident Command System

An ICS provides a standard, professional, organized approach to managing emergency incidents. The use of an ICS enables an emergency response agency to operate more safely and effectively. A standardized approach facilitates and coordinates the use of resources from multiple agencies, working toward common objectives. It also eliminates the need to develop a special approach for each situation.

Effective management of incidents requires an organizational structure to provide both a hierarchy of authority and responsibility and formal channels for communications. Through the use of command, the specific responsibilities and authority of everyone in the organization are clearly stated, and all relationships are well defined.

Jurisdictional Authority

Jurisdictional authority is usually not a problem at an incident with a single focus. Matters can become more complicated when several jurisdictions are involved or multiple agencies within a single jurisdiction have authority for various aspects of the incident. When there are overlapping responsibilities, the ICS may employ a **unified command**. This approach brings representatives of different agencies together to work on one plan and ensures that all actions are fully coordinated. *Command*, although the chosen term of the ICS system, is perhaps misleading. It is important to remember that incidents are managed; personnel are commanded. *Incident command*, whether conducted by an individual or through unified command, is a management and leadership position. It is responsible for setting strategic objectives and maintaining a comprehensive understanding of the impact of an incident as well as identifying the strategies required to manage it effectively. The command function is structured in one of two ways: single or unified.

Single command is the most traditional perception of the command function and is the genesis of the term **incident commander**. When an incident occurs within a single jurisdiction, and when there is no jurisdictional or functional agency overlap, a single incident commander should be identified and designated with overall incident management responsibility by the appropriate jurisdictional authority. This does not mean that other agencies do not respond or do not have a role in supporting the management of the incident.

Single command is best used when a single discipline in a single jurisdiction is responsible for the strategic objectives associated with managing the incident. Single command also is appropriate in the later stages of an incident that was initially managed through unified command. Over time, as many incidents stabilize, the strategic objectives become increasingly focused in a single jurisdiction or discipline. In this situation, it is appropriate to transition from unified command to single command.

It is also acceptable, if all agencies and jurisdictions agree, to designate a single incident commander in multiagency and multijurisdictional incidents. In this situation, however, command personnel should be carefully chosen. The incident commander is responsible for developing the strategic incident objectives on which the **incident action plans (IAPs)** will be based. An IAP is an oral or written plan containing general objectives reflecting the overall strategy for managing an incident. The incident commander is responsible for the IAP and all requests pertaining to the ordering and releasing of incident resources.

When multiple agencies with overlapping jurisdictions or legal responsibilities are involved in the same incident, unified command provides several advantages. In this approach, representatives from each agency cooperate to share command authority. They work together and are directly involved in the decision-making process. Unified command helps ensure cooperation, avoids confusion, and guarantees agreement on goals and objectives.

All-Risk and All-Hazard System

The ICS has evolved into an all-risk, all-hazard system that can be applied to manage resources at fires, floods, tornadoes, plane crashes, earthquakes, hazardous materials incidents, or any other type of emergency situation. This kind of system has also been used to manage many nonemergency events, such as large-scale public events, that have similar requirements for command, control, and communications. The flexibility of the ICS enables the management structure to expand as needed, using whatever components are required. The operations of multiple agencies and organizations can be integrated smoothly in the management of the incident.

Everyday Applicability

An ICS can and should be used for everyday operations as well as major incidents. Command should be established at every incident. Regular use of the system ensures familiarity with standard procedures and terminology. It also increases the users' confidence in the system. Frequent use of ICS for routine situations makes it easier to apply to larger incidents.

Unity of Command

Unity of command is a management concept in which each person has only one direct supervisor. All orders and assignments come directly from that supervisor, and all reports are made to the same supervisor. This approach eliminates the confusion that can result when a person receives orders from more than one boss. Unity of command reduces delays in solving problems as well as the potential for life and property losses. By ensuring that each person has only one supervisor, unity of command can increase overall accountability, prevent freelancing, improve the flow of communication, assist with the coordination of operational issues, and enhance the safety of the entire situation. An ICS is not necessarily a rank-oriented system. The best-qualified person should be assigned at the appropriate level for each situation, even if that means a lower-ranking individual is temporarily assigned to a higher-level position. This concept is critical for the effective application of the system and must be embraced by all participants. Additionally, a critical and developing component of NIMS will be a national credentialing standard for ICS positions such as command and section chiefs in the operations, planning, logistics, and finance/administration sections.

Span of Control

Span of control refers to the number of subordinates who report to one supervisor at any level within the organization. Span of control relates to all levels of ICS—from the strategic level to the operational/tactical level and to the task level.

In most situations, one person can effectively supervise only three to seven people or resources. Because of the dynamic nature of emergency incidents, an individual who has command or supervisory responsibilities in an ICS normally should not directly supervise more than five people. The actual span of control should depend on the complexity of the incident and the nature of the work being performed. For example, at a complex incident involving hazardous materials, the span of control might be only three; during less intense operations, the span of control could be as high as seven.

Modular Organization

The ICS is designed to be flexible and modular. The ICS organizational structure—command, operations, planning, logistics, and finance/administration—is predefined, ready to be staffed and made operational as needed. Indeed, an ICS has often been characterized as an organizational toolbox, where only the tools needed for the specific incident are used. In an ICS, these tools consist of position titles, job descriptions, and an organizational structure that defines the relationships between positions. Some positions and functions are used frequently, whereas others are needed only for complex or unusual situations. Any position can be activated simply by assigning someone to it.

Common Terminology

ICS promotes the use of common terminology both within an organization and among all agencies involved in emergency incidents. Common terminology means that each word has a single definition, and no two words used in managing an emergency incident have the same definition. Everyone uses the same terms to communicate the same thoughts, so everyone understands what is meant. Each job comes with one set of responsibilities, and everyone knows who is responsible for each duty.

Integrated Communications

Integrated communications ensures that everyone at an emergency can communicate with both supervisors and subordinates. The ICS must support communication up and down the chain of command at every level. A message must be able to move efficiently through the system from command down to the lowest level, and from the lowest level up to the command level.

Consolidated Incident Action Plans

An ICS ensures that everyone involved in the incident is following one overall plan. Different components of the organization may perform different functions, but all of their efforts contribute to the same goals and objectives. Everything that occurs is coordinated with everything else. At smaller incidents, command develops an action plan and communicates the incident priorities, objectives, strategies, and tactics to all of the operating units. Representatives from all participating agencies meet regularly to develop and update the plan. In both large and small incidents, those involved in the incident understand what their specific roles are and how they fit into the overall plan.

Designated Incident Facilities

Designated incident facilities are assigned locations where specific functions are always performed. For example, command will always be based at the incident command post. The staging area, rehabilitation area, casualty collection point, treatment area, base of operations, and helispot are all designated areas where particular functions take place. The facilities required for the specific incident are established according to the specific IAP or a predefined ICS plan.

Resource Management

Resource management entails the use of a standard system of assigning and keeping track of the resources involved in the incident. The resource management system of the ICS keeps track of the various resource assignments. At large-scale incidents, units are often dispatched to a **staging area**, rather than going directly to the incident location. A staging area is a location close to the incident scene where a number of units can be held in reserve, ready to be assigned if needed.

Organization of the Incident Command System

The ICS structure identifies a full range of duties, responsibilities, and functions that are performed at emergency incidents. It defines the relationships among all these different components. Some components are used on almost every incident, whereas others apply to only the largest and most complex situations. The five major components of an ICS organization are command, operations, planning, logistics, and finance/administration.

An ICS organization chart may be quite simple or very complex. Each block on an ICS organization chart refers to a function area or a job description. Positions are staffed as they are needed. The only position that must be filled at every incident is incident command. Incident command decides which additional components are needed for the given situation and activates those positions by assigning someone to perform those tasks.

Command

On an ICS organization chart, the first component is **command** (**Figure 19-7**). Command is the only position in the ICS that must always be filled for every incident, because there must always be someone in charge. Command is established when the first unit arrives on the scene and is maintained until the last unit leaves the scene.

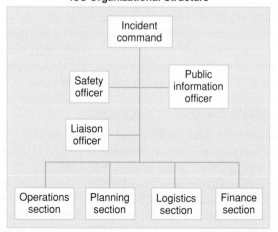

ICS Organizational Structure

Figure 19-7 The ICS organization chart.

In the ICS structure, command (either single or unified) is ultimately responsible for managing an incident and has the necessary authority to direct all activities at the incident scene. Command is directly responsible for the following tasks:

- Determining strategy
- Selecting incident tactics
- Setting the action plan
- Developing the ICS organization
- Managing resources
- Coordinating resource activities
- Providing for scene safety
- Releasing information about the incident
- Coordinating with outside agencies

Incident Command Post

The **incident command post (ICP)** is the headquarters for the incident. Command functions are centered in the ICP; thus command and all direct support staff should always be located at the ICP. The location of the ICP should be broadcast to all units as soon as the ICP is established.

Relative to the incident scene, ICP should be in a nearby, protected location. Often, the ICP for a major incident is located in a special vehicle or building. This location enables the command staff to function without needless distractions or interruptions. For large incidents that are geographically spread out, the command post may be some distance from part of the emergency incident.

Command Staff

Individuals on the **command staff** perform functions that report directly to command and cannot be delegated to other major sections of the organization. The safety officer, liaison officer, and public information officer are always part of the command staff. In addition, aides, assistants, and advisors may be assigned to work directly for members of the command staff.

Safety Officer. The **safety officer** is responsible for ensuring that safety issues are managed effectively at the incident scene. He or she is the eyes and ears of command in terms of safety—identifying and evaluating hazardous conditions, watching out for unsafe practices, and ensuring that safety procedures are followed. The safety officer is appointed early during an incident. As the incident becomes more complex and the number of resources present at the scene increases, additional qualified personnel can be assigned as assistant safety officers.

Liaison Officer. The **liaison officer** is a representative of command who serves as a point of contact for representatives from outside agencies. This member of the command staff is responsible for exchanging information with representatives from those agencies. During an active incident, command may not have time to meet directly with everyone who comes to the ICP. The liaison officer functions as the representative of command under these circumstances, obtaining and providing information, or directing people to the proper location or authority. The liaison area should be adjacent to, but not inside, the ICP.

Public Information Officer. The **public information officer (PIO)** is responsible for gathering and releasing incident information to the news media and other appropriate agencies. At a major incident, the public will want to know what is being done. Because command must make managing the incident the top priority, the PIO serves as the contact person for media requests, which frees up command to concentrate on the incident. A media headquarters should be established near—but not within—the ICP. The information presented to the media by the PIO needs to be approved by the incident commander.

General Staff Functions

The incident commander has the overall responsibility for the entire incident command organization, although some elements of the incident commander's responsibilities can be handled by the command staff. When the incident is too large or too complex for just one person to manage effectively, the incident commander may appoint someone to oversee parts of the operation. Everything that occurs at an emergency incident can be divided among the major functional components within ICS:

- Operations
- Planning
- Logistics
- Finance/administration

The chiefs of these four sections are known as the **ICS general staff**. Command decides which (if any) of these four positions need to be activated, when to activate them, and who should be placed in each position. Recall that the blocks on the ICS organization chart refer to functional areas or job descriptions, not to positions that must always be staffed.

The four section chiefs on the ICS general staff, when they are assigned, may run their operations from the main ICP, although this structure is not required. At a large incident, the four functional organizations may operate from different locations, but will always be in direct contact with command.

Operations

The **operations section** is responsible for the management of all actions that are directly related to controlling the incident. The operations section rescues any trapped individuals, treats any injured patients, and does whatever else is necessary to alleviate the emergency situation.

For most smaller incidents, command directly supervises the functions of the operations section. At complex incidents, a separate **operations section chief** takes on this responsibility so that command can focus on overall strategy while the operations section chief focuses on the tactics that are required to get the job done.

Operations are conducted in accordance with an IAP that outlines what the strategic objectives are and how emergency operations will be conducted. At most incidents, the IAP is relatively simple and can be expressed in a few words or phrases. The IAP for a large-scale incident can be a lengthy document that is regularly updated and used for daily briefings of the command staff.

Planning

The **planning section** is responsible for the collection, evaluation, dissemination, and use of information relevant to the incident. The planning section works with preincident plans, building construction drawings, maps, aerial photographs, diagrams, reference materials, and status boards. It is also responsible for developing and updating the IAP. The planning section develops what needs to be done by whom and identifies which resources are needed.

Command activates the planning section when information needs to be obtained, managed, and analyzed. The **planning section chief** reports directly to command. Individuals assigned to planning examine the current situation, review available information, predict the probable course of events, and prepare recommendations for strategies and tactics. The planning section also keeps track of resources at large-scale incidents and provides command with regular situation and resource status reports.

Logistics

The **logistics section** is responsible for providing supplies, services, facilities, and materials during the incident. The **logistics section chief** reports directly to command and serves as the supply officer for the incident. Among the responsibilities of this section are keeping vehicles fueled, providing food and refreshments for emergency responders, and arranging for specialized equipment.

Finance/Administration

The **finance/administration section** is the fourth major ICS component managed directly by command. This section is responsible for the accounting and financial aspects of an incident, as well as any legal issues that may arise in its aftermath. This function is not staffed at most incidents, because cost and accounting issues are typically addressed after the incident. Nevertheless, a finance/administration section may be needed at large-scale and long-term incidents that require immediate fiscal management, particularly when outside resources must be procured quickly. A finance/administration section may also be established during a natural disaster or during a hazardous materials incident where reimbursement may come from the shipper, carrier, chemical manufacturer, or insurance company.

Medical Response to Disasters

The effective response to an MCI depends upon the initiation of a series of actions, which, when combined, will help to minimize the mortality and morbidity of victims of the event. Although these actions will be discussed sequentially in this chapter, it is important to remember that during an actual disaster many of the actions will occur simultaneously (**Figure 19-8**).

Initial Response

The first step is notification and activation of the EMS response system. This is usually performed by witnesses to the event who then call the local emergency dispatch center seeking response by appropriate police, fire, and emergency medical agencies.

The first prehospital care providers to arrive at the scene have a number of important functions to fulfill that will set the stage for the entire emergency medical response to the incident. Most importantly, these actions do not include initiating care to the most critically injured patients, as would be the case in most non-MCI situations. Before beginning the process of providing emergency medical assistance, the first prehospital care providers must take the time to perform an overall scene assessment. The goals of this assessment are to evaluate any potential

hazards, estimate the potential number of casualties, determine what additional medical resources will be needed at the scene, evaluate whether any specialized equipment or personnel, such as search-and-rescue teams, will be required, and, depending on the incident, determine the likelihood or potential for a secondary device designed to harm emergency responders.

Once this assessment is complete, the next step is to communicate the overall assessment to the dispatch center, where the process of acquiring and dispatching the needed resources can be performed. After this, the prehospital care providers should identify appropriate locations to perform triage, to collect casualties, and to stage incoming ambulances, personnel, and supplies so as not to impede rapid ingress and egress or expose responding assets to potential hazards from the event.

In addition to providing for the emergency medical response to the disaster scene, it is essential that the responding EMS agency notify the likely receiving hospitals in the community so that they can activate their disaster plans to prepare to receive casualties. EMS agencies must remember that the field component of the disaster response is the first link in the overall chain of medical care for a disaster patient and that they are responsible for notifying and activating the other components of the health care system.

Search and Rescue

At this point, the on-scene process of initiating patient care can begin. Generally, this will start with a search-and-rescue effort to identify and evacuate casualties from the impacted site to a safer location. The local population near a disaster site, as well as survivors themselves if they are able, are often the immediate search-and-rescue resource and may have already begun to search for victims before the arrival of any public safety personnel.[6] Experience has demonstrated that the local community will respond to a disaster site and begin the process of aiding victims.

Many countries and communities have developed formal, specialized search-and-rescue teams as an integral part of their national and local disaster-response plans. Members of these teams receive specialized training in confined-space environments and are activated as needed for a particular event. These search-and-rescue units generally include the following:

- A cadre of medical specialists
- Technical specialists knowledgeable in hazardous materials, structural engineering, heavy equipment operation, and technical search-and-rescue methods (e.g., listening equipment, remote cameras)
- Trained canines and their handlers

Local construction companies may provide valuable search-and-rescue assets by providing equipment, tools, and wooden planks that can be used at the disaster site to assist in moving heavy debris.

Figure 19-8 The Basic Steps in Medical Response to Disasters

Medical response to a disaster involves the following basic steps:

1. Notification and activation of EMS
2. Initial response
3. EMS response to the scene
4. Assessment of the situation
   a. Cause
   b. Number of casualties
   c. Additional resources
      i. Medical
      ii. Other
5. Communication of the situation and needs
6. Activation of the medical community
   a. Notify receiving facilities.
7. Search and rescue
8. Triage (treatment of airway and hemorrhage life threats)
9. Casualty collection
10. Treatment
11. Transport
12. Retriage

Triage

As patients are identified and evacuated, they are brought to the triage site, where they can be assessed and a triage category assigned (**Figure 19-9**). The term triage is a French word that means "to sort." From a medical perspective, triage means sorting casualties based on the severity of their injuries. This process was first described in the early 1800s by Baron Dominique Larrey, who was surgeon-in-chief to Napoleon and was most famous for developing the prototype ambulance during the Napoleonic Wars. Larrey stated:

> Those who are dangerously wounded should receive the first attention, without regard to rank or distinction. They who are injured in a less degree may wait until their brethren in arms, who are badly mutilated, have been operated on and dressed, otherwise the latter would not survive many hours; rarely, until the succeeding day.[7]

This concept, which has been further expanded upon since Larrey, serves to prioritize the patient's need for medical care and transport to the hospital.

Triage is one of the most important missions of any disaster medical response. As noted previously, the objective of conventional triage in the nondisaster setting is to do the greatest good for the individual patient. This imperative usually means finding and treating the sickest patient. The objective of mass-casualty triage is to do the greatest good for the greatest number of people. Mass-casualty triage in the field must be overseen by a trained triage officer. A **triage officer** should have a wide breadth of clinical experience in the assessment and management of field injuries, as potentially difficult decisions may have to be made about patients who will be deemed critical versus those who will be classified as mortally wounded with little chance of survival. A paramedic with significant field experience usually meets this requirement. A trained physician with experience in the field may also function in this capacity.[8,9]

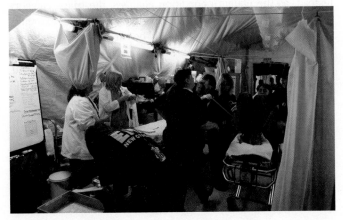

Figure 19-9 Triage and initial stabilization at a makeshift medical treatment facility—Hurricane Katrina, Louisiana, 2005.
Source: © Bill Haber/AP Images.

A number of different methodologies exist for evaluating and assigning the triage category.[10] One method involves a rapid physiologic and mental status evaluation. This triage process is referred to as the **START triage algorithm** (**s**imple **t**riage **a**nd **r**apid **t**reatment). This system evaluates the respiratory status, perfusion status, and mental status of the patient in making a prioritization for initial transfer to definitive care facilities (see pages 132–133 in the Scene Assessment chapter).[9,11] Other triage systems include the MASS (**m**ove, **a**ssess, **s**ort, **s**end), Smart, and Sacco triage methods.

In an effort to provide national guidance and bring uniformity to the triage process, the Centers for Disease Control and Prevention (CDC) in the United States convened a multidisciplinary group of experts to develop a consensus-based triage system, now known as SALT (see page 134 in the Scene Assessment chapter).[9] This triage system involves **s**orting the patient based upon the patient's ability to move, **a**ssessing the patient for the need for **l**ifesaving interventions, performing those interventions, and **t**reating and **t**ransporting.

Regardless of the exact triage method used, all triage systems ultimately classify patients into one of (usually) four injury-severity categories. Highest priority patients are those who are identified as having critical, but likely survivable, injuries and are usually categorized as *immediate* and color-coded *red*. Patients with moderate injuries who can potentially tolerate a short delay in care are categorized as *delayed* patients and color-coded *yellow*. Patients with relatively minor injuries, often referred to as the "walking wounded," are classified as *minimal* victims and color-coded *green*. Patients who have expired on the scene or whose injuries are so severe that death is imminent or likely are categorized as *dead* or *expectant*, respectively, and color-coded *black*. Of note, some triage systems, particularly SALT, specifically separate those patients classified as mortally wounded from those who are dead, color coding the expectant as *gray*.

All these color codes refer to the use of "disaster tags," which are used at disaster scenes and attached to patients once they have been triaged. The color code provides an immediate visual reference to the patient's triage category. Some triage systems also use a classification system in which immediate, delayed, minimal, and dead or expectant patients are referred to as Class I, Class II, Class III, and Class IV, respectively.

It is important that all triage personnel keep in mind that they must avoid the temptation to stop performing triage in favor of treating a critically injured patient whom they encounter. As mentioned earlier, the primary principle involved in dealing with an MCI is to do the most good for the most people. During this initial triage phase, medical interventions are limited to those actions that are performed easily and rapidly and that are not labor intensive. Generally, this means performing only procedures such as manual airway opening, needle chest decompression, administration of a chemical antidote, and external hemorrhage control. Interventions such as bag-mask ventilation and closed chest compression involve the use of significant personnel and are not performed.

Once patients have been triaged, they are brought together at **casualty collection points** according to their triage priority. Specifically, all the immediate patients (red) are grouped, as are the delayed (yellow) and minimal (green) patients. Casualty collection points should be located close enough to the disaster site that the victim can be easily carried to them and treatment rapidly provided, but far enough away from the impact site to be safe from any ongoing hazard. Important considerations include the following:

- Proximity to the disaster site
- Safety from hazards and uphill and upwind from contaminated environments
- Protection from climatic conditions (when possible)
- Easy visibility for disaster victims and assigned personnel
- Convenient entry and exit routes for ground, air, and water evacuation
- Safe distance from staging ambulance exhaust fumes

As additional medical staff and resources arrive and become available on scene, medical care and interventions are provided at the casualty collection points according to the triage priority. These are appropriate locations to which physicians responding to the scene may be assigned to further evaluate and treat injured patients.

Finally, as transportation resources become available, patients are transported for definitive care according, once again, to their triage priority (**Figure 19-10**). Immediate patients are not held on scene for the provision of further medical care if transport is available (**Figure 19-11**). Needed medical interventions should be conducted during transport to the definitive care facility.

Because of visible, critical injuries, emergency responders often tend to move individual patients forward for immediate treatment and transport and to bypass the triage process. This tendency must be avoided so that all victims can be

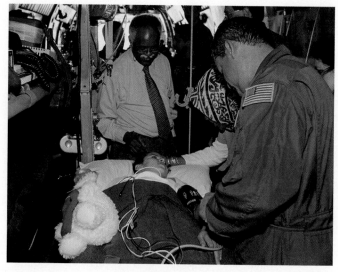

Figure 19-11 Interior of a military transport plane converted for medical evacuation with patient litters.
Source: © Evan Vucci/AP Images.

evaluated, the most life-threatening victims can be treated first, and the best care can be provided for the majority of victims. However, bypassing the triage process is indicated in certain situations. These conditions include:

1. Risk, as in bad weather
2. Potential impending darkness without the capabilities of lighting resources
3. The continued risk of injury as a result of natural or unnatural events
4. No triage facility or triage officer immediately available
5. Any tactical situation in a law enforcement scenario in which the victims are rapidly moved from the impact site to the collection point for transport[11,12]

Lastly, triage is not a static process; it is dynamic and ongoing. Once a patient is evaluated and categorized, the patient does not carry that triage category for the remainder of his or her care. Instead, as the patient's condition changes, the triage category may change as well. For example, a patient with a major extremity wound and hemorrhage may initially be categorized as an immediate patient; however, after pressure is applied to the wound and the bleeding is controlled, the patient may be retriaged as delayed. Alternatively, a patient initially categorized as immediate could deteriorate and subsequently be retriaged as expectant.

Retriage should occur on the scene while patients are waiting for transport resources. In addition, patients will undergo retriage upon arrival at the receiving destination and again as they are prioritized for surgery.

Treatment

Since the number of patients will initially exceed the available resources, treatment on the scene is generally limited to manually opening the airway, correcting tension pneumothorax,

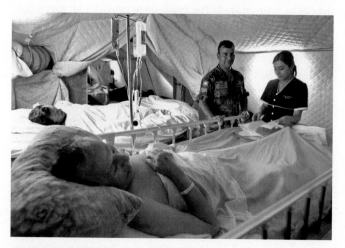

Figure 19-10 Definitive medical care at a U.S. field hospital—Bam, Iran, earthquake, 2005.
Source: © Cristobel Fuentes/AP Images.

controlling external hemorrhage, and administering chemical agent antidote. Only when adequate resources have arrived on scene or during transport to the hospital will additional interventions be provided, such as intravenous access and splinting of fractures.

Transport

The transport and tracking of patients from an MCI to the receiving hospitals involves a coordinated effort using a variety of transport vehicles. Immediate and delayed patients will be taken to the hospital in ambulances or helicopters (if available and conditions permit). Those incidents that result in huge numbers of patients, particularly patients in the minimal category, may require the use of nontraditional transport vehicles such as buses and vans, and in some cases, patients may be transported to nonhospital sites for evaluation and treatment. It is important to remember, however, that when such alternate transport mechanisms are used, prehospital care providers with adequate supplies and equipment must be assigned to accompany the casualties in that vehicle. Each patient's movement and destination should be accurately recorded on a patient tracking log or via commercially available tracking systems.

Another important issue in effectively responding to an MCI relates to the decision-making process for patient destination once transport is initiated.[13] Recent events have demonstrated that patients with non-life-threatening injuries will often depart the disaster site using any available means of transportation and make their own way to the hospital.[6] Often this results in large numbers of "walking wounded" arriving at the hospital closest to the disaster site. In fact, approximately 70% to 80% of patients will get to a hospital without EMS ambulance transport.

Prehospital care providers must understand that the hospital closest to a disaster scene may be overwhelmed with patients even before the arrival of the first transporting ambulance. Before taking a patient to the closest hospital, contact should be made to ascertain the status of the emergency department (ED) and its ability to accept and treat patients transported by ambulance. If the closest hospital is overwhelmed, the EMS system should transport patients to more distant facilities when possible. Although the transport time will be longer, the patient's care will not be complicated by the presence of numerous other patients. Dispersal of patients to multiple institutions will ultimately better preserve the ability of all the receiving hospitals to optimize the patient care that they can provide.

Even if the closest medical facility is not overwhelmed with self-transported patients, it is imperative that prehospital care providers do not overwhelm the nearest hospital with patients transported by ambulance. Often, the natural desire is to transport a patient to the closest hospital so that the ambulance and its crew can quickly return to the disaster scene to pick up and transport another patient. Transferring the MCI from the disaster site to the closest hospital will negatively impact the hospital's ability to provide the "most good for the most patients."

However, in those communities that have limited numbers of hospitals, EMS will have no option but to transport patients to the nearest hospital.

Medical Assistance Teams

If the disaster is of significant proportion that additional on-scene resources are needed, some hospitals have developed disaster-response teams to help augment the EMS field response and provide on-site care, thus allowing prehospital care providers to be freed from the task of providing medical care at casualty collection points and, instead, perform patient transport (**Figure 19-12**). If outside resources are needed from the state or federal government, other emergency medical response teams are available in many municipalities.

As a result of the Metropolitan Medical Response System (MMRS) in the United States, MMRS task forces or strike teams have been created in many cities. The MMRS was developed and funded by the U.S. Department of Health and Human Services (DHHS) to help respond to terrorist or public health emergencies. The goal is to help integrate the various local response agencies and services together to enhance the response to such an event. These response assets comprise medical personnel from emergency medicine, trauma surgery, surgical subspecialties, and nursing. MMRS task forces can respond with resources that have been purchased through state and federal funds. These strike teams can be used to augment and backfill medical facilities or to staff mobile medical facilities that are established to provide surge capacity and medical care to patients.

On a larger-scale basis, the U.S. government has capabilities through the National Disaster Medical System to mobilize disaster medical assistance teams (DMATs). DMATs are able to provide field care as well as create mobile medical facilities, some of which have the capability to perform surgical interventions and meet the critical care needs of patients, when

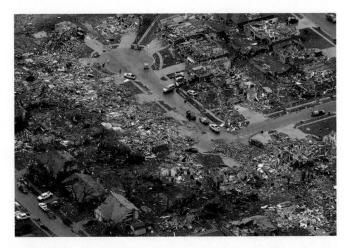

Figure 19-12 An aerial view of the destruction caused by a tornado in Oklahoma in 2013.
Source: © Tony Gutierrez/AP Images.

local resources have been overwhelmed. A request for DMATs must come through the appropriate channels, usually from the local emergency manager to the state emergency management authority and the governor's office through the federal government to the DHHS, which houses the National Disaster Medical System's response program.

Threat of Terrorism and Weapons of Mass Destruction

Terrorism may present one of the most challenging MCIs for emergency responders. The spectrum of terrorist threats is limitless, ranging from suicide bombers to conventional weapons or explosives to military weapons to WMDs (chemical, biologic, radiologic, and nuclear). Terrorist events have the greatest potential of all man-made disasters to generate large numbers of casualties and fatalities (see the Explosions and Weapons of Mass Destruction chapter for detailed information about specific weapons).

Terrorists have demonstrated their ingenuity and capacity to not be limited by conventional technology or weaponry. During the terrorist attacks on September 11, 2001, the terrorists used passenger jets full of fuel as "flying bombs," generating massive destruction of life and property.

One of the unique features of a terrorist threat, especially involving WMDs, is that psychological casualties usually predominate. Terrorists do not need to kill a large number of people to achieve their goals; they only need to create a climate of fear and panic to overwhelm the medical infrastructure. In the March 1995 sarin attacks in Tokyo, 5,000 casualties presented to hospitals. Of these, fewer than 1,000 had physical effects from the sarin gas; the remaining presented with psychological stress. The 2001 anthrax incidents in the United States also dramatically increased the number of individuals presenting to EDs with non-specific respiratory symptoms that ultimately did not result from actual anthrax infection.

Explosions and bombings continue to be the most frequent cause of mass casualties in disasters caused by terrorists worldwide, both as a primary event and when secondary devices are planted to injure or kill emergency responders. The majority of these bombings consist of relatively small explosives that produce low mortality rates. However, when strategically placed in buildings, pipelines, or moving vehicles, their impact can be much greater (**Figure 19-13**). The high morbidity and mortality rates are related not only to the intensity of the blast but also to the subsequent structural damage that leads to collapse of the targeted buildings. A greater threat will be disasters caused by conventional explosives in combination with a chemical, biologic, or radiologic agent, such as a "dirty bomb" that combines a conventional explosive with radioactive material.

The WMDs that create contaminated environments may prove to be the greatest disaster challenge. Emergency responders will not be able to bring victims into hospitals because of the risk of further contaminating medical facilities. Prehospital care providers must be prepared and equipped to perform triage, not

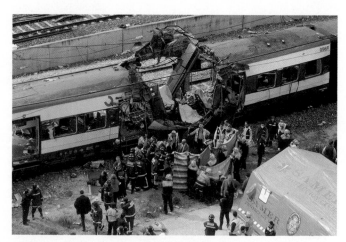

Figure 19-13 Madrid terrorist bombing, 2004.
Source: © Paul White/AP Images.

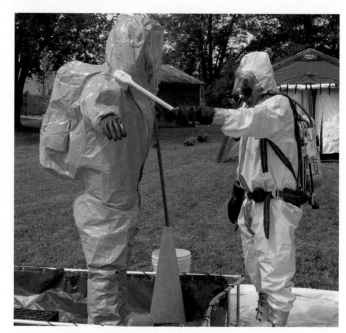

Figure 19-14 Decontamination in the "warm zone" by personnel in level B personal protective equipment.
Source: © Jones & Bartlett Learning.

only to determine the extent of the injuries but also to assess the potential for contamination and need for decontamination and initial stabilization. At the same time, prehospital care providers need to take appropriate steps to protect themselves from potential contamination.

Decontamination

Decontamination is an important consideration for all disasters involving hazardous materials and WMDs (**Figure 19-14**). Terrorist events, with their large number of victims, unknown substances, and multitude of "worried well," significantly increase the possibility of contaminated or potentially contaminated casualties (see the Explosions and Weapons of Mass Destruction chapter for additional information). As a general rule, patients being transported by ambulance should be decontaminated prior to the transport to avoid contaminating the receiving EDs.

Treatment Area

When responding to a disaster involving hazardous materials and WMDs, it is critical that the triage and casualty collection points be appropriately positioned upwind and uphill of the contaminated area (300 yards [275 meters]).

Psychological Response to Disasters

Psychological trauma and other adverse psychological **sequelae** are frequently the side effects of events such as natural disasters and unintentional disasters caused by humans.[14] In contrast, one of the objectives of terrorism is to inflict psychological pain, trauma, and disequilibrium. Maintaining good mental health is just as important as maintaining good physical health for all emergency responders.

Characteristics of Disasters That Affect Mental Health

Not all disasters have the same level of psychological impact. Disaster characteristics that seem to have the most significant mental health impact include the following:

- Little or no warning
- Serious threat to personal safety
- Potential unknown health effects
- Uncertain duration of the event
- Human error or malicious intent
- Symbolism related to the terrorist target

Factors Impacting Psychological Response

Everyone who experiences a disaster, either as a victim or as an emergency responder, is affected by it in some fashion. Fortunately, this does not mean that most individuals will develop a mental health disorder. It does mean, however, that all affected individuals, both victims and emergency responders, will have some type of psychological or emotional response to the event, and, in some cases, it can be career ending.

Similarly, there are both individual and collective reactions that interact with each other as individuals and communities recover from these extraordinary events. Factors affecting individual response to disasters include the following:

- Physical and psychological proximity to the event
- Exposure to gruesome or grotesque situations

- Diminished health status before or because of the disaster
- Magnitude of loss
- History of previous trauma

Factors impacting collective response to trauma include:

- Degree of community disruption
- Predisaster family and community stability
- Community leadership
- Cultural sensitivity of recovery efforts

Psychological Sequelae of Disasters

Postdisaster psychological responses are wide ranging, from mild stress responses to full-blown **posttraumatic stress disorder (PTSD)**, major depression, or acute stress disorder.[14] PTSD is a mental health condition that results from exposure to a horrific or terrifying event and leads to flashbacks to the incident, nightmares, anxiety, and uncontrollable thoughts about the incident. Although many people may exhibit signs of psychological stress, relatively few (typically 15% to 25%) of those most directly impacted will subsequently develop a diagnosable mental disorder.

Interventions

A number of relatively simple actions can help individuals to minimize the psychological effects of an event and assist them in returning to normal function.

- Individuals should return to normal activities as soon as possible.
- In persons with no diagnosed mental disorder, it is helpful to provide educational materials that help them understand what they and their families are experiencing.
- Crisis counseling should be provided, followed by referral when treatment is indicated.
- When a mental disorder is diagnosed, therapeutic interventions can be helpful, including cognitive-behavioral therapy and psychiatric medications.

Emergency Responder Stress

Emergency responders can also become secondary victims of stress and other psychological sequelae. These consequences can adversely affect their functioning during and after an event. They can also adversely impact their personal well-being and their family and work relationships. Supervisory personnel and colleagues should be alert for the development or manifestations of stress and psychological distress in those individuals who were involved in an incident response.

A number of intervention strategies are often used in an effort to help prevent and manage stress after an incident. These include debriefing, defusing, and grief management sessions. Collectively, these processes have been referred to as **critical incident stress management (CISM)**. The value of CISM has been questioned in recent years, particularly in those instances where CISM has been a mandated intervention for emergency responders. CISM can be offered as an option to those emergency responders who feel a need to participate but should not be mandated for all emergency responders.

Signs of Stress in Workers

Some common signs of stress in emergency responders include physiologic, emotional, cognitive, and behavioral elements.

Physiologic Signs

- Fatigue, even after rest
- Nausea
- Fine motor tremors
- Tics
- **Paresthesia**
- Dizziness
- Gastrointestinal upset
- Heart palpitations
- Choking or smothering sensations

Emotional Signs

- Anxiety
- Irritability
- Feeling overwhelmed
- Unrealistic anticipation of harm to self or others

Cognitive Signs

- Memory loss
- Decision-making difficulties
- Anomia (inability to name common objects or familiar people)
- Concentration problems or distractibility
- Reduced attention span
- Calculation difficulties

Behavioral Signs

- Insomnia
- Hypervigilance
- Crying easily
- Inappropriate humor
- Ritualistic behavior

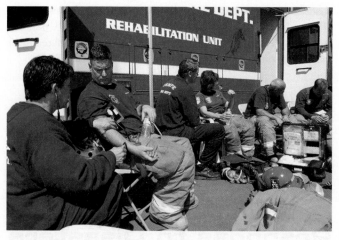

Figure 19-15 Fatigue contributes greatly to stress.
Source: © Jones and Bartlett Learning. Courtesy of MIEMSS.

Managing Stress On-Site

The following on-site interventions can assist in reducing stress:

- Limited exposure to traumatic stimuli
- Reasonable operational hours
- Adequate rest and sleep (**Figure 19-15**)
- Reasonable diet
- Regular exercise program
- Private time
- Talking to somebody who understands
- Monitoring signs of stress
- Identifiable endpoint for involvement

Disaster Education and Training

The development and implementation of a formal educational and training program will improve the prehospital care provider's ability to respond efficiently and effectively to an MCI. The prehospital care provider may fulfill a variety of roles in disaster and mass-casualty management, including mitigation and preparedness, search and rescue, triage, acute medical care, transport, and postevent recovery. Preparedness with regard to education and learning can be accomplished in various structured, as well as unstructured, learning environments. Each has its individual advantages and disadvantages, as measured by educational impact and comparative cost.

Independent learning is the foundation of disaster preparedness. A multitude of resources are available through printed literature as well as via the Internet. The CDC, public health agencies, FEMA, the Center for Domestic Preparedness, and the military forces all offer Internet-based learning opportunities and resources to individuals. Courses can be completed on an independent basis on a time-flexible schedule. The limitation of this modality of learning is that it does not allow for an interactive learning experience.

Group training is directed at specific response teams with regard to disaster response. Training programs are broadly available and include understanding incident command structure and WMD preparedness. Numerous professional and paraprofessional organizations have developed training programs and modules specific to their scope of professional practice, including public health, emergency medicine, critical care, and surgical and medical specialties, as well as all levels of prehospital care providers.

Simulations provide a training opportunity that brings together many individuals from varied backgrounds who are essential to the implementation of a disaster response. These exercises come in two specific forms: a tabletop exercise and a fully active field-training exercise. Tabletop exercises are cost-effective and highly useful methods to test and evaluate a disaster response. As the name suggests, these exercises are conducted around a table with the various participants verbally indicating what the expected response actions would be. A starting point with focused-incident goals and accomplishments and an order for completion of the exercise are usually established in advance. Tabletop exercises allow for real-time communications and interaction between multidisciplinary agencies. These activities require direction in the form of an experienced facilitator guiding the participants through the objective and critical evaluation of the results at the conclusion.

Field exercises are the most realistic training events, involving the actual execution and performance of the community disaster-response plan. The field exercise allows for a real-time assessment of the physical capacity to meet the objectives as defined in writing. Ideally, the exercises will involve moving victims from the point of impact and injury through the EMS response system and into definitive care at medical facilities. These events, however, are labor intensive, long in duration, and expensive.

For optimal learning from educational exercises, it is imperative that interdisciplinary training events be conducted often to include all the appropriate agencies and participants in a disaster response. In this way, each agency will have the opportunity to learn about and understand the roles, responsibilities, and capabilities of the co-responding services.

Common Pitfalls of Disaster Response

Numerous studies performed after significant MCIs have identified several consistent shortcomings in the medical response to these events. Identification of these deficiencies has resulted from subsequent evaluations of the response to these incidents as well as from communities that have performed risk, vulnerability, and needs assessments mandated by the U.S. government in order to receive funding to enhance the disaster-response infrastructure.

Preparedness

As emergency responders in a community, prehospital care providers prepare for the devastation that can occur in a mass-casualty event and plan for such events in a variety of ways. Although a tabletop drill can be a valuable method of preparing, it does not truly test the ability of the prehospital care provider to perform the necessary duties or the ability of the EMS agency to bring resources and assets to the site in a timely and efficient manner. Realistic functional disaster drills—during which victims are triaged, evaluated, "treated," transported, and tracked through the emergency medical response system to a hospital facility's doors in a realistic fashion—better test the emergency medical response that will be required. The ability to provide for *surge capacity* (the ability to expand services to meet a sudden influx of patients) and for supplying the large number of staff, ambulances, and other equipment needed for victims must be appropriately addressed by the entire medical response community.

Unfortunately, few agencies have actually tested a surge-capacity response in real time and, instead, have relied on tabletop drills as a measure of their ability to respond. Only through communitywide drills that involve multiple EMS agencies and ambulance services can the true level of preparedness to respond to an MCI as a community be assessed.

Communications

Many events have demonstrated that the lack of a unified communication system significantly hinders the ability to mount a coordinated response to an MCI. Individual communication systems are effective, but relying on a single system for communication is doomed to failure. The use of cellular phones became impossible when the central communication center located in the World Trade Center in New York City no longer existed. Also, the inability of police, fire, and EMS agencies to communicate with each other because of different radio technologies or frequencies is a serious deficiency that significantly reduces the ability to respond to MCIs effectively.

Redundancy in the system is of paramount importance, regardless of the chosen source for primary communications. Landlines, hardwired phone systems, cellular phone systems, satellite phone systems, VHF radios, and 800- to 900-MHz frequency systems all have some degree of vulnerability and could be compromised by an incident. Therefore, having multiple communications options is crucial in ensuring ongoing communications.

The following two principles are essential to maintain communications capability:

1. A unified communication system must exist to which all pertinent emergency responders in the community have access.
2. There must be system redundancy such that if one modality of communication fails or is disabled another source can be used efficiently and effectively as a backup.

Another common problem is the use of codes as a form of communication shorthand. Unfortunately, there is no single, agreed-upon set of codes for all agencies to use; thus, a responding agency may find itself at a scene with other agencies, all of whom are using codes that have the same terminology but different meanings. It is for this reason that ICS and NIMS recommend the use of plain English during an incident to avoid any confusion in meaning.

Scene Security

Scene security has become an ever-increasing problem in MCIs. Scene security is important for the following reasons:

1. To protect the emergency response teams from a second incident, resulting in further casualties.
2. To provide for the safe ingress and egress of emergency responders and victims unencumbered by onlookers at the disaster.
3. To protect and assist in securing the scene and physical evidence.

Scene security becomes a significant challenge during a disaster event because, by definition, all resources are stretched to the maximum of their capabilities and limits. Coordination with local law enforcement leaders is essential for the prehospital and medical community to ensure that security will be available.

Self-Dispatched Assistance

In many MCIs, public safety and EMS agencies (as well as medical responders of all types) from adjacent and even distant communities have responded to the scene without any formal request for assistance from the impacted jurisdiction.[5] These self-dispatched emergency responders, although well intentioned, often serve only to further complicate and confuse an already chaotic situation. With self-dispatched assistance, coordinated rescue efforts are impossible because of the lack of participation in the incident command structure, and communications issues are often made more difficult by incompatible radio systems brought by the self-dispatched emergency responders.

Ideally, public safety and EMS agencies should respond to a disaster site only if they have been specifically requested to do so by the responsible jurisdiction and the incident commander.[15] In addition, it is extremely helpful if access to the scene is controlled and a staging area is established as soon as possible to which all responding units and volunteers can be directed to be credentialed and better incorporated into the incident response.

Supply and Equipment Resources

Most EMS agencies have plans for the routine utilization of supplies and have purchased supplies based on the expected daily demand. Events of large magnitude will rapidly exhaust these resources and may disrupt conventional supply lines. Having a seamless plan and backup plan for the reconstitution of supplies during a disaster is essential for the ongoing mission of treating victims. Supplies must be available in a timely fashion, and appropriate mechanisms must be in place for distribution. Distribution plans cannot include the prehospital care providers in the field, who will already be fully occupied.

The EMS agency must have a plan for pharmaceutical replenishment in place. In those communities that have been designated to receive Metropolitan Medical Response System (MMRS) funds, community stockpiles of pharmaceuticals have been or are being purchased in preparation for such events.

Failure to Notify Hospitals

In the confusion of responding to and assessing an MCI as well as performing the numerous tasks that must be accomplished in initiating the prehospital medical response to such an event, it is often easy for EMS agencies to overlook the need to contact hospitals and have them activate their internal disaster plans. Numerous actual events have demonstrated that unless hospital notification and activation are integral parts of the EMS agency's MCI plan, hospitals may be left on their own to discover that an incident has occurred, either when patients self-transport and report the event or when the first ambulance arrives to an unprepared facility. It is essential that EMS agencies include hospital notification as part of their MCI plan so that a coordinated seamless transition from field care to hospital care can occur.

In addition, ongoing communication from the field to the hospital and from the hospital to the field is important for monitoring the status of the event and the patient load at hospitals.

Media

The media are often seen as a detriment to the physical and operational process of disaster response. However, EMS agencies are encouraged to partner with the media because these outlets can be an asset during a disaster response. The media can provide for the dissemination of appropriate and accurate information to the general population, giving them directions as to what actions they can take to maintain personal safety and where to report to obtain information or to reunite with family members, as well as communicating other needed information. It is inevitable that the media will broadcast information to the public, and as emergency responders, prehospital care providers have the responsibility to partner with the media to ensure that the information provided is timely and accurate as well as helpful to the response process.

Having a designated public information officer (PIO) who is trained to deal with the media and authorized to speak about the incident is an important method of communicating with the various media representatives seeking information about the incident. Of particular importance is the recognition that each responding agency will likely have a PIO present. Under the unified command concept, ideally one consistent message needs to be delivered by a single PIO; however, any messages given out by the various agencies' PIOs must be consistent with each other.

Summary

- Disasters result from natural climactic or geologic events; however, they may also result from intentional or unintentional acts of humans.
- Although disasters may be unpredictable, adequate preparation can turn an unthinkable event into a manageable situation.
- Implementation of the incident command system allows multiple agencies to collaborate in the disaster response.
- Despite the fact that disasters occur in varying sizes and result from many different causes, common pitfalls have been identified that hinder management of such an event, including:
  - Inadequate preparedness
  - Communications failures
  - Inadequate scene safety measures
  - Self-dispatched assistance
  - Supply and equipment shortages
  - Poor media relations
- Disaster response may take a heavy psychological toll on those involved, both victims and emergency responders.
- The best outcomes in response to MCIs result from the creation of a well-devised disaster plan that has been rehearsed, tested, and critiqued to identify and improve problem areas.

SCENARIO RECAP

You are dispatched to a local high school that has been placed into service as a shelter following community-wide flooding from a large weather event. Your community's mayor and other dignitaries are in attendance at the school to address the community's concerns about closed roads and the lack of electrical power.

While en route to the scene, dispatch updates you that there are multiple reports of many casualties following the structural collapse of elevated bleachers in the gym that were being used as seating during a storm update. Police and fire resources are also en route to the scene but have limited available resources due to other ongoing, storm-related public safety incidents.

- What safety and security concerns would you expect to encounter?
- What triage system should be utilized?
- How should the response to this incident be organized?

SCENARIO SOLUTION

While still en route to the high school, preplanned mutual aid resources are summoned to assist. The local hospitals are also updated that you are responding to an MCI. As the first-arriving EMS unit, you report to the incident command post where a unified command structure is being assembled. As practiced, you conduct an overall assessment of the scene and the medical needs and relay that information back to dispatch.

Triage team leaders begin sorting through the casualties. Treatment areas are established a safe distance from the collapse. As casualties arrive at the treatment areas, they are organized by acuity of injuries. Prehospital care providers begin appropriate care and secondary triage of the injured. As mutual aid resources arrive at staging areas, they are assigned tasks and placed into service. Transport vehicles arrive and the injured are transported to hospitals. All patients are tracked and accounted for through each step of this process.

Once all casualties have left the scene, fire services, code inspectional services, and police begin to investigate the origin of the collapse.

References

1. World Health Organization. Definitions: emergencies. http://www.who.int/hac/about/definitions/en/index.html. Accessed January 26, 2013.

2. Noji EK. *The Public Health Consequences of Disasters.* New York, NY: Oxford University Press; 1997.

3. Noji EK, Siverston KT. Injury prevention in natural disasters: a theoretical framework. *Disasters.* 1987;11:290.

4. Cuny SC. Introduction to disaster management. Lesson 5: technologies of disaster management. *Prehosp Disaster Med.* 1993;6:372.

5. U.S. Department of Health and Human Services, Agency for Healthcare Research and Quality. Mass medical care with scarce resources: a community planning guide. AHRQ Publication No. 07-0001, February 2007. http://www.ahrq.gov/research/mce/. Accessed January 4, 2014.

6. Auf der Heide E. The importance of evidence-based disaster planning. *Ann Emerg Med.* 2006;47:34-49.

7. Larrey DJ. *Memoires de Chirurgie Militaire, et Campagnes.* Vols 1-4. Paris, France: J. Smith, Publisher; 1812-1817.

8. Burkle FM, ed. *Disaster Medicine: Application for the Immediate Management and Triage of Civilian and Military Disaster Victims.* New Hyde Park, NY: Medication Examination Publishing; 1984.

9. Burkle FM, Hogan DE, Burstein JL. *Disaster Medicine.* Philadelphia, PA: Lippincott, Williams & Wilkins; 2002.

10. Lerner EB, Schwartz RB, Coule PL, et al. Mass casualty triage: an evaluation of the data and development of a proposed national guideline. *Disaster Med Public Health Preparedness.* 2008;2(suppl 1):S25-S34.

11. Super G. *START: A Triage Training Module.* Newport Beach, CA: Hoag Memorial Hospital Presbyterian; 1984.

12. Burkle FM, Newland C, Orebaugh S, et al. Emergency medicine in the Persian Gulf. Part II. Triage methodology lessons learned. *Ann Emerg Med.* 1994;23:748.

13. Bloch YH, Schwartz D, Pinkert M, et al. Distribution of casualties in a mass-casualty incident with three local hospitals in the periphery of a densely populated area: lessons learned from the medical management of a terrorist attack. *Prehosp Disast Med.* 2007;22:186-192.

14. Hick JL, Ho JD, Heegaard WG, et al. Emergency medical services response to a major freeway bridge collapse. *Disaster Med Public Health Preparedness.* 2008; 2(suppl 1):S17-S24.

15. Asaeda G, Cherson A, Richmond N, Clair J, Guttenberg M. Unsolicited medical personnel volunteering at disaster scenes. A joint position paper from the National Association of EMS Physicians and the American College of Emergency Physicians. *Prehosp Emerg Care.* 2003;7:147-148.

Suggested Reading

Briggs SM, Brinsfield KH. *Advanced Disaster Medical Response: Manual for Providers.* Boston, MA: Harvard Medical International; 2003.

De Boer J, Dubouloz M. *Handbook of Disaster Medicine: Emergency Medicine in Mass Casualty Situations.* Utrecht, The Netherlands: Van der Wees; 2000.

Eachempati SR, Flomenbaum N, Barie PS. Biological warfare: current concerns for the health care provider. *J Trauma.* 2002;52:179.

Emerg Med Clin North Am. 1996;14(2), (entire issue).

U.S. Department of Homeland Security, Federal Emergency Management Agency. www.fema.gov. Accessed January 7, 2014.

Feliciano DV, Anderson GV Jr., Rozycki GS, et al. Management of casualties from the bombing at the centennial olympics. *Am J Surg.* 1998;176(6):538.

Hirshberg A, Holcomb JB, Mattox KL. Hospital trauma care in multiple-casualty incidents: a critical view. *Ann Emerg Med.* 2001;37(6):647.

Hogan DE, Burstein, JL, eds. *Disaster Medicine.* 2nd ed. Philadelphia, PA: Lippincott, Williams & Wilkins; 2007.

Slater MS, Trunkey DD. Terrorism in America: an evolving threat. *Arch Surg.* 1997;132(10):1059.

Stein M, Hirshberg A. Medical consequences of terrorism: the conventional weapon threat. *Surg Clin North Am.* 1999;79(6):1537.

www.fema.gov

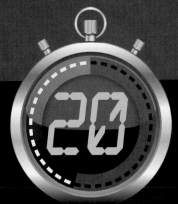
Explosions and Weapons of Mass Destruction

CHAPTER OBJECTIVES

At the completion of this chapter, the reader will be able to do the following:

- Discuss the essential considerations regarding mitigation of a weapon of mass destruction (WMD) event:

  - Scene assessment
  - Incident command
  - Personal protective equipment
  - Patient triage
  - Principle of decontamination

- Describe the mechanisms of injury, evaluation and management, and transport considerations associated with specific categories of WMD agent:

  - Explosive agents
  - Incendiary agents
  - Chemical agents
  - Biologic agents
  - Radiologic agents

- Know how to access and utilize resources for further study.

SCENARIO

It is a warm summer evening and you are dispatched to the scene of a reported explosion outside of a popular café. You know that this café is usually quite busy and that it typically has patrons both inside and outside on the patio. Dispatch tells you that at this point the number of victims is unknown but that they have received multiple emergency calls. Other public safety agencies have also been dispatched to the location.

Upon arrival at the location, you note that you are the first prehospital care provider on scene. No incident command has yet been established. Dozens of people are running about the scene. Many are screaming for you to assist victims who are obviously bleeding. Other victims are lying on the ground.

- What will you do first?
- What are your priorities as you determine your course of action?
- How will you care for so many people?

Introduction

Preparing to manage an incident that potentially involves a weapon of mass destruction (WMD) is a daily challenge for emergency medical services (EMS) systems. Part of the reason that WMDs are so prevalent is that they can be made from a great variety of materials. Although a number of different mnemonics are used to recall the various types of WMDs, perhaps the easiest to remember is BNICE, which stands for **b**iologic, **n**uclear, **i**ncendiary, **c**hemical, and **e**xplosive. Clearly, a person or organization intent on harming a large group of people does not have to look far for an effective means of inflicting damage or casualties.

Recent history has demonstrated that these events can occur at any time and in any location.

- The 1993 World Trade Center bombing in New York City resulted in 6 deaths and 548 casualties, with more than 1,000 people requiring or seeking assistance from EMS. Emergency responders became casualties as well, with 105 fire fighters reporting injuries.
- The 1995 bombing of the Murrah Federal Building in Oklahoma City resulted in 168 deaths and 700 casualties. Eighty percent of the deaths resulted from the collapse of the building, rather than the direct effects of the explosive. One-third of the patients brought to one Oklahoma City hospital were transported by EMS. Sixty-four percent of these transported patients required admission to the hospital, whereas only 6% of self-referred patients to the emergency department (ED) required admission.
- The September 11, 2001, World Trade Center attacks in which terrorists used passenger aircraft as flying bombs resulted in over 1,100 injured survivors, with almost one-third of those casualties transported to the hospital by prehospital care providers. Emergency responders accounted for 29% of the casualties.
- The multiple train bombings in Madrid, Spain, in 2004 caused 190 deaths and 2,051 injuries.
- The mass transit attack in London in 2005 in which bombs exploded in three subway trains and one double-decker bus caused 52 deaths and more than 779 injuries.
- The Boston Marathon bombings in 2013 resulted in 3 deaths and approximately 264 injuries.

Although conventional explosives are the most commonly used and most likely form of WMD event, EMS systems worldwide have also been challenged by chemical and biohazard events. The 1994 sarin gas attack in Matsumoto, Japan, killed 7 people and injured more than 300. The 1995 sarin gas attack in the Tokyo subway system killed 12, and more than 5,000 people sought medical attention, many of whom were asymptomatic but concerned about possible exposure. The Tokyo Fire Department sent 1,364 fire fighters to the 16 affected subway sites, and 135 emergency responders (10%) were affected by direct or indirect exposure to the nerve agent.

No life-threatening bioterrorism assault in the United States has yielded a large number of casualties, but this does not mean that EMS systems have not been challenged to prepare for bioterrorism threats. During 1998 and 1999, almost 6,000 persons across the United States were affected by a series of anthrax-related hoaxes in more than 200 incidents. The letters containing anthrax delivered in the fall of 2001 resulted in only 22 cases of clinical anthrax but generated countless calls for public safety agencies to respond to suspicious packages and powders.

Although not a bioterrorist event, severe acute respiratory syndrome (SARS), a naturally occurring infectious disease outbreak, seriously challenged the Toronto EMS system in 2003. During the epidemic, 526 paramedics had to be quarantined, mostly due to potential unprotected exposure to the virus. This loss of key resources seriously strained Toronto's ability to mitigate the crisis.

The threat that EMS may one day have to respond to a radiologic WMD event grows, with increasing speculation that terrorists may detonate a radiologic dispersal device ("dirty bomb") that will generate injuries and panic about radioactive contamination.

General Considerations

Scene Assessment

The ability of the prehospital care provider to assess the scene properly is crucial to ensuring personal safety and the safety of other emergency responders. WMD events pose significant threats to responding emergency services. In the case of a high-explosives detonation, there may be fire, spilled hazardous materials, power line hazards, and risk of falling debris or *subsidence* (the creation of craters). One emergency responder was killed by falling debris in response to the Oklahoma City bombing.[1] Many emergency responders were killed in the 2001 World Trade Center attack, including 343 fire fighters, 15 emergency medical technicians, and 3 law enforcement officers when the buildings collapsed.

Chemical attacks potentially expose the prehospital care provider to the offending agent not only from the primary source— the weapon—but also from secondary exposure to contamination of victims' skin, clothing, and personal belongings. Biologic agents, depending on the form of their delivery, pose a risk of illness from the offending agent (e.g., aerosolized anthrax spores) or from transmission of a communicable disease (e.g., plague or smallpox). A further risk to prehospital care providers and patients alike is the possibility of additional devices. For example, a second bomb could be placed at the scene of the incident, set to explode after arrival of emergency responders, with the intention of increasing not only injury but also confusion and panic.

All of these factors must be taken into consideration when dispatched to the scene of a possible explosive or WMD event and when evaluating the scene. Before entering any such scene, all responding units from all involved agencies should approach from an upwind and uphill direction and stage at a safe distance from the incident site. Approaching from an upwind direction is important because many of the WMDs, particularly the chemical and biologic agents, pose an inhalation risk, and inadvertent exposure is more likely at a downwind location. An uphill location is chosen to avoid exposure to runoff at an incident involving the release of liquid chemical.

Prehospital care providers should then conduct a critical evaluation, ideally with binoculars, of the scene looking for clues that would warn them of potential hazards. The presence of visible vapors, spilled liquid, or possibly ongoing dispersion should be noted; such observations are indicative of an active danger. Looking to see how patients are presenting must be included as part of the scene assessment, with particular attention to the clues, such as seizures in multiple casualties, suggesting a possible chemical or biologic agent release. Prehospital care providers need to communicate their observations through the chain of command so that proper steps can be taken to mount an appropriate response, to increase the protective measures for the emergency responders, and to ensure the delivery of care to patients.

Access to and egress from the potentially contaminated site must be controlled. Concerned bystanders and well-meaning volunteers must not be allowed to enter the scene, as they may contribute to the casualty count if they expose themselves to the agent. Victims of the incident must also be contained as they seek to evacuate the scene, since self-transport may further disseminate a dangerous chemical or substance to unsuspecting contacts or hospital EDs. Similar to a hazardous materials incident, scene control zones (hot, warm, cold) should be established with controlled access points and transit corridors to prevent spread of the contaminants and inadvertent exposure and to provide safe areas for patient assessment and management (**Figure 20-1**) (see the Personal Protective Equipment section).

Incident Command System

The National Incident Management System describes the framework to be used for response to a major incident or disaster, particularly when there are multiple agencies and jurisdictions involved in the response. The incident command system (ICS) defines the chain of command through which the response to a scene is organized and structured and how communication takes place. The ICS is the model tool for command, control, and coordination. It was developed to mitigate the recurring failures of response to disasters, which include the following:

1. Nonstandard terminology used by responding agencies
2. Nonstandard and nonintegrated command structures of responding agencies
3. Lack of capability to expand and contract as required by the situation
4. Nonstandard and nonintegrated communications
5. Lack of consolidated incident action plans
6. Lack of designated facilities

ICS offers a management structure that coordinates all available resources to ensure an effective response. All incidents, regardless of size or complexity, will have a designated incident commander, who may be the first responding prehospital care provider until relieved by some other

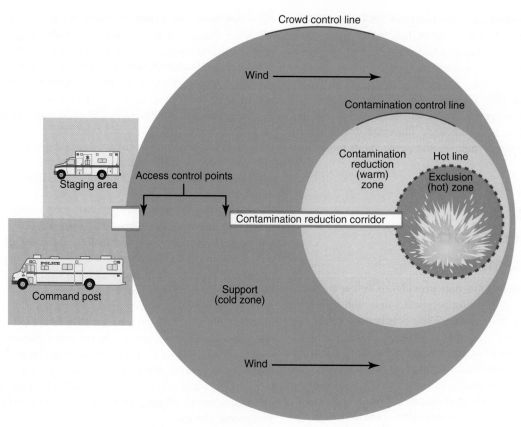

Figure 20-1 The scene of a WMD or hazardous materials incident is generally divided into hot, warm, and cold zones.

competent authority. It is essential that prehospital care providers are familiar with and have the opportunity to practice implementation of the ICS (see the Scene Assessment and the Disaster Management chapters for a detailed discussion of ICS).

Personal Protective Equipment

When responding to WMD events, the proper personal protective equipment (PPE) needs to be worn. Requirements for PPE may range from the standard daily uniform to a fully encapsulated suit with **self-contained breathing apparatus (SCBA)** depending upon the specific agent involved and the specific role and training level of the prehospital care provider. This equipment is designed to protect the emergency responder from exposure to offending agents by providing defined levels of protection of the respiratory tract, skin, and other mucous membranes. When dealing with hazardous substances of any type, PPE has generally been described in terms of the following levels (**Figure 20-2**):

- *Level A.* This level offers the highest amount of respiratory and skin protection. The respiratory tract is protected by a SCBA or **supplied air respirator (SAR)** delivering air to the emergency responder with positive

pressure. A chemical-resistant barrier that completely encapsulates the wearer protects the skin and mucous membranes. It takes considerable time to don this protection, thus delaying the provider's ability to access and help patients. Patience on the part of the prehospital care providers responding to the chaos of this type of event is essential. Additional resources also need to be committed to assist emergency responders with donning and doffing this level of protection. The amount of time that a trained emergency responder can spend in level A protection is also limited by both the available air supply and the buildup of heat and humidity within the enclosed suit.

- *Level B.* The respiratory tract is protected in the same manner as in Level A protection, with positive-pressure-supplied air. Nonencapsulated chemical-resistant garments, including suit, gloves, and boots, which provide splash protection only, protect the skin and mucous membranes. The highest respiratory protection is afforded, with a lower level of skin protection. Similar to level A protection, level B protection takes time to don and doff, and work time within the suit is again limited.

- *Level C.* The respiratory tract is protected by an **air-purifying respirator (APR)**. This may be a

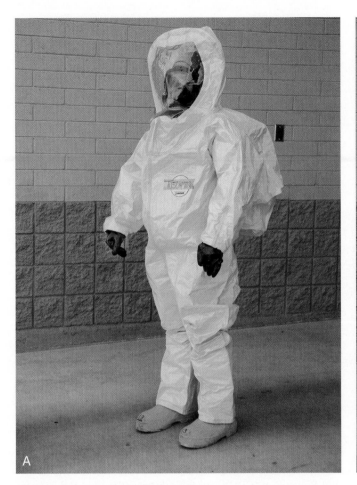

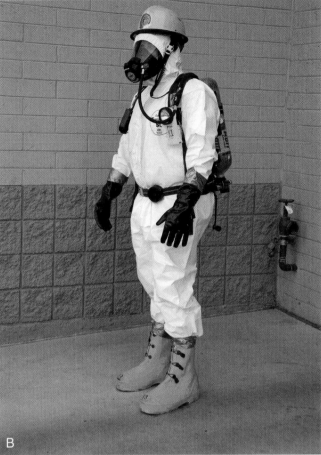

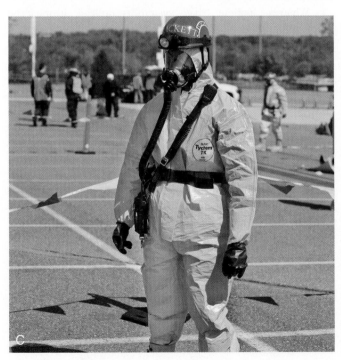

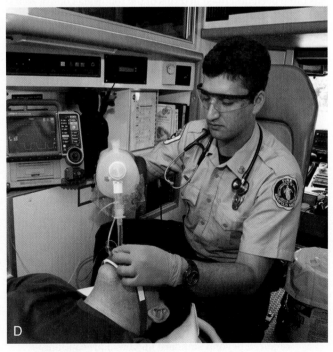

Figure 20-2 Personal protective equipment. **A.** Level A. **B.** Level B. **C.** Level C. **D.** Level D.
Source: Courtesy of Rick Brady.

powered air-purifying respirator (PAPR), which draws ambient air through a filter canister and delivers it under positive pressure to a face mask or hood, or a nonpowered APR, which relies on the wearer to draw ambient air through a filter canister by breathing through a properly fitted mask. The skin protection is the same as for level B.

- *Level D.* This level represents standard work clothes (i.e., standard uniform for the emergency responder) and may also include a gown, gloves, and surgical mask. Level D provides minimal respiratory protection and minimal skin protection.

It might be concluded that the best protective posture for a prehospital care provider is always to respond in the highest level of protection, level A, regardless of the threat. This is, however, not a reasonable response. Level A protection is cumbersome, often making manual tasks difficult to perform. Significant training and experience are required when using an SCBA. Level A protection puts the wearer at risk for heat stress and physical exhaustion. It can make communication between emergency responders and victims difficult. Appropriate PPE must be selected based on the presumed threat, the level of training, and the operational responsibilities of the prehospital care provider. Most importantly, the prehospital care provider must be trained and practiced in the use of the PPE selected.

Control Zones

PPE is selected based on the known (or suspected) hazards of the environment and proximity to the threat. Proximity to the threat has often been described in terms of the following control zones:

- The *hot zone* is the area where there is immediate threat to health and life. This includes an environment contaminated with a hazardous gas, vapor, aerosol, liquid, or powder. PPE adequate to protect the emergency responder is determined based on potential routes of exposure to the substance and the likely agent. Level A protection is most often used in the hot zone.
- The *warm zone* is characterized as an area where the concentration of the offending agent is limited. In the case of a WMD scene, this is the area to which victims are brought from the hot zone and where any decontamination takes place. The prehospital care provider is still at risk for exposure if working in this area as the agent is carried from the hot zone on victims, emergency responders, and equipment. PPE is recommended based on potential routes of exposure to the substance.
- The *cold zone* is the area outside the hot and warm zones that is not contaminated, where there is no risk of exposure, and thus no specific level of PPE is required beyond standard universal precautions.

It is important to note that it is often difficult to define these control zones and that they may be dynamic rather than static.

Factors that contribute to the dynamics of the control zones include the activity of the victims and emergency responders and ambient conditions. For example, unless completely incapacitated, contaminated victims might walk toward prehospital care providers in the cold zone or leave the scene completely, either in panic or with the intention of seeking medical aid at a nearby hospital. By design, warm zones and cold zones are designated upwind of the hot zone, but if wind direction changes, prehospital care providers would be at risk of exposure if they were unable to don the proper PPE or to rapidly retreat. These contingencies must be anticipated when planning for or responding to a WMD event.

Patient Triage

Prehospital care providers will potentially face a large and overwhelming number of victims who will require evaluation and treatment after a WMD event. Every EMS system should identify and rehearse a mechanism for rapidly triaging victims. The objective of patient triage in a WMD incident is to do the greatest good for the greatest number of victims.

Field triage is typically based on easily measurable physiologic criteria that assign patients to severity categories in order to identify those victims who require treatment and transport to a medical treatment facility most urgently.[2] Several triage schemes and criteria are available.[3] Triage systems include the START (**s**imple **t**riage **a**nd **r**apid **t**reatment) system, the MASS (**m**ove, **a**ssess, **s**ort, **s**end) system, and the SALT (**s**ort by ability to move, **a**ssess need for **l**ifesaving interventions, **t**riage and **t**ransport) system advocated by the Centers for Disease Control and Prevention (CDC)[4] (for more information, see the Disaster Management chapter).

Whatever patient triage system is utilized, it must be employed in routine EMS operations to promote familiarity and to ensure recognition among prehospital care providers at all levels of care, including the hospital or trauma center.

Principles of Decontamination

Patients and prehospital care providers alike may require decontamination after exposure to agents that may pose a risk to health. These individuals should have decontamination procedures performed in the field in a designated decontamination area. Decontamination areas are typically upwind and uphill of the affected area when conditions allow. Known exposure to only vapor or gases does not require decontamination to prevent secondary contamination, although the victim's clothing should be removed.

Decontamination is a two-step process that first involves removal of all clothing, jewelry, and shoes, which are bagged, tagged, and secured for later identification. These items may serve as evidence in incident investigation and may be returned to the owner if successfully decontaminated. The simple act of removing clothing achieves removal of 70% to 90% of contamination. Any remaining solid contaminant should be carefully brushed away and any liquid contamination should be blotted off. The second step involves washing the skin surfaces with water or water and a mild detergent to ensure removal of all substances from the skin. Avoid using harsh detergents or bleach solutions on skin and scrub gently. Chemically or physically aggravating the skin may contribute to increased absorption of the offending agent. When washing, skin folds, axillae, groin, buttocks, and feet must receive special attention because contaminants can collect in these areas and may be overlooked.

Decontamination should be performed in a systematic manner to avoid missing areas of contaminated skin. Contact lenses should be removed from the eyes, and the mucous membranes should be irrigated with copious amounts of water or saline, especially if the patient is symptomatic. Ambulatory patients should be able to perform their own decontamination under instruction from prehospital care providers. Nonambulatory patients will require the assistance of emergency responders properly outfitted with appropriate PPE to decontaminate patients on litters.

Expeditious decontamination may be warranted in the effort to decrease exposure time to various life-threatening substances. All prehospital care providers need to be familiar with a hasty decontamination procedure that may be executed even before arrival of the formal hazardous materials/decontamination team, to minimize exposure time for both patients and emergency responders.

When planning for and setting up a decontamination area, the issues to consider include:

- Offering privacy for males and females required to disrobe
- Having warm water available when possible for irrigation and showering
- Providing a suitable substitute for clothing at the completion of decontamination
- Ensuring victims that their personal belongings will be secure until a final disposition is made regarding their return or necessary disposal
- Collecting effluent, if practical

After the victim has been decontaminated, there must be a method in place for documenting that the patient has undergone decontamination. At this point, the victim is not released but is instead observed for a period to note whether signs of toxicity occur or reoccur, indicating incomplete removal of the offending agent and the need for repeat washing and treatment.

Explosions and Explosives

Understanding injury from explosives is essential for all prehospital care providers in both civilian and military settings. Prehospital care providers need to understand the pathophysiology of injury resulting from unintentional and industrial explosive devices and from the wide range of antipersonnel explosive devices such as letter bombs, shaped warheads from rocket-propelled grenades, antipersonnel land mines, aerial-delivered cluster bombs, enhanced blast weapons, and improvised explosive devices

(IEDs). A study of the 36,110 bombing incidents in the United States reported by the Bureau of Alcohol, Tobacco, and Firearms (ATF) between 1983 and 2002 concluded that "the U.S. experience reveals that materials used for bombings are readily available [and] healthcare providers . . . need to be prepared."[5]

Explosions occur in homes (primarily due to gas leaks or fires) and are an occupational hazard of many industries, including mining and those involved in demolition, chemical manufacturing, or the handling of fuel or dust-producing substances such as grain. Industrial explosions result from chemical spills, fires, faulty equipment maintenance, or electrical/machinery malfunctions and may produce toxic fumes, building collapse, secondary explosions, falling debris, and large numbers of casualties. Another common cause of explosion is the rupture of a pressurized containment vessel, such as boiler, when the internal pressure exceeds the capability of the container to withstand the elevated pressure.

As a whole, however, unintentional explosions are responsible for relatively few injuries and deaths (e.g., 150 in the United States in 2004[6]) compared with the large numbers of injuries and deaths produced by explosives used by terrorists and military adversaries worldwide.

Terrorists worldwide are increasingly using bombs, especially IEDs, against civilian targets. These devices are inexpensive, are made from easily obtained materials, and result in the devastating havoc that focuses international exposure on their efforts. An emergency responder is much more likely to encounter injury from conventional explosives than from a chemical, biologic, or nuclear attack. Several databases compile statistics on terrorist events and the nature of the incidents. In one database, it is reported that only 56 of 23,000 incidents involved the use of a chemical, biologic, or radiologic weapon; in another database, 41 of 69,000 reportedly involved these types of weapons.[7]

Because both civilian and military emergency responders may be called upon during a bomb attack on civilian populations, all prehospital care providers need to be familiar with their roles during these increasingly frequent occurrences.

Review of the U.S. State Department's historical data on terrorist incidents worldwide between 1961 and 2003 reveals a significant increase beginning in 1996 and an exponential increase after the attacks of September 11, 2001.[8] In past decades, there has been a shift from bomb attacks occurring largely in certain "trouble spots," such as Northern Ireland (1970s) or Beirut, Lebanon (1980s), to incidents occurring in all regions of the world, from Atlanta to Jerusalem to Nairobi. In recent years, however, primary trouble spots have been Iraq, where 60% of the fatalities (a total of 13,606) caused by terrorist attacks occurred in 2007, Afghanistan, Pakistan, and Syria.[9]

At present, although the United States is not typically exposed to as many bomb attacks as other countries, bomb-related incidents, including the theft/recovery of explosives, accidental explosions, and so forth, in 2012 totaled 4,033. These incidents resulted in 37 injuries and 1 fatality (**Figure 20-3**).[10]

Worldwide, a total of 10,283 terrorist attacks were reported in 2011, which resulted in 25,903 injuries and 12,533 deaths, a 5% and 18% decrease, respectively, from 2010.[11,12] A majority

(~70%) of the victims were civilians.[13] Continuing the trend from previous years, most attacks were carried out by terrorists using bombs and small arms.[13] Of note, in 2007, terrorists coordinated secondary attacks to target emergency responders and intensified their enhancement of IEDs with chlorine gas to create clouds of toxic fumes.[13] In recent years, however, the number of terror attacks and their associated injuries and deaths have declined (**Figure 20-4**).[14]

Categories of Explosives

Prehospital care providers need to consider the type of explosive device and its location when evaluating casualties of terrorist blast incidents.[15] Explosives fall into one of two categories based on the velocity of detonation: high explosives and low explosives.

High Explosives

High explosives react almost instantaneously. Because they are designed to detonate and release their energy very quickly, high explosives are capable of producing a shock wave, or **overpressure phenomenon**, which can result in primary blast injury. The initial explosion creates an instantaneous rise in pressure, creating a *shock wave* that travels outward at supersonic speed (1,400–9,000 miles per second, or 2,250–14,500 kilometers (km) per second).[16] Overpressures from high explosions can exceed 4 million pounds per square inch (psi), compared with 14.7 psi ambient pressure. The shock wave is the leading front and an integral component of the *blast wave*, which is created on the rapid release of enormous amounts of energy, with subsequent propulsion of fragments, generation of environmental debris, and often intense thermal radiation (**Figure 20-5**). The shock wave or pressure wave propagates from the point of origin, rapidly dissipating as the distance from the point of detonation increases. This wave is not to be confused with wind generated by a blast.

Common examples of high explosives are 2,4,6-trinitrotoluene (TNT), nitroglycerin, dynamite, ammonium nitrate-fuel oil, and the more recent polymer-bonded explosives that have 1.5 times the power of TNT, such as gelignite and the plastic explosive Semtex. High explosives have a sharp,

Figure 20-3   Explosives-Related Incidents in the United States

Year	Number of Explosives Incidents	Number of Injuries	Number of Fatalities
2012	4,033	37	1
2011	5,219	36	5
2010	4,897	99	22
2009	3,886	57	4
2008	3,558	118	23
2007	2,772	60	15
2006	3,445	135	14
2005	3,722	148	18
2004	3,790	263	36

Figure 20-4   Terrorist Attacks Worldwide with Associated Injuries and Deaths: 2007–2011

	2007	2008	2009	2010	2011
Attacks worldwide	14,415	11,663	10,968	11,641	10,283
People killed as a result of terrorism, worldwide	22,720	15,709	15,311	13,193	12,533
People injured as a result of terrorism, worldwide	44,103	33,901	32,660	30,684	25,903

Source: Data from http://www.state.gov/j/ct/rls/crt/2011/195555.htm#footnote1. Accessed 07/03/2013.

Figure 20-5 Explosion Terminology

- **Blast wave:** A blast wave results from the sudden conversion of a high explosive from a solid (or liquid) to a gas. This event produces an almost instantaneous rise in atmospheric pressure in the area around the detonation, resulting in highly compressed air molecules that travel faster than the speed of sound. This wave will dissipate rapidly over time and distance.
- **Shock wave:** The leading edge of a blast wave is the shock wave. This high-velocity wave travels at supersonic speeds (10,000–26,000 feet per second, or 3,000–8,000 meters per second). The shock wave carries energy that will strike and pass through objects in its path, causing damage.
- **Stress wave:** Stress waves are high-frequency, supersonic, longitudinal pressure waves that create high local forces with small, rapid distortions of tissue. Longitudinal waves are waves in which the particle displacement occurs in the same direction as the wave is travelling. They cause microvascular injury and are reinforced/reflected at tissue interfaces, thereby enhancing injury potential, especially in gas-filled organs such as the lungs, ears, and intestines. They cause injury via pressure differentials across delicate

structures such as alveoli, rapid compression/re-expansion of gas-filled structures, and reflection of the tension wave (a component of the compressive stress wave) at the tissue–gas interface.
- **Shear wave:** Shear waves are low-frequency, transverse waves with a lower velocity and longer duration than stress waves. Transverse waves are waves in which the displaced particles move perpendicular to the direction in which the wave is travelling. They cause asynchronous movement of tissues. The degree of damage depends on the extent to which the asynchronous motions overcome inherent tissue elasticity, resulting in tearing of tissue and possible disruption of organ attachments.
- **Blast wind:** After the detonation of a high explosive, the force of the explosion pushes all of the air out of the area immediately around the detonation site, creating a sudden vacuum. Once the force of the explosion has been spent, all of the air that was pushed out comes rushing back in response to the vacuum. The result is a powerful wind that can cause objects and debris to be sucked back in toward the site of the explosion.

shattering effect (*brisance*) that can pulverize bone and soft tissue, create blast overpressure injuries (*barotrauma*), and propel debris at ballistic speeds (*fragmentation*). It is also important to note that a high explosive may result in a low-order explosion, particularly if the explosive has deteriorated as a result of age (Semtex) or in some cases become wet (dynamite). The reverse, however, is not true; a low explosive cannot produce a high-order explosion.

Low Explosives

Low explosives (e.g., gunpowder), when activated, change relatively slowly from a solid to a gaseous state (in an action more characteristic of burning than of detonation), generally creating a blast wave that moves less than 6,500 feet per second (2,000 meters per second). Examples of low explosives include pipe bombs, gunpowder, and pure petroleum-based bombs such as Molotov cocktails.[17] Explosions resulting from container rupture and ignition of volatile compounds fall into this category as well. Because they release their energy much more slowly, low explosives are not capable of producing overpressure.

The type and amount of explosive will determine the size of the blast associated with detonation of the device. This fact makes the approach to the scene and the location for staging emergency responders and equipment a critical decision. When responding to a scene that involves either a suspicious device or a potential secondary device, all emergency responders must stage at a safe distance from the site in the event of a detonation

(see the Scene Assessment chapter). **Figure 20-6** provides guidelines for safe distances depending on the possible size of the explosion.

Mechanisms of Injury

Traumatic injury after explosions has generally been divided into three categories: primary, secondary, and tertiary blast injury.[18] In addition to the injuries that result directly from the blast, additional categories of injuries classified as quaternary and quinary have been described and result from complications or toxic effects that are related to the explosive or contaminants. Although these injuries are described separately, they may occur in combination in victims of explosions. **Figure 20-7** shows the effects of explosions on the human body.

Primary Blast Injury

Primary blast injury results from high-order explosive detonation and the interaction of the blast overpressure wave with the body or tissue to produce stress and shear waves. **Stress waves** are supersonic, longitudinal pressure waves that (1) create high local forces with small, rapid distortions; (2) produce microvascular injury; and (3) are reinforced and reflected at tissue interfaces, thereby enhancing injury potential, especially in gas-filled organs such as the lungs, ears, and intestines. Injuries from the stress waves are caused by (1) pressure differentials across delicate structures such as the alveoli of the lung,

BOMB THREAT STAND-OFF CHART

Threat Description Improvised Explosive Device (IED)	Explosives Capacity[1] (TNT Equivalent)	Building Evacuation Distance[2]	Outdoor Evacuation Distance[3]
Pipe Bomb	5 LBS	70 FT	1200 FT
Suicide Bomber	20 LBS	110 FT	1700 FT
Briefcase/Suitcase	50 LBS	150 FT	1850 FT
Car	500 LBS	320 FT	1500 FT
SUV/Van	1,000 LBS	400 FT	2400 FT
Small Moving Van/ Delivery Truck	4,000 LBS	640 FT	3800 FT
Moving Van/ Water Truck	10,000 LBS	860 FT	5100 FT
Semi-Trailer	60,000 LBS	1570 FT	9300 FT

1. These capacities are based on the maximum weight of explosive material that could reasonably fit in a container of similar size.
2. Personnel in buildings are provided a high degree of protection from death or serious injury; however, glass breakage and building debris may still cause some injuries. Unstrengthened buildings can be expected to sustain damage that approximates five percent of their replacement cost.
3. If personnel cannot enter a building to seek shelter they must evacuate to the minimum distance recommended by Outdoor Evacuation Distance. These distance is governed by the greater hazard of fragmentation distance, glass breakage or threshold for ear drum rupture.

Figure 20-6 Explosives Safe Distance Stand-off Chart.
Source: Courtesy of U.S. Department of Homeland Security.

(2) rapid compression of and subsequent re-expansion of gas-filled structures, and (3) reflection of the wave at the tissue–gas interface. Depending on the proximity of the victim to the explosion, as well as shielding from or augmentation to the shock wave if the explosion occurs in a closed space, a victim may suffer primary blast injury.

Shear waves are transverse waves with a lower velocity and longer duration that cause asynchronous movement of tissues. The degree of damage depends on the extent to which the asynchronous motions overcome inherent tissue elasticity, resulting in tearing of tissue and possible disruption of attachments. However, muscle, bone, and solid-organ injury are much more likely to result from the tertiary and quaternary effects of the explosion than from the shock wave alone.[19,20]

Primary blast injury occurs in gas-filled organs such as the lung, bowel, and middle ear. The injury to the tissue occurs at the gas–fluid interface, presumably from a rapid compression of the gas in the organ, causing violent collapse of that organ, followed by an equally rapid and violent expansion, resulting in tissue injury. Damage to the lung manifests as pulmonary contusions, or possibly *hemopneumothoraces*, resulting in hypoxemia if the patient does not immediately succumb to the injuries (**Figure 20-8**). The alveolar–capillary interface can also become disrupted, resulting in arterial gas emboli, which may

cause cerebral or cardiac embolic complications. Damage to the bowel may include petechiae or hematomas of the bowel wall or even perforation of the bowel. Tympanic membrane rupture or disruption of the middle ear ossicles also may occur. Loss of hearing is common after an explosion and may be temporary or permanent.

Evidence of primary blast injury to the lung (or blast lung injury) is found more often in patients who die minutes after the explosion from associated injuries than those who survive; however, pulmonary primary blast injury has been noted with greater frequency among surviving victims of confined-space explosions.[21-23] Primary blast injury has also been associated with other severe injuries and is indicative of increased mortality risk in survivors of the initial event. After an open-air explosion in Beirut, only 0.6% of survivors had evidence of primary blast injury, and 11% of those died.[13] In a confined-space explosion in Jerusalem, 38% of survivors had evidence of primary blast injury, with a similar mortality rate of approximately 9%.[24] Similarly, two of the three bombs that were detonated in the London subway system exploded in wide tunnels, resulting in six and seven fatalities, respectively. The third device detonated in the subway system was exploded in a narrow tunnel, causing 26 fatalities. This difference in mortality between open- and closed-space bombings results from the reflection of the blast wave back onto

Figure 20-7   Blast Injury Categories

Effect	Impact	Mechanism of Injury	Typical Injuries
Primary	Direct blast effects (over- and underpressurization)	■ Contact of blast shockwave with body ■ Stress and shear waves occurring in tissues ■ Waves reinforced/reflected at tissue density interfaces ■ Impact with gas-filled organs (lungs, ears, etc.), which are at particular risk	■ Tympanic membrane rupture ■ Blast lung ■ Eye injuries ■ Concussion
Secondary	Projectiles propelled by explosion	Ballistic wounds produced by: ■ Primary fragments (pieces of exploding weapon) ■ Secondary fragments (environmental fragments [e.g., glass])	■ Penetrating injuries ■ Traumatic amputations ■ Lacerations ■ Concussion
Tertiary	Propulsion of body onto hard surface or object, or propulsion of objects onto individuals	■ Whole-body translocation ■ Crush injuries caused by structural damage and building collapse	■ Blunt injuries ■ Crush syndrome ■ Compartment syndrome ■ Concussion
Quaternary	Heat and/or combustion fumes	■ Burns and toxidromes from fuel and metals ■ Septic syndromes from soil and environmental contamination	■ Burns ■ Inhalation injury ■ Asphyxiation
Quinary	Additives such as radiation or chemicals (e.g., dirty bombs)	Contamination of tissue from: ■ Bacteria, radiation, or chemical agents ■ Allogeneic bone fragments	■ Variety of health effects, depending on agent

Source: Data from Department of Defense Directive: Medical Research for Prevention, Mitigation, and Treatment of Blast Injuries. Number 6025.21E. http://www.dtic.mil/whs/directives/corres/pdf/602521p.pdf. Accessed April 19, 2014

the victims rather than the dispersal of the blast wave into the surrounding area.

Secondary Blast Injury

Secondary blast injury is caused by flying debris and bomb fragments. Secondary blast injury (fragment [fragmentation] injury or secondary injury) is the most common category of injury in terrorist bombings and low explosions. These projectiles may be components of the bomb itself, as in military weapons designed to fragment, or may be parts of improvised bombs augmented with nails, screws, and bolts. Secondary blast injury is also caused by debris that is carried by the *blast wind*. The force required to create enough overpressure to

rupture 50% of exposed tympanic membranes (approximately 5 psi) can briefly generate blast winds of 145 miles per hour (233 km per hour). Blast winds associated with an overpressure resulting in significant primary blast injury may exceed 831 miles per hour (1,337 km per hour).[18] Although brief in duration, these blast winds can propel debris with great force and for great distances, causing both penetrating and blunt trauma.

Tertiary Blast Injury

Tertiary blast injury is caused by the blast wind throwing the victim's body, resulting in tumbling and collision with stationary objects. This can result in the whole spectrum of injuries

Figure 20-8   Blast Lung Injury: What Prehospital Care Providers Need to Know

Current patterns in worldwide terrorist activity have increased the potential for casualties related to explosions, yet few civilian prehospital care providers in the United States have experience treating patients with explosion-related injuries. **Blast lung injury (BLI)** presents unique triage, diagnostic, and management challenges and is a direct consequence of the blast wave from high-explosive detonations upon the body. Persons in enclosed space explosions or those in close proximity to the explosion are at a higher risk. BLI is a clinical diagnosis characterized by respiratory difficulty and hypoxia. BLI can occur, although rarely, without obvious external injury to the chest.

Clinical Presentation

- Symptoms may include dyspnea, hemoptysis, cough, and chest pain.
- Signs may include tachypnea, hypoxia, cyanosis, apnea, wheezing, decreased breath sounds, and hemodynamic instability.
- Victims with greater than 10% body surface area burns, skull fractures, and penetrating torso or head injuries may be more likely to have BLI.
- Hemothoraces or pneumothoraces may occur.
- Due to tearing of the pulmonary and vascular tree, air may enter the arterial circulation (*air emboli*) and result in embolic events involving the central nervous system, retinal arteries, or coronary arteries.
- Clinical evidence of BLI is typically present at the time of initial evaluation; however, it has been reported to occur over the course of 24 to 48 hours after an explosion.
- Other injuries are often present.

Prehospital Management Considerations

While scene safety is always a major consideration for prehospital care providers, incidents such as these often require emergency responders of all types to enter the scene before it can be declared completely secure. Prehospital care providers must remain aware of their surroundings, be observant for possible additional devices, and consider other hazards that may have resulted as a consequence of the primary explosion. Patient assessment and management steps are as follows:

- Initial triage, trauma resuscitation, and transport of patients should follow standard protocols for multiple injured patients or mass casualties, including assessment and treatment of the ABCDEs (airway, breathing, circulation, disability, and expose/environment) and immediate control of exsanguinating hemorrhage.
- Note the patient's location and the surrounding environment. Explosions in a confined space result in a higher incidence of primary blast injury, including lung injury.
- All patients with suspected or confirmed BLI should receive supplemental high-flow oxygen sufficient to prevent hypoxemia.
- Impending airway compromise requires immediate intervention.
- If ventilatory failure is imminent or occurs, patients should be intubated; however, prehospital care providers must realize that mechanical ventilation and positive pressure may increase the risk of alveolar rupture, pneumothorax, and air embolism in BLI patients.
- High-flow oxygen should be administered if air embolism is suspected, and the patient should be placed in a prone, semileft lateral, or left lateral position.
- Clinical evidence of or suspicion for a hemothorax or pneumothorax warrants close observation. Chest decompression should be performed for patients clinically presenting with a tension pneumothorax. Close observation is warranted for any patient with suspicion of BLI who is transported by air.
- Fluids should be administered judiciously, as overzealous fluid administration in the patient with BLI may result in volume overload and the worsening of pulmonary status.
- Patients with BLI should be transported rapidly to the nearest, appropriate facility, in accordance with community response plans for mass-casualty events.

Source: Data from Centers for Disease Control and Prevention, Atlanta.

associated with blunt trauma and even penetrating trauma, such as an impalement.

Quaternary and Quinary Effects

Following the blast itself, **quaternary effects** may be seen.[17] These injuries include burns and toxicities from fuel, metals, trauma from structural collapse, septic syndromes from soil, and environmental contamination.

The increasing threat of radiation-, chemical-, or biologic-enhanced explosives (i.e., "dirty bombs") has given rise to a fifth (*quinary*) category of effects, which includes injuries caused by radiation, chemicals, or biologic agents and projectiles such as bone fragments of a suicide bomber.[25,26]

Injury Patterns

The prehospital care provider will be confronted with a combination of familiar penetrating, blunt, and thermal injuries and possibly survivors with primary blast injury.[27] The numbers and types of injury will depend on multiple factors, including explosion magnitude, composition, environment, and location and number of potential victims at risk.

Various mortality rates have been associated with different types of bombing. One study that examined terrorist bombings showed that 1 of 4 victims died immediately after structural-collapse bombings, 1 of 12 died immediately in closed-space bombings, and 1 of 25 died immediately after open-space bombings.[15,28] Additional studies have found that mortality is higher when an explosion occurs in an enclosed space.[29,30] Soft-tissue injuries, orthopedic trauma, and traumatic brain injury are predominant among survivors (**Figure 20-9**).

For example, of 592 survivors of the Oklahoma City bombing, 85% had soft-tissue injuries (lacerations, puncture wounds, abrasions, contusions), 25% had sprains, 14% had head injuries, 10% had fractures/dislocations, 10% had ocular injuries (9 with ruptured globes), and 2% had burns.[10] The most common location for soft-tissue injury was the extremities (74%), followed by head and neck (48%), face (45%), and chest (35%). Eighteen survivors had severe soft-tissue injuries, including carotid artery and jugular vein lacerations, facial and popliteal artery lacerations, and severed nerves, tendons, and ligaments. Seventeen survivors had serious internal organ injury, including partial bowel transection, lacerated kidney, spleen, and liver, pneumothorax, and pulmonary contusion. Of patients with fractures, 37% had multiple fractures. Of those diagnosed with a head injury, 44% required admission to the hospital.[30]

Figure 20-9 Terrorist Bombings: Patterns of Injury

- Most wounds are noncritical soft-tissue or skeletal injuries.
- Head injury predominates among casualties who die (50%–70%).
- Most head injury survivors (98.5%) have noncritical injuries.
- Head injuries are disproportionate to exposed total body surface area.
- Most casualties with blast lung injury die immediately.
- Survivors have a low incidence of abdominal and chest wounds, burns, traumatic amputations, and blast lung injury, although specific mortalities are high (10%–40%).

Source: Data from Frykberg ER, Tepas JJ III: Terrorist bombings: lessons learned from Belfast to Beirut, Ann Surg 208:569, 1988.

Evaluation and Management

The general evaluation and management of trauma victims are applicable to the casualty from a WMD and are addressed in other chapters. Unique to this patient population, however, is the possibility of primary blast injury. Primary blast injuries might increase the likelihood that prehospital care providers will encounter patients with hemoptysis and pulmonary contusions, pneumothorax or tension pneumothorax, or even arterial gas embolism. Among survivors of primary blast injury, clinical manifestations may be present immediately[31,32] or may have a delayed onset of 24 to 48 hours.[33] Intrapulmonary hemorrhage and focal alveolar edema result in frothy bloody secretions and lead to ventilation–perfusion mismatch, increased intrapulmonary shunting, and decreased compliance. Hypoxia results, with increased work of breathing, pathophysiologically similar to pulmonary contusions induced by other mechanisms of nonpenetrating thoracic trauma.[34] The presence of rib fractures should increase suspicion of tertiary or quaternary injury to the thorax.

Primary blast injuries are not immediately apparent, and, therefore, care at the scene should include (1) monitoring for frothy secretions and respiratory distress, (2) sequential oxygen saturation (SpO_2) measurements, and (3) provision of oxygen. Decreased SpO_2 is a "red flag" for early blast lung injury even before symptoms begin. Fluid administration must be carefully managed, with care taken to avoid fluid overload.[1]

The likelihood of multisystem trauma is increased in bomb victims.[35] The management principles for these patients are similar to those for trauma from other mechanisms.

Transport Considerations

Patients requiring transport must be brought to an appropriate medical treatment facility for further evaluation and management. These patients will often require the services of a designated trauma center. Prehospital care providers should be aware of the epidemiology of patient transport after an explosives event. Patient arrival at hospitals is usually *bimodal*, with ambulatory patients arriving first and more critically ill patients arriving later by ambulance.

This bimodal patient transport was demonstrated in the Oklahoma City bombing. Patients began to arrive in the EDs 5 to 30 minutes after the bombing, with patients more seriously injured taking longer to arrive. Also, the geographically closest hospitals in Oklahoma City received the majority of victims, as seen with other disasters. Nearby hospitals that are overwhelmed by the first wave of patients may experience some difficulty managing the critically ill patients that arrive in the second wave. In Oklahoma City, the aggregate peak arrival rate of patients to EDs was 220 per hour at 60 to 90 minutes; 64% of patients visited EDs within a 1.5-mile radius of the event. Prehospital care providers should consider this latter fact when determining the destination of patients transported by ambulance from the bomb scene.[1]

Incendiary Agents

Incendiary agents are typically encountered in the military and are used to burn equipment, vehicles, and structures. The three incendiaries most often recognized are thermite, magnesium, and white phosphorus. All three are highly flammable compounds that burn at extremely high temperatures.

Thermite

Thermite is powdered aluminum and iron oxide that burns furiously at 3,600°F (1,982°C) and scatters molten iron.[36] Its primary mechanism of injury is partial-thickness or full-thickness burns. The primary and secondary assessments are performed with intervention directed at treating burns. Thermite wounds can be irrigated with copious amounts of water and any residual particles or material subsequently removed.

Magnesium

Magnesium is also a metal in powdered or solid form that burns furiously hot. In addition to its ability to cause partial-thickness or full-thickness burns, magnesium can react with tissue fluid and cause alkali burns. The same chemical reaction produces hydrogen gas, which can cause the wound to bubble or can result in subcutaneous emphysema. Inhalation of magnesium dust can produce respiratory symptoms, including cough, tachypnea, hypoxia, wheeze, pneumonitis, and airway burns. Residual magnesium particles in a wound will react with water, so irrigation is discouraged until the wounds can be debrided and the particulates removed. If irrigation is required for other reasons, such as decontamination of another suspected material, care should be taken to ensure flushing or removal of magnesium particles from the wound.[36]

White Phosphorus

White phosphorus (WP) is a solid that spontaneously ignites when exposed to air, causing a yellow flame and white smoke. WP that comes in contact with skin can quickly result in partial-thickness or full-thickness burns. WP can become embedded in the skin, propelled by the blast of WP munitions. The substance will continue to burn in the skin if exposed to air. Prehospital care providers can decrease the likelihood of combustion in the skin by immersing the affected areas in water or applying saline-soaked dressings to the area. Oily or greasy dressings are avoided in these patients because WP is lipid soluble, and application of these dressings may increase the likelihood of systemic absorption and toxicity. Copper sulfate has historically been used to neutralize WP and facilitate its removal because the reaction results in a black compound, which is easier to identify in the skin. Copper sulfate has fallen out of favor, however, because of complications from its use—specifically, intravascular hemolysis (breakdown or rupture of red blood cells within blood vessels).[37]

Chemical Agents

Many scenarios could expose the prehospital care provider to chemical agents, including an industrial complex accident, a spilled tanker truck or railway car, unearthed military ordnance, or a terrorist attack (**Figure 20-10**). The 1984 Union Carbide industrial accident in Bhopal, India, and the sarin gas attack in Tokyo in 1995 are examples of such incidents.

Physical Properties of Chemical Agents

The physical properties of a substance are affected by its chemical structure, the environmental temperature, and ambient pressure. These factors will determine whether a substance exists as a solid, liquid, or gas. Understanding the physical state of a chemical agent is important for the prehospital care provider because it gives clues as to the likely route of exposure and the potential for transmission and contamination.

A solid is in a state of matter that has a fixed volume and shape; a powder is an example of a solid. When heated to its melting point, solids become liquids. Liquids that are heated to their boiling point become a gas. Solid particles and liquid particles can become suspended in the air, similar to a dust particle or a liquid mist. This is considered an **aerosol**. A **vapor** is simply a solid or liquid that is in a gaseous state, but technically would be expected to be found as a solid or liquid at standard temperature and pressure, defined as 32°F (0°C) and normal atmospheric pressure (1 atmosphere, 14.7 psi). Some solids and liquids can, therefore, emit vapors at room temperature. The process of solids emitting vapors, bypassing the liquid state, is

Figure 20-10 Classification of Chemical Agents

- Cyanides (blood agents or asphyxiants)
  - Hydrogen cyanide, cyanogen chloride
- Nerve agents
  - Tabun (GA), sarin (GB), soman (GD), cyclosarin (GF), VX
- Lung toxicants (choking or pulmonary agents)
  - Chlorine, phosgene, diphosgene, ammonia
- Vesicants (blistering agents)
  - Mustard, lewisite
- Incapacitating agents
  - BZ (3-quinuclidinyl benzilate)
- Lacrimating agents (riot control agents)
  - CN, CS (tear gas agents), Oleoresin Capsicum (OC or pepper spray)
- Vomiting agents
  - Adamsite

called **sublimation**. The likelihood that solids or liquids vaporize into a gaseous form at room temperature is defined as the **volatility** of the substance. Highly volatile substances easily convert into a gas at room temperature.

These physical properties have implications for primary and secondary contamination and possible routes of exposure. **Primary contamination** is defined as exposure to the chemical agent at its point of release. For example, primary contamination occurs, by definition, in the hot zone. Gases, vapors, liquids, solids, and aerosols can all play a role in primary contamination.

Secondary contamination is defined as exposure to a chemical agent after it has been carried away from the point of origin, whether by a victim, an emergency responder, or a piece of contaminated equipment or debris. Secondary contamination generally occurs in the warm zone, although it may happen at more remote locations if the exposed victim is able to self-evacuate. Solids and liquids (and sometimes aerosols) generally contribute to secondary contamination. Gases and vapors do not typically play a role in secondary contamination because they cause injury by inhalation of the substance and do not deposit on skin. However, vapors can become trapped in clothing and then off-gas to potentially expose others to the hazard.

Volatility plays a significant role in the risk of secondary contamination. More volatile substances are considered "less persistent," meaning that because they vaporize, the likelihood of long-lasting physical contamination is unlikely. These chemical agents will readily disperse and be carried away by the wind. Less volatile substances are considered "more persistent." These substances do not vaporize, or do so at a very slow rate, thereby remaining on exposed surfaces for a long time, increasing the risk of secondary contamination. For example, the nerve agent sarin is a nonpersistent agent, whereas the nerve agent VX is a persistent agent.[38]

Personal Protective Equipment

PPE is selected based on the threat of exposure to the chemical agent. Level A is appropriate for emergency responders entering the hot zone.

Evaluation and Management

After ensuring the safety of the scene, the prehospital care provider will first confirm that victims are undergoing decontamination. Patients with likely skin exposure to the liquid form of a chemical will require decontamination with water. If available, soap may be used as well, but showering with copious amounts of water will generally suffice. Exposure to a gas only does not mandate decontamination by shower, but does mandate removal from any ongoing exposure as well as removal of any clothing that may have trapped residual vapors, which can subsequently off-gas and pose a hazard to care providers in the field or in the hospital.

Once the victim has been properly decontaminated, the prehospital care provider will likely encounter patients with signs and symptoms of exposure to a hazardous substance that has not yet been specifically identified. Victims of chemical agents can manifest signs and symptoms of exposure that affect:

- The respiratory system, affecting oxygenation and ventilation
- The mucous membranes, causing eye and upper airway injury
- The nervous system, resulting in seizures or coma
- The gastrointestinal (GI) tract, causing vomiting or diarrhea
- The skin, causing burning and blistering

It is important to evaluate the presenting signs and symptoms and whether they are improving or progressing. Patients with worsening clinical findings likely had incomplete cleansing of the contaminant and should undergo repeat decontamination to assure complete removal.

Patients will require a primary assessment to determine what lifesaving intervention may be immediately required. A secondary assessment may then assist in the identification of symptom constellations that might indicate the nature of the chemical agent and suggest a specific antidote. This constellation of clinical signs and symptoms suggesting exposure to a certain class of chemical or toxin is called a **toxidrome**.[39]

The *irritant gas toxidrome* will include mucous membrane burning and inflammation, coughing, and difficulty breathing. Agents responsible might include chlorine, phosgene, or ammonia.

The *asphyxiant toxidrome* is caused by cellular oxygen deprivation. This can result from inadequate oxygen availability, as in an oxygen-poor atmosphere; inadequate oxygen delivery to the cells, as in carbon monoxide poisoning; or inability to utilize oxygen at the cellular level, as in cyanide poisoning. Signs and symptoms include shortness of breath, chest pain, dysrhythmias, syncope, seizures, coma, and death.

The *cholinergic toxidrome* is characterized by rhinorrhea, respiratory secretions, difficulty breathing, nausea, vomiting, diarrhea, profuse sweating, pinpoint pupils and possible altered mental status, seizures, and coma. Pesticides and nerve agents can cause these cholinergic signs and symptoms.[40,41]

Most often, prehospital care providers will initiate supportive therapy without knowing the specific chemical cause of the injury. If the offending agent is properly identified, or if its identity is suggested by the toxidrome or clinical presentation, therapy specific to the agent may be delivered. Cyanide and nerve agent victims are examples of patients who can benefit from agent-specific antidote therapy.

Transport Considerations

Contaminated patients should not be transported until they have been decontaminated. Transporting contaminated patients results in cross-contamination of the transporting vehicle and personnel, thus taking them out of service until they have been decontaminated. This leads to compromise of the response capability of the ambulance service and may prolong the scene time and management of ill or injured patients. This same concern about not transporting contaminated patients applies to air-medical services as well.

Patients must be brought to an appropriate medical treatment facility for further evaluation and management. Transporting to the optimal facility is particularly important because some chemical toxic effects may not become apparent for 8 to 24 hours. Communities may identify preferred hospitals for the management of chemical casualties. These facilities may be more capable of managing these patients by virtue of specialized training or availability of critical care services and specific antidotes. Considerations similar to those previously noted for explosive incidents regarding transport epidemiology also apply to these patients.

Nearby EDs may become overwhelmed by ambulatory, self-evacuated, self-transported patients. Of the 640 patients presenting to one hospital in Tokyo after the sarin incident, 541 arrived without EMS assistance.[42] Hospitals closest to the event will likely receive the largest number of ambulatory patients. These factors should be considered in determining the destination of patients transported via ambulance.

Selected Specific Chemical Agents
Cyanides

Most commonly, prehospital care providers might encounter cyanides when responding to a fire in which certain plastics are burning or in certain industrial complexes, where it is found in large quantities and used in chemical syntheses, electroplating, mineral extraction, dyeing, printing, photography, and agriculture, and in the manufacture of paper, textiles, and plastics. However, cyanide has been inventoried in military stockpiles and some terrorist websites have provided the instructions for making a cyanide dispersal device.

Hydrogen cyanide is a highly volatile liquid and, thus, will most often be encountered as a vapor or gas. Therefore, it has greater potential for mass casualties in a confined space with poor ventilation than if released outdoors. Although a smell of bitter almonds has been associated with this agent, this is not a reliable indicator of hydrogen cyanide exposure. It is estimated that as much as 40% to 50% of the general population is incapable of detecting the odor of cyanide.

Cyanide's mechanism of action is arrest of metabolism or respiration at the cellular level, quickly resulting in cell death. Cyanide binds in the mitochondria of cells, preventing oxygen usage in cellular metabolism. Victims of cyanide poisoning actually are able to inhale and absorb oxygen into the blood, but are unable to use it at the cellular level. Thus, patients who are ventilating will present with evidence of acyanotic hypoxia.

The organs most affected are the central nervous system (CNS) and the heart. Symptoms of mild cyanide poisoning include headache, dizziness, drowsiness, nausea, vomiting, and mucosal irritation. Severe cyanide poisoning includes alteration of consciousness, dysrhythmias, hypotension, seizures, and death. Death can occur within a few minutes after inhalation of high levels of cyanide gas.

Management

Supportive therapy is important, including high-concentration oxygen delivery, correction of hypotension with fluids or vaso-pressors, and management of seizures. Cyanide antidote kits are available for patients with known or suspected cyanide poisoning. The traditional cyanide antidote treatment involved treatment with two medications, a nitrite followed by thiosulfate. The administration of inhaled amyl nitrite, or preferably intravenous (IV) sodium nitrite, creates methemoglobin (itself a poison that in high enough concentrations can kill), which binds cyanide in the bloodstream, making it less available to poison the patient's cellular respiration. The nitrite is followed by IV administration of sodium thiosulfate to assist the body in the conversion of cyanide to harmless thiocyanate, which is excreted by the kidneys.

In late 2006, the U.S. Food and Drug Administration (FDA) approved the use of hydroxocobalamin for treatment of cyanide poisoning. This medication has been used in Europe for over a decade for cyanide therapy. Hydroxocobalamin given intravenously binds with cyanide to form cyanocobalamin (vitamin B_{12}), which is nontoxic. Hydroxocobalamin has become the preferred antidote for cyanide poisoning because it is easy to use, it involves a single medication administration instead of two, and it does not create an intermediate chemical that is itself a poison.

Nerve Agents

Nerve agents were originally developed as insecticides, but once their effects on humans were recognized, numerous different types were developed in the early to mid-1900s. These deadly chemicals can be found in the military stockpiles of many nations. The most recent known use in a military conflict was in the Syrian civil war in 2013. Nerve agents have also been produced and used by terrorist organizations, the most notorious releases occurring in Matsumoto, Japan, in 1994 and in the Tokyo, Japan, subway system in 1995. Commonly available pesticides (e.g., malathion, carbaryl [Sevin]) and common therapeutic drugs (e.g., physostigmine, pyridostigmine) share properties with nerve agents, causing similar clinical effects.

Nerve agents are usually liquids at room temperature. Sarin is the most volatile of the group. VX is the least volatile and is found as an oily liquid. The main routes of intoxication are through inhalation of the vapor (usually the volatile or nonpersistent agents) and absorption through the skin (usually VX). Nerve agents can injure or kill at very low doses. A single, small drop the size of a pinhead of VX, the most potent nerve agent developed, placed on the skin could kill a victim. Because nerve agents are liquids, they pose a risk for secondary contamination from contact with contaminated clothes, skin, and other objects.

The mechanism of action of nerve agents is inhibition of the enzyme acetylcholinesterase. This enzyme is necessary to inhibit the action of acetylcholine. **Acetylcholine** is a neurotransmitter that stimulates cholinergic receptors. These receptors are found in smooth muscles, skeletal muscles, the CNS, and most exocrine (secretory) glands. Some of these cholinergic receptors are termed **muscarinic sites** (because experimentally they are stimulated by muscarine), mostly found in smooth muscles and glands. Others are termed **nicotinic sites** (because experimentally they are stimulated by nicotine), mostly found in skeletal muscle. The mnemonic **DUMBELS** (**d**iarrhea, **u**rination, **m**iosis, **b**radycardia, **b**ronchorrhea, **b**ronchospasm, **e**mesis, **l**acrimation, **s**alivation, **s**weating) represents the constellation of symptoms associated with the muscarinic effects of nerve agent toxicity. The mnemonic **MTWHF** (**m**ydriasis [rarely seen], **t**achycardia, **w**eakness, **h**ypertension, **h**yperglycemia, **f**asciculations) represents the constellation of symptoms associated with stimulation of nicotinic receptors (**Figure 20-11**). The CNS effects, a result of both muscarinic and nicotinic receptors, include confusion, convulsions, and coma.

The clinical effects depend on the dose and route of nerve agent exposure (inhalation or dermal) and whether the muscarinic or nicotinic effects predominate. Small amounts of vapor exposure primarily cause irritation to eyes, nose, and airways. Large amounts of vapor exposure can quickly lead to loss of consciousness, seizures, apnea, and muscular flaccidity. *Miosis* (constricted pupils) is the most sensitive marker of exposure to vapor. Symptoms of dermal exposure also vary according to dose and time of onset. Small doses may not result in symptoms for up to 18 hours. Fasciculations of the underlying muscles and localized sweating at the site of the skin exposure may occur, followed by GI symptoms, nausea, vomiting, and diarrhea. Large dermal doses will result in onset of symptoms in minutes, with effects similar to a large vapor exposure.

Clinical symptoms of the nerve agents include *rhinorrhea* (runny nose), chest tightness, miosis (pupil is pinpoint, and patient complains of blurry or dim vision), shortness of breath, excessive salivation and sweating, nausea, vomiting, abdominal cramps, involuntary urination and defecation, muscle fasciculations, confusion, seizures, flaccid paralysis, coma, respiratory failure, and death.

Management

Management of nerve agent poisoning includes decontamination (**Figure 20-12**), a primary assessment, administration of antidotes, and supportive therapy. Ventilation and oxygenation of the patient may be difficult because of bronchoconstriction and copious secretions. The patient will likely require frequent suctioning. These symptoms improve after the antidote is administered. The three therapeutic drugs for the management of nerve agent poisoning are atropine, pralidoxime chloride, and diazepam.

Atropine is an anticholinergic drug that reverses most of the muscarinic effects of the nerve agent but has little effect on the nicotinic sites. Atropine is indicated for exposed victims with pulmonary complaints. Miosis alone is not an indication for atropine, and furthermore, atropine will not correct the ocular abnormalities. Atropine is given according to local system protocols. It is titrated until the patient's ability to breathe or ventilate is improved or there is drying of pulmonary secretions. In moderate to severe exposures, it is not unusual to start with an initial dose of 4 to 6 milligrams (mg) and give as much as 10 to 20 mg of atropine over a few hours.

Pralidoxime chloride (2-PAM chloride) is an oxime. Pralidoxime works by uncoupling the bond between the nerve agent and acetylcholinesterase, thereby reactivating the enzyme and helping to reduce the effects of the nerve agent, primarily on nicotinic receptors. The oxime therapy needs to be initiated within minutes to a few hours of the exposure to be effective, depending on the nerve agent released; otherwise, the bond between acetylcholinesterase and the nerve agent will become permanent ("aging"), delaying recovery of the patient.

Figure 20-11 Mnemonics

The mnemonic DUMBELS (**d**iarrhea, **u**rination, **m**iosis, **b**radycardia, **b**ronchorrhea, **b**ronchospasm, **e**mesis, **l**acrimation, **s**alivation, **s**weating) represents the constellation of symptoms associated with the muscarinic effects of nerve agent toxicity. The mnemonic MTWHF (**m**ydriasis [rarely seen], **t**achycardia, **w**eakness, **h**ypertension, **h**yperglycemia, **f**asciculations) represents the constellation of symptoms associated with stimulation of nicotinic receptors.

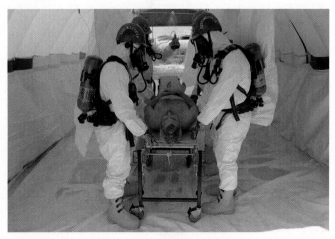

Figure 20-12 Decontamination from nerve agents.
Source: © Jones and Bartlett Learning. Photographed by Glen E. Ellman.

Diazepam (Valium) is a benzodiazepine and anticonvulsant. If patients develop seizures after significant exposure, benzodiazepine therapy is initiated to manage the seizures and help to reduce the brain injury and other life-threatening effects associated with status epilepticus. Diazepam given intramuscularly has erratic absorption; therefore, the preferred route for patients who are actively seizing is intravenous if access is available. In addition, diazepam administration is recommended for all patients with signs of severe nerve agent poisoning, whether or not they have begun to seize. There are no data in either humans or animals for rectal administration of diazepam.[43] Lorazepam (Ativan) has been studied in animal models and found to be less effective than diazepam.[43] Midazolam (Versed), on the other hand, has been shown to be effective in animal models and, in the future, may become the first-line medication for nerve agent–induced seizures.[44]

All three of these medications are available and packaged as autoinjectors. Atropine and pralidoxime come packaged together in a single autoinjector called DuoDote (**Figure 20-13**). The dose of atropine is 2.1 mg, and the dose of pralidoxime is 600 mg. This autoinjector is intended for rapid intramuscular injection in the event of a nerve agent exposure. Total dosage is determined by protocol and titration of these drugs to effect. In the past, the atropine and pralidoxime were supplied in individual autoinjectors marketed as the Mark-1 kit. These kits have largely been supplanted by the single autoinjector containing both antidotes. Diazepam for seizures is also available as an autoinjector.

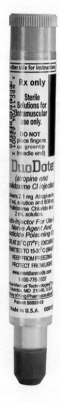

Figure 20-13 DuoDote.
Source: Courtesy of Pfizer, Inc.

Lung Toxicants

Lung toxicants, including chlorine, phosgene, ammonia, sulfur dioxide, and nitrogen dioxide, are present in numerous industrial manufacturing applications. Phosgene has been stockpiled for military applications and was the most lethal chemical warfare agent used in World War I.

Lung toxicants that are chemical pulmonary agents may be gases, vapors, aerosolized liquids, or solids. The properties of the agent influence its ability to cause injury. For example, aerosolized particles of 2 micrometers (μm) or smaller readily access the alveoli of the lung, causing injury there, whereas larger particles are filtered out before reaching the alveoli. Water solubility of an agent also affects the injury pattern. Ammonia and sulfur dioxide, which are highly water soluble, cause irritation and injury to the eyes, mucous membranes, and upper airways. Phosgene and nitrogen oxides, which have low water solubility, tend to cause less immediate irritation and injury to the eyes, mucous membranes, and upper airways, thus providing little warning to the victim and allowing for prolonged exposure to these agents. Prolonged exposure makes it more likely that the alveoli will be injured, resulting not only in upper-airway injury, but also in alveolar collapse and noncardiogenic pulmonary edema. Moderately water-soluble agents, such as chlorine, can cause both upper airway and alveolar irritation.

The mechanisms of injury vary among the lung toxicants. Ammonia, for example, combines with the water in the mucous membranes to form a strong base, ammonium hydroxide. Chlorine and phosgene, when combined with water, produce hydrochloric acid, causing injury to the tissues. Lung toxicants are not systemically absorbed but compromise the victim by damaging components of the pulmonary system, from the upper airway to the alveoli.

The agents with high water solubility cause burning of the eyes, nose, and mouth. Tearing, rhinorrhea, coughing, dyspnea, and respiratory distress secondary to glottic irritation or laryngospasm are possible. Bronchospasm can result in coughing, wheezing, and dyspnea. Agents with low water solubility, causing injury to the alveoli, can immediately injure the alveolar epithelium in the case of a large exposure, leading to death from acute respiratory failure, or, with less massive exposure, can result in a delayed onset (24 to 48 hours) of respiratory distress, secondary to development of mild noncardiogenic pulmonary edema to fulminant acute respiratory distress syndrome, depending on the dose.

Management

Management of lung toxicants includes removal of the patient from the offending agent, decontamination with copious irrigation (if solid, liquid, or aerosol exposure, especially for ammonia), primary assessment, and supportive therapy, which will likely require interventions to maximize ventilation and oxygenation. Eye irritation can be managed with copious irrigation using normal saline. Contact lenses should be removed. Expect to manage profuse airway secretions, which will require suctioning. Bronchospasm may respond to inhaled beta-adrenergic agonists. Hypoxia will require correction with high-flow oxygen and possibly intubation with positive-pressure ventilation. Prehospital care providers need to be prepared to encounter difficult airway management secondary to copious secretions, inflammation of glottic structures, and laryngeal spasm. All victims exposed to phosgene should be transported for evaluation because of the likelihood of delayed symptoms.

Vesicant Agents

The vesicants include sulfur mustard, nitrogen mustards, and lewisite. These agents have been stockpiled for military operations by many countries. Sulfur mustard was first introduced to the battlefield in World War I. It was reportedly used by Iraq against its Kurdish population and also in its conflict with Iran in 1980. It is relatively easy and inexpensive to manufacture.

Sulfur mustard is an oily, clear to yellow-brown liquid that can be aerosolized by a bomb blast or a sprayer. Its volatility is low, allowing it to persist on surfaces for a week or more. This persistence allows for easy secondary contamination. The agent is absorbed through the skin and mucous membranes, resulting in direct cellular damage within 3 to 5 minutes of the exposure, although clinical symptoms and signs may take 1 to 12 hours (usually 4 to 6 hours) after exposure to develop. The delayed onset of symptoms often makes it difficult for the victim to recognize that the exposure occurred and, therefore, increases the potential for secondary contamination. Warm, moist skin increases the likelihood of skin absorption, making the groin and axillary regions particularly susceptible. The eyes, skin, and upper airways can develop a range of findings, from erythema and edema to vesicle development to full-thickness necrosis. Upper airway involvement can result in cough and bronchospasm. High-dose exposures can result in nausea and vomiting, as well as bone marrow suppression.

Management for sulfur mustard involves decontamination using soap and water, primary assessment, and supportive therapy; no antidote exists for the effects of mustard agents. In fact, it is important to note that because the cellular damage from sulfur mustard occurs within several minutes of the exposure, decontamination will not change the clinical course of the exposed patient. It is primarily intended to prevent inadvertent cross-contamination. Eyes and skin should be decontaminated with copious amounts of water as soon as exposure is recognized to minimize further absorption of the agent and prevent secondary contamination. The fluid in resulting vesicles and blisters is not a source of secondary contamination. Pulmonary bronchoconstriction may benefit from nebulized beta-agonists. Skin wounds should be treated as burns, with regard to local wound care.

Lewisite has a similar constellation of symptoms, but the onset of action is much quicker than with sulfur mustard, resulting in immediate pain and irritation to the eyes, skin,

and respiratory tract. Unlike mustard, lewisite does not cause bone marrow suppression. Also unique to this agent is "lewisite shock," the result of intravascular volume depletion secondary to capillary leak.

As with sulfur mustard, prehospital management of these exposed patients involves decontamination, primary assessment, and supportive care. British anti-lewisite is an antidote available for the in-hospital treatment of lewisite-exposed patients. It is administered intravenously for patients with hypovolemic shock or pulmonary symptoms. Applied topically, British anti-lewisite ointment has been reported to prevent mucous membrane and skin injury.

Biologic Agents

Biologic agents in the form of contagious disease exposure represent a threat to prehospital care providers on a daily basis (**Figure 20-14**). Proper infection control procedures must be in place to prevent the contraction or transmission of tuberculosis, influenza, human immunodeficiency virus (HIV), methicillin-resistant staphylococci (MRSA), SARS, meningococcus, and a myriad of other organisms.

Preparing for bioterrorist events increases the complexity of EMS system preparation. An intentional terrorist act might include delivery of a biologic agent with the potential to cause disease or illness, such as aerosolized spores, aerosolized live organisms, or an aerosolized biologic toxin. Patients with pathogens not typically seen by prehospital care providers, such as

Figure 20-14 Classification of Biologic WMD Agents

- Bacterial agents
  - Anthrax
  - Brucellosis
  - Glanders
  - Plague
  - Q fever
  - Tularemia
- Viral agents
  - Smallpox
  - Venezuelan equine encephalitis
  - Viral hemorrhagic fevers
- Biologic toxins
  - Botulinum
  - Ricin
  - Staphylococcal enterotoxin B
  - T-2 mycotoxins

plague, anthrax, and smallpox, might be encountered, requiring appropriate PPE and precautions. Familiar infection control procedures will be effective in the safe management of these potentially contagious patients. If the prehospital care provider is responding to an overt release event, appropriate precautions regarding decontamination of victims and PPE are required, similar to other hazardous materials events.

Concentrated Biohazard Agent Versus Infected Patient

Prehospital care providers can experience bioterrorism in two ways. The first scenario involves the overt release of a material that is either identified as, or thought to be, a biologic agent. The anthrax hoaxes of 1998 and 1999 and the anthrax letters of 2001 are good examples. Prehospital care providers responded on countless occasions to individuals covered in "white powder" or suspected anthrax. In this situation, the prehospital care provider will encounter an environment or a patient contaminated with a suspicious substance. EMS systems may be summoned to suspicious activity, such as a device delivering an unknown aerosol agent. The nature of the threat at these events is usually unknown and precautions for personal safety should always be paramount. These incidents must be respected and treated as a WMD incident until proven otherwise. If the suspicious substance is in fact a concentrated aerosol of an infectious organism or toxin, PPE appropriate for the biologic agent and decontamination are required.

In this situation, prehospital care providers will be caring for victims contaminated with suspected biologic agent on their skin or clothing. Any person, patient, or prehospital care provider coming in direct physical contact with a suspected biologic agent should remove all exposed articles of clothing and perform a thorough washing of exposed skin with soap and water.[45] Clinically significant re-aerosolization of material from victims' skin or clothing is unlikely, and the risk to the prehospital care provider is negligible.[46] However, as a matter of routine practice, potentially contaminated clothing normally removed by pulling the item over the face and head should instead be cut off to minimize any risk of inadvertent inhalation of contaminant. Decontamination may then proceed using water or soap and water. Consultation with appropriate public health and law enforcement officials will then determine the need for antibiotic prophylaxis.

The second scenario involves a response to a patient who is a victim of a remote, covert bioterrorist event. Perhaps the patient inhaled anthrax spores after a covert attack at work and now, several days later, is manifesting signs of pulmonary anthrax. Perhaps a terrorist has inoculated himself or herself with smallpox, and you are summoned to assist the victim with a suspicious rash. In these cases, personal and public safety can be ensured by knowledge of proper infection control procedures and the proper donning and removal of PPE appropriate for the biohazard (**Figures 20-15** and **20-16**). Decontamination of the

patient in this scenario is not necessary because the exposure occurred several days in the past.

All prehospital care providers should be familiar with PPE for infection-control purposes. Different types of PPE are recommended, depending on the potential for transmission and the likely route of transmission. **Transmission-based PPE** is used in addition to the standard precautions, which are used in the care of all patients. These include contact, droplet, and aerosol precautions.

Contact Precautions

This level of protection is recommended to reduce the likelihood of transmission of microorganisms by direct or indirect contact. Contact precautions include the use of gloves and a gown.

Commonly encountered organisms that require contact precautions include viral conjunctivitis, MRSA, scabies, and herpes simplex or zoster virus. Organisms that require strict contact precautions that might be encountered as a result of bioterrorism include bubonic plague or the viral hemorrhagic fevers, such as Marburg or Ebola, as long as the patient does not have pulmonary symptoms or profuse vomiting and diarrhea, in which case airborne precautions should also be taken.

Figure 20-15   Sequence for Donning PPE

The type of PPE used will vary based on the level of precautions required (e.g., standard precautions and contact, droplet, or airborne infection isolation).

1. Gown
   - Fully cover torso from neck to knees, arms to end of wrists, and wrap around the back.
   - Fasten in back of neck and waist.
2. Mask or respirator
   - Secure ties or elastic bands at middle of head and neck.
   - Fit flexible band to nose bridge.
   - Fit snug to face and below chin.
   - Fit/check respirator.
3. Goggles or face shield
   - Place over face and eyes and adjust to fit.
4. Gloves
   - Extend to cover wrist of isolation gown.

Use safe work practices to protect yourself and limit the spread of contamination:

- Keep hands away from face.
- Limit surfaces touched.
- Change gloves when torn or heavily contaminated.
- Perform hand hygiene.

Source: From Centers for Disease Control and Prevention, Atlanta.

Figure 20-16 Sequence for Removing PPE

Except for the respirator, remove PPE at the doorway or in an anteroom of the involved room. Remove the respirator after leaving the contaminated room and closing the door.

1. Gloves
   - The outside of the glove is contaminated!
     - Grasp outside of glove with opposite gloved hand; peel off.
     - Hold removed glove in gloved hand.
     - Slide fingers of ungloved hand under remaining glove at wrist.
     - Peel glove off over first glove.
     - Discard gloves in waste container.
2. Goggles
   - The outside of the goggles or face shield is contaminated!
     - To remove, handle by headband or ear pieces.
     - Place in designated receptacle for reprocessing or in waste container.
3. Gown
   - The gown front and sleeves are contaminated!
     - Unfasten gown ties.
     - Pull away from neck and shoulders, touching inside of gown only.
     - Turn gown inside out.
     - Fold or roll into a bundle and discard.
4. Mask or respirator
   - The front of the mask/respirator is contaminated— do not touch!
     - Grasp bottom, then top ties or elastics, and remove.
     - Discard in waste container.

Once PPE is removed, wash the hands.

Source: From Centers for Disease Control and Prevention, Atlanta.

Droplet Precautions

This level of protection is recommended to reduce the likelihood of transmission of microorganisms that are known to be transmitted by large droplet nuclei (greater than 5 μm) expelled by an infected person in the course of talking, sneezing, or coughing or during routine procedures, such as suctioning. These droplets infect by landing on the exposed mucous membranes of the eyes, nose, and mouth. Because the droplets are large, they do not remain suspended in air, and therefore, contact must be in close proximity, usually defined as 3 feet (0.9 meter) or less. Droplet precautions include the contact precautions of gloves and gown and add eye protection and a surgical mask. Because the droplets do not remain suspended

in air, no additional respiratory protection or air filtration is required.

Typically encountered organisms in this category include influenza, *Mycoplasma pneumoniae*, and invasive *Haemophilus influenzae* or *Neisseria meningitidis*, causing sepsis or meningitis. Pneumonic plague is an example of a possible agent encountered as a result of a bioterrorist event.

Aerosol Precautions

This level of protection is recommended to reduce the likelihood of transmission of microorganisms by the airborne route. Some organisms can become suspended in the air attached to small droplet nuclei (less than 5 μm) or attached to dust particles. In this case, microorganisms can become widely dispersed by air currents immediately around the source or more distant from the source, depending on environmental conditions. To avoid such dispersion, these patients are kept in negative-pressure isolation rooms in a hospital in which the exhaust ventilation can be filtered.

Aerosol precautions include gloves, gown, eye protection, and a fit-tested high-efficiency particulate air (HEPA) filter mask, such as the N-95 (**Figure 20-17**). Examples of illnesses typically encountered that would require aerosol precautions include tuberculosis, measles, chickenpox, and SARS. Smallpox and viral hemorrhagic fever with pulmonary symptoms are examples that could possibly be related to a bioterrorist event.

Selected Agents
Anthrax

Anthrax is a disease caused by the bacterium *Bacillus anthracis*. *B. anthracis* is a spore-forming bacterium and, thus, can exist as a vegetative cell or as a spore. The vegetative cell lives well in a host organism but cannot survive long

Figure 20-17 Biologic Agent Precautions

Note that many illnesses associated with biologic events require no additional protection beyond standard precautions, provided there is no risk of exposure to a concentrated agent. Examples include patients with inhalational anthrax or a biologic toxin such as botulinum. However, in most cases, the specific biologic agent will likely not be identified for several days. Although some agents, such as anthrax, are not spread from person to person, prehospital care providers must assume the worst—that the biologic agent is contagious—and use all available precautions, including aerosol precautions.

outside the body, unlike the spore, which can be viable in the environment for decades.

The disease is naturally occurring, contracted most often by persons in contact with infected animals or anthrax-contaminated animal products resulting in the cutaneous form of the disease. The spores have been weaponized and are known to be inventoried in several nations' military stockpiles. The accidental release of aerosolized anthrax spores from a Soviet military facility at Sverdlovsk in 1979 resulted in approximately 79 cases of pulmonary anthrax with 68 reported deaths. Letters contaminated with anthrax spores were sent through the U.S. Postal Service in 2001 to prominent legislators and media outlets. Although only 22 cases (11 pulmonary, 11 cutaneous) and 5 deaths resulted, thousands of people required prophylaxis with antibiotics. An efficient release of 220 pounds (100 kilograms [kg]) of anthrax spores over Washington, DC, is reported to be capable of causing 130,000 to 3 million deaths.[47]

Routes of exposure to anthrax include the respiratory tract, the GI tract, and breaks in the skin. Exposure to anthrax through the respiratory tract leads to inhalational or pulmonary anthrax. Exposure through the GI tract causes gastrointestinal anthrax, and skin infection causes cutaneous anthrax.

Gastrointestinal anthrax is rare and would result from ingesting food substances contaminated with spores. Patients would have nonspecific symptoms of nausea, vomiting, malaise, bloody diarrhea, and acute abdomen; mortality is approximately 50%. Cutaneous anthrax follows deposition of spores or organisms into a break in the skin. This results in a papule, which subsequently ulcerates and causes a dry, black eschar with local edema. If not treated with antibiotics, mortality approaches 20%; with antibiotics, mortality is less than 1%.

For maximal effectiveness in a terrorist attack, anthrax would likely be disseminated in its spore form. Anthrax spores are approximately 1 to 5 μm in size, which allows the spores to be suspended in air as an aerosol. Aerosolized spores can be inhaled into the lungs and deposited in the alveoli. They are then consumed by macrophages and carried to the mediastinal lymph nodes, where they germinate, manufacture toxins, and cause *acute hemorrhagic mediastinitis* (bleeding into the lymph nodes in the middle of the chest cavity) and often death. The onset of symptoms after inhalation of spores varies, with most victims developing symptoms within 1 to 7 days, although there may be a latency period as long as 60 days. Symptoms initially are nonspecific, including fever, chills, dyspnea, cough, chest pain, headache, and vomiting. After a few days, symptoms improve, followed by a rapidly deteriorating course of fever, dyspnea, diaphoresis, shock, and death.[45,48,49] Before the 2001 anthrax attacks, mortality from inhalational anthrax was thought to be 90%, but recent experience suggests that with early antibiotic therapy and critical care services, mortality may be less than 50%.[50]

Inhalational anthrax is not contagious and does not pose a risk to the prehospital care provider. Only exposure to aerosolized spores poses a risk of infectivity. Caring for patients known to be infected with inhalational anthrax requires only standard precautions; however, if the specific agent is unknown, aerosol precautions are warranted. The prehospital care provider will provide supportive therapy and transport ill patients to facilities in which critical care services are available.

Management

Prophylaxis with antibiotics is required only for individuals who have been exposed to spores. Local public health officials will determine the appropriate antibiotic and length of prophylactic treatment. The latest recommendations suggest 60 days of therapy with oral doxycycline or a quinolone antibiotic.

An anthrax vaccine does exist, and an immunization program for U.S. military forces was instituted in 1998. The current regimen requires a series of six initial shots and annual boosters. It is currently recommended only for military personnel and for laboratory and industrial workers at high risk for exposure to spores. The CDC has purchased tens of thousands of doses of the anthrax vaccine for the Strategic National Stockpile that would be made available to emergency responders in the event of an anthrax incident with risk of exposure.

Plague

Plague is a disease caused by the bacterium *Yersinia pestis*. It is naturally occurring, found in fleas and rodents. If an infected flea bites a human, the person can develop *bubonic plague*. If this local infection goes untreated, the patient can become systemically ill, resulting in septicemia and death. A number of patients may proceed to develop pulmonary symptoms (*pneumonic plague*). Plague was responsible for the Black Death of 1346, which killed 20 to 30 million people in Europe, approximately one-third of its population at that time. *Y. pestis* has been weaponized for military stockpiles with techniques developed to aerosolize the organism directly, bypassing the animal vector. The World Health Organization reports that in a worst-case scenario, 110 pounds (50 kg) of *Y. pestis*, released as an aerosol over a city of 5 million, would result in 150,000 cases of pneumonic plague and 36,000 deaths.[51]

Naturally occurring plague, resulting from the bite of an infected flea, will cause symptoms in 2 to 8 days, with onset of fever, chills, weakness, and acutely swollen lymph nodes (buboes) in the neck, groin, or axilla. Untreated patients can deteriorate to systemic illness and death. Twelve percent have been described as developing pneumonic plague, with complaints of chest pain, dyspnea, cough, and hemoptysis, and these patients can also succumb from systemic illness.

Plague occurring from terrorist deployment of a weapon would likely result from aerosolized organisms, and thus, it would clinically present as the pneumonic form of the disease. Inhalation of *Y. pestis* aerosol will result in symptoms in 1 to 6 days. Patients will present with fever, cough, and dyspnea, with bloody or watery sputum. They may also develop nausea, vomiting, diarrhea, and abdominal pain. Buboes are not typically present. Without antibiotics, death occurs in 2 to 6 days after development of respiratory symptoms.[52]

Currently, no vaccine is available to protect from pneumonic plague. Treatment of the disease includes antimicrobial and supportive therapy, often requiring critical care services. Antibiotic regimens are also recommended for individuals with unprotected close exposure to patients with known pneumonic plague.

Patients with plague represent a communicable disease risk. If patients present with only cutaneous signs and symptoms (bubonic plague), contact precautions are adequate to protect the prehospital care provider. If patients present with pulmonary signs of plague (pneumonic plague), a more likely scenario after a terrorist attack, prehospital care providers will be required to wear PPE suitable for respiratory droplet protection. Droplet precautions include a surgical mask, eye protection, gloves, and a gown. Responders to the scene of an overt *Y. pestis* aerosol delivery, which would not likely be a recognized event, would require level A PPE suitable for a hazardous environment if entering the hot zone or warm zone.

Management

Plague victims are treated in the field with supportive therapy. Communication with the receiving facility is vital before arrival to ensure that the pneumonic plague patient can be properly isolated in the ED and that staff are prepared with the appropriate PPE. Asking the patient to wear a surgical mask, if tolerated, may also decrease the likelihood of secondary transmission.

Decontamination of the vehicle and equipment is similar to that required after transport of any patient with communicable disease. Contact surfaces should be wiped down with disinfectant approved by the Environmental Protection Agency (EPA) or 1:1,000 diluted bleach solution. There is no evidence to suggest that *Y. pestis* poses a long-term environmental threat after dissolution of the primary aerosol.[52] The organism is sensitive to heat and sunlight and does not last long outside the living host. *Y. pestis* does not form spores.

Smallpox

Smallpox is also known as *variola major* and *variola minor*, depending on the severity of the illness. This naturally occurring viral disease was eradicated in 1977 but still exists in at least two laboratories—Russia's Institute of Virus Preparations and the CDC. It was alleged that the Soviet government began a program in 1980 to produce large quantities of smallpox virus for use in bombs and missiles, as well as to develop more virulent strains of the virus for military purposes. There is concern that smallpox virus may have changed hands after the dissolution of the Soviet Union.[53]

The smallpox virus infects its victim by entering the mucous membranes of the oropharynx or respiratory mucosa. After a 12- to 14-day incubation period, the patient develops fever, malaise, headache, and backache. The patient then develops a **maculopapular rash** that starts on the oral mucosa and quickly progresses to a generalized skin rash with characteristic round, tense vesicles and pustules. The rash tends to affect the head and extremities more densely than the trunk (centrifugal), with the stage of the lesions appearing uniform (**Figure 20-18**). This

presentation distinguishes smallpox from *varicella*, or chickenpox (**Figure 20-19**), which begins on and is more dense on the trunk (centripetal) and has lesions at various stages of development (new lesions appear with older, crusted lesions) (**Figure 20-20**). Mortality from naturally occurring smallpox was approximately 30%. Little is known about the natural course of the disease in immunocompromised patients, such as those with HIV.

Smallpox is a contagious disease that is primarily spread by droplet nuclei projected from the oropharynx of infected patients and by direct contact. Contaminated clothing and bed linens can also spread the virus. Patients are contagious beginning slightly before the onset of the rash, although this might not always be obvious if the rash is subtle in the oropharynx. When managing a patient with smallpox, prehospital care providers must wear PPE appropriate for contact and aerosol precautions. This includes N-95 mask, eye protection, goggles, and gown. Ideally, persons managing patients with smallpox will have been immunized.[54]

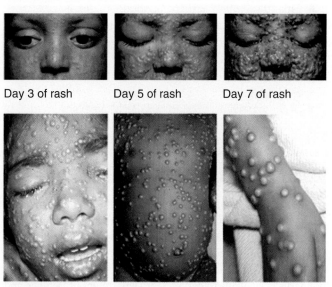

Day 3 of rash   Day 5 of rash   Day 7 of rash

On any part of the body, all lesions are in the same stage of development.

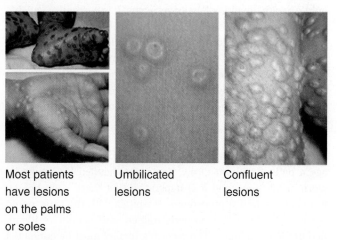

Most patients have lesions on the palms or soles

Umbilicated lesions

Confluent lesions

Figure 20-18 Smallpox.

Source: Courtesy Centers for Disease Control and Prevention, Atlanta.

Figure 20-19 Differentiating Chickenpox From Smallpox

Chickenpox (varicella) is the most likely condition to be confused with smallpox. Characteristics of chickenpox include the following:

- There is no prodrome or mild prodrome.
- Lesions are superficial vesicles: "dewdrop on a rose petal."
- Lesions appear in crops; on any one part of the body, there are lesions in different stages (papules, vesicles, crusts).
- Distribution is centripetal, with the greatest concentration of lesions on the trunk, and the fewest lesions on distal extremities. Lesions may involve the face/scalp; occasionally, the entire body is equally affected.
- First lesions appear on the face or trunk.
- Patients are rarely toxic or moribund.
- Lesions evolve rapidly, from macules to papules to vesicles to crusts (less than 24 hours).
- Palms and soles are rarely involved.
- Patient lacks a reliable history of varicella or varicella vaccination.
- Of these patients, 50% to 80% recall an exposure to chickenpox or shingles 10 to 21 days before rash onset.

Source: Courtesy Centers for Disease Control and Prevention, Atlanta.

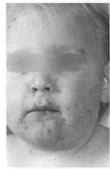
Healthy child with varicella

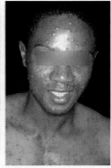
Healthy adult with varicella

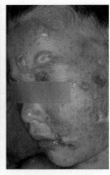
Bacterial super-infection of lesions

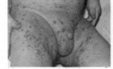
Note centripetal distribution of rash

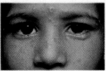
Day 3 of rash

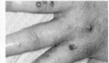
Lesions are in different stages of development

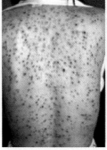
Healthy adult with varicella

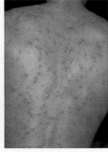
Healthy adult with varicella

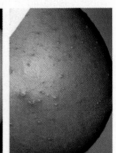
Pregnant woman with varicella

Figure 20-20 Chickenpox.
Source: Courtesy Centers for Disease Control and Prevention, Atlanta.

The smallpox vaccination program in the United States was stopped in 1972. The residual immunity provided by this vaccination program is unknown, and it is suggested that individuals whose last immunization was 40 years ago will likely now be susceptible to contracting smallpox.[53] Vaccination for the smallpox virus is available to certain U.S. Department of Defense and State Department members. It was also made available under a Department of Health and Human Services program to develop public health Smallpox Response Teams. It is currently available to the general public only for participants in clinical trials. In case of a public health emergency, the United States has stockpiles of vaccine that can be released for mass immunization of the public. Vaccination within 4 days of the exposure has been shown to offer some protection against contracting the illness and substantial protection against a fatal outcome.[53]

Management

Prehospital care providers will provide supportive care to manage a patient with smallpox. The recommended PPE must be worn at all times, and it is imperative that there is no breach in infection-control procedures. Hospitals with the appropriate isolation facilities and properly trained staff should be identified in the community. The receiving facility must be contacted to inform the staff of the intention to transport the confirmed or suspected case of smallpox to their facility so that proper precautions can be taken to prevent transmission of the virus. The identification of a patient with smallpox would be considered a public health emergency of enormous significance.

Proper removal of PPE without breach in infection control procedures is important for the safety of the prehospital care provider. All contaminated disposable medical waste must be properly bagged, labeled, and disposed of as other regulated medical waste. Reusable medical equipment must be cleaned after use according to standard protocol, either by autoclaving or by subjecting the equipment to high-level disinfection. Environmental surfaces need to be cleaned by an approved EPA-registered detergent-disinfectant. Air decontamination or fumigation of the emergency vehicle is not required.[55]

Botulinum Toxin

Botulinum toxin is produced by the bacterium *Clostridium botulinum* and is the most poisonous substance known. It is

15,000 times more toxic than the nerve agent VX and 100,000 times more toxic than sarin.[56] Botulinum toxin has been weaponized for military use by the United States, the former Soviet Union, Iraq, and probably Iran, Syria, and North Korea.[57] The Aum Shinrikyo cult, responsible for the Tokyo subway sarin attack, attempted to deliver an aerosol of botulinum toxin without success in 1995. Despite the reported difficulty of concentrating and stabilizing the toxin for dissemination, it is estimated that a terrorist point-source delivery of botulinum aerosol could incapacitate or kill 10% of persons downwind 0.3 mile (0.5 km). The toxin could also be introduced into the food supply in an attempt to poison large numbers of people.

Three forms of botulism exist naturally. *Wound botulism* occurs when toxins are absorbed from a dirty wound, often with devitalized tissue, in which *C. botulinum* is present. *Food-borne botulism* occurs when improperly prepared or home-canned foods allow the bacteria to grow and produce toxin, which is ingested by the victim. *Intestinal botulism* occurs when toxin is produced and absorbed within the GI tract. In addition to these three naturally occurring forms, a man-made form of botulism, called *inhalational botulism*, is a result of aerosolized botulinum toxin.

Regardless of the route, botulinum toxin is carried to the neuromuscular junction where it binds irreversibly, preventing normal release of the neurotransmitter acetylcholine and causing a descending flaccid paralysis. Onset of symptoms is several hours to a few days. All patients will present with diplopia (double vision) and multiple cranial nerve deficits, causing difficulty with sight, speech, and swallowing. The extent and rapidity of the descending paralysis depend on the dose of the toxin. Patients become fatigued, lose the ability to control the muscles of the head and neck, may lose their gag reflex, or may progress to paralysis of the muscles of respiration and develop respiratory failure, requiring intubation and months of mechanical ventilation. Untreated patients usually die of mechanical upper airway obstruction or inadequate ventilation. The classic triad of botulinum toxicity is (1) descending symmetric flaccid paralysis with cranial nerve deficits, (2) lack of fever, and (3) a clear sensorium. After weeks to months, patients may recover as new axon buds develop to innervate the denervated muscles.

Management

Care for the patient with botulism is supportive, with administration of antitoxin in the hospital. Early use of antitoxin will minimize further deterioration but cannot reverse existing paralysis. This antitoxin is available from the CDC.

Prehospital care providers caring for victims of botulism would need to be vigilant about airway compromise and inadequate ventilation. Patients may not be able to manage their secretions or maintain a patent airway. Because of diaphragm paralysis, patients may not be able to generate an adequate tidal volume. This may be exacerbated by having the patient in a supine or semi-recumbent position. Patients experiencing respiratory difficulty should be intubated and adequately ventilated.

Standard precautions are adequate for the management of patients experiencing the effects of botulinum toxicity because it is not a contagious disease. Botulism aerosols degrade readily in the environment, and it is anticipated that after delivery in a terrorist incident, substantial inactivation will occur after 2 days. Responders to an overt aerosol dissemination event would require level A PPE suitable for a hazardous environment if working in the hot zone or warm zone.

Because the aerosol can persist for approximately 2 days under average weather conditions, victims who have been exposed to botulinum aerosol require decontamination by clothing removal and washing with soap and water. Equipment can be decontaminated using a 0.1% hypochlorite bleach solution.[58] Patients will not require isolation after arrival at the hospital, but critical care services may be needed for patients requiring mechanical ventilation.

Radiologic Disasters

Since the terrorist attacks of September 11, 2001, new consideration has been given to the likelihood of EMS systems needing to manage a radiologic emergency. Historically, planning has focused on civil-defense preparation for a strategic exchange of military nuclear weapons or the rare occurrence of a nuclear power plant accident. Currently, however, there is increasing awareness of the possibility that terrorists could deploy an improvised nuclear detonation device, or perhaps more likely a radiologic dispersal device, that uses conventional explosives to disseminate radioactive material into the environment.

Although radiologic accidents are rare, there have been 243 radiation accidents since 1944 in the United States, with 1,342 casualties that met criteria for significant exposure. Worldwide, 403 accidents have occurred, with 133,617 victims, 2,965 with significant exposure, and 120 fatalities. The Chernobyl disaster of 1986 was responsible for 116,500 to 125,000 exposed casualties and close to 50 deaths as of 2005, although it is estimated that the total number of deaths could reach as many as 4,000 as additional cancer victims succumb.[59,60] The Fukushima nuclear power plant in Japan was seriously damaged after a nearby earthquake and tsunami in 2011, resulting in the destruction of several reactors and the release of radiation into the environment. It will take years and even decades before the health impact of this incident on the surrounding population and environment can be fully evaluated.

Radiation disasters have the potential to generate fear and confusion in both victims and emergency responders. Familiarization with the hazard and management principles will help to ensure an appropriate response and help to reduce panic and disorder (**Figure 20-21**).

Exposure to ionizing radiation and radioactive contamination may result from several different scenarios: (1) detonation of a nuclear weapon, whether high grade or an improvised low-yield device; (2) detonation of a "dirty bomb" or radiation dispersion device, in which there is no nuclear detonation, but rather conventional explosives are detonated to disperse a *radionuclide* (radioactive material); (3)

Figure 20-21   Principles of Management of a Radiologic Disaster

1. Assess the scene for safety.
2. All patients should be medically stabilized from their traumatic injuries before radiation injuries are considered. Patients are then evaluated for their external radiation exposure and contamination.
3. An external source of radiation, if great enough, can cause tissue injury, but it does not make the patient radioactive. Patients with even lethal exposures to external radiation are not a threat to prehospital care providers.
4. Patients can become contaminated with radioactive material deposited on their skin or clothing. More than 90% of surface contamination can be removed by removal of clothing. The remainder can be washed off with soap and water.
5. Prehospital care providers should protect themselves from radioactive contamination by observing, at a minimum, standard precautions, including protective clothing, gloves, and a mask.
6. Patients who develop nausea, vomiting, or skin erythema within 4 hours of exposure have likely received a high external radiation exposure.
7. Radioactive contamination in wounds should be treated as dirt and irrigated as soon as possible. Avoid handling any metallic foreign body.
8. Potassium iodide (KI) is only of value if there has been a release of radioactive iodine. KI is not a general radiation antidote.
9. The concept of time/distance/shielding is key in the prevention of untoward effects from radiation exposure. Radiation exposure is minimized by decreasing time in the affected area, increasing distance from a radiation source, and using metal or concrete shielding.

Source: Modified from Department of Homeland Security Working Group on Radiological Dispersion Device Preparedness/Medical Preparedness and Response Subgroup, 2004, http://www1.va.gov/emshg/docs/Radiologic_Medical_Countermeasures_051403.pdf.

sabotage or accident at a nuclear reactor site; and (4) mishandled nuclear waste.

Medical Effects of Radiation Catastrophes

The injuries and risks associated with a radiologic catastrophe would be multifactorial. In the case of a nuclear detonation, casualties would be produced by the explosion, resulting in primary, secondary, and tertiary blast injuries, thermal injury, and structural collapse. Victims may be further subjected to radiation injury from *irradiation*, in which radiation passes through the body causing damage but does not result in contamination (similar to getting an x-ray); from external radioactive contamination, which can be deposited on skin and clothing from fallout; or from internal radiation through radioactive particulate contamination, which victims may inhale, ingest, or have deposited in wounds.

Accidents at nuclear reactors could generate large doses of ionizing radiation, without a nuclear detonation, especially under circumstances in which the reactor reaches a point of "criticality." Explosions, fire, and gas release could also result in radioactive gas or particulate matter, which could expose emergency responders to the risk of exposure to contamination with radioactive particles.

Radiation dispersion devices (RDDs) typically would not deliver enough radiation to cause immediate injury. However, RDDs would complicate management for prehospital care providers by distributing radioactive particulates that could contaminate victims and emergency responders and make it difficult to manage the injuries caused by the conventional explosive. RDDs could cause confusion and panic in the public and among emergency responders concerned about radioactivity, hindering efforts to assist victims.

Ionizing radiation causes injury to cells by interacting with atoms and depositing energy. This interaction results in **ionization**, which can either damage the cell nucleus directly, causing cell death or malfunction, or indirectly, damaging cell components by interacting with water in the body and resulting in toxic molecules. Acute exposure to large doses of penetrating ionizing radiation (irradiation with gamma rays and neutrons) in a short time can result in acute radiation illness. Types of ionizing radiation include alpha particles, beta particles, gamma rays, and neutrons.

Alpha particles are relatively large and cannot penetrate even a few layers of skin. Intact skin or a uniform offers adequate protection from external contamination emitting alpha particles. Ionizing radiation from alpha particles is a concern only if it is internalized in the body by inhaling or ingesting alpha-particle emitters. When internalized, alpha-particle radiation can cause significant local cellular injury to adjacent cells.

Beta particles are small charged particles that can penetrate more deeply than alpha particles and can affect deeper layers of the skin with the ability to injure the base of the skin, causing a *beta burn*. Beta-particle radiation is found most frequently in nuclear fallout. Beta particles also result in local radiation injury.

Gamma rays are similar to x-rays and can easily penetrate tissue. Gamma rays are emitted with a nuclear detonation and with fallout. They could also be emitted from some radionuclides

Figure 20-22 Terrorism with Ionizing Radiation: General Guide

Diagnosis

Be alert to the following:

1. The acute radiation syndrome follows a predictable pattern after substantial exposure or catastrophic events (Figure 20-23).
2. Individuals may become ill from contaminated sources in the community and may be identified over much longer periods based on specific syndromes (Figure 20-24).
3. Specific syndromes of concern, especially with a 2- to 3-week prior history of nausea and vomiting, are:
   - Thermal burnlike skin effects without documented thermal exposure
   - Immunologic dysfunction with secondary infections
   - Tendency to bleed (epistaxis, gingival bleeding, petechiae)

- Marrow suppression (neutropenia, lymphopenia, and thrombocytopenia)
- Epilation (hair loss)

Understanding Exposure

Exposure may be known and recognized or clandestine and may occur by the following means:

1. Large recognized exposures, such as a nuclear bomb or damage to a nuclear power station
2. Small radiation source emitting continuous gamma radiation, producing group or individual chronic intermittent exposures (e.g., radiologic sources from medical treatment devices, environmental water or food pollution)
3. Internal radiation from absorbed, inhaled, or ingested radioactive material (internal contamination)

Source: Modified from Department of Veterans Affairs pocket guide produced by Employee Education System for Office of Public Health and Environmental Hazards. This information is not meant to be complete, but to be a quick guide; please consult other references and expert opinion.

that might be present in an RDD. Gamma radiation can result in what is termed *whole-body exposure*. Whole-body exposure can result in acute and chronic radiation illnesses (**Figures 20-22, 20-23,** and **20-24**).

Neutrons can penetrate tissue easily, with 20 times the destructive energy of gamma rays, disrupting the atomic structure of cells. Neutrons are released during a nuclear detonation but are not a fallout risk. Neutrons also contribute to whole-body radiation exposure and can result in acute radiation illness. Neutrons can convert stable metals into radioactive isotopes. This ability has significance in patients with metal hardware or those in possession of metal objects at the time of exposure.

Whole-body exposure is measured in terms of the *gray* (Gy). The *rad* (radiation absorbed dose) was a familiar dose unit that was replaced by the gray; 1 Gy equals 100 rad. The rem (radiation equivalent–man) describes the dose in rad multiplied by a "quality factor," which takes into account the intrinsic special deposition pattern of different types of radiation. The rem has been replaced with the *sievert* (Sv); 1 Sv equals 100 rem.

Radiation affects rapidly dividing cells most readily, resulting in injury to the bone marrow and GI tract where high cell turnover rates occur. Higher doses can affect the CNS directly. The dose of whole-body exposure determines the medical consequences of the exposure. Patients receiving up to 1 Gy of whole-body irradiation would typically not exhibit signs of injury. At 1 to 2 Gy, less than half of patients will develop nausea and vomiting, many will subsequently develop *leukopenia* (decreased white blood cell count), and deaths will be minimal. Most victims

receiving greater than 2 Gy will become ill and require hospitalization; at greater than 6 Gy, mortality becomes high. At doses greater than 30 Gy, neurologic signs are manifest, and death is most likely.[19]

Acute radiation syndrome generally follows a defined progression that first manifests in a prodromal phase characterized by malaise, nausea, and vomiting. This is followed by a latent phase, in which the patient is essentially asymptomatic. The length of the latent phase depends on the total absorbed dose of radiation. The greater the dose of radiation, the shorter the latent phase. The latent phase is followed by the subsequent illness phase, manifested by the organ system that has been injured. Damage to the bone marrow occurs with total doses of 0.7 to 4.0 Gy and results in decreasing levels of white blood cells and decreased immunity to infection over several days to weeks. Decreased platelets can result in easy bruising and bleeding. Decreased red blood cells will result in anemia. At 6 to 8 Gy, the GI tract will also be affected, resulting in diarrhea, volume loss, and hematochezia (bloody stools). Above 30 Gy, the patient will manifest symptoms of the neurovascular syndrome, experiencing the prodromal phase of nausea and vomiting, a short latent phase lasting only a few hours, followed by a rapid deterioration of mental status, coma, and death, sometimes accompanied by hemodynamic instability. Doses this high can occur after a nuclear detonation, but the victim will most likely have been killed by injuries associated with the blast. Victims could also be exposed to these high doses at a nuclear power facility where no blast has occurred, but a reactor core has reached criticality.[19]

Figure 20-23 Acute Radiation Syndrome

Feature	Effects of Whole-Body Irradiation or Internal Absorption, by Dose Range in rad (1 rad = 1 centigray; 100 rad = 1 gray)					
	0–100 (0–1 Gy)	100–200 (1–2 Gy)	200–600 (2–6 Gy)	600–800 (6–8 Gy)	800–3000 (8–30 Gy)	> 3000 (>30 Gy)
PRODROMAL PHASE OF SYNDROME						
Nausea, vomiting	None	5–50%	50–100%	75–100%	90–100%	100%
Time of onset	—	3–6 hr	2–4 hr	1–2 hr	< 1 hr	N/A
Duration	—	< 24 hr	< 24 hr	< 48 hr	48 hr	N/A
Lymphocyte count	Unaffected	Minimally decreased	< 1000 at 24 hr	< 500 at 24 hr	Decreases within hours	Decreases within hours
CNS function	No impairment	No impairment	Routine task performance Cognitive impairment for 6–20 hr	Simple, routine task performance Cognitive impairment for > 24 hr	Rapid incapacitation; May have a lucid interval of several hours	
LATENT PHASE OF SYNDROME						
No symptoms	> 2 wk	7–15 d	0–7 d	0–2 d	None	None
MANIFEST ILLNESS						
Signs/symptoms	None	Moderate leukopenia	Severe leukopenia, purpura, hemorrhage, pneumonia, hair loss after 300 rad		Diarrhea, fever, electrolyte disturbance	Convulsions, ataxia, tremor, lethargy
Time of onset	—	> 2 wk	2 d to 4 wk	2 d to 4 wk	1–3 d	1–3 d
Critical period	—	None	4–6 wk; greatest potential for effective medical intervention		2–14 d	1–46 hr
Organ system	None	—	Hematopoietic; respiratory (mucosal) systems		GI tract Mucosal systems	CNS
Hospitalization duration	0%	< 5% 45–60 d	90% 60–90 d	100% 100+ d	100% Weeks to months	100% Days to weeks
Mortality	None	Minimal	Low with aggressive therapy	High	Very high; significant neurologic symptoms indicate lethal dose	

CNS, central nervous system; d, day(s); hr, hour(s); N/A, not available; wk, week(s).

Source: Modified from Armed Forces Radiobiology Research Institute: Medical management of radiological casualties, Bethesda, MD, 2003.

Not all radiation accidents or terrorist events will result in high-dose radiation exposure. Low-dose radiation exposure, as would most likely occur after an RDD detonation, probably would not produce acute injury secondary to radiation. Dependent on dose, the patient may have an increased future risk of developing cancer. The acute effects of RDD detonation, besides the effects of the detonation of the conventional explosive, will likely be psychological, including stress reactions, fear, acute depression, and psychosomatic complaints, which would significantly strain the EMS agencies and medical infrastructure.

Figure 20-24 Symptom Clusters as Delayed Effects After Radiation

1	2	3	4
Headache Fatigue Weakness	Anorexia Nausea Vomiting Diarrhea	Partial-thickness and full-thickness skin damage Epilation (hair loss) Ulceration	Lymphopenia Neutropenia Thrombocytopenia Purpura Opportunistic infections

Source: Modified from Armed Forces Radiobiology Institute, Medical management of radiological casualties, Bethesda, MD, 2003.

Patients can become contaminated with material that emits alpha, beta, and even gamma radiation, but the most common contaminants will emit alpha and beta radiation. Only gamma radiation contributes to whole-body irradiation, as previously described. Alpha and beta radiation have limited ability to penetrate, but still can cause local tissue injury. Patients can easily be decontaminated by clothing removal and washing with water or soap and water. It is impossible for a patient to be so contaminated as to be a radiologic hazard to prehospital care providers caring for the individual, so management of traumatic life-threatening injury is an immediate priority and should not be delayed pending decontamination.[19]

As described, radioactive particles can be inhaled, ingested, or absorbed through the skin or contaminated wounds. This type of exposure to radiation will not result in acute effects of radiation exposure but can result in delayed effects. Any victims or emergency responders who operate in an area at risk for airborne radioactive particles without the benefit of respiratory protection would require subsequent evaluation to identify internal contamination, which could require medical intervention to dilute or block the effects of the inhaled radionuclide.

Personal Protective Equipment

Prehospital care providers would be operating in an environment with risk of exposure to ionizing radiation after a radiologic disaster. The radiation risk would depend greatly on the type of radiologic event.

The PPE available to prehospital care providers for use in chemical and biologic hazards will offer some protection from radioactive particulate contamination. However, it will not provide protection from high-energy radiation sources, such as a damaged reactor or nuclear blast at ground zero.

Radioactivity can be present in gases, aerosols, solids, or liquids. If radioactive gases are present, SCBA will offer the highest protection. If aerosols are present, an APR may be adequate to prevent internal contamination caused by inhalation of contaminated particles. An N-95 mask will offer some protection from inhaled particulates. A standard splash-resistant suit will protect against particulates that emit alpha radiation and will offer some protection from beta radiation, but will provide no protection from gamma radiation or neutrons. This type of barrier protection will assist in the decontamination of particulate matter from an individual, but it does not protect against the risks of acute radiation illness when the person is exposed to high-energy sources of external radiation.

None of the typical PPE carried by prehospital care providers protects from a high-energy point source of radiation. This type of radiation is encountered during the first minute of a nuclear detonation, in a critical reactor core, or with a high-energy radiation source such as cesium-137, which may be dispersed in an RDD. The best protection from these sources is decreased time of exposure, increased distance from the source, and shielding. Some new materials that may offer some protection from low-level gamma radiation for emergency responder PPE are under investigation.

Unlike insufficient PPE worn to protect against chemical agents, the inhalation, ingestion, or skin absorption of radiation-emitting gas or particulate will not immediately incapacitate a prehospital care provider or victim. All prehospital care providers who operated in an environment potentially contaminated with radioactive material would have to undergo a radiation survey to determine if internal contamination had occurred and undergo active management if warranted.

Dose rate meters or alarms should be worn if available. Standards exist for acceptable doses of ionizing radiation in the occupational environment under normal and emergency conditions.[20] Dose rates of ionizing radiation can be measured to prevent emergency responders from putting themselves at risk for acute radiation illness or an unacceptably higher incidence of cancer. The incident commander should be approached for guidance on radiation-exposure readings and limits.

Assessment and Management

Patients who have been injured in a radiologic catastrophe should receive primary and secondary assessments as dictated by the mechanism of injury. Prehospital care providers can expect to evaluate patients who have sustained blast injury and thermal injury in the case of a nuclear detonation, or from the conventional high explosive detonation of an RDD (**Figure 20-25**). Priority should be given to management of traumatic injuries with the radiologic aspects of the case receiving secondary consideration. Decontamination of the victim is recommended to eliminate radioactive particulate contamination but should not delay the care of patients requiring immediate intervention for their traumatic injuries. If the patient does not show signs of serious injury requiring immediate intervention, the patient can be decontaminated first.

If radioiodine is present in the environment, as might be encountered in a nuclear reactor, following a spent fuel rod accident, or following detonation of a nuclear device, then giving potassium iodide to emergency responders and victims may help prevent accumulation of radioiodine in the thyroid, where it can increase the likelihood of cancer. Other *blocking* and *decorporation therapy* may be recommended by the hospital or federal assistance agencies when more information about the catastrophe is available. Blocking therapy is designed to interfere with the effects of the radiologic agent, whereas decorporation treatment is targeted at removing the agent from the body using medications that combine with the agent and allow for its elimination.

Transport Considerations

Patients should be transported to the nearest appropriate medical center that is capable of managing trauma and radiation injuries. All hospitals are required to have a plan for management of a radiologic emergency, but communities may have identified institutions that have decontamination facilities, are capable of managing trauma, and have staff trained to deal effectively with possible external or internal radioactive contamination, as well as the complications of whole-body exposure to ionizing radiation.

Figure 20-25 Treatment and Decontamination Considerations for Radiation Exposure

Treatment Considerations
- If trauma is present, treat.
- If external radioactive contaminants are present, decontaminate (after treatment of life-threatening problems).
- If radioiodine (e.g., reactor accident) is present, consider giving prophylactic potassium iodide (Lugol's solution) within first 24 hours only (ineffective later).
- See http://www.afrri.usuhs.mil or http://www.orau.gov/reacts/guidance.htm.

Decontamination Considerations
- Exposure without contamination requires no decontamination.
- Exposure with contamination requires standard (universal) precautions, removal of patient clothing, and decontamination with water.
- Internal contamination will be determined at the hospital.
- Treating contaminated patients before decontamination may contaminate the facility; plan for decontamination before arrival.
- For a patient with a life-threatening condition, *treat*, then decontaminate.
- For a patient with a non-life-threatening condition, *decontaminate*, then treat.

Source: Modified from Armed Forces Radiobiology Institute: Medical management of radiological casualties, Bethesda, MD, 2003.

Summary

- Weapons of mass destruction manufactured by terrorist regimes pose a significant threat to civilized society.
- Prehospital care providers may also come in contact with explosions and with chemical and radiologic material as the result of industrial mishaps.
- The safety of prehospital care providers is paramount. They should possess a working knowledge of levels of personal protective equipment and the fundamentals of decontamination.
- Explosive agents have predominated in recent terrorist attacks. High explosives produce primary blast injuries in survivors who are in close proximity to the blast, and secondary injuries result from flying debris.
- Chemical agents may not only injure the skin and pulmonary system but may also result in systemic illness, manifesting as a specific toxidrome that yields clues to the agent. Antidotes are used for some of these agents.
- Biologic agents can be highly virulent bacteria or viruses, or toxins produced by living organisms. The types of protective precautions used by providers vary with the specific agents.
- Several types of radiation exist. Exposure to these agents may result in acute radiation illness, which is typically a function of the type of radiation and the length of exposure.

SCENARIO RECAP

It is a warm summer evening and you are dispatched to the scene of a reported explosion outside of a popular café. You know that this café is usually quite busy and that it typically has patrons both inside and outside on the patio. Dispatch tells you that at this point the number of victims is unknown but that they have received multiple emergency calls. Other public safety agencies have also been dispatched to the location.

Upon arrival at the location, you note that you are the first prehospital care provider on scene. No incident command has yet been established. Dozens of people are running about the scene. Many are screaming for you to assist victims who are obviously bleeding. Other victims are lying on the ground.

- What will you do first?
- What are your priorities as you determine your course of action?
- How will you care for so many people?

SCENARIO SOLUTION

As always, the first priority is safety. Assess the scene. Look for evidence of a secondary device that may pose a threat to emergency responders. Are there other hazards? Look for hanging debris, downed or exposed power lines, or hazardous materials spills. Carefully observe the crowd for evidence of a toxidrome. Is there an unusually high proportion of respiratory difficulty? Are victims vomiting and seizing? Is there evidence of agent dispersal in addition to the explosive blast? Don PPE appropriate for the incident.

Communicate with your chain of command and use the incident command system (ICS). As the first emergency responder to the scene, the communications center will be relying on you for information. Describe pertinent details of the scene, observed hazards, numbers of victims, and likely number of resources required to manage the scene and victims. Based on your observations, the communications center and the on-duty supervisor can apprise other units and agencies of your situation and dispatch the necessary resources. A predefined disaster response plan may be activated.

Once the personal safety of all emergency responders has been ensured and information has been communicated, prepare to serve as the incident commander until relieved by another competent authority.

As soon as is feasible, approach the victims with the intention of triaging them for treatment and transport using the START algorithm. Without engaging in the medical management of victims initially, sort the victims into immediate, urgent, delayed, and expectant categories. Remember, blast victims may not be able to hear directions or questions from emergency responders. As other assistance arrives, direct personnel to assume roles of the ICS until supervisory personnel arrive to assume command and control functions.

References

1. Hogan DE, Waeckerle JF, Dire DJ, et al. Emergency department impact of the Oklahoma City terrorist bombing. *Ann Emerg Med.* 1999;34:160.
2. Kennedy K, Aghababian R, Gans L, et al. Triage: techniques and applications in decision making. *Ann Emerg Med.* 1996; 28(2):136.
3. Garner A, Lee A, Harrison K. Comparative analysis of multiple-casualty incident triage algorithms. *Ann Emerg Med.* 2001;38:541.
4. Lerner EB, Schwartz RB, Coule PL, et al. Mass casualty triage: an evaluation of the data and development of a proposed national guideline. *Disaster Med Public Health Preparedness.* 2008;2(suppl 1):S25–S34.
5. Kapur GB, Hutson HR, Davis MA, Rice PL. The United States twenty-year experience with bombing incidents: implications for terrorism preparedness and medical response. *J Trauma.* 2005;59:1436–1444.
6. Hall JR Jr. Deaths due to unintentional injury from explosions. Quincy, MA: National Fire Protection Association, Fire Analysis and Research Division; 2008.
7. Mohtadi H, Murshid A. A global chronology of incidents of chemical, biological, radioactive and nuclear attacks: 1950–2005. http://www.ncfpd.umn.edu/Ncfpd/assets/File/pdf/GlobalChron.pdf. Accessed September 21, 2013.
8. U.S. Department of State, Office of the Historian, Bureau of Public Affairs. Significant terrorist incidents, 1961–2003: a brief chronology, Washington, DC: U.S. Department of State; 2004.
9. National Counterterrorism Center. *2007 Report on Terrorism: 30 April 2008.* http://www.fbi.gov/stats-services/publications/terror_07.pdf. Accessed January 10, 2014.
10. U.S. Bomb Data Center (USBDC). Explosive incidents 2007. 2007 USBDC explosives statistics. Washington, DC: USBDC; 2007.
11. U.S. Department of State. Country Reports on Terrorism 2011. http://www.state.gov/j/ct/rls/crt/2011/195555.htm. Accessed February 25, 2013.

12. National Counterterrorism Center. *2006 Report on Terrorist Incidents: 30 April 2007*. http://www.fbi.gov/stats-services/publications/terror_06.pdf. Accessed January 10, 2014.

13. Frykberg ER, Tepas JJ, Alexander RH. The 1983 Beirut Airport terrorist bombing: injury patterns and implications for disaster management. *Am Surg*. 1989;55:134.

14. U.S. Department of State. Bureau of Counterterrorism. Country Reports on Terrorism 2011. http://www.state.gov/documents/organization/195768.pdf. Accessed January 10, 2014.

15. Arnold J, Halpern P, Tsai M. Mass casualty terrorist bombings: a comparison of outcomes by bombing type. *Ann Emerg Med*. 2004;43:263.

16. DePalma RG, Burris DG, Champion HR, et al. Blast injuries. *N Engl J Med*. 2005; 352(13):1335–1342.

17. Centers for Disease Control and Prevention. Explosions and blast injuries: a primer for clinicians. http://www.bt.cdc.gov/masscasualties/explosions.asp. Updated May 9, 2003. Accessed January 10, 2014.

18. Wightman JM, Gladish JL. Explosions and blast injuries. *Ann Emerg Med*. 2001;37:664.

19. Armed Forces Radiobiology Research Institute. (AFRRI). Medical management of radiological casualties. Bethesda, MD: AFRRI; 2003.

20. U.S. Department of Veterans Affairs. Department of Homeland Security Working Group on Radiological Dispersion Device Preparedness/Medical Preparedness and Response Subgroup. http://www.acr.org/~/media/ACR/Documents/PDF/Membership/Legal%20Business/Disaster%20Preparedness/Counter%20Measures. Accessed January 10, 2014.

21. Almogy G, Mintz Y, Zamir G, et al. Suicide bombing attacks: can external signs predict internal injuries? *Ann Surg*. 2006;243(4):541–546.

22. Garner MJ, Brett SJ. Mechanisms of injury by explosive devices. *Anesthesiol Clin*. 2007;25(1):147–160.

23. Avidan V, Hersch M, Armon Y, et al. Blast lung injury: clinical manifestations, treatment, and outcome. *Am J Surg*. 2005;190(6):927–931.

24. Katz E, Ofek B, Adler J, et al. Primary blast injury after a bomb explosion in a civilian bus. *Ann Surg*. 1989;209:484.

25. Kluger Y, Nimrod A, Biderman P, et al. Case report: the quinary pattern of blast injury. *J Emerg Mgmt*. 2006;4(1):51–55.

26. Sorkine P, Nimrod A, Biderman P, et al. The quinary (Vth) injury pattern of blast (Abstract). *J Trauma*. 2007;56(1):232.

27. Nelson TJ, Wall DB, Stedje-Larsen ET, et al. Predictors of mortality in close proximity blast injuries during Operation Iraqi Freedom. *J Am Coll Surg*. 2006;202(3):418–422.

28. Mallonee S, Shariat S, Stennies G, et al. Physical injuries and fatalities resulting from the Oklahoma City bombing. *JAMA*. 1996;276:382.

29. Arnold JL, Tsai MC, Halpern P, et al. Mass-casualty, terrorist bombings: epidemiological outcomes, resource utilization, and time course of emergency needs (Part I). *Prehosp Disaster Med*. 2003;18(3):220–234.

30. Halpern P, Tsai MC, Arnold JL, et al. Mass-casualty, terrorist bombings: implications for emergency department and hospital emergency response (Part II). *Prehosp Disaster Med*. 2003;18(3):235–241.

31. Caseby NG, Porter MF. Blast injury to the lungs: clinical presentation, management and course. *Injury*. 1976;8:1.

32. Leibovici D, Gofrit ON, Shapira SC. Eardrum perforation in explosion survivors: is it a marker of pulmonary blast injury? *Ann Emerg Med*. 1999;34:168.

33. Coppel DL. Blast injuries of the lungs. *Br J Surg*. 1976;63:735.

34. Cohn SM. Pulmonary contusion: review of the clinical entity. *J Trauma*. 1997;42:973.

35. Peleg K, Limor A, Stein M, et al. Gunshot and explosion injuries: characteristics, outcomes, and implications for care of terror-related injuries in Israel. *Ann Surg*. 2004;239(3):311.

36. Tappan J. Magnesium and thermite poisoning. http://emedicine.medscape.com/article/833495-overview. Accessed January 10, 2014.

37. Irizarry L. White phosphorus exposure. http://emedicine.medscape.com/article/833585-overview. Accessed January 10, 2014.

38. Sidell FR, Takafuji ET, Franz DR, eds. Medical aspects of chemical and biological warfare, TMM series, Part 1, Warfare, weaponry and the casualty, Washington, DC: Office of the Surgeon General, TMM Publications; 1997.

39. Walter FG, ed. *Advanced HAZMAT Life Support*. 2nd ed. Tucson, AZ: Arizona Board of Regents; 2000.

40. U.S. Army, Medical Research Institute of Chemical Defense. *Medical Management of Chemical Casualties Handbook*. 3rd ed. Aberdeen Proving Ground, MD: US Army Research Institute; 2000.

41. Greenfield RA, Brown BR, Hutchins JB, et al. Microbiological, biological and chemical weapons of warfare and terrorism. *Am J Med Sci*. 2002;323(6):326.

42. Okumura T, Takasu N, Ishimatsu S, et al. Report on 640 victims of the Tokyo subway sarin attack. *Ann Emerg Med*. 1996;28(2):129.

43. Rotenberg JS, Newmark J. Nerve-agent attacks on children: diagnosis and management. *Pediatrics*. 2003;112:648.

44. McDonough JH, Capacio BR, Shih TM. Treatment of nerve-agent-induced status epilepticus in the nonhuman primate. In: *U.S. Army Medical Defense—Bioscience Review, June 2–7*. Hunt Valley, MD: U.S. Army Medical Research Institute; 2002.

45. Ingelsby TV, Henderson DA, Bartlett JG, et al. Anthrax as a biological weapon: medical and public health management. *JAMA*. 1999;281(18):1735.

46. Keim M, Kaufmann AF. Principles for emergency response to bioterrorism. *Ann Emerg Med*. 1999;34(2):177.

47. U.S. Congress, Office of Technology Assessment. Proliferation of weapons of mass destruction, Pub No OTA-ISC-559. Washington, DC: U.S. Government Printing Office.

48. Inglesby TV, O'Toole T, Henderson DA, et al. Anthrax as a biological weapon, 2002: updated recommendations for management. *JAMA*. 2002;287:2236–2252.

49. Kman NE, Nelson RN. Infectious agents of bioterrorism: a review for emergency physicians. *Emerg Med Clin North Am*. 2008;26:517–547.

50. Bell DM, Kozarsky PE, Stephens DS. Conference summary: clinical issues in the prophylaxis, diagnosis and treatment of anthrax. *Emerg Infect Dis*. 2002;8(2):222.

51. World Health Organization (WHO). *Health Aspects of Chemical and Biological Weapons*. Geneva: WHO; 1970.

52. Inglesby TV, Dennis DT, Henderson DA. Plague as a biological weapon: medical and public health management. *JAMA*. 2000;283(17):2281.

53. Henderson DA, Inglesby TV, Bartlett JG. Smallpox as a biological weapon: medical and public health management. *JAMA*. 1999;281(22):2127.

54. Centers for Disease Control and Prevention (CDC). *Smallpox Response Plan and Guidelines*. Version 3.0, Guide C, Part 1. Atlanta: CDC; 2008:1–13.

55. Centers for Disease Control and Prevention (CDC). *Smallpox Response Plan and Guidelines*. Version 3.0, Guide F. Atlanta: CDC; 2003:1-10.

56. Franz DR, Jahrling PB, Friedlander AM, et al. Clinical recognition and management of patients exposed to biological warfare agents. *JAMA*. 1997;278(5):399.

57. Arnon SS, Schechter R, Inglesby TV, et al. Botulinum toxin as a biological weapon. Medical and public health management. *JAMA*. 2001;285:1059–1070.

58. Arnon SS, Schechter R, Inglesby TV, et al. Botulinum toxin as a biological weapon: medical and public health management. *JAMA*. 2001;285(8):1059.

59. Hogan DE, Kellison T. Nuclear terrorism. *Am J Med Sci*. 2002;323(6):341.

60. World Health Organization, International Atomic Energy Agency, United Nations Development Programme. Chernobyl: the true scale of the accident. http://www.who.int/mediacentre/news/releases/2005/pr38/en/index.html. Accessed January 10, 2014.

Suggested Reading

Centers for Disease Control and Prevention Emergency Preparedness and Response Site: http://www.bt.cdc.gov/

U.S. Army Medical Research Institute of Infectious Diseases: http://www.usamriid.army.mil/

U.S. Army Public Health Command: http://phc.amedd.army.mil/home/

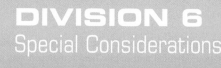

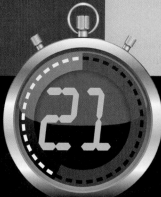

CHAPTER

21

Environmental Trauma I: Heat and Cold

CHAPTER OBJECTIVES

At the completion of this chapter, the reader will be able to do the following:

- Explain why heatstroke is considered an emergent life-threatening condition.

- Identify the similarities and differences between heatstroke and exercise-associated hyponatremia.

- Describe the two most effective and rapid cooling procedures for heatstroke.

- List the five factors that place prehospital care providers at risk for heat illness.

- Discuss the fluid hydration guidelines and how they can be applied to prevent dehydration in warm or cold environments.

- Identify the differences in the management of mild hypothermia from that of severe hypothermia.

- List the signs of mild, moderate, and severe frostbite and discuss how to prevent its progression.

- Explain reasons for actively warming hypothermic patients in cardiopulmonary arrest.

It is a hot summer afternoon with temperatures reaching 102°F (38.9°C). Over the past 30 days, it has been very humid, with temperatures reaching over 100°F (37.8°C) daily. The ambient temperature has resulted in many heat-related injuries that have required emergency medical services (EMS) personnel to transport numerous patients to the emergency departments (EDs) of the inner city.

At 1700 hours, your ambulance unit responds to a dispatch for an unresponsive male patient in a vehicle. As your ambulance unit arrives on scene, you observe a 76-year-old man who appears to be unconscious in a vehicle parked outside a department store. Your rapid assessment of the patient's airway, breathing, and circulation (ABCs) and level of consciousness reveals that the patient is verbal, but he is saying things that are illogical and irrational.

- What are the potential causes for this patient's decreased level of consciousness?
- What hallmark signs support a heat-related diagnosis?
- How would you emergently manage this patient at the scene and en route to the ED?

Introduction

This chapter focuses on recognizing and treating exposure to both hot and cold temperatures. The most significant morbidity and mortality in the United States from all environmental traumas are caused by thermal trauma.[1-5]

Environmental extremes of heat and cold have a common outcome of injuries and potential death that can affect many individuals during the peak summer and winter months. It is critical to know that mortality increases significantly when a traumatized patient presents in the hospital with either hypothermia (core body temperature less than 96.8°F [36°C]) or hyperthermia (core body temperature greater than 100.4°F [38°C])[6] (**Figure 21-1**). Individuals who are especially susceptible to both highs and lows of temperature are very young persons, the elderly population, people living in urban areas and in poverty, individuals who take specific medications, patients with chronic illnesses, and persons with alcoholism.[3-5,7-10] The majority of emergency medical services (EMS) responses in the United States for heat and cold injuries are for patients with hyperthermia or hypothermia in an urban setting. However, expanding interest in recreational and high-risk adventure activities in the wilderness backcountry during periods of environmental extremes places more individuals at risk for heat-related and cold-related injuries and fatalities.[11-14]

Epidemiology

Heat-Related Illness

During a 20-year period (1979 to 1999) in the United States, 8,015 heat-related deaths from all causes were recorded.[2] Currently, an average of 1,300 people in the United States die from heat-related incidents each year. By the end of this century, that number is expected to increase to an average of 4,500 per year due to climate change. The year 2012 was documented as the warmest year in recorded history according to the U.S. National Oceanic and Atmospheric Administration. More deaths were caused by heat stress than by hurricanes, lightning, tornadoes, floods, and earthquakes combined. Of the 8,015 deaths previously mentioned, 3,829 (48%) were related to high ambient temperatures and includes an average of about 182 heat-related deaths per month during the four warmest months (May through August). The greatest percentage of deaths (1,891, or 45%) occurred in those who are 65 years of age and older.

Furthermore, morbidity and mortality can be extremely high when periodic seasonal heat waves occur (more than 3 consecutive days of air temperatures 90°F [32.2°C] or higher). The Centers for Disease Control and Prevention reported a total of 3,442 deaths (1999 to 2003) resulting from exposure to extreme heat (annual mean of 688). In 2,239 (65%) of the deaths recorded, the underlying cause was exposure to excessive heat, whereas in the remaining 1,203 (35%), hyperthermia was recorded as a contributing factor. Males accounted for 66% of deaths and outnumbered deaths among females in all age groups. Of the 3,401 decedents for whom age information was available, 228 (7%) were aged less than 15 years; 1,810 (53%) were aged 15 to 64 years; and 1,363 (40%) were aged 65 years and older.[3]

In July of 1995, a record heat wave occurred during a 17-day period in Chicago, Illinois.[15,16] The Chicago Medical Examiner's office reported 1,177 heat-related deaths during this short period. These cases included deaths in which heat was determined to be the underlying (primary) cause of death and in which cardiovascular disease was listed as the cause of death and heat as a contributing factor (secondary). Compared with the same period in 1994, this was an 84% increase in heat-related deaths. Of these 1,177 cases, heat was the primary cause of death in 465 (39.5%).[16]

Figure 21-1	Conversion of Temperature Between Fahrenheit and Centigrade (Celsius)
Fahrenheit	**Centigrade**
110	43.3
109	42.8
108	42.2
107	41.7
106	41.1
105	40.6
104	40.0
103	39.4
102	38.9
101	38.3
100	37.8
99	37.2
98.6	**37.0**
98	36.7
97	36.1
96	35.6
95	35.0
94	34.4
93	33.9
92	33.3
91	32.8
90	32.2
88	31.1
86	30.0
84	28.9
82	27.8
80	26.7

Note: To convert from °F to °C: $°C = (°F - 32) \times 5/9$
To convert from °C to °F: $°F = (°C \times 9/5) + 32$

Cold-Related Illness

Mild to severe cold weather conditions cause an average of 689 deaths per year in the United States. Almost one-half of these deaths occurred in persons 65 years of age and older.[4] When adjusted for age, death from hypothermia occurred approximately 2.5 times more often in men than in women. The incidence of hypothermia-related deaths progressively increases with age and is three times higher in males than in females after age 15 years. From 1999 through 2011, the CDC reports an average of 1.301 deaths were reported from exposure to cold weather in the United States; of these deaths, 67% were males and 51% were older than 65 years of age.[8] Major contributing factors for accidental hypothermia are urban poverty, socioeconomic conditions, alcohol intake, malnutrition, and age (very young and senior citizens).[4,8]

While hypothermia is typically associated with cool or colder weather, it may occur in conditions that one would ordinarily not consider cold, but that allow the body's temperature to fall below 96°F (35.6°C). For example, the elderly and infants may develop hypothermia in summertime if the air conditioning in their home is too cold for their limited adaptive mechanisms. Swimmers and surfers can become hypothermic in the summer when exposed to water that is cooler than body temperature. Hypothermia is not just a cold weather disease.

Anatomy

The Skin

The skin, the largest organ of the body, interfaces with the external environment and serves as a layer of protection. It prevents the invasion of microorganisms, maintains fluid balance, and regulates temperature. Skin is composed of three tissue layers: the epidermis, dermis, and subcutaneous tissue (**Figure 21-2**). The outermost layer, the epidermis, is made up entirely of epithelial cells, with no blood vessels. Underlying the epidermis is the thicker dermis. The dermis is 20 to 30 times thicker than the epidermis. It is made up of a framework of connective tissues that contain blood vessels, blood products, nerves, sebaceous

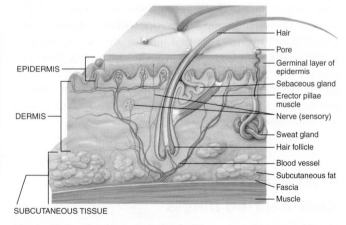

Figure 21-2 The skin is composed of three tissue layers—epidermis, dermis, and subcutaneous layer—and associated muscle. Some layers contain structures such as glands, hair follicles, blood vessels, and nerves. All these structures are interrelated to the maintenance, loss, and gain of body temperature.

glands, and sweat glands. The innermost layer, the subcutaneous layer, is a combination of elastic and fibrous tissue as well as fatty deposits. Below this layer is skeletal muscle. The skin, nerves, blood vessels, and other underlying anatomic structures have major roles in regulating body temperature.

Physiology

Thermoregulation and Temperature Balance

Humans are considered **homeotherms**, or warm-blooded animals. A key feature of homeotherms is that they are able to regulate their own internal body temperature independent of varying environmental temperatures.

The human body is essentially divided into a warmer, inner core and an outer shell. The brain and the thoracic and abdominal organs are included in the inner core, and the skin and subcutaneous layer make up the outer shell. The outer shell plays a critical role in the regulation of the body's **core temperature**. The core temperature is regulated through a balance of heat-production and heat-dissipation mechanisms. The temperature of the skin's surface and the "thickness" of the outer shell depend on the **environmental temperature**. The outer shell becomes "thicker" in colder temperatures and "thinner" in warmer temperatures based on the shunting of blood away from or to the skin, respectively. This outer shell or tissue insulation, as induced by vasoconstriction, has been estimated to offer about the same level of protection as wearing a light business suit.

Metabolic heat production will vary based on activity levels. Independent of the variation of external temperature, the body normally functions within a narrow temperature range, known as **steady-state metabolism**, of about 1°F on either side of 98.6°F (37°C ± 0.6°C). Normal body temperature is maintained in a narrow range by homeostatic mechanisms regulated in the hypothalamus, which is located in the brain. The **hypothalamus** is known as the **thermoregulatory center** and functions as the body's thermostat to control neurologic and hormonal regulation of body temperature. As noted in preceding chapters, trauma to the brain can disrupt the hypothalamus, which in turn causes an imbalance in the regulation of the body temperature.

Humans have two systems to regulate body temperature: **behavioral regulation and physiologic thermoregulation**. Behavioral regulation is governed by the individual's thermal sensation and comfort, and the distinguishing feature is the conscious effort to reduce thermal discomfort (e.g., adding clothing, seeking shelter in cold environments). The processing of sensory feedback to the brain of thermal information in behavioral regulation is not well understood, but the feedback of thermal sensation and comfort responds more quickly than physiologic responses to changes in environmental temperature.[17]

Heat Production and Thermal Balance

Basal metabolic rate is the heat produced primarily as a by-product of metabolism, mostly from the large organs of the core and from skeletal muscle contraction. The heat generated is transferred throughout the body by blood in the circulatory system. Heat transfer and its dissipation from the body by the cardiopulmonary system are important in the assessment and management of heat illness, as discussed later in the chapter.

Shivering increases the metabolic rate by increasing muscle tension, which leads to repeated bouts of muscular contraction and relaxation. There are some individual differences, but typically shivering starts when the core temperature drops to between 94°F and 97°F (34.4°C to 36.1°C) and continues until the core temperature is 88°F (31.1°C).[15] With maximal shivering, heat production is increased by five to six times the resting level.[18,19]

The physiologic thermoregulation systems that control heat production and heat loss responses are well documented.[17,19,20] Two principles in thermoregulation are key to understanding how the body regulates core temperature: **thermal gradient** and **thermal equilibrium**. A thermal gradient is the difference in temperature (high vs. low temperature) between two objects. Thermal equilibrium is the state at which two objects in contact with one another are at the same temperature; it is achieved by the transfer of heat from a warmer object to a colder object until the objects are the same temperature.

When body temperature rises, the normal physiologic response is to increase skin blood flow and to begin sweating. The majority of body heat is transferred to the environment at the skin surface by conduction, convection, radiation, and evaporation. Because heat is transferred from greater temperature to lower temperature, the human body can gain heat by radiation and conduction during hot weather conditions.

Methods to maintain and dissipate body heat are important concepts for prehospital care providers. They must understand how both heat and cold are transferred to and from the body so that they can effectively manage a patient who has hyperthermia or hypothermia (**Figure 21-3**). The methods of heat and cold transfer are described as follows:

- **Radiation** is the loss or gain of heat in the form of electromagnetic energy; it is the transfer of energy from a warm object to a cooler one. A patient with heat illness can acquire additional body heat from the hot ground or directly from the sun. These sources of heat will increase body temperature and impede interventions to cool the patient until the prehospital care provider eliminates these sources of radiant heat when assessing and treating the patient.
- **Conduction** is the transfer of heat between two objects in direct contact with each other, such as a patient lying on a frozen lawn after a fall. A patient will generally lose heat faster when lying on the cold ground than when exposed to cold air. Therefore, prehospital care providers need to lift the patient off the ground in cold temperatures rather than merely covering the patient with a blanket.
- **Convection** is the transfer of heat from a solid object to a medium that moves across that solid object, such as air or water over the body. The movement of cool air or

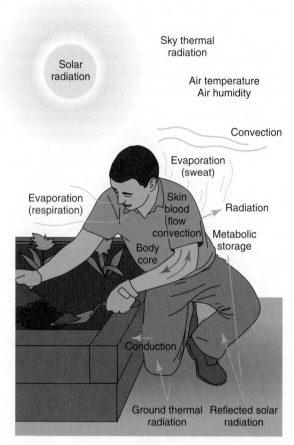

Figure 21-3 How humans exchange thermal energy with the environment.

water across the warmer skin provides for the continuous elimination of heat from the body. The body will lose heat 25 times faster in water than in air of the same temperature. A patient with wet clothing will lose body heat rapidly in mild to cold temperatures, so prehospital care providers should remove wet clothing and keep a patient dry to maintain body heat. When prehospital care providers effectively manage a patient with heat illness, they use the principle of convective heat loss by moistening and fanning the patient to dissipate body heat quickly.

■ **Evaporation** of sweat from a liquid to a vapor is an extremely effective method of heat loss from the body, depending on the relative humidity or moisture in the air. A **basal level** of both water and accompanying heat loss from exhaled air, skin, and mucous membranes is called **insensible loss** and is caused by evaporation. This insensible loss is normally about 10% of basal heat production, but when the body temperature rises, this process becomes more active (sensible), and sweat is produced. Evaporative heat loss increases in cool, dry, and windy conditions (e.g., deserts). Collectively, convection and evaporation are more important than other methods of heat transfer

because they are regulated by the body to control core temperature.[5]

Increases (*hyperthermia*) and decreases (*hypothermia*) in body temperature beyond the steady-state range (98.6°F ± 1°F [37°C ± 0.6°C]) can result from different internal and external causes, and return to steady-state temperature can occur without complications.[20] Hyperthermia occurs primarily in one of three ways:

■ As a normal response to sustained exercise, in which the heat produced elevates core temperature and is the stimulus for heat-dissipating responses (e.g., sweating, increased blood flow in skin)
■ When the sum of heat production and heat gained from the environment is greater than the body's heat dissipation capability
■ From a fever

Unlike the first two ways, fever usually occurs in response to inflammation because of a change in the *thermoregulatory set point* (body temperature setting) of the brain, and the body responds by elevating body temperature to a higher value (100°F to 106°F [37.8°C to 41.1°C]). Heat production increases only temporarily to achieve a new thermoregulatory set point temperature in an attempt to make the environment less hospitable for the invading infection.[20]

Homeostasis

All of these anatomic structures and physiologic systems are interacting so that the body functions properly when exposed to temperature changes. The body is in a constant state of neurologic feedback from peripheral and internal regions to the thermoregulatory center and other regions in the brain—all in an effort to maintain constant, stable internal conditions, or homeostasis, in the body. However, at times, this does not occur. For example, when an imbalance occurs in the cardiovascular and thermoregulatory adjustments to eliminate excessive body heat, one outcome is the loss of excessive body fluid through sweating, which causes acute dehydration and may lead to signs and symptoms of heat illness.

Risk Factors in Heat Illness

Many studies on humans have demonstrated large individual differences in their tolerance to hot environments.[21] These differences can be partially explained by both physical characteristics and medical conditions that are associated with an increased risk for heat illness (**Figure 21-4**). It is important to realize that any situation in which heat production exceeds the body's ability to dissipate heat may result in heat injury.

Figure 21-4 Heat Illness Risk Factors

Conditions

- Cardiovascular disease
- Dehydration
- Autonomic neuropathies (nerve dysfunction involving the sympathetic, parasympathetic, or both systems)
- Parkinsonism
- Dystonias (abnormal, involuntary muscle movements or contractions)
- Skin disorders: psoriasis, sunburn, burns
- Endocrine disorders (hyperthyroidism, pheochromocytoma)
- Fever
- Delirium tremens (alcohol withdrawal)
- Psychosis
- Neonates, elderly persons
- History of **heatstroke**
- Obesity
- Low fitness

Toxins/Drugs

- Increase heat production
  - Thyroid hormone
  - Cyclic antidepressants
  - Hallucinogens (e.g., LSD)
  - Cocaine
  - Amphetamines

- Decrease thirst
  - Haloperidol
  - Angiotensin-converting enzyme (ACE) inhibitors
- Decrease sweating
  - Antihistamines
  - Anticholinergics
  - Phenothiazines
  - Glutethimide
  - Beta blockers
- Increase water loss
  - Diuretics
  - Ethanol
  - Nicotine

Behavior

- Injudicious exertion (e.g., excessive exercise in hot conditions)
- Inappropriate clothing
- Poor acclimatization
- Poor fluid intake
- Poor supervision
- High motivation (e.g., working too hard in hot conditions)
- Athletic profile
- Military recruit profile

Source: This article was published in Emerg Med Clin North Am 10(2), Tek D, Olshaker JS: Heat illness, p. 299, Copyright Elsevier 1992.

Key risk factors that contribute to the onset of heat illness are alcohol consumption, medications, dehydration, higher body mass index, obesity, inadequate diet, improper clothing, low fitness, sleep loss, extremes of age, cardiovascular disease, skin injuries, previous heat-related illness, sickle cell trait, cystic fibrosis, sunburn, viral illness, and exercise during the hottest hours of day.[22,23] Transient conditions include those affecting individuals who travel from cooler climates and are not heat-acclimatized to warmer climates on arrival. Other transient factors that place individuals at risk for heat illness are common illnesses, including colds and other conditions that cause fever, vomiting, and diarrhea, along with poor dietary and fluid intake.[24,25]

Factors considered to be chronic conditions that place individuals at greater risk for heat illness are fitness level, body size, age, medical condition, and medication use.

Fitness and Body Mass Index

Low levels of physical fitness caused by genetic factors or a sedentary lifestyle with inadequate daily physical activity will reduce tolerance to heat exposure. Physical fitness provides a cardiovascular reserve to maintain cardiac output as needed to sustain thermoregulation. Individuals who are overweight have a normal response to heat exposure—vasodilation of skin blood vessels and increased sweating; however, the combination of low fitness, lack of heat acclimatization, and higher body mass index increases the energy cost of movement, placing them at greater risk for heat illness.

Age

Thermoregulatory capacity and tolerance to heat diminish with age, particularly in those individuals 65 years or older. These individuals can improve their heat tolerance by maintaining a low body weight and obtaining an improved level of physical fitness.

Special consideration must be given for infants and young children since their body surface area makes up a much greater proportion of their overall weight compared to an adult, causing them to face a much greater risk of heat-related illness. Furthermore, infants have an immature thermoregulatory capacity that cannot adequately maintain body temperature when exposed to high heat.

Gender

A long-held belief was that women are less tolerant of heat than men are. Although wide variation was reported previously, these differences resulted from women who were less physically fit and had less exposure to heat compared with men in conditions that would induce full heat acclimatization. More recent studies have controlled for differences in physical fitness and **heat acclimatization** between men and women and indicate that women demonstrate equal work tolerance in heat and, in some studies, are more tolerant of heat than men are.

Medical Conditions

Underlying medical conditions such as diabetes mellitus, thyroid disorders, and renal disease can increase the risk for heat intolerance and heat illness. Cardiovascular disease and circulatory problems that increase cutaneous blood flow and circulatory demand are aggravated by heat exposure. In these extreme environmental conditions, heart disease and pulmonary diseases may be the presenting signs and symptoms aggravated by high ambient temperatures. A mild form of heat illness seen in individuals is "prickly heat rash," which has been shown to cause reduced heat tolerance.

Medications

The use of specific prescription or over-the-counter medications can place individuals at a greater risk for heat illness (see Figure 21-4). Certain medications can increase metabolic heat production, suppress body cooling, reduce cardiac reserve, and alter renal electrolyte and fluid balance. Sedative and narcotic drugs will affect mental status and can affect logical reasoning and judgment, suppressing decision-making ability, when the individual is exposed to heat.

Dehydration

Body water is the largest component of the human body, representing 45% to 70% of body weight. For example, a 165-pound (75-kilogram [kg]) man contains approximately 45 liters of water, representing 60% of body weight. Excessive changes in the normal body water balance (*euhydration*) resulting from either overconsumption of water (*hyperhydration*) or fluid loss (causing acute dehydration) alter homeostasis, producing specific signs and symptoms. Acute dehydration can be a serious outcome of both heat and cold exposure, but it is also seen as a dangerous side effect of diarrhea, vomiting, and fever.

Dehydration is a common finding in many cases of heat illness occurring over many days, as seen in geriatric patients, or during physical activity, as seen with profuse sweating in athletes. Generally, these individuals consume no fluid or low volumes of fluid during daily activities, not replacing the depleted body water. Children (younger than 15 years) and persons older than 65 years are particularly susceptible to dehydration.

Body water is lost daily through sweat, tears, urine, and stool. Normally, drinking fluids and eating foods that contain water replace body water. When a person becomes sick with fever, diarrhea, or vomiting, or an individual is exposed to heat, dehydration occurs. Occasionally, drugs that deplete body fluids and electrolytes, such as diuretics, can cause dehydration.

During heat exposure, body water is primarily lost as sweat. Individuals can sweat 0.8 to 1.4 liters per hour (liters/hour), and it has been reported that some elite athletes who are heat-acclimatized can sweat up to 3.7 liters/hour during competition in hot environments.[26] The keys to avoiding the onset of heat illness are to maintain a body fluid balance and to minimize dehydration during daily activities, particularly during any physical activity in moderate to high heat exposure. Individuals normally do not perceive thirst until a deficit of approximately 2% of body weight has resulted from sweating.[27] Thirst provides a poor indicator of body water needs during rest or physical activity.

With mild to moderate levels of acute dehydration (2% to 6% body weight), individuals experience fatigue, headache, decreased heat tolerance, and cognitive deterioration, along with reductions in strength and aerobic physical capacity.[28,29] People will consistently underconsume fluids and remain dehydrated at approximately 1% to 2% of body weight without some form of fluid hydration guidelines to direct them regarding the amount of fluids to consume per hour when exposed to mild or high heat exposure. The underconsumption of fluid to restore normal water balance is currently known as *voluntary dehydration*.[23]

When individuals are encouraged to drink fluids frequently during heat exposure, the rate at which fluids can be replaced by mouth is limited by the rate of gastric emptying and the rate of fluid absorption in the small intestine.[30] Fluids empty from the stomach to the small intestine, where absorption occurs into the bloodstream, at a maximal rate of approximately 1 to 1.2 liters/hour.[29] Furthermore, gastric emptying rates are decreased approximately 20% to 25% when sweat-induced weight loss causes dehydration of 5% of total body weight (e.g., 5% of a 200-pound male = 10-pound weight loss).[31]

The important message is that once dehydration occurs, it becomes more challenging to rehydrate the individual adequately with oral fluids. In addition, rapid oral administration of fluids may lead to nausea and vomiting, further exacerbating the dehydration problem. The key to minimizing dehydration during heat exposure is to begin consuming oral fluids before heat exposure and to maintain fluid intake frequently during and after heat exposure. The goal of oral hydration throughout daily activity is to prevent excessive dehydration (less than 2% body weight loss) and excessive changes in electrolytes (e.g., sodium, potassium, and chloride).[32]

Signs and Symptoms of Dehydration

The following are the most common signs and symptoms of dehydration in infants, children, and adults, although each individual may experience symptoms differently:

- Less frequent urination and dark color urine
- Thirst
- Dry skin
- Fatigue
- Light-headedness
- Headache
- Dizziness
- Confusion
- Dry mouth and mucous membranes
- Increased heart rate and breathing

In infants and children, additional symptoms may include the following:

- Dry mouth and tongue
- No tears when crying
- No wet diapers for more than 3 hours
- Sunken abdomen, eyes, or cheeks
- High fever
- Listlessness
- Irritability
- Skin that does not flatten when pinched and released (*skin tenting*)

Injuries Caused by Heat

Heat-related disorders can range from minor to severe in patients with heat illness.[23,33] It is important to note that prehospital care providers may or may not see a progression of signs and symptoms, starting with minor syndromes (e.g., heat rash or muscle cramps) and advancing to major heat-related illness (e.g., classic heatstroke). In the majority of heat exposures, the patient is able to dissipate core body heat adequately and maintain core temperature within the normal range. However, when heat-related conditions result in a call for EMS assistance, the minor heat-related conditions may be apparent to the prehospital care provider during patient assessment, along with signs and symptoms of a major heat illness (**Figure 21-5**).

Minor Heat-Related Disorders

The minor heat-related disorders include heat rash, heat edema, heat tetany, muscle (heat) cramps, and heat syncope. These are not life-threatening problems but require assessment and treatment.

Heat Rash

Heat rash, also known as "prickly heat" and *miliaria rubra*, is a red, *pruritic* (itchy), *papular* (raised bumps) rash normally seen on the skin in areas of restrictive clothing and heavy sweating (**Figure 21-6**). This condition is caused by inflammation of the sweat glands that blocks the sweat ducts. As a result, affected areas cannot sweat, putting individuals at increased risk of heat illness, depending on the amount of skin surface involved.

Management

Treatment begins by cooling and drying the affected area(s) and by preventing further conditions that cause sweat in these areas. For example, get the patient out of the heat and humidity and into a cooler, dryer environment.

Heat Edema

Heat edema is a mild, dependent edema in the hands, feet, and ankles seen during early stages of heat acclimatization when plasma volume is expanding to compensate for the increased need for thermoregulatory blood flow. This form of edema does not indicate excessive fluid intake or cardiac, renal, or hepatic disease. In the absence of other diseases, this condition is of no clinical significance and is self-limited. Heat edema is observed more often in females.

Management

Treatment consists of loosening any constricting clothes, removing any tight or constricting jewelry, and elevating the legs. Diuretics are not indicated and may increase risk of heat illness.

Heat Tetany

Heat tetany is a rare and self-limited condition that may occur in patients acutely exposed to short, intense heat conditions. The hyperventilation that results from these conditions is considered to be the principle cause of the symptoms that develop, including numbness and tingling; spasm of the hands, fingers, and toes (carpopedal spasm); and muscle spasms.

Management

Treatment consists of removal from the source of heat and controlling hyperventilation. Dehydration is not a common occurrence with these short heat exposures. Heat tetany may be seen along with signs and symptoms of heat exhaustion and heatstroke.

Muscle (Heat) Cramps

Muscle cramps are manifested by short-term, painful muscle contractions frequently seen in the calf (gastrocnemius) muscles, but also in the voluntary muscles of the abdomen and extremities, and are commonly observed following prolonged physical activity, often in warm to hot temperatures. These cramps occur in individuals during exercise that produces profuse sweating or during the exercise-recovery period. Smooth muscle, cardiac,

Figure 21-5 Common Heat-Related Disorders

Disorder	Cause/Problem	Signs/Symptoms	Treatment
Muscle (heat) cramps	Failure to replace sodium chloride (salt, or NaCl) lost through sweating; electrolyte and muscle problems	Painful muscle cramps, usually in legs or abdomen	Move to cool place; massage/stretch muscle; encourage drinking sport drinks or drinks with NaCl (e.g., tomato juice). Transport those with signs or symptoms listed below.
Dehydration	Failure to replace sweat loss with fluids	Thirst, nausea, excessive fatigue, headache, hypovolemia, decreased thermoregulation; reduces physical and mental capacity	Replace sweat loss with lightly salted fluids; rest in cool place until body weight and water losses are restored. In some patients, IV rehydration is necessary.
Heat exhaustion	Excessive heat strain with inadequate water intake; cardiovascular problems with venous pooling, decreased cardiac filling time, reduced cardiac output; untreated, may progress to heatstroke	Low urine output, tachycardia, weakness, unstable gait, extreme fatigue, wet clammy skin, headache, dizziness, nausea, collapse	Remove from heat source and place in cooler location; cool body with water and fanning; encourage drinking lightly salty fluids (e.g., sport drinks); administer intravenous (IV) 0.9% NaCl or lactated Ringer's solution.
Heatstroke	High core temperatures > 105°F (40.6°C); cellular disruption; dysfunction of multiple organ systems common; neurologic disorder with thermoregulatory center failure	Mental status changes; irrational behavior or delirium; possible shivering; tachycardia initially, then bradycardia late; hypotension; rapid and shallow breathing; dry or wet, hot skin; loss of consciousness; seizures and coma	Emergency: Apply rapid, immediate cooling by water immersion, or wet patient or wrap in cool wet sheets and fan vigorously. Continue until core temperature is < 102°F (38.9°C). Treat for shock if necessary once core temperature is lowered. Immediately transport to emergency department.
Exercise-associated hyponatremia (also referred to as water intoxication)	Low plasma sodium concentration; typically seen in individuals during prolonged activity in hot environments; drinking water (> 4 liters/hour) that exceeds sweat rate; failure to replace sodium loss in sweat	Nausea, vomiting, malaise, dizziness, ataxia, headache, altered mental status, polyuria, pulmonary edema, signs of intracranial pressure, seizures, coma; core temperature < 102°F (38.9°C); mimics signs of heat illness	Restrict water intake; give salty foods/saline. Unresponsive patients receive "ABC" standard care, 15 liters/minute oxygen by nonrebreathing mask. If available, provide IV hypertonic saline 100-ml bolus of 3% hypertonic saline, which can be repeated twice at 10-minute intervals. Transport immediately with alert patient in sitting position or left-lateral position if unresponsive.

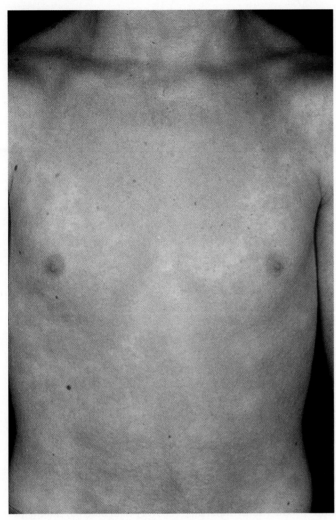

Figure 21-6 Heat rash.
Source: © Wellcome Images Library / Custom Medical Stock Photo

diaphragm, and *bulbar* muscles (muscles involved with speech, chewing, and swallowing) are not involved. Muscle cramps can occur alone or in association with heat exhaustion.

The cause of muscle cramping is unknown, but it is believed to be related to muscle fatigue commonly from exercise, body water loss, and large sodium and other electrolyte losses. It is more commonly seen when individuals exercise in hot and humid environments. Salt supplementation in the diet has been shown to reduce the incidence of muscle cramps.

Management

Treatment consists of rest in a cool environment, prolonged stretching of the affected muscle, and consuming oral fluids and food containing sodium chloride (i.e., 1/8 to 1/4 teaspoon of table salt added to 10 to 16 ounces [300 to 500 ml] of fluids or sport drinks, 1 to 2 salt tablets with 10 to 16 ounces of fluid, bullion broth, or salty snacks). Intravenous (IV) fluids are rarely needed, but prolonged and severe diffuse muscle cramps can be resolved more rapidly with IV normal saline (NS). Avoid the use of salt

tablets by themselves because these can cause gastrointestinal (GI) distress.

Heat Syncope

Heat syncope is seen with prolonged standing in warm environments and is caused by low blood pressure that results in fainting or feeling faint or light-headed. Heat exposure causes vasodilation and venous blood pooling in the legs, causing low blood pressure. The effects are commonly experienced on transition from sitting to standing.

Management

After removal to a cool environment, patients rest in a recumbent position and are provided oral or IV rehydration. If a fall occurred, patients should be thoroughly evaluated for any injury. Patients with a significant history of cardiac or neurologic disorders need further evaluation for the cause of their syncopal episode. Monitoring of vital signs and the electrocardiogram (ECG) during transport is essential.

Major Heat-Related Disorders

The major heat-related disorders include exertion-associated collapse, heat exhaustion, and heatstroke (classic and exertional forms) and may pose a life threat if allowed to progress.

Exertion-Associated Collapse

This disorder occurs when an individual collapses after strenuous exercise.[34-39] During exercise, contraction of the muscles of the lower extremities assists in augmenting venous blood return to the heart. When exercise stops, such as at the end of a jog, the muscle contraction that assisted blood return to the heart slows significantly. This in turn causes venous blood return to the heart to decrease, resulting in a decreased cardiac output to the brain.

Assessment

Signs and symptoms include nausea, light-headedness, collapse, or syncope. Patients may feel better when lying down but become light-headed when they attempt to stand or sit (*orthostatic hypotension*). Profuse sweating is not unusual. Ventilations and pulse rates may be rapid. The patient's core body temperature may be normal or slightly elevated. It is difficult to rule out dehydration, but this type of postexercise collapse is not from hypovolemia. In contrast, collapse that occurs during exercise requires immediate evaluation for other causes (e.g., cardiovascular).

Management

The patient is removed to a cool environment and rests in a recumbent position. IV rehydration is provided if truly needed for moderate to severe dehydration; otherwise provide cool fluids by mouth. Since many of these patients experienced collapse because of the decreased venous return at the end of exercise and not from dehydration, it is highly recommended to withhold IV therapy until further assessment is completed following recumbent rest (Trendelenburg position) and passive "cool down." As with any form of collapse, further evaluation is necessary to rule out other disorders (e.g., exercise-associated hyponatremia, cardiac or neurologic causes). Monitoring of vital signs and ECG during transport is essential to detect cardiac dysrhythmias.

Heat Exhaustion

Heat exhaustion is the most common heat-related disorder seen by prehospital care providers. This condition can develop over days of exposure, as in elderly persons living in poorly ventilated spaces, or acutely, as in athletes. Heat exhaustion results from cardiac output that is insufficient to support the increased circulatory load caused by competing demands of thermoregulatory heat dissipation, increased skin blood flow, reduced plasma volume, reduced venous return to the heart from vasodilation, and sweat-induced depletion of salt and water.[25] Patients with heat exhaustion normally present with a rectal temperature less than 104°F (40°C), but this is a guide and not always a reliable finding.[38]

Another form of heat exhaustion is known as exertional heat exhaustion. This occurs with physical exercise or heavy exertion in all temperatures. It is defined as the inability to continue the exercise or exertion and may or may not be associated with physical collapse.[23] The key predisposing factors are dehydration and high body mass index that place an individual at greater risk for exertional heat exhaustion.

Distinguishing severe heat exhaustion from heatstroke often may be difficult, but a quick mental status assessment will determine the level of neurologic involvement. If heat exhaustion is not effectively treated, it may lead to heatstroke, a life-threatening form of heat illness. Heat exhaustion is a *diagnosis of exclusion* when there is no evidence of heatstroke. These patients will need further physical and laboratory evaluation in the ED.

Assessment

Signs and symptoms of heat exhaustion are neither specific nor sensitive. They include low fluid intake, decreased urine output, frontal headache, drowsiness, euphoria, nausea, vomiting, light-headedness, anxiety, fatigue, irritability, decreased coordination, heat sensation on head and neck, chills, and apathy. Patients may feel better when lying down but may become light-headed when they attempt to stand or sit (orthostatic hypotension). During the acute stage of heat exhaustion, the blood pressure is low, and the pulse and ventilatory rates are rapid. The radial pulse may feel thready. The patient generally appears sweaty, pale, and ashen. The patient's core body temperature may be either normal or slightly elevated, but generally below 104°F (40°C).

It is important to obtain a good history of prior heat illness and the current heat exposure incident because these patients may display signs and symptoms of other conditions of fluid and sodium loss (e.g., hyponatremia; see later discussion). Reassessment is critical since heat exhaustion may progress to heatstroke. Continuously look for any changes in mentation and personality (i.e., confusion, disorientation, irrational or unusual behavior). Any such change should be taken as a progressive sign of hyperthermia indicating heatstroke—*a life-threatening condition!*

Management

Immediately remove the patient from the hot environment (e.g., sun, hot pavement, hot vehicle) to a cooler location either in the shade or air-conditioned space (i.e., ambulance). Place the patient in a supine resting position. Remove clothing and anything restricting heat dissipation, such as a hat or any excess clothing. Assess the patient's heart rate, blood pressure, ventilatory rate, and rectal temperature (if a thermometer is available and conditions permit), and be alert particularly for central nervous system status changes as an early indicator of life-threatening heatstroke.

Oral rehydration should be considered for any patient who can take fluids by mouth and who is not at risk of aspirating, using sport electrolyte fluids diluted to half-strength. Large amounts of oral fluids may increase bloating, nausea, and vomiting. Normally IV fluids are not needed as long as blood pressure, pulse, and rectal temperature are normal. However, in patients who are not able to consume fluids by mouth, IV fluids provide rapid recovery from heat exhaustion.[23] If IV fluids are needed, lactated Ringer's (LR) solution or NS should be used. IV solutions produce more rapid fluid recovery than fluids by mouth due to delays in gastric emptying and absorption in the small intestine caused by dehydration.

In exertional heat exhaustion, most exercising patients recover with recumbent rest and oral fluids. Before any decision is made for IV therapy in these patients, there needs to be a thorough assessment for signs and symptoms of dehydration, *orthostatic* (postural) pulse, blood pressure changes, and the ability to ingest oral fluids. Ongoing mental status changes should prompt further evaluation for hyponatremia, hypoglycemia, and other medical problems. In the exertional heat exhaustion patient, the recommended IV fluids are NS or 5% dextrose in NS for patients who are mildly hypoglycemic. However, caution should be used to ensure that large amounts of IV fluids are not administered to a patient who has been participating in prolonged exercise (greater than 4 hours), especially individuals who do not have obvious clinical signs of dehydration, or in a collapsed athlete with suspected heat exhaustion who has been drinking a large amount of water. This type of patient may have exercise-associated hyponatremia (low serum sodium level), and providing oral and/or IV fluids will cause further *dilutional hyponatremia*, potentially causing a life-threatening condition.[40,41] See the discussion on exercise-associated hyponatremia for information on how best to correctly assess the patient for heat-related illness or exercise-associated hyponatremia.

Because heat exhaustion may be difficult to distinguish from heatstroke and because patients with heatstroke should be cooled rapidly to reduce core temperature, the best course of action is to provide some active cooling procedures to all patients with heat exhaustion. Active cooling can be done simply and quickly by wetting the head and upper torso with water or a wet cloth and then fanning or positioning the patient into the wind to increase convective body heat dissipation. Body-cooling procedures will also improve mental status. Transport all patients who are unconscious, who do not recover rapidly, or who have a significant medical history. Proper environmental temperature control and monitoring of vital signs and mental status are essential during transport.

Heatstroke

Heatstroke is considered the most emergent and life-threatening form of heat illness. Heatstroke is a form of hyperthermia resulting in failure of the thermoregulatory system—a failure of the body's physiologic systems to dissipate heat and cool down. Heatstroke is characterized by an elevated core temperature of 104°F (40°C) or greater and central nervous system dysfunction, resulting in delirium, convulsions, or coma.[31,36,42]

The most significant difference in heatstroke compared with heat exhaustion is neurologic disability, which presents to the prehospital care provider as mental status changes. Pathophysiologic changes often result in multiple organ failure.[33,43] These pathophysiologic changes occur when organ tissue temperatures rise above a critical level. Cell membranes are damaged, leading to disruption in cell volume, metabolism, acid–base balance, and membrane permeability that causes cellular and a whole organ dysfunction with ultimate cell death and organ failure.[23] The degree of complications in patients with heatstroke is not entirely related to the magnitude of core temperature elevation.

This whole-body pathophysiologic dysfunction is the underlying reason for the need for early heatstroke recognition by prehospital care providers. With early recognition, prehospital care providers can quickly provide aggressive whole-body cooling in an effort to rapidly reduce core temperature and decrease the associated heatstroke morbidity and mortality too frequently seen in the emergency department (ED).

Morbidity and mortality are directly associated with the duration of elevated core temperature, and a positive patient outcome is directly related to how fast the core temperature can be decreased below 102°F (38.9°C). Even with aggressive prehospital intervention and in-hospital management, heatstroke can be fatal, and many patients who survive have permanent neurologic disability.

Heatstroke has two different clinical presentations: classic heatstroke and exertional heatstroke (**Figure 21-7**).

Classic heatstroke is a disorder of infants, febrile children, poor people, the elderly, alcoholic persons, and sick patients, which may be compounded by the risk factors listed in Figure 21-4 (e.g., medications). A classic presentation is a patient who is exposed to elevated humidity and high room temperatures over several days without air conditioning, leading to dehydration and high core temperature. Often this patient's sweating mechanism has stopped, known as **anhidrosis**. This is especially common in large cities during summer heat waves, when effective home ventilation is either not possible or not used.[15] Scene assessment will provide information helpful in the identification of classic heatstroke.

Exertional heatstroke (EHS) is a preventable disorder often seen in those individuals with poor physical fitness or lack of heat acclimatization who are involved in short-term, strenuous physical activity (e.g., industrial workers, athletes, military recruits, fire fighters, and other public safety personnel) in a hot, humid environment. These conditions can rapidly elevate internal heat production and limit the body's ability to dissipate heat. Almost all EHS patients exhibit sweat-soaked and pale skin at

Figure 21-7	Classic Versus Exertional Heatstroke	
	Classic	**Exertional**
Patient characteristics	Elderly	Men (15 to 45 years)
Health status	Chronically ill	Healthy
Concurrent activity	Sedentary	Strenuous exercise
Drug use	Diuretics, antidepressants, antihypertensives, anticholinergics, antipsychotics	Usually none
Sweating	May be absent	Usually present
Lactic acidosis	Usually absent; poor prognosis if present	Common
Hyperkalemia	Usually absent	Often present
Hypocalcemia	Uncommon	Frequent
Hypoglycemia	Uncommon	Common
Creatine	Mildly elevated	Greatly elevated
Rhabdomyolysis	Mild	Frequently severe

Source: Modified from Knochel JP, Reed G. Disorders of heat regulation. In: Kleeman CR, Maxwell MH, Narin RG, eds. *Clinical Disorders of Fluid and Electrolyte Metabolism.* New York, NY: McGraw-Hill; 1987.

time of collapse as compared to dry, hot, and flushed skin in the classic heatstroke patient.[23] Even though drinking fluids can slow the rate of dehydration during strenuous activity and reduce the rate at which core temperature rises, hyperthermia and EHS may still occur in the absence of significant dehydration.

With aggressive treatment, no one should die from EHS if prompt care begins within 10 minutes of collapse. Some of the common reasons that death from EHS may occur are listed in **Figure 21-8**.[34-36] The motto to "cool first, transport second" is meant to avoid any delays in initiating the lowering of core temperature.

Assessment

The appearance of signs and symptoms depends on the degree and duration of hyperthermia.[28] Patients with heatstroke typically present with hot, flushed skin. They may or may not be sweating, depending on where they are found and whether they have classic or exertional heatstroke. Blood pressure may be elevated or diminished, and the radial pulse is usually tachycardic and thready; 25% of these patients are hypotensive. The patient's level of consciousness can range from confused to unconscious, and seizure activity may also be present, particularly during cooling.[44] As confirmed in hospitals, rectal temperature may range from 104° to 116°F (40°C to 46.7°C).[33,44]

The keys to distinguishing heatstroke from one of the other heat-related conditions are the elevation in body temperature and altered mental status. Any patient who is warm to the touch with an altered mental status (confused, disoriented, combative, or unconscious) should be suspected of having heatstroke and managed immediately and aggressively to reduce core temperature.

Management

Heatstroke is a true emergency. Immediately remove the patient from the source of heat. Cooling the patient should begin immediately in the field by one prehospital care provider as another provider assesses and stabilizes the patient's ABCs. Cooling of the patient begins immediately with whatever means are available (e.g., garden hose, fire hose, bottled water, IV saline liter bags), even before removing clothing. Application of ice or cold-water immersion are the fastest two methods of cooling, but these approaches are generally limited in the prehospital setting.[35,45-47]

Since the late 1950s, it has been thought that cold- or ice-water immersion will cause vasoconstriction sufficient to decrease heat loss from the body and cause the onset of shivering so that internal heat is produced, thus limiting the exchange of heat. Empirical evidence now refutes this concern that cooling rates in these patients are blunted. Therefore, this form of cooling, if available, should not be withheld from a patient with heatstroke.[39]

If cold water and ice are not immediately available, remove the patient's excess clothing, wet down the patient head to toe, and provide continuous fanning of the skin. It is essential that this procedure begin immediately and not be delayed before preparing to transport the patient from the scene to the ambulance. Patient wetting and fanning is the next most effective cooling technique, causing evaporation and convective heat loss.[45] Individuals who rapidly become lucid during whole-body cooling usually have the best prognosis. *The most important intervention prehospital care providers can deliver to a patient with heatstroke (along with ABCs) is immediate and rapid whole-body cooling to reduce core temperature.*

During transport, the patient should be placed in a prepared, air-conditioned ambulance. It is an error to place a patient with heatstroke in a hot internal cabin of the ambulance even if it is a short transfer time to the hospital. Remove any additional clothing, cover the patient with a sheet, and wet down the sheet with irrigation fluids along with providing continuous fanning, ideally by powered fans from the cabin overhead. Ice packs, if available and time allows, can be placed in the groin area, in the axillae, and around the anterior-lateral neck because blood vessels are closest to the skin surface in these areas. The widespread

---

Figure 21-8   Common Causes of Death from Exertional Heatstroke (EHS)

1. *Inaccurate temperature assessment or misdiagnosis.* This is often due to the inability to rule out other similar medical conditions. Oral, axillary, and tympanic temperature measurements may underestimate the degree of temperature elevation; therefore, prehospital care providers should rely only on the rectal temperature to determine the degree of hyperthermia.

2. *No care or a treatment delay.* Failing to recognize the potential for EHS and delaying the response to provide effective care can have disastrous results.

3. *Inefficient whole-body cooling techniques.* The goal to reduce core temperature rapidly below 104°F (40°C) within 30 minutes is critical. This is recognized as the "golden half-hour" of heatstroke management and is the standard to meet with rapid whole-body cooling.

4. *Immediate transport.* With EHS it is critical to begin whole-body cooling to reduce the core temperature at the scene and not to transport until this treatment gets started. Cooling should continue during transport with rectal temperature assessment to ensure core temperature drops below 104°F (40°C).

recommendation of using ice packs alone is a much inferior core cooling technique. They are completely insufficient to rapidly lower core body temperature and should be considered only as an extra cooling method and not a priority in patient care.[4,44,45]

If possible, the patient's rectal temperature should be measured every 5 to 10 minutes during transport to ensure effective cooling. Other means to assess the patient's temperature (e.g., oral, skin, axillary) should not be used for treatment decisions since they do not adequately reflect the patient's core temperature.[23]

Active cooling should stop when the patient's rectal temperature reaches 101.5°F to 102°F (38.6°C to 38.9°C) since the core temperature will continue to drop even after cooling procedures stop and could end up below 98°F (36.7°C).[38,47] Provide high-flow oxygen, support ventilations with a bag-mask device as needed, and monitor the patient's cardiac rhythm.

Patients with heatstroke generally do not require extensive fluid resuscitation and typically are initially given IV fluids consisting of 1.0 to 1.5 liter of NS. Provide a 500-milliliter (ml) fluid challenge and assess vital signs. Fluid volume should not exceed 1 to 2 liters in the first hour, or follow local medical protocol. Monitor blood glucose because these patients are frequently hypoglycemic and may require a bolus of 50% dextrose IV. Seizures can be managed with 5 to 10 milligrams (mg) of diazepam or other benzodiazepines as per local protocol. Transport the patient in a right or left lateral recumbent position to maintain an open airway and to avoid aspiration.

Exercise-Associated Hyponatremia

Exercise-associated hyponatremia (EAH), also known as exertional hyponatremia or water intoxication, is a life-threatening condition that has been increasingly described after prolonged physical exertion in recreational hikers, marathoners, ultra-marathoners, triathletes, adventure racers, and military infantry personnel.[48-52] With the increasing popularity of these outdoor activities, the incidence of mild to severe EAH has steadily increased since it was first reported in the mid-1980s.[51] It is now known to be one of the most severe medical complications of endurance activities and is an important cause of event-related fatalities.[40,41]

EAH is commonly associated with excessive consumption of water (1.5 quarts [1.4 liters] or greater per hour) during prolonged activities.[52] Two major pathogenic mechanisms largely account for the development of EAH: (1) excessive fluid intake and (2) impaired urinary water excretion due largely to persistent secretion of *arginine vasopressin (AVP)*, also referred to as antidiuretic hormone (ADH).[40,41] EAH can take two forms, mild or severe, depending on presenting symptoms.

In the severe form, low plasma sodium concentration disturbs the osmotic balance across the blood–brain barrier, resulting in the rapid influx of water into the brain, which causes cerebral edema.[40,41,51,52] In similar fashion to the signs and symptoms of increased intracranial pressure in head trauma (see the Head Trauma chapter), a progression of neurologic symptoms from hyponatremia will occur, including headache, vomiting,

malaise, confusion, and seizures to coma, permanent brain damage, brain stem herniation, and death.[40,41,51] These individuals are said to have **exercise-associated hyponatremic encephalopathy (EAHE)**.[40,41,51]

Symptomatic EAHE patients generally have a serum sodium concentration below 126 milliequivalents (mEq)/liter (normal range, 135 to 145 mEq/liter) with rapidly developing (less than 48 hours) hyponatremia, as seen frequently in prolonged endurance activities.[40,41,48,52] Alternatively, the milder form of EAH generally presents with isolated serum sodium levels of 135 to 128 mEq/liter, without easily discernable symptoms (i.e., weakness, nausea/vomiting, headache, or no symptoms), and is self-limiting with rest, food, and electrolyte fluids. Even with the initial presenting mild signs and symptoms of EAH, a patient can progress into EAHE. It has been suggested that there is an acute drop in serum sodium concentration at the end of an endurance event caused by the absorption of water retained in the GI tract.[40,41] This may account for a transient lucid period after finishing an endurance activity followed by the acute development of clinic signs of EAHE within about 30 minutes following the cessation of the activity.

Studies have reported that 18% to 23% of ultra-marathoners and 29% of the Hawaiian Ironman Triathlete finishers had EAH.[38,43-56] In 2003, 32 cases of EAH were reported in hikers in the Grand Canyon National Park, requiring extensive rescue efforts by park rangers and paramedics in many cases.[57]

EAH can occur in the following situations:

1. Excessive sodium and water loss in sweat throughout an endurance event, resulting in dehydration and sodium depletion
2. Overhydration solely with water while maintaining plasma sodium, creating a dilution of sodium concentration
3. Combination of excessive sodium and fluid loss in sweat and an excessive overhydration with water only

The evidence indicates that EAH is a result of fluid retention in the extracellular space (*dilutional*) rather than fluid remaining unabsorbed in the intestine.[48] Typically, these patients have not consumed sport electrolyte drinks, have consumed energy food supplements containing no salt, or have consumed salt in insufficient quantity to balance the loss of sodium in sweat or the dilution from excessive water intake.

The following are a few key risk factors that have been linked to the development of EAH[34,35,58]:

1. Activity or exercise duration (greater than 4 hours) or slow running/exercise pace
2. Female gender (may be explained by lower body weight)
3. Low or high body mass index
4. Excessive drinking (greater than 1.5 liters/hour) during an event or activity
5. Use of nonsteroidal anti-inflammatory drugs (NSAIDs), which decrease renal filtration

EAH has been described as the "other heat-related illness" because the symptoms are nonspecific and are similar to those exhibited in minor and major heat-related disorders.[57] Many endurance events and multiday adventure activities are conducted in warm to hot environments; therefore, it is assumed that the signs and symptoms of EAH are some form of heat illness, and patients are managed with standard protocols that address the presumed hypovolemia and excessive body heat. Standard protocols that provide body cooling and IV fluid challenge to correct hyperthermia, sweat-induced dehydration, and mental status changes can complicate the dilutional hyponatremia and place the patient at further risk for seizure and coma. Treating a patient with EAH with fluids and rest will worsen the patient's condition, unlike the heat exhaustion patient.

This "other heat-related disorder" is becoming more widely recognized and correctly treated today by EMS and ED personnel, largely because of an increased effort to educate medical personnel and the public in its prevention, early recognition, and management (**Figure 21-9**). Prehospital care providers directly supporting or responding to calls at physical endurance events in the cities or in the wilderness settings need to be aware that EAH is more frequently reported today. It is important to remember that, in general, dehydration is more common in prolonged exertional activities and that it can lead to impaired performance during exercise or work-related tasks and to serious heat illness; however, symptomatic hyponatremia brought on by overdrinking is more dangerous and potentially a life-threatening illness.[58]

Assessment

A wide range of signs and symptoms may be found in the endurance-athlete population with hyponatremia (see Figure 21-5). Core temperature is usually normal but can be low or slightly elevated, depending on the ambient temperature, body heat dissipation, and recent exercise intensity at assessment. Heart rate and blood pressure can be low, normal, or elevated, depending on core temperature, exercise intensity, hypovolemia, or shock. Ventilatory rate ranges from within normal limits to slightly elevated. Hyperventilation observed with EAH can account for vision disturbances, dizziness, tingling in hands, and paresthesias in the extremities. The hallmark assessment and findings are mental status changes, fatigue, malaise,

headache, and nausea. Other forms of neurologic changes include slowed speech, ataxia, and cognitive changes, including irrational behavior, combativeness, and fear. These patients also often report that they have a sense of "impending doom."

Management

The first step in treatment is recognizing the disorder and determining the severity. Management is based on the severity of EAH and what portable diagnostic tools are available to measure serum sodium.[59] **Figure 21-10** provides an algorithm for assessing patients to determine whether EAH or a heat-related illness is present. Mild symptoms should be managed conservatively by observing the patient to ensure no further progression to EAHE and waiting for normal diuresis of excessive fluid.

Symptomatic patients should be placed in an upright position to maintain their airway and to minimize any positional effect on intracranial pressure. These patients are known to have projectile vomiting when transported. Place unconscious patients in the left lateral recumbent position, anticipate vomiting, and consider active airway management. Provide high-flow oxygen, establish IV access at the keep vein open (KVO) rate, and monitor for seizures.

As needed, administer anticonvulsant therapy (e.g., titrate benzodiazepine IV, per medical protocol). Check with medical control for volume of NS fluid, if any, to be administered, depending on patient severity and transport time to hospital. Because these patients are already fluid-overloaded, infusion of IV hypotonic fluids is contraindicated, as this can worsen the degree of hyponatremia and fluid overload.[60,61]

Patients with extensive signs and symptoms of EAHE (i.e., cerebral edema and pulmonary edema) need to have their plasma sodium concentration increased. The current consensus for management in the prehospital setting is to provide a 100-ml bolus infusion of 3% hypertonic saline over 10 minutes to acutely reduce brain edema. Each dose will raise sodium by 2 to 3 mEq/L, if this solution is available.[60,61] If no clinical improvement is noted, up to two additional 100-ml, 3% bolus infusions can be given per medical protocol.[59,60] These severe cases of EAHE have a poor outcome if they do not receive hypertonic saline.[62] Keep the patient calm while en route to the ED, and continue to monitor for mental status changes or seizures.

Figure 21-9 Guidelines for Managing EAH and EAHE

Recently, the Wilderness Medical Society published practice guidelines for managing EAH and EAHE, with an emphasis on how patients competing in endurance events should be managed in the prehospital environment by a medical director and staff or by responding EMS personnel.[59]

Prevention of Heat-Related Illness

Because heat stress is a significant public health factor in the United States, methods for preventing heat illness are vital to any community, particularly for those individuals who must work in high-heat occupational settings. For example, from 2002 to 2011, fire fighter (volunteer, career, wildland) deaths in the United States from all causes totaled 1,054,[61] for a yearly average of 105 fire fighter deaths. The lowest fire fighter all-cause mortality total was recorded in 2011, at 83 deaths (downward trend 2009 to 2011). Of these total deaths, 50 fire fighter deaths (60%)

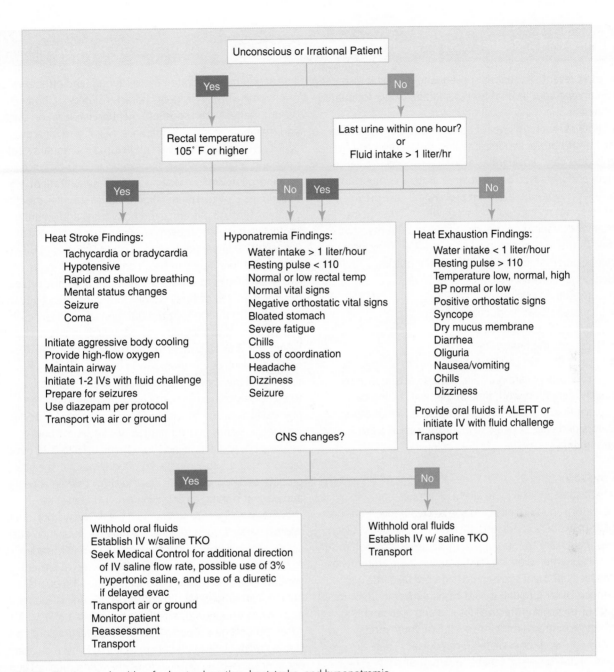

Figure 21-10 Treatment algorithm for heat exhaustion, heatstroke, and hyponatremia.

occurred at the scene due to stress/overexertion, which includes heat illness as a cause of death in this category.[61]

Prehospital care providers and their EMS agencies are a good resource as partners for community education on heat stress prevention strategies in many different formats, including workshops, educational handouts, agency website or newsletter, community presentations, and local newspaper.

As with the general public, it may not be possible to prevent all forms of heat-related illness in prehospital care providers; therefore, EMS and other public safety personnel need to use prevention strategies and prepare for exposure to high ambient temperature and high occupational exposures. These

strategies, which include administrative policies, procedures, engineering controls, use of equipment, and medical surveillance programs, are designed to help minimize the overall impact from acute or chronic heat exposure. The implementation of simple preventive procedures can have a dramatic impact on lowering the incidence of heat illness, but individuals in an organization often do not consider these strategies. **Figure 21-11** provides an overview of heat stress prevention strategies for prehospital care providers, fire fighters, and other public safety personnel.[63]

A complex interaction of factors that combine to exceed the tolerance limits for individual heat exposure can eventually lead

Figure 21-11 Prevention of Heat-Related Disorders in Prehospital Care Providers

You can prevent the serious consequences of heat disorders by improving your level of fitness and becoming acclimated to the heat.

Maintaining a high level of aerobic fitness is one of the best ways to protect yourself against heat stress. The fit prehospital care provider has a well-developed circulatory system and increased blood volume. Both are important to regulate body temperature. Fit prehospital care providers start to sweat sooner, so they work with a lower heart rate and body temperature. They adjust to the heat twice as fast as the unfit prehospital care provider. They lose acclimatization more slowly and regain it quickly.

Heat acclimatization occurs in 5 to 10 days of heat exposure as the body:

- Increases sweat production
- Improves blood distribution
- Decreases the heart rate
- Lowers the skin and body temperatures

As a prehospital care provider, you can acclimatize by gradually increasing work time in the heat, taking care to replace fluids, and resting as needed. Acclimatization is maintained with periodic work or exercise in a hot environment.

On the Job

The heat stress index (Figure 21-12) illustrates how temperature and humidity combine to create moderate-heat or high-heat stress conditions. Be alert for heat stress when radiant heat from the sun or nearby flames is high, when the air is still, or when working hard, creating large amounts of metabolic heat. Heat stress indexes do not take into account the effects of long hours of hard work, dehydration, or the impact of personal protective clothing and equipment.

When heat stress conditions exist, you must modify the way you work or exercise. Pace yourself. There are individual differences in fitness, acclimatization, and heat tolerance. Push too hard and you will become a candidate for a heat disorder.

When possible, you should:

- Avoid working close to heat sources
- Do harder work during cooler morning and evening hours
- Change tools or tasks to minimize fatigue
- Take frequent rest breaks

Most important, maintain hydration by replacing lost fluids.

Hydration

Maintaining body fluids is essential for sweating and the removal of internal heat generated during physical activities. To minimize dehydration and the risk of heat illness, you must hydrate before, during, and after exercise or physical work. Individual characteristics (e.g., body weight, genetic predisposition, heat acclimatization state, and metabolic state) will influence sweat rate for a given activity. These factors will result in large individual sweat rates and total sweat loss. For example, long-distance running is known to cause an average sweat rate of 1.5 to 2 quarts (1.4 to 1.9 liters) per hour in summer months, whereas football players (large body mass and wearing protective gear) are known to sweat on average over 2 quarts (1.9 liters) per hour and up to 9 quarts (8.5 liters) per day.[48] There needs to be a commitment to frequent hydration breaks to ensure dehydration does not exceed greater than 2% of body weight (based on preactivity nude body weight) throughout the duration of physical activity.

Before work, you should take extra fluids to prepare for the heat. Drink 8 to 16 ounces (0.2 to 0.5 liters) of water, juice, or a sport drink before work. Avoid excess caffeine; it hastens fluid loss in the urine. There is no physiologic advantage to excessively consuming large amounts of fluid prior to physical activity. The American College of Sports Medicine now recommends prehydrating slowly for several hours before a physical activity and consuming 0.16 to 0.24 ounces (approximately 5 to 7 ml) per kg of body weight. The goal is to produce urine output that is clear to straw color in appearance and prevent starting an activity in a dehydrated state.

While working, take several fluid breaks every hour, drinking approximately 1 quart (0.9 liter) of fluid per hour. Individual sweat rates will vary, as will the amount of water needed to consume per hour. Caution should be used to prevent consumption of excessive fluids greater than 1.5 quarts/hour (1.4 liters/hour) for prolonged periods unless you have determined your individualized sweat loss rate per hour. The American College of Sports Medicine now recommends a starting point of 14 to 28 ounces (0.4 to 0.8 liters) on average per hour for exercise activities (e.g., marathon running) and adjusting the amount consumed based on individual lower or higher sweat rates for activities in cool or warm temperature conditions, and for lighter or heavier individuals.[48]

Water is the body's greatest need during work in the heat. Studies show that workers drink more when lightly flavored beverages are available. Providing a portion of fluid replacement with a carbohydrate/electrolyte sport beverage will help to retain fluids and maintain energy and electrolyte levels. Unfortunately, many sport drinks contain large amounts of sugar, which can actually slow absorption of ingested fluid.

After work, you need to continue drinking to replace fluid losses. To achieve rapid and complete recovery for

(Continues on next page)

Figure 21-11 Prevention of Heat-Related in Prehospital Care providers (*Continued*)

activities resulting is large sweat loss (i.e., firefighting), drink approximately 24 ounces for each pound of body weight loss (1.5 liters for each kilogram of body weight loss).[48] *Thirst always underestimates fluid needs*, so you should drink more than you think you need. Rehydration is enhanced when fluids contain sodium and potassium or when foods with these electrolytes are consumed along with the fluid.

Sodium lost in sweat is easily replaced at meals with liberal use of the salt shaker. Unacclimatized prehospital care providers lose more salt in the heat, so they need to pay particular attention to salt replacement. Do not overdo salt intake; too much salt impairs temperature regulation. Excessive salt can cause stomach distress, fatigue, and other problems.

Make potassium-rich foods such as bananas and citrus fruits a regular part of your diet, and drink lots of lemonade, orange juice, or tomato juice. Limit the amount of caffeine drinks such as coffee and colas because caffeine increases fluid loss in the urine. Avoid alcoholic drinks because they also cause dehydration. To avoid common viruses, avoid sharing water bottles except in emergencies.

Hydration can be reassessed by observing your urine's volume, color, and concentration. Low volumes of dark, concentrated urine and painful urination indicate a serious need for rehydration. Other signs of dehydration include a rapid heart rate, weakness, excessive fatigue, and dizziness. Rapid loss of several pounds of body weight is a certain sign of dehydration. Rehydrate before returning to work. Continuing to work in a dehydrated state can lead to serious consequences, including heatstroke, muscle breakdown, and kidney failure.

Clothing

Personal protective clothing strikes a balance between protection and comfort. Australian researchers have concluded that *the task for personnel wearing personal protective equipment is not to keep heat out, but to let it out*. About 70% of the heat load comes from within, from metabolic heat generated during hard work. Only 30% comes from the environment. Wear loose-fitting garments to enhance air movement. Wear cotton T-shirts and underwear to help sweat evaporate. Avoid extra layers of clothing that insulate, restrict air movement, and contribute to heat stress.

Individual Differences

Individuals differ in their response to heat. Some emergency responders, such as fire fighters, are at greater risk for heat disorders. The reasons include inherited differences in heat tolerance and sweat rate; excess body weight, which raises metabolic heat production; and illness, illicit drugs, and medications, which can also influence the body's response to work in a hot environment. Check with your physician or pharmacist if you are using prescription or over-the-counter medications, or if you have a medical condition.

You should always train and work with a partner who can help in the event of a problem. Remind each other to drink lots of fluids, and watch each other. If your partner develops a heat disorder, start treatment immediately.

Summary
Prevention
- Improve or maintain aerobic fitness.
- Acclimate to the heat.

On the Job
- Be aware of conditions (temperature, humidity, air movement).
- Take frequent rest breaks.
- Avoid extra layers of clothing.
- Maintain a steady pace.

Hydrate
- The hydration goal is to prevent dehydration (sweat loss) of greater than 2% of nude body weight.
- Before work, drink several cups of water, juice, or a sport drink.
- During work, take frequent fluid breaks.
- After work, keep drinking to ensure rehydration.
- Remember, "Only you can prevent dehydration."

Partners
- Always work or train with a partner.

Drinks
- Sport drinks with carbohydrates (no more than 6% to 8%; ~30 to 60 grams/hour) and electrolytes (e.g., sodium 460 to 1150 mg/liter or 20 to 50 mEq/liter) encourage fluid intake, provide energy, and diminish urinary water loss. The carbohydrates also help maintain immune function and mental performance during prolonged, arduous work. Drinks with caffeine and alcohol interfere with rehydration by increasing urine production.

Source: Modified from U.S. Department of Agriculture, U.S. Forest Service. Heat stress brochure, http://www.fs.fed.us/fire/safety/fitness/heat_stress/hs_pg1.html. Accessed January 11, 2014. See also: American College of Sports Medicine, Sawka MN, Burke LM, et al. American College of Sports Medicine position stand: exercise and fluid replacement. *Med Sci Sports Exerc.* 2007;39(2):377.

to the onset of signs and symptoms of heat-related illness. The capacity of humans to work in moderate to hot environments can be maximized through advanced preparation of physical fitness, heat acclimatization, living and working conditions, personal hygiene, and use of food and beverages to maintain and replace electrolytes and water in the body. Environment, fluid hydration, physical fitness, and heat acclimatization are essential factors to understand.

Environment

Prehospital care providers and other public safety personnel are subjected to high heat environments as part of their occupational requirements. During training or an emergency response, many personnel will encounter high levels of heat stress while working in personal protective equipment (PPE) (impermeable clothing), such as turnout gear, hazardous material suit, or chemical/biologic protective garment. This heat stress is further compounded by the need to enter poorly ventilated or confined spaces or to work on a multivehicle crash in the sun on a hot, humid day.

PPE compromises the body's ability to dissipate body heat and prevents the evaporation of sweat during a heavy workload. With high sweat rates from internal heat production during physically demanding tasks and the external heat exposure, personnel are at a high risk of dehydration and heat illness. Thus, the use of PPE diminishes the physiologic advantage gained through heat acclimatization and physical fitness.

These risks can be minimized by measuring the environmental heat conditions and, when applicable, following the recommended work/rest and hydration guidelines for work in highly thermal environments.[21,64]

One traditional method for measuring the thermal load is by use of the **heat stress index** (**see Figure 21-12**). This index uses the combination of ambient temperature (read on a thermometer) and relative humidity. This is a better method of predicting potential systemic heat injury than the ambient temperature alone. If working in direct sunlight, near surfaces that radiate large amounts of heat, or in heavy protective clothing, 10°F (~5.5°C) should be added to the value in the table.

A more widely used method for measurement of environmental heat strain used in many industrial and military settings is the *wet-bulb globe temperature* (WBGT) *index*[21,65] (**Figure 21-13**). This index uses the combination of a dry bulb for ambient temperature, wet bulb for humidity measurement, black globe for radiant heat, and air movement to provide a more accurate impact of the environmental conditions. Integrated in the five-level WBGT index range of temperatures are hourly work/rest (minutes) and hydration (quarts) guidelines. A color flag (no flag, green, yellow, red, or black) represent each of the five WBGT ranges of temperatures. The WBGT can be monitored hourly and the corresponding color flag placed on a flagpole outdoors for all personnel to see throughout the day. When applicable, the appropriate adjustments of clothing, physical activity, work/rest cycles, and fluid intake can then be made based on these WBGT conditions. This integrated WBGT system and related policies can easily be developed at various public safety locations and training sites to ensure that effective heat illness prevention programs are in use to reduce fatigue, injuries, and heat illness.

Hydration

If the WBGT flag system is not used to provide guidelines for hydration, another excellent resource is published by the American College of Sports Medicine, based on years of research.[58] These guidelines are easily applied to any individual engaged in physical activity. Hydration guidelines should be established within an agency in an effort to prevent excessive dehydration (greater than 2% body weight loss) by creating easy access to water and sport electrolyte drinks, particularly during activity in warm environments (**Figure 21-14**). Studies show that the average individual does not drink sufficient quantities of fluids before, during, and after work or exercise to recover body fluids lost from sweating, even though these individuals believe they are consuming enough fluids.[58] Although overconsumption of fluids can

Temperature (°F) versus Relative Humidity (%)						
	90%	80%	70%	60%	50%	40%
80	85	84	82	81	80	79
85	101	96	92	90	86	84
90	121	113	105	99	94	90
95		133	122	113	105	98
100			142	129	118	109
105				148	133	121
110						135

High	Possible Heat Disorder
80°F - 90°F	Fatigue possible with prolonged exposure and physical activity.
90°F - 105°F	Sunstroke, heat cramps, and heat exhaustion possible.
105°F - 130°F	Sunstroke, heat cramps, and heat exhaustion likely, and heat stroke possible.
130°F or greater	Heat stroke highly likely with continued exposure.

Due to the nature of the heat index calculation, the values in the tables have an error +/− 1.3° F.

Figure 21-12 Heat stress index.

Source: Courtesy of the National Weather Service, Pueblo, Colorado (http://www.crh.noaa.gov/pub/heat.htm).

Figure 21-13 Fluid Replacement Guidelines for Warm-Weather Training

Heat Category	WBGT Index (°F)	Easy Work		Moderate Work		Hard Work	
		Work/Rest (minutes)	Water Intake (qt/hour)	Work/Rest (minutes)	Water Intake (qt/hour)	Work/Rest (minutes)	Water Intake (qt/hour)
1	78 to 81.9	NL	1/2	NL	3/4	40/20	3/4
2	82 to 84.9	NL	1/2	50/10	3/4	30/30	1
3	85 to 87.9	NL	3/4	40/20	3/4	30/30	1
4	88 to 89.9	NL	3/4	30/30	3/4	20/40	1
5	> 90	50/10	1	20/40	1	10/50	1

		Easy Work	Moderate Work	Hard Work
		Walking on hard surface at 2.5 mph, less than 31-lb load.	Walking on hard surface at 3.5 mph, less than 41-lb load. Walking in loose sand at 2.5 mph, no load. Calisthenics.	Walking on hard surface at 3.5 mph, greater than 40-lb load. Walking in loose sand at 2.5 mph with load.

lb, pound; mph, miles per hour; NL, no limit to work time; WBGT, wet-bulb globe temperature.
The work/rest times and fluid replacement volumes will sustain performance and hydration for at least 4 hours of work in the specified heat category. Individual water needs will vary. Rest means minimal physical activity (sitting or standing), accomplished in shade if possible.
Caution: Hourly fluid intake should not exceed 1.5 quarts. Daily fluid intake should not exceed 12 quarts. When wearing body armor: Add 5°F (~2.75°C) to WBGT index in humid climates. When wearing PPE over garment: Add 10°F (~5.5°C) to WBGT index for easy work and 20°F (~11°C) for moderate and hard work.
Source: Current version of WBGT, hydration, and work/rest guidelines as updated by U.S. Army Research Institute for Environmental Medicine (USARIEM) and published by Montain SJ, Latzka WA, Sawka MN. *Mil Med.* 1999;164:502.

lead to hyponatremia (see the preceding Exercise-Associated Hyponatremia section), it is more common for individuals to become dehydrated (greater than 2% of body weight) during a given physical activity. Ideally, fluid-replacement programs should be customized based on individualized sweat rate loss, body mass, and exercise intensity as determined from a pre- or post-physical activity nude body weight loss measurement.

Fitness

To increase heat tolerance effectively in high-heat conditions, prehospital care providers should increase their aerobic fitness through individualized programs (e.g., walking, jogging, biking, swimming, stair stepping, using elliptical exercise machines).[65] These programs will provide the cardiac reserve to sustain the cardiac output required to meet the competing demands of physical (muscular) work and heat dissipation mechanisms (thermoregulation) in a high-temperature environment.[66,67] The American College of Sports Medicine, American Heart Association, and Department of Health and Human Services have collaborated recently to establish updated nationwide physical activity recommendations to maintain health and well-being.[67]

Heat Acclimatization

A policy and protocol for heat acclimatization should be provided within a public safety organization.[68] Heat acclimatization can be achieved with 60 to 90 minutes of exercise a day in hot conditions for approximately 7 to 14 days.[69] The benefits of heat acclimatization are increased work performance, heat tolerance, and reduced physiologic strain. These adjustments include increased blood volume, increased stroke volume, decreased heart rate at a given activity level, reduced sodium concentration in sweat, sodium conserved in the body, earlier onset of sweating, and increased sweat volume rate (**Figure 21-15**). These changes improve the transfer of body heat from the core to the skin in an effort to increase the heat transfer from the skin to the environment. Although heat tolerance is improved in these individuals (e.g., endurance athletes, military infantry personnel) and is considered desirable, the greater sweat-volume production (1 to 2 liters/hour) results in large fluid losses, leading to dehydration. Consequently, the greater volume of sweat loss in heat-acclimatized individuals increases the hydration requirements during heat exposure, particularly when the person does not adhere to a rigorous oral hydration schedule. **Figure 21-16** provides an overview of heat acclimatization guidelines.

Figure 21-14   Hydration Guidelines to Minimize Dehydration

General Principles

It is important to maintain hydration, especially when exercising or performing activities that involve heavy physical exertion. A person's hydration needs will differ depending on how heavily the person sweats. General principles to remember include:

1. Drink before and during exertion.
2. Use water and electrolyte drinks to replace lost fluids.
3. Note your weight before and after exertion to help track whether your fluid intake is sufficient, deficient, or excessive.

Make sure you drink sufficiently even when not exercising. If you postpone drinking during your regular day, your body may dehydrate more quickly once you exert yourself.

Weight

Weight is a factor used to determine hydration (or dehydration). It is important to replace fluid lost during physical exertion. If a person does not replace this fluid, he or she will weigh less after exertion. Conversely, if a person drinks excessive amounts during physical exertion, he or she may gain weight due to the fluid intake. Ideally, a person will weigh approximately the same before and after exercise; this indicates that the person maintained the appropriate fluid level.

When you do not drink enough during exertion, be sure to replenish fluids afterwards. Also remember: do not use dehydration as a weight loss technique.

Type of Drink

In addition to remembering to drink sufficient amounts, it is important to know what type of fluid to drink. Drinking only water during heavy exertion can lead to electrolyte imbalance. Sport electrolyte drinks are designed to replace electrolytes lost through sweat. During exercise, stay alert for swelling of the hands and feet, headache, and bloating, which could indicate hyponatremia.

In addition, if you are an athlete or work in a profession that requires heavy exertion, include a moderate amount of salt in your diet to help fulfill your body's increased need for sodium chloride.

Fluid Intake Recommendations

Recommendations for replacing fluid (with water and sports electrolyte drinks) are as follows:

Time frame	Quantity
2-3 hours before exertion	2-3 cups
30 minutes before exertion	5-10 oz.
During exertion	5-10 oz. every 10-20 min.

Source: Data from: Murray B, Eichner ER, Stofan J. Hyponatremia in athletes. *Sports Sci Exchange.* 2003;16(1):88.

Figure 21-15   Benefits of Heat Acclimatization

1. Thermal comfort: improved
2. Core temperature: reduced
3. Skin blood flow: earlier
4. Heart rate: lowered
5. Salt losses (sweat and urine): reduced
6. Exercise performance: improved
7. Sweating: earlier and greater
8. Body heat production: lower
9. Thirst: improved
10. Organ protection: improved

Emergency Incident Rehabilitation

In 1992, the U.S. Fire Administration (USFA) stated the following:

The physical and mental demands of EMS, firefighting and emergency operations that are associated with extreme heat and humidity create conditions that can have an adverse impact upon the safety and health of the individual emergency responder. Members who are not provided adequate rest and rehydration during emergency operations and training exercises are at increased risk for illness, and may jeopardize the safety of others on the incident scene. When emergency responders become fatigued, their ability to operate safely is impaired. As a result, their reaction time is reduced, and their ability to make critical decisions diminishes. Rehabilitation is

Figure 21-16 Heat Acclimatization Guidelines

The following is a modified version of the heat acclimatization guidelines designed for healthy and physically fit infantry personnel in preparation for physical activity in hot environments.

Should You Be Concerned About Hot Weather?

If you are used to working in cool or temperate climates, exposure to hot weather will make it much more difficult to complete your advanced training course. Hot weather will make you feel fatigued, make it more difficult to recover, and increase your risk of becoming a casualty to heat. Individuals with the same abilities but who are used to training in hot weather will have a greater heat tolerance and physical ability during heat exposure.

What Is Heat Acclimatization?

Heat acclimatization refers to biologic adaptations that reduce physiologic strain (e.g., heart rate, body temperature), improve physical work capabilities, improve comfort, and protect vital organs (brain, liver, kidneys, muscles) from heat injury. The most important biologic adaptation from heat acclimatization is an earlier and greater sweating response, and for this response to improve, it needs to be invoked.

Heat acclimatization is specific to the climate (desert) and physical activity level. However, acclimatization to desert climates greatly improves the ability to work in other climates. Individuals who perform only light or brief physical work will achieve the level of heat acclimatization needed to perform that task. If they attempt a more strenuous or prolonged task, additional acclimatization and improved physical fitness will be needed to perform that task successfully in the heat.

How Do You Become Heat Acclimatized?

Heat acclimatization occurs when repeated heat exposures are sufficiently stressful to elevate body temperature and provoke profuse sweating. Resting in the heat, with physical activity limited to that required for existence, results in only partial acclimatization. Physical exercise in the heat is required to achieve optimal heat acclimatization for that exercise intensity in a given hot environment.

Generally, about 2 weeks of daily heat exposure is needed to induce heat acclimatization. Heat acclimatization requires a minimum daily heat exposure of about 2 hours (can be broken into two 1-hour exposures) combined with physical exercise that requires cardiovascular endurance (e.g., jogging) rather than strength training. Gradually increase the exercise intensity or duration each day. Work up to an appropriate physical training schedule adapted to the required physical activity.

The benefits of heat acclimatization will be retained for about 1 week and then decay, with about 75% lost by about 3 weeks, once heat exposure ends. One or 2 days of intervening cool weather will not interfere with acclimatization to hot weather.

How Quickly Can You Become Heat Acclimatized?

For the average individual, heat acclimatization requires about 2 weeks of heat exposure and progressive increases in physical work. By the second day of acclimatization, significant reductions in physiologic strain are observed. By the end of the first week and second week, greater than 60% and greater than 80% of the physiologic adaptations are complete, respectively. Less fit individuals or those unusually susceptible to heat exposure may require several days or weeks more to fully acclimatize.

Physically fit individuals should be able to achieve heat acclimatization in about 1 week. However, several weeks of living and working in the heat (seasoning) may be required to maximize tolerance to high body temperatures.

What Are the Best Heat Acclimatization Strategies?

1. Maximize physical fitness and heat acclimatization before hot weather exposure. Maintain physical fitness with maintenance programs tailored to the environment, such as physical training in the cooler morning or evening hours.
2. Integrate training and heat acclimatization. Train in the coolest part of the day and acclimatize in the heat of the day. Start slowly by reducing your usual training intensity and duration (compared to what you could achieve in temperate climates). Increase training and heat exposure volume as your heat tolerance permits. Use interval training to modify your activity level.
3. If the new climate is much hotter than what you are accustomed to, recreational activities may be appropriate for the first 2 days with periods of run/walk. By the third day, you should be able to integrate training runs (20 to 40 minutes) at a reduced pace.
4. Consume sufficient water to replace sweat losses. Sweat rates of more than 1 quart (0.9 liter) per hour are common. Heat acclimatization increases the sweating rate and, therefore, increases water requirements. As a result, heat-acclimatized individuals will dehydrate faster if they do not consume fluids. Dehydration negates many of the thermoregulatory advantages conferred by heat acclimatization and high physical fitness.

For the complete report, visit http://www.usariem.army.mil/assets/docs/partnering/HeatAcclimatizationGuide.pdf.

an essential element on the incident scene to prevent more serious conditions such as heat exhaustion or heatstroke from occurring.

Due to the importance of rehabilitation for emergency responders, the USFA created a standardized approach for evaluating and rehabilitating fire fighters and emergency personnel during environmental extremes (**Figure 21-17**). NFPA 1584, *Standard on the Rehabilitation Process for Members During Emergency Operations and Training Exercises*, complements the USFA standard and the standards set by other agencies (e.g., the Occupational Safety and Health Administration). The 2008 edition of NFPA 1584 reflects current science and knowledge on rehabilitation and upgrades the previous document from a recommended practice to a standard.[70-72] The introduction of NFPA 1584 as a standard means that every fire department and EMS agency must have standardized procedures outlining how they provide rehabilitation at incidents and training exercises.

The nine key components of rehabilitation required by NFPA 1584 are:

1. *Relief from climactic conditions*. An area free of smoke, away from vehicle exhaust fumes, and sheltered from extreme heat or cold is provided. This might be a nonfire floor in a high-rise building, a shaded area upwind from a brush fire, or the heated fire apparatus cab during cold winter months. The theme is providing shelter from environmental extremes and on-scene hazards.

2. *Rest and recovery*. Emergency responders are afforded the ability to rest for at least 10 minutes or as long as needed to recover work capacity.

3. *Cooling or rewarming*. Emergency responders who feel hot should be able to remove their PPE and drink water and should have the means to cool off. Emergency responders who are cold should be able to add clothing and wrap in blankets and should have the means to warm themselves.

4. *Rehydration (fluid replacement)*. Fluid volume requirements were eliminated from the standard with the exception of prehydration with 16 ounces (500 ml) of fluids consumed 2 hours prior to scheduled events. On-scene, potable fluids must be provided so members can satisfy their thirst. Fluids should also be provided to encourage continued hydration after the incident.

5. *Calorie and electrolyte replacement*. This component is intended for longer duration events, such as incidents exceeding 3 hours or situations in which emergency responders are likely to work for more than 1 hour. Of note, whenever food is available, means for emergency responders to wash their hands and faces must also be provided.

6. *Medical monitoring*. This component specifies a minimum of six conditions that EMS must assess in each emergency responder during rehabilitation:

   a. Presence of chest pain, dizziness, shortness of breath, weakness, nausea, or headache.

   b. General complaints such as cramps or aches and pains.

   c. Symptoms of heat- or cold-related stress.

   d. Changes in gait, speech, or behavior.

   e. Alertness and orientation to person, place, and time.

   f. Any vital signs considered abnormal in local protocol. The specific vital signs and the definitions of "normal" are entirely up to local medical control and department medical authorities. Vital signs listed in the NFPA 1584 annex include temperature, pulse, respirations, blood pressure, pulse oximetry, and carbon monoxide assessment, using either an exhaled breath carbon monoxide monitor or a pulse carbon monoxide-oximeter (i.e., a pulse oximeter designed to measure carboxyhemoglobin).

7. *EMS treatment in accordance with local protocol*. Services must be available on scene for emergency responders who require treatment or transport. Note that medical monitoring is documented in the fire department data collection system. When EMS treatment or transport is provided, a medical report must be generated and included in the emergency responder's employee medical record.

8. *Accountability*. A personnel accountability system must track emergency responders assigned to rehabilitation by incident command as they enter and leave.

9. *Release*. Prior to leaving rehabilitation, EMS must confirm that emergency responders are able to safely perform full duty.[61]

EMS Drug Storage in Thermal Extremes

Prehospital care providers work in regions within the United States and elsewhere where annual weather extremes range from below freezing to high heat and humidity. Their vehicles, including mobile intensive care units, paramedic units, and medical helicopters, and the medications stored in those vehicles, are also subjected to the environmental extremes unless a temperature-controlled storage device is on board. Medications used by prehospital care providers are intended for storage at controlled room temperature according to recommendations of the drug manufacturers. The U.S. Pharmacopeia (USP) has oversight responsibilities in the United States for establishing drug standards intended to ensure the quality of medications, and the USP defines controlled room temperature as follows:

A temperature maintained thermostatically that encompasses the usual and customary working environment of 68°F to 77°F (20°C to 25°C); that results in a mean kinetic temperature calculated to be not more than 77°F (25°C); and allows for excursions between 59°F to 86°F (15°C to 30°C) that are experienced in pharmacies, hospitals and warehouses. Provided

Figure 21-17   U.S. Fire Administration (USFA) Standard Operating Procedure on Emergency Incident Rehabilitation

Purpose

To ensure that the physical and mental conditions of members operating at the scene of an emergency or a training exercise do not deteriorate to a point that affects the safety of each member or that jeopardizes the safety and integrity of the operation.

Scope

This procedure will apply to all emergency operations and training exercises in which strenuous physical activity or exposure to heat or cold exists.

Responsibilities

The incident commander will consider the circumstances of each incident and make adequate provisions early in the incident for the rest and rehabilitation for all members operating at the scene. These provisions will include medical evaluation, treatment, and monitoring; food and fluid replenishment; mental rest; and relief from extreme climatic conditions and the other environmental parameters of the incident. The rehabilitation will include the provision of EMS at the basic life support (BLS) level or higher. The incident commander will establish a rehabilitation sector or group when conditions indicate rest and rehabilitation is needed for persons operating at the incident scene or training evaluation.

Guidelines

Climatic or environmental conditions of the emergency scene should not be the sole justification for establishing a rehabilitation area. Any activity or incident that is large in size, long in duration, or labor intensive will rapidly deplete the energy and strength of personnel and, therefore, merits consideration for rehabilitation. Climatic or environmental conditions that indicate the need to establish a rehabilitation area are a heat stress index above 90°F (32.2°C) (see Figure 21-12) or windchill index below 10°F (−12.2°C) (see Figure 21-30).

Hydration

During heat stress, the member should consume at least 1 quart (0.9 liter) per hour and should not exceed 1.5 quarts (1.4 liters) per hour. The rehydration should be a 50/50 mixture of water and a commercially prepared activity beverage (sport electrolyte beverage) and should be administered at about 40°F (4.4°C). Alcohol and caffeine beverages should be avoided before and during heat stress because both interfere with the body's water conservation mechanisms. Carbonated beverages should also be avoided.

Nourishment

The department will provide food at the scene of an extended incident when units are engaged for 3 or more hours. A cup of soup, broth, or stew is highly recommended because it is digested much faster than sandwiches and fast-food products.

Rest

The "two-bottle rule," or 45 minutes of work time, is recommended as an acceptable level before mandatory rehabilitation. Members will rehydrate (at least 8 ounces [250 ml]) while self-contained breathing apparatus (SCBA) cylinders are charged. Fire fighters having worked for two full 30-minute-rated bottles, or 45 minutes, will be immediately placed in the rehabilitation area for rest and evaluation. Rest will not be less than 10 minutes and may exceed an hour, as determined by the rehabilitation officer.

Recovery

Members in the rehabilitation area should maintain a high level of hydration. Certain drugs impair the body's ability to sweat, and extreme caution must be exercised if the member has taken antihistamines, such as Actifed or Benadryl, or has taken diuretics or stimulants.

Medical Evaluation

EMS should be staffed and provided by the most highly trained and qualified prehospital care providers on the scene (at a minimum of BLS level). They will evaluate vital signs, examine members, and make proper disposition (return to duty, continued rehabilitation, or treatment and transport to medical facility). Continued rehabilitation should consist of additional monitoring of vital signs, providing rest, and providing fluids for rehydration. Prehospital care providers will be assertive in an effort to find potential medical problems early; considerations include the following:

- If a member's heart rate exceeds 110 beats/minute, an oral temperature should be taken.
- If the member's temperature exceeds 100.6°F (38.1°C), he or she should not be permitted to wear protective equipment.
- If it is below 100.6°F and heart rate remains above 110 beats/minute, rehabilitation time should be increased.
- If the heart rate is less than 110 beats/minute, the chance of heat stress is negligible.
- EMS should document all medical evaluations.

the mean kinetic temperature remains in the allowed range, transient spikes up to 104°F (40°C) may be permitted if the manufacturer so instructs.[73]

Manufacturers will guarantee a medication's stability, quality, and potency only when the drugs are stored within the recommended temperature range. In many cases across the country, EMS vehicles have been shown periodically to have stored medications at temperatures outside the USP-recommended range.[74-77] These studies have examined thermal exposure of drugs in both field and laboratory settings for short (1 to 4 weeks) and long (12 to 26 weeks) durations.[74] What remains unclear is the effect of these thermal fluctuations on the bioavailability of many common prehospital drugs. Laboratory assessment shows that the majority of these drugs remain stable, except for epinephrine, which significantly degrades in extreme cold and heat.[74,78,79]

To improve compliance with the USP standards and manufacturers' recommendations, some states have implemented specific rules regarding storage of medication. For example, the New Jersey Office of Emergency Medical Services (Department of Health and Senior Services) passed regulations requiring the following:

> Each vehicle and cabinet or other storage place for medications shall be sufficiently climate controlled so that the medications and solutions are kept within temperature range recommended by the manufacturer. Each vehicle shall have a temperature recording device which shall, at least, record the highest and lowest temperature during a specified time period.[80]

EMS agencies need to consider how they will deal with this concern for the efficacy of the medications used in their vehicles to assure that these drugs always work as intended when used by the EMS personnel. The cost for implementing environmentally controlled storage for all advanced life support (ALS) units, as recommended by each drug manufacturer and the USP, is certainly not insignificant, but to take no action based on these studies is unacceptable as well. It is suggested that each EMS agency develop a policy to investigate the thermal conditions in the vehicle medication storage area and consider a medication rotation system during periods of extreme cold and heat, or some other system to minimize the exposure of medications to thermal extremes in their region.[74]

Injuries Produced by Cold

Dehydration

Dehydration occurs very easily in the cold, particularly with increased physical activity. This occurs for three primary reasons:

- Evaporation of sweat
- Increased respiratory heat and fluid losses caused by the dryness of cold air
- Cold-induced diuresis

Cold-induced diuresis is a normal physiologic response resulting from skin vasoconstriction from prolonged cold exposure. This is the body's response to reduce body heat loss by shunting blood away from the colder periphery to deeper veins of the body. This response causes a central blood volume expansion, which results in a rise in the mean arterial pressure, stroke volume, and cardiac output.[71] The expanded blood volume can produce a diuresis, manifested by frequent urination. Cold-induced diuresis can reduce plasma volume by 7% to 15%, resulting in hemoconcentration and acute dehydration from almost a twofold fluid loss over normal.

As with exposure to heat, adherence to fluid hydration guidelines while working in cold environments is necessary to minimize dehydration along with the associated fatigue, and physical and cognitive changes. Because thirst is suppressed in cold environments, dehydration is a significant risk.

Minor Cold-Related Disorders

Contact Freeze Injury

When cold material comes into contact with unprotected skin, it can produce local **frostbite** immediately. Do not touch any metal surface, alcohol, gasoline, antifreeze, ice, or snow with the hands. (See the Frostbite section for assessment and management.)

Frostnip

Frostnip is a precursor to frostbite and produces reversible signs of skin blanching and numbness in localized tissue. It is typically seen on the face, nose, and ears. Frostnip is a self-limited tissue injury as long as cold exposure does not continue; it does not require prehospital care provider intervention and transport.

Cold Urticaria

Cold urticaria ("hives") is a disorder characterized by the rapid onset (within minutes) of itchiness, redness, and swelling of the skin after exposure to cold. The sensation of burning may be a prominent feature. This condition, caused by a local release of histamine, is sometimes observed when ice is applied directly to the skin during cold therapy for sprains and strains. Individuals with a history of cold urticaria are advised to avoid cold-water immersion, which could potentially cause death from systemic anaphylaxis. Treatment includes avoiding the cold and possibly taking antihistamines.

Chilblains (Pernio)

Chilblains are small skin lesions that are itchy and tender, appearing as red or purple bumps that occur on the extensor skin surface of the finger or any skin surface (e.g., ears, face) from chronic cold exposure. Chilblains occur several hours after exposure to the cold in temperate humid climates. They are sometimes aggravated by sun exposure. Cold causes constriction of the small arteries and veins in the skin, and rewarming results in leakage of blood into the tissues and swelling of the skin.

Chilblains are more likely to develop in those with poor peripheral circulation. Some contributing factors are a familial tendency, peripheral vascular disease caused by diabetes, smoking, hyperlipidemia (increased serum lipid levels), poor nutrition (e.g., anorexia nervosa), connective tissue disease, and bone marrow disorders. Each chilblain comes up over a few hours as an itchy, red swelling and subsides over the next 7 to 14 days. In severe cases, blistering, pustules, scabs, and ulceration can occur. Occasionally the lesions may be ring shaped. They may become thickened and persist for months.

Symptoms will subside with removal of the individual from the cold. Management involves protection from cold with appropriate gloves and clothing.

Solar Keratitis (Snow Blindness)

Without protection from dry air and from exposure to bright reflections on snow, the risk of ultraviolet burns to skin and eyes increases. This risk is greatly enhanced at higher altitudes. **Solar keratitis** is insidious during the exposure phase, with corneal burns occurring within 1 hour, but not becoming apparent until 6 to 12 hours after exposure.

Management of snow blindness is based on symptoms, which include excessive tearing, pain, redness, swollen eyelids, pain when looking at light, headache, a gritty sensation in the eyes, and decreased (hazy) vision. Prehospital care providers need to consider patching affected eyes if there is no other method to prevent further ultraviolet exposure (e.g., sunglasses), then transport the patient. Topical ophthalmic anesthetic drops, if available, may be used to provide symptomatic relief. Medical attention is required to determine the level of severity and the need for antibiotics and analgesics.

Major Cold-Related Disorders
Localized Cutaneous Cold Injury

Cold injuries occur at peripheral sites on the body and are classified as either freezing (e.g., frostbite) or nonfreezing (e.g., immersion foot) injuries. Localized cold injuries are preventable with proper preparation for cold exposure, early recognition of cold injury, and effective medical care. However, frostbite, potentially the most serious form of freezing injury because of the risk of limb loss, is the primary injury of concern in this section.

It is imperative to recognize, manage, and prevent further tissue freezing in mild to severe forms of freezing injury. Nicotine, alcohol intoxication, homelessness, and major psychiatric disorders remain important predisposing factors.[81] When comparing cold weather injuries by ethnicity, African Americans are reported to be at greater risk for cold weather injuries, including frostbite. This relationship is related to the greater susceptibility of pigmented cells to freeze compared with nonpigmented cells.[82,83] Tight or constricting clothes, too many socks, and tight-fitting footwear are predicable factors in the onset of

frostbite. With an increase in adventure sports and other recreational activities conducted in the winter season, localized cold injuries are now seen more often.

Prehospital care providers need to prevent body heat loss and protect exposed skin from frostbite in patients during prolonged exposure to cold conditions. For example, in patients needing vehicular extrication, in scenarios resulting in the inability to move the patient, and in patients in cold environments with soft-tissue swelling, impaired circulation can lead to an increased incidence of localized cold injury.

Nonfreezing Cold Injury

Nonfreezing cold injury (NFCI), a syndrome also called immersion foot and trench foot, results from damage to peripheral tissues caused by prolonged (hours to days) wet/cold exposure.[84-86] NFCI does not involve freezing of tissue but may coexist with freezing injury such as frostbite. This syndrome involves primarily the feet and is reflected in two types of NFCI. **Trench foot** occurs primarily in military personnel during infantry operations and is related to the combined effects of prolonged cold exposure and restricted circulation in the feet; it does not involve immersion in water.[84] **Immersion foot** is caused by prolonged immersion of extremities in moisture that is cool to cold. Prehospital care providers may see immersion foot in persons who are homeless, persons with alcoholism, or elderly persons; in hikers and hunters; in multiday adventure sport athletes; and in ocean survivors.[84,87,88] Frequently, this syndrome goes unrecognized during assessment of individuals who have been exposed to cold or wet conditions because of the lack of formal medical training in NFCI.[84]

This syndrome occurs as a result of many hours of cooling of the lower extremities in temperatures ranging from 32°F to 65°F (0°C to 18.3°C). Soft-tissue injury occurs to the skin of the feet, known as **maceration**. The breakdown of the skin will predispose individuals to infection as well. The greatest injury is seen to the peripheral nerves and blood vessels, caused by secondary ischemic injury. Mild NFCI is self-limited initially, but with continued prolonged cold exposure, it becomes irreversible. When the feet are wet and cold, they are at increased risk and the injury's course is accelerated because wet socks insulate poorly, and water cools more effectively than air at the same temperature. Any factors that reduce circulation to the extremities also contribute to the injury, such as constrictive clothing, boots, prolonged immobility, hypothermia, and crouched posture.

NFCI is classified in four degrees of severity, as follows:

- *Minimal.* Hyperemia or engorgement caused by an increase in blood flow to the feet and slight sensory change will remain 2 to 3 days after injury. Condition is self-limited, and no signs of injury remain after 7 days. Occasionally, cold sensitivity will remain.
- *Mild.* Edema, hyperemia, and slight sensory change remain 2 to 3 days after injury. Seven days after injury, anesthesia is found on the plantar surface of the foot and tips of the toes and lasts 4 to 9 weeks. Blisters and

skin loss are not observed. Ambulation is possible when walking does not cause pain.

- *Moderate.* Edema, hyperemia, blisters, and mottling are present 2 to 3 days after injury. At 7 days, anesthesia to touch is present to both dorsal and plantar surface and toes. Edema persists 2 to 3 weeks, and pain and hyperemia last up to 14 weeks. Some blister sloughing occurs, but no loss of deep tissue. Some patients will have permanent injury.

- *Severe.* Severe edema, blood forced into surrounding tissues (*extravasation*), and gangrene are present 2 to 3 days after injury. Complete anesthesia of the entire foot remains at 7 days, with paralysis and muscle wasting in the affected extremities. The injury goes beyond the foot into the lower leg. This severe injury produces significant tissue loss, resulting in *autoamputation* (nonsurgical amputation of dead tissue). Gangrene is a constant risk until tissue loss is complete. The patient is expected to have prolonged convalescence and a permanent disability. [84]

Assessment. Because the patient has experienced mild or moderate cold exposure, it is essential to rule out hypothermia and assess for dehydration. Even though this is not a freezing injury, NCFI still is an insidious and potentially disabling injury; the common finding with these two localized cold injuries is that the extremity is cooled to the point of anesthesia or numbness while the injury is occurring.

The key to management of NFCI is detection and recognition during assessment. During the primary assessment, injured tissue appears macerated, edematous, pale, anesthetized, pulseless, and immobile, but not frozen. Patients complain of clumsiness and stumbling when attempting to walk. After removal from cold, and during or after rewarming, peripheral blood flow increases as reperfusion of ischemic tissue begins. Extremities change color from white to mottled pale blue while remaining cold and numb. The diagnosis of trench foot or immersion foot is generally made when these signs have not changed after passive rewarming of the feet. From 24 to 36 hours after rewarming, a marked hyperemia develops, along with severe burning pain and reappearance of sensation proximally, but not distally. This is caused by venous vasodilation. Edema and blisters develop in the injured areas as perfusion increases. Skin will remain poorly perfused after hyperemia appears, and the skin is likely to slough as the injury evolves. Any pulselessness after 48 hours in the injured extremity suggests severe, deep injury and a greater chance of substantial tissue loss.

Management. Once a possible NFCI is detected, the priorities are to eliminate any further cooling, prevent further trauma to the extremity, and transport the patient. Do not allow the patient to walk on an injured extremity. Carefully remove the footwear and socks. Cover the injured part or extremity with a loose, dry, sterile dressing; protect it from the cold; and begin passive rewarming of injured tissue during transport. The affected area may be aggravated by the weight of a blanket. No active rewarming is

necessary. Do not massage the affected area because doing so may cause further tissue damage. As needed, treat the patient for dehydration with a bolus of IV fluids, and reassess. Depending on length of transport, severe pain may develop during passive rewarming as tissues begin to reperfuse, and it may be necessary to manage the discomfort with adequate opiate analgesia (e.g., begin with 5 mg morphine IV as needed).

Freezing Cold Injury

On the continuum of further peripheral cold tissue exposure beginning with frostnip (no tissue loss), frostbite ranges from mild to severe tissue destruction and possibly the loss of tissue due to intense vasoconstriction.[8,9,13] The most susceptible body parts for frostbite are those tissues with large surface-to-mass ratios, such as the ears and nose or areas farthest from the body's core, such as the hands, fingers, feet, toes, and male genitalia. These structures are most susceptible to cold injury because they contain many arteriovenous capillary **anastomoses** (connections) that easily shunt blood away during vasoconstriction. The body's normal response to lower-than-desirable temperatures is to reduce blood flow to the skin surface to reduce heat exchange with the environment. The body accomplishes this by vasoconstriction of peripheral blood vessels in an attempt to shunt warm blood to the body's core to maintain a normal body temperature. Reduction of this blood flow greatly reduces the amount of heat delivered to the distal extremities.

The longer the period of exposure to the cold, the more the blood flow is reduced to the periphery. The body conserves core temperature at the expense of extremity and skin temperature. The heat loss from the tissue becomes greater than the heat supplied to that area.

When an extremity is cooled to 59°F (15°C), maximal vasoconstriction and minimal blood flow occur. If cooling continues to 50°F (10°C), vasoconstriction is interrupted by periods of **cold-induced vasodilation (CIVD)**, known as the "hunting response," and an associated increase in tissue temperature caused by an increase in blood flow. CIVD recurs in 5- to 10-minute cycles to provide some protection from the cold. Individuals show differences in susceptibility to frostbite when exposed to the same cold conditions, which may be explained by the amount of CIVD.

Tissue does not freeze at 32°F (0°C) because cells contain electrolytes and other solutes that prevent tissue from freezing until skin temperature reaches approximately 28°F (−2.2°C). In cases of below-freezing temperatures, when the extremities are left unprotected, the intracellular and extracellular fluids can freeze. This results in the formation of ice crystals. As the ice crystals form, they expand and cause damage to local tissues. Blood clots may also form, further impairing circulation to the injured area.

The type and duration of cold exposure are the two most important factors in determining the extent of freezing injury. Frostbite is classified by depth of injury and clinical presentation.[13] The degree of injury in many cases will not be known for at least 24 to 72 hours after thawing, except in very minor or severe exposures. Skin exposure to cold that is short in duration but very intense will create a superficial injury, whereas severe frostbite to a whole extremity can occur during prolonged exposures. Direct cold injury is usually reversible, but permanent tissue damage occurs during rewarming. In more severe cases, even with appropriate rewarming of tissue, microvascular thrombosis can develop, leading to early signs of gangrene and necrosis. If the injured site freezes, thaws, and then refreezes, the second freezing causes a greater amount of severe thrombosis and vascular damage and tissue loss. For this reason, prehospital care providers need to prevent any frozen tissue that thaws during initial field treatment from refreezing.

Traditional methods of frostbite classification present four degrees of injury (similar to burns) based on initial physical findings after freezing and advanced imaging in the hospital after rewarming (**Figures 21-18** and **21-19**), as follows:

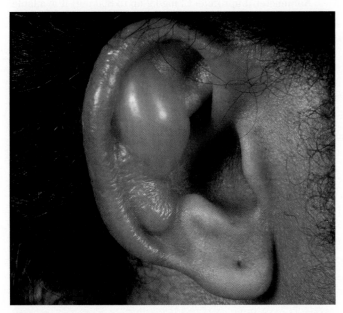

Figure 21-18 Edema and blister formation 24 hours after frostbite injury.
Source: © J. Barabe / Custom Medical Stock Photo.

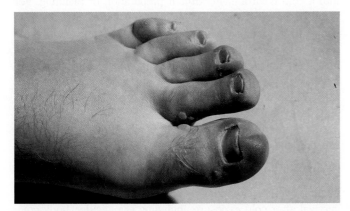

Figure 21-19 Deep second-degree and third-degree frostbite with hemorrhagic blebs, one day after thawing.
Source: © ANT Photo Library / Science Source.

- **First-degree frostbite**. This epidermal injury is limited to skin that has brief contact with cold air or metal. The skin appears white or as yellowish plaque at the site of injury. There is no blister or tissue loss. Skin thaws quickly, feels numb, and appears red with surrounding edema; healing occurs in 7 to 10 days.
- **Second-degree frostbite**. This degree of injury involves all the epidermis and superficial dermis. It initially appears similar to first-degree injury; however, frozen tissues are deeper. Tissue feels stiff to the touch, but tissue beneath gives way to pressure. Thawing is rapid; after thawing, superficial skin blister or vesiculation occurs, with clear or milky fluid after several hours, surrounded by erythema and edema. There is no permanent loss of tissue. Healing occurs in 3 to 4 weeks.
- **Third-degree frostbite**. This degree of injury involves the epidermis and dermis layers. Frozen skin is stiff, with restricted mobility. After tissue thaws, skin swells along with a blood-filled blister (*hemorrhagic bulla*), indicating vascular trauma to deep tissues; swelling restricts mobility. Skin loss occurs slowly, leading to mummification and sloughing. Healing is slow.
- **Fourth-degree frostbite**. At this level, frozen tissue involves full thickness completely through the dermis, with muscle and bone involvement. There is no mobility when frozen and passive movement when thawed, with no intrinsic muscle function. Skin perfusion is poor, and blisters and edema do not develop. Early signs of necrotic tissue are evident. A slow mummification process will occur along with sloughing of tissue and autoamputation of nonviable tissue.

Although traditional classification of frostbite is by the four degrees of injury, it is easiest for prehospital care providers in the prehospital setting to classify as either superficial or deep.[89-91] **Superficial frostbite** (first and second degree) affects the skin and subcutaneous tissues, resulting in clear blisters when rewarmed. **Deep frostbite** (third and fourth degree) affects skin, muscle, and bone, and the skin has hemorrhagic blisters when rewarmed. The level of severity and anticipated tissue loss may vary within a single extremity.[92]

In special situations, frostbite may occur rapidly, and prehospital care providers may respond to the following:

- Hydrocarbon fluid spills on skin (e.g., Gasoline will cause rapid evaporation and conduction in below-freezing temperatures.)
- Touching extremely cold metal with warm skin
- Intense windchill on exposed skin caused by rotary wind from a medical helicopter

Assessment. On arrival, assess scene safety and then the patient for ABCs. Remove the patient from the cold, and place in an area protected from moisture, cold, and wind. Many frostbite victims may have additional associated medical conditions, such as dehydration, hypovolemia, hypothermia, hypoglycemia, and traumatic injury. Remove any wet clothing to minimize further body heat loss. When in doubt, treat hypothermia first. Superficial frostbite is usually assessed through a combination of recognizing the environmental conditions, locating the patient's chief complaint of pain or numbness, and observing discolored skin in the same area. The environmental conditions during exposure must be below freezing.

Frostbite injuries are insidious because the patient may have no pain at the injury site when skin is frozen and covered by a glove or footwear. Detection of the affected area requires direct visual inspection of highly suspect body regions, as previously listed. Gentle palpation of the area can determine if the underlying tissue is compliant or hard. Ensure that the patient or prehospital care provider does not rub or massage the affected skin, because this will cause further cellular damage to frozen tissues. The patient with superficial freezing will usually complain of discomfort during the manipulation of the frostbitten area. In patients with deep frostbite, the frozen tissue will be hard and usually is not painful when touched. After inspection of the affected area, a decision is necessary about the method of rewarming, which is usually based on transport time to the ED.

The State of Alaska EMS protocol for frostbite rewarming in the prehospital phase states[93]:

1. If transport time is short (1 to 2 hours at most), then the risks posed by improper rewarming or refreezing in the prehospital phase outweigh the risks for delaying treatment for deep frostbite.
2. If transport time will be prolonged (more than 1 to 2 hours), frostbite will often thaw spontaneously. It is more important to prevent hypothermia than to rewarm frostbite rapidly in warm water. This does not mean that a frostbitten extremity should be kept in the cold to prevent spontaneous rewarming. Anticipate that frostbitten areas will rewarm as a consequence of keeping the patient warm and protect them from refreezing at all costs.

Management. Patients with superficial frostnip or frostbite should be placed with the affected area against a warm body surface, such as covering the patient's ears with warm hands or placing affected fingers into armpits, axillae, or groin regions. Superficial frostbite only needs to be warmed at normal body temperatures.

Management of deep frostbite in the prehospital setting includes first assessing and treating the patient for hypothermia, if present.[92] Provide supportive care and appropriate shelter for the patient and the affected part to minimize heat loss. Do not allow the patient to walk on affected feet. Protect fragile tissues from further trauma during patient movement. Assess the frostbite area. Remove any clothing and jewelry from the affected area and check for loss of sensation.

If there is frostbite distal to a fracture, attempt to align the limb unless there is resistance. Splint the fracture in a manner that does not compromise distal circulation.

Air dry the affected area 'rand do not rub the tissues. Cover the affected area with a loose, dry, bulky sterile dressing that is noncompressive and nonadherent. Fingers and toes should be individually separated by and protected with sterile cotton gauze. Do not drain any blisters. Hands and feet should be splinted and elevated to reduce edema.

IV opiate analgesics are usually required for pain relief and should be initiated before the tissues have thawed. Initiate IV NS with a 250-ml bolus to treat dehydration and reduce blood viscosity and capillary sludging. Ensure early transport to an appropriate facility.

Attempts to begin rewarming of deep frostbite patients in the field can be hazardous to the patient's eventual recovery and are not recommended unless prolonged transport times (over 2 hours) are involved. If prolonged transport is involved, thaw the affected part in a warm water bath at a temperature no greater than 98.6°F to 102°F (37°C to 38.9°C) on the affected area until the area becomes soft and pliable to the touch (~30 min). If refreezing is a concern, do not thaw.

Administer ibuprofen (12 mg/kg up to 800 mg) if available. Nonsteroidal medications such as ibuprofen help decrease inflammation and pain and inhibit the production of substances that cause vasoconstriction.

During transport, hydrate the patient by providing something warm (and nonalcoholic) if it is available, depending on the patient's level of consciousness and other injuries. Tobacco use (smoking, chewing, using nicotine patches) should be discouraged because nicotine causes further vasoconstriction.

Accidental Hypothermia

Hypothermia is defined as the condition in which the core body temperature is below 95°F (35°C), as measured by a rectal thermometer probe placed at least 6 inches (15 cm) into the rectum.[14] Hypothermia can be viewed as a decrease in core temperature that renders a patient unable to generate sufficient heat production to return to homeostasis or normal bodily functions.

Hypothermia can occur in many different situations, resulting from cold ambient air, cold-water immersion, or cold-water submersion (cold-water near-drowning), and can be intentionally induced during surgery.[14,94,95] Immersion ("head out") hypothermia typically occurs when an individual is accidentally placed into a cold environment without preparation or planning. For example, a person who has fallen into ice water is immediately in danger of becoming a submersion casualty, resulting from "cold shock" gasp reflex, loss of motor skills, hypothermia, and drowning. These unique aspects of submersion incidents can lead to hypoxia and hypothermia (see later discussion and the chapter titled Environmental Trauma II: Drowning, Lightning, Diving, and Altitude).

The progression of hypothermia in cold air or cold water can be delayed as long as the metabolic heat production can match the loss of heat. Surviving an overwhelming cold exposure is possible, with many reported cases of survival at sea and in other extreme situations.[96,97] Many factors are known to affect survival after cold exposure, including age, gender, body composition (e.g., body surface area to body mass ratio), onset and intensity of shivering, level of physical fitness, nutritional state, and alcohol consumption.

Hypoglycemia can occur during progressive phases of hypothermia and may be more common in immersion hypothermia. This occurs due to the rapid depletion of the fuel sources blood glucose and muscle glycogen by the contracting muscles during the shivering process. As the blood glucose stores are depleted through shivering, the brain's hypothalamus, which acts as the body's thermoregulatory center, is deprived its primary fuel. Consequently, a person who has consumed alcohol is at greater risk for hypothermia since alcohol blocks the production of glucose in the body and inhibits maximal shivering for heat production.[14] Thus, rapid assessment and effective management of low blood glucose in the patient with hypothermia are essential to achieve effective increase in metabolism and shivering during rewarming.

Unlike frostbite, hypothermia leading to death can occur in environments with temperatures well above freezing. **Primary hypothermia** generally occurs when healthy individuals are in adverse weather conditions, they are unprepared for overwhelming acute or chronic cold exposure, and there is an involuntary drop of core temperature (below 95°F [35°C]). Deaths by primary hypothermia are a direct result of cold exposure and are documented by the medical examiner as accident, homicide, or suicide.[13]

Secondary hypothermia is considered a normal consequence of a patient's systemic disorders, including hypothyroidism, hypoadrenalism, trauma, carcinoma, and sepsis. See **Figure 21-20** for a wide variety of medical conditions associated with secondary hypothermia. If unrecognized or improperly treated, hypothermia can be fatal, in some cases within 2 hours. Death in patients with secondary hypothermia is often caused by the underlying disease and is potentiated by hypothermia. Mortality is greater than 50% in cases of secondary hypothermia caused by complications of other injuries and in severe cases in which the core body temperature is below 89.6°F (32°C).[14]

Rapid attention to preventing further body heat loss in the traumatic patient is needed by the prehospital care provider since mild hypothermia is very common following injury in all weather conditions.

Hypothermia and the Trauma Patient

It is all too common to receive patients with hypothermia arriving at a trauma center and to have further body heat loss during the primary assessment.[98,99] The development of hypothermia that begins in the prehospital setting is related to the effect of trauma on thermoregulation and the inhibition of shivering as a primary mechanism for heat production.[100] In many patients,

Figure 21-20 Conditions Associated with Secondary hypothermia

Impaired Thermoregulation
- Central failure
- Anorexia nervosa
- Cerebrovascular accident
- Central nervous system trauma
- Hypothalamic dysfunction
- Metabolic failure
- Neoplasm
- Parkinson's disease
- Pharmacologic effects
- Subarachnoid hemorrhage
- Toxins
- Peripheral failure
- Acute spinal cord transection
- Decreased heat production
- Neuropathy
- Endocrinologic failure
- Alcoholic or diabetic ketoacidosis
- Hypoadrenalism
- Hypopituitarism
- Lactic acidosis
- Insufficient energy

- Extreme physical exertion
- Hypoglycemia
- Malnutrition
- Neuromuscular compromise
- Recent birth and advanced age with inactivity
- Impaired shivering

Increased Heat Loss
- Dermatologic disorder
- Burns
- Medications and toxins
- Iatrogenic cause
- Emergency childbirth
- Cold infusions
- Heat-stroke treatment
- Other associated clinical states
- Carcinomatosis
- Cardiopulmonary disease
- Major infection (bacterial, viral, parasitic)
- Multisystem trauma
- Shock

Source: Data from the 2005 Cardiopulmonary Resuscitation and Emergency Cardiovascular Care Guidelines and 2010 American Heart Association Guidelines for Cardiopulmonary Resuscitation and Emergency Cardiovascular.

further heat loss continues after arrival at the hospital due to a multitude of reasons: an exposed patient in a cold ED or trauma center, administration of cool resuscitation fluids, open abdominal or thoracic cavities, the use of anesthetic and neuromuscular blocking agents that prevent heat-producing shivering, and further cold exposure in an operating room environment.[101,102]

In the prehospital setting, the trauma patient should be moved off of cold ground as soon as possible and placed in a warm ambulance. The temperature in the ambulance should be adjusted to minimize heat loss from the patient and not for the comfort of the prehospital care provider. Warmed (100°F to 108°F [37.8°C to 42.2°C]) IV fluids will also help to maintain the patient's body temperature.

One cause of higher mortality in hypothermic trauma patients is related to the lethal combination of *hypothermia*, *acidosis*, and *coagulopathy* (inability of blood to clot normally). This is known as the *lethal triad* in trauma patients.[103] It is essential to assess and treat patients for both trauma and hypothermia because the coagulopathy is reversible with patient rewarming.[99] In one study, 57% of the trauma patients admitted to a level I trauma center were hypothermic at some point in the continuum of care. The mortality rate has been reported to range from 40% to 100% when core temperature falls below 90°F (32.2°C) in a trauma patient. This rate is in contrast to a mortality of 20% in a primary hypothermic (nontraumatic) patient at moderate core temperature levels (82°F to 90°F [28°C to 32.2°C]).[102] Consequently, the mortality rate associated with hypothermia in the trauma victim is very significant, such that the definition of mild, moderate, and severe hypothermia in the trauma patient has resulted in a special classification[103,104] (**Figure 21-21**).

This relationship of trauma, hypothermia, and increased mortality has been reported for decades, including recently in combat casualty patients.[105] However, recent clinical studies have reported that hypothermia is not an independent risk factor for mortality in trauma patients, but is more closely related to injury severity or multiple organ dysfunction syndrome.[106-109] One study reported that certain prehospital care practices can influence the severity of hypothermia in trauma patients. These practices include anticipating hypothermia, avoiding undressing patients, taking frequent temperature measurements, maintaining warm mobile cabin temperatures, and maintaining and providing only warm IV fluids.[108] The potential therapeutic benefits of intentionally induced hypothermia are currently under study (**Figure 21-22**).

Immersion Hypothermia

During immersion, if there is no heat gain or heat loss by the body, water temperature is considered *thermoneutral*. Thermoneutral water temperature is 91°F to 95°F (32.8°C to 35°C), at which temperatures a naked individual passively standing in neck-level water can maintain a nearly constant core temperature for at least 1 hour.[102,114] Individuals in thermoneutral water are at almost no risk for the initial immersion cold shock and hypothermia experienced in sudden cold-water exposure.[115]

When immersion occurs in water temperature colder than the lower thermoneutral limit, the immediate physiologic changes are a rapid decline in skin temperature, peripheral vasoconstriction resulting in shivering, and increased metabolism, ventilation, heart rate, cardiac output, and mean arterial pressure. To offset any heat loss in water, heat production must occur by increasing physical activity, shivering, or both. If not, core temperature continues to fall and shivering ceases, and these physiologic responses decrease proportionally with the fall in core temperature.[95]

The greatest risk of immersion hypothermia usually begins in water temperature less than 77°F (25°C).[116] Because the heat dissipation capacity of water is 24 times greater than that of air, individuals are at risk for more rapid hypothermia in water. However, continued physical activity (i.e., swimming to keep warm) in cold water will eventually become a detriment by increasing convective heat loss to the colder water surrounding the body, resulting in a faster onset of hypothermia. This understanding has led to the recommendation for individuals to minimize heat loss during cold-water immersion by using the *heat escape lessening posture* (HELP) or the *huddle position* when multiple immersion victims are together[116] (**Figure 21-23**).

Figure 21-21 Ranges of Severity of Hypothermia: Trauma Versus Accidental Hypothermia

Classification	Traditional	Trauma
Mild hypothermia	95–89.6°F (35–32°C)	96.8–93.2°F (36–34°C)
Moderate hypothermia	89.6–82.4°F (32–28°C)	93.2–89.6°F (34–32°C)
Severe hypothermia	82.4–68°F (28–20°C)	< 89.6°F (32°C)
Profound hypothermia	68–57.2°F (20–14°C)	
Deep hypothermia	< 57.2°F (14°C)	

Source: Surgical Clinics of North America 75(2), Gentilello et al, Advances in management of hypothermia, pp. 243–256, Copyright Elsevier 1995.

Figure 21-22 Therapeutic Hypothermia

It is well established that the detrimental *lethal triad* in trauma victims increases mortality. However, there is mounting evidence showing that intentionally induced hypothermia has a beneficial role in shock, organ transplantation, nontraumatic cardiac arrest, and control of intracranial pressure from traumatic brain injury.[104,110] The fastest growing application of therapeutic hypothermia treatment in the prehospital setting is for victims of sudden nontraumatic cardiac arrest.[104,111,112] It is well known that the outcome following cardiac arrest is very poor, with only 3% to 27% of all cardiac arrest patients surviving to discharge. However, based on the growing amount of evidence for increased survival rate with therapeutic hypothermia in the past decade, the International Liaison Committee on Resuscitation and other organizations published an advisory statement in 2003, as did Nolan in 2008 and Noland et al. in 2010, on the role of hypothermia following nontraumatic cardiac arrest. These statements recommended intentional cooling of the patient to 89.6°F to 93.2°F (32°C to 34°C) for 12 to 24 hours in unconscious adults with spontaneous circulation after an out-of-hospital non-traumatic cardiac arrest.[110,112,113] Currently, there is no evidence to support therapeutic hypothermia in the multiple trauma patient.

The lowest recorded core temperature for an infant with an intact neurologic recovery from accidental hypothermia is 59°F (15°C).[117] In an adult, 56.6°F (13.7°C) is the lowest recorded core temperature for a survivor of accidental hypothermia. This occurred in a 29-year-old female who struggled to self-rescue for more than 40 minutes before symptoms of severe hypothermia affected muscular contraction.[97] She was immersed for more than 80 minutes before a rescue team arrived and cardiopulmonary resuscitation (CPR) was initiated during transport to a local hospital. After 3 hours of continuous rewarming, her core temperature returned to normal, and she survived with normal physiologic function.

Because vital signs may have decreased to a nearly imperceptible level, the initial impression of a hypothermic patient may be that he or she is dead. Prehospital care providers managing patients with hypothermia should not stop treatment interventions and declare the patient deceased until the patient has been rewarmed to over 95°F (35°C) and still has no evidence of cardiorespiratory and neurologic function. The 29-year-old hypothermia survivor is only one example of a patient being discharged from the hospital with full neurologic function after prolonged CPR in the field. The lesson from this case, and others with a similar outcome, is that although the initial impression of a hypothermic patient may be that he or she is dead, this impression is not sufficient justification to withhold basic or advanced life support. Keep the following phrase in mind: *Patients are not dead until they are warm and dead.*

Whether intentional or unintentional, cold-water immersion (head out) occurs throughout the year in the United States as a

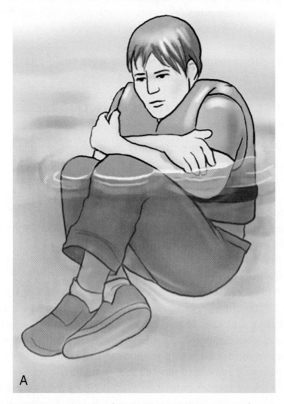

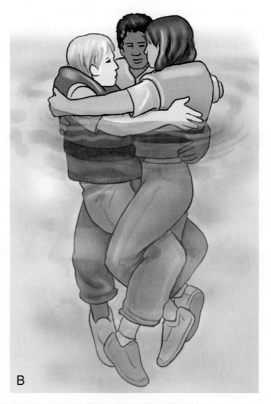

Figure 21-23 Techniques for decreasing cooling rates of survivors in cold water. **A.** Heat escape lessening posture (HELP). **B.** Huddle technique.

result of recreational and industrial activities, as well as from accidents. If the individual survives the initial submersion incident without drowning, he or she is at risk for hypothermia, depending on the water temperature. It is important to note that the public generally underestimates the amount of time required to become hypothermic in very cold water, thinking that it occurs and results in death rapidly. However, rapid death from immersion is the result of panic leading to aspiration of water and drowning, not of hypothermia. The key points to understand are that cold shock is initially the greatest threat and that the victim should focus more on controlling the gasp reflex and his or her breathing to survive this initial physiologic response (**Figure 21-24**). The body's responses to cold-water immersion can be divided into the following four phases leading to death. It is important to note that deaths have been reported to occur in all four phases[116]:

- *First phase—cold shock response.* This phase begins with a cardiovascular reflex known as *cold shock response* that occurs quickly (within 0 to 2 minutes) after immersion (may occur in water colder than 68°F [20°C]). It begins with rapid skin cooling, peripheral vasoconstriction, a gasp reflex and the inability to breath-hold, hyperventilation, and tachycardia.[81,94] The gasp response may lead to aspiration and drowning, depending on the individual's head location above or below water. These responses can lead to immediate sudden death or death within minutes following immersion because of several conditions in this setting, including syncope or convulsions resulting in drowning, vagal arrest, and ventricular fibrillation.[95,118-120]
- *Second phase—cold incapacitation.* If a victim survives the cold shock phase, significant cooling of peripheral tissues, especially in the extremities, occurs over the next 5 to 15 minutes of immersion. This cooling has a deleterious effect on gross and fine motor skills of the

extremities, causing finger stiffness, poor coordination, and loss of muscle power, making it nearly impossible to swim, grasp a rescue line, or perform other survival motor skills.[95,116]

- *Third phase—onset of hypothermia.* Surviving the first two phases without drowning places an individual at risk of hypothermia from continued heat loss and core temperature reduction from immersion longer than 30 minutes. If the victim is not able to remain above the water surface because of fatigue and hypothermia, he or she is at risk of becoming a submersion casualty, leading to aspiration and drowning.[81,98] How long an individual can survive in cold water depends on many factors. It has been estimated that a submersion victim cannot survive for more than 1 hour at a water temperature of 32°F (0°C), and at a water temperature of 59°F (15°C), survival is uncommon after 6 hours.[121]
- *Fourth phase—circum-rescue collapse.* In this phase, fatalities have been observed during all periods of survivor rescue (before, during, and after) despite the apparent stable and conscious condition. Symptoms range from apparent fainting to cardiac arrest and have been referred to as rewarming shock or postrescue collapse. Deaths are reported to occur up to 90 minutes postrescue, during transport, and up to 24 hours after rescue. The three proposed reasons for circum-rescue collapse are (1) afterdrop of core temperature, (2) collapse of arterial blood pressure, and (3) changes in hypoxia, acidosis, or rapid changes in pH that induce ventricular fibrillation. It is noted that up to 20% of those who are recovered alive during the fourth phase will die due to circum-rescue collapse.[116]

For more information about surviving cold-water immersion, see **Figures 21-25** and **21-26**.

Pathophysiologic Effects of Hypothermia on the Body

Whether from exposure to a cold environment or immersion, the influence of hypothermia on the body affects all major organ systems, particularly the cardiac, renal, and central nervous systems. As the body's core temperature decreases to 95°F (35°C), maximal rate of vasoconstriction, shivering, and metabolic rate occurs, with increases in heart rate, respiration, and blood pressure. Cerebral metabolism oxygen demand decreases by 6% to 10% per 1.8°F (~1°C) drop in core temperature, and cerebral metabolism is preserved.

When core temperature falls to between 86°F (30°C) and 95°F (35°C), cognitive function, cardiac function, metabolic rate, ventilatory rate, and shivering rate are all significantly decreased or completely inhibited. At this point, the limited physiologic defensive mechanisms to prevent heat loss from the body are overwhelmed and core temperature falls rapidly.

At a core temperature of 85°F (29.4°C), cardiac output and metabolic rate are reduced approximately 50%. Ventilation and perfusion are inadequate and do not keep up with the metabolic

---

Figure 21-24   The 1-10-1 Principle

If you fall into ice-cold water, remember that you have 1 minute—10 minutes—1 hour.*

- You have 1 minute to get your breathing under control, so don't panic.
- You have 10 minutes of meaningful movement to get out of the water or to attain a stable situation.
- You have up to 1 hour until you become unconscious from hypothermia if you don't panic or struggle unnecessarily. If you are wearing a personal flotation device, you may have another hour until your heart stops beating as a result of hypothermia.

*Times are subject to individual variability and factors such as body size, water temperature, and the amount of body immersed.[98]

Figure 21-25 Cold Water Survival Guidelines

The U.S. Coast Guard and other search-and-rescue organizations use guidelines to assist in estimating how long individuals can survive in the cold water. These guidelines are mathematical models that estimate core temperature cooling rate based on the influence of the following variables:

- Water temperature and sea state
- Clothing insulation
- Body composition (amount of fat, muscle, and bone)
- Amount of the body immersed in water
- Behavior (e.g., excessive movement) and posture (e.g., HELP, huddle) of the body in the water
- Shivering thermogenesis[122-124]

Figure 21-26 Self-Rescue

Early studies in the 1960s to 1970s suggested that during accidental immersion in cold water, it was a better option not to self-rescue by attempting to distance-swim to safety, but to stay in place, float still in lifejackets, or hang on to wreckage and not swim around to keep warm. More recent research has suggested that self-rescue swimming during accidental immersion in cold water (50°F to 57°F [10°C to 13.9°C]) is a viable option based on the following conditions:

- The victim has initially survived the cold-shock phase within the first few minutes of cold-water exposure.
- The victim has decided early to attempt self-rescue or wait for rescue since decision-making ability will become impaired as hypothermia progresses.
- There is a low probability for rescue by emergency responders in the area.
- The victim can reach shore within 45 minutes of swimming based on his or her fitness level and swimming ability.
- On average, a cold-water immersion victim wearing a personal flotation device should be able to swim approximately a half mile (800 meters) in 50°F (10°C) water before incapacitation due to muscle cooling and fatigue of the arms, rather than general hypothermia, occurs.
- Cold water swim distance is about one-third of the distance covered in warmer water.[125]

demand, causing cellular hypoxia, increased lactic acid, and an eventual metabolic and respiratory acidosis. Oxygenation and blood flow are maintained in the core and brain.

Bradycardia occurs in a large percentage of patients as a direct effect of cold on the depolarization of cardiac pacemaker cells and their slower propagation through the conduction system. It is important to note that the use of atropine, as well as other cardiac medications, is often ineffective to increase the heart rate when the myocardium is cold.[8] When core temperature falls below 86°F (30°C), the myocardium becomes irritable. The PR, QRS, and QTC intervals are prolonged. ST-segment and T-wave changes and J (or Osborne) waves may be present and may mimic other ECG abnormalities, such as an acute myocardial infarction. The J waves are a striking ECG feature in hypothermic patients and are seen in approximately one-third of moderately to severely hypothermic patients (less than 90°F [32.2°C]). The J wave is described as a "humplike" deflection between the QRS complex and the early part of the ST segment.[126] The J wave is best viewed in the aVL, aVF, and left lateral leads (**Figure 21-27**).

Atrial fibrillation and extreme bradycardia develop and may continue between 83°F and 90°F (28.3°C to 32.2°C). When the core temperature reaches 80°F to 82°F (26.7°C to 27.8°C), any physical stimulation of the heart can cause ventricular fibrillation (VF). CPR or rough handling (patient assessment and movement) of the patient could be sufficient to cause VF. At these extremely low core temperatures, pulse and blood pressure are not detectable, and the joints are stiff. The pupils become fixed and dilated at extremely low core temperatures. Remember, a patient should not be assumed to be dead until he or she is rewarmed and still has no signs of life (ECG, pulse, ventilation, and central nervous system function).

With acute cold exposure, renal blood flow increases because of the shunting of blood during vasoconstriction. This may result in a phenomenon known as *cold diuresis* in which patients produce more urine and may, as a result, become dehydrated. At 81°F to 86°F (27.2°C to 30°C), renal blood flow is depressed by 50%. At this moderate to severe hypothermic level, the decrease in cardiac output causes a fall in renal blood flow and glomerular filtration rate, which in turn results in acute renal failure.

Assessment

It is imperative to assess scene safety on arrival. All emergency responders need to ensure their safety and protection from cold exposure while working in this environment. There should be a high suspicion for hypothermia even when the environmental conditions are not highly suggestive (e.g., wind, moisture, temperature).

Assess the patient's ABCs. Take up to 60 seconds to carefully evaluate the patient's pulse, which may present as very weak or absent in a patient with moderate to severe hypothermia. Some patients who are alert may present with vague complaints of fatigue, lethargy, nausea, vomiting, and dizziness. Neurologic

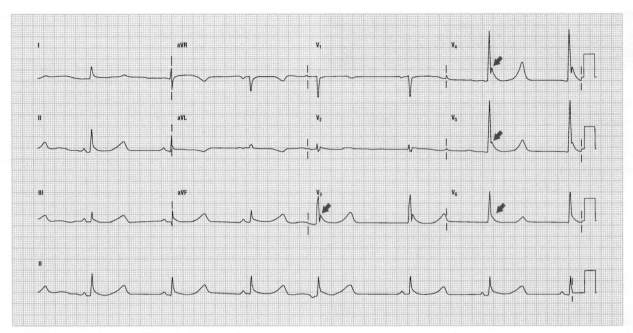

Figure 21-27   Osborne or J wave in hypothermic patient.
Source: From 12 Lead ECG: The Art of Interpretation, Courtesy of Tomas B.Garcia, MD.

function is assessed and monitored frequently. Patients with severe hypothermia generally present with bradypnea, stupor, and coma.

To accurately measure hypothermic temperatures, a low-range rectal thermometer is often necessary. However, rectal temperatures are not usually assessed in the field or widely used as a vital sign in most prehospital systems. Ambulances that do have access to a thermometer usually carry a standard-range oral or rectal (for infants) thermometer with a lower limit of 96°F (35.6°C). Electronic thermometers are not useful in hypothermic situations for accurate readings. Tympanic membrane infrared temperature measurement is generally accurate if careful technique is used to assure aiming the probe at the tympanic membrane and not the ear canal, which can affect the reading. In addition, the ear must be clear of cerumen (ear wax) and blood. Therefore, prehospital care providers need to rely on scene size-up, patient mental status, skin vitals, and ABCS.

Figure 21-28 provides the anticipated physiologic responses with decreasing core temperature.

Signs of shivering and mental status change are important in the assessment of suspected hypothermia. Patients with mild hypothermia (core temperature greater than 90°F [32.2°C]) will be shivering and usually show signs of altered level of consciousness (e.g., confusion, slurred speech, altered gait, clumsiness). They will be slow in their actions and are usually found in a nonambulatory state, sitting or lying. Law enforcement personnel and prehospital care providers may misinterpret this condition as drug or alcohol intoxication or, in geriatric patients, as cerebrovascular accident (stroke). However, a patient's level of consciousness is not a reliable indicator of the degree of hypothermia; some patients have remained conscious at core temperature below 80°F (26.7°C).

When the patient's core temperature falls below 90°F (32.2°C), moderate hypothermia is present, and the patient will probably not complain of feeling cold. Shivering will be absent, and the patient's level of consciousness will be greatly decreased, possibly to the point of unconsciousness and coma. The patient's pupils will react slowly or may be dilated and fixed. The patient's palpable pulses may be diminished or absent, and systolic blood pressure may be low or indeterminate. The patient's ventilations may have slowed to as few as 2 breaths/minute. An ECG may show atrial fibrillation, the most common dysrhythmia. As the myocardium becomes progressively colder and more irritable at about 82°F (27.8°C), VF is observed more often.

Because of the changes in cerebral metabolism, evidence of *paradoxical undressing* may be observed before the patient loses consciousness. This is an attempt by the patient to remove the clothing while in the cold environment, and it is thought to represent a response to an impending thermoregulatory failure.

The clinical management of hypothermia is based on the following three ranges of rectal body temperature as presented by the American Heart Association for the use of advanced cardiac life support[127]:

- *Mild hypothermia* is above 93°F to below 97°F (33.9°C to 36.1°C).
- *Moderate hypothermia* is 86° to 93°F (30°C to 33.9°C).
- *Severe hypothermia* is below 86°F (below 30°C).

Figure 21-28   Physiologic Characteristics of Hypothermia

Stage	°C	°F	Characteristics
Mild	37.6	99.7 ±1	Normal rectal temperature
	37.0	98.6 ±1	Normal oral temperature
	36.0	96.8	Increase in metabolic rate and blood pressure and pre-shivering muscle tone
	35.0	95.0	Urine temperature 34.8° C; maximum shivering thermogenesis
	34.0	93.2	Amnesia, dysarthria, and poor judgment develop; maladaptive behavior; normal blood pressure; maximum respiratory stimulation; tachycardia, then progressive bradycardia
	33.3	91.4	Ataxia and apathy develop; linear depression of cerebral metabolism; tachypnea, then progressive decrease in respiratory minute volume; cold diuresis
Moderate	32.0	89.6	Stupor; 25% decrease in oxygen consumption
	31.0	87.8	Extinguished shivering thermogenesis
	30.0	86.0	Atrial fibrillation and other arrhythmias develop; poikilothermia; pupils and cardiac output two thirds of normal; insulin ineffective
	29.0	84.2	Progressive decrease in level of consciousness, pulse, and respiration; pupils dilated; paradoxical undressing
Severe	28.0	82.4	Decreased ventricular fibrillation threshold; 50% decrease in oxygen consumption and pulse; hypoventilation
	27.0	80.6	Loss of reflexes and voluntary motion
	26.0	78.8	Major acid–base disturbances; no reflexes or response to pain
	25.0	77.0	Cerebral blood flow one third of normal; loss of cerebrovascular autoregulation; cardiac output 45% of normal; pulmonary edema may develop
	24.0	75.2	Significant hypotension and bradycardia
	23.0	73.4	No corneal or oculocephalic reflexes; areflexia
	22.0	71.6	Maximum risk of ventricular fibrillation; 75% decrease in oxygen consumption
Profound	20.0	68.0	Lowest resumption of cardiac electromechanical activity; pulse 20% of normal
	19.0	66.2	Electroencephalographic silencing
	18.0	64.4	Asystole
	15.0	59.0	Lowest infant accidental hypothermia survival
	13.7	56.7	Lowest adult accidental hypothermia survival
	10.0	50.0	92% decrease in oxygen consumption
	9.0	48.2	Lowest therapeutic hypothermia survival

Source: Modified from Danzl DF: Accidental hypothermia. In Auerbach PS: Wilderness medicine, ed 6, St. Louis, 2012, Mosby Elsevier.

Management

Prehospital care of the patient with hypothermia consists of preventing further heat loss, gentle handling, initiating rapid transport, and rewarming. This includes moving the patient away from any cold source to a warm ambulance or to a warm shelter if transportation is not immediately available (see the Prolonged Transport section). After assessing pulse and if no signs of life are present, CPR should immediately be started.[127] Any wet clothing should be removed by cutting with trauma shears to avoid unnecessary movement and agitation of the patient. Concern for initiating ventricular dysrhythmia based on the handling of the patient should not delay any critical interventions. This concern becomes more realistic in severe hypothermic patients (core temperature below 86°F [30°C]). The patient's head and body should be insulated from the cold ground and covered completely with warm blankets or sleeping bags, followed by an outer windproof layer to prevent conductive, convective, and evaporative heat loss.

If the patient is conscious and alert, he or she should avoid drinks containing alcohol or caffeine. Anticipate hypoglycemia and assess the patient's blood glucose level. For the patient with mild hypothermia with normal glucose levels, provide warm, high-caloric or glucose fluids. For patients with moderate hypothermia with low blood glucose concentration, establish IV fluids and administer 50% dextrose (D_{50}) IV per local medical protocol, and repeat glucose determination every 5 minutes to determine the need for an additional D_{50} bolus.

Hypothermic patients need high-flow oxygen because they have decreased oxygen delivery to the tissues; the oxyhemoglobin dissociation curve shifts to the left with a decrease in core temperature. High-flow oxygen should be delivered using a non-rebreathing mask or bag-mask device. Ideally, the patient may benefit more if the oxygen can be warmed and humidified (108°F to 115°F [42.2°C to 46.1°C]). If possible, warmed oxygen administered before movement may prevent VF during transport.

In unresponsive hypothermic patients, passive rewarming will be insufficient to increase core temperature. These patients will need an airway adjunct to protect the airway, and this should be initiated depending on jaw rigidity. The prehospital care provider should not hesitate to definitively support the airway since there is a low risk of triggering a fatal dysrhythmia during an advanced airway procedure.[98] If endotracheal intubation cannot be successfully achieved without rough handling, continue ventilation with a bag-mask device and consider another advanced airway device (e.g., King supraglottic airway, laryngeal mask airway, nasal intubation). At a minimum, use an oral or nasal pharyngeal airway with bag-mask ventilation.

Intravenous NS, ideally with 5% dextrose, should be warmed to 109°F (42.8°C) and administered without agitating the patient. *The patient with hypothermia should not be given "cold" (room-temperature) fluids* because this could make the patient colder or could delay rewarming. When NS and dextrose solutions are unavailable, any warm crystalloid solution is satisfactory. Provide a fluid challenge of 500 to 1,000 ml, and prevent the solution from freezing or becoming colder by placing the IV bag under the patient to infuse warm fluids under pressure. The rewarming effect of warmed IV fluids is minimal at best, and the prehospital care provider should use good judgment to decide whether fluids (orally or IV) are worth the risks of aspiration, coughing, and painful stimuli to the patient. Hot packs or massaging of the patient's extremities are not recommended.

Typically, active external rewarming occurs only to the thoracic region, with no active rewarming of the extremities. This approach will prevent increased peripheral circulation, causing an increased amount of colder blood returning from the extremities to the thorax before central core rewarming. Increased return of peripheral blood can increase acidosis and hyperkalemia and can actually decrease the core temperature ("afterdrop"). This complicates resuscitation and may precipitate VF.

2010 American Heart Association Guidelines for Cardiopulmonary Resuscitation and Emergency Cardiovascular Care Science

Cardiac Arrest in Special Situations— Accidental Hypothermia

Guidelines for resuscitation of a patient with hypothermia have evolved over many decades. The most recent revision of the emergency cardiovascular care guidelines by the American Heart Association (AHA) were published by the AHA in the journal *Circulation* in November 2010.[127]

The victim with hypothermia can present many challenges to the prehospital care provider, particularly the unconscious patient with moderate to severe hypothermia. Because severe hypothermia is defined by a core temperature of less than 86°F (30°C), the patient can present as clinically dead with no detectable pulse or respiration because of the reduced cardiac output and decreased arterial pressure. Historically, the challenge has been to determine whether to initiate BLS or ALS interventions on these patients based on the viability of the patient. Furthermore, it may be difficult to determine from bystanders whether these patients had a primary hypothermic exposure or a medical event or traumatic injury that preceded the hypothermia. Other concerns for a prehospital care provider are protecting the hypothermic patient with a potential irritable myocardium from any rough handling and initiating chest compression for the patient with nondetectable pulse, in whom both these interventions may initiate VF.[127]

Independent of any scenario that created the primary or secondary hypothermia, lifesaving procedures should generally not be withheld on the basis of clinical presentation, whether in an urban setting with short transport distances or in the backcountry environment with potentially significant delays in transport, in which scenario extended patient care may be necessary (see later discussion).

Basic Life Support Guidelines for Treatment of Mild to Severe Hypothermia

Patients with hypothermia should be kept in a horizontal position at all times to avoid aggravating hypotension because these patients are often volume-depleted from cold diuresis. It may be difficult to feel or detect respiration and a pulse in the patient with hypothermia. Therefore, it is recommended initially to assess for breathing and then a pulse up to 60 seconds to confirm one of the following:

- Respiratory arrest
- Pulseless cardiac arrest (asystole, ventricular tachycardia, VF)
- Bradycardia (requiring CPR)

If the patient is not breathing, start rescue breathing immediately unless the victim is obviously dead (e.g, decapitation, rigor mortis). Start chest compressions immediately in any patient with hypothermia who is pulseless and has no detectable signs of circulation.[127] If there is a doubt about detecting a pulse, begin compressions. Never withhold BLS interventions until the patient is rewarmed. If the patient is determined to be in cardiac arrest, use the current BLS guidelines.

An automated external defibrillator (AED) should be used if pulseless ventricular tachycardia or VF is present. The current emergency cardiovascular care guidelines (see Figure 21-29) recommend that these patients be treated by providing up to five cycles (2 minutes) of CPR (one cycle is 30 compressions to 2 breaths) before checking the ECG rhythm and attempting to shock when an AED arrives.[128] If a shockable rhythm is determined, give one shock, then continue five cycles of CPR. If the patient with hypothermia does not respond to one shock with a detectable pulse, further attempts to defibrillate the patient should be deferred and efforts directed toward effective CPR with an emphasis on rewarming the patient to above 86°F (30°C) before attempting further defibrillation.[128]

When performing chest compressions in a patient with hypothermia, a greater force is required because chest wall elasticity is decreased when cold.[129] If core temperature is below 86°F (30°C), the conversion to normal sinus rhythm does not normally occur until rewarming above this core temperature is accomplished.[130]

The importance of not declaring a patient dead until the patient has been rewarmed and remains unresponsive cannot be overemphasized. Studies of victims of hypothermia indicate that cold exerts a protective effect on the vital organs.[130,131]

Advanced Cardiac Life Support Guidelines for Treatment of Hypothermia

The treatment of severe hypothermia in the field remains controversial.[127] However, the guidelines for administering advanced cardiovascular life support (ACLS) procedures are different than with a normothermic patient. Unconscious patients with hypothermia need a protected airway and should be intubated. Do not delay airway management based on the concern of initiating VF. As noted earlier, if a shockable rhythm is detected, defibrillate once at 120 to 200 biphasic joules or 360 monophasic joules, resume CPR, and then defer cardiac drugs and subsequent defibrillation attempts until core temperature is above 86°F (30°C). If possible, initiate active rewarming procedures with warm, humid oxygen and warm IV solutions, and package the patient for transport by preventing further heat loss. It is important to note that passive rewarming is adequate for patients with mild hypothermia. However, patients with moderate to severe hypothermia need active rewarming that is generally limited to procedures performed in an ED or critical care unit. Passive rewarming procedures alone for these patients are totally inadequate to increase core temperature in the prehospital setting, and EMS personnel should focus on effective techniques in preventing further heat loss.[14]

The challenge with ACLS procedures in a patient with hypothermia is that the heart may be unresponsive to ACLS drugs, pacing, and defibrillation.[132] Furthermore, ACLS drugs (e.g., epinephrine, amiodarone, lidocaine, procainamide) can accumulate to toxic levels in the circulation with repeated administration in the patient with severe hypothermia, particularly when the patient rewarms.[127] Consequently, it is recommended to withhold IV medications in patients with a core temperature below 86°F (30°C). If a patient with hypothermia initially presents with a core temperature above 86°F (30°C), or if a patient with severe hypothermia has been rewarmed above this temperature, IV medications may be administered. However, longer intervals between drug administration are recommended than with standard drug intervals in ACLS.[127] The use of repeated defibrillation is indicated if the core temperature continues to rise above 86°F (30°C), consistent with the current ACLS guidelines.[128]

Finally, BLS/ACLS procedures performed in the field should be withheld only if the patient's injuries are incompatible with life, if the body is frozen such that chest compressions are impossible, or if the mouth and nose are blocked with ice.[14,127] **Figure 21-29** provides an algorithm of mild, moderate, and severe hypothermia guidelines for both patients with a pulse and pulseless patients.[108]

Prevention of Cold-Related Injuries

The prevention of cold injuries in patients, yourself, and other prehospital care providers is vital when on the scene. Recommendations to prevent cold-related injuries include the following:

1. Note the risk factors generally associated with for cold injury:
   - Fatigue
   - Dehydration

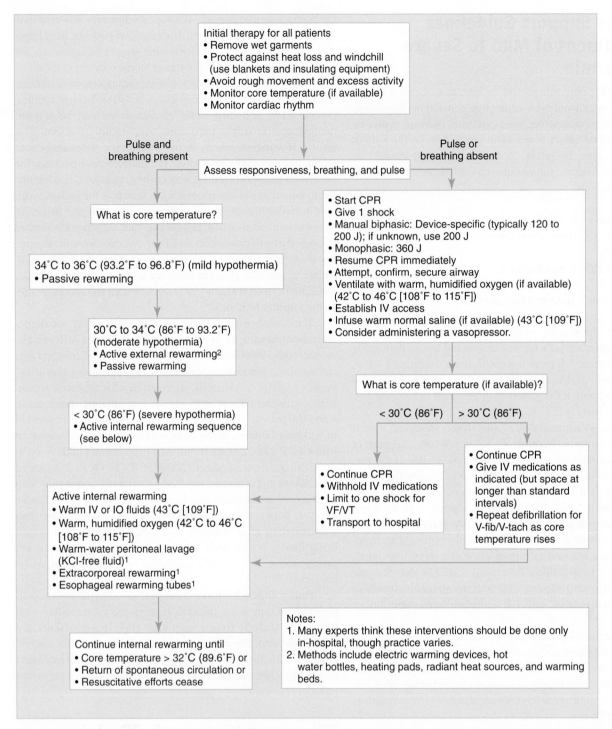

Figure 21-29 Modified from American Heart Association (AHA) hypothermia algorithm from the 2005 Cardiopulmonary Resuscitation and Emergency Cardiovascular Care guidelines and 20120 American Heart Association Guidelines for Cardiopulmonary Resuscitation and Emergency Cardiovascular Care. Note: Peritoneal lavage, extracorporeal rewarming, and esophageal rewarming tubes are usually hospital-only procedures.

Source: Data from: American Heart Association: Handbook of emergency cardiovascular care for healthcare providers, Chicago, 2006, AHA.

- Undernutrition
- Lack of cold weather experience
- African ancestry
- Tobacco use
- Windchill

2. When you cannot stay dry under conditions of cold, wet, and wind, end your session outdoors and seek shelter as soon as possible.

3. Remember that individuals with a history of cold injury are at a greater risk of a subsequent cold injury.

4. Avoid dehydration.

5. Avoid alcohol in cold environments.

6. Use the huddle technique with others if accidental water immersion in cold water occurs. You are more likely to survive if you remain still in cold water less than 68°F (20°C) and do not attempt to swim to shore unless it is nearby.

7. Increase your likelihood of survival in cold environments by:
   - Maintaining a will to survive
   - Being adaptable and improvising
   - Staying optimistic and believing that the event is only a temporary situation
   - Maintaining a calm outlook and a sense of humor

8. Use body heat to warm extremities that are cold or nearly frozen by placing fingers in the armpits or groin area. Toes and feet can be placed on another person's stomach.

9. Keep protective cold weather clothing (e.g., boots, socks, gloves, winter hat, insulated pants and jacket, windproof outer shell) in your car for unexpected car emergencies during cold weather months. Avoid clothing that absorbs moisture, as wet clothing will exacerbate heat loss (i.e., use wool or fleece).

10. Always wear gloves. Frostbite can occur rapidly when touching metal objects in the cold with your bare hands. Mittens are more effective at trapping warm air around all fingers than are five-finger gloves.

11. Understand that the windchill index (**Figure 21-30**) is composed of wind speed and air temperature, and dress for extreme cold with insulated clothing and a windproof garment.

12. Keep feet dry with socks that transfer moisture from your feet to the footwear.

13. Do not walk through snow with low-cut shoes. If you lack appropriate shoes and protective clothes, attempt to stay in a protected area.

14. Do not lie or rest directly on snow. Lie on tree boughs, a sleeping pad, or a poncho. Use a sleeping bag outdoors.

15. Do not wear clothing that will absorb and retain sweat; any sweat retained in your clothes will increase heat loss and cause shivering.

16. When using lotion, use an oil-based one (e.g., ChapStick, Vaseline). Water-based lotions on the face, hands, and ears will increase the risk for frostnip and frostbite.

17. When protecting the lower extremities from cold weather, be sure to protect the genital region. Use

Wind Chill Chart

Temperature (°F)

Calm	40	35	30	25	20	15	10	5	0	-5	-10	-15	-20	-25	-30	-35	-40	-45
5	36	31	25	19	13	7	1	-5	-11	-16	-22	-28	-34	-40	-46	-52	-57	-63
10	34	27	21	15	9	3	-4	-10	-16	-22	28	-35	-41	-47	-53	-59	-66	-72
15	32	25	19	13	6	0	-7	-13	-19	-26	-32	-39	-45	-51	-58	-64	-71	-77
20	30	24	17	11	4	-2	-9	-15	-22	-29	-35	-42	-48	-55	-61	-68	-74	-81
25	29	23	16	9	3	-4	-11	-17	-24	-31	-37	-44	-51	-58	-64	-71	-78	-84
30	28	22	15	8	1	-5	-12	-19	-26	-33	-39	-46	-53	-60	-67	-73	-80	-87
35	28	21	14	7	0	-7	-14	-21	-27	34	-41	-48	-55	-62	-69	-76	-82	-89
40	27	20	13	6	-1	-8	-15	-22	-29	-36	-43	-50	-57	-64	-71	-78	-84	-91
45	26	19	12	5	-2	-9	-16	-23	-30	-37	-44	-51	-58	-65	-72	-79	-86	-93
50	26	19	12	4	-3	-10	-17	-24	-31	-38	-45	-52	-60	-67	-74	-81	-88	-95
55	25	18	11	4	-3	-11	-18	-25	-32	-39	-46	-54	-61	-68	-75	-82	-89	-97
60	25	17	10	3	-4	-11	-19	-26	-33	-40	-48	-55	-62	-69	-76	-84	-91	-98

Wind (MPH)

Frostbite Times: ☐ 30 minutes ☐ 10 minutes ☐ 5 minutes

$$\text{Wind Chill (°F)} = 35.74 + 0.6215T - 35.75(V^{0.16}) + 0.4275T(V^{0.16})$$
Where, T = Air temperature (°F) V = Wind speed (mph)

Figure 21-30 Windchill index.

Source: Courtesy of the National Weather Service.

sweatpants, long underwear, Lycra tights, Gore-Tex pants, or any combination of these garments.

18. To prevent frostbite:

- Do not wear tight clothing, gloves, or boots that restrict circulation.
- Exercise fingers, toes, and face periodically to keep them warm and to detect numb areas.
- Work or exercise with a partner, who watches for warning signs of cold injury and hypothermia.
- Wear properly insulated clothing, and keep it dry; carry extra undergarments, socks, and shoes at all times.
- Watch for numbness and tingling.[133]

Prolonged Transport

At times, the location of a patient will result in a delay in transport or a prolonged transport to an appropriate facility, necessitating extended prehospital care. Consequently, prehospital care providers may need to consider management options beyond what would be used with a rapid transport. How the patient is managed will depend on the time to definitive care, approved medical protocols, equipment and supplies on hand, additional personnel and resources, and location of the patient and severity of the injuries.

Some extended care considerations for moderately to severely injured patients from each of the environments discussed in this chapter are provided here. As with all patient care, it is understood that the first priorities are scene safety, ABCDEs (airway, breathing, circulation, disability, expose/environment), and the use of standard assessment and management procedures appropriate to these environments. If medical control is available, always obtain a consult early, and communicate routinely throughout the extended care period. Any of the procedures listed that fall outside an individual's scope of practice are to be used only by other, credentialed medical providers.

Also, it is important to know that all agencies have established guidelines for discontinuation of CPR. The AHA published a discussion on the ethical issues arising from withholding or withdrawing BLS or ALS resuscitation efforts.[128] The Wilderness Medical Society recommends that once CPR is initiated, it should be continued until resuscitation is successful with an awake patient, until rescuers are exhausted, until rescuers are placed in danger, until the patient is turned over to more definitive care, or until the patient does not respond to prolonged (30 minutes) resuscitative efforts.[134] The National Association of EMS Physicians also provides guidelines for the termination of CPR in the prehospital environment (see the Patient Assessment and Management chapter).[135] If medical control is available, begin patient consult early, if possible, for consideration of CPR termination after a total time of 20 minutes, depending on special patient circumstances (see the chapter titled Environmental Trauma II: Drowning, Lightning, Diving,

and Altitude for additional situations [e.g., cold-water submersion, lightning strike] in which CPR may be extended longer than 20 to 30 minutes).[134]

Heat-Related Illness

Heatstroke

Provide whole-body cooling as quickly as possible. Think about using any available access to water. Immerse the body to neck level in cool water (maintain body control and protect the airway), or spray the whole body with water (e.g., IV fluids, saline, water bottles, water from hydration backpacks), and provide a source of continuous wind current (e.g., natural wind current, fanning with towel, fire ventilation fans). When possible, stay in contact with medical control to keep them informed of the patient's status and to receive further medical directions. Stop body cooling when rectal temperature reaches 102°F (38.9°C). Then protect the patient from shivering and hypothermia.

As you are cooling the patient, manage the airway in unresponsive patients and initiate good ventilation with a bag-mask device with high-flow oxygen. Insert an IV line, provide a 500-ml NS fluid challenge, and assess vital signs. Patients should have vital signs assessed after every 500 ml. Total fluid volume should not exceed 1 to 2 liters in the first hour. An additional liter can be considered during the second hour if prehospital care is extended.

The next priorities are to manage any seizure activity and hypoglycemia per medical protocol with diazepam and dextrose, respectively. Place the patient in the recovery position, and continue the assessment to include level of consciousness, vital signs, rectal temperature, and blood glucose. Provide supportive care and basic bodily needs throughout the remaining extended care period.

Exercise-Associated Hyponatremia

Correct the presumed low blood sodium concentration. If the patient can take food by mouth and if such food is available, provide potato chips, pretzels, or other salty food, or a sport electrolyte or other sodium-containing beverage. An oral sodium solution has been demonstrated to be an appropriate hypertonic saline treatment.[136] In the field, this solution could be prepared by dissolving three to four bouillon cubes in a half cup of water (125 ml) (~9% saline). Salt tablets given alone are not recommended; additional fluid must accompany the tablets, and there is the risk of increasing sodium levels too much.

Next, establish an IV line and start NS with a flow rate set to KVO. Check with medical control to consider a flow rate of 250 or greater ml/hour based on the estimated delay in transporting the patient to the hospital or the presence of severe dehydration or **rhabdomyolysis**. Do not use hypotonic IV fluids because they will exacerbate cerebral edema and could potentiate the condition, leading to seizure, coma, and death. In a patient with severe signs or symptoms (seizure or coma), consider administration of furosemide (a diuretic, if available) to reduce extracellular body water content while providing some sodium by infusing NS, 250 to 500 ml/hour IV.

Assess cerebral edema and increased intracranial pressure. Establish a baseline Glasgow Coma Scale score, and reassess every 10 minutes as an indicator of progressive cerebral edema and increased intracranial pressure (manage per recommendations for cerebral edema; see the Head Trauma chapter).

Be prepared to manage nausea and projectile vomiting. Take one side of a large trash bag and make a hole for the patient's head about 12 inches (30 centimeters) below the rim of the bag. Place the patient's head through the hole so that the patient can look down into the center of the bag. Also be prepared to manage urine when diuresis begins. Use a large trash bag as a diaper or use a bucket or other container.

Give supplemental oxygen (2 to 4 liters/min by nasal cannula) if the patient shows signs of pulmonary distress or for lethargic or obtunded patients. Manage the airway of unresponsive patients, and initiate good ventilation with a bag-mask device (no hyperventilation; see the Head Trauma chapter), with oxygen at 10 breaths/minute.

Assess the patient's blood glucose level, and provide IV dextrose per protocol to hypoglycemic patients. Monitor for seizures, and administer an anticonvulsant (e.g., diazepam, initially 2 to 5 mg IV/intramuscular, and titrate per medical protocol). Place unconscious patients in a left lateral recumbent position. Continue ongoing assessment of the patient.

Cold-Related Illness

Frostbite

Start IV fluids KVO before initiation of rewarming procedures. If a vein cannot be accessed, the intraosseous route is an alternative. In a situation of significant transport delay, active rewarming should be considered. Rapid, active rewarming can reverse the direct injury of ice crystals in tissues, but it may not change the injury severity. It is critical to keep the thawed tissue from refreezing because this significantly worsens the outcome compared with passive thawing. When and where to begin active rewarming are key considerations, if active rewarming is to be done at all.

A standard rewarming procedure is to immerse the affected extremity in circulating water warmed to between a temperature no greater than 98.6°F and 102°F (37°C and 38.9°C) in a large enough container to accommodate the frostbitten tissues without them touching the sides or bottom of the container.[93] Water should feel warm, but not hot, to the normal hand. (Note that the temperature range given here is lower than that previously recommended; this temperature range decreases pain for the patient while only slightly slowing the

rewarming phase.) If available, an oral or rectal thermometer should be used to measure water temperature. A temperature below that recommended will thaw tissue but is less beneficial for rapid thawing and for tissue survival. Any greater temperature will cause greater pain and may cause a burn injury. Avoid active rewarming with intense sources of dry heat (e.g., placing near campfire). Continue immersion until tissue is soft and pliable, which may take up to 30 minutes. Active motion of the extremity during immersion is beneficial, without directed rubbing or massaging of the affected part. If immersion warming is not available, the affected parts may be wrapped in loose, bulky sterile dressings.

Extreme pain is experienced during rapid thawing. Treat with morphine, 5 to 10 mg IV, and titrate as needed. Provide ibuprofen, 400 mg orally every 12 hours, alone or in combination with morphine. Aspirin may be given if ibuprofen is not available, although the optimal dosage regimen has not been determined. (Aspirin is contraindicated in pediatric patients because of the risk of Reye's syndrome.)

The return of normal skin color, warmth, and sensation in the affected part are all favorable signs. Dry all affected parts with warm air (do not towel dry affected parts), and ideally, apply topical aloe vera on skin, place sterile gauze between toes or fingers, bandage, splint, and elevate the extremity. Cover any extremity with insulating material, and wrap a windproof and waterproof material (e.g., trash bag) as the outer layer, particularly if continuing patient extraction outdoors to a transport location.

Hypothermia

Start active rewarming procedures. The key point is to prevent further heat loss. Administer heated IV fluids (104°F to 109°F [40°C to 42.8°C]).

Shivering is the single best way for rewarming patients with mild hypothermia in the prehospital setting compared with external methods of rewarming. Patients with hypothermia who are able to shiver maximally can increase their core temperature by up to 6°F to 8°F (~3°C to 4°C) per hour. External heat sources are often used but may provide only minimal benefit.[84] For the patient with moderate to severe hypothermia, these heat sources remain important considerations in the extended-care situation when used in combination with the hypothermia insulation wrap. Some considerations regarding external heat sources include the following:

- Warmed (maximum 108°F [42.2°C]), humidified oxygen by mask can prevent heat loss during ventilation and provide some heat transfer to the chest from the respiratory tract.
- Body-to-body contact has merit for heat transfer, but many studies fail to show any advantage except in patients with mild hypothermia.

- Electric and portable heating pads provide no additional advantage.
- Forced-air warming has some benefit in minimizing postcooling core temperature ("afterdrop"); it provides an effective warming rate comparable to shivering for patients with mild hypothermia.

Insulate all patients with hypothermia in the remote setting to minimize heat loss. Prepare a multilayer hypothermia wrap. Place a large, waterproof plastic sheet on the floor or ground. Add an insulation layer of blankets or a sleeping bag on top of the waterproof layer. Lay the patient on top of the insulation layer along with any external heat sources. Add a second insulating layer on top of the patient. The left side of the hypothermia wrap is folded over the patient first, then the right side. The patient's head is covered to prevent heat loss, keeping an opening at the face to allow patient assessment.

Assess the patient for hypoglycemia. Providing dextrose will ensure that adequate fuel (sugar) is available for muscular metabolism during shivering and will prevent further hypoglycemia. Alert patients can consume warm, sugary fluids by mouth.

Summary

- Prehospital care providers will inevitably be faced with environmental encounters such as those described in this chapter.
- Basic knowledge of common environmental emergencies is necessary to provide rapid assessment and treatment in the prehospital setting.
- It is not easy to remember this type of information because these problems are infrequently encountered, so remember the general principles involved.
- For heat-related illness, treat patients with heatstroke with effective, rapid, whole-body cooling to reduce core temperature quickly.
- For cold-related illness, manage all patients with moderate to severe hypothermia gently, taking the time to remove them from the cold environment, and begin passive rewarming while monitoring core temperature. The key is to prevent further body heat loss.
- Remember, drugs and defibrillation are generally ineffective when core temperature is less than 86°F (30°C).
- Patients are not dead until they are warm and dead.
- Remember that you must maintain your own safety. In too many cases, prehospital care providers have lost their lives as a result of attempting a rescue.

SCENARIO RECAP

It is a hot summer afternoon with temperatures reaching 102°F (38.9°C). Over the past 30 days, it has been very humid, with temperatures reaching over 100°F (37.8°C) daily. The ambient temperature has resulted in many heat-related injuries that have required EMS personnel to transport numerous patients to the EDs of the inner city.

At 1700 hours, your ambulance unit responds to a dispatch for an unresponsive male patient in a vehicle. As your ambulance unit arrives on scene, you observe a 76-year-old man who appears to be unconscious in a vehicle parked outside of a department store. Your rapid assessment of the patient's ABCs and level of consciousness reveals that the patient is verbal, but he is saying things that are illogical and irrational.

- What are the potential causes for this patient's decreased level of consciousness?
- What hallmark signs support a heat-related diagnosis?
- How would you emergently manage this patient at the scene and en route to the ED?

SCENARIO SOLUTION

This 76-year-old male victim has been waiting in his car for his spouse to return from the shopping center. He has been exposed to high heat without effective hydration to offset fluid loss (sweat) and is dehydrated. The patient has a body mass index over 30, placing him at greater risk of heat-related illness because of obesity.

On the wife's return, she provided additional history indicating that he is taking a diuretic for hypertension, a beta blocker for coronary heart disease, and an anticholinergic for Parkinson's disease. All three medications are known risk factors for heat-related illness. This patient needs quick assessment of his ABCs and level of consciousness using the AVPU (**a**lert, responds to **v**erbal stimulus, responds to **p**ainful stimulus, **u**nresponsive) scale, as he was found in a non-air-conditioned car. Due to his irrational and illogical verbal statements, his age, and the location, you have a high suspicion for heatstroke.

You rapidly assess for blunt or penetrating trauma and find none. Next, geriatric patients must be assessed for exacerbation of any underlying medical disease, such as cardiac disease or a neurologic disorder (e.g., stroke). All three of his medical conditions are known to be made worse with hyperthermia, thereby increasing his mortality risk. It is essential that this patient receive whole-body cooling immediately.

You move the patient out of the direct sunlight on the front seat and remove any excess clothing. You use the saline water bottles from the trauma bag to begin wetting him down from his head to toes. You have your partner start the fan and place the air conditioning on high to increase airflow across the patient's body to increase convective heat transfer. The stretcher is readied to transfer the patient to the ambulance. Ice water and cool moist towels are readied in the back of the ambulance for this patient with hyperthermia.

You quickly transfer the patient from his vehicle to the ambulance. The patient's whole body is wetted down with cold wet towels, and the overhead fans are directed at the patient. The patient is placed on high-flow oxygen, ECG is monitored, and an IV is established at a KVO rate initially. You are prepared to evaluate rectal temperature to confirm hyperthermia (greater than or equal to 104°F [40°C]). If confirmed, you will provide a 500-ml saline IV bolus. You take a set of vital signs and inform medical control to prepare for a 76-year-old male patient with heatstroke.

References

1. National Center for Health Statistics. *Compressed Mortality File.* Hyattsville, MD: U.S. Department of Health and Human Services, Centers for Disease Control and Prevention; 2002.

2. Centers for Disease Control and Prevention. Heat-related deaths— Chicago, Illinois, 1996–2001, and United States, 1979–1999. *MMWR.* 2003;52(26):610.

3. Centers for Disease Control and Prevention. Heat-related deaths— United States, 1999–2003. *MMWR.* 2006;55(29):796.

4. Centers for Disease Control and Prevention. Hypothermia-related deaths—Utah, 2000, and United States, 1979–1998. *MMWR.* 2002;51(4):76.

5. Centers for Disease Control and Prevention. Hypothermia-related deaths—United States, 2003. *MMWR.* 2004;53(08);172.

6. Wade CE, Salinas J, Eastbridge BJ, et al. Admission hypo- or hyperthermia and survival after trauma in civilian and military environments. *Int J of Emerg Med.* 2011;4:35.

7. Lugo-Amador NM, Rothenhaus T, Moyer P. Heat-related illness. *Emerg Med Clin North Am.* 2004;22:315.

8. Ulrich AS, Rathlev NK. Hypothermia and localized injuries. *Emerg Med Clin North Am.* 2004;22:281.

9. Centers for Disease Control and Prevention. Hypothermia-related deaths—United States, 2003. *MMWR.* 2004;53(8):172.

10. Brown DJA, Brugger H, Boyd J, et al. Accidental hypothermia. *N Engl J Med.* 2012;367(20);1930.

11. Leon LR, Kenefick RW. Pathophysiology of heat-related illnesses. In: Auerbach PS, ed. *Wilderness Medicine.* 6th ed. St. Louis, MO: Mosby Elsevier; 2012.

12. O'Brien KK, Leon LR, Kenefick RW. Clinical management of heat-related illnesses. In: Auerbach PS, ed. *Wilderness Medicine.* 6th ed. St. Louis, MO: Mosby Elsevier; 2012.

13. Freer L, Imray CHE. Frostbite. In: Auerbach PS, ed. *Wilderness Medicine.* 6th ed. St. Louis, MO: Mosby Elsevier; 2012.

14. Danzl, DF. Accidental hypothermia. In: Auerbach PS, ed. *Wilderness Medicine.* 6th ed. St. Louis, MO: Mosby Elsevier; 2012.

15. Semenza JC, Rubin CH, Flater KH, et al. Heat-related deaths during the July 1995 heat wave in Chicago. *N Engl J Med.* 1996;335(2):84.

16. Centers for Disease Control and Prevention. Heat related mortality—Chicago, July 1995. *MMWR.* 1995;44 (21):577.

17. Hardy JD. Thermal comfort: skin temperature and physiological thermoregulation. In Hardy JD, Gagge AP, Stolwijk JAJ, eds. *Physiological and Behavioral Temperature Regulation.* Springfield, IL: Charles C. Thomas; 1970.

18. Pozos RS, Danzl DF. Human physiological responses to cold stress and hypothermia. In: Pandolf KB, Burr RE, eds. *Medical Aspects of Harsh Environments.* Vol 1. Washington, DC: Office of the Surgeon General, Borden Institute/TMM Publications; 2001: 351–382.

19. Stocks JM, Taylor NAS, Tipton MJ, Greenleaf JE. Human physiological responses to cold exposure. *Aviat Space Environ Med.* 2004;75:444.

20. Wenger CB. The regulation of body temperature. In Rhoades RA, Tanner GA, eds. *Medical Physiology*. Boston, MA: Little, Brown; 1995.

21. Nunnelely SA, Reardon MJ. Prevention of heat illness. In: Pandolf KB, Burr RE, eds. *Medical Aspects of Harsh Environments*. Vol 1. Washington, DC: Office of the Surgeon General, Borden Institute/TMM Publications; 2001:209–230.

22. Yeo T. Heat stroke: a comprehensive review. *AACN Clin Issues*. 2004;15:280.

23. Wenger CB. Section I: human adaption to hot environments. In: Pandolf KB, Burr RE, eds. *Medical Aspects of Harsh Environments*. Vol 1. Washington, DC: Office of the Surgeon General, Borden Institute/TMM Publications; 2001:51–86.

24. Sonna LA. Practical medical aspects of military operations in the heat. In: Pandolf KB, Burr RE, eds. *Medical Aspects of Harsh Environments*. Vol 1. Washington, DC: Office of the Surgeon General, Borden Institute/TMM Publications; 2001:293–309.

25. Tek D, Olshaker JS. Heat illness. *Emerg Med Clin North Am*. 1992;10(2):299.

26. Armstrong LE, Hubbard RW, Jones BH, Daniels JT. Preparing Alberto Salazar for the heat of the 1984 Olympic marathon. *Phys Sportsmed*. 1986;14:73.

27. Hubbard RW, Sandick BL, Matthew WT. Voluntary dehydration and alliesthesia for water. *J Appl Physiol*. 1984;57:868.

28. Johnson RF, Kobrick JL. Psychological aspects of military performance in hot environments. In: Pandolf KB, Burr RE, eds. *Medical Aspects of Harsh Environments*. Vol 1. Washington, DC: Office of the Surgeon General, Borden Institute/TMM Publications; 2001.

29. Sawka MN, Pandolf KB. Physical exercise in hot climates: physiology, performance, and biomedical issues. In: Pandolf KB, Burr RE, eds. *Medical Aspects of Harsh Environments*. Vol 1. Washington, DC: Office of the Surgeon General, Borden Institute/TMM Publications; 2001.

30. Dutchman SM, Ryan AJ, Schedl HP, et al. Upper limits of intestinal absorption of dilute glucose solution in men at rest. *Med Sci Sport Exerc*. 1997;29:482.

31. Neufer PD, Young AJ, Sawka MN. Gastric emptying during exercise: effects of heat stress and hypohydration. *Eur J Appl Physiol*. 1989;58:433.

32. American College of Sports Medicine. Position stand: exertional heat illness during training and competition. *Med Sci Sports Exerc*. 2007;39(3):556.

33. Bouchama A, Knochel JP. Medical progress: heatstroke. *N Engl J Med*. 2002;346(25):1978–1988.

34. Adams T, Stacey E, Stacey S, Martin D. Exertional heat stroke. *Br J Hosp Med (London)*. 2012;73(2):72–78.

35. Case DJ, Armstrong LE, Kenny GP, O'Connor FG, Huggins RA. Exertional heat stroke: new concepts regarding cause and care. *Curr Sports Med Rep*. 2012;11(3):115–123.

36. Casa DJ, McDermott BP, Lee E, Yeargin SW, Armstrong LE, Maresh CM. Cold-water immersion: the gold standard for exertional heat stroke treatment. *Exerc Sport Rev*. 2007;35(3):141–149.

37. Holtzhausen LM, Noakes TD. Collapsed ultra-endurance athlete: proposed mechanisms and an approach to management. *Clin J Sport Med*. 1997;7(4):292.

38. Gardner JW, Kark JA. Clinical diagnosis, management and surveillance of exertional heat illness. In: Pandolf KB, Burr RE, eds. *Medical Aspects of Harsh Environments*. Vol 1. Washington, DC: Office of the Surgeon General, Borden Institute/TMM Publications; 2001:231–279.

39. Asplune CA, O'Connor FG, Noakes TD. Exercise-associated collapse: an evidence-based review and primer for clinicians. *Br J Sports Med*. 2011;45:1157–1162.

40. Rosner MH. Exercise-associated hyponatremia. *Semin Nephrol*. 2009;29(3):271–281.

41. Rosner M, Bennett B, Hoffman M, Hew-Butler T. Exercise induced hyponatremia. In: Simon E, ed. *Hyponatremia: Evaluation and Treatment*. New York, NY: Springer; 2013.

42. Leon LR, Helwig BG. Heat stroke: role of the systemic inflammatory response. *J Appl Physiol*. 2010;109(6):1980–1988.

43. Gaffin SL, Hubbard RW. Pathophysiology of heatstroke. In: Pandolf KB, Burr RE, eds. *Medical Aspects of Harsh Environments*. Vol 1. Washington, DC: Office of the Surgeon General, Borden Institute/TMM Publications; 2001:161–208.

44. Knochel JP, Reed G. Disorders of heat regulation. In: Narins RE, ed. *Maxwell & Kleenman's Clinical Disorders of Fluid and Electrolyte Metabolism*. 5th ed. New York, NY: McGraw-Hill; 1994.

45. Armstrong LE, Crago AE, Adams R, et al. Whole-body cooling of hyperthermic runners: comparison of two field therapies. *Am J Emerg Med*. 1996;14:335.

46. Costrini A. Emergency treatment of exertional heatstroke and comparison of whole-body cooling techniques. *Med Sci Sports Exerc*. 1984;22:15.

47. Gaffin SL, Gardner J, Flinn S. Current cooling method for exertional heatstroke. *Ann Intern Med*. 2000;132:678.

48. Speedy DB, Noakes TD. Exercise-associated hyponatremia: a review. *Emerg Med*. 2001;13:17.

49. Backer HD, Shopes E, Collins SL, Barkan H. Exertional heat illness and hyponatremia in hikers. *Am J Emerg Med*. 1999;17(6):532.

50. Gardner JW. Death by water intoxication. *Mil Med*. 2002;164(3):432.

51. Noakes TD, Goodwin N, Rayner BL, et al. Water intoxication: a possible complication during endurance exercise. *Med Sci Sports Exerc*. 1985;17:370.

52. Rosner MH, Kirven J. Exercise-associated hyponatremia. *Clin J Am Soc Nephrol*. 2007;2:151.

53. Adrogue HJ, Madias NE. Hyponatremia. *N Engl J Med*. 2000;342(21):1581.

54. Hiller WDB. Dehydration and hyponatremia during triathlons. *Med Sci Sports Exerc*. 1989;21:S219.

55. Speedy DB, Noakes TD, Rodgers IR. Hyponatremia in ultra-distance triathletes. *Med Sci Sports Exerc*. 1999;31:809.

56. Laird RH. Medical care at ultra-endurance triathlons. *Med Sci Sports Exerc*. 1989;21:S222.

57. Collins S, Reynolds B. The other heat-related emergency. *JEMS*. July 2004.

58. American College of Sports Medicine. Position stand on exercise and fluid replacement. *Med Sci Sports Exerc*. 2007;39(2):377.

59. Bennett BL, Hew-Butler T, Hoffman M, Rogers I, Rosner M. Wilderness Medicine Society practice guidelines for treatment of exercise-associated hyponatremia. *Wilderness Environ Med*. 2013;24(3):228–240.

60. Hew-Bulter T, Ayus JC, Kipps C, et al. Statement of Second International Exercise-Associated Hyponatremia Consensus Development Conference, New Zealand, 2007. *Clin J Sport Med*. 2008;18:111.

61. U.S. Fire Administration. Fire fighter fatalities in the United States in 2011. Federal Emergency Management Agency. July 2012.

http://www.usfa.fema.gov/downloads/pdf/publications/ff_fat11.pdf. Accessed January 24, 2014.

62. Ayus JC, Arieff A, Moritz ML. Hyponatremia in marathon runners. *N Engl J Med.* 2005;353:427.

63. U.S. Department of Agriculture, U.S. Forest Service. Heat stress brochure. http://www.fs.fed.us/fire/safety/fitness/heat_stress/hs_pg1.html. Accessed January 24, 2014

64. Montain SJ, Latzka WA, Sawka MN. Fluid replacement recommendations for training in hot weather. *Mil Med.* 1999; 164(7):502.

65. Parson KC. International standards for the assessment of the risk of thermal strain on clothed workers in hot environments. *Ann Occup Hyg.* 1999;43(5):297.

66. American College of Sports Medicine. Position stand on the recommended quantity and quality of exercise for developing and maintaining cardiorespiratory and muscular fitness, and flexibility in adults. *Med Sci Sports Exerc.* 1998;30(6):975.

67. Haskell WL, Lee IM, Pate RR, et al. Physical activity and public health: updated recommendation for adults from the American College of Sports Medicine and the American Heart Association. *Med Sci Sports Exerc.* 2007;39(8):1423.

68. Heat acclimatization guide. http://www.usariem.army.mil/assets/docs/partnering/HeatAcclimatizationGuide.pdf. Accessed January 24, 2014.

69. Eichna LW, Park CR, Nelson N, et al. Thermal regulation during acclimatization in a hot, dry (desert type) environment. *J Appl Physiol.* 1950;163:585.

70. McEnvy M. Making a rehab a requirement: NFPA 1584. FireRescue1. http://www.firerescue1.com/firerehab/articles/327047-Making-Rehab-a-Requirement-NFPA-1584/. Published December 10, 2007. Accessed January 13, 2014.

71. Hostler D. First responder rehab: good, better, best. *JEMS.* 2007;32(12).

72. Federal Emergency Management System, U.S. Fire Administration. Emergency Incident Rehabilitation. http://www.usfa.fema.gov/downloads/pdf/publications/fa_314.pdf. Published February 2008. Accessed January 24, 2014.

73. *U.S. Pharmacopeia, National Formulary (USP-25/NF-20).* Rockville, MD: U.S. Pharmacopeia Convention; 2000.

74. Brown LH, Krumperman K, Fullagar CJ. Out of hospital medical storage temperature. *Prehosp Emerg Care.* 2004;8:200.

75. Mehta SH, Doran JV, Lavery RF, Allegra JR. Improvements in prehospital medication storage practices in response to research. *Prehosp Emerg Care.* 2002;6:319.

76. Allegra JR, Brennan J, Lanier V. Storage temperatures of out-of-hospital medications. *Acad Emerg Med.* 1999;6:1098.

77. Palmer RG, Zimmerman J, Clawson JJ. Altered states: the influence of temperature on prehospital drugs. *J Emerg Med Serv.* 1985;10(12):29.

78. Johansen RB, Schafer NC, Brown PI. Effects of extreme temperature on drugs for prehospital ACLS. *Am J Emerg Med.* 1993;11:450.

79. Church WH, Hu SS, Henry AJ. Thermal degradation of injectable drugs. *Am J Emerg Med.* 1994;12:306.

80. New Jersey Department of Health and Senior Services. Suppl Section 8:41–43.12, paragraph (f), August 17, 1998.

81. Ulrich AS, Rathlev NK. Hypothermia and localized injuries. *Emerg Med Clin North Am.* 2004;22:281.

82. Chandler W, Ivey H. Cold weather injuries among U.S. soldiers in Alaska: a five-year review. *Mil Med.* 1997;162:788.

83. DeGroot DW, Castellani JW, Williams JO, Amoroso PJ. Epidemiology of U.S. Army cold-weather injuries, 1980–1999. *Mil Med.* 2003; 74:564.

84. Thomas JR, Oakley EHN. Nonfreezing cold injury. In: Pandolf KB, Burr RE, eds. *Medical Aspects of Harsh Environments.* Vol 1. Washington, DC: Office of the Surgeon General, Borden Institute/TMM Publications; 2001:467–490.

85. Montgomery H. Experimental immersion foot: review of the physiopathology. *Physiol Rev.* 1954;34:127.

86. Francis TJR. Nonfreezing cold injury: a historical review. *J R Nav Med Serv.* 1984;70:134.

87. Wrenn K. Immersion foot: a problem of the homeless in the 1990s. *Arch Intern Med.* 1991;151:785.

88. Ramstead KD, Hughes RB, Webb AJ. Recent cases of trench foot. *Postgrad Med J.* 1980;56:879.

89. Biem J, Koehncke N, Classen D, Dosman J. Out of cold: management of hypothermia and frostbite. *Can Med Assoc J.* 2003;168(3):305.

90. Vogel JE, Dellon AL. Frostbite injuries of the hand. *Clin Plast Surg.* 1989;16:565.

91. Mills WJ. Clinical aspects of freezing injury. In: Pandolf KB, Burr RE, eds. *Medical Aspects of Harsh Environments.* Vol 1. Washington, DC: Office of the Surgeon General, Borden Institute/TMM Publications; 2001.

92. McIntosh SE, Hamonko M, Freer L, et al. Wilderness Medical Society Practice guidelines of the prevention and treatment of frostbite. *Wilderness Environ Med.* 2011;22;156–166.

93. Gilbertson J, Mandsager R. State of Alaska cold injuries guidelines. Department of Health and Social Services, Juneau, Alaska, 2005 (revision). dhss.alaska.gov/dph/Emergency/Documents/ems/assets/Downloads/AKColdInj2005.pdf. Accessed January 13, 2014.

94. Sessler DI. Mild preoperative hypothermia. *N Engl J Med.* 1997;336:1730.

95. Giesbrecht GG. Cold stress, near drowning and accidental hypothermia: a review. *Aviat Space Environ Med.* 2000;71:733.

96. Stocks JM, Taylor NAS, Tipton MJ, Greenleaf JE. Human physiological responses to cold exposure. *Aviat Space Environ Med.* 2004;75:444.

97. Gilbert M, Busund R, Skagseth A, et al. Resuscitation from accidental hypothermia of 13.7°C with circulatory arrest. *Lancet.* 2000;355:375.

98. Danzl DF, Pozos RS, Auerbach PS. Multicenter hypothermia survey. *Ann Emerg Med.* 1987;16:1042.

99. Tsuei BJ, Kearney PA. Hypothermia in the trauma patient. *Injury Int J Care Injured.* 2004;35:7.

100. Stoner HB. Effects of injury on the responses to thermal stimulation of the hypothalamus. *J Appl Physiol.* 1972;33:665.

101. Ferrara A, MacArthur J, Wright H. Hypothermia and acidosis worsen coagulopathy in the patient requiring massive transfusion. *Am J Surg.* 1990;160:515.

102. Epstein M. Renal effects of head-out immersion in man: implications for understanding volume homeostasis. *Physiol Rev.* 1978; 58:529.

103. Jurkovich G. Hypothermia in the trauma patient. *Adv Trauma.* 1989;4:111.

104. Jurkovich GJ. Environmental cold-induced injury. *Surg Clin N Am.* 2007;87:247.

105. Arthurs Z, Cuadrado D, Beekley A, Grathwohl K. The impact of hypothermia on trauma care at the 31st combat support hospital. *Am J Surg.* 2006;191(5):610–614.

106. Beilman GJ, Blondett JJ, Nelson AB. Early hypothermia in severely injured trauma patients is a significant risk factor of multiple organ dysfunction syndrome but not mortality. *Ann Surg.* 2009;249:845–850.

107. Mommsen P, Andruszkow H, Fromke C, et al. Effects of accidental hypothermia on posttraumatic complications and outcome in multiple trauma patients. *Injury.* 2013;44(1):86–90.

108. Lapostolle F, Sebbah JL, Couvreur J. Risk factors for the onset of hypothermia in trauma victims: the Hypotrauma study. *Crit Care.* 2012;16(4):R142.

109. Trentzsch H, Huber-Wagner S, Hildebrand F, et al. Hypothermia for prediction of death in severely injured blunt trauma patients. *Shock.* 2012;37(2):131.

110. Nolan JP, Morley PT, Vanden Hoek TL, et al. Therapeutic hypothermia after cardiac arrest. An advisory statement by the Advance Life Support Task Force of the international liaison committee on resuscitation, *Circulation.* 2003;108:118.

111. Alzaga AG, Cerdan M, Varon J. Therapeutic hypothermia. *Resuscitation.* 2006;70:369.

112. Nolan JP, Neumar RW, Adrie C, et al. Post-cardiac arrest syndrome: epidemiology, pathophysiology, treatment, and prognostication. A scientific statement from the International Liaison Committee on Resuscitation; the American Heart Association Emergency Cardiovascular Care Committee; the Council on Cardiovascular Surgery and Anesthesia; the Council on Cardiopulmonary, Perioperative, and Critical Care; the Council on Clinical Cardiology; the Council on Stroke. *Resuscitation.* 2008;79:350.

113. Nolan JP, Hazinski MF, Billi JE, et al. Part 1: executive summary: 2010 International Consensus on Cardiopulmonary Resuscitation and Emergency Cardiovascular Care Science With Treatment Recommendations. *Resuscitation.* 2010;81S:e1–e25.

114. Carlson LD. Immersion in cold water and body tissue insulation. *Aerospace Med.* 1958;29:145.

115. Wittmers LE, Savage M. Cold water immersion. In: Pandolf KB, Burr RE, eds. *Medical Aspects of Harsh Environments.* Vol 1. Washington, DC: Office of the Surgeon General, Borden Institute/ TMM Publications; 2001:531–552.

116. Giesbrecht GG, Steinman AM. Immersion into cold water. In: Auerbach PS, ed. *Wilderness Medicine.* 6th ed. St. Louis, MO: Mosby Elsevier; 2012.

117. Nozaki R, Ishibashi K, Adachi N, et al. Accidental profound hypothermia. *N Eng J Med.* 1986;315:1680 (letter).

118. Tipton MJ. The initial responses to cold-water immersion in man. *Clin Sci.* 1989;77:581.

119. Keatinge WR, McIlroy MB, Goldfien A. Cardiovascular responses to ice-cold showers. *J Appl Physiol.* 1964;19:1145.

120. Mekjavic IB, La Prairie A, Burke W, Lindborg B. Respiratory drive during sudden cold water immersion. *Respir Physiol.* 1987; 70:21.

121. Cushing TA, Hawkins SC, Sempsrott J, Schoene RB. Submersion injuries and drowning . In: Auerbach PS. *Wilderness Medicine.* 6th ed. St. Louis, MO: Mosby Elsevier; 2012.

122. Wissler EH. Probability of surviving during accidental immersion in cold water. *Aviat Space Environ Med.* 2003;74:47.

123. Tikuisis P. Predicting survival time at sea based on observed body cooling rates. *Aviat Space Environ Med.* 1997;68:441.

124. Hayward JS, Errickson JD, Collis ML. Thermal balance and survival time prediction of man in cold water. *Can J Physiol Pharmacol.* 1975;53:21.

125. Ducharme MB, Lounsbury DS. Self-rescue swimming in cold water: the latest advice. *Appl Physiol Nutr Metab.* 2007;32:799.

126. Van Mieghem C, Sabbe M, Knockaert D. The clinical vales of the ECG in noncardiac conditions. *Chest.* 2004;125:1561.

127. Vanden Hoek TL, Morrison LJ, Shuster M, et al. Part 12.9: cardiac arrest in special situations: accidental hypothermia. In: *2010 American Heart Association Guidelines for Cardiopulmonary Resuscitation and Emergency Cardiovascular Care. Circulation.* 2010;122:S829–S861.

128. Morrison LJ, Kierzek G, Diekema DS, et al. Part 3: Ethics. In: *2010 American Heart Association Guidelines for Cardiopulmonary Resuscitation and Emergency Cardiovascular Care. Circulation.* 2010;122:S665–S675.

129. Danzl DF, Lloyd EL. Treatment of accidental hypothermia. In: Pandolf KB, Burr RE, eds. *Medical Aspects of Harsh Environments.* Vol 1. Washington, DC: Office of the Surgeon General, Borden Institute/TMM Publications; 2001:491–529.

130. Southwick FS, Dalglish PH. Recovery after prolonged asystolic cardiac arrest in profound hypothermia: a case report and literature review. *JAMA.* 1980;243:1250.

131. Bernard MB, Gray TW, Buist MD, et al. Treatment of comatose survivors of out-of-hospital cardiac arrest with induced hypothermia. *N Engl J Med.* 2002;346(8):557.

132. Reuler JB. Hypothermia: pathophysiology, clinical setting, and management. *Ann Intern Med.* 1978;89:519.

133. Armstrong LE. Cold, windchill, and water immersion. In: *Performing in Extreme Environments.* Champaign, IL: Human Kinetics; 2000.

134. Wilderness Medical Society. Myocardial infarction, acute coronary syndromes, and CPR. In: Forgey WW, ed. *Practice Guidelines for Wilderness Emergency Care.* 5th ed. Guilford, CT: Globe Pequot Press; 2006.

135. Siegel AJ, d'Hemecourt P, Adner MM, Shirey T, Brown JL, Lewandrowski KB. Exertional dysnatremia in collapsed marathon runners: a critical role for point-of-care testing to guide appropriate therapy. *Am J Clin Pathol.* 2009;132(3):336–340.

136. Position paper of the National Association of EMS Physicians: termination of resuscitation in nontraumatic cardiac arrest. *Prehosp Emerg Care.* 2011;15:545.

Suggested Reading

Auerbach PS, ed. *Wilderness Medicine.* 6th ed. St. Louis, MO: Mosby Elsevier; 2012.

Pandolf KB, Burr RE, eds. *Medical Aspects of Harsh Environments.* Vol 1. Washington, DC: Office of the Surgeon General, Borden Institute/ TMM Publications; 2001.

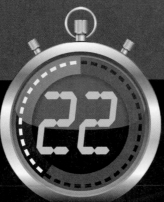
Environmental Trauma II: Lightning, Drowning, Diving, and Altitude

CHAPTER OBJECTIVES

At the completion of this chapter, the reader will be able to do the following:

- Explain why there is no safe place outdoors from lightning.

- Describe the use of "reverse" triage for multiple lightning casualties.

- Identify the key risk factors for high-altitude illness.

- Explain the new recommendation during the initial ABC (airway, breathing, and circulation) management of a drowning incident.

- Describe three signs or symptoms that can occur in a patient after a drowning incident.

- Identify five methods for preventing a drowning incident.

- Contrast the signs and symptoms of Type I and Type II decompression sickness.

- Describe two primary treatment interventions for Type II decompression sickness and arterial gas embolism.

- Discuss the similarities and differences between acute mountain sickness and high-altitude cerebral edema.

SCENARIO

In a coastal town, a family of four was strolling on the beach with their dog during a chilly winter day. The son tossed a rubber ball toward the water's edge, and the dog gave chase. In an instant, a large shore-breaking wave swallowed up the dog in the rough surf. The 17-year-old son was first into the water to attempt to save the dog, only to be overtaken by the water. He was seen struggling in the rough surging surf by his parents and sister.

The boy's father and mother both followed him into the surf in an effort to help. Their 19-year-old daughter remained on shore and called for help on her cell phone. The dog eventually made it back to the shore. The parents were able to pull their son out of the cold water after finding him submerged and unresponsive. Your paramedic unit arrives to the scene within 7 minutes of the daughter's call.

As you exit the ambulance, you observe an unconscious teenage boy lying partially facedown in sand with surging water close by. He is still in the surf zone and could be submersed by a wave. You team up with arriving fire department emergency responders to approach the victim.

- How should you approach the patient in this setting?
- If the patient has no pulse or respirations, what is the next immediate intervention?
- What other concerns do you have for the patient that need to be addressed on scene?

Introduction

Each year in the United States, significant morbidity and mortality are caused by a variety of environmental conditions, including lightning strikes, submersion incidents, recreational scuba diving, and high-altitude climbing (see the Environmental Trauma I: Heat and Cold chapter for heat and cold conditions). Prehospital care providers must know the major and minor disorders associated with each type of environment; understand the anatomy, physiology, and pathophysiology involved; and know how to rapidly perform patient assessment and management. At the same time, they must know how to prevent injury to themselves and other public safety personnel.

Lightning-Related Injuries

Lightning is the most widespread threat to people and property during the thunderstorm season and is second only to floods in causing storm-related death in the United States since 1959.[1] The National Weather Service estimates that 100,000 thunderstorms occur each year in the United States and that lightning is present in all storms. Lightning is reported to start approximately 75,000 forest fires annually and starts 40% of all fires.[2] The most destructive form of lightning is the cloud-to-ground strike (**Figure 22-1**). Based on real-time lightning-detection systems, it is estimated that cloud-to-ground lightning strikes occur approximately 20 million times per year, with as many as 50,000 flashes per hour during a summer afternoon.[3,4] In the United States, lightning occurs most frequently from June through August, but occurs in Florida and along the southeastern coast of the Gulf

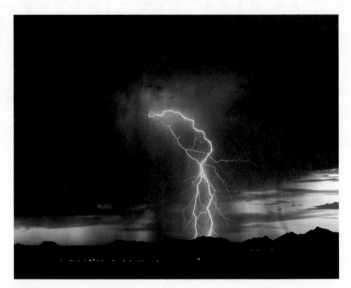

Figure 22-1 A cloud-to-ground lightning strike, with streak lightning pattern.
Source: © Jhaz Photography/ShutterStock, Inc.

of Mexico throughout the year (see **Figure 22-2** for distribution of lightning flashes in the United States and worldwide).[5] Internationally, lightning strikes occur approximately 50 times per second, and it is estimated that one-fifth of these strike the ground.[6,7] Worldwide, rural populations are at the greatest risk due to the lack of lightning safe structures and prevention education. Consequently, it is estimated that 24,000 fatalities occur annually and about 10 times more injuries worldwide.[8,9]

Since the 1950s, the number of deaths from lightning in the United States has decreased, possibly because of fewer people working outdoors in rural areas, improved warning systems for approaching storms, increased public education on lightning

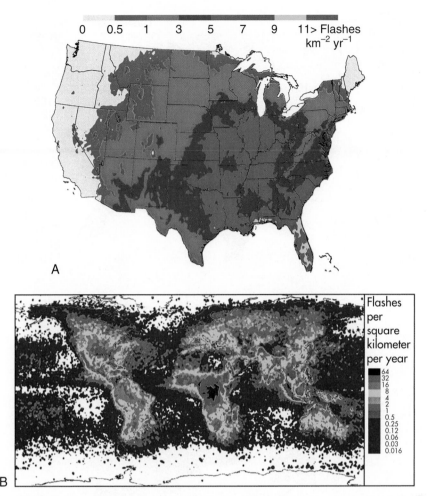

Figure 22-2 **A.** Distribution of lightning ground strikes in the United States, with the heaviest concentration in the southeast region. **B.** Distribution of lightning ground strikes worldwide.

Source: Huffines GR, Orville RE: Lightning ground flash density and thunderstorm duration in the continental United States, 1989–1996. *J Appl Meteorol* 38:1013, 1999.

safety, and improved medical care.[6] Latest reports indicate that lightning kills 50 to 300 individuals each year and injures about 1,000.[2,10]

The greatest life threats from lightning strikes are neurologic and cardiopulmonary injuries. A recently published practice guideline from the Wilderness Medical Society is available for the prevention and treatment of lightning injuries for prehospital and in-hospital care.[11,12] These recommendations for medical management are graded, based on the quality of the supporting evidence (see the chapter titled The Science, Art, and Ethics of Prehospital Care Principles, Preferences, and Critical Thinking).

Epidemiology

Based on the National Oceanic and Atmospheric Administration (NOAA) publication called *Storm Data*, 3,529 deaths (average 98 deaths per year), 9,818 injuries, and 19,814 property-damage reports occurred during the 36-year period from 1959 to 1994 due to lightning.[1] **Figure 22-3** shows the ranking of lightning injuries and deaths by state from 1959 to 1994.

There were 1,318 lightning deaths between 1980 and 1995 in the United States, on review of medical examiners' death

certificates listing lightning as the cause of death.[13] Of those who died during this 16-year period, 1,125 (85%) were male, and 896 (68%) were 15 to 44 years of age. The highest death rate from lightning occurred among those 15 to 19 years of age (6 deaths per 10,000,000). Analysis shows that about 30% die and 74% of the survivors have permanent disabilities. Furthermore, victims with cranial or leg burns are at a greater risk for death.[12] Of the individuals who died from a lightning strike, 52% were outside (25% of whom were at work). Death occurred within 1 hour in 63% of the lightning victims.[6]

Mechanism of Injury

Injury from lightning can result from the following five mechanisms[11,12]:

- *Direct strike* occurs when a person is in an open environment unable to find shelter. It accounts for only 3% to 5% of lightning strikes involving people.
- *Side flash* or *splash contact* occurs when lightning hits an object (e.g., ground, building, tree) and splashes onto a victim or multiple victims. The current will jump

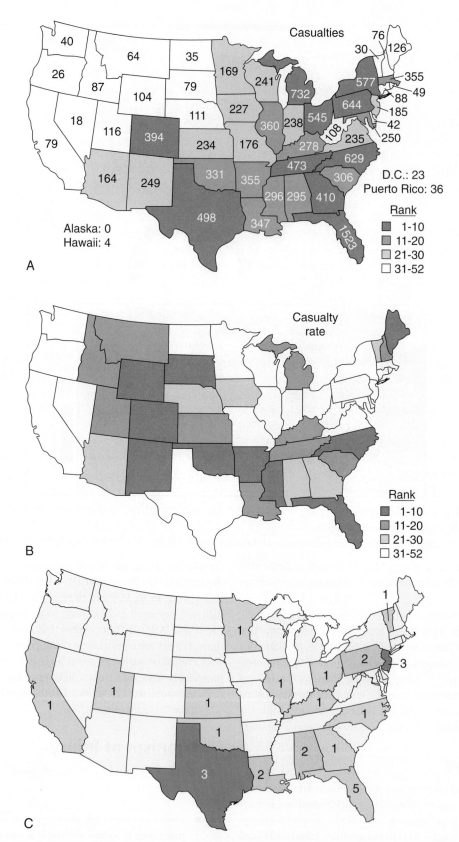

Figure 22-3 Rank of each state in lightning casualties (deaths and injuries combined) from 1959 to 1994. **A.** Casualties per state.
B. Casualties weighted by state population. **C.** 2012 lightning fatalities.

Source: A., B. Data from Curran EB, Holle RL, Lopez RE: Lightning fatalities, injuries, and damage reports in the United States from 1959–1994. NOAA Tech Memo NWS
SW-193, 1997. C. Data from: http://www.lightningsafety.noaa.gov/fatalities.htm Accessed Jan 7, 2013.

from the primary strike object and can splash over to a person. Splashes occur from person to person, tree to person, and even indoors from telephone wire to a person talking on the phone.

■ *Contact* occurs when a person is in direct contact with an object that is struck directly or by a splash. It accounts for one-third of all lightning injuries.

■ *Step voltage* occurs when lightning hits the ground or a nearby object and the current spreads outward radially, passing through a person's body in the process. Human tissue provides less resistance than the ground, and the current will travel, for example, up one leg and down the other, following the path of least resistance. Ground current accounts for over 50% of lightning injuries. Step voltage is also known as *stride voltage* or *ground current*.

■ *Upward streamer* occurs when current passes up from the ground and through the victim, but does not connect with the downward lightning streamer. The energy in this streamer is less as compared to a full lightning strike and accounts for approximately 1% to 15% of lightning injuries. Upward streamer is a newer form of lightning contact that has been recently identified.

Blunt trauma can occur from a shock wave produced by lightning, which can propel a person up to 10 yards. In addition, injuries can result from lightning that causes forest fires, building fires, and explosions.[2,14,15]

There are six known factors that determine the injury severity from electrical and lightning current:

■ Type of circuit
■ Duration of exposure
■ Voltage
■ Amperage
■ Resistance of tissue
■ The pathway of current

Once lightning or other high-voltage electrical source contacts the human body, the heat generated within the body is directly proportional to the amount of current, tissue resistance, and duration of contact. As resistance of various tissues increases (e.g., from nerve < blood < muscle < skin < fat < bone), so does the heat generated by the passage of current.

It is easy to assume that lightning injuries are similar to high-voltage electrical injuries. However, significant differences exist between the two mechanisms of injury. A lightning strike is direct current (DC) as opposed to alternating current (AC), which is responsible for industrial and household electrical injuries. Lightning produces millions of volts of electrical charge, with currents ranging from 30,000 to 50,000 amps, and the duration of exposure to the body is instantaneous (10 to 100 milliseconds). The temperature of lightning varies with the diameter, but the average temperature is approximately 14,430°F (8,000°C).[10] In comparison, high-voltage electrical exposure tends to be a much lower voltage than lightning. However, the key factor that distinguishes lightning injury from high-voltage electrical injury is the duration of current exposure within the body.[14] **Figure 22-4** lists differences between lightning and generator-produced, high-voltage electrical injuries.

At times, lightning can show injury patterns similar to those seen with high-voltage electricity because of a rare lightning pattern that produces a prolonged strike lasting up to 0.5 second. This type of lightning, called *hot lightning*, is capable of causing deep burns, exploding trees, and setting fires. Lightning can show entry and exit wounds on the body, but a more common pathway of lightning once it strikes a victim is to pass over the body. This is referred to as a *flashover* current. A flashover current can also enter the eyes, ears, nose, and mouth. It is theorized that the flashover current flow is the reason why many victims survive lightning strikes. It is also known that a flashover current may vaporize moisture on skin or blast a part of clothing or shoes off a victim. The immense flashover current generates large magnetic fields, which in turn can induce secondary electric currents within the body and are thought to cause cardiac arrest and other internal injuries.[16,17]

Figure 22-4 Comparison of Lightning and High-Voltage Electrical Injuries

Factor	Lightning	High Voltage
Energy level	30 million volts; 50,000 amperes	Usually much lower
Time of exposure	Brief, instantaneous	Prolonged
Pathway	Flashover, orifice	Deep, internal
Burns	Superficial, minor	Deep, internal
Cardiac	Primary and secondary arrest, asystole	Ventricular fibrillation
Renal	Rare myoglobinuria or hemoglobinuria	Myoglobinuric renal failure common
Fasciotomy	Rarely if ever necessary	Common, early, and extensive
Blunt injury	Explosive thunder effect	Falls, being thrown

Source: Modified table from Cooper MA, Holle RL, Andrews CJ, Blumenthal R: Lightning injuries. In Auerbach PS: Wilderness medicine, ed 6, St. Louis, 2012, Mosby Elsevier.

Injuries From Lightning

Lightning injuries range from minor superficial wounds to major multisystem trauma and death. **Figure 22-5** lists common signs and symptoms of lightning injury. As a tool to determine the likely recovery or prognosis from lightning strikes, victims can be placed in one of three injury categories: minor, moderate, and severe.[11,18]

Minor Injury

Patients with minor injury are awake and report an unpleasant and abnormal sensation (*dysesthesia*) in the affected extremity or extremities. In a more serious lightning strike, victims report they have been hit in the head or state that an explosion hit them, because they are unsure of the source. A patient may present at the scene with the following:

- Confusion (short term or hours to days)
- Amnesia (short term or hours to days)
- Temporary deafness
- Blindness
- Temporary unconsciousness
- Temporary paresthesia
- Muscular pain
- Cutaneous burns (rare)
- Transient paralysis

Victims present with normal vital signs or with mild, transient hypertension, and recovery is usually gradual and complete.

Moderate Injury

Victims with moderate injury have progressive, single or multisystem injuries, some of which are life threatening. Some patients in this category also have a permanent disability. Patients may present at the scene with the following:

- **Immediate effects**
  - Neurologic signs
  - Seizures
  - Deafness
  - Cardiac arrest and cardiac injuries
  - Pulmonary injuries
  - Confusion, amnesia
  - Blindness
  - Dizziness
  - Contusion from shockwave
  - Blunt trauma (e.g., fractures)
  - Chest pain, muscle aches
  - Tympanic membrane rupture
  - Headache, nausea, postconcussion syndrome
- **Delayed effects**
  - Neurologic symptoms and signs
  - Memory deficits
  - Attention deficits
  - Neuropsychological changes
  - Coding and retrieval problems
  - Distractibility
  - Personality changes
  - Irritability
  - Chronic pain
  - Seizures

Depending on the location of the lightning strike, a strike affecting the respiratory center of the brain can result in prolonged respiratory arrest that may lead to secondary cardiac arrest as a result of hypoxia.[12] Victims in this category may experience immediate cardiopulmonary arrest, although the inherent automaticity of the heart may produce a spontaneous

Figure 22-5	Lightning Injury: Common Signs, Symptoms, and Treatment	
Injuries	**Signs/Symptoms**	**Treatment**
Minor	Feeling of strange sensation in extremity; confusion; amnesia; temporary unconsciousness, deafness, or blindness; tympanic membrane rupture	Scene safety; ABCDEs; medical history and secondary assessment; monitor ECG; give oxygen and transport all patients with mild injuries.
Moderate	Disorientation, combativeness, paralysis, fractures, blunt trauma, absent pulses in lower extremities, spinal shock, seizures, temporary cardiorespiratory arrest, comatose	Scene safety; ABCDEs; medical history and secondary assessment; monitor ECG; CPR (CAB) early when needed; give oxygen and transport all patients.
Severe	Any of the above, otorrhea (fluid leak) in ear canal, cardiac fibrillation or cardiac asystole	CPR (CAB) and advanced lifesaving procedures; use "reverse" triage with multiple patients.

Note: ABCDE, airway, breathing, circulation, disability, expose/environment; CAB, circulation, airway, breathing; CPR, cardiopulmonary resuscitation; ECG, electrocardiogram.
Source: Data from O'Keefe GM, Zane RD: Lightning injuries. Emerg Med Clin North Am 22:369, 2004; and Cooper MA, Holle RL, Andrews CJ, Blumenthal R: Lightning injuries. In Auerbach PS: Wilderness medicine, ed 6, St. Louis, 2012, Mosby Elsevier.

return to normal sinus rhythm.[12] Because immediate cardio-pulmonary arrest is the greatest threat, prehospital care providers need to assess the CABs (circulation, airway, breathing) quickly in all lightning-strike victims and continuously monitor the electrocardiogram (ECG) for secondary cardiac events.

Severe Injury

The mechanism for sudden death from lightning strike is simultaneous cardiac and respiratory arrest. Victims with severe injury from a direct lightning strike (cardiovascular or neurologic injuries) or delays in cardiopulmonary resuscitation (CPR) have a poor prognosis. On arrival at the scene, the prehospital care provider may find the patient in cardiac arrest with asystole or ventricular fibrillation. Lightning causes a massive DC countershock, which simultaneously depolarizes the entire myocardium.[16] The American Heart Association (AHA) recommends vigorous resuscitation measures for those who appear dead on initial evaluation. This is based on many reports of excellent recovery after lightning-induced cardiac arrest and on the fact that victims in this category are typically young and without heart disease.[15]

It is not uncommon to observe the initial cardiac arrest with spontaneous recovery of electrical activity following the lightning strike, but any ongoing respiratory arrest due to a paralyzed medullary respiratory center may cause secondary hypoxic cardiac arrest.[15,19] If prolonged cardiac and neurologic ischemia has occurred, it may be very difficult to resuscitate these patients.[10] Other common findings are tympanic membrane rupture with cerebrospinal fluid and blood in the ear canal, ocular injuries, and various forms of blunt trauma from falls, including soft-tissue contusions and fractures of the skull, ribs, extremities, and spine. Many patients in this category have no evidence of burns. In those patients presenting with cutaneous burns caused by lightning, it is generally reported to be less than 20% total body surface area.

Injury to the central nervous system (CNS) is common in a lightning victim and has been classified into four groups of CNS injuries[12]:

- Group 1 CNS effects (Immediate and Transient): Loss of consciousness (75%); paresthesias (80%); weakness (80%); confusion, amnesia, and headaches
- *Group 2 CNS effects* (immediate and prolonged): Hypoxic ischemic neuropathy; intracranial hemorrhage; postarrest cerebral infarction
- *Group 3 CNS effects* (possible delayed neurologic syndromes): Motor neuron diseases and movement disorders
- *Group 4 CNS effects* (trauma from fall or blast): Subdural and epidural hematomas and subarachnoid hemorrhage

Assessment

On arrival at the scene, as with any other call, the priority is the safety of the prehospital care providers and other public safety personnel. Emergency responders must determine whether there is still a chance of lightning in the area. As a storm approaches or has passed, there still is a source of danger that is not always apparent since lightning remains a very real threat as far as 10 miles away—hence its nickname, the "bolt from the blue."[12]

The mechanism of injury may be unclear without a witness because lightning can strike during a sunny day. When in doubt about the mechanism of injury, immediately assess for ABCDEs (airway, breathing, circulation, disability, expose/environment) and any life-threatening conditions, as for any emergency. These patients do not carry an electrical charge and touching them poses no risk in providing patient care. Assess the victim's heart rhythm with the ECG. It is common to see nonspecific ST-segment and T-wave changes such as QT interval prolongation and transient T-wave inversions, but more specific evidence of myocardial infarction with Q-wave or ST-segment elevation is rarely seen.[20]

Once the patient is stable, a detailed head-to-toe assessment is necessary to identify the wide range of injuries that can occur with this type of trauma. Assess the patient's situational awareness and the neurologic function of all extremities because the upper and lower extremities may experience transient paralysis (known as *keraunoparalysis*). Lightning victims are known to have an autonomic dysfunction causing dilated pupils, which will mimic head trauma.[19] Assess the eyes because 55% of victims have some form of ocular injury. Look for blood and cerebrospinal fluid in the ear canals; 50% of these victims will have one or two ruptured tympanic membranes. All victims of lightning injury have a high probability of blunt trauma from being thrown against a solid object or being struck by falling objects. Cervical spine precautions are needed during the assessment to minimize further injury.

Assess the skin for signs of any burns, ranging from superficial to full thickness. Lightning burns may or may not be apparent in the field since they develop within the first few hours. Burns occur in less the one-half of lightning survivors and in most cases are superficial.[11,12] It is common to see a feathering appearance in the skin, known as **Lichtenberg's figures**, but these patterns are not burns and resolve in 24 hours (**Figure 22-6**). It is more common to see burns secondary to igniting of clothes and heating of jewelry or other objects.

If the incident involves multiple victims, the principles of triage should be implemented immediately. The normal rules of triage are to focus limited personnel and resources on patients with moderate and severe injuries and quickly bypass those patients without respiration and circulation. However, with multiple lightning-strike patients, the rule changes to use "reverse" triage and "resuscitate the dead," because these patients are either in respiratory arrest or cardiac arrest and have a high probability of recovery if managed expeditiously.[12,21] In contrast,

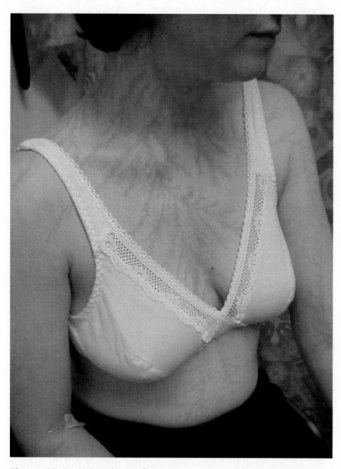

Figure 22-6 Lichtenberg's figures.

Source: © British Association of Plastic, Reconstructive and Aesthetic Surgeons.

other patients who have survived a lightning strike have little likelihood of deteriorating, unless there is associated trauma and occult hemorrhage.

Management

The priorities for managing a lightning victim are to ensure scene safety for yourself and your crew and to assess any victim for CAB. If spontaneous respiration or circulation is absent, initiate effective CPR up to five cycles (2 minutes), and evaluate the heart rhythm with an automated external defibrillator (AED) or cardiac monitor based on current guidelines.[15] Use ALS measures to manage lightning-induced cardiopulmonary arrest based on current AHA guidelines for advanced cardiovascular life support (ACLS) and pediatric advanced life support (PALS), as discussed elsewhere.[15] Evaluate and treat for shock and hypothermia. Apply high-flow oxygen for all moderately and severely injured patients. Intravenous fluids should be started at a keep-vein-open (KVO) rate since patients who have been injured by lightning, unlike conventional high-voltage electrical-injured patients, do not have massive tissue destruction and burns requiring a larger amount of fluids. Patients who show unstable vital signs or who have sustained associated trauma may have their fluids titrated as appropriate.

Stabilize any fractures, and package the blunt trauma patient for cervical spine immobilization. Lightning-strike victims with minor to severe injuries need to be transported to an emergency department (ED) for further evaluation and observation. Transport the patient by either ground or air, as determined by availability, distance, and time to the hospital and overall risk to the flight crew and benefit to patient.

As mentioned previously, lightning-strike victims have a higher probability of a positive outcome from early and effective resuscitation. However, there is little evidence to suggest that these patients can regain a pulse from prolonged basic life support (BLS) or advanced life support (ALS) procedures lasting longer than 20 to 30 minutes.[2] Before terminating resuscitation, all efforts should be made to stabilize the patient by establishing an airway, supporting ventilation, and correcting any hypovolemia, hypothermia, and acidosis.

Prevention

With numerous thunderstorms throughout the year, lightning ground strikes are common. Both prehospital care providers and the general public must be educated about prevention and the many lightning myths and misconceptions (**Figure 22-7**). Numerous lightning-prevention resources are provided by such agencies as the National Weather Service/NOAA, National Lightning Safety Institute, American Red Cross, and Federal Emergency Management Agency.[22-24]

Official guidelines are published for lightning-injury prevention and treatment by both national and international medical commissions and organizations, including the Wilderness Medical Society, the AHA, and the International Commission for Mountain Emergency Medicine and Medical Commission of the International Mountaineering and Climbing Federation (**Figure 22-8**).[11,15,25]

Prehospital care providers and other public safety personnel should establish procedures for a severe weather watch that provides storm warnings updated throughout the day as one method of safety prevention. There is no place that is 100% safe outdoors. The ambulance is the safest shelter if the prehospital care providers are near it when no large building is available.

One public education motto used is, "If you see it, flee it; if you hear it, clear it." Another useful rule is the "30–30 rule." When the time between seeing lightning and hearing thunder is 30 seconds or less, individuals are in danger and need to seek appropriate shelter. Following this rule, it is recommended to resume outdoor activity only after 30 minutes following the last lightning or thunder, because a passing thunderstorm still is a threat and lightning can strike up to 10 miles after the storm passes.[26,27] Another measure of lightning proximity is the "flash-to-bang" rule, which states that 5 seconds = 1 mile; that is, following lightning, for every 5 seconds until the sound of thunder, the lightning is 1 mile away.

For more information about preventing lightning strike, see **Figure 22-9**. See **Figure 22-10** for information about support for lightning strike survivors.

Figure 22-7 Myths and Misconceptions About Lightning

General Myths

All of the following common beliefs about lightning are false:

- Lightning strikes are invariably fatal.
- A major cause of death is burns.
- A victim struck by lightning bursts into flames or is reduced to ashes.
- Victims remain charged or electrified after they are struck.
- Individuals are only at risk for being struck when there are storm clouds overhead.
- Occupying a building during the storm affords 100% protection from lightning.
- Lightning never strikes the same place twice.
- Wearing rubber-soled shoes and a raincoat will protect a person.
- Rubber tires in a vehicle are what protect a person from injury.
- Wearing metal jewelry increases the risk of attracting lightning.
- Lightning always hits the highest object.
- There is no danger from lightning unless it is raining.
- Lightning can occur without thunder.

Misconceptions Regarding Patient Care

Some myths and misconceptions held by prehospital care providers can adversely affect the care and outcome of their patients.

- If the victim is not killed by lightning, he or she will be okay.
- If the victim has no outward signs of injury, the damage cannot be that serious.
- Lightning injuries should be treated similar to other high-voltage electrical injuries.
- Lightning victims who undergo resuscitation efforts for several hours might still recover successfully.

Source: Modified from O'Keefe GM, Zane RD: Lightning injuries. Emerg Med Clin North Am 22:369, 2004; and Cooper MA, Andrews CJ, Holle RL, Lopez RE: Lightning injuries. In Auerbach PS: *Wilderness medicine*, ed 5, St. Louis, 2007, Mosby Elsevier.

Figure 22-8 Prevention Guidelines for Prehospital Care Providers in Mountainous Regions

Prehospital care providers servicing mountainous regions are at greater risk for lightning strike, especially those who serve as park rangers, search and rescue members, and other public safety personnel in high-altitude and remote areas. Some general prevention guidelines for these prehospital care providers include the following:

- Take note of the weather forecast since thunder and lightning in the mountains occur mainly during summer months in the late afternoons and night. Thus, the saying, "Up by noon and down by 2:00 p.m." is used to remind individuals to return to lower elevations by the middle to late afternoon to decrease the risk for lightning strike.
- The best place to get out of a lightning storm in the mountains is a hut or mountain refuge. Stay away from open doors and windows.
- Tents do not provide any protection from lightning strike, and tent poles may act as lightning rods.
- Larger caves and valleys are protective, but small caves provide little protection if the person is near the opening and sidewalls.
- Wet stream beds are more dangerous than open areas.
- Stay off mountain ridges and summits, power lines, and ski lifts.
- Stay clear of the base of taller trees since lightning will travel down the trunk to the base. In a forest, it is best to get into a cluster of smaller trees.
- If caught in the open, do not sit or lie flat. It is best to crouch down with feet or knees together and keep contact with as small an area of the ground as possible to minimize injury from ground current. Prehospital care providers should try to use some insulation between themselves and the ground, such as a dry pack on which to kneel or sit.
- If in a group, stay apart from each other, but within sight, to reduce the number of people injured by ground current or side flashes between persons.
- Consider the use of small, portable lightning detectors so that advance warning is received and prevention steps can be implemented before the storm arrives.

Drowning

Drowning incidents that lead to injury are all too common in the United States, accounting for approximately 3,880 deaths annually. It is the third leading cause of unintentional death worldwide.[28] Drowning remains a leading cause of preventable death across all age groups, but is an epidemic in children.[28-31] The World Health Organization estimates that there are approximately 400,000 deaths annually from unintentional submersion incidents, not including deaths from drowning resulting from floods, suicide, or homicide.[32] Submersion injuries have a substantial cost to society; an estimated $3.25 billion

Figure 22-9 Lightning Safety Guidelines

The following are guidelines for lightning safety as a storm develops:

- Find a lightning-safe vehicle or a lightning-safe structure.[22,26]
  - An automobile that is a fully enclosed metal vehicle is a lightning-safe shelter. Other all-metal mobile transportation-related vehicles such as airplanes, buses, vans, and construction equipment with enclosed mostly metal cabs are also safe. A cautionary note, however, will emphasize that the "outer metal shield" of a vehicle should not be compromised. This means:
    - Windows need to be rolled up.
    - Contact must not be made with any interior objects such as radio dials, metal door handles, two-way radio microphones, etc., that connect with external objects.
  - All other objects that penetrate from inside to outside should be avoided.
  - Unsafe vehicles include those made of fiberglass and other plastics, plus small riding machinery or vehicles without enclosed canopies, such as motorcycles, farm tractors, golf cars, and all-terrain vehicles.
  - Metal buildings are lightning-safe places. So, too, are large permanent structures made of masonry and wood. Once again, the caveat is to not become part of the pathway conducting lightning. This means avoiding all electrical circuits, switches, powered equipment, metal doors and windows, hand rails, and so on. Small post-supported structures, such as bus stops, picnic shelters, or baseball field dugouts are not safe.

The following are guidelines for lightning safety when indoors:

- Seek a building and stay away from windows, open doors, fireplaces, bath and shower, and metal objects such as sinks and appliances.
- Turn off the radio and computer and avoid hardwired telephones; use a telephone only in an emergency.
- Turn off all faucets, electrical appliances, and devices before a storm arrives.

The following are guidelines for lightning safety when outdoors:

- Avoid using handheld radios, cell phones, or other electronic signal/communication devices if possible.
- Avoid metal objects such as bikes, tractors, and fences.
- Avoid tall objects such as trees, and make yourself small.
- Avoid areas near pipelines, power lines, and ski lifts.
- Avoid open fields.
- Avoid open shelters (e.g., carport, bus shelter), depending on overall size, because side flashes or ground strikes can occur.
- Drop ski poles and golf clubs, which may attract lightning.
- In large public outdoor events, seek out nearby buses or minivans.
- Seek to make the smallest contact with ground, if possible, to minimize ground contact. In the "lightning position", the individual squats with the feet together, hands covering the ears; a ground pad, backpack, or some insulation material is placed under the feet. An alternative position of comfort is to kneel or sit cross-legged.
- Do not stand, hug, squat, or huddle near tall trees; seek out a low area of lower trees or saplings.
- Seek out ditches unless there is contact with water.
- If on water, seek shore immediately and move inland, away from the water. Avoid swimming, boating, or being near the tallest object on water.[1,10]

Figure 22-10 Survivors of Lightning Injury

Support for survivors of lightning injury is available from Lightning Strike & Electric Shock Survivors International, Inc. (LS&ESSI, Inc.). This nonprofit support group is comprised of survivors, their families, and other interested parties. There are members throughout the United States and in more than 13 other countries (http://www.lightning-strike.org/).

or more is spent on these patients each year in the United States alone.[33]

The terminology describing these patients continues to evolve. Thirty-five years ago, *drowning* was defined as the process by which air-breathing mammals succumb on submersion in a liquid, and *near-drowning* was defined as submersion with at least temporary survival.[34] The term *secondary drowning* was used to describe patients who recovered initially from a submersion injury, but then died from respiratory failure secondary to submersion.[35,36] However, this latter term has come under question lately, and some suggest that it should not be used.[35] Any submersion or immersion incident without evidence of respiratory impairment should be considered a water rescue and not a drowning. Older and more archaic terms such as near-drowning, dry drowning, wet drowning, secondary drowning, and passive drowning have all been abandoned.

The more accepted definitions adopted by the World Health Organization are[37]:

- **Drowning**: The process of experiencing respiratory impairment from submersion/immersion in liquid. The victim may live or die after this process, but it is known as a drowning incident. The drowning process begins with respiratory impairment as the person's airway goes below the surface of the water or that water splashes over the face.[38]
- **Submersion**: The entire body, including the airway, has gone under water.
- **Immersion**: Water has splashed or washed over the face and airway and allows for drowning to occur by aspiration.

Epidemiology

Death by unintentional drowning is the seventh leading cause of death for all ages, the leading cause of death for ages 1 to 4 years, the second leading cause of death for ages 4 to 14 years, and the third leading cause of death of infants (less than 1 year of age).[29] Infants are at risk from drowning in bathtubs, buckets, and toilets.[39] The incidence of submersion incident may be 500 to 600 times the rate of drowning.[40] The Centers for Disease Control and Prevention (CDC) reported that from 2005 to 2009 there were an average of 3,880 cases of unintentional fatal drowning in the United States each year, and an estimated 5,789 cases were treated in U.S. hospital EDs each year for nonfatal drowning (**Figure 22-11**).[29,30] An additional 347 people died each year from drowning in boating-related incidents.[29]

For every child who drowned, three others survived and required emergency care for their submersion incident. Each week, approximately 40 children die from drowning, 115 are hospitalized, and 12 have irreversible brain injury.[31]

The CDC reported an average of 9,669 submersion casualties (fatal and nonfatal) annually from 2005 to 2009.[29] Of these, fatal incidents occurred in bathtubs (10%), pools (18%), and natural water settings such as lakes, rivers, and oceans (51%). In comparison, unintentional nonfatal submersion incidents treated in EDs in the United States were highest for pools (58%), with natural water settings accounting for 25% and bathtubs 10%.

Figure 22-11 Unintentional Drowning—United States, 2005–2009

Characteristic	Nonfatal*	Fatal*
Age (in years)		
Newborn to 4	3057	513
5 to 14	1012	252
≥ 15	1718	3107
Unknown	2	9
Gender		
Male	3486	3057
Female	2301	823
Location		
Bathtub	534	403
Pool	3341	683
Natural water (ocean, lakes, rivers)	1460	1982
Other	484	813
Disposition		
Treated/released	2540	—
Hospitalized	2908	—
Other	340	—
Total	5789	3880

*Estimated number.
Source: Data from Centers for Disease Control and Prevention: Annual average Nonfatal and fatal drownings in recreational water settings—United States, 2005–2009. *MMWR* 61(19):345, 2012.

The nonfatal and fatal injury rates were the highest for children 4 years of age or younger and for males of all ages. The nonfatal rate for males was almost twice that of females, whereas the fatal rate for males was almost four times that of females.

Submersion Factors

Specific factors place individuals at an increased risk for submersion incidents.[34,35,39,41,42] Recognizing these factors will increase awareness and assist in the creation of preventive strategies and policies to minimize these occurrences. For infants and young children, the major risk factor is inadequate supervision, and for adolescents and adults, it is risky behavior and use of drugs or alcohol.[39]

Submersion factors include the following:

- *Ability to swim.* Swimming ability is not consistently related to drowning. White males have a higher incidence of drowning than white females, even though they are reported to have better swimming ability.[34] One study reported that nonswimmers or beginners accounted for 73% of drownings in home swimming pools and 82% of incidents in canals, lakes, and ponds.[43]

- *Shallow-water blackout.* In an effort to increase their underwater swim distance, some swimmers will intentionally hyperventilate immediately before going underwater. They do this in an effort to lower the partial pressure of arterial carbon dioxide ($PaCO_2$). Since the body's carbon dioxide level provides the stimulus to breathe in patients without chronic obstructive pulmonary disease,[44] a decrease in $PaCO_2$ decreases the feedback to the respiratory center in the hypothalamus to take a breath during breath holding. However, these swimmers are at risk of a submersion incident because the partial pressure of arterial oxygen (PaO_2) does not change significantly with hyperventilation. As the individual continues to swim underwater, PaO_2 will decrease significantly and cause a possible loss of consciousness and cerebral hypoxia.

- *Accidental cold-water immersion.* Another situation that places individuals at greater risk of drowning is cold-water immersion (*head out*). The physiologic changes that occur with cold-water immersion can have either a disastrous outcome or a protective effect on the body, depending on many circumstances. Adverse outcomes are more common, resulting from both cardiovascular collapse and sudden death within minutes of cold-water immersion (see the Environmental Trauma I: Heat and Cold chapter for more information).

- *Age.* Drowning is recognized as a young person's accident, with toddlers as the largest group, based on their inquisitive nature and a lack of parental supervision. Children under 1 year of age have the highest drowning rate.[29,45]

- *Gender.* Males account for more than half of submersion victims, with two age-related peak incidences. The first peak incidence occurs in males at age 2 years, decreases until age 10 years, and then rises rapidly to peak again at age 18 years. Older males may be more at

risk for drowning because of higher exposure rates to aquatic activities, higher alcohol consumption while at the waterfront, and more risk-taking behavior.[34,46]

- *Race.* Due to the history of segregation in the United States, many older African Americans were denied access to pools and swimming lessons. If a grandparent or parent does not swim, swimming lessons for children may become a lower priority for the family. Today, African American children experience more submersion incidents than white children. African American children tend to drown in ponds, lakes, and other natural sources of water.[28] The drowning rate of African American male children has been estimated to be as high as three times that of white males.[47]

- *Location.* Submersion incidents typically occur in backyard swimming pools and in the ocean, but also occur in buckets.[35] Houses in rural areas with open wells increase the risk of a young child drowning by sevenfold.[34] Other hazardous locations are water barrels, fountains, and underground cisterns.

- *Alcohol and drugs.* Alcohol is the primary drug associated with submersion incidents,[48,49] most likely because it causes a loss of sound judgment.[46] As many as 20% to 30% of adult boating fatalities and submersion incidents involve alcohol use in which the occupants used poor judgment, were speeding, failed to wear life jackets, or handled the watercraft recklessly.[34,50]

- *Underlying disease or trauma.* The onset of illness from underlying disease can account for submersion victims. Hypoglycemia, myocardial infarction, cardiac dysrhythmia, depression and suicidal thoughts, and syncope predispose individuals to drowning incidents.[39] A recent study reported that the risk of drowning in people with epilepsy is raised 15- to 19-fold compared to people in the general population.[51] Cervical spine injuries and head trauma should be suspected in all unwitnessed incidents and injuries involving body surfers, board surfers, and victims diving in shallow water or water with submerged objects such as rocks or trees (**Figures 22-12** and **22-13**).

- *Child abuse.* A high incidence of child abuse from submersion incidents is reported, particularly in bathtubs. A study of children sustaining bathtub submersion between 1982 and 1992 found that 67% had historical or physical findings compatible with a diagnosis of abuse or neglect.[42] Consequently, it is highly recommended that any suspicious child-submersion bathtub incident be reported to local social services for appropriate investigation.

- *Hypothermia.* Drowning may result directly from prolonged immersion leading to hypothermia. (See the Cold-Related Disorders sections in the Environmental Trauma I: Heat and Cold chapter for further discussion of accidental hypothermia.) Hypothermia is defined as a core (central) body temperature less than 96.8°F (36°C). Immersion into water allows for rapid loss of body heat into the usually cooler water, thus precipitating hypothermia.

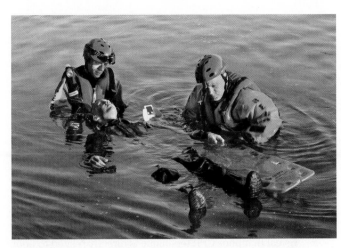

Figure 22-12 Spine board immobilization in water. First the prehospital care providers bring a spine board to place underneath the patient.
Source: Courtesy of Rick Brady.

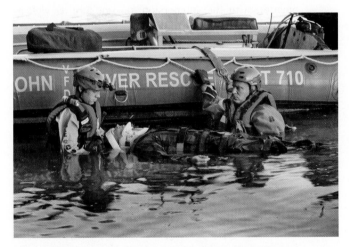

Figure 22-13 Spine board immobilization in water. A cervical collar is placed on the patient to assist in spinal immobilization.
Source: Courtesy of Rick Brady.

Mechanism of Injury

A common scenario of *head-out immersion* in water or a whole-body submersion incident begins with a situation that creates a panic response, leading to breath holding, air hunger, and increased physical activity in effort to stay or get above the water surface. According to most bystander reports, submersion victims are rarely seen screaming and waving for assistance while struggling to stay above the surface of the water. Rather, they are seen either floating on the surface or in a motionless position, or they dive underwater and fail to come up. As the submersion incident continues, a reflex inspiratory effort draws water into the pharynx and larynx, causing a choking response and laryngospasm. The onset of laryngospasm represents the first step in suffocation and brain hypoxia, which in turn causes the victim to lose consciousness and submerge underwater even further.[38]

Over the years, controversies have surrounded the pathophysiology of drowning, mostly about the differences between drowning in freshwater versus saltwater and whether water entered or did not enter the lungs.[35,37,39] Approximately 15% of drownings are termed *dry drowning* because the severe laryngospasm prevents the aspiration of fluid into the lungs. The remaining 85% of submersion incidents are considered *wet drownings*, in which the laryngospasm relaxes, the glottis opens, and the victim aspirates water into the lungs.[52]

Theoretically, there are different effects on the pulmonary system when freshwater (hypotonic) versus saltwater (hypertonic) enters the lung. In freshwater drowning, the hypotonic fluid enters the lung and then moves across the alveolus into the intravascular space, causing a volume overload and dilutional effect on serum electrolytes and other serum components. Conversely, in saltwater aspiration, the hypertonic fluid enters the lung, which in turn causes additional fluid from the intravascular space to enter the lung across the alveolus, causing pulmonary edema and hypertonicity of serum electrolytes.

It has since been shown that no real differences exist between wet and dry drowning and freshwater and saltwater aspiration.[39,53,54] For prehospital care providers, the common denominator in any of these four submersion scenarios is brain hypoxia caused by either laryngospasm or water aspiration. The whole drowning process from immersion or submersion to hypoxemia, apnea, loss of consciousness that leads to cardiac arrest, pulseless electrical activity, and asystole usually occurs in seconds to a few minutes.[38] For those victims who survive, the scene management should be aimed at quickly reversing hypoxia in these patients, thereby preventing cardiac arrest.

Surviving Cold-Water Submersion

There are four phases that describe the body's responses and mechanisms of death during cold-water immersion. These phases correlate to the 1-10-1 principle[55]:

1. *Initial immersion and the cold shock response.* The victim has 1 minute to get his or her breathing under control.
2. *Short-term immersion and the loss of performance.* The victim has 10 minutes of meaningful movement to get out of the water.
3. *Long-term immersion and the onset of hypothermia.* The victim has up to 1 hour until he or she become unconscious from hypothermia.
4. *Circum-rescue collapse just before, during, or after rescue.* If the victim survives the first three phases, up to 20% may experience this type of collapse during rescue.

In each of these phases, there is wide individual variation due to body size, water temperature, and amount of the body that is immersed. Each phase is accompanied by specific survival hazards for the immersion victim that originate from or are influenced by a variety of pathophysiologic mechanisms. Deaths have occurred during all four phases of immersion.

In rare cases of prolonged submersion—one case for as long as 66 minutes—patients have presented to the hospital with severe hypothermia and recovered with either partial or full neurologic function.[56,57] In these submersion incidents, the lowest recorded core temperature of a survivor is 56.6°F (13.7°C) in an adult female.[58] In another case, a child survived fully intact after submersion in ice water for 40 minutes, with a core temperature of 75°F (23.9°C). After 1 hour of resuscitation, spontaneous circulation returned.[59]

No explanation exists for such cases, but hypothermia is thought to be protective. Immersion in cold water may lead to hypothermia within an hour depending on many factors, as listed below, because of increased surface heat loss and core cooling. In addition, swallowing or aspiration of cold water may contribute to rapid cooling. Rapid onset of hypothermia during freshwater drowning may result from core cooling caused by pulmonary aspiration and rapid absorption of cold water and subsequent brain cooling.

Another factor that may explain why some young children survive is the mammalian diving reflex. The **mammalian diving reflex** slows heart rate, shunts blood to the brain, and closes the airway. Recent evidence suggests that the diving reflex present in various mammals is active in only 15% to 30% of human subjects, so while it cannot be considered the lone explanation of why some children survive, it still may explain part of this phenomenon.[34]

Every submersion patient should have full resuscitation efforts made, regardless of the presence or absence of any of these factors. The following factors appear to influence the outcome of a cold-water submersion patient.

- *Age.* Many successful infant and child resuscitations have been well documented in the United States and Europe. The smaller mass of a child's body cools faster than an adult's body, thus permitting fewer harmful by-products of anaerobic metabolism to form and causing less irreversible damage (see the Physiology of Life and Death chapter).
- *Submersion time.* The shorter the duration of submersion, the lower the risk for cellular damage caused by hypoxia. Accurate information concerning submersion time needs to be obtained. Submersion longer than 66 minutes is probably fatal. Therefore, a reasonable approach to resuscitation of a submersion victim is that efforts should be initiated if the duration of submersion is less than 1 hour.
- *Water temperature.* Water temperatures of 70°F (21.1°C) and below are capable of inducing hypothermia. The colder the water, the better the chance of survival, probably because of the rapid decrease in brain temperature and metabolism when the body is quickly chilled.
- *Struggle.* Submersion victims who struggle less have a better chance of resuscitation (unless their struggling efforts are successful in avoiding drowning). Less struggling means less hormonal release (e.g., epinephrine) and less muscle activity; this translates to less heat (energy) production and less vasodilatation.

These factors in turn cause decreased muscular oxygen demand, which results in smaller muscle oxygen deficit, and less carbon dioxide and lactic acid production. Thus, the rate of cooling of the patient is increased, which may improve resuscitation chances.
- *Cleanliness of water.* Patients generally do better after resuscitation if they were submerged in clean rather than muddy or contaminated water.
- *Quality of CPR and resuscitative efforts.* Patients receiving adequate and effective CPR, combined with proper rewarming and ALS measures, generally do better than patients receiving one or more substandard measures. Immediate initiation of CPR is a key factor for submersion-hypothermia patients. Past and current studies reveal that poor CPR technique is directly related to poor resuscitation outcome.[60,61] See the current BLS guidelines as outlined in the AHA hypothermia algorithm in the Environmental Trauma I: Heat and Cold chapter.[62]
- *Associated injuries or illness.* Patients with an existing injury or illness, or who become ill or injured in combination with the submersion, do not fare as well as otherwise healthy individuals.

Water Rescue

Many water safety organizations recommend the use of highly skilled professionals who regularly train for water rescue, retrieval, and resuscitation. If no professional water rescue teams are available, however, prehospital care providers must consider their own safety and the safety of all emergency responders before attempting an in-water rescue. The following guidelines are recommended to safely rescue a victim out of the water:

- *Reach.* Attempt to perform the water rescue by reaching out with a pole, stick, paddle, or anything so that the rescuer stays on land or on a boat. Use caution to avoid being inadvertently pulled into the water.
- *Throw.* When reaching is not possible, throw something to a victim, such as a life preserver or rope so that it floats to the victim.
- *Tow.* Once the victim has a rescue line, tow the victim to safety.
- *Row.* If water entry is necessary, it is preferable to use a boat or paddleboard to reach the victim and wear a personal flotation device if entering the water in a boat or to swim.[34]

Swimming rescues are not recommended unless the prehospital care provider has been trained appropriately to manage a victim who can rapidly turn violent from panic, creating a potential double drowning. Too many well-intentioned emergency responders have become additional victims because their own safety was not the priority. See **Figure 22-14** for a few options for in-water rescue systems, equipment for a submersion and/or trauma victim (C-spine precaution), and movement when in deep water.

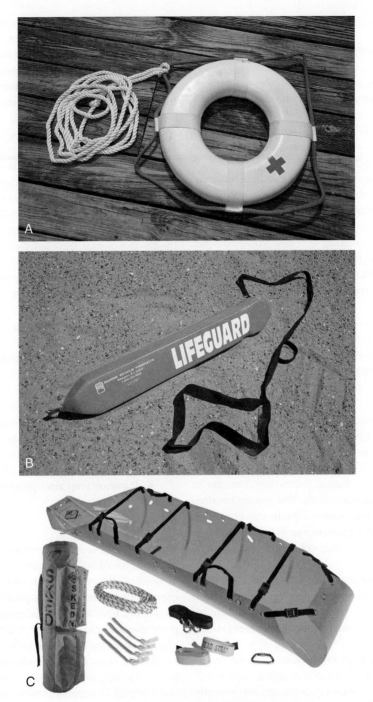

Figure 22-14 Options for in-water rescue equipment and patient packaging. **A.** Rescue throw lines. **B.** Tow device. **C.** In-water patient packing equipment.
Source: Courtesy of Rick Brady.

Predicators of Survival

The following are important facts and predicators of outcome in resuscitation of a person who has drowned.[38]

1. Early BLS and ALS are crucial.
2. During drowning, a reduction of brain temperature by 10°C (~18°F) decreases adenosine triphosphate (ATP) consumption by 50%, doubling the duration of time a brain can survive.
3. The greater the duration of submersion, the greater the risk of death or severe neurologic impairment after hospital discharge:
   - 0 to 5 minutes = 10%
   - 6 to 10 minutes = 56%
   - 11 to 25 minutes = 88%
   - Greater than 25 minutes = 100%
4. Signs of brain stem injury predict death or severe neurologic impairment and deficits.

Assessment

The initial priorities for any submersion patient include[34,38]:

1. Prevent injuries to the patient and emergency responders.
2. Initiate plans early for water extraction and rapid transport to the ED.
3. Conduct a safe water rescue (consider a possible diving-related cause and the need for spine immobilization).
4. Due to hypoxia, assess the ABCs (airway, breathing, circulation) using the traditional approach, not CAB (circulation, airway, breathing).
5. Reverse hypoxia and acidosis with five rescue breaths initially, followed by 30 chest compressions, and continue with two breaths thereafter (30:2). Watch for regurgitation, which is the most common complication during rescue breathing (65%) and during CPR (86%).
6. CPR with only chest compression is not advised in persons who have drowned.
7. Restore or maintain cardiovascular stability.
8. Prevent further loss of body heat and initiate rewarming efforts in hypothermic patients.

Initially, it is safest to presume that the submersion patient is hypoxic and hypothermic until proved otherwise. Consequently, all efforts should be made to establish effective respirations during water rescue since cardiac arrest from drowning is the result primarily of lack of oxygen. Submersion patients in respiratory arrest usually respond after a few rescue breaths. Attempts to provide chest compressions when in water too deep to stand are ineffective, so taking time to assess for the presence of a pulse is meaningless and will only delay getting the patient to land.

Remove the patient from the water safely. Once on land, the patient should be placed in a supine position with the trunk and head in the same position, which is usually parallel to the shore. Check for responsiveness and continue rescue breathing as needed.

If the patient is breathing, place the patient in the recovery position and monitor for effective respirations and pulse. Quickly assess the patient for any other life threats, and evaluate for head trauma and cervical spine injuries, particularly if there is suspicion of trauma associated with the submersion incident (e.g., falls, boat accidents, diving into water with underwater hazards). However, it has been shown that the typical submersion casualty has a low chance of traumatic injury, unless the victim dove into the water.[63]Acquire the vital signs, and assess all lung fields of submersion patients because they present with a wide range of pulmonary distress, including shortness of breath, rales, rhonchi, and wheezing. Submersion patients can present without symptoms initially and then deteriorate rapidly with signs of pulmonary edema.

Assess the patient's oxygen saturation with pulse oximetry and monitor the end-tidal carbon dioxide levels. Assess for cardiac rhythm disturbances, since submersion patients often have dysrhythmias secondary to hypoxia and hypothermia. Assess for altered mental status and neurologic function of all extremities because many submersion patients develop sustained neurologic damage. Determine the patient's blood glucose level, as hypoglycemia may have been the cause for the submersion incident. Acquire a baseline Glasgow Coma Scale (GCS) score and continue to assess for trends. Always suspect hypothermia and minimize further heat loss. Remove all wet clothing and assess rectal temperature (if the appropriate thermometers are available and the situation permits) to determine the level of hypothermia, and initiate steps to minimize further heat loss (see the Environmental Trauma I: Heat and Cold chapter for management of hypothermia).

The following variables are predictive of a more favorable outcome in submersion patients:

- Children age 3 years and older
- Female sex
- Water temperature less than 50°F (10°C)
- Duration of submersion less than 10 minutes
- No aspiration
- Time to effective BLS less than 10 minutes
- Rapid return of spontaneous cardiac output
- Spontaneous cardiac output on arrival in ED
- Core temperature less than 95°F (35°C)
- No coma on arrival and GCS score greater than 6
- Pupillary responses present

Management

Figure 22-15 presents a management tool for persons who have drowned based on a six-grade classification system and a guide of medical intervention for each grade.[38] A patient who has experienced some form of submersion incident, but who is not presenting with any signs or symptoms at the time of the primary assessment, still needs follow-up care in a hospital after assessment at the scene due to the potential for delayed onset of symptoms. Many asymptomatic patients (Grade 2) are released in 6 to 8 hours, depending on clinical findings in the hospital. In one study of 52 swimmers who experienced a submersion incident and were all initially asymptomatic immediately after the incident, 21 (40%) went on to develop shortness of breath and respiratory distress due to hypoxemia within 4 hours.[64] In general, all symptomatic patients are admitted to the hospital for at least 24 hours for supportive care and observation because the initial clinical assessment can be misleading. It is critical to obtain a good history of the incident detailing the estimate of submersion time and any past medical history.

All suspected submersion patients should receive high-flow oxygen (15 liters/minute) independent of their initial breathing status or oxygen saturation, based on the concern for delayed

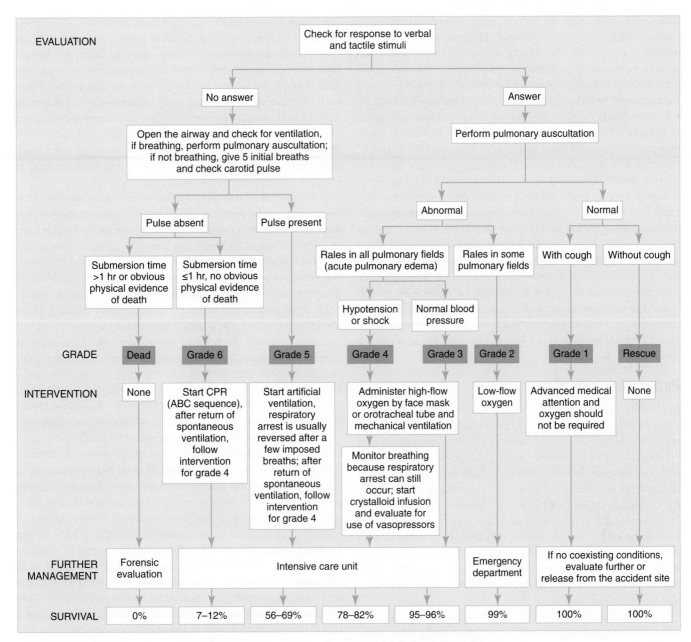

Figure 22-15 Drowning management system based on six classification grades for level of severity.

Source: From Ref. 9 Szpilman D, Bierens JLM, Handley A, Orlowshi JP. Drowning. *New Engl J Med* 366:2102–10;2012.

pulmonary distress, particularly if the patient develops shortness of breath. Monitor and maintain the patient's oxygen saturation greater than 90%. Apply and monitor the ECG, particularly for pulseless electrical activity or asystole. Obtain intravenous (IV) access and provide normal saline (NS) or lactated Ringer's (LR) solution at a KVO rate unless the patient is hypotensive, then provide a 500-milliliter (ml) fluid bolus and reassess vital signs.

Transport all submersion patients to the ED for evaluation. Because many submersion patients are asymptomatic, some may refuse transport because they have no immediate chief complaint. If so, take the time necessary to provide good patient education about the delayed signs and symptoms in a drowning incident,

explaining that many victims develop secondary complications from pulmonary injury. Firm and persistent persuasion is needed for them to agree to be transported or for them to report to the closest ED for further evaluation and observation. If the patient is adamant about refusing care, the patient must be informed of the potential ramifications of refusing care, and a signed refusal of care against medical advice must be obtained.

A symptomatic patient with a history of submersion who presents with signs of distress (e.g., anxiety, rapid respirations, difficulty breathing, coughing) is considered to have a submersion pulmonary injury until hospital evaluation has proved otherwise. Emphasis should be placed on correcting hypoxia, acidosis, and hypothermia. Provide cervical spine immobilization in all patients with suspicion of trauma. In unresponsive patients, use suction to clear the airway and keep the airway open with an airway adjunct. Hypoxia and acidosis can be corrected with effective ventilation support. Patients who are apneic should be supported with bag-mask ventilation. Intubation should be considered early to protect the airway in patients who are apneic or cyanotic or who have decreased mental status, since submersion patients swallow large amounts of water and are at risk of vomiting and aspirating stomach contents. Although the value of the Sellick maneuver (cricoid pressure) has been questioned, it may be applied during manual ventilation with a bag-mask and intubation in an effort to prevent or minimize regurgitation and aspiration in this group of patients who are at high risk. If ventilations are impaired, the amount of pressure applied should be modified to improve the ease of ventilation. Monitor the ECG for rate and rhythm disturbances and investigate for evidence of a cardiac event that might have preceded or followed the submersion incident. Provide 100% oxygen (15 liters/minute) with a nonrebreathing mask. Obtain IV access and provide NS or LR solution at a KVO rate. Provide transport to the local ED.

Patient Resuscitation

Rapid initiation of effective BLS and standard ALS procedures for submersion patients in cardiopulmonary arrest is associated with the best chance of survival.[35] Patients may present in asystole, pulseless electrical activity, or pulseless ventricular tachycardia/ventricular fibrillation. Follow the current version of the AHA guidelines for pediatric and adult ALS and ACLS for managing these rhythms.[62,65] As briefly presented in the Environmental Trauma I: Heat and Cold chapter, it is currently recommended to use therapeutic hypothermia in patients who remain in a coma from cardiac arrest caused by ventricular fibrillation; it might be equally effective for other causes of cardiac arrest, but it has not been proven beneficial to induce hypothermia for submersion patients.[65]

Routine stabilization of the cervical spine during in-water rescue is not necessary unless the reasons leading to the submersion indicate that trauma is likely (e.g., diving, use of water slide, signs of injury, alcohol use).[65] When these indicators are not present, spinal injury is unlikely. Routine cervical stabilization and other means to immobilize the spine during a water rescue can cause delays in opening the airway so that rescue breathing can begin.

The use of CPR during in-water rescue is not recommended for a number of reasons. Firstly, the depth of chest compressions is ineffective in water. Besides delaying effective CPR out of water, attempting to provide CPR in water puts rescuers at risk from fatigue, cold water, wave, surge, and current dangers. Place a greater emphasis on establishing an open airway and providing rescue breathing for patients who are apneic as soon as possible, depending on the patient's in-water position, number of rescuers, and rescue equipment (e.g., in-water backboard).

When a beach rescue (or any location) involves sloping terrain, it is no longer recommended to place a patient in a head-down (or head-up) position in an effort to drain the airway. Resuscitation efforts are shown to be more successful when the patient is placed supine on the ground, parallel to the water, with effective ventilation and chest compressions. Maintaining a level position on the ground will prevent a decrease in forward blood flow during chest compressions in the head-up position or an increase in intracranial pressure in the head-down position. Furthermore, no evidence suggests that lung drainage is effective with any particular maneuver.

The Heimlich maneuver has been previously suggested for use in submersion patients. However, the Heimlich maneuver is designed for airway obstruction and does not remove water from the airway or lungs. Rather, it may induce vomiting in submersion patients and place them at greater risk for aspiration. Currently, the AHA and the Institute of Medicine advise against the Heimlich maneuver except when the airway is blocked with foreign material.[66] If the patient recovers with spontaneous breathing, he or she should be placed in a lateral recumbent position with head slightly lower than the trunk to reduce the risk of aspiration if the patient vomits. (The Environmental Trauma I: Heat and Cold chapter outlines ALS procedures regarding resuscitation of a hypothermic patient. See Figure 21-29 of that chapter for the hypothermia algorithm. These guidelines are the same for all hypothermic patients regardless of the source of cold exposure.)

Use the regional EMS medical protocol for established guidelines that determine the criteria for an obviously dead individual. Acceptable guidelines for an obviously dead victim are a normal rectal temperature in a patient who presents with asystole, apnea, postmortem lividity, rigor mortis, or other injuries incompatible with life. A patient who has been recovered from warm water without vital signs or unsuccessful resuscitative efforts lasting 30 minutes may be considered dead on the scene.[34,67] Consult local medical control early for any individual recovered from cold-water submersion. As stated previously, many individuals have fully recovered from more than 60 minutes of cold-water submersion. These submersion patients should be managed as a hypothermic patient, based on the rectal temperature.

Prevention of Submersion-Related Injuries

Prevention strategies are vital in the effort to lower the rates of submersion incidents in the United States. It is estimated that 85% of all cases of drowning can be prevented by supervision, swimming instruction, technology regulations, and public education.[38] Many education programs are emphasizing the reduction of unintentional water entry of infants and children by encouraging the installation of various types of barriers around pools (e.g., isolation fences, pool covers, alarms) and the use of personal flotation devices such as life vests.[41] Furthermore, CPR initiated by a bystander before the arrival of prehospital care personnel is associated with improved patient prognosis.[40]

Figure 22-16 Submersion Patient: Summary of Assessment and Management

History	Examination	Intervention
Asymptomatic Patient		
Time submerged	Appearance	Administer oxygen by face mask at 8–10 liters/minute.
Description of incident	Vital signs	Initiate IV line at KVO rate.
Complaints	Head and neck trauma Chest examination: lung fields	Re-examine patient as needed.
Past medical history	ECG monitor	Transport patient to ED.
Symptomatic Patient		
Description of incident	General appearance	Administer oxygen by nonrebreathing mask at 12 to 15 liters/minute.
Time submerged, water temperature, water contamination, vomiting, type of rescue	Level of consciousness (AVPU)	Initiate IV line at KVO rate; intubate early as needed.
Symptoms	Vital signs; monitor ECG	Transport patient to ED.
On-scene field resuscitation	Assess ABCDEs; vital signs; AED or ECG monitor	Initiate CPR early; intubate; 100% oxygen at 12 to 15 liters/minute via bag-valve mask; consider NG tube for gastric distension; use ACLS procedures for VF and asystole; use ACLS hypothermia algorithm.

Note: ABCDEs, airway, breathing, circulation, disability, expose/environment; ACLS, advanced cardiovascular life support; AED, automated external defibrillator; AVPU, alert, responds to verbal stimulus, responds to painful stimulus, unresponsive; CPR, cardiopulmonary resuscitation; ECG, electrocardiogram; ED, emergency department; IV, intravenous; KVO, keep vein open; NG, nasogastric; VF, ventricular fibrillation.
Source: Modified from Schoene RB, Nachat A, Gravatt AR, Newman AB: Submersion incidents. In Auerbach PS: *Wilderness medicine*, ed 6, St. Louis, 2012, Mosby Elsevier.

Prehospital care providers have great opportunities to be advocates of water safety and education in their respective communities, with an emphasis on communication of the risk factor areas previously identified. Furthermore, prevention should be emphasized to prehospital care providers and other public safety personnel who arrive on the scene so that they do not become additional submersion victims. A panicked and struggling victim can be a danger to an unprepared in-water rescuer, potentially resulting in a double drowning. Prehospital care providers need to assess the problem quickly, control the scene to prevent bystanders from entering the water, and ensure their own safety.

Community education regarding submersion incidents should include the following recommendations:

- **Beaches**
  - Always swim near a lifeguard.
  - Ask a lifeguard about a safe place to swim.
  - Always swim with others.
  - Do not overestimate your swimming capability.
  - Always watch your children.
  - Swim away from piers, rocks, and stakes.
  - Avoid drinking alcohol and having a heavy meal before swimming.
  - Take lost children to the nearest lifeguard tower.
  - Be aware that 85% of ocean drownings occur in rip currents.
  - Know the weather conditions before going into water.
  - Never try to rescue someone without knowing what you are doing; many people have died in such attempts.
  - If you are fishing on rocks, be cautious with waves that may sweep you into the ocean.
  - Always enter shallow water feet first.

- Do not dive in shallow water; injury to the cervical spine could result.
- Keep away from marine animals.
- Read and heed signs and flags posted on the beach.
- **Residential pools and other water sources**
  - Adult supervision is necessary, closely observing all children.
  - Set rules for water safety.
  - Never leave a child alone near a pool or a source of water, such as a bathtub or bucket.
  - Install a four-sided fence that is at least 4 feet (1.2 meters [m]) tall around the pool with a self-closing and self-latching gate.
  - Do not allow children to use arm buoys or other air-filled swim aids.
  - Know how to use an approved life jacket.
  - Avoid toys that will attract children around pools.
  - Turn off pump filters when using pools.
  - Use cordless or cell phones near pool to prevent leaving the poolside to answer the telephone elsewhere.
  - Keep rescue equipment (e.g., shepherd's hook, life preserver) and a telephone by the pool.
  - Do not try or allow hyperventilation to increase underwater swim time.
  - Do not dive in shallow water.
  - Provide swimming lessons for all children by age 4 years.[68]
  - After the children have finished swimming, secure the pool so they cannot return (locks or audible alarms on gates are recommended).
  - All family members and others watching children should learn first aid and CPR.[12]

Recreational Scuba-Related Injuries

Recreational diving using **self-contained underwater breathing apparatus (scuba)** is a common activity enjoyed by many age groups. The popularity of this activity continues to grow, with more than 400,000 new certified divers each year, now totaling over five million scuba divers in the United States.[69,70] Relative to the increasing number of new divers each year, the injury rate is low, but the concern for medical fitness to dive has increased because of the diversity of divers, increasing age, low physical fitness, and underlying medical conditions. Water is an unforgiving environment when problems occur. Currently, there are medical guidelines that indicate relative and temporary health risks and absolute contraindications for scuba diving.[70-74]

Injuries to divers occur from many underwater hazards (e.g., shipwrecks, coral reefs) or from handling hazardous marine life. However, more often, prehospital care providers respond to scuba-related injuries and fatalities caused by **dysbarism**, or altered environmental pressure, which accounts for the majority of the serious diving medical disorders. The mechanism of injury is based on the principles of gas laws when breathing compressed gases (e.g., oxygen, carbon dioxide, nitrogen) at varying underwater depths and pressures, as will be described in detail in subsequent sections.

The associated causes for diving fatalities have not changed significantly in recent history. The most frequently cited problem is insufficient gas (air) or running out of gas. Other common factors included entrapment or entanglement, buoyancy control, equipment misuse or problems, rough water, and emergency ascent. The principal injuries or causes of death included drowning or asphyxia due to inhalation of water, air embolism, and cardiac events. Older divers were at greater risk of cardiac events, with men at higher risk than women, although the risks were equal at age 65.[75]

Most scuba-related injuries caused by dysbarism present with signs (e.g., ear squeeze on descent) and symptoms either immediately or within 60 minutes after surfacing, but some symptoms are delayed up to 48 hours after individuals depart the dive site and return home. Consequently, with the increasing number of scuba divers today flying to and from popular dive sites in the United States, Caribbean, and other remote locations, there is a greater possibility of responding to diving-related injuries at locations distant from the actual dive site. Prehospital care providers need to recognize these scuba-related disorders, provide initial treatment, and initiate plans early for transport to the local ED or for treatment at the closest recompression chamber.[73]

Epidemiology

Divers Alert Network (DAN) compiles an extensive morbidity and mortality database based on casualty data provided from participating recompression chambers in North America. In 2000, they published a report summarizing 11 years (1987 to 1997) of data.[75] They also publish annual reports, which can be found on their website.[76] The majority of scuba-related diving injuries occur in the United States and North America during the months of May to September, with August as the peak month. Europe comes in a distant second in reported deaths. Three to four times more male divers are injured than female divers. The primary cause of diving-related injury is decompression sickness. From 1970 to 2006, the number of diving-related deaths ranged from 66 to 147 per year.[75] In 2007, the most recent year for which data are available at the time of this publication, almost 85% of the deaths occurred in males, with most of the deaths in divers 40 to 59 years of age. The causes of death were drowning (86%), cardiovascular factors (9%), arterial gas embolism (3%), and decompression sickness (1%). Even though drowning was the leading cause of fatalities, it is unclear what led to the drowning, such as equipment issues, lack of air, entanglement, narcosis, panic, disorientation, hypothermia, heart attack, or arterial gas embolism.

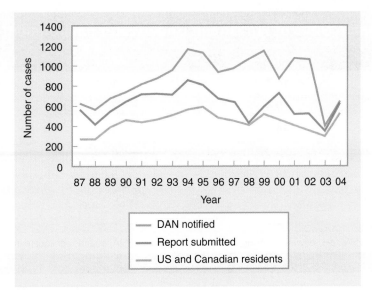

Figure 22-17 Annual diving injuries.

Source: Data courtesy of Divers Alert Network® (DAN®).

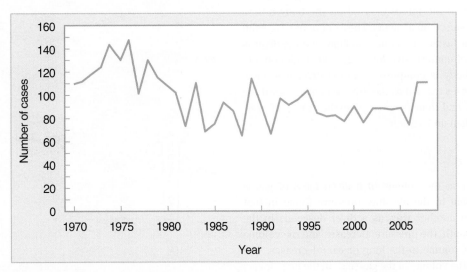

Figure 22-18 Annual number of U.S. and Canadian diving fatalities. The number of U.S. and Canadian fatalities recorded annually has varied substantially from year to year from 1970 to 2007.

Source: Data courtesy of Divers Alert Network® (DAN®).

Many drowning deaths during scuba diving are actually arterial gas embolism leading to secondary drowning.[75] See **Figures 22-17** and **22-18** for a summary of annual diving injuries and fatalities from the DAN 2008 annual report.[77]

Mechanical Effects of Pressure

Scuba-related diving injuries incurred by the changing atmospheric pressure, or dysbarism, can be separated into two types: (1) the conditions when a change in pressure from the underwater environment results in tissue trauma or barotrauma in closed air spaces in the body (e.g., ears, sinuses, intestines, lungs) and (2) the problems that occur from breathing compressed gases at elevated partial pressure, such as decompression sickness.

Barotrauma associated with scuba diving relates directly to the pressure effects of air and water on the diver. When standing at sea level, the atmospheric pressure is 760 torr, which is essentially the same as 760 millimeters of mercury [mm Hg]) or 14.7 pounds per square inch (psi) on the body. This amount of pressure is also known as 1 atmosphere (1 atm). As a diver descends deeper in water, the absolute pressure increases 1 atm for every 33 feet (10 m) of seawater. Consequently, a depth of 33 feet of seawater is equivalent to 2 atm (air [1 atm] and 33 feet of water [1 atm]) of pressure on

Figure 22-19   Common Units of Pressure in Underwater Environment

Depth (FSW)	PSIA	ATA	Torr or mm Hg (absolute)
Sea level	14.7	1	760
33	29.4	2	1520
66	44.1	3	2280
99	58.8	4	3040
132	73.5	5	3800
165	88.2	6	4560
198	102.9	7	5320

Note: ATA, atmosphere absolute; FSW, feet seawater; mm Hg, millimeters of mercury; PSIA, pounds per square inch absolute.

the body. **Figure 22-19** lists common units of pressure in the underwater environment.

When a diver descends under the increasing pressure of seawater, the effect of the forces exerted on the body differs depending on the tissue compartments. The force applied to solid tissue acts in similar fashion to a fluid medium, and the diver is generally unaware of compressive force. The air in air-containing spaces of the body is compressed as the diver descends. Conversely, these gases expand as the diver ascends toward the surface. Boyle's law and Henry's law explain the effects of pressure on the body when underwater.

Boyle's Law

Boyle's law states that the volume of a given mass of gas is inversely proportional to the absolute pressure found in that environment. Stated another way, as a diver descends in the water to a greater depth, the pressure increases and the volume of the gas (e.g., the volume in the lung or ear) decreases. The reverse is also true, the volume of the gas (e.g., in the lung or ear) increases in size when the diver returns toward the surface. This is the principle behind the effects of barotrauma and arterial gas embolism in the body. **Figure 22-20** shows the effects of pressure on the volume and diameter of a gas bubble.

Henry's Law

At a constant temperature, the amount of gas that will dissolve in a liquid is directly proportional to the partial pressure of that gas outside the liquid. Henry's law is fundamental in the understanding of how gas from a compressed air cylinder (scuba tank) behaves in the body as the diver descends in the water. For example, the increasing partial pressure of nitrogen will cause it to dissolve in the fluids of the body's tissues as the pressure increases during descent. On return toward the surface, nitrogen will bubble out of the fluid solution in the tissues. Henry's law describes the principle that explains why decompression sickness occurs.

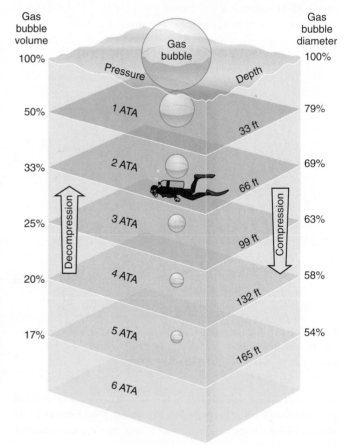

Figure 22-20   Boyle's law. The volume of a given quantity of gas at constant temperature varies inversely with pressure.

Barotrauma

Barotrauma, also known as *squeeze*, is the most common form of scuba-related diving injury.[78] Although many forms of barotraumas cause pain, most resolve spontaneously and do not require EMS involvement or recompression chamber therapy.

However, some pulmonary overpressurization injuries are very serious. During scuba diving, barotrauma occurs within noncompressible, gas-filled body cavities (e.g., sinuses). If the pressure in these spaces cannot equalize during a dive as ambient pressure increases, vascular engorgement, hemorrhage, and mucosal edema result from decreasing air volume when the diver descends, and tissue disruption results from increasing air volume when the diver ascends. The various forms of barotraumas are described next.

Barotrauma of Descent

Mask Squeeze

This form of barotrauma generally occurs in inexperienced or inattentive divers who fail to equalize the pressure in their face mask by increasing the external water pressure during their descents. Examine the soft tissue around the patient's eyes and conjunctival tissues for capillary rupture. Signs and symptoms of mask squeeze include skin ecchymoses and conjunctival hemorrhage. Mask barotrauma is self-limited and treatment is no diving until the tissue damage clears. Management includes providing a cold compress over the eyes, encouraging the patient to rest, and providing pain medication as needed.

Tooth Squeeze

A very infrequent finding, this form of barotrauma occurs in divers when gas is trapped in the interior portion of a tooth after receiving a dental filling, recent tooth extractions, or a root canal, or with defective dental restorations. During descent, the tooth can fill with blood or can implode with increasing external pressure. During ascent, any air forced into the tooth will expand, causing either pain or explosion of the tooth. To prevent tooth squeeze, it is recommended that divers do not dive for 24 hours after any dental treatment.

Examine the affected tooth to see if it is intact. Signs and symptoms of tooth squeeze include pain and a fractured tooth. Refer the patient for dental evaluation and give pain medication as needed.

Middle-Ear Squeeze

This type of squeeze occurs in 40% of scuba divers and is considered the most common diving injury.[79] Ear squeeze occurs near the surface of the water, when the greatest changes in pressure occur as the diver descends. Divers need to begin equalizing their middle ear early as they start to descend so a pressure differential across the tympanic membrane (TM) leading to rupture of the eardrum does not occur. The diver will experience pain and vertigo if the TM ruptures, allowing water to enter the middle ear. Divers with upper respiratory infection or allergies may have difficulty equalizing their middle ear during a dive.

Examine the ear canal for blood caused by ruptured TM. Signs and symptoms of middle-ear squeeze include pain, vertigo, conductive hearing losses with TM rupture, and vomiting.

No pressure changes are permitted (e.g., diving or flying) in patients with middle-ear squeeze. Patients may need decongestants if the TM has not ruptured to open up the eustachian tube and allow the pressure to equalize. Antiemetics such as prochlorperazine (Compazine) or ondansetron (Zofran) may be necessary for vertigo and vomiting. Transport the patient in an upright position or position of comfort. Antibiotics may be prescribed with ruptured TM to prevent infection. The patient should be referred for audiometric evaluation to assess possible hearing loss.

Sinus Squeeze

Normally, pressure in the sinuses equalizes easily as the diver is descending and ascending. Pressure develops by the same mechanism as the middle ear squeeze, but sinus squeeze is not as common. As a diver descends, there is an inability to maintain pressure in the sinuses, and a vacuum develops in the sinus cavity, causing intense pain, mucosal wall trauma, and bleeding in the sinus cavity. This squeeze may be caused by congestion, sinusitis, *mucosal hypertrophy* (enlargement or thickening), rhinitis, or nasal poyps.[78] A reverse sinus squeeze during ascent can occur as well (see later discussion on Sinus Barotrauma).

Examine the patient's nose for discharge. Signs and symptoms of sinus squeeze include severe pain over the affected sinus or bloody discharge, usually from frontal sinuses.

No specific management is needed at the scene unless extensive bleeding is observed, in which case, treat the patient for epistaxis (nosebleed) by pinching firmly on the fleshy part of the patient's nostrils just below the nasal bones. Transport in a position of comfort.

Internal-Ear Barotrauma

Although much less common than middle-ear squeeze, this is the most serious form of ear barotrauma because it may lead to permanent deafness.[79] Internal-ear barotrauma occurs when a diver descends and has failed attempts to equalize the middle ear. Further forceful attempts can result in a large rise in middle-ear pressure and can rupture the round window structure.

Examine the ear canal for any discharge. Signs and symptoms include roaring tinnitus, vertigo, hearing loss, a feeling of fullness or "blockage" in the affected ear, nausea, vomiting, pallor, diaphoresis (sweating), disorientation, and ataxia (loss of muscular coordination).

The patient should avoid strenuous activities and loud noises, with no pressure changes (e.g., diving or flying). Transport the patient in an upright position. Early medical consultation with DAN or an ED is recommended because it may be difficult to determine if this is inner-ear decompression sickness and if there is an immediate need for recompression chamber therapy.

Barotrauma of Ascent (Reverse Squeeze)

Alternobaric Vertigo

This is an unusual form of barotrauma in that it occurs as expanding gas moves through the eustachian tube and unequal pressure develops in the middle ear, which can cause vertigo.

Although the symptoms are brief, vertigo can trigger panic in divers, leading to other forms of injury caused by a rapid ascent to the surface (e.g., air embolism, drowning).

Examine the ear canal for any discharge; assess any hearing loss. Signs and symptoms of alternobaric vertigo are short in duration, resulting in transient vertigo, pressure in the affected ear, tinnitus, and hearing loss.

No specific intervention is required; diving is not recommended until any hearing loss returns. Provide decongestants as needed and according to the EMS system's policies and procedures. No transport to the ED is needed if symptoms resolve quickly, and the patient may follow up with his or her primary care provider. If symptoms persist, transport for evaluation is appropriate.

Sinus Barotrauma

This form of sinus squeeze can occur on ascent when some form of blockage in the sinus openings prevents expanding gas from escaping. The expanding gas puts pressure on the mucosal lining of the sinus, causing pain with hemorrhage. Sinus barotrauma occurs in divers with upper respiratory infections or allergies. It is common for divers to take a decongestant before a dive as a preventive measure to help equalize the middle ear when diving. However, the vasoconstrictive benefits can wear off at depth, causing mucosal tissue expansion and forming a sinus blockage of expanding gas during the return to the surface.

Examine the nose for discharge. Signs and symptoms of sinus barotrauma include severe pain over the affected sinus and bloody discharge, usually from the frontal sinuses.

No specific management is needed at the scene unless extensive bleeding is observed, in which case treat for epistaxis by pinching firmly on the fleshy part of the patient's nostrils, just below the nasal bones. Transport the patient in a position of comfort.

Gastrointestinal Squeeze

This type of barotrauma occurs when expanding gas in the gut becomes trapped as the diver surfaces. Gastrointestinal (GI) barotrauma occurs in novice divers who frequently perform Valsalva maneuvers in the head-down position, which forces air into the stomach. It can also occur in divers who chew gum when diving or who have consumed carbonated beverages or other gas-producing foods before diving.

Examine the abdominal quadrants. Signs and symptoms of GI squeeze include abdominal fullness, belching, and flatulence.

GI squeeze normally resolves on its own and rarely needs medical attention. If the pain and fullness do not resolve, transport for evaluation is appropriate. Only in severe cases is recompression chamber therapy needed.

Pulmonary Overinflation Barotrauma

Pulmonary overinflation is a serious form of barotrauma resulting from the expansion of gas in the lungs during ascent. Normally the diver eliminates expanding gas with normal exhalations when returning to the surface. If the expanding gas does not escape, there is a rupture of the alveoli, which in turn causes one of many forms of injury, depending on the amount of air that escapes outside the lung and its final location. A common scenario is a diver who has a rapid and uncontrollable ascent to the surface caused by running out of air, panic, or a dropped weight belt. These types of injuries are collectively called pulmonary overpressurization syndrome (POPS), or *burst lung*.

The five forms of POPS are:

1. Overdistension with local injury
2. Mediastinal emphysema
3. Subcutaneous emphysema
4. Pneumothorax
5. Arterial gas embolism

Overdistension with Local Injury. This is the mildest form of POPS, with only a small, isolated lung barotrauma. Auscultate the lung fields for diminished breath sounds. Chest pain may or may not be present. Blood is often seen in the sputum (hemoptysis).

Ensure that the patient rests in a position of comfort, and treat the patient's symptoms as needed. Monitor the patient's vital signs and oxygen saturation with pulse oximetry; provide oxygen at 2 to 4 liters/minute with nasal cannula. Transport the patient in position of comfort. The patient needs further medical evaluation to rule out a more severe form of POPS and should avoid further pressure exposure (e.g., diving or commercial flying).

Mediastinal Emphysema. This is the most common form of POPS, caused by escaping gas from ruptured alveoli entering the interstitial space to the mediastinum. This condition is usually benign. Examine the lung fields for diminished breath sounds. Signs and symptoms include hoarseness, neck fullness, and minor substernal chest pain; often a dull ache or tightness worsens with breathing and coughing. Examine the patient's chest and neck for subcutaneous emphysema. In severe cases, the diver presents with chest pain, dyspnea, and difficulty swallowing.

Ensure that the patient rests in a position of comfort. Monitor the patient's vital signs and oxygen saturation with pulse oximetry; provide oxygen at 2 to 4 liters/minute with nasal cannula. Usually, mediastinal emphysema requires no specific treatment or recompression therapy. Rare cases need to be medically evaluated to rule out other causes of chest pain and severe forms of POPS. Transport the patient in a supine position. The patient should avoid further pressure exposure (e.g., diving or commercial flying).

Subcutaneous Emphysema. With subcutaneous emphysema, air escaping from ruptured alveoli continues to move superiorly into the neck and clavicle regions of the chest. Examine the lung fields for diminished breath sounds. Signs and symptoms of subcutaneous emphysema include swelling, crepitus, hoarseness, sore throat, and difficulty swallowing.

No specific treatment is required besides rest. Monitor the patient's vital signs and oxygen saturation with pulse oximetry, and provide oxygen by nasal cannula at 2 to 4 liters/minute. The patient needs further medical evaluation to rule out more severe forms of POPS. Transport the patient in the supine position. The patient should avoid further pressure exposure (e.g., diving or commercial flying).

Pneumothorax. Pneumothorax is seen in less than 10% of POPS cases because air must escape through the visceral pleura around the lung, which presents greater resistance than air escaping through the interstitial space between the lung and visceral pleura. If the diver is at depth when a pulmonary rupture occurs, a tension pneumothorax can result as the volume of escaping gas expands as the diver continues toward the surface. Examine the lung fields for diminished breath sounds. Signs and symptoms will vary based on the size of the pneumothorax and include sharp chest pain, diminished breath sounds, breathlessness, subcutaneous emphysema, and dyspnea.

Provide ongoing assessment to monitor for conversion from simple to tension pneumothorax. Ensure rest in a position of comfort. Monitor the patient's vital signs and oxygen saturation with pulse oximetry and provide oxygen by nasal cannula at 2 to 4 liters/minute. Provide standard ALS management of tension pneumothorax with 14-gauge needle thoracostomy as necessary. Transport the patient in a position of comfort. The patient needs further medical evaluation to rule out more severe forms of POPS and should avoid further pressure exposure (e.g., diving or commercial flying). Recompression therapy is generally not necessary.

Arterial Gas Embolism. This is the most feared complication of POPS and, after drowning, is a leading cause of death in divers, accounting for about 30% of fatalities.[80] Arterial gas embolism (AGE) can occur from any of the four POPS conditions previously presented as a result of air escaping and forming an air embolism. AGE typically occurs in divers who have an uncontrolled ascent to the surface without appropriate exhalation, causing an overinflation pulmonary injury. However, AGE can occur in divers who surface slowly without underlying lung pathology. During ascent, once the pulmonary overinflation bursts alveoli, air enters the pulmonary venous capillary circulation; the gas bubbles enter the left atrium and left ventricle, then exit the heart through the aorta, and are distributed to the cerebral, coronary, and other systemic vasculature. Gas bubbles can enter the coronary circulation, causing an occlusion resulting in cardiac dysrhythmia, cardiac arrest, or myocardial infarction.[81] If gas bubbles enter the cerebral circulation, the diver presents with signs and symptoms similar to an acute stroke.

Unlike decompression sickness, which can present with delayed symptoms hours after diving, symptoms of AGE appear either immediately at the water surface or typically within 2 minutes. Any loss of consciousness once a diver surfaces must be presumed to be AGE until proved otherwise.[81] The primary treatment for AGE is recompression chamber (hyperbaric) therapy.

Historically, it was recommended that patients with AGE be placed in the Trendelenburg position for transport, based on the belief that this would help keep bubbles from circulating in the systemic vasculature. However, recent evidence has shown that the head-down position does not prevent systemic circulation of nitrogen bubbles, makes it more difficult to oxygenate the patient, and may worsen cerebral edema.[82] Currently, it is recommended that all AGE patients be placed in a supine position in the field and during transport. The supine position also provides a greater rate of nitrogen bubble washout.[83,84]

Decompression Sickness

Decompression sickness (DCS) is directly related to Henry's law. When scuba divers breathe compressed air containing oxygen (21%), carbon dioxide (0.03%), and nitrogen (79%), the amount of gas that will be dissolved in liquid is directly proportional to the partial pressure of gas in contact with liquid. Oxygen is used in the body for tissue metabolism when in solution and does not form gas bubbles during ascent from depth.

Nitrogen, an inert gas not used for metabolism, is the primary source of concern in DCS. Nitrogen is five times more soluble in fat than in water and becomes dissolved in tissue proportionately to the increasing ambient pressure. Consequently, the deeper underwater the diver goes and the longer the diver stays at depth, the greater the amount of nitrogen that dissolves into tissue. As the diver ascends toward the surface, the absorbed nitrogen must be eliminated. If there is inadequate time to eliminate nitrogen during ascent, nitrogen comes out of solution in the tissues in the form of intravascular gas bubbles, causing obstruction of the vascular and lymphatic systems and tissue distension, and activating inflammatory responses.[85]

Most divers experience DCS within the first hour after surfacing, although some will present with symptoms up to 6 hours after surfacing. Only 2% of divers will have delayed symptoms between 24 and 48 hours after surfacing. Traditionally, symptoms of DCS are categorized as Type I, a mild form involving cutaneous, lymphatic, and musculoskeletal systems, or Type II, a severe form involving neurologic and cardiopulmonary systems (**Figure 22-21**). Mild symptoms of DCS include fatigue and malaise. However, mild symptoms can be precursors to more severe signs and symptoms, such as numbness, weakness, and paralysis.

Studies now suggest that it is more important clinically to describe DCS by the region of the body affected and not as Type I or Type II.[70] This suggestion is applicable for prehospital care providers to ensure that even patients with mild DCS symptoms are treated aggressively with 100% oxygen and an early consult for recompression therapy. Many divers with the mild form of DCS will not have a medical evaluation. Divers may delay up to 32 hours before seeking medical care for DCS because denial of DCS is a common finding in the scuba diving population.[88]

Figure 22-21   Decompression Illnesses

The term decompression illness (DCI) has been proposed to encompass Type I and Type II DCS and AGE.[86,87]

Several factors predispose a diver to DCS.[89,90] Some risk factors are known to enhance the uptake of nitrogen in tissues during descent and slow the release of nitrogen during ascent. Certain host and environmental factors, as well as equipment failures and improper technique, increase the risk for DCS (**Figure 22-22**).

Figure 22-22   Factors Related to Decompression Sickness (DCS)

Host Factors
- Lack of fitness
- Advancing age
- Female sex
- Hypothermia
- Alcohol or drug use
- Patent foramen ovale (hole in the wall between the right and left atria)
- Obesity
- Sleep deprivation
- Dehydration
- Inadequate nutrition
- Heavy exertion at depth or fatigue
- Underlying medical illness (e.g., asthma)
- Prior history of DCS

Environmental Factors
- Extremes of temperature
- Rough seas
- Flying after diving
- Heavy exercise at depth
- Nitrogen narcosis (state of confusion/euphoria similar to alcohol intoxication from nitrogen entering the blood under pressure)
- Elevated arterial carbon dioxide tension
- Low water temperature

Equipment Failures and Improper Technique
- Violating the decompression tables
- Difficulty with buoyancy
- Rapid ascent
- Running out of air
- Regulator malfunction
- Unfamiliar or improper equipment

Source: From Barratt DM. Harch PG. Van Meter K: Decompression illness in divers: A review of the literature. Neurologist 8:186, 2002. Reprinted by permission of Lippincott Williams & Wilkins.

Limb Pain (Type I DCS)

This form of DCS results from bubble formation in the musculo-skeletal system, typically occurring in one or more joints. The most common joints involved are the shoulder and elbow, followed by the knee, hip, wrist, hand, and ankle.[69] This pain is described as a severe tendonitis, joint pain with a grating sensation on movement. The pain starts gradually, presenting as a deep, dull ache of mild to severe intensity. Victims often attempt to relieve their pain by flexion of their joints, hence the common name for this condition—the *bends*. Although this form of DCS is not life threatening, it indicates that bubbles are present in the venous circulation. It can lead to more severe forms if left untreated.

Cutaneous and Lymphatic (Type I DCS)

This form of DCS is uncommon. It represents inadequate elimination of bubbles forming in the skin or lymphatic systems. Cutaneous *skin bends* are uncommon and usually not serious, but signs of mottling and marbling are considered precursors of delayed neurologic problems.[61] Symptoms include an intense rash that progresses to a red patchy or bluish discoloration of the skin.[83] Lymphatic obstruction can result in swelling and an orange-peel appearance (*peau d'orange*).

Cardiopulmonary (Type II DCS)

This severe form of DCS is referred to as the *chokes* and results when venous bubbles overwhelm the pulmonary capillary system. Hypotension can occur from a massive venous air embolism in the lung. Symptoms include nonproductive cough, substernal chest pain, cyanosis, dyspnea, shock, and cardiopulmonary arrest. This disorder resembles acute respiratory distress syndrome (see the Airway and Ventilation chapter).[91]

Spinal Cord (Type II DCS)

The white matter of the spinal cord is vulnerable to bubble formation, and nitrogen is highly soluble in spinal cord tissue (*myelin*). The most common site for this form of DCS is the lower thoracic spine, followed by the lumbar/sacral and cervical regions.[88] Common signs and symptoms include low back pain and "heaviness" in the legs. With this form of DCS, the patient often gives a vague statement in an effort to describe "strange sensations," or paresthesia, which can progress to weakness, numbness, and paralysis. Bowel and bladder dysfunction, leading to urinary retention, also has been reported.[92]

Assessment of AGE and DCS

A standardized approach for patients with AGE and DCS is provided to ensure that consistent care is given. It is recommended that all patients with scuba-related diving injuries be examined for signs and symptoms of AGE and DCS because the primary and essential lifesaving treatment is recompression chamber therapy.

Arterial Gas Embolism

About 5% of all AGE patients present with immediate apnea, unconsciousness, and cardiac arrest. Others present with signs and symptoms similar to acute stroke, with loss of consciousness, stupor, confusion, hemiparesis, seizure, vertigo, visual changes, sensory changes, and headache.

Decompression Sickness

Type I DCS is characterized by deep pain in a joint, including minor forms of cutaneous pruritus (severe itching) and obstruction of lymph vessels (lymphedema). Type II DCS is characterized by symptoms involving the CNS, ranging from weakness and numbness to paralysis.

Obtain a dive profile and medical history of the events that led to the diving-related injury from a fellow diver, including:

- Time of onset of signs and symptoms
- Source of breathing medium (e.g., air or mixed gases; heliox)
- Dive profile (dive activity, depth, duration, dive frequency, surface interval, interval between dives)
- Dive location and water conditions
- Dive risk factors
- Underwater medical and equipment problems on ascent and descent
- Whether the diver was attempting a no-decompression dive or a decompression dive
- Rate of ascent
- Decompression stop(s)
- Postdive activity level
- Postdive aircraft travel, with type and duration
- Past and present medical history (especially a history of previous DCS)
- Medication use
- Current use of alcohol or illicit drugs[93]

Management

Ensure the ABCs, protect the patient's airway, and initiate BLS or ALS procedures as required. Initiate 100% oxygen at 12 to 15 liters/minute, and give NS or LR (no dextrose) IV fluid therapy (1 to 2 ml/kg/hour). Monitor the patient's vital signs, pulse oximetry, and ECG. Check and treat the patient's blood glucose as required. Control any seizures. Protect the patient from hypothermia, and consult early with local medical control or DAN for the closest recompression chamber (primary treatment) (see **Figure 22-23** for DAN contact information). Standard recompression therapy with 100% hyperbaric oxygen is given according to the U.S. Navy treatment tables.[94] Transport the patient in a supine

Figure 22-23 Divers Alert Network (DAN) Contact Information for Emergency and Nonemergency Consult

Diving Emergencies (Remember: Call local EMS first, then DAN!)
1-919-684-9111
Nonemergency Medical Questions
1-800-446-2671 or 1-919-684-2948
Monday–Friday, 8:30 a.m. to 5:00 p.m. (EST)
All Other Inquiries
1-800-446-2671 or 1-919-684-2948
1-919-490-6630 (fax)
Contact Information to Send a Letter
Divers Alert Network
The Peter B. Bennett Center
6 West Colony Place
Durham, NC 27705 USA

Source: Data courtesy of Divers Alert Network® (DAN®).

position. For any scuba-related diving injury, if air evacuation is provided by helicopter or other nonpressurized aircraft, it is recommended to fly as low as possible (e.g., 500 feet [150 m]), but not to exceed 1,000 feet (300 m) to minimize further expansion of air bubbles (Boyle's law) and further dysbarism trauma.[70,84]

Definitive treatment for specific barotraumas, including AGE and DCS, is to administer 100% oxygen by mask at two to three times the atmospheric pressure at sea level in a recompression chamber.[94] (For further discussion of recompression chamber treatment methods for scuba-related diving injuries, see the U.S. Navy Diving Manual or other sources.[70,94]) The patient immediately benefits, based on the principles of Boyle's law, by increasing the ambient pressure and decreasing the size of bubbles formed and increasing the oxygen concentration in tissues. **Figure 22-24** describes recompression and hyperbaric oxygen therapy.

Figure 22-25 summarizes signs and symptoms of barotrauma and its treatment. **Figure 22-26** summarizes signs and symptoms of DCS and its treatment.

Prevention of Scuba-Related Diving Injuries

Millions of certified scuba divers need frequent skill refresher training to prevent and recognize scuba-related dive injuries. Many scuba professionals in the United States, such as

Figure 22-24 Recompression Therapy for Scuba-Related Diving Injuries

The goals of recompression therapy for scuba-related diving injuries caused by pulmonary overinflation barotrauma and decompression sickness (DCS) are to compress the bubbles and increase oxygen delivery to tissues. Recompression therapy includes the following mechanisms:

- Reduces volume of the bubbles where they are circulated to the pulmonary capillaries and filtered out
- Promotes reabsorption of bubbles in solution
- Increases oxygen delivery to the tissues
- Corrects hypoxia
- Provides an increased diffusion gradient for nitrogen
- Reduces edema
- Reduces blood vessel permeability

All divers with arterial gas embolism (AGE) and DCS must be considered early for recompression in a hyperbaric treatment facility because the treatment is more successful if started within 6 hours after the onset of symptoms. Divers are not always near a recompression chamber when symptoms occur, and there can be considerable delays getting to a chamber by ground or by arranging for air transport. Contact the Diver's Alert Network (DAN) to consult for diving medical assistance and to determine the closest recompression chamber (see Figure 22-23).

In the meantime, place the patient in a supine position. Nitrogen washout can be increased by providing 100% oxygen by mask and by starting an IV fluid line with normal saline or lactated Ringer's solution at 1 to 2 ml/kg/hr to ensure adequate intravascular volume and capillary perfusion. During recompression treatment, patients with AGE or DCS normally will receive recompression treatment at 2.5 to 3.0 atm for 2 to 4 hours while breathing 100% oxygen. Longer and repeated treatment will be necessary if the patient has no clinical improvement of symptoms.

Recompression treatment principles include the following:

- Any painful or neurologic signs or symptoms occurring within 24 hours of a dive are caused by DCS until proved otherwise.
- Any painful or neurologic signs or symptoms occurring within 48 hours of flying after diving are caused by DCS until proved otherwise.
- Contact the DAN 24-hour emergency hotline for consultation at 919-684-9111.
- Every diver with signs or symptoms of DCS should receive recompression treatment.
- Never fail to treat doubtful cases.
- Early treatment improves outcomes, whereas delayed treatment worsens outcomes.
- Long delays should never preclude treatment because divers respond to recompression therapy days to weeks after injury.
- Monitor the patient closely for signs of relief from or progression of symptoms.
- Inadequate treatment can lead to a recurrence.
- Continue to treat until clinical plateau.

Source: Modified from: Tibbles PM, Edelsberg JS: Hyperbaric oxygen therapy. N Engl J Med 334(25):1642, 1996; from Barratt DM, Harch PG, Van Meter K: Decompression illness in divers: A review of the literature. Neurologist 8:186, 2002; and from Van Hoesen KB, Bird NH: Diving medicine. In Auerbach PS: Wilderness medicine, ed 6, St. Louis, 2012, Mosby Elsevier.

lifeguards, fire and law enforcement personnel, search and rescue members, Coast Guard members, and Department of Defense employees, depend on local prehospital care providers to provide initial and follow-up medical care and transport to local hospitals or recompression chambers. Collaboration among dive teams and local EMS agencies to develop medical scenarios during dive training is strongly encouraged. This should include frequent scuba training in varying underwater conditions and locations, along with in-water rescue scenarios and initial medical care, which are paramount to responding safely and effectively for in-water swimmer/diver rescues and recoveries. Scuba training coordination among medical dive team members and local prehospital care providers will ensure effective communication and appropriate continuity of field care. This training should include scenario-based consults with local medical control and DAN.

Medical Fitness to Dive

Prehospital care providers responding to diving-related incidents must assess divers, in all ages groups, not only for primary diving disorders related to a submersion incident (e.g., DCS, AGE) but also for underlying medical conditions (e.g., cardiac, pulmonary, neurologic, endocrine, psychiatric, or a combination of both medical and dysbaric disorders). Ideally, all new divers should be cleared medically before the start of scuba

Figure 22-25 Barotrauma: Common Signs, Symptoms, and Treatment

Type	Signs/Symptoms	Treatment*
Mask squeeze	Corneal injection, conjunctival hemorrhage	Self-limited; rest, cold compresses, pain medication
Sinus squeeze	Pain, bloody nasal discharge	Pain medication, decongestants, antihistamines
Middle-ear squeeze	Pain, vertigo, tympanic membrane rupture, hearing loss, vomiting	Decongestants, antihistamines, pain medication; may need antibiotics; avoid diving and flying
Internal-ear barotraumas	Tinnitus, vertigo, ataxia, hearing loss	Bed rest; elevate head; avoid loud noises; stool softeners; avoid strenuous activity; no diving or flying for months
External-ear barotraumas	Difficulty with Valsalva maneuver, earache, bloody discharge, possible tympanic membrane rupture	Maintain dry ear canal; antibiotics may be needed for infection
Tooth squeeze	Tooth pain while diving	Self-limited; pain medication
Alternobaric vertigo	Pressure, pain in affected ear, vertigo, tinnitus	Usually short lived; decongestants; prohibit diving until resolution with normal hearing
Pulmonary barotraumas	Substernal pain, voice change, dyspnea, subcutaneous emphysema	Assess ABCs, neurologic functions; 100% oxygen 12 to 15 liters/minute nonrebreathing mask; transport patient lying supine; need to rule out AGE
Subcutaneous emphysema	Substernal pain and crepitus, brassy voice, neck swelling, dyspnea, bloody sputum	Rest; avoid diving and flying; oxygen and recompression therapy only in severe cases
Pneumothorax	Sharp chest pain, dyspnea, diminished breath sounds	100% oxygen 12 to 15 liters/minute nonrebreathing mask; monitor pulse oximetry; transport in position of comfort; assess for tension pneumothorax
Tension pneumothorax	Cyanosis, distended neck veins, tracheal deviation	14-gauge needle thoracentesis; 100% oxygen 12 to 15 liters/minute nonrebreathing mask; monitor pulse oximetry
Arterial gas embolism (AGE)	Unresponsiveness, confusion, headache, visual disturbances, seizure	Assess ABCs, neurologic functions; initiate BLS/ALS; control seizures; 100% oxygen 12 to 15 liters/minute nonrebreathing mask; transport patient lying supine; glucose-free IV fluid therapy (1 to 2 ml/kg /hr); monitor ECG; consult DAN (919-684-8111) for closest recompression chamber (primary treatment)

*Good patient education on scene for minor barotrauma injuries is important because some of these injuries are self-limiting and others need physician evaluation; others need patient referral to the family physician or emergency department and will not necessitate EMS transport.
ABCs, airway, breathing, circulation; ALS, advanced life support; BLS, basic life support; DAN, Divers Alert Network; ECG, electrocardiogram.
Source: From Clenney TL, Lassen LF: Recreational scuba diving injuries. *Am Fam Physician* 53(5):1761, 1996; Salahuddin M, James LA, Bass ES. SCUBA Medicine: A First-Responder's Guide to Diving Injuries. Curr Sports Med Reports 10(3):134-139, 2011. and Van Hoesen KB and Bird NH: Diving medicine. In Auerbach PS: Wilderness medicine, ed 6, St. Louis, 2012, Mosby Elsevier.

Figure 22-26 Decompression Sickness (DCS): Common Signs, Symptoms, and Treatment

Condition	Signs/Symptoms	Treatment
DCS Type I		
Skin bends	Intense itching (pruritus); red rash patches over shoulders and upper chest; skin marbling may precede burning sensation and itching over shoulders and torso; localized cyanosis and pitting edema.	Self-limiting; resolves on its own; observe for delayed signs of limb-pain DCS.
Limb-pain DCS	Large joint tenderness; mild to severe joint or extremity pain; pain is usually steady but may throb and present in 75% of cases; grating sensation on joint motion; worse with movement. DCS Type I may progress to DCS Type II.	Mild pain only often resolves on its own; observe 24 hours; moderate to severe pain. Start with 100% oxygen, 12 to 15 liters/minute nonrebreathing mask; transport all patients in supine position; glucose-free IV fluid therapy (1 to 2 ml/kg/hr); early consult DAN (919-684-8111) for closest recompression chamber for definitive treatment.
DCS Type II		
Cardiopulmonary "chokes"	Substernal pain, mild cough, dyspnea, nonproductive cough, cyanosis, tachypnea, tachycardia, shock and cardiac arrest	ABCs; 100% oxygen, 12 to 15 liters/minute nonrebreathing mask; BLS or ALS as needed; glucose-free IV fluid therapy (1 to 2 ml/kg/hr); transport all patients in supine position; early consult DAN (919-684-8111) for closest recompression chamber for definitive treatment.
Neurologic		
Brain	Many visual changes, headache, confusion, disorientation, nausea and vomiting	
Spinal cord	Back pain, heaviness or weakness, numbness, paralysis, urine retention, fecal incontinence	
Inner ear	Vertigo, ataxia	

ABCs, airway, breathing, circulation; ALS, advanced life support; BLS, basic life support; DAN, Divers Alert Network; IV, intravenous.
Source: From Barratt DM, Harch PG, Van Meter K: Decompression illness in divers: A review of the literature. Neurologist 8:186, 2002; and Van Hoesen KB, Bird NH: Diving medicine. In Auerbach PS: Wilderness medicine, ed 6, St. Louis, 2012, Mosby Elsevier.

training. Five general medical screening recommendations for identifying individuals who are at an increased risk for a diving-related problem are listed below. These recommendations are based on consensus of medical diving specialists.[70,95] Also refer to **Figure 22-27** for the severe risk (absolute contraindications), relative risk, and temporary risk conditions of concern for scuba diving.[70] Recommendations include the following:

- Inability to equalize pressure in one or more of the body's air spaces increases the risk for barotrauma.
- Medical or psychiatric conditions may manifest underwater or at a remote diving site and can endanger the diver's life because of the condition itself, because it occurs in the water, or because inadequate medical help is available.
- Impaired tissue perfusion or diffusion of inert gases increases the risk of DCS.
- Poor physical condition increases the risk of DCS or exertion-related medical problems. The factors compromising physical condition may be physiologic or pharmacologic.
- In women who are pregnant, the fetus may be at increased risk of dysbaric injury.

Figure 22-27	Fitness to Dive: Guidelines for Medical Clearance for Recreational Diving		
System	**Severe Risk Conditions**	**Relative Risk Conditions**	**Temporary Risk Conditions**
Neurologic	Seizures Transient ischemic attack or cerebrovascular accident Serious decompression sickness with residual deficits	Complicated migraine Head injury with sequelae Herniated disc Peripheral neuropathy Multiple sclerosis Spinal cord or brain injury Intracranial tumor or aneurysm	Arterial gas embolism without residual, in which pulmonary air trapping has been excluded and probability of recurrence is low
Cardiovascular	Intracardiac right-to-left shunt (atrial septal defect) Hypertrophic cardiomyopathy Valvular stenosis	Coronary artery bypass grafting Percutaneous transluminal coronary angioplasty or coronary artery disease History of myocardial infarction Congestive heart failure Hypertension Dysrhythmias Valvular regurgitation	Pacemaker: if problem necessitating pacing does not preclude diving; pacemakers must be certified by manufacturer to withstand pressure
Pulmonary	Spontaneous pneumothorax Impaired exercise performance due to respiratory disease	Asthma or reactive airway disease Exercise-induced bronchospasm Solid, cystic, or cavitating lesions Pneumothorax caused by surgery, trauma, previous overinflation Immersion pulmonary edema Interstitial lung disease	
Gastrointestinal	Gastric outlet obstruction Chronic or recurrent small bowel obstruction Severe gastroesophageal reflux Paraesophageal hernia	Inflammatory bowel disease Functional bowel disorders	Unrepaired hernias of the abdominal wall Peptic ulcer disease associated with obstruction or severe reflux
Metabolic and endocrine	Pregnancy	Insulin- or noninsulin-dependent diabetes mellitus	
Otolaryngologic	Open tympanic membrane perforation Tube myringotomy Middle ear or inner ear surgery Tracheostomy	Recurrent otitis externa, otitis media or sinusitis Eustachian tube dysfunction History of tympanic membrane perforation, tympanoplasty, or mastoidectomy Significant conductive or sensorineural hearing loss History of round or oval window rupture	Acute upper respiratory infection Acute sinusitis Acute otitis media
Orthopedic		Amputation Scoliosis with impact on respiratory performance Aseptic necrosis	Back pain

(Continues on next page)

Figure 22-27	Fitness to Dive: Guidelines for Medical Clearance for Recreational Diving (*Continued*)		
System	**Severe Risk Conditions**	**Relative Risk Conditions**	**Temporary Risk Conditions**
Hematologic		Sickle cell disease Leukemia Hemophilia Polycythemia vera	
Behavioral health	Inappropriate motivation to dive Claustrophobia Acute psychosis Untreated panic disorder	Use of psychotropic medications Previous psychotic episodes	

Source: *From Van Hoesen KB, Bird NH: Diving medicine. In Auerbach PS: Wilderness medicine, ed 6, St. Louis, 2012, Mosby Elsevier.

For many years, diabetics have questioned the diving medical experts about scuba diving waivers for individuals who have control of their blood sugar. In June 2005, an international workshop was held in the United States that was jointly sponsored by the Undersea and Hyperbaric Medical Society (UHMS) and DAN. They brought together over 50 medical and research experts from around the world to develop guidelines for recreational divers with diabetes.[96] The panel indicated that dive candidates who use medication (oral hypoglycemic agents or insulin) to treat diabetes, but who are otherwise qualified to dive may undertake recreational scuba diving. However, they stated that strict criteria need to be met before diving. The panel agreed that those diabetics using dietary control will easily meet the new guidelines. The consensus guidelines (**Figure 22-28**) consist of 19 points, under the categories of selection and surveillance, scope of diving, and glucose management on the day of diving.

Figure 22-28   Guidelines for Recreational Diving With Diabetes

Selection and Surveillance

- Individual must be at least 18 years of age (16 years if in special training program).
- Diving will be delayed after starting/changing medication, as follows:
  - Three months with oral hypoglycemic agents
  - One year after initiation of insulin therapy
- There must be no episodes of hypoglycemia or hyperglycemia requiring intervention from a third party within at least 1 year.
- There must be no history of hypoglycemia unawareness.
- A glycated hemoglobin (HbA1c) test result of ≤ 9% must be recorded no more than 1 month prior to initial assessment and at each annual review.
  - Values > 9% indicate the need for further evaluation and possible modification of therapy.

- There must be no significant secondary complications from diabetes.
- A physician/diabetologist should carry out an annual review and determine that the diver has a good understanding of the disease and the effect of exercise in consultation with an expert in diving medicine, as required.
- An evaluation for silent cardiac ischemia for candidates older than 40 years of age must be performed.
  - After initial evaluation, periodic surveillance for silent cardiac ischemia can be in accordance with accepted local/national guidelines for the evaluation of diabetics
- Candidate must document intent to follow protocol for divers with diabetes and to cease diving and seek medical review for any adverse events during diving possibly related to diabetes.

(*Continues on next page*)

Figure 22-28   Guidelines for Recreational Diving With Diabetes (*Continued*)

Scope of Diving

- Diving should be planned to avoid:
  - Depths > 100 feet (30 m) seawater
  - Durations > 60 minutes
  - Compulsory decompression stops
  - Overhead environments (e.g., cave, wreck penetration)
  - Situations that may exacerbate hypoglycemia (e.g., prolonged cold and arduous dives)
- Individuals must have a dive buddy/leader informed of diver's condition and steps to follow in case of problem.
  - Dive buddy should not have diabetes.

Glucose Management on the Day of Diving

- Individuals should perform a general self-assessment of fitness to dive.
- Blood glucose must be ≥ 150 mg·dl^{-1} (8.3 mmol·l^{-1}), stable or rising, before entering the water.

- Complete a minimum of three predive blood glucose tests to evaluate trends at 60 minutes, 30 minutes, and immediately prior to diving.
- Alterations in dosage of oral hypoglycemic agent or insulin on evening prior or day of diving may help.
- Delay dive if blood glucose is:
  - < 150 mg·dl^{-1} (8.3 mmol·l^{-1})
  - > 300 mg·dl^{-1} (16.7 mmol·l^{-1})
- Rescue medication considerations include:
  - Carry readily accessible oral glucose during all dives.
  - Have parenteral glucagon available at the surface.
- If hypoglycemia is noticed underwater, the diver should surface (with buddy), establish positive buoyancy, ingest glucose, and leave the water.
- Check blood sugar frequently for 12 to 15 hours after diving.
- Ensure adequate hydration on days of diving.
- Log all dives, including blood glucose test results and all information pertinent to diabetes management.

Source: Data courtesy of Divers Alert Network® (DAN®)

Figure 22-29   Current Guidelines Recommended by Diver's Alert Network for Flying Safely After Diving

The following guidelines are the consensus of attendees at the 2002 Flying After Diving Workshop. They apply to dives followed by flights at cabin altitudes of 2,000 to 8,000 feet (610 to 2438 m) for divers who do not have symptoms of decompression sickness (DCS). The recommended preflight surface intervals do not guarantee avoidance of DCS. Longer surface intervals will reduce DCS risk further.

- For a single no-decompression dive, a minimum preflight surface interval of 12 hours is suggested.

- For multiple dives per day or multiple days of diving, a minimum preflight surface interval of 18 hours is suggested.

For dives requiring decompression stops, there is little evidence on which to base a recommendation, and a preflight surface interval substantially longer than 18 hours appears prudent.

Source: Data courtesy of Divers Alert Network® (DAN®)

Flying After Diving

Because diving is conducted at many popular dive locations in the United States and at remote locations outside the United States, persons may dive the day before flying. Because of Boyle's principle, flying too soon after a dive can increase the risk of DCS during flight or after arriving at the destination because of the reduced atmospheric pressure in either a pressurized or a nonpressurized commercial aircraft. **Figure 22-29** lists the current guidelines recommended by DAN for flying safely after diving.[70]

High Altitude Illness

In the United States, more than 40 million people each year travel above 8,202 feet (2,500 m) without acclimatization to participate in activities that include snowboarding, alpine skiing, hiking, camping, concerts, and festivals. Thus, many people are at risk for altitude-related illness, which can develop within hours to days after they arrive at altitude.[97] Prehospital care providers and ED staff need to become familiar with the predisposing factors, signs and symptoms, medical management, and education and prevention techniques to reduce the morbidity and mortality of high-altitude illness. See **Figure 22-30** for a wide range of acute medical problems experienced by visitors and residents at high altitudes.

This section presents three medical conditions directly caused by high-altitude environments and highlights specific underlying medical conditions that worsen as a result of high-altitude-induced hypoxia (altitude-exacerbated pre-existing medical conditions).

Epidemiology

High-altitude illness is a term that encompasses two cerebral and one pulmonary syndrome: (1) acute mountain sickness, (2) high-altitude cerebral edema, and (3) high-altitude pulmonary edema. Even though the risks of acquiring high-altitude illness are low, once it develops, progression can be fatal.[98,99]

Acute mountain sickness (AMS) is a mild form of high-altitude illness, rarely experienced at altitudes below 6,540 feet (2,000 m), but the incidence increases to 1.4% to 25% with increasing altitudes of 6,754 to 8,000 feet (2,060 to 2,440 m).[100,101]

AMS develops in 20% to 25% of cases above 8,200 feet (2,500 m) and in 40% to 50% of cases at 14,000 feet (4,267 m). The incidence of AMS is greater than 90% when the rate of ascent to approximately 14,000 feet (4,267 m) occurs over hours versus days.[102] Furthermore, a small number of AMS cases (5% to 10%) progress from mild symptoms to become high-altitude cerebral edema, a severe form of AMS.[99] **High-altitude cerebral edema (HACE)** is a severe neurologic form of high-altitude illness and has a low incidence rate of 0.01% in the general population at an altitude above 8,200 feet (2,500 m); this rate increases to 1% to 2% in more physically active individuals.[97]

High-altitude pulmonary edema (HAPE) is rare but accounts for the most deaths from high-altitude illness and is easily reversed if recognized early and managed correctly. HAPE typically presents within 2 to 5 days after arrival at altitude.[99] The incidence rate for HAPE is 0.01% to 0.1% at 8,200 feet (2,500 m) in the general population and increases to 2% to 6% in climbers at an altitude of 13,120 feet (4,000 m). The overall mortality for HAPE is 11% and increases to 44% when no treatment interventions are made.[103] Forty-seven cases of HAPE were reported in Vail, Colorado, from 1975 to 1982. These were young, healthy males who skied at an average altitude of 7,644 feet (2,330 m).[104]

Hypobaric Hypoxia

There are three defined levels of altitude. **High altitude** is defined as an elevation of 5,000 to 11,480 feet (1,500 to 3,500 m). This is a common altitude in the western mountain ranges of the United States, where high-altitude illness is reported with greater frequency than in other regions.[104] **Very high altitude** is defined

---

Figure 22-30   Medical Problems of High Altitude

Lowlanders on Ascent to Altitude
- Acute hypoxia
- High-altitude headache
- Acute mountain sickness
- High-altitude cerebral edema
- Cerebrovascular syndromes
- High-altitude pulmonary edema
- Symptomatic pulmonary hypertension
- High-altitude deterioration
- Organic brain syndrome (extreme altitude)
- Peripheral edema
- Retinopathy (engorgement of retinal veins; may be associated with vitreous hemorrhage and swelling of the optic disc, leading to vision impairment)

- Disordered sleep
- Periodic breathing disturbances during sleep
- High-altitude pharyngitis, bronchitis, and cough
- Ultraviolet keratitis (snow blindness)
- Exacerbation of pre-existing conditions

Lifelong or Long-Term Residents of Altitude
- Chronic mountain sickness (chronic mountain polycythemia)
- Symptomatic high-altitude pulmonary hypertension with or without right heart failure
- Problems of pregnancy: preeclampsia, hypertension, and low-birth weight infants
- Exacerbation of lung disease and congenital heart disease

Source: Modified from Hackett PH, Roach RC: High-altitude medicine. In Auerbach PS: Wilderness medicine, ed 6, St. Louis, 2012, Mosby Elsevier.

as an elevation of 11,480 to 18,045 feet (3,500 to 5,500 m) and is the more common altitude for serious forms of high-altitude illness.[105] **Extreme altitude** is defined as elevations higher than 18,045 feet (5,500 m).[99] With a progressive increase in altitude, the environment becomes very hostile to an individual not acclimatized to the decreased availability of oxygen, causing a condition known as **hypobaric hypoxia**.

High altitude is a unique environment because there is a decreased availability of oxygen for respiration, which results in cellular hypoxia. Even though the concentration of oxygen remains at 21% at all altitudes, decreased atmospheric pressure at higher altitude results in a decreased partial pressure of oxygen (PO_2). For example, PO_2 is 160 mm Hg at sea level (1 atm) and 80 mm Hg at 18,045 feet (0.5 atm at 5,500 m), resulting in less oxygen available during respiration. **Figure 22-31** shows that as altitude increases from sea level to extreme altitude, there is a proportional decrease in barometric pressure, arterial blood gases, and arterial oxygen saturation (SaO_2). It is worth noting that SaO_2 remains, on average, above 91% in healthy, acclimatizing adults until reaching an altitude above 9,200 feet (2,810 m). Prehospital care providers are trained to provide aggressive ventilatory support with 100% oxygen for all patients who are symptomatic with a pulse oximetry reading of 91% SaO_2, because this is indicative of moderate hypoxia (86% to 91%).

This relationship between increasing altitude and progressive hypoxia forms the basis for the acute physiologic adjustments in ventilatory rate and cardiac output and biochemical changes.[106] Consequently, it is the hypobaric hypoxia and hypoxemia that set up nonacclimatized individuals for high-altitude illness.[98]

Factors Related to High-Altitude Illness

The major development of high-altitude illness depends on many factors specific to each high-altitude exposure, but key factors include rapid ascent, poor acclimatization, physical exertion at altitude, young age, and history of prior altitude illness (**Figure 22-32**). Additional factors include:

- *Increased altitude and ascent rate.* The incidence and severity of high-altitude illness are primarily related to the speed of ascent, altitude reached, and length of stay, because these three factors increase the hypoxic stress in the body.[98,106]
- *Previous history of high-altitude illness.* A documented history of high-altitude illness is a valuable predicator of who is susceptible for subsequent high-altitude illness when returning to the same altitude at the same ascent rate.[107] Incidence rates for HAPE increase from 10% to 60% for those with a previous history of HAPE who abruptly ascend to an altitude of 14,960 feet (4,560 m).[108]
- *Preacclimatization.* Having a permanent residence above 2,950 feet (900 m) provides some preacclimatization and is associated with a lower rate of and severity of high-altitude illness when ascending to higher altitudes. However, this protection is limited if the ascent rate is rapid or reaches an extreme altitude.[106,107]
- *Age and gender.* Age, but not gender, is a factor in developing AMS; the incidence is lower in those older than 50 years. HAPE occurs more frequently and with

Figure 22-31 Relationship of Altitude, Barometric Pressure (Pb), Arterial Blood Gases, and Oxygen Saturation*

Altitude (meters)	Altitude (feet)	Pb (mm Hg)	PaO$_2$ (mm Hg)	SaO$_2$ (%)	PaCO$_2$ (mm Hg)
Sea level	Sea level	760	100	98.0	40.0
1646	5400	630	73.0	95.1	35.6
2810	9200	543	60.0	91.0	33.9
3660	12,020	489	47.6	84.5	29.5
4700	15,440	429	44.6	78.0	27.1
5340	17,500	401	43.1	76.2	25.7
6140	20,140	356	35.0	65.6	22.0

*Data are mean values for subjects age 20 to 40 years.

PaO$_2$, Arterial oxygen partial pressure; SaO$_2$, arterial oxygen saturation; PaCO$_2$, arterial carbon dioxide partial pressure.

Source: Modified from Hackett PH, Roach RC: High-altitude medicine. In Auerbach PS: Wilderness medicine, ed 6, St. Louis, 2012, Mosby Elsevier.

Figure 22-32 Common Medical Conditions That Worsen at High Altitude Without Supplemental Oxygen[113]

Probably No Extra Risk	Caution	Contraindicated
Young and old	Moderate COPD	Sickle cell anemia (with history of crises)
Fit and unfit	Compensated congestive heart failure (CHF)	Severe COPD
Obesity	Sleep apnea syndromes	Pulmonary hypertension
Diabetes	Troublesome arrhythmias	Uncompensated CHF
After coronary artery bypass grafting (without angina)	Stable angina/coronary artery disease	
Mild chronic obstructive pulmonary disease (COPD)	High-risk pregnancy	
Asthma	Sickle cell trait	
Low-risk pregnancy	Cerebrovascular diseases	
Controlled hypertension	Any cause for restricted pulmonary circulation	
Controlled seizure disorder	Seizure disorder (not receiving medication)	
Psychiatric disorders	Radial keratotomy (surgery of the cornea to improve near-sightedness)	
Neoplastic diseases		
Inflammatory conditions		

Source: From Hackett PH, Roach RC: High-altitude medicine. In Auerbach PS: Wilderness medicine, ed 6, St. Louis, 2012, Mosby Elsevier.

greater severity in children and young adults and is reported in equal proportions of males and females in these age groups.[98,109]

- *Physical fitness and exertion.* The onset and severity of high-altitude illness is independent of physical fitness; fitness does not accelerate altitude acclimatization. A high level of fitness does allow individuals to exert themselves more, but vigorous exertion on arrival at high altitude further exacerbates hypoxemia and hastens the onset of high-altitude illness.[104,110]

- *Medications and intoxicants.* Any substance that depresses ventilation and disrupts sleep patterns at altitude should be avoided because this will further exacerbate altitude-induced hypoxemia. These substances include alcohol, barbiturates, and opiates.[99,111]

- *Cold.* Exposure to cold ambient temperatures increases the risk for HAPE because cold increases the pulmonary arterial pressure.[112]

Pre-existing medical conditions are another factor related to high-altitude illness. It is important to note that when clinical studies are used to determine effective dose of medication for altitude illness, they generally include only healthy individuals without underlying medical problems. However, today many more high-altitude travelers and those who move their residence to higher altitudes have underlying diseases such as diabetes, hypertension, heart disease, or depression. The current medication recommendations for managing altitude illness may not be appropriate for these patients due to the potential for drug interactions and for those patients with renal and/or hepatic insufficiencies. A discussion of these issues can be found in a review article of the medications for the prevention and treatment of altitude illness (i.e., AMS, HAPE, and HACE) for healthy individuals and the drug selection and dosing for patients with underlying medical conditions.[112]

Figure 22-33 lists conditions that increase the likelihood of developing high altitude illness. Additionally, specific medical conditions known to increase susceptibility to high-altitude illness include:

- Cardiopulmonary congenital abnormalities: absent pulmonary artery, primary pulmonary hypertension, congenital heart defects
- Carotid artery surgery: irradiation or abolishing carotid bodies

High-Altitude Illness
Acute Mountain Sickness

AMS is a self-limited, nonspecific syndrome that is easily mistaken for a number of other conditions because of common symptoms, including influenza, hangover, exhaustion, and dehydration. A consensus panel defined AMS as the presence of headache in an unacclimatized person who has recently arrived at an altitude above 8,202 feet (2,500 m) and has one or more symptoms of AMS.[114] However, AMS can occur at levels as low as 6,562 feet (2,000 m). AMS has been viewed as a mild form of cerebral

Figure 22-33	Risk Categories of High Altitude Illness
Risk Category	**Description**
Low	■ Individuals with no prior history of altitude illness and ascending < 9,200 ft (2,800 m) ■ Individuals taking ≥ 2 day to arrive at 8,200 to 10,000 ft (2,500 to 3,000 m) with subsequent increases in sleeping elevation of less than 1,600 ft (500 m) per day
Moderate	■ Individuals with prior history of AMS and ascending to 8,200 to 9,100 ft (2,500 to 2,800 m) in 1 day ■ No history of AMS, but ascending > 9,100 ft (2,800 m) in 1 day ■ All individuals ascending > 1,600 ft (500 m) per day at altitudes above 10,000 ft (3,000 m)
High	■ History of AMS and ascending to ≥ 9,100 ft (2,800 m) in 1 day ■ All individuals with prior history of HAPE or HACE ■ All individuals ascending to > 11,500 ft (3,500 m) in 1 day ■ All individuals ascending > 1,600 ft (500 m) per day at altitudes above 11,500 ft (3,500 m) ■ Very rapid ascents

AMS, acute mountain sickness; HACE, high-altitude cerebral edema; HAPE, high-altitude pulmonary edema.
Source: Modified from Luk AM, McIntosh SE, Grissom et al. Wilderness Medical Society consensus guidelines for the prevention and treatment of acute altitude illness. Wilderness Environ Med 21:146-55;2010.

edema, often preceding both HACE and HAPE. At the other end of the spectrum, HACE is viewed as a severe form of AMS.[115,116] The majority of AMS cases do not progress to more severe forms of high-altitude illness unless there is continued exposure to higher altitude.

The hallmark symptom of AMS is a mild to severe, protracted headache believed to be caused by hypoxia-induced cerebral vasodilation.[117] Patients describe their headache as throbbing, as located in the occipital or temporal regions, and as worsening at night or on awakening. Other symptoms include nausea, vomiting, insomnia, dizziness, *lassitude* (weariness), fatigue, and difficulty sleeping. Malaise and lack of appetite may be present along with a decrease in urine output. It is important to recognize early symptoms of AMS so that continued ascent does not cause a preventable condition to progress into a severe form of HACE.

The onset of symptoms in AMS can occur as early as 1 hour after arriving at high altitude but typically occurs after 6 to 10 hours of exposure. Symptoms usually peak in 24 to 72 hours and subside in 3 to 7 days. If the onset of symptoms occurs beyond 3 days after arriving at altitude and does not include headache, and if oxygen therapy provides no benefit, the condition is probably not AMS.[98]

Assessment

If patients are alert, the key is to obtain a good medical history, including the onset and severity of symptoms, rate of ascent, duration of exposure, use of medications that may cause dehydration, use of alcohol, and level of physical exertion. Obtain vital signs, including pulse oximetry. Also, assess the status of any underlying medical condition, as determined by the medical history.

Because a headache is the most common finding with AMS, assess for location and quality. Cheyne-Stokes respirations are a common finding in individuals who have ascended above 10,000 feet (3,000 m). Findings of a dry cough and dyspnea on exertion are common at altitude and may not always be specific for AMS. Auscultate all lung fields because crackles are common with AMS. Assess neurologic function, and assess specifically for ataxia and excessive lethargy, as these symptoms are indicative of HACE.

Management

Descending 1,640 to 3,280 feet (500 to 1,000 m) will provide the quickest resolution of symptoms. Mild AMS will resolve on its own, but patients should avoid further ascent and any exertion until symptoms resolve. Provide analgesics for headache and antiemetics for nausea per local protocols. For moderate symptoms, descend to lower altitude and provide oxygen at 2 to 4 liters/minute by nasal cannula initially. Assess pulse oximetry for SaO_2 greater than 90%. If lower than 90%, titrate oxygen by 1 to 2 liters/minute and reassess. For patients with neurologic symptoms, see management of HACE. Patients with underlying medical problems exacerbated by altitude should be transported on oxygen for medical evaluation of their primary illness and the secondary development of high-altitude illness.

See **Figure 22-34** for a summary of the signs and symptoms, management, and prevention of AMS. See **Figure 22-35** for dosing recommendations for children with AMS.

High-Altitude Cerebral Edema

HACE is a very serious neurologic syndrome that can develop in individuals with AMS or HAPE. At altitudes above 8,000 feet (2,438 m), cerebral blood flow increases as a result of

Figure 22-34 High-Altitude Illness (AMS, HACE, HAPE): Signs, Symptoms, Treatment, and Prevention

Signs/Symptoms	Treatment	Prevention
Acute Mountain Sickness (AMS)		
Mild: Headache, nausea, dizziness, and fatigue in first 12 hours	Oxygen 1 to 2 liters/minute by nasal cannula, and/or descend 1700 to 3300 feet (500 to 1000 m); avoid further ascent until symptoms resolve; consider acetazolamide (125 mg PO bid) to speed acclimatization; give analgesics and antiemetics as needed	Ascend at slow rate; spend night at intermediate altitude; avoid overexertion; avoid direct transport to 9000 feet (2750 m) Consider acetazolamide 125 mg PO bid, starting day before ascent and continued for 2 days at maximum altitude Treat AMS early
Moderate: Moderate to severe headache, marked nausea, vomiting, decreased appetite, dizziness, insomnia, fluid retention for ≥ 12 hours	Descend, consider dexamethasone (4 mg PO/IM every 6 hours) and/or acetazolamide (250 mg PO bid); if unable to descend, vigilant observation for deterioration; oxygen (1 to 2 liters/minute) and/or portable hyperbaric therapy (2 to 4 psi) for a few hours if available	Same as listed above. Dexamethasone 2 mg q 6 hours, or 4 mg q 12 hours PO, starting day of ascent and discontinued cautiously after 2 days at maximum altitude
High-Altitude Cerebral Edema (HACE)		
AMS for ≥ 24 hours, ataxia, confusion, bizarre behavior, severe lassitude	Immediately descend or evacuate ≥ 3300 foot (1000 m); give oxygen 2 to 4 liters/minute; titrate to maintain SaO_2 ≥ 90% with pulse oximetry; dexamethasone (8 mg IV/IM/PO initially, then 4 mg q 6 hours); hyperbaric therapy if cannot descend	As listed above for AMS
High-Altitude Pulmonary Edema (HAPE)		
Dyspnea at rest, moist cough, rales, severe exercise limitation, cyanosis, drowsiness, tachycardia, tachypnea, desaturation	Start oxygen 4 to 6 liters/minute, then titrate to maintain SaO_2 ≥ 90% with pulse oximetry; minimize exertion; keep warm; descend or evacuate 1700 to 3300 feet (500 to 1000 m); consider nifedipine (30 mg sustained-release PO q 12 hours or 20 mg of sustained-release every 8 hours) if no HACE; consider inhaled beta-agonists (salmeterol, 125 mcg inhaled q 12 hours, or albuterol); consider EPAP mask; dexamethasone only if HACE develops	Ascend at a slow rate; avoid overexertion; consider nifedipine (30-mg sustained-release dose every 12 hours bid PO or 20 mg sustained-release every 8 hours) in person with repeated episodes of HAPE; start 1 day prior to ascent and continue for 2 days at maximum altitude

bid, twice daily; EPAP, expiratory positive airway pressure; IM, intramuscular; IV, intravascular; m, meter; mcg, microgram; mg, milligram; PO, by mouth; psi, pounds per square inch; q, every; SaO_2, arterial oxygen saturation.
Source: Modified from Luk AM, McIntosh SE, Grissom et al. Wilderness Medical Society consensus guidelines for the prevention and treatment of acute altitude illness. Wilderness Environ Med 21:146-55;2010.

hypoxia-induced vasodilation. The mechanism of injury appears to be related to a combination of sustained cerebral vasodilation, increased capillary permeability across the blood–brain barrier, and the inability to compensate sufficiently for the excess cerebral edema.[118]

HACE can occur within 3 to 5 days after arrival at 9,022 feet (2,750 m), but generally it occurs at altitudes above 12,000 feet (3,600 m), with an onset of symptoms within hours. Some mild to moderate symptoms of AMS may be present, but the hallmark features of HACE are altered level of

| **Figure 22-35** | **Drug Dosing for Children With Altitude Illness[113]** |

In 2001, the International Society for Mountain Medicine published a consensus statement recommending that adult treatment algorithms (for AMS, HACE, and HAPE) be followed with adjustments for pediatric drug dosages.

AMS	Acetazolamide 2.5 mg/kg/dose PO q 12 hours (maximum 125 mg per dose)
	Dexamethasone 0.15 mg/kg/dose PO q 6 hours up to 4 mg
HACE	Acetazolamide 2.5 mg/kg/dose PO q 12 hours (maximum 125 mg per dose)
HAPE	Dexamethasone 0.15 mg/kg/dose PO q 6 hours up to 4 mg

kg, kilogram; mg, milligram; PO, by mouth; q, every.
Source: From Pollard AJ, Niermeyer S, Barry PB, Bartsch P, Berghold F, Bishop RA, et al: Children at high altitude: An international consensus statement by an ad hoc committee of the International Society for Mountain Medicine. High Alt Med Biol 2001:2:389–401.); Luk AM, McIntosh SE, Grissom et al. Wilderness Medical Society consensus guidelines for the prevention and treatment of acute altitude illness. Wilderness Environ Med 21:1146–55;2010

consciousness and ataxia, along with drowsiness, stupor, and irrational behavior progressing to coma. Death results from brain herniation.[119]

Assessment

If patients are alert, as with AMS, the key in patients with HACE is to obtain a good medical history, including the onset and severity of symptoms, rate of ascent, duration of exposure, and level of physical exertion. Obtain the patient's vital signs, including pulse oximetry. Also, assess the status of any underlying medical condition, as determined by the patient's medical history. It is important to assess the patient's lung sounds because a strong association exists between HACE and HAPE.

Management

Do not delay planning for treatment and evacuation at the first signs or symptoms of HACE. The highest priority for any patient with HACE is immediate descent, along with initiation of high-flow oxygen (15 liters/minute) by nonrebreathing mask and monitoring of SaO$_2$ until 90% or greater. Unconscious patients should be managed as a patient with head injury (see the Airway and Ventilation and the Head Trauma chapters), including intubation and other ALS procedures.[111]

See **Figure 22-34** for a summary of the signs and symptoms, management, and prevention of HACE. See **Figure 22-35** for dosing recommendations for children with HACE.

High-Altitude Pulmonary Edema

The onset of HAPE follows a pattern similar to that seen with AMS and HACE, occurring in unacclimatized individuals after a rapid ascent to high altitude. This high-altitude illness has a different mechanism of injury than AMS and HACE, however, because HAPE is induced by hypobaric hypoxia. HAPE is a form of noncardiogenic pulmonary edema associated with pulmonary hypertension and elevated capillary pressure.[107] More than 50% of patients with HAPE have AMS, and 14% have HACE.[120] The signs and symptoms generally appear during the second night (onset

of 1 to 3 days) and rarely occur 4 days after arriving at a given altitude.[121] The development of HAPE and the rate of progression are hastened by cold exposure, vigorous exertion, and continued ascent. Compared with the other two high-altitude illnesses, HAPE accounts for the greatest number of fatalities.

Assessment

Patient assessment, including vital signs, lung sounds, and medical history, are vital in the determination of HAPE, which is defined by at least two or more symptoms (e.g., dyspnea at rest, cough, weakness, or decreased exertion performance; chest tightness or congestion) and at least two signs (e.g., crackles or wheezing, central cyanosis, tachypnea, or tachycardia).[122] Rales are generally present in the lung fields, starting in the right axilla and eventually becoming bilateral. Assess the patient for fever, which is a common sign with HAPE. Late findings as HAPE progresses are resting tachycardia, tachypnea, and blood-tinged sputum. If treatment interventions are not provided, symptoms will progress over hours to days to include audible gurgling, respiratory distress, and eventually death.

Management

Descending to a lower altitude by at least 1,640 to 3,280 feet (500 to 1,000 m) provides the fastest recovery, but initially patients show good improvement with rest and oxygen. Keep patients warm, and prevent any exertion. These patients need to improve their arterial oxygenation, so start oxygen at 4 to 6 liters/minute or titrate oxygen flow until SaO$_2$ is 90% or greater. Reassess the patient's vital signs after starting oxygen because improved arterial oxygenation decreases the tachycardia and tachypnea. As HAPE is a form of noncardiogenic pulmonary edema, diuretics have not been shown to be helpful. Anecdotal case reports have suggested favorable results with the use of continuous positive airway pressure (CPAP) for serious cases of HAPE; however, specific research is lacking and such equipment is often not available in the environment most likely to be associated with HAPE.[123,124]

See **Figure 22-34** for a summary of the signs and symptoms, management, and prevention of HAPE. See **Figure 22-35** for dosing recommendations for children with HAPE.

Prevention

Acute high-altitude illness in unacclimatized individuals is preventable. The common factor for the onset of AMS, HACE, and HAPE is the rate of ascent to higher altitude. Altitude illness may be experienced by skiers who travel by commercial airlines and take an early morning flight from cities at sea level, arrive at high altitude around noon, and begin skiing by early afternoon at about 7,000 to 14,000 feet (2,100 to 4,500 m). Another scenario with risk of high-altitude illness is a call for mutual aid to various public safety personnel living below 3,300 feet (1,000 m). They assemble quickly and then arrive at 9,000 feet (2,750 m) or higher to assist local volunteer search-and-rescue teams trekking to higher altitudes in search of a missing backcountry hiker. Prehospital care personnel, whether ground crew or flight crew, who have responsibilities at high altitude for patient transfer to another hospital or for medical evacuation from the backcountry need to possess the knowledge to minimize the risk of high-altitude illness for their own safety and the safety of coworkers (**Figures 22-36** and **22-37**).

Medications as Prophylaxis for High-Altitude Illness

For the prevention of AMS and HACE, individuals traveling from sea level to over 9,850 feet (3,000 m) as their sleeping altitude in 1 day or individuals who have a history of AMS should consider prophylactic treatment. The drug of choice is oral acetazolamide (Diamox), 125 to 250 mg twice daily, beginning 1 day before ascent and continuing for 2 days at maximum altitude. The alternative drug is dexamethasone (Decadron), 2 mg orally or intramuscularly (IM) every 6 hours and continuing for 2 days at maximum altitude. The combination of both drugs has been shown to be more effective than either drug alone.[111,112] Aspirin (325 mg) taken every 4 hours for three doses reduced the incidence of headache from 50% to 7%.[115]

Recent research clearly demonstrated the advances of prophylactic use of ibuprofen 600 mg three times per day beginning 6 hours before ascending from 4,100 feet (1,250 m) up to 12,570 feet (3,800 m) as compared to a placebo treatment. The study reported that 43% of the participants in the ibuprofen group reported the development of AMS compared with 69% in the placebo group. Also, the placebo group reported that the severity of AMS was worse than reported in the ibuprofen group.[125] The benefit for using ibuprofen is that it provides a second-choice medication and can be taken the same day of ascent with no or low side effects when compared to the traditional use of acetazolamide for the prevention of AMS.[125]

For the prevention of HAPE in individuals with a history of repeated episodes, prophylaxis with oral nifedipine, 20 to 30 mg

Figure 22-36   Altitude Acclimatization Procedures

The following are key points for acclimatizing to high altitude:

- Ascend high enough to induce adaptions, but not so high as to develop altitude illness.
- Unacclimatized individuals should not ascend above 7,800 feet (2,400 m).
- Stage for 7 to 14 days between 4,600 and 6,500 feet (1,400 to 2,000 m).
- Stage for 4 to 6 days between heights of 6,500 and 7,800 feet (2,000 to 2,400 m).
- Staging reduces AMS incidence for altitudes 3,300 to 6,500 feet (1,000 to 2,000 m) above the staging altitude.
- Graded ascents above 7,800 feet (2,400 m) should not exceed 1,000 feet/day (300 m/day).
- Graded ascents greater than 1,000 feet/day (300 m/day) should include a rest day at each higher altitude.
- Avoid heavy exertion for the first 3 days.
- Keep well hydrated with water.
- Avoid alcohol, sleeping pills, and other sedatives.
- Eat a high-carbohydrate diet.
- Avoid overexertion.
- Avoid smoking.
- Physical training is not preventive for high-altitude illness.

Figure 22-37   Golden Rules of High-Altitude Illness

The "golden rules" of high-altitude illness are as follows:

1. If you are ill at altitude, your symptoms are caused by the altitude until proved otherwise.
2. If you have altitude symptoms, do not go any higher.
3. If you are feeling ill or are getting worse, or if you cannot walk heel to toe in a straight line, descend immediately.
4. A person ill with altitude illness must always be accompanied by a responsible companion who can accomplish or arrange for descent should it become necessary.[111]

(extended-release formulation) every 12 hours, is recommended. Currently, prophylactic treatment should be avoided as a method to prevent altitude illness in children because of insufficient clinical studies.[126]

Prolonged Transport

Drowning

Asymptomatic patients can become symptomatic in an extended-care situation with a delay of 4 hours before pulmonary symptoms. Initiate CPR for a drowning victim with five continuous breaths using the traditional ABC approach, not CAB, to begin correcting hypoxia. Obtain a pulse oximetry reading before and after administration of oxygen. Provide high-flow oxygen via a nonrebreathing mask at 15 liters/minute.

Any patient with pulse oximetry values less than 90%, altered mental status, apnea, or coma may require early active airway management to protect from aspiration. Any patient who continues to be hypoxic with pulse oximetry readings less than 85% after administration of high-flow oxygen is a candidate for CPAP or rapid-sequence intubation protocol. Liberal use of suction through the endotracheal tube is necessary to remove pulmonary secretions and water aspirated during submersion. Consult with medical control, if available, to sedate and paralyze the patient (if permitted by protocols) to ensure successful intubation, oxygenation, and effective ventilation.

Another effective method to ensure effective oxygenation and ventilation is the use of positive end-expiratory pressure (PEEP) in apneic submersion patients.[34,39] PEEP increases the diameter of small and large airways and improves the ventilatory–perfusion ratio and arterial oxygenation.

Determine the patient's GCS score and assess routinely for trends because it is predictive of patient outcome. Monitor for hypothermia and hypoglycemia. Any comatose patient should have his or her blood glucose measured or, if unable, receive IV dextrose. The placement of a nasogastric tube may be needed to reduce gastric content and water swallowed during submersion.

Lightning Injury

Victims of lightning maybe in respiratory arrest, cardiac arrest, or both. Following CAB assessment, initiate CPR rapidly. When in an extended-care situation with multiple victims, use *reverse triage* and resuscitate those who appear dead first. However, prolonged (multiple hours) CPR on these victims has a poor patient outcome, and there is little benefit from CPR or ACLS procedures lasting longer than 20 to 30 minutes. All measures to stabilize the patient to correct for hypoxia, hypovolemia, hypothermia, and acidosis should be attempted before terminating resuscitative efforts.[2]

Assess the patient for cerebral edema and increased intracranial pressure (ICP). Establish a baseline GCS score, and reassess the patient every 10 minutes as an indicator of progressive cerebral edema and increased ICP (manage per recommendation for cerebral edema; see the Head Trauma chapter).

Recreational Scuba-Related Diving Injuries

The standard treatment protocol for scuba-related injuries causing pulmonary overpressurization syndrome (e.g., AGE, DCS) is to provide high-flow oxygen (15 liters/minute via nonrebreathing mask) at the scene and continue oxygen therapy during transport of the patient to the closest recompression chamber for hyperbaric oxygen (HBO) therapy. Conduct an extensive neurologic evaluation, and reassess the patient frequently for progression of signs and symptoms. Use analgesics for pain control per local protocols. Also consider giving aspirin (325 or 650 mg) for its antiplatelet activity.[70]

Use Divers Alert Network (DAN, telephone 919-684-9111) and local medical control for the closest location of a functional recompression chamber. Before transporting a patient for HBO therapy, contact the chamber directly because the status of chamber readiness can change without notification. When transporting by air, use aircraft that can preferably maintain sea-level atmosphere during flight. Any nonpressurized aircraft should maintain an altitude below 1,000 feet (300 m) en route to the chamber site.

High-Altitude Illness

Mild to moderate AMS can be managed with low-volume oxygen at 2 to 4 liters/minute by nasal cannula, titrated by 1 to 2 liters/minute (greater than 90% SaO_2), with a combination of analgesics (e.g., aspirin, 650 mg; acetaminophen, 650 to 1,000 mg; ibuprofen, 600 mg) for headache and prochlorperazine (5 to 10 mg IM) for nausea. Other medications used for treating mild to moderate AMS include oral acetazolamide (250 mg twice daily) and dexamethasone (4 mg orally [PO] or IM every 6 hours) until symptoms resolve.

Treat HACE with descent to a lower level, oxygen at 2 to 4 liters/minute by nasal cannula, to maintain greater than 90% SaO_2, and with dexamethasone (8 mg PO, IV, or IM initially, then 4 mg every 6 hours). Consider using oral acetazolamide (250 mg twice daily) with prolonged delays to descent.

If a severe form of HACE develops and the patient is comatose, manage according to recommendations for cerebral edema (see the Shock chapter). Prolonged management of HAPE primarily consists of administering oxygen at 4 to 6 liters/minute by nasal cannula (greater than 90% SaO_2) until improvement of symptoms, then 2 to 4 liters/minute for conserving oxygen. If oxygen is not available, give oral nifedipine (10 mg initially, then 30 mg extended-release dose every 12 to 24 hours). If the patient acquires HACE, add dexamethasone (8 mg PO or IM every 6 hours).

Use of portable hyperbaric chambers, such as the Gamow bag (Altitude Technologies), has been successful for treating high-altitude illness.[99] These lightweight, fabric pressure bags simulate descending to a lower altitude with or without the use of supplemental oxygen or medication (e.g., acetazolamide, dexamethasone, nifedipine). They inflate with manual pumps up to 2 psi, which is equivalent to descending 5,250 feet (1,600 m), depending on the initial altitude. The use of these chambers for 2 to 3 hours can effectively improve symptoms. This is an ideal use of technology while waiting for transportation to definitive care.

Summary

- Prehospital care providers will inevitably be faced with unpredictable environmental encounters, such as those described in this chapter.
- Basic knowledge of common environmental emergencies is necessary so that rapid assessment and treatment in the prehospital setting can be provided.
- It is not easy to remember this type of information because these problems are not frequently encountered. Therefore, remember the general principles involved, as follows:
    - *Drowning.* Assume all drowning patients have pulmonary distress until proved otherwise; correct hypoxia, acidosis, and hypothermia as indicated.
    - *Lightning.* Patients with severe lightning injury need rapid assessment of cardiopulmonary status. Use the *reverse triage* principle for multiple victims. Initiating CPR early is the key to survival.
    - *Recreational scuba-related diving injuries.* Patients with severe decompression sickness and arterial gas embolism need high-flow oxygen and rapid treatment in a recompression chamber for the best outcome. Consult early with medical control and Divers Alert Network (919-684-9111).
    - *High-altitude illness.* Key interventions for acute mountain sickness and high-altitude cerebral or pulmonary edema are to descend at least 1,640 to 3,280 feet in altitude (500 to 1,000 m) and provide rest and oxygen.
- In every case, remember that personal safety must be maintained. There are too many cases in which prehospital care providers and other emergency responders have lost their lives as a result of attempting a rescue.

SCENARIO RECAP

In a coastal town, a family of four was strolling on the beach with their dog during a chilly winter day. The son tossed a rubber ball toward the water's edge, and the dog gave chase. In an instant, a large shore-breaking wave swallowed up the dog in the rough surf. The 17-year-old son was first into the water to attempt to save the dog, only to be overtaken by the water. He was seen struggling in the rough surging surf by his parents and sister.

The boy's father and mother both followed him into the surf in an effort to help. Their 19-year-old daughter remained on shore and called for help on her cell phone. The dog eventually made it back to the shore. The parents were able to pull their son out of the cold water after finding him submerged and unresponsive. Your paramedic unit arrives to the scene within 7 minutes of the daughter's call.

As you exit the ambulance, you observe an unconscious teenage boy lying partially facedown in sand with surging water close by. He is still in the surf zone and could be submersed by a wave. You team up with arriving fire department emergency responders to approach the victim.

- How should you approach the patient in this setting?
- If the patient has no pulse or respirations, what is the next immediate intervention?
- What other concerns do you have for the patient that need to be addressed on scene?

SCENARIO SOLUTION

Your plan is to have one fire fighter serve as a lookout for a threat of oncoming surf and for you, your partner, and two other fire fighters to approach the victim to pick him up by all four extremities and quickly carry him away from the surging waves.

As the lead prehospital care provider, you direct the team to place the victim supine, parallel to the shore, so that the head and trunk are at the same level and then immediately check for responsiveness. The other emergency responders begin staging the emergency medical gear near the victim as you check the ABCs. The patient may be apneic and need only rescue breathing or may need full CPR. In either situation, you know that the recommendation for drowning is now to provide five rescue breaths initially followed by 30 chest compressions and then to continue two breaths and 30 compressions until signs of life appear.

The initial approach to the ABCs in drowning victims is essential to address the hypoxia. High-flow oxygen is provided using a bag-mask device. You start an IV with crystalloids. In this case, spinal immobilization is not needed since there was no mechanism of injury to suspect spinal trauma. Early intubation or mechanical ventilation (e.g., CPAP) may be indicated if the victim shows signs of deterioration with SpO_2 less than 90%. You transport the patient and his parents to the hospital for continued treatment and evaluation.

References

1. Curran EB, Holle RL, Lopez RE. Lightning fatalities, injuries and damage reports in the United States, 1959–1994. NOAA Tech Memo NWS SR-193, 1997.

2. Gatewood MO, Zane RD. Lightning injuries. *Emerg Med Clin North Am.* 2004;22:369.

3. Huffins GR, Orville RE. Lightning ground flash density and thunderstorm duration in the contiguous United States. *J Appl Meteorol.* 1999;38:1013.

4. Cummins KL, Krider EP, Malone MD. A combined TOA/MDF technology upgrade of the U.S. National Lightning Detection Network. *J Geophys Res.* 1998;103:9035.

5. MacGorman, DR, Rust WD. Lightning strike density for the contiguous United States from thunderstorm duration records, Pub No NUREG/CR03759. Washington, DC: Office of Nuclear Regulatory Research; 1984.

6. Dulcos PJ, Sanderson LM, Klontz KC. Lightning-related mortality and morbidity in Florida. *Pub Health Rep.* 1990;105:276.

7. National Oceanic and Atmospheric Administration. Severe Weather 101. Lightning. http://www.nssl.noaa.gov/education/svrwx101/lightning/faq/ Accessed January 24, 2014.

8. Holle R. Annual rates of lightning fatalities by country, 2008. Tucson, AZ: International Lighting Detection Conference; 2008. http://www.vaisala.com/Vaisala%20Documents/Scientific%20papers/Annual_rates_of_lightning_fatalities_by_country.pdf. Accessed January 17, 2014.

9. Cherington M, Walker J, Boyson M, Glancy R, Hedegaard H, Clark S. Closing the gap on the actual numbers of lightning casualties and deaths. 11th Conference on Applied Climatology. Dallas, TX: American Meterological Society; 1999:379–380.

10. Cooper MA, Holle RL, Andrews CJ, Blumenthal R. Lightning injuries. In: Auerbach PS, ed. *Wilderness Medicine.* 6th ed. St. Louis, MO: Mosby Elsevier; 2012.

11. Davis C, Engeln A, Johnson E, et al. The Wilderness Medical Society practice guidelines for the prevention and treatment of lightning injuries. *Wilderness & Environ Med.* 2012;23:260–269.

12. Cooper MA. Lightning injuries: prognostic signs of death. *Ann Emerg Med.* 1980;9:134.

13. Centers for Disease Control and Prevention. Lightning associated deaths: 1980–1995. *MMWR.* 1998;47(19):391.

14. Andrews CJ, Darveniza M, Mackerras D. Lightning injury: a review of the clinical aspects, pathophysiology and treatment. *Adv Trauma.* 1989;4:241.

15. Vanden Hoek TL, Morrison LJ, Shuster M, et al. 2010 American Heart Association guidelines for cardiopulmonary resuscitation and emergency cardiovascular care: Part 12.12: Cardiac arrest associated with electric shock and lightning strikes. *Circulation.* 2010;122:848.

16. Ritenour AE, Morton MJ, McManus JG, Barillo DJ, Cancio LC. Lightning injury: a review. *Burns.* 2008;34:585.

17. Beir M, Chen W, Bodnar E, Lee RC. Biophysical injury mechanisms associated with lightning injury. *Neurorehabilitation.* 2005;20(1):53.

18. Cooper MA. Electrical and lightning injuries. *Emerg Med Clin North Am.* 1984;2:489.

19. Casten JA, Kytilla J. Eye symptoms caused by lightning. *Acta Ophthalmol.* 1963;41:139.

20. Kleiner JP, Wilkin JH. Cardiac effects of lightning stroke. *JAMA.* 1978240:2757.

21. Taussig HB. Death from lightning and the possibility of living again. *Ann Intern Med.* 1968;68:1345.

22. Zimmerman C, Cooper MA, Holle RL. Lightning safety guidelines. *Ann Emerg Med.* 2002;39:660.

23. National Lightning Safety Institute. Personal lightning safety. http://www.lightningsafety.com/nlsi_pls.html. Accessed January 17, 2014.

24. National Weather Service. Lightning risk reduction outdoors. http://www.lightningsafety.noaa.gov/outdoors.htm. Accessed January 17, 2014.

25. Zafren K, Durrer B, Henry JP, Brugger H. Lightning injuries: prevention and on-site treatment in mountains and remote areas—official guidelines of the International Commission for Mountain Emergency Medicine and Medical Commission of the International Mountaineering and Climbing Federation (ICAR and UIAA MEDCOM). *Resuscitation.* 2005;65:369.

26. National Oceanic and Atmospheric Administration. Lightning safety myths and truths. http://www.lightningsafety.noaa.gov/myths.htm Accessed January 24, 2014

27. National Oceanic and Atmospheric Administration. Lightning risk reduction outdoors. http://www.lightningsafety.noaa.gov/outdoors.htm. Accessed January 24, 2014.

28. Peden M, Oyegbite K, Ozanne-Smith J, et al., eds. World report on child injury prevention. Geneva, Switzerland: World Health Organization; 2008.

29. Centers for Disease Control and Prevention. Nonfatal and fatal drowning in recreational water settings—United States, 2005–2009. *MMWR*. 2012;61(19):345.

30. Centers for Disease Control and Prevention. Drowning—United States, 2005–2009. *MMWR*. 2012;61(19);344–347.

31. Zuckerman GB, Conway EE Jr. Drowning and near-drowning. *Pediatr Ann*. 2000;29:6.

32. World Health Organization. Facts about injuries: drowning. http://www.who.int/violence_injury_prevention/publications/other_injury/en/drowning_factsheet.pdf. Accessed January 17, 2014.

33. University of Minnesota. Unintentional drowning. http://blog.lib.umn.edu/spon0024/unintentional_drowning/01-introduction.html. Accessed September 18, 2013.

34. Cushing TA, Hawking SC, Sempsrott J, Schoene RB. Submersion injuries and drowning. In: Auerbach PS, ed. *Wilderness Medicine*. 6th ed. St. Louis, MO: Mosby Elsevier; 2012.

35. DeNicola LK, Falk JL, Swanson ME, Kissoon N. Submersion injuries in children and adults. *Crit Care Clin*. 1997;13(3):477.

36. Olshaker JS. Near-drowning. *Emerg Med Clin North Am*. 1992;10(2):339.

37. Van Beeck EF, Branche CM, Szpilman D, et al. A new definition of drowning: towards documentation and prevention of a global public health program. *Bull World Health Organ*. 2005;83:853–856.

38. Szpilman D, Bierens JLM, Handley A, Orlowshi JP. Drowning. *New Engl J Med*. 2012;366:2102-2110.

39. Olshaker JS. Submersion. *Emerg Med Clin North Am*. 2004;22:357.

40. Kyriacou DN, Arcinue EL, Peek C, Kraus JF. Effect of immediate resuscitation on children with submersion injury. *Pediatrics*. 1994;94:137.

41. Moran K, Quan L, Franklin R, Bennett E. Where the evidence and expert opinion meet: a review of the open-water recreational safety messages. *Int J Aquatic Res Educ*. 2011;5:251–270.

42. Lavelle JM. Ten-year review of pediatric bathtub near-drownings: evaluation for child abuse and neglect. *Ann Emerg Med*. 1995;25:344.

43. Rowe MI, Arango A, Allington G. Profile of pediatric drowning victims in a water-oriented society. *J Trauma*. 1977;17:587.

44. Craig AB Jr. Underwater swimming and loss of consciousness. *JAMA*. 1961;176:255.

45. Jensen LR, Williams SD, Thurman DJ, Keller PA. Submersion injuries in children younger than 5 years in urban Utah. *West J Med*. 1992;157:641.

46. Howland J, Smith GS, Mangione TW, et al. Why are most drowning victims men? Sex differences, aquatic skills and behaviors. *Am J Public Health*. 1996;86:93.

47. Schuman SH, Rowe JR, Glazer HM, et al. The iceberg phenomenon of near-drowning. *Crit Care Med*. 1976;4:127.

48. Howland J, Mangione T, Hingson R, et al. Alcohol as a risk factor for drowning and other aquatic injuries. In: Watson RR, ed. *Alcohol and Accidents: Drug and Alcohol Abuse Reviews*. Vol 7. Totowa, NJ: Humana Press, Inc; 1995.

49. Howland J, Hingson R. Alcohol as a risk factor for drownings: a review of the literature (1950–1985). *Accid Anal Prev*. 1988;20(1):19–25.

50. Howland J, Smith GS, Mangione T, et al. Missing the boat on drinking and boating. *JAMA*. 1993;270:91.

51. Bell GS, Gaitatzis A, Bell CL, Johnson AL, Sander JW. Drowning in people with epilepsy. *Neurology*. 2008;71:578.

52. Karch KB. Pathology of the lung in near-drowning. *Am J Emerg Med*. 1986;4(1):4.

53. Orlowski JP. Drowning, near-drowning, and ice water submersion. *Pediatr Clin North Am*. 1987;34(1):75.

54. Modell JH, Moya F. Effects of volume of aspirated fluid during chlorinated fresh-water drowning. *Anesthesiology*. 1966;27:663.

55. Giesbrecht GG, Steinman AM. Immersion into cold water. In: Auerbach PS, ed. *Wilderness Medicine*. 6th ed. St. Louis, MO: Mosby Elsevier; 2012.

56. Bolte RG, Black PG, Bowers RS. The use of extracorporeal rewarming in a child submerged for 66 minutes. *JAMA*. 1988;260:377.

57. Lloyd EL. Accidental hypothermia. *Resuscitation*. 1996;32:111.

58. Gilbert M, Busund R, Skagseth A. Resuscitation from accidental hypothermia of 13.7°C with circulatory arrest. *Lancet*. 2000;355:375.

59. Siebke H, Breivik H, Rod T, et al. Survival after 40 minutes submersion without cerebral sequelae. *Lancet*. 1975;1:1275.

60. Abella BS, Alvarado JP, Myklebust H, et al. Quality of cardiopulmonary resuscitation during in-hospital cardiac arrest. *JAMA*. 2005;293(3):305.

61. Wik L, Kramer-Johansen J, Myklebust H, et al. Quality of cardiopulmonary resuscitation during out-of-hospital cardiac arrest. *JAMA*. 2005;293(3):299.

62. Sayre MR, Koster RW, Botha M, et al. Part 5: adult basic life support. In: *2010 International Consensus on Cardiopulmonary Resuscitation and Emergency Cardiovascular Care Science With Treatment Recommendations. Circulation*. 2010;122:S298–S324.

63. Hwang V, Frances S, Durbin D, et al. Prevalence of traumatic injuries in drowning and near-drowning in children and adolescents. *Arch Pediatr Adolesc Med*. 2003;157(1):50–53.

64. Pratt FD, Haynes BE. Incidence of "secondary drowning" after saltwater submersion. *Ann Emerg Med*. 1986;15(9):1084.

65. Berg RA, Hemphill R, Abella BS, et al. Part 5: adult basic life support. In: *2010 American Heart Association Guidelines for Cardiopulmonary Resuscitation and Emergency Cardiovascular Care. Circulation*. 2010;122:S685–S705.

66. Rosen P, Stoto M, Harley J. The use of the Heimlich maneuver in near-drowning: Institute of Medicine report. *J Emerg Med*. 1995;13:397.

67. Wilderness Medical Society. Submersion injuries. In: Forgey WW. Practice Guidelines for Wilderness Emergency Care. 5th ed. Helena, MT: Globe Pequot Press; 2006.

68. http://www.aap.org/en-us/about-the-aap/aap-press-room/Pages/AAP-Gives-Updated-Advice-on-Drowning-Prevention.aspx Accessed January 24, 2014

69. Melamed Y, Shupak A, Bitterman H. Medical problems associated with underwater diving. *N Engl J Med*. 1992;326:30.

70. Van Hoesen KB, Bird NH. Diving medicine. In: Auerbach PS, ed. *Wilderness Medicine*. 6th ed. St. Louis, MO: Mosby Elsevier; 2012.

71. Salahuddin M, James LA, Bass ES. SCUBA medicine: a first-responder's guide to diving injuries. *Curr Sports Med Rep*. 2011;10(3):134–139.

72. Lynch JA, Bove AA. Diving medicine: a review of the current evidence. *J Am Board Fam Med*. 2009;22:399–407.

73. Strauss MB, Borer RC Jr. Diving medicine: contemporary topics and their controversies. *Am J Emerg Med*. 2001;19:232.

74. Morgan WP. Anxiety and panic in recreational scuba divers. *Sports Med.* 1995;20(6):398.

75. Divers Alert Network (DAN). Eleven-year trends (1987–1997) in diving activity: the DAN annual review of recreational SCUBA diving injuries and fatalities based on 2000 data. In: *Report on Decompression Illness, Diving Fatalities and Project Dive Exploration.* Durham, NC: Divers Alert Network; 2000:17–29.

76. Divers Alert Network. *Annual Diving Report.* Durham, NC: Divers Alert Network; 2008.

77. Divers Alert Network (DAN). *Report on Diving Fatalities: 2008 Edition.* Durham, NC: Divers Alert Network; 2008.

78. Hardy KR. Diving-related emergencies. *Emerg Med Clin North Am.* 1997;15(1):223.

79. Green SM. Incidence and severity of middle-ear barotraumas in recreational scuba diving. *J Wilderness Med.* 1993;4:270.

80. Kizer KW. Dysbaric cerebral air embolism in Hawaii. *Ann Emerg Med.* 1987;16:535.

81. Cales RH, Humphreys N, Pilmanis AA, Heilig RW. Cardiac arrest from gas embolism in scuba diving. *Ann Emerg Med.* 1981;10(11):589.

82. Butler BD, Laine GA, Leiman BC, et al. Effect of Trendelenburg position on the distribution of arterial air emboli in dogs. *Ann Thorac Surg.* 1988;45(2):198.

83. Moon RE. Treatment of diving emergencies. *Crit Care Clin.* 1999;15:429.

84. Van Meter K. Medical field management of the injured diver. *Respir Care Clin North Am.* 1997;5(1):137.

85. Francis TJ, Dutka AJ, Hallenbeck JM. Pathophysiology of decompression sickness. In: Bove AA, Davis JC, eds. *Diving Medicine.* 2nd ed. Philadelphia, PA: Saunders; 1990.

86. Neuman TS. DCI/DCS: does it matter whether the emperor wears clothes? *Undersea Hyperb Med.* 1997;24:2.

87. Bove AA. Nomenclature of pressure disorders. *Undersea Hyperb Med.* 1997;24:1.

88. Spira A. Diving and marine medicine review. Part II. Diving diseases. *J Travel Med.* 1999;6:180.

89. Clenney TL, Lassen LF. Recreational scuba diving injuries. *Am Fam Physician.* 1996;53(5):1761.

90. Kizer KW. Women and diving. *Physician Sportsmed.* 1981;9(2):84.

91. Francis TJ, Dutka AJ, Hallenbeck JM. Pathophysiology of decompression sickness. In: Bove AA, Davis JC, eds. *Diving Medicine.* 2nd ed. Philadelphia, PA: Saunders; 1990.

92. Greer HD, Massey EW. Neurologic injury from undersea diving. *Neurol Clin.* 1992;10(4):1031.

93. Kizer KW. Management of dysbaric diving casualties. *Emerg Med Clin North Am.* 1983;1:659.

94. Department of the Navy. *U.S. Navy Diving Manual.* Vol 1, Rev 4. Washington, DC: U.S. Government Printing Office; 1999.

95. Davis JC. Hyperbaric medicine: critical care aspects. In: Shoemaker WC, ed. *Critical Care: State of the Art.* Aliso Viejo, CA: Society of Critical Care Medicine; 1984.

96. Pollock NW, Uguccioni DM, Dear GdeL, eds. Diabetes and recreational diving: guidelines for the future. Proceedings of the Undersea and Hyperbaric Medical Society/Divers Alert Network. June 19, 2005, Workshop. Durham, NC: Divers Alert Network; 2005.

97. Gallagher SA, Hackett PH. High-altitude illness. *Emerg Med Clin North Am.* 2004;22:329.

98. Hackett PH, Roach RC. High-altitude illness. *N Engl J Med.* 2001;345(2):107.

99. Hackett PH, Roach RC. High-altitude medicine. In: Auerbach PS, ed. *Wilderness Medicine.* 6th ed. St. Louis, MO: Mosby Elsevier; 2012.

100. Houston CS. High-altitude illness disease with protean manifestations. *JAMA.* 1976;236:2193.

101. Montgomery AB, Mills J, Luce JM. Incidence of acute mountain sickness at intermediate altitude. *JAMA.* 1989;261:732.

102. Gertsch JH, Seto TB, Mor J, Onopa J. Ginkgo biloba for the prevention of severe acute mountain sickness (AMS) starting day one before rapid ascent. *High Alt Med Biol.* 2002;3(1):29.

103. Tso E. High-altitude illness. *Emerg Clin North Am.* 1992;10(2):231.

104. Honigman B, Theis MK, Koziol-McLain J, et al. Acute mountain sickness in a general tourist population at moderate altitudes. *Ann Intern Med.* 1993;118(8):587.

105. Zaphren K, Honigman B. High-altitude medicine. *Emerg Clin North Am.* 1997;15(1):191.

106. Hultgren HN. *High-Altitude Medicine.* Stanford, CA: Hultgren Publications; 1997.

107. Schneider M, Bernasch D, Weymann J, et al. Acute mountain sickness: influence of susceptibility, pre-exposure, and ascent rate. *Med Sci Sports Exerc.* 2002;34(12):1886.

108. Bartsch P. High-altitude pulmonary edema. *Med Sci Sports Exerc.* 1999;31(suppl 1):S23.

109. Roach RC, Houston CS, Honigman B. How well do older persons tolerate moderate altitude? *West J Med.* 1995;162(1):32.

110. Roach RC, Maes D, Sandoval D, et al. Exercise exacerbates acute mountain sickness at simulated high altitude. *J Appl Physiol.* 2000;88(2):581.

111. Roeggla G, Roeggla H, Roeggla M, et al. Effect of alcohol on acute ventilation adaptation to mild hypoxia at moderate altitude. *Ann Intern Med.* 1995;122:925.

112. Luks AM, Swenson ER. Medication and dosage considerations in the prophylaxis and treatment of high-altitude illness. *Chest.* 2008;133:744.

113. Luk AM, McIntosh SE, Grissom CK, et al. Wilderness Medical Society consensus guidelines for the prevention and treatment of acute altitude illness. *Wilderness Environ Med.* 2010;21:1146–1155.

114. Roach RC, Bartcsh P, Oelz O, Hackett PH, Lake Louise Scoring Committee. The Lake Louise Acute Mountain Sickness Scoring System. In: Sutton JR, Houston CS, Coates G, eds. *Hypoxia and Molecular Medicine.* Burlington, VT: Charles S. Houston; 1993.

115. Muza SR, Lyons TP, Rock PB. Effect of altitude on exposure on brain volume and development of acute mountain sickness (AMS). In: Roach RC, Wagner PD, Hackett PH, eds. *Hypoxia: Into the Next Millennium: Advances in Experimental Medicine and Biology.* Vol 474. New York, NY: Kluwer Academic/Plenum; 1999.

116. Hacket PH. High-altitude cerebral edema and acute mountain sickness: a pathological update. In: Roach RC, Wagner PD, Hackett PH, eds. *Hypoxia: Into the Next Millennium: Advances in Experimental Medicine and Biology.* Vol 474. New York, NY: Kluwer Academic/Plenum; 1999.

117. Sanchez del Rio M, Moskkowitz MA. High-altitude headache: lessons from aches at sea level. In: Roach RC, Wagner PD, Hackett PH, eds. *Hypoxia: Into the Next Millennium: Advances in Experimental Medicine and Biology.* Vol 474. New York, NY: Kluwer Academic/Plenum; 1999.

118. Hackett PH. The cerebral etiology of high-altitude cerebral edema and acute mountain sickness. *Wilderness Environ Med.* 1999;10(2):97.

119. Yarnell PR, Heit J, Hackett PH. High-altitude cerebral edema (HACE): the Denver/Front Range experience. *Semin Neurol.* 2000;20(2):209.

120. Hultgren HN, Honigman B, Theis K, Nicholas D. High-altitude pulmonary edema at ski resort. *West J Med.* 1996;164:222.

121. Stenmark KR, Frid M, Nemenoff R, et al. Hypoxia induces cell-specific changes in gene expression in vascular wall cells: implications for pulmonary hypertension. In: Roach RC, Wagner PD, Hackett PH, eds. *Hypoxia: Into the Next Millennium: Advances in Experimental Medicine and Biology.* Vol 474. New York, NY: Kluwer Academic/Plenum; 1999.

122. The Lake Louise Consensus on the Definition and Quantification of Altitude Illness. In: Sutton JR, Coates G, Houston C, eds. *Hypoxia and Mountain Medicine.* Burlington, VT: Queen City Press; 1992.

123. Luks AM. Do we have a "best practice" for treating high-altitude pulmonary edema? *High Alt Med Biol.* 2008;9:111–114.

124. Koch RO, Burtscher M. Do we have a "best practice" for treating high-altitude pulmonary edema? Letter to the Editor. *High Alt Med Biol.* 2008;9:343–344.

125. Lipman G. Ibuprofen prevents altitude illness: randomized controlled trial for prevention of altitude illness with nonsteroidal anti-inflammatories. *Ann Emerg Med.* 2012;59(6):484–490.

126. Pollard AJ, Niermeyer S, Barry PB, et al. Children at high altitude: an international consensus statement by an ad hoc committee of the International Society for Mountain Medicine. *High Alt Med Biol.* 2001;2:389.

Suggested Reading

Auerbach PS, ed. *Wilderness Medicine.* 6th ed. St. Louis, MO: Mosby Elsevier; 2012.

Bennett P, Elliott D. *The Physiology and Medicine of Diving.* 4th ed. Philadelphia, PA: Saunders; 1993.

Bove AA. *Bove and Davis' Diving Medicine.* 5th ed. Philadelphia, PA: Saunders; 2003.

Sutton JR, Coates G, Remmers JE, eds. *Hypoxia: The Adaptations.* Philadelphia, PA: BC Dekker; 1990.

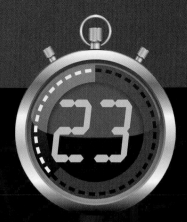

Wilderness Trauma Care

CHAPTER OBJECTIVES

At the completion of this chapter, the reader will be able to do the following:

- Explain four factors that distinguish the *wilderness* and *street* emergency medical services (EMS) contexts.

- List the five critical selection criteria for clearing a spine in the wilderness.

- Discuss the reasons for the dictum, "Every wilderness patient is hypothermic, hypoglycemic, and hypovolemic until proven otherwise."

- Describe updated ways to manage bleeding wounds in the wilderness.

- Discuss the symptoms and signs of common bites and stings and medical management in the wilderness.

- Describe when, in the wilderness context, an attempt at cardiopulmonary resuscitation (CPR) is appropriate and when it is not appropriate.

SCENARIO

Your search and rescue (SAR) team is called out at 2130 hours to support the county's volunteer fire fighters in the technical rescue of a trauma victim in a remote location. Early reports indicate that one member of a three-person rock climbing group, a 31-year-old man, fell at around 2030 hours from the cliff edge to the rocky floor 80 feet (24 meters) below, sustaining multiple long-bone fractures. One member of the group ran back to his truck, grabbed a sleeping bag to keep the patient warm, and instructed the other climber to go get help.

The volunteer technical rescue team includes a paramedic and an emergency department (ED) nurse. They arrive at the incident command post at about 2230 hours. Following an incident briefing, the initial rescue team comprised of six personnel drive several miles on a trail using all-terrain vehicles and then hike for 60 minutes up a creek bed with gear to arrive at the scene. When you arrive after midnight, it is raining lightly and the ambient temperature is 50°F (10°C). You and the initial rescue team find the patient at the bottom of the cliff sitting up with his back against a rock.

- How would you begin managing this patient in this wilderness setting with limited resources?
- What are the major concerns when treating this patient's injuries?
- What will be the best way to evacuate this patient?

Proper Care Depends on Context

Although our medical knowledge, understanding, and technology change from month to month, the principles of medical care change little over the years and independent of the patient's location. PHTLS has long advocated that the critically injured patient be transported as quickly as possible to an appropriate destination, without detailed physical examination and treatment of noncritical conditions.[1]

However, *proper* care is still somewhat context dependent. The definition of *detailed physical examination* and *noncritical conditions* may be different on an urban street than when deep in the wilderness (**Figure 23-1**). This concept is introduced in the chapter titled The Science, Art, and Ethics of Prehospital Care: Principles, Preferences, and Critical Thinking, showing how situation, knowledge level, skill, scene conditions, and equipment available may alter management of the trauma patient.[1]

Consider a patient with a complex fracture–dislocation of the shoulder. What is the proper care in the operating room (OR)? In many cases it involves an open reduction and internal fixation (ORIF). However, proper care in the OR may *not* be proper care in the emergency department (ED), where it would not be proper to attempt an open reduction. In the ED, the patient needs to have x-ray films taken to evaluate the fracture–dislocation, a short-acting pain medication is given, and a *closed* reduction of the dislocation is performed to reduce pain and swelling, to realign the bones grossly, and to decrease pressure on nerves and blood vessels. The definitive ORIF will occur later, in the OR.

Likewise, proper care in the ED may not be proper care in the field. The prehospital care providers may not have the advantage of a large, warm, dry area to perform an assessment

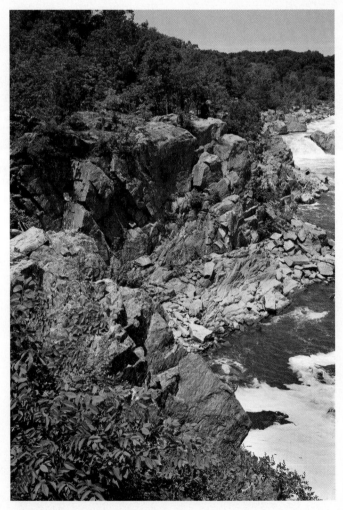

Figure 23-1 Wilderness terrain.
Source: Courtesy of Rick Brady.

and provide treatment. They may be working in the rain, where the patient is hanging upside down inside a crushed vehicle while a rescue crew uses power tools to cut and remove metal to reach the patient. Once the patient is free, the prehospital care provider will assess the patient for other injuries, check the distal neurovascular status in the arm, immobilize the patient's shoulder, provide some pain medication, and transport the patient rapidly to the ED. Similarly, on the street, it would not be proper care to attempt a closed or open reduction to reduce the fracture–dislocation. Finally, proper care on the street may not be proper care in the wilderness (**Figure 23-2**). What if a patient falls off a rope a half-mile into a limestone cave, requiring a multihour evacuation through cave passages, followed by a several-hour drive to the nearest hospital?

For most conditions, however, proper care is proper care whether it is performed in the OR, in the ED, on the street, or in the wilderness. Given a good fund of knowledge, critical-thinking skills, and understanding of key principles, prehospital care providers can make reasoned decisions regarding patient care in all of the various situations in which they will encounter patients.

For a small but significant number of situations, great differences exist between proper street emergency medical services (EMS) care and proper wilderness EMS care. Such situations bring up the following important questions:

- Is street EMS care always optimal in the wilderness?
- If street EMS care is not optimal, how does the prehospital care provider know what the optimal care is? Is this written down as a set of protocols?
- How does the prehospital care provider deal with situations in the field when unsure precisely what the patient's injury might be? For example, in the previous case, how does the wilderness medicine provider determine that a fracture–dislocation is present when examining a patient who is hanging upside down from a rope deep within a cave?
- How does the prehospital care provider decide, for a particular patient in a particular situation, which is *more* proper, street or wilderness care?
- What makes a situation *wilderness* or *street*? What about all the in-between cases?

Definitive answers to all the questions cannot be provided. Often the answer is "it depends." But at least good background information can be provided so that prehospital care providers may, as needed in a particular patient care situation, answer the questions. The Prehospital Trauma Life Support (PHTLS) philosophy has always been that, given a good fund of knowledge and key principles, prehospital care providers are capable of making reasoned decisions regarding patient care.

Several wilderness issues are critical for optimal wilderness patient care and are common wilderness problems for which management is different than on the street. This chapter provides an overview of the many issues involved in wilderness-related medical emergencies. Prehospital care providers who will be functioning in a formal capacity in the wilderness setting as wilderness medicine providers should obtain specific training in managing these patients (**Figure 23-3**). In addition, medical direction by a knowledgeable physician should be an integral component of wilderness medicine activities.[2] However, in many regions of the United States there is no medical direction for wilderness medicine providers on many search and rescue teams.[3,4]

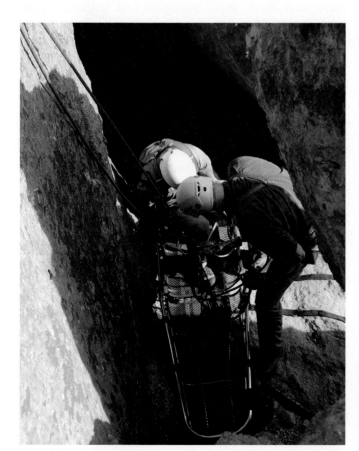

Figure 23-2 Trauma care in the wilderness is often hampered by adverse environmental conditions, mud, underbrush, and confined spaces.
Source: Courtesy of Tom Pendley/Desert Rescue Research.

Figure 23-3   Wilderness EMS Training

Those prehospital care providers who may provide EMS in the wilderness as wilderness medicine providers or who regularly travel in the backcountry are advised to take a specialized course.

The Wilderness EMS Context

Many terms are used to describe areas far from civilization, including wilderness, remote, backcountry, isolated, and austere. EMS personnel tend to lump these together under the rubric *wilderness* and to speak of *wilderness EMS*. According to the dictionary, the following definitions apply to *wilderness*[5]:

- A tract or region uncultivated and uninhabited by human beings
- An area essentially undisturbed by human activity together with its naturally developed life community
- An empty or pathless area or region

Because EMS is focused on *patient care*, the EMS definition of wilderness differs from the preceding definitions. The EMS definition is really the answer to a question: "When should we think about wilderness EMS?" That is, "When should we think and work differently from what we do on the street?"

The answer to this question goes beyond simple geography and involves the following considerations:

- Access to the scene
- Weather
- Daylight
- Terrain
- Special transport and handling needs
- Access and transport times
- Available personnel
- Communications
- Hazards present
- Medical and rescue equipment available
- Injury patterns for the specific environment

Numerous potential examples exist besides the traditional view of wilderness. For example:

1. In a city after an earthquake, it may be very difficult to access those who are injured or trapped, there may be no road for transport, and local EMS systems may be out of commission. In this situation, patients are likely to remain in their location for a considerable amount of time. They will have the same care requirements as a hiker who has fallen in the mountains and is hours or days away from a hospital.

2. A person who has fallen into a suburban landfill site late in the evening during an ice storm is at risk from the same factors as a patient suffering the same type of fall in the wilderness. The patient may need a rescue team with ropes, ice axes, and crampons, and prehospital care providers who can anticipate and cope with issues such as hypothermia, toileting needs, prevention of pressure sores, wound management, and food and fluid requirements.

We often talk of *wilderness EMS*, but in reality, *all* of EMS lies on a spectrum. At one end of the spectrum is an incident half a block from a level I trauma center, and at the other end of the spectrum is an incident in the deepest part of the Mammoth–Flint Ridge cave system in Kentucky. In the final analysis, where does *the street* end and *the wilderness* begin? The answer is, "It depends." It depends on the distance from the ambulance and the ED. It depends on the weather. It depends on the terrain. Even more importantly, it depends on the nature of the injury and the capabilities of the EMS and rescue personnel on scene.

Wilderness Injury Patterns

As mentioned in the PHTLS: Past, Present, and Future chapter, death from trauma has a trimodal (three-peaked) distribution. The **first peak of death** is within seconds to minutes of injury. Deaths occurring during this period are usually caused by lacerations of the brain, brain stem, high spinal cord, heart, aorta, or other large vessels and can best be managed by preventive measures such as helmets and seat belts. Only a few of the patients can be saved, and then only in large urban areas where rapid emergency transport is available.

The **second death peak** occurs within minutes to a few hours after injury. Rapid assessment and resuscitation are carried out to reduce this second peak of trauma deaths. Deaths occurring during this period are usually caused by subdural and epidural hematomas, hemopneumothoraces, a ruptured spleen, lacerations of the liver, pelvic fractures, or multiple injuries associated with significant blood loss. The fundamental principles of trauma care (hemorrhage control, airway management, balanced fluid resuscitation, and transport to an appropriate facility) can best be applied to these patients. The **third death peak** occurs several days or weeks after the initial injury and is almost always caused by sepsis and organ failure.

Prehospital care providers focus mostly on saving patients from the second death peak. In the wilderness, most of those who survive to be rescued have already weathered the first peak of death and usually most of the second. However, the presence of medically trained individuals on a search and rescue (SAR) rescue team may also prevent deaths related to the second death peak.[6,7] Often, this wilderness care focuses on, "What can we do *now* that will keep the patient from dying or having major complications later?" Wilderness medicine providers need to make sure the patient does not develop problems such as kidney failure from dehydration, overwhelming infection from poor resistance due to starvation, pulmonary embolism from deep venous thrombosis (blood clots in the legs breaking off and going to the lungs), and infections from *decubiti* (bedsores).

Safety

In the wilderness, even more so than on the street, scene safety is paramount.[8] An injured or dead wilderness medicine provider distracts from the care of the patient and limits the possibility of a successful rescue mission. Street scene safety considerations still apply even in the wilderness. In the wilderness, scene dangers are usually much less obvious than on the street; they tend to slowly "sneak up" on unwary wilderness medicine providers.

The wilderness medicine provider and patient will be exposed to the weather, and changes in weather, such as an incoming cold front with freezing rain, which may complicate the operation or even injure or kill the wilderness medicine provider and patient. If a rescue lasts for hours, the lack of food and water may cause debilitation. The wilderness terrain is often rugged, and poisonous plants and wildlife may complicate patient care (**Figure 23-4**). Wilderness medicine providers need to be aware of dangers specific to the environment, such as rockfall, avalanche risk, rising waters, high altitudes or altitude exposure, and recirculating eddies at the base of waterfalls.

It is essential that appropriate preparations and precautions are taken to ensure the safety, health, and well-being of the SAR team. All members of the SAR team must be educated about the hazards and dangers of the specific environment in which they will be working. Each member of the SAR team must know their limitations and not exceed their capabilities trying to rescue an injured patient. Each member of the SAR team must be appropriately prepared with the necessary clothing and equipment for the environmental conditions and rescue at hand. Lastly, ensuring that the medical needs of the SAR team are met must be an integral component of the response effort. Appropriate supplies to address potential illness or injury of an SAR team member as well as enforcement of work–rest cycles will help maintain a well-functioning SAR team.

The Wilderness Is Everywhere

In the rest of this chapter, *wilderness EMS*, *in the wilderness*, and *wilderness patients* will be discussed. However, remember that *the wilderness* might be a short distance from the road if it is dark and the weather is bad, or even *on* the road if a disaster has made roads impassable or made nearby hospitals unable to accept patients.

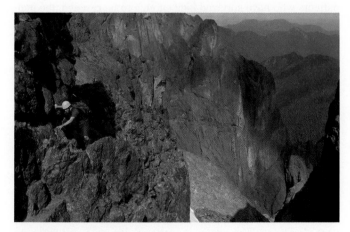

Figure 23-4 Steep slopes and uneven footing are a danger in wilderness rescue.
Source: © Danny Warren/iStock/Thinkstock.

EMS Decision Making: Balancing Risks and Benefits

Experienced physicians, nurses, and prehospital care providers know that procedures such as airway management and wound management are the easy part of medicine. The difficult part is in knowing *when* to do *what*: critical thinking. Even more often than on the street, in the wilderness one risk needs to be weighed carefully against another and against the potential benefits. For this particular patient, in *this* particular setting, and with *these* particular resources, and with *this* particular likelihood of *this* particular help arriving at *this* particular time in the future, what are the potential risks? What are the potential benefits? Wilderness EMS is largely the art of compromise: balancing the particular risks and benefits for each patient. To illustrate the wilderness EMS decision-making process, consider the following example:

> A healthy 22-year-old woman was rock climbing along a river gorge when she fell 65 feet (20 meters [m]). All her chocks (anchors placed in cracks in the cliff) came out one by one, so she fell all the way to the ground, but was slowed by each anchor as it failed. She was wearing a helmet but struck her head and experienced a brief loss of consciousness. After an hour-long hike up the river gorge from where they parked the ambulance at the end of the road, a wilderness medicine provider and partner find the patient conscious and alert, complaining of only a mild headache, with a normal neurologic examination and a normal physical examination. It is late fall, it is getting dark, the nearest helicopter landing zone is back at the road an hour away, and the forecast is for a blizzard to start tonight. Does the patient need to undergo spinal immobilization? Does the wilderness medicine provider need to call for an SAR team with a Stokes litter and a long backboard, or can the patient be walked out to the ambulance?

Street Cervical Spine Management History

Spinal immobilization for severely injured trauma patients became the standard of care decades ago. Even if unstable cervical spine fractures were rare in alert trauma patients, and even if no evidence indicated that spinal immobilization was effective at preventing paralysis in alert patients, strapping a patient to a board seemed unlikely to hurt anyone. Over the ensuing years, prehospital care providers used spinal immobilization for more and more patients. It has since been recognized that patients experience gradually increasing pain from the long backboard. Studies show moderate pain at 30 minutes and severe pain after about 45 minutes.[9]

As EMS training became more widely used by wilderness SAR teams, the practice of strapping every patient to a long backboard after an accident did not seem to make sense, especially if the patient was on the side of a mountain in a snowstorm and the nearest long backboard was 10 miles away and 10,000 feet (3,000 m) down. So SAR teams in cooperation with the physicians working with them developed guidelines, based on the available literature, for when *not* to immobilize trauma patients in the wilderness.[10-12] Recently the Wilderness Medical Society published a practice guideline for managing spine injuries in the wilderness.[13] That guideline is available on their website.

Implications of the NEXUS Study

A large and important multicenter study called *NEXUS* (short for National Emergency X-radiography Utilization Study) showed that, in the hospital, many trauma patients can have their spinal column *cleared* without the need for x-ray films, if the following selection criteria are used[14]:

- Absence of tenderness at the posterior midline of the cervical spine
- Absence of a focal neurologic deficit
- Normal level of alertness
- No evidence of intoxication
- Absence of clinically apparent pain that might distract the patient from the pain of a cervical spine injury

Although the NEXUS study was not a prehospital study, variants of these criteria have been used by many EMS systems to guide the need for spinal immobilization. A few studies suggest some problems with using these criteria in the field. The wording of some EMS *selective spinal-immobilization protocols* deviates significantly from the previous wording, raising concerns about whether they really reflect the NEXUS criteria. However, it is generally accepted that the NEXUS criteria, when properly applied, are a reasonable guide for the selection of patients who do not need to be strapped to a long backboard, whether on the street or in the wilderness. Although NEXUS may be useful for inference in the EMS setting, one should remember that the study was not designed as a prehospital spinal-immobilization trial, but rather an evaluation of the need for cervical spine x-rays in-hospital.

The problem in the wilderness, however, is not as simple. What if a patient does not quite meet these criteria? Does that mean that the patient *has* to be immobilized? As discussed earlier, wilderness EMS is the art of compromise, and nowhere is this more apparent than in making decisions about spinal immobilization.

What if the patient has a potential spine injury and it is a 2-hour walk from the nearest road, and no spinal-immobilization equipment is at hand? Is it necessary to send someone on the 4-hour round-trip hike back to the ambulance for it? What if the patient is in a cave, with the water level rising? Could the patient and rescuers be cut off from an escape route and drown if the SAR team delays? What if the patient is in the mountains, far from the ambulance, and a storm is moving in? What are the risks to the patient and rescuers if they are forced to spend the night on the mountain?

In each of these situations, wilderness medicine providers at the scene are faced with the following two options:

- Stay and wait for the spinal-immobilization equipment to arrive.
- Start an improvised evacuation without spinal immobilization.

Neither option is ideal; however, wilderness medicine providers need to choose. To make this choice intelligently, the following questions must be asked and answered:

- What are the risks of an improvised evacuation without spinal immobilization, and what are the risks of waiting for spinal-immobilization equipment to arrive, *for this particular patient in this particular situation*?
- What are the benefits of moving without waiting for spinal immobilization versus waiting for spinal-immobilization equipment to arrive, *for this particular patient in this particular situation*?

The benefits of spinal immobilization depend on the likelihood that this particular patient has an unstable spinal injury. In the NEXUS study, even those who did not meet the NEXUS criteria, and who could not be "cleared," still had a very low risk of unstable spinal fracture, as follows[14]:

- 2% of those who *failed* the NEXUS "clearing" protocol had "clinically significant" fractures.
- Of that 2%, only a small fraction likely required specific treatment.
- Of *that* small fraction, only a small fraction likely had injuries that might endanger the spinal cord if not immobilized, and most of those were in patients with multiple major fractures and multiple life-threatening injuries.

Therefore, it seems likely that, for wilderness trauma patients who have survived long enough to be rescued, the incidence of unstable spinal injury will be less than 1%.

In the end, wilderness medicine providers at the scene need to assess these potential risks and benefits to make an informed decision for their patient.

Improvised Evacuations

When discussing spinal injury in the wilderness context, consider the idea of starting an improvised evacuation rather than waiting for a litter and spinal-immobilization equipment.[15]

Carrying patients in the wilderness is an extremely difficult, time-consuming, and potentially dangerous activity for both the patient and those doing the carrying. Those with no SAR experience generally underestimate the time and difficulty of a wilderness evacuation by at least half, or sometimes up to

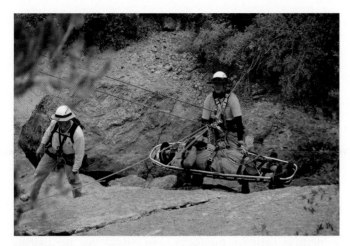

Figure 23-5 Because of uneven terrain, creativity and technical rescue skills may be needed to evacuate patients safely out of the wilderness.
Source: Courtesy of Tom Pendley/Desert Rescue Research.

a factor of five for more difficult evacuations, especially cave rescues.

If someone without SAR experience says, "It'll take us about 2 hours to get the patient out of here," the time should be tripled. Wilderness medicine providers should expect it to take 6 hours or longer if the patient is in a cave, if the SAR team is short on people, if the terrain is particularly difficult, or if the weather is bad. This is especially important to remember if darkness is approaching or the weather is deteriorating.

Walking a patient out, even with a couple of people helping, is almost always much faster. If the patient is able to and starts moving now, rather than waiting for a litter or spinal immobilization, the evacuation will be much, much faster and completed much earlier. If the patient cannot walk (e.g., because of an ankle fracture), it may be possible to do a piggyback carry or to make an improvised stretcher out of sticks and rope (**Figure 23-5**).

Patient Care in the Wilderness

Elimination Needs

The truth described in a popular children's book *Everyone Poops*[16] applies to wilderness patients as well. Given the relatively short transport times in an urban setting, most patients do not have an elimination need. Trauma patients almost never defecate during their prehospital and ED care. However, if you are caring for a patient who has been in the wilderness for a day or more and it takes you several hours to get to the patient, it is much more likely that the patient will need to urinate or defecate.

Having patient care supplies that include *blue pads* (Chux) for placing under the patient, having some toilet paper, improvising a large trash bag as an outer layer diaper, or even stopping to let the patient urinate or defecate are all reasonable measures

(**Figure 23-6**). It is possible for men and women to urinate even while immobilized in a Stokes litter (**Figure 23-7**) with a full-body vacuum splint, if packaging is planned carefully and the litter is tipped up on the foot end. For women, a small funnel device, often carried by women when backpacking, will be needed to assist in elimination.

Patients who are lying on their backs for a long time tend to develop decubiti (bedsores). These sores may end up requiring surgery or debridement, resulting in a longer hospital admission. Some patients will die from infection and other complications of the decubiti. Lying in one's own urine and feces for a long time (just hours, not even days) may make decubiti more likely. If patient care occurs for only a few minutes during a short transport, urine and feces are not a major issue. However, if a wilderness medicine provider has been taking care of a patient for several hours and then delivers the patient to the ED lying in his or her own feces, the likelihood of decubiti and resulting sepsis is much greater.

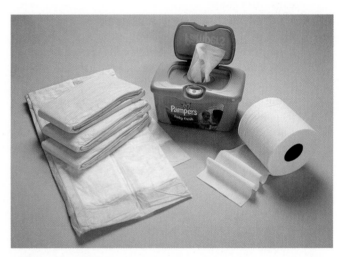

Figure 23-6 Elimination supplies.

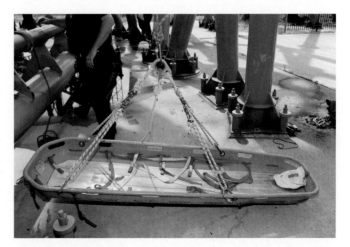

Figure 23-7 Stokes litter.
Source: Courtesy of Rick Brady.

Long Backboard Use

Other important preventive measures for wilderness patients, especially those who face prolonged evacuation, include prevention of decubiti as follows[15,17]:

- Allow (and assist) the patient to turn from side to side in the litter.
- Keep the patient's *sacrum* (buttocks) clean and dry.
- Provide adequate padding.

If the patient truly needs spinal immobilization, prevention of decubiti is even more important, although correspondingly more difficult. Techniques to avoid decubiti during spinal immobilization include the following:

- Put the patient in a full-body vacuum splint rather than on a long backboard. Vacuum mattresses provide excellent spinal immobilization and are much less likely to cause decubiti.[18-21]
- If no full-body vacuum splint is available, pad the long backboard well and add support under the lumbar spine, knees, and neck. Studies show that immobilization on an unpadded long backboard causes even uninjured people to experience excruciating pain in about 45 minutes and skin necrosis (cell death) in about 90 minutes.[9, 22-25]
- Carry the litter first on one side, then the other, so that pressure alternates between the two hips rather than always on the sacrum.

To prevent deep venous thrombosis and pulmonary embolism, do the following:

- Package patients so that they can move their legs; do not tie them down tight.
- Consider rest stops to allow patients to get out of the litter to stretch their legs.

If there is mild suspicion of a cervical spine injury but not a lumbar spine injury, it might be appropriate to allow an alert patient to get out of the litter, still wearing a cervical collar, and, with many trained hands to help, allow the patient to stretch his or her legs and take care of any elimination needs. Speaking with a physician knowledgeable with wilderness EMS first might be reassuring if this is contemplated.

Food and Water Needs

Every wilderness patient should be considered to be cold, hungry, and thirsty; that is, he or she should be considered hypothermic, starved, and dehydrated—or at a slight expense of accuracy, *hypothermic, hypoglycemic,* and *hypovolemic.*

Starvation is much more than just hypoglycemia (low blood sugar), and not all starving patients are significantly hypoglycemic. Dehydration is more than just hypovolemia, which refers only to intravascular volume within the blood vascular system. Patients who are dehydrated have also lost water from their cells and the interstitial spaces between the cells.

On the street, water and food are generally *not* given to patients. There are many reasons not to feed patients on the street. If the patient needs to go to the OR, having food or fluid in the stomach is harmful; it increases the likelihood of vomiting or, more likely, passive regurgitation leading to possible aspiration when under anesthesia. Also a patient will not starve or dehydrate in the time it takes to get to the hospital.

In the wilderness, if a rescued patient needs to go to the OR, it will take time to transport the patient to the hospital, to be evaluated in the ED, and to be prepared for the OR. With wilderness patients, the focus is to ensure that the patient does not die right after admission to the hospital. Starving patients is seldom good for injured bodies. Feeding the patient today will make the patient better tomorrow. Since the stomach needs to be empty for only a few hours before anesthesia, the wilderness medical provider may provide food and water to any reasonably alert wilderness patient who can safely swallow.[26,27]

Vomiting and aspiration are always a danger, and careful attention to the patient's airway is always important (e.g., positioning on the side for long transports, even if the patient needs spinal immobilization). Wilderness medicine providers may still attempt to provide food and water for wilderness patients, even though they have vomited once or twice, as long as their airway is protected.

Sun Protection

The ultraviolet (UV) rays of the sun can damage the skin—acutely, sometimes severely, and in a delayed fashion. Acute injury can include partial-thickness and full-thickness sunburns seen in some victims of exposure, and such severe sunburn can cause shock or death. Delayed injury is manifested as increased risk for skin cancer. Avoiding exposure to direct sunlight, especially from 10 a.m. to 3 p.m. when UV radiation from the sun is strongest, decreases but does not eliminate the risk of sunburn.

Topical sunscreens usually contain combinations of organic chemicals that absorb various wavelengths of UV light. UV light comes in two frequencies, A and B (UVA and UVB). UVA was once thought to be harmless, but now we know that it works synergistically with UVB to cause sunburn. UVB is responsible for most of the *erythema* (redness) of sunburn. UVA has been implicated in the development of phototoxicity and photoaging.[28] Thus, sun-blocking materials or creams must block both UVA and UVB to be effective. Seek the term board-spectrum sun protection factor (SPF) on the product label to ensure coverage for both UVA and UVB.

Sun protection is measured by SPF (**Figure 23-8**). The SPF is a numeric measure of how much the clothing or cream increases the minimum dose of UV light to make the skin red. For example, a sunscreen lotion with a rating of SPF 45 provides protection from sunburn for about 45 times longer than without the sunscreen. An SPF of 10 blocks 90% of UVB radiation, an SPF of 15 blocks 93%, an SPF of 30 blocks 97%, and an SPF of 50 blocks 98%. Consequently, the Food and Drug Administration does not allow sunscreen products to have an SPF label greater than 50 due to the limited benefit added for protection. The degree of protection against UVA is hard to quantify and is usually much less than protection against UVB.[29]

It is advisable to wear protective clothing, such as wide-brimmed hats, pants, and long-sleeved shirts, and to apply sunscreen to exposed skin. To check clothing for SPF, hold a piece of clothing up against a light bulb. If an image of the light bulb is seen through it, the SPF is slightly below 15. If light is seen through it but not the image of the light bulb, the SPF is in the range of 15 to 60 SPF.

Protective lotions with a minimum SPF of 15 should be applied to exposed skin to minimize the potential injury from sun exposure. For prolonged evacuations, lotion with an SPF of 30 should be used, but little benefit can be claimed with an SPF 30 alone unless it is reapplied every 90 minutes. Ideally, sunscreens should be applied 15 to 30 minutes before going out into the sun. Most people do not apply a thick enough layer to achieve the claimed SPF. A minimum of 1 ounce (about a shot glass full) should be used on all exposed areas. With profuse sweating or water immersion, sunscreen should be reapplied frequently depending on the product label. Generally, water-resistant SPF will be effective up to either 40 or 80 minutes per product directions. Further considerations regarding the application of sunscreen are included in **Figures 23-9** and **23-10**.

Sunburn is treated as any other burn, and the care is essentially the same in the wilderness as on the street

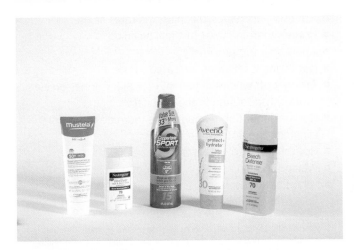

Figure 23-8 Sunscreen.
Source: Jones & Bartlett Learning. Photographed by Darren Stahlman.

Figure 23-9 Factors That Decrease SPF Effectiveness

Wind, heat, humidity, and altitude can all decrease the effective sun protection factor (SPF) of a sunscreen. Also, it is now known that the combined application of insect repellents that contain DEET (N,N-diethyl-meta-toluamide) also decreases SPF effectiveness.[28]

Figure 23-10 Allergic Reactions

Some patients may have an acute allergic reaction if the lotion contains para-amino benzoic acid (PABA); therefore PABA-free products are recommended.

Figure 23-11 Sunburn Treatment

Sunburn Treatments

Pain Control
- Acetylsalicylic acid
- Nonsteroidal anti-inflammatory drugs

Skin Care
- Cool soaks and compresses
- Nonmedicated moisturizers
- Topical anesthetics
  - Pramoxine (Prax) lotion
  - Menthol plus camphor (Sarna) anti-itch lotion
  - Anti-itch concentrated lotion (Pramoxine) plus camphor plus calamine (Aveeno)
  - Lidocaine plus camphor (Neutrogena Norwegian Formula) soothing relief moisturizer

Steroids
- Topical (e.g., triamcinolone 0.1% cream applied twice daily when erythema first appears)
- Systemic

Source: From Krakowski AC and Kaplan LA. Exposure to Radiation from the Sun. Auerbach PS, editor: Wilderness medicine, ed 6, Philadelphia, 2012, Elsevier Mosby.

(**Figure 23-11**).[30] The only major difference is that in the wilderness, the prehospital care provider needs to be aware of and treat the potential fluid loss, dehydration, or sometimes even shock, and to recognize that patients with sunburn are at higher risk for hypothermia.

Specifics of Wilderness EMS

This section reviews a few of the most important situations in which proper wilderness trauma care differs from care on the street. Issues covered include wound management, joint dislocations, cardiopulmonary arrest, and bites and stings.

Wound Management

Wound management encompasses the following:

- *Hemostasis* (stopping bleeding)
- *Antisepsis* (preventing infection)
- Restoration of function (returning the skin to its protective function, and restoring a limb or other body part to normal function)
- *Cosmesis* (ensuring pleasant appearance)

In the wilderness, prevention of infection and restoration of function assume great importance.

Hemostasis

Control of bleeding is part of the primary assessment. On the street, arterial bleeding can kill. In the wilderness, even venous bleeding can kill if it continues for a sufficient amount of time. Remember, every red blood cell counts. Bleeding control, including standard measures such as direct pressure, is as important or more important in the wilderness. Unless medical personnel are part of the actual injured party's group, severe bleeding that is not stopped will probably result in the patient's demise prior to the SAR team's arrival (**Figure 23-12**).

Training programs for those venturing into wilderness situations should address these lifesaving skills:

- Direct digital pressure should be applied for 10 to 15 minutes directly on the bleeding site followed by a pressure bandage.
- Hemostatic agents may be useful in wilderness care in the control of severe bleeding. Wilderness medicine providers may encounter injured patients who have had hemostatic agents already applied by others in their group. Many of these agents are available for sale to the general public; however, training on how to effectively apply them is still recommended. It is important to remember that even if hemostatic agents are used, direct pressure on the wound remains part of the treatment process.
- Tourniquets may be used when all other methods to control the hemorrhage have failed and the priority is life preservation over limb preservation. The tourniquet should be applied above the wound as close to the wound as possible (**Figure 23-13**). (For more about hemostatic agents, tourniquets, and other hemorrhage control principles and preferences, see the Shock chapter.)

Prevention of Infection

After injury in the wilderness, it may be a long time before the wound receives definitive treatment in an ED. Routine wound care in the ED includes appropriate cleaning to prevent infection. Wounds contaminated by dirt or caused by

---

Figure 23-12 Updated Hemorrhage Control Principles

Recently, an international consensus panel, convened by the American Heart Association, updated first aid skills, including hemorrhage control principles.[31] It is now recommended to control severe bleeding by manual direct pressure, gauze and a pressure dressing, hemostatic agents, and a tourniquet. The traditional methods of using pressure points and extremity elevation are no longer recommended due to the lack of any evidence supporting their effectiveness.

Figure 23-13 Tourniquet Mistakes to Avoid

- Not using one when the injury indicates its use
- Using a tourniquet for minimal bleeding
- Applying it too proximally
- Not taking it off when indicated
- Taking it off when the patient is in shock or has only a short transport time to the hospital
- Not making it tight enough (The tourniquet should eliminate the distal pulse.)
- Not using a second tourniquet if needed
- Waiting too long to apply the tourniquet
- Periodically loosening the tourniquet to allow blood flow to the injured extremity

Source: Adapted from the Department Defense Lessons Learned from the Committee on Tactical Combat Casualty Care. See Chapter 27 in the eighth edition of *PHTLS: Prehospital Trauma Life Support, Military Edition.*

penetration from a dirty object are cleaned with high-pressure irrigation. Uncontaminated wounds are cleaned with low-pressure irrigation.

High-pressure irrigation may cause swelling of wounds, but in the case of contaminated wounds full of dirt and bacteria, the benefit of removing bacteria outweighs the risks from wound swelling.[32,33] Infection may set in quickly. After a wound has been open for about 8 hours, bacteria have spread from the skin deep into the wound, and suturing a wound is likely to create a deep wound infection. Deep wound infections develop pressure, which keeps out white blood cells, the body's normal defense mechanism against infection.

Routine wound care on the *street* does not include cleansing the wound because it makes sense to delay wound cleansing for a few minutes until the patient reaches the ED, which is better suited for wound cleansing and evaluating the patient's wound. The ED can determine if the patient has a tendon or nerve laceration, an associated fracture, a spleen laceration, or a subdural hematoma in the head.

Delaying wound care does not make sense in the wilderness. If it will take hours to get to the ED, the wound should be cleaned. In extremely remote areas, the wound could even become infected before the patient arrives at the ED several days later.

Studies have shown that early irrigation is essential to removing bacteria and reducing wound infections.[34-36] It is not necessary or practical to carry sterile solutions for wound irrigation. There is no need to add an antiseptic to the water.[37] Water that is good enough to drink is good enough to irrigate a wound. Water from streams or melted snow can be treated with any standard wilderness drinking water treatment and used to cleanse a wound.[32, 38-42]

When cleaning an uncontaminated wound, for example, a laceration sustained from a football player banging his forehead against a teammate's helmet, it is only necessary to wash the laceration out with water poured through the wound. A bulb syringe, usually available in the ED, is commonly used, but squirting some clean available water from a drinking-water bottle or a hydration bladder-backpack system, for example, will do as well.

If the wound is contaminated, it must be irrigated with enough pressure to clean out the bacteria. The original studies showed that a 35-milliliter (ml) syringe with an 18-gauge needle provided an appropriate amount of pressure (5 to 15 pounds per square [psi]).[43-45] Squirt the water, at high pressure, throughout the wound. This procedure, however, is a major bloodborne pathogen risk; protection from the spray of blood with a gown or a clean trash bag or rain poncho when irrigating is necessary. Eye protection and gloves are essential.

Sometimes it is necessary to use a gauze pad or clean cloth with gloved fingers to clean out some gross dirt or foreign material. The patient's pain may need to be treated before the wound can be cleaned. Lidocaine applied topically to the wound or injected subcutaneously for local anesthesia can provide relief in most cases. Narcotic analgesics may impair the patient's ability to ambulate and thus delay the evacuation. Once the irrigation is complete, dress and bandage the wound. Reapply a clean dressing at least daily or sooner if the bandage gets wet.

If the wound is gaping open, a wet dressing will prevent tissue damage as a result of drying out; change or at least rewet the dressing with clean water several times a day. However, because the wound will be mostly closed by bandaging, a dry dressing can be used in most cases.

Early antibiotic administration is commonly used upon arrival at the ED for patients with significant trauma. Antibiotics are not given in most civilian prehospital emergency medical systems because of the very short transport times encountered in the urban environment. However, definitive care may be significantly delayed in wilderness settings due to the longer distances to be covered and rescue considerations in rugged terrain.

Antibiotics must be given as soon as possible after injury to maximize their ability to prevent wound infections. Intramuscular benzylpenicillin begun within 1 hour of injury was found to be effective in preventing streptococcal infections in a swine model of wound infection. If administration was delayed until 6 hours after injury, the medication was not effective.[46]

A recent military review of antibiotic use on the battlefield recommended that antibiotics be used if arrival at a medical treatment facility was anticipated to be 3 hours or longer.[47] The U.S. Department of Defense's Tactical Combat Casualty Care Course (TCCC) advocates for the early administration of antibiotics for any open wounds at the point of wounding. TCCC cites multiple case studies where no wound infections developed when service men and women received battlefield antibiotics. TCCC further recommends that oral antibiotics be given to casualties once a day if the casualty has the ability to swallow. Although no comparable studies have been done in the civilian setting, these recommendations make sense for application in the wilderness environment if the physician medical director agrees.

Restoration of Function and Cosmesis: Closing Wilderness Wounds

Because of the lack of good lighting, x-ray films, and a warm, dry place to work, it does not make sense to perform definitive wound closure in the wilderness. It is recommended to simply cleanse the wound, dress and bandage, ensure good wound care for 4 days, and then have a **delayed primary closure** performed in the ED. As long as the wound is not infected, it is safe to suture the wound 4 days later as if it had just occurred. Although bacteria move into the wound soon after injury, eventually enough of the body's defenses (e.g., white blood cells) have entered the wound and make it safe to close. If a physician or someone else experienced at wound closure is present, the wound may be closed at the scene. However, it is still reasonable to only cleanse, dress, and bandage the wound and allow closure to occur later.

Closing a wilderness wound may be important in one situation: when bleeding cannot be controlled in any other way.

These situations are uncommon and usually involve a scalp laceration. For this reason, some wilderness medicine providers are trained to use disposable surgical staplers to repair scalp wounds. However, wound repair is complex and should not be attempted without sufficient training and experience.

Dislocations

A healthy 20-year-old man was kayaking along a white-water stream when the top of his kayak paddle hit a low-hanging tree branch. Now his right shoulder is swollen, deformed, and painful. He cannot bring his right arm across his chest. Distal pulses, capillary refill, sensation, and movement are intact. From the ambulance, the wilderness medicine provider and partner hike a mile through the woods to get to the stream. Should they "splint it as it lies" or try to reduce what looks like an anterior shoulder dislocation?

The common practice for fractures and dislocations on the street is to "splint it as it lies" and transport for definitive treatment. The only exception is the patient whose distal pulse is not palpable, in which case the extremity is realigned anatomically in an effort to restore circulation.

Although "splint it as it lies" is a good general rule for the street, "make it look normal" is a better general rule for the wilderness patient. It is certainly appropriate for both fractures and dislocations when transport is delayed.

There are many types of dislocations—finger, toe, shoulder, patella, knee, elbow, hip, ankle, and jaw—and all have been successfully reduced in the wilderness, some more easily than others. It is usually very easy to reduce dislocations of the ankle (which are almost always fracture–dislocations), patella, toe, or finger, except the proximal interphalangeal joint of the index finger in some cases. Elbow, knee, and hip dislocations are usually quite difficult. All are much easier with training and practice; in particular, it takes training or experience to know, without a radiograph, when a joint is likely dislocated and to attempt reduction.

EMS training courses seldom provide training in dislocation reduction. However, because wilderness dislocations are so common, dislocation reduction is covered in almost all wilderness emergency responder and wilderness EMS training or at orthopedic workshops at wilderness medicine conferences. Those who might provide EMS in the wilderness or who regularly travel in the backcountry are advised to take one of these courses.

Cardiopulmonary Resuscitation in the Wilderness

Traumatic cardiac arrest on the street has a poor prognosis, even if the scene is within minutes of a level I trauma center. No person survives more than a few minutes of cardiopulmonary resuscitation (CPR) after traumatic arrest.[48-51] This reality is recognized in many EMS protocols. For traumatic cardiac arrest, initiate CPR with cervical spine stabilization if:

1. Cardiac arrest occurs in the presence of EMS personnel.
2. A victim of penetrating trauma had signs of life within 15 minutes of the arrival of EMS personnel.

Wilderness Traumatic Arrest

A few signs can be uniformly equated with nonsurvivability:

- Decapitation
- Transection of the torso
- Patient is frozen so hard that the patient's chest cannot be compressed
- Patient's rectal temperature is very cold and the same as the environment
- Well-progressed decomposition

The following presumptive signs of death may be of use to wilderness medicine providers, although no one sign by itself is reliable:

- **Rigor mortis.** Postmortem rigidity is well known but not always present, and similar rigidity is often observed in hypothermic patients.
- **Dependent lividity.** This finding is common in corpses but can also be found, along with pressure necrosis and frostbite, in some patients exposed to the elements for a long time.
- **Decomposition.** This finding is usually self-evident.
- *Lack of presumptive signs of life.* Hypothermia can mimic death, in that pulses may not be palpable, respirations may be undetectable, and pupils may be dilated and unreactive with no signs of consciousness. However, some such severely hypothermic patients have occasionally been resuscitated, with full neurologic recovery.

Therefore, in the wilderness context, CPR is inappropriate for traumatic arrest. It is appropriate for wilderness medicine providers and the SAR team members to examine the patient, then gently but firmly tell the companions that the victim is dead and there is no reason to initiate resuscitation. Although it is oftentimes difficult to use the word "dead," euphemisms often lead to misunderstanding and misinterpretation of what is actually being said.

Wilderness Medical Arrest

The term medical cardiac arrest applies to a patient who has a contributing, underlying medical condition or suffers an acute medical condition (chest pain, shortness of breath, diabetes, etc.) and then sustains a cardiac arrest. Again, in the wilderness context, the chances of survival are poor or nonexistent when the patient is more than a few minutes from CPR or defibrillation.[52-58] It is possible that an SAR team might be carrying out a patient when the patient sustains a cardiac arrest. Although some lightweight defibrillators are now being manufactured, the weight-to-need-for-use ratio of defibrillators is so poor that they are seldom carried by SAR teams.

Recently a position statement was released on the Termination of Resuscitation of Nontraumatic Cardiopulmonary Arrest by the National Association of EMS Physicians (NAEMSP).[57] This statement, which is available on the NAEMSP website, can provide some guidance on when to consider termination of a cardiac arrest resuscitation effort.

There are a variety of other causes of cardiac arrest in the wilderness, such as ventricular fibrillation (VF) cardiac arrest secondary to hypothermia or cardiac arrest secondary to pulmonary embolism. For such cardiac arrests, survival is even less likely than with a cardiac arrest secondary to a myocardial infarction.

However, "nontraumatic" wilderness cardiac arrest might be survivable in the following situations:

- Hypothermia[58]
- Cold-water submersion[59-62]
- Lightning strike[63]
- Electrocution
- Drug overdose
- Avalanche burial[64]

In all these cases, a patient may appear to be in cardiac arrest but still might be resuscitated by basic CPR. For hypothermia in particular, there is a saying that "Nobody is dead until they are warm and dead" (see the Environmental Trauma I: Heat and Cold chapter). A significant minority of those who appear dead from the mechanisms listed can be resuscitated. There are special considerations for each of these situations—for example, scene safety for those who have been electrocuted and are still attached to a power line, or the fact that external cardiac compression can actually induce a VF cardiac arrest in a hypothermic patient whose heart is beating just enough to keep the patient alive.[65-68] Although appropriate in a wilderness EMS course, detailed discussion of these topics is beyond the scope of this chapter (see the Environmental Trauma I: Heat and Cold and the Environmental Trauma II: Drowning, Lightning, Diving, and Altitude chapters).

Two simple and standard wilderness CPR rules are:

- If the patient appears to be in cardiac arrest from causes other than trauma, attempt CPR for 15 to 30 minutes; if, at the end of this period of time, the patient has not been resuscitated, stop CPR and consider the patient dead.
- Do not start CPR if it will put rescuers at risk and decrease their chances of retreating from the scene safely, given concerns about daylight, terrain, weather, and available nearby shelter.

Bites and Stings

Bites and stings are common wilderness problems. The exact type of bite or sting likely in a wilderness area depends on the specific locale.

Bee Stings

The most widespread, common, and deadly sting is that of the common honeybee, at least to those who are allergic. Most reactions to bee stings are severe (although brief) local pain, and in some cases local swelling and redness persist for 1 or 2 days; these latter reactions are likely directly related to injected toxins and are not an indication of allergy.

Some individuals who are stung will progress within a few minutes to a generalized allergic reaction. This may range from *urticarial* (hives) to a full-blown anaphylactic reaction. Although the exact spectrum of generalized allergic reaction depends on the contents of the injected toxin (which varies among the many species of bees and wasps) and the allergic history of the patient, one or more of the following are usually seen:

- Urticaria (hives) (**Figure 23-14**)
- Lip swelling
- Hoarseness or stridor
- Wheezing and/or shortness of breath
- Abdominal cramping, vomiting, or diarrhea
- Tachycardia or bradycardia
- Hypotension
- Syncope
- Shock

Those individuals with a history of a generalized allergic reaction to a sting are more likely to have another generalized reaction to the next sting. However, venom among different

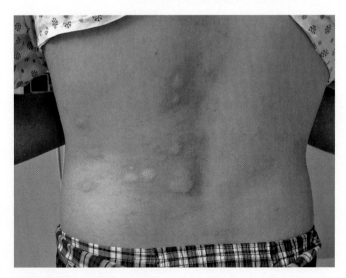

Figure 23-14 Allergic urticaria.
Source: © Chuck Stewart, MD.

species varies enough that, despite a history of generalized allergy in the past, a patient might have no generalized reaction to the next sting.

A patient with mild urticaria after a sting will probably do well. If a patient with hives after a sting progresses to *real* anaphylaxis, however, the best early sign is hoarseness. The major cause of death after bee sting allergic reaction is airway obstruction from hives in the airway, and hoarseness is usually the first sign of airway swelling. Any patient with a generalized reaction to a bee sting needs treatment immediately.

Basic life support interventions generally involve keeping the patient flat or in a position of comfort, performing standard airway management, and providing oxygen.

Honey bee stingers usually remain in the skin when the insect leaves because the stinger is barbed. Venom from the stinger and venom sac will continue to enter the skin for 45 to 60 seconds if the stinger is not removed; thus it is important to remove the stinger quickly. There has been a great deal of discussion about the proper way to remove a bee stinger, but recent information indicates it really does not matter how it gets out as long as it is removed as soon as possible. Fingernails, a knife blade edge, or a credit card edge are all effective tools for removing an embedded stinger. If a stinger is removed within 15 seconds of the sting, the severity of the sting is reduced.

The main medications used to treat allergic reactions to bee stings include the following:

1. Epinephrine (adrenalin). Although epinephrine acts only for a few minutes, it can be lifesaving.
2. Antihistamines (e.g., diphenhydramine [Benadryl]). Anyone who requires epinephrine for a bee sting allergy should receive an antihistamine.
3. Steroids (e.g., prednisone). Most people who require epinephrine also require steroids.

Some wilderness SAR teams carry drugs for bee sting allergic reactions in their medical kits; the SAR team's wilderness medicine providers have special training in their use. Oftentimes, some people with a history of bee sting allergy will carry these medications in their personal first-aid kits.

The most important drug is epinephrine, which acts rapidly to reverse the acute reaction. Epinephrine is available as a pen-sized autoinjector (e.g., EpiPen), which is often prescribed to any patient who has had a generalized allergy to bee stings (**Figure 23-15**). These autoinjectors are found in many wilderness first-aid kits. The Wilderness Medical Society has recently published a practice guideline on the use of epinephrine in the wilderness.[69] This guideline recommends the administration of epinephrine by wilderness instructors who are trained to recognize acute anaphylaxis and to give epinephrine.

Figure 23-15 Autoinjectors

Warning: There is another autoinjector medication on the market that has the appearance of an EpiPen autoinjector. The drug is Alsuma, a sumatriptan autoinjector prescribed to treat migraines. This autoinjector could be used by mistake on an anaphylactic patient since there is no warning that it is not epinephrine and has the identical size, color, and cap appearance as the EpiPen released in 2010.[70]

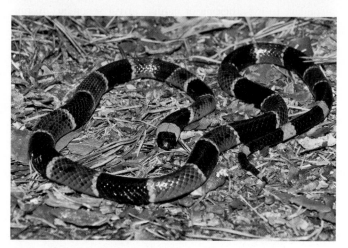

Figure 23-16 Coral snake.
Source: © Jason Ondreicka/Thinkstock.

Snakebite

There are approximately 3,000 species of snakes, of which some 600 are poisonous but only 200 are considered to be medically significant venomous types.[71,72] Few are found in northern latitudes. Most reside naturally in tropical areas, and many are deadly. Although many snakes have venom glands, there are only two types of snakes in North America with venom strong enough to cause more than minor irritation to humans.

Coral snakes are small snakes found in the southern parts of North America. They have venom that is neurotoxic and causes paralysis (**Figure 23-16**). These snakes are small, have small fangs, cannot open their mouths very far compared to larger snakes, and have to chew to allow the venom to penetrate; therefore, serious envenomations are not common.

Pit vipers are found throughout large portions of North America and include *rattlesnakes* of various types (**Figure 23-17**), copperheads (**Figure 23-18**), and *water moccasins*, or *cottonmouths* (**Figure 23-19**). The majority of pit viper bites do not occur in the wilderness, but rather in rural, suburban, or even urban areas. A classic example is the intoxicated man who was kissing his pet rattlesnake when he was bitten on the lips or tongue.

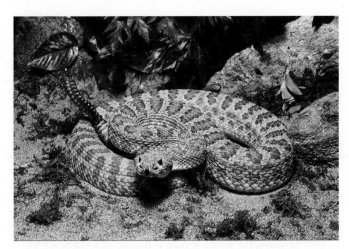

Figure 23-17 Rattlesnake.
Source: © Patrica Vargas/Photos.com/Thinkstock.

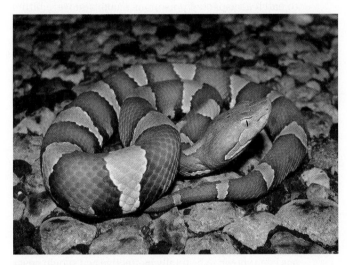

Figure 23-18 Copperhead snake.
Source: © Matt Jeppson/ShutterStock, Inc.

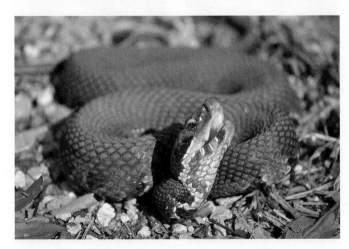

Figure 23-19 Water moccasin (cottonmouth) snake.
Source: © James DeBoer/ShutterStock, Inc.

Snakebites are not as rare as one might think. In the United States, almost 10,000 patients are treated each year for snakebites, and 5 die.[73] It is estimated that worldwide there are approximately 421,000 envenomations annually, resulting in 20,000 deaths, although this number could be much higher because of poor death records in many countries.[72]

Historically, there have been a variety of prehospital treatments attempted by patients, bystanders, or sometimes EMS personnel. The only treatment shown to be effective for envenomated pit viper bites is antivenin (antivenom), which is very expensive (thousands of U.S. dollars for a single treatment) and, thus, not routinely carried in first-aid kits. The only street care proven to be helpful is transport to the hospital.[74]

The first step in treating snakebite is to *watch for signs of envenomation* (i.e., determine that venom was injected). Only a fraction of bites by pit vipers actually result in envenomation (20% to 25% are dry bites), and the signs of envenomation are fairly distinct. Although signs and symptoms of envenomation usually develop in a few minutes, sometimes they are delayed by 6 to 8 hours or perhaps even longer, so starting to the hospital after a suspected poisonous snakebite is appropriate. Signs of envenomation include the following:

- Severe local redness, swelling, bruising, and pain
- Continued nonsignificant bleeding from the bite
- Paresthesias in the fingers and toes (Paresthesia is unusual sensation, usually caused by damage to nerves or biochemical abnormalities; a feeling of "pins and needles" is a common paresthesia.)
- Metallic taste in the mouth
- Feeling of severe anxiety ("impending doom")
- Nausea, vomiting, and abdominal pain

Prehospital Treatment of Suspected Pit Viper Envenomation[73,74]

When managing a patient with a suspected envenomation, the initial care is similar to any other seriously ill or injured patient: Support the ABCs (airway, breathing, circulation), provide oxygen to maintain an adequate oxygen saturation, apply a cardiac monitor, start intravenous therapy (to keep vein open), and take the patient's vital signs.

Assess the bite site for signs of envenomation, including erythema, swelling, ecchymoses, tenderness, and the development of blisters or soft-tissue necrosis. Any jewelry or tight clothing on the involved extremity should be removed.

The leading edge of the swelling should be marked with a black pen every 15 minutes to determine the severity of the swelling and rate of progression. The involved extremity should also be immobilized and elevated to help minimize any swelling. Major joints such as the elbow should be maintained in relative extension (less than 45 degrees of flexion).

If the patient requires pain relief, opiates are preferred for pain relief over nonsteroidal anti-inflammatory drugs because of the risk of bleeding associated with some envenomations and with nonsteroidal use.

Do not attempt to kill the snake. A killed or decapitated snake still offers a risk of envenomation to EMS personnel. If circumstances permit, take a photo of the snake from a safe distance.

While a litter rescue is preferred, if necessary the patient can be slowly walked for evacuation, with frequent rest stops and reassurance to help keep the patient calm. Transport the patient rapidly to an appropriate destination with notification of the situation while en route so that the receiving hospital can make preparations to receive and treat the patient.

Extremity Immobilization

Pressure immobilization has been used effectively in Australia for field management of *elapid* (cobra, mambas, North American Coral) snakebites, but newer evidence indicates that this procedure may be beneficial with pit viper bites in the United States (**Figure 23-20**).[75] This technique involves immediately wrapping the entire bitten extremity with an elastic wrap or crepe bandage as tightly as would be done for a sprain, and then splinting and immobilizing the extremity. This technique resulted in significantly longer survival, but higher intracompartmental pressures after artificial, intramuscular western diamondback rattlesnake envenomation in a pig model.

If the patient is more than 2 hours from medical attention, and the bite is on an arm or leg, use the pressure immobilization technique. Place a 2- by 2-inch (5- by 5-centimeter [cm]) cloth pad over the bite site. Next, apply an elastic wrap firmly around the involved limb directly over the padded bite site with a margin of at least 4 to 6 inches (10 to 15 cm) on either side of the wound. Take care to check for adequate circulation in the fingers and toes (normal pulses, feeling, and color). An alternative method is to simply wrap the entire limb as tightly as for a sprain with an elastic bandage. The wrap is meant to impede absorption of venom into the general circulation by containing it within the compressed tissue and microscopic blood and lymphatic vessels near the limb surface. Finally, splint the limb to prevent motion. If the bite is on a hand or arm, also apply a sling.

It should be noted that this recommendation is controversial, in that some experts believe that localizing venom in a single area might lead to an increased chance for local tissue damage.

The following are treatments that have been recommended over the years but are not supported by the literature and should not be performed:

1. *Rest.* Some recommendations insist that those who have been bitten should always avoid exertion. Deaths from North American snakebite are very rare,[76] and it is very unlikely that the exertion of hiking out from a wilderness area will make a victim of a snakebite significantly more ill. If the victim can be carried out, that is ideal. However, if waiting for a carryout will delay the victim's arrival at a hospital, the victim should walk out with whatever assistance can be given.

2. *Catching the snake and bringing it to the hospital.* There are numerous reports of bystanders who tried to catch a suspected poisonous snake and were bitten during the attempt. A single antivenin is used for all pit viper venoms in the United States, and treatment is based on clinical degree of envenomation, relying on the previous signs and symptoms. Therefore, identifying a domestic snake is of minor importance compared with the dangers of attempting to catch the snake. A digital photograph of the snake might be useful, but identification is not worth the risk of an additional bite.

3. *Suction or incision.* Suction, with or without cutting, has been shown to be useless for poisonous snakebite. Snakebite kits consisting of suction devices should be left out of all first-aid kits and should never be used.[77,78]

4. *Electric shock.* Electric shock applied to the snakebite has been shown to be totally ineffective and should never be used.[79,80]

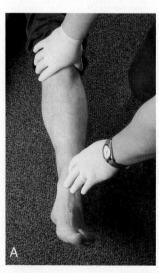 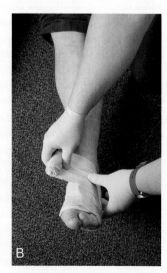 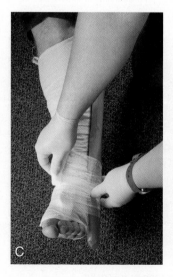 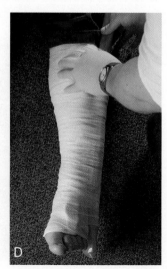

Figure 23-20 Pressure immobilization technique.
Source: © Jones & Bartlett Learning. Photographed by Darren Stahlman.

5. *Cold packs*. Cold packs have been shown to increase tissue damage from North American pit viper bites and should not be used.[81]

6. *Splinting, arterial or venous tourniquets, lymph constrictors, or elastic bandages*. Although widely recommended, none of these treatments has been shown to be effective and may worsen local damage to the bite area.[81,82]

The *Wilderness EMS* Context Revisited

At the beginning of this chapter, we asked when EMS is *wilderness EMS*. "When should we think about wilderness EMS; that is, when should we think and work differently from what we do on the street?" The short answer: "It depends."

Time, distance, weather, and terrain all enter into the decision. The decision that a particular patient, in a particular situation, with a particular set of injuries, needs *wilderness* care rather than *street* care is a medical decision—one best made by the prehospital care provider directly attending the patient. If the prehospital care provider at the scene can contact a knowledgeable EMS physician, especially one with wilderness EMS experience or training, the advice is definitely worth seeking. Ultimately, the decision is up to the prehospital care provider at the scene.

PHTLS believes that, given a good fund of knowledge and key principles, prehospital care providers are capable of making reasoned decisions regarding patient care.

Summary

- While many of the principles of *wilderness* EMS are the same as *street* EMS, preferences and practice may change because of the unique circumstances.
- Wilderness patients seldom need more or different invasive procedures; they do usually need prehospital care providers with keen critical-thinking skills.
- Clinical situations in which wilderness care is different include clearing the cervical spine, irrigating wounds, reducing dislocations, and terminating CPR.
- Managing patients in the wilderness setting requires that the wilderness medicine providers have a good understanding of environmental medical issues (see the Environmental Trauma I: Heat and Cold and the Environmental Trauma II: Drowning, Lightning, Diving, and Altitude chapters).
- When managing patients in the wilderness, the wilderness medicine providers have to also consider food and water requirements and elimination needs.
- A basic principle of wilderness care is that all patients are hypothermic, hypoglycemic, and hypovolemic.

SCENARIO RECAP

Your SAR team is called out at 2130 hours to support the county's volunteer fire fighters in the technical rescue of a trauma victim in a remote location. Early reports indicate that one member of the three-person rock climbing group, a 31-year-old man, fell at around 2030 hours from the cliff edge to the rocky floor 80 feet (24 m) below, sustaining multiple long-bone fractures. One member of the group ran back to his truck, grabbed a sleeping bag to keep the patient warm, and instructed the other climber to go get help.

The volunteer technical rescue team includes a paramedic and an ED nurse. They arrive at the incident command post at about 2230 hours. Following an incident briefing, the initial rescue team comprised of six personnel drive several miles on a trail using all-terrain vehicles and then hike for 60 minutes up a creek bed with gear to arrive at the scene. When you arrive after midnight, it is raining lightly and the ambient temperature is 50°F (10°C). You and the initial rescue team find the patient at the bottom of the cliff sitting up with his back against a rock.

- How would you begin managing this patient in this wilderness setting with limited resources?
- What are the major concerns when treating this patient's injuries?
- What will be the best way to evacuate this patient?

SCENARIO SOLUTION

As with street EMS, good medicine and optimal care can be provided in an austere environment with the right training and preparation. First and foremost you should be concerned about scene safety. One member of the SAR team should be designated safety lookout as the wilderness medicine providers start to stage gear and begin the patient assessment process.

The victim's face appears severely traumatized, with his jaw broken on both sides. A rapid trauma assessment reveals that the patient has multiple fractures to the face, both upper and lower extremities, and a suspected pelvis fracture. Your concerns include hypothermia, internal bleeding, hypotension, and shock. Your next challenge is protecting his airway. Initially it is best to leave him in the seated position against the rock wall as found. Besides the sleeping bag covering him, some additional insulation, if available, can be placed under and behind him to protect him from conductive heat loss to the rock.

The next concern is to determine his hemodynamic stability with a quick assessment of his radial pulse, ventilatory rate, and level of consciousness. Asking the patient about neck pain, in this case, is not a reliable assessment due to his many distracting injuries. You need to start an intravenous line, which can prove to be difficult due to hypotension and ongoing blood loss. Alternatively, intravenous fluid management can be started with an intraosseous device, but this may not be the best choice due to his many fractures. For this patient, the best option may be an external jugular vein if another peripheral vein cannot be found.

You realize the patient cannot be transported in the litter supine over rough terrain for any distance without a secure airway device because his mandible fracture, blood, and tissue will collapse back, obstructing his airway. You can attempt to place a nasopharyngeal airway initially, but you may be hesitant due to concern for potential basal skull fracture. Attempting a supraglottic airway and endotracheal intubation without sedation is out of the question due to his alert level of consciousness, and many of these advanced supraglottic airways require intact airway anatomy. You determine that the best way to manage the airway will either be with rapid sequence intubation or a surgical airway. Once the airway is controlled, the patient can be placed in the supine position. As additional personnel arrive from the staging point, the patient can be safely rolled onto a backboard and lifted into the Stokes litter for the long ground evacuation. You assign one paramedic and a nurse to remain at the patient's head to monitor vital signs, airway, and level of sedation during the long evacuation.

References

1. Salomone JP, Pons PT, McSwain NE, eds. The science and art of prehospital care: principles, preferences and critical thinking. In: *Prehospital Trauma Life Support.* 7th ed. St. Louis, MO: Elsevier Mosby; 2011.

2. Lifrig JR, McStay CM. Wilderness medicine education. In: Auerbach PS, ed. *Wilderness Medicine.* 6th ed. Philadelphia, PA: Elsevier Mosby; 2012.

3. Bennett BL. A time has come for wilderness emergency medical service: a new direction. *Wilderness Environ Med.* 2012;23(1):5–6.

4. Warden CR, Millin MG, Hawkins SC, et al. Medical direction of wilderness and other operational emergency services programs. *Wilderness Environ Med.* 2012;23(1):37–43.

5. *Merriam-Webster's Collegiate Dictionary.* 11th ed. Springfield, MA: Merriam-Webster; 2007.

6. Goodman T, Iserson KV, Strich H. Wilderness mortalities: a 13-year experience. *Ann Emerg Med.* 2001;37:279–283.

7. Gentile DA, Morris JA, Schimelpfenig T, Bass SM, Auerback PS. Wilderness injuries and illnesses. *Ann Emerg Med.* 1992;21:853–861.

8. Singletary E, Markenson DS. Injury prevention: decision making, safety, and accident avoidance In: Auerbach PS, ed. *Wilderness Medicine.* 6th ed. Philadelphia, PA: Elsevier Mosby; 2012.

9. Chan D, Goldberg R, Tascone A, et al. The effect of spinal immobilization on healthy volunteers. *Ann Emerg Med.* 1994;23(1):48.

10. Conover K. EMTs should be able to clear the cervical spine in the wilderness (editorial). *J Wild Med.* 1992;3(4):339.

11. Vaillancourt C, Stiell IG, Beaudoin T, et al. The out-of-hospital validation of the Canadian C-Spine Rule by paramedics. *Ann Emerg Med.* 2009;54(5):663–671.

12. Ahn H, Singh J, Nathens A, et al. Pre-hospital care management of a potential spinal cord injured patient: a systematic review of the literature and evidence-based guidelines. *J Neurotrauma.* 2011;28:1341–1361.

13. Quinn R, Williams J, Bennett BL, Stiller G, Islas A, McCord S. Wilderness Medical Society practice guidelines for spine immobilization in the austere environment. *Wilderness Environ Med.* 2013;24(3):241–252.

14. Hoffman JR, Mower WR, Wolfson AB, Todd KH, Zucker MI. Validity of a set of clinical criteria to rule out injury to the cervical spine in patients with blunt trauma. National Emergency X-radiography Utilization Study Group. *N Engl J Med.* 2000;343:94–99.

15. Zafren K, McCurley LH, Shimanski C, Smith W. Technical rescue, self-rescue, and evacuation. In: Auerbach PS, ed. *Wilderness Medicine.* 6th ed. Philadelphia, PA: Elsevier Mosby; 2012.

16. Gomi T. *Everyone Poops.* Brooklyn, NY: Kane/Miller Book Publishers; 1993.

17. Cooper DC, Mier TP. Litters and carries. In: Auerbach PS, ed. *Wilderness Medicine.* 6th ed. Philadelphia, PA: Elsevier Mosby; 2012.

18. Goldberg R, Chan D, Mason J, Chan L. Backboard versus mattress splint immobilization: a comparison of symptoms generated. *J Emerg Med*. 1996;14(3):293.

19. Hamilton RS, Pons PT. The efficacy and comfort of full-body vacuum splints for cervical-spine immobilization. *J Emerg Med*. 1996;14(5):553.

20. Johnson DR, Hauswald M, Stockhoff C. Comparison of a vacuum splint device to a rigid backboard for spinal immobilization. *Am J Emerg Med*. 1996;14(4):369.

21. Lovell ME, Evans JH. A comparison of the spinal board and the vacuum stretcher, spinal stability and interface pressure. *Injury*. 1994;25(3):179.

22. Cordell WH, Hollingsworth JC, Olinger ML, et al. Pain and tissue-interface pressures during spine-board immobilization. *Ann Emerg Med*. 1995;26(1):31.

23. Delbridge TR, Auble TE, Garrison HG, Menengazzi JJ. Discomfort in healthy volunteers immobilized on wooden backboards and vacuum mattress splints. *Prehosp Disaster Med*. 1993;8(suppl 2).

24. Linares HA, Mawson AR, Suarez E. Association between pressure sores and immobilization in the immediate postinjury period. *Orthopedics*. 1987;10:571.

25. Mawson AR, Bundo JJ, Neville P. Risk factors for early occurring pressure ulcers following spinal cord injury. *Am J Phys Med Rehab*. 1988;67:123.

26. Askew W. Nutrition, malnutrition and starvation. In: Auerbach PS, ed. *Wilderness Medicine*. 6th ed. Philadelphia, PA: Elsevier Mosby; 2012.

27. Kenefick RW, Cheuvront SN, Leon LR, Obrien K. Dehydration, rehydration and hyperhydration. In: Auerbach PS, ed. *Wilderness Medicine*. 6th ed. Philadelphia, PA: Elsevier Mosby; 2012.

28. Prevention and treatment of sunburn. *Med Lett Drugs Ther*. 2004;46:45.

29. Stern RS. Clinical practice. Treatment of photoaging. *N Engl J Med*. 2004;350:1526.

30. Krakowski AC, Kaplan LA. Exposure to radiation from the sun. In: Auerbach PS, ed. *Wilderness Medicine*. 6th ed. Philadelphia, PA: Elsevier Mosby; 2012.

31. Markenson D, Ferguson JD, Chameides L. Part 17: first aid: 2010 American Heart Association and American Red Cross Guidelines for First Aid. *Circulation*. 2010;122;S934–S946.

32. Edlich RF, Rodeheaver GT, Morgan RF, et al. Principles of emergency wound management. *Ann Emerg Med*. 1988;17(12):1284.

33. Edlich RF, Thacker JG, Buchanan L, Rodeheaver GT. Modern concepts of treatment of traumatic wounds. *Adv Surg*. 1979;13:169.

34. Bhandari M, Thompson K, Adili A, Shaughnessy SG. High and low pressure irrigation in contaminated wounds with exposed bone. *Int J Surg Invest*. 2000;2(3):179.

35. Bhandari M, Adili A, Lachowski RJ. High pressure pulsatile lavage of contaminated human tibiae: an in vitro study. *J Orthop Trauma*. 1998;12(7):479.

36. Bhandari M, Schemitsch EH, Adili A, et al. High and low pressure pulsatile lavage of contaminated tibial fractures: an in vitro study of bacterial adherence and bone damage. *J Orthop Trauma*. 1999;13(8):526.

37. Anglen JO. Wound irrigation in musculoskeletal injury. *J Am Acad Orthop Surg*. 2001;9(4):219.

38. Valente JH, Forti RJ, Freundlich LF, et al. Wound irrigation in children: saline solution or tap water? *Ann Emerg Med*. 2003;41(5):609.

39. Backer HD. Field water disinfection. In: Auerbach PS, ed. *Wilderness Medicine*. 6th ed. Philadelphia, PA: Elsevier Mosby; 2012.

40. Griffiths RD, Fernandez RS, Ussia CA. Is tap water a safe alternative to normal saline for wound irrigation in the community setting? *J Wound Care*. 2001;10(10):407.

41. Moscati R, Mayrose J, Fincher L, Jehle D. Comparison of normal saline with tap water for wound irrigation. *Am J Emerg Med*. 1998;16(4):379.

42. Moscati RM, Reardon RF, Lerner EB, Mayrose J. Wound irrigation with tap water. *Acad Emerg Med*. 1998;5(11):1076.

43. Rodeheaver GT, Pettry D, Thacker JG, et al. Wound cleansing by high pressure irrigation. *Surg Gynecol Obstet*. 1975;141(3):357.

44. Edlich RF, Reddy VR. Revolutionary advances in wound repair in emergency medicine during the last three decades: a view toward the new millennium. 5th Annual David R. Boyd, MD, Lecture. *J Emerg Med*. 2001;20(2):167.

45. Singer AJ, Hollander JE, Subramanian S, et al. Pressure dynamics of various irrigation techniques commonly used in the emergency department. *Ann Emerg Med*. 1994;24(1):36.

46. Mellor SG, Cooper GJ, Bowyer GW. Efficacy of delayed administration of benzylpenicillin in the control of infection in penetrating soft tissue injuries in war. *J Trauma*. 1996;40(3 Suppl):S128–134.

47. Hospenthal DR, Murray CK, Andersen RC, et al. Guidelines for the prevention of infection after combat-related injuries. *J Trauma*. 2008;64(3 suppl):S211–S220.

48. Fulton RL, Voigt WJ, Hilakos AS. Confusion surrounding the treatment of traumatic cardiac arrest. *J Am Coll Surg*. 1995;181:209.

49. Pasquale MD, Rhodes M, Cipolle MD, et al. Defining "dead on arrival": impact on a level I trauma center. *J Trauma*. 1996;41:726.

50. Mattox KL, Feliciano DV. Role of external cardiac compression in truncal trauma. *J Trauma*. 1982;22:934.

51. Shimazu S, Shatney CH. Outcomes of trauma patients with no vital signs on admission. *J Trauma*. 1983;23(3):213.

52. Forgey WW, Wilderness Medical Society. *Practice Guidelines for Wilderness Emergency Care*. 5th ed. Guilford, CN: Globe Pequot Press; 2006.

53. Goth P, Garnett G, Rural Affairs Committee, National Association of EMS Physicians. Clinical guidelines for delayed/prolonged transport. I. Cardiorespiratory arrest. *Prehosp Disaster Med*. 1991;6(3):335.

54. Eisenberg MS, Bergner L, Hallstrom AP. Cardiac resuscitation in the community: importance of rapid provision and implications of program planning. *JAMA*. 1979;241:1905.

55. Kellermann AL, Hackman BB, Somes G. Predicting the outcome of unsuccessful prehospital advanced cardiac life support. *JAMA*. 1993;270(12):1433.

56. Bonnin MJ, Pepe PE, Kimball KT, Clark PS. Distinct criteria for termination of resuscitation in the out-of-hospital setting. *JAMA*. 1993;270(12):1457.

57. Millin MG, Khandker SR, Malki A. Termination of resuscitation of nontraumatic cardiopulmonary arrest: resource document for the National Association of EMS Physicians position statement. *Prehosp Emerg Care*. 2011;15(4):547–554.

58. Leavitt M, Podgorny G. Prehospital CPR and the pulseless hypothermic patient. *Ann Emerg Med*. 1984;13:492.

59. Keatinge WR. Accidental immersion hypothermia and drowning. *Practitioner*. 1977;219:183.

60. Olshaker JS. Near drowning. *Emerg Med Clin North Am*. 1992;10(2):339.

61. Bolte RG, Black PG, Bowers RS, et al. The use of extracorporeal rewarming in a child submerged for 66 minutes. *JAMA*. 1988;260(3):377.

62. Orlowski JP. Drowning, near-drowning, and ice-water drowning. *JAMA*. 1988;260(3):390.

63. Cooper MA. Lightning injuries. In: Auerbach PS, Geehr EC, eds. *Wilderness Medicine: Management of Wilderness and Environmental Emergencies*. 2nd ed. St. Louis, MO: Mosby; 1989.

64. Durrer B, Brugger H. Recent advances in avalanche survival. Presented at the Second World Congress on Wilderness Medicine. Aspen, CO; 1995.

65. Steinman AM. Cardiopulmonary resuscitation and hypothermia. *Circulation*. 1986;74(6, pt 2):29.

66. Zell SC. Epidemiology of wilderness-acquired diarrhea: implications for prevention and treatment. *J Wild Med*. 1992;3(3):241.

67. Lloyd EL. *Hypothermia and Cold Stress*. Rockville, MD: Aspen Systems; 1986.

68. Maningas PA, DeGuzman LR, Hollenbach SJ, et al. Regional blood flow during hypothermic arrest. *Ann Emerg Med*. 1986;15(4):390.

69. Gaudio F, Lamery J, Johnson D. Recommendations on the use of epinephrine in outdoor education and wilderness settings. *Wilderness Environ Med*. 2010;21:185–187.

70. Hawkins S, Weil C, Fitzpatrick D. Letter to the editor: epinephrine autoinjector warning. *Wilderness Environ Med*. 2012;23:371–378.

71. Paw Nation. Snake bite death statistics worldwide. http://animals.pawnation.com/snake-bite-death-statistics-worldwide-2431.html. Accessed September 15, 2013.

72. Kasturiratne A, Wickremasinghe AR, de Silva N, et al. The global burden of snakebite: a literature analysis and modelling based on regional estimates of envenoming and deaths. *PLoS Med*. 2008;5(11):e218.

73. O'Neil ME, Mack KA, Gilchrist J, Wozniak EJ. Snakebite injuries treated in United States emergency departments, 2001–2004. *Wilderness Environ Med*. 200718(4):281–287.

74. Lavonas EJ, Ruha AM, Banner W, et al. Unified treatment algorithm for the management of crotaline snakebite in the United States: results of an evidence-informed consensus workshop. *BMC Emerg Med*. 2011;11:2.

75. Norris R, Bush S, Cohen-Smith J. Bites by Venomous Reptiles in Canada, the United States and Mexico. In: Auerbach PS, ed. *Wilderness Medicine*. 6th ed. Philadelphia, PA: Elsevier Mosby; 2012.

76. Curry SC, Kunkel DB. Death from a rattlesnake bite. *Am J Emerg Med*. 1985;3(3):227.

77. Bush SP. Snakebite suction devices don't remove venom: they just suck. *Ann Emerg Med*. 2004;43(2):187.

78. Alberts MB, Shalit M, LoGalbo F. Suction for venomous snakebite: a study of "mock venom" extraction in a human model. *Ann Emerg Med*. 2004;43(2):181.

79. Davis D, Branch K, Egen NB, et al. The effect of an electrical current on snake venom toxicity. *J Wild Med*. 1992;3(1):48.

80. Howe NR, Meisenheimer JL Jr. Electric shock does not save snake-bitten rats. *Ann Emerg Med*. 1988;17(3):254.

81. Gill KA Jr. The evaluation of cryotherapy in the treatment of snake envenomation. *South Med J*. 1968;63:552.

82. Norris RL. A call for snakebite research. *Wilderness Environ Med*. 2000;11(3):149.

Suggested Reading

Auerbach PS, ed. *Wilderness Medicine*. 6th ed. Philadelphia, PA: Elsevier Mosby; 2012.

Goth P, Garnett G. Clinical guidelines for delayed or prolonged transport: II. Dislocations. Rural Affairs Committee, National Association of Emergency Medical Services Physicians. *Prehosp Disaster Med*. 1993;8(1):77.

Goth P, Garnett G. Clinical guidelines for delayed or prolonged transport: IV. Wounds. Rural Affairs Committee, National Association of Emergency Medical Services Physicians. *Prehosp Disaster Med*. 1993;8(3):253.

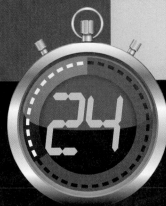

CHAPTER 24

Introduction to Tactical Combat Casualty Care

CHAPTER OBJECTIVES

At the completion of this chapter, the reader will be able to do the following:

- State the three goals of Tactical Combat Casualty Care (TCCC).

- List the three phases of TCCC and describe the tactical situation that defines each phase.

- Describe the composition of the Committee on Tactical Combat Casualty Care (CoTCCC).

- List the two U.S. civilian medical entities that endorse the TCCC guidelines.

SCENARIO

You are the only medic traveling in a 10-person, four-vehicle convoy through a small village in eastern Iraq. As you pull out on open road at the end of the village, an improvised explosive device (IED) explodes under the second vehicle. There is no follow-up hostile fire, so the unit sets up a secure perimeter. You proceed to assess the three major casualties at the scene.

Casualty 1 is a soldier with femoral arterial bleeding from a large wound on the right thigh, as well as a right hand amputation with blood oozing from the stump. He is conscious and has a good radial pulse.

Casualty 2 is a soldier with a large open head wound in which mangled gray matter is clearly visible. He is unresponsive, and his breathing is agonal.

Casualty 3 is a civilian bystander with penetrating injury to his right lower abdomen. He is conscious and in great pain.

Casualty Evacuation (CASEVAC) by helicopter is available in 20 minutes, and the flight to the nearest medical treatment facility will take approximately 30 minutes.

1. What are some of the considerations in managing these casualties that are not present in most civilian settings?

Introduction

Prehospital trauma care on the battlefield varies in many respects from prehospital trauma care as practiced in the civilian sector. The types and severity of the injuries are different from those encountered in civilian settings, and combat medical personnel face multiple additional challenges in caring for their wounded teammates in tactical settings. They must provide care while under hostile fire, often working in the dark, with multiple casualties and limited equipment. They must also often contend with prolonged evacuation times as well as the need for tactical maneuvers superimposed upon their efforts to render medical care. Treatment guidelines developed for the civilian setting do not necessarily translate well to the battlefield. Preventable deaths and unnecessary additional casualties may result if the tactical environment is not considered when developing battlefield trauma care strategies **(Figure 24-1)**.

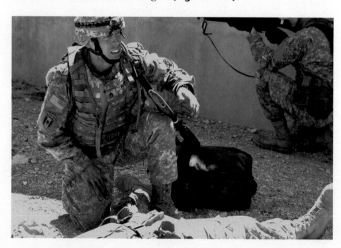

Figure 24-1 Prehospital medicine in the civilian setting differs from the battlefield due to the nature of the environment.
Source: Courtesy of Mr. Jerry Harben/U.S. Army

The above considerations notwithstanding, at the onset of hostilities in Afghanistan, most U.S. combat medical personnel were being trained using the following civilian-based principles of trauma care[1]:

- To render care with no structured consideration of the evolving tactical situation
- <u>Not</u> to use tourniquets to control extremity hemorrhage
- To manage external hemorrhage with prolonged direct pressure, thereby precluding the medic from attending to other injuries or rendering care to other casualties
- No use of hemostatic dressings
- Two large-bore intravenous (IV) lines started on all casualties with significant trauma
- Treatment of hypovolemic shock with large-volume crystalloid fluid resuscitation
- No special considerations made for traumatic brain injury (TBI) with respect to avoiding hypotension or hypoxia
- Management of the airway in facial trauma or unconscious casualties with endotracheal intubation
- No specific techniques or equipment to prevent hypothermia and secondary coagulopathy in combat casualties
- Management of pain in combat casualties with intramuscular (IM) morphine, a battlefield analgesic that dates back to the Civil War
- No intraosseous access techniques
- No prehospital electronic monitoring techniques
- No effective nonparenteral analgesic medications
- No prehospital antibiotics
- No delineation of which casualties might benefit most from supplemental oxygen in the Tactical Evacuation (TACEVAC) phase of care
- Spinal precautions applied broadly to casualties with significant trauma, without consideration of tactical concerns or mechanism of injury

The need for reconsideration of trauma care guidelines in the tactical setting has long been recognized.[2-4] The Tactical Combat Casualty Care (TCCC) project was initiated by the Naval Special Warfare Command in 1993 and later continued by the U.S. Special Operations Command (USSOCOM). This effort culminated in a set of tactically appropriate battlefield trauma care guidelines that were published as a supplement to *Military Medicine* in 1996.[5] The TCCC guidelines provide combat medics and corpsmen with trauma management strategies that combine good medicine with good small-unit tactics. TCCC has three goals for trauma care in the tactical environment: (1) *Treat the casualty*, (2) *prevent additional casualties*, and (3) *complete the mission*. The trauma care measures proposed in the original TCCC guidelines included:

- A three-phase approach to tactical trauma care
- Tourniquets
- Battlefield antibiotics
- Tactically appropriate fluid resuscitation
- Improved battlefield analgesia (IV vs. IM morphine)
- Nasopharyngeal airways as first-line airway devices
- Surgical airways for maxillofacial trauma with obstructed airway
- Aggressive diagnosis and treatment of tension pneumothorax
- Combat medical personnel input into the TCCC guidelines
- Scenario-based TCCC training
- Combining good tactics with good medicine

As the name implies, TCCC is used when casualties are sustained during combat missions. Prehospital trauma care in the military is most commonly provided by enlisted combat medical personnel: medics in the Army, corpsmen in the Navy and Marine Corps, and both medics and pararescuemen (PJs) in the Air Force.

TCCC is divided into three phases: **Care Under Fire**, **Tactical Field Care**, and **Tactical Evacuation Care**. In the Care Under Fire phase, combat medical personnel and their units are under effective hostile fire, and the care they can provide is very limited. In the Tactical Field Care phase, combat medical personnel and their casualties are no longer under effective hostile fire, and more extensive care can be provided. In the Tactical Evacuation phase, casualties are transported to a medical facility by an aircraft, ground vehicle, or boat, and there is an opportunity to provide additional medical personnel and equipment to further increase the level of care rendered. Each of these phases of care will be discussed in greater detail in the respective Care Under Fire, Tactical Field Care, and Tactical Evacuation Care chapters.

The first TCCC course was taught in 1996 in the Undersea Medical Officer course sponsored by the Navy Bureau of Medicine and Surgery (BUMED). Shortly thereafter, this training was mandated for all Navy Sea, Air, and Land (SEAL) corpsmen.[6]

Since that time, TCCC has been gradually gaining acceptance in U.S.[7-13] and allied[14] military forces. It has also found acceptance in the civilian law enforcement medical community.[15]

The incorporation of the TCCC guidelines in the *Prehospital Trauma Life Support* (*PHTLS*) manual was an important milestone in the TCCC transition process. The fourth edition of *PHTLS*, published in 1999, contained a chapter on military medicine for the first time, and TCCC was included as part of this chapter.[16] The recommendations contained in the *PHTLS* textbook carry the endorsement of the American College of Surgeons Committee on Trauma, the National Association of Emergency Medical Technicians (NAEMT) and the U.S. Department of Defense. TCCC is the only set of battlefield trauma care guidelines ever to have received this triple endorsement.

The Committee on Tactical Combat Casualty Care (CoTCCC)

The need for periodic updates to the TCCC guidelines was recognized early in the development of TCCC. The original TCCC paper recommended that the TCCC guidelines be updated as needed by a Department of Defense–sponsored committee established for this purpose.[5] This concept was endorsed by the USSOCOM, and the Committee on Tactical Combat Casualty Care (CoTCCC) was subsequently funded as a 2001/2002 USSOCOM biomedical research project. The command chosen to execute the project, the Naval Operational Medicine Institute, subsequently conducted the necessary coordination with Navy Medicine leadership to ensure that there would be long-term support of this effort. BUMED programmed for financial and personnel support of the CoTCCC beginning in fiscal year 2004. In fiscal years 2007 through 2009, the Office of the Surgeon General of the Army and the U.S. Army Institute of Surgical Research also provided substantial support for the Committee.

CoTCCC Membership

Since the goal of TCCC is to provide the best possible medical care consistent with good small-unit tactics, it was and still is essential that the membership of the CoTCCC included combat medical personnel as well as physicians. Additionally it was also critical to have tri-service representation present. This representation ensures that differences in doctrine and experience among the Army, Navy, and Air Force medical departments are identified and best practices from each are incorporated into TCCC. The combat medics selected included Navy SEAL corpsmen, Navy corpsmen assigned to

Marine units, Ranger medics, Special Forces 18-D medics, Air Force PJs, Air Force aviation medics, and Coast Guard health specialists. Physician membership included representatives from the trauma surgery, emergency medicine, critical care, and operational medicine communities. Physician assistants, medical planners, and medical educators were also represented.

CoTCCC Alignment

In 2007, due to the increasing visibility of TCCC in the Global War on Terrorism, the Navy Medical Support Command proposed that the CoTCCC be considered for realignment at a more senior joint command. This proposal was briefed to the offices of the Assistant Secretary of Defense for Health Affairs and the Surgeon for the Joint Chiefs of Staff.

In March 2008, the CoTCCC was relocated to function as a working group of the Trauma and Injury Subcommittee of the Defense Health Board, which has a charter to provide independent advice and recommendations to the Secretary of Defense, through the Undersecretary of Defense for Personnel and Readiness, and the Assistant Secretary of Defense for Health Affairs on medical issues, to include the care of U.S. service members wounded in combat operations.

On February 21, 2013, by direction of the Acting Undersecretary of Defense for Personnel and Readiness, the CoTCCC was moved once more, this time to the Joint Trauma System to be co-located with the rest of the trauma system organization in the Department of Defense.

TCCC Guideline Updates

Since 2001, the CoTCCC has monitored advances in prehospital trauma care and technology. It uses this information to update the TCCC guidelines as needed. These updates were initially performed on a 3- to 4-year cycle that was matched to the publication of the *PHTLS* textbook. However, the CoTCCC realized that the guidelines needed to be updated on a more frequent basis, and updates are now posted on both the PHTLS and the Military Health System websites after they are approved.

The CoTCCC updates the guidelines based upon (1) ongoing review of the published civilian and military prehospital trauma literature; (2) ongoing interaction with military combat casualty care research laboratories; (3) direct input from experienced combat corpsmen, medics, and PJs; (4) input from the service medical lessons-learned centers; (5) case reports discussed at the weekly Joint Theater Trauma System process improvement video-teleconferences; and (6) expert opinion from both military and civilian trauma experts **(Figure 24-2)**.

Figure 24-2 Guideline Updates

U.S. combat medics, corpsmen, and pararescuemen are now taught battlefield trauma care techniques based on the TCCC guidelines. These guidelines are reviewed quarterly and updated as needed by the CoTCCC.[1] Proposed changes to the TCCC guidelines must be approved by a two-thirds majority of the CoTCCC to be accepted. Changes recommended by the CoTCCC are then forwarded to the Director of the Joint Trauma System for approval. Once approved, updated versions of the TCCC guidelines are posted on both the Military Health System and the PHTLS section of the NAEMT website. At 3- to 4-year intervals, the TCCC guidelines are also published in updates to the military version of the *PHTLS* manual.

Battlefield Trauma Care Today

TCCC-based training is now provided to all U.S. combat medical personnel and includes[17]:

- Phased care in the tactical environment to ensure that good medicine is combined with good small-unit tactics. The three defined phases of care are:
    - Care Under Fire
    - Tactical Field Care
    - Tactical Evacuation (TACEVAC) Care
- Casualty and medic actions during the Care Under Fire phase that focus on gaining and maintaining the tactical advantage, with only tourniquets recommended as standard medical care in this phase
- Aggressive use of tourniquets to control life-threatening extremity hemorrhage
- The use of Combat Gauze™ to control life-threatening hemorrhage from external bleeding at sites that are not amenable to tourniquet use
- The use of nasopharyngeal airways to maintain a patent airway when there is no airway obstruction from direct maxillofacial or neck trauma
- Initial management of the airway in maxillofacial trauma by having the casualty sit up and lean forward if possible, thus allowing blood to simply drain out of the oropharynx, clearing the airway
- Surgical airways for maxillofacial or neck trauma when airway compromise is present and the sit-up-and-lean-forward position is not feasible or not successful
- Aggressive needle thoracostomy for tension pneumothorax

- A different approach to spinal precautions—they are not emphasized for casualties with penetrating trauma only, but are still recommended, if tactically feasible, when blunt trauma is present
- IV access only when required for medications or fluid resuscitation
- The preferential use of a saline lock for IV access as opposed to an IV catheter running fluids at a keep-vein-open rate
- The use of intraosseous devices when vascular access is needed but difficult to obtain
- Hypotensive resuscitation with Hextend™ for casualties in shock
- More aggressive fluid resuscitation and supplemental oxygen as needed to avoid hypotension and hypoxia in casualties with TBI
- More rapid and effective battlefield analgesia through the use of IV morphine, oral transmucosal fentanyl citrate (OTFC) lozenges, and ketamine
- Prevention of hypothermia and secondary coagulopathy with improved technology to prevent heat loss
- The use of moxifloxacin, ertapenem, or cefotetan on the battlefield to reduce preventable deaths and morbidity from wound infections
- Combat scenario–based trauma training emphasizing that trauma care on the battlefield must be consistent with good small-unit tactics
- Resuscitation with 1:1 plasma and packed red blood cells when feasible during the TACEVAC phase for casualties who are in shock
- Better identification of casualties likely to derive the most benefit from supplemental oxygen during TACEVAC[18]
- The use of tranexamic acid to help prevent death from noncompressible and junctional hemorrhage
- The use of the Combat Ready Clamp™, the Junctional Emergency Treatment Tool, and the SAM Junctional Splint to help prevent death from junctional hemorrhage
- Strategies for management of wounded hostile combatants
- Rules of thumb and specific examples of injury patterns for determining evacuation priorities[19,20]

Battlefield Experience With TCCC in Iraq and Afghanistan

Holcomb and coauthors examined the first 82 Special Operations fatalities in Iraq and Afghanistan.[21] They found that 8 of the 12 individuals who died from injuries that were potentially survivable might have been saved simply by the proper application of TCCC principles.

Numerous reports published in the medical literature and collected from combat medical personnel have documented

that TCCC is saving lives on the battlefield and is improving the tactical flow of missions on which casualties have been sustained. Tarpey[22] described the use of TCCC by elements of the Third Infantry Division in the initial phase of the war in Iraq. He reported:

> The adoption and implementation of the principles of TCCC by the medical platoon of Task Force 1-15 in OIF 1 [Operation Iraqi Freedom 1] resulted in overwhelming success. In over 25 days of continuous combat with 32 friendly casualties, many of them serious, we had 0 Killed in Action and 0 Died of Wounds, while simultaneously caring for a significant number of Iraqi civilian and military casualties.

Gresham[23] noted that the 101st Airborne Division:

> … by teaching and using [TCCC] ideas, has achieved one of the highest casualty survival rates in combat of any unit in the Army.

In an article in *Tip of the Spear*, the official publication of the USSOCOM, Bottoms[24] stated:

> Multiple reports from SOF First Responders have credited TCCC techniques and equipment with saving lives on the battlefield.

General Doug Brown, Commander of USSOCOM, sent a letter of appreciation to the Army Surgeon General for the outstanding work done by the U.S. Army Institute of Surgical Research (USAISR) in establishing a pilot program called the TCCC Transition Initiative (described by Butler and Holcomb[25]). This program was established to fast-track new TCCC training and equipment to deploying Special Operations Forces (SOF) units and to collect data about the success of these measures. General Brown stated in his letter[26] that the USAISR's TCCC program had:

> … produced remarkable advances in our force's ability to successfully manage battlefield trauma.

A team from Madigan Army Medical Center used TCCC-based training to prepare 1,317 combat medics for deployment to Iraq or Afghanistan. Of the 140 combat medics who subsequently deployed to Iraq for 1-year periods:

> 99% indicated that the principles taught in the TCCC course helped with the management of injured casualties during their deployment.[27]

Master Sergeant Ted Westmoreland, one of the senior enlisted medics in the Army Special Missions Unit, accumulated extensive experience using TCCC to treat combat casualties in the first few months of the conflict in Afghanistan. In a presentation to the Special Operations Medical Association in December 2005, he made the following recommendation:

> Implement TCCC into all service medical training NOW.[7]

In a paper titled "Understanding Combat Casualty Care Statistics," Holcomb and his coauthors[28] documented that combat casualties of American forces in Iraq and Afghanistan were experiencing the highest casualty survival rate in U.S. history. They identified TCCC as one of the major factors responsible for this landmark achievement.

In their discussion of the newly developed Joint Theater Trauma System, the Director, Colonel Brian Eastridge, and coauthors[29] recognized the strong positive impact of Tactical Combat Casualty Care and similar courses of instruction on the battlefield trauma care training the United States provides to its combat medical personnel.

Beekley, Starnes, and Sebesta[30] reviewed major surgical lessons learned from the conflicts in Iraq and Afghanistan. Nine of the 19 advances that they highlighted were battlefield trauma management strategies pioneered primarily by TCCC.

Perhaps the most successful TCCC intervention has been the widespread reintroduction of tourniquet use on the battlefield. Despite deploying initially to Afghanistan and Iraq without modern tourniquets, U.S. military troops now routinely carry well-made tourniquets into combat. Tourniquets have proven remarkably effective at saving lives in casualties with extremity hemorrhage, with very few complications.[31-35] Other TCCC recommendations such as moving away from large volume crystalloid fluid resuscitation, using nasopharyngeal airways instead of endotracheal tubes in Tactical Field Care, and using needle decompression initially to treat tension pneumothorax instead of chest tubes have not only proven effective, but have helped to reduce the medical equipment load carried by combat medical personnel and their training requirements.[7]

Mabry and McManus[35] recently noted that:

> ... the new concept of Tactical Combat Casualty Care has revolutionized the management of combat casualties in the prehospital tactical setting.

In 2008, Dr. Jeffrey Salomone, the Prehospital Trauma Chair for the American College of Surgeons Committee on Trauma, wrote to the Assistant Secretary of Defense for Health Affairs:

> I am writing to offer my congratulations for the recent dramatic advances in prehospital trauma care delivered by the U.S. military. Multiple recent publications have shown that Tactical Combat Casualty Care is saving lives on the battlefield.[36]

Sergeant Major Mike Hetzler and Master Sergeant Justin Ball, two combat-experienced Special Forces medics, confirmed that:

> TCCC's identification of causes of combat mortality and essential procedures for their treatment (i.e., tourniquets, needle decompression, etc.) has greatly assisted the medic in focusing the cube space of his gear to the most relevant life threats.[37]

Colonel Andy Pennardt reported no potentially preventable deaths among the 201 casualties (including 12 fatalities) sustained by his USSOCOM unit during the conflicts in Afghanistan and Iraq through 2009.[38] All nonmedical personnel in this command had been trained in TCCC beginning prior to 2001.

Through the course of hostilities in Afghanistan and Iraq, TCCC has gone from being used by only a few USSOCOM and 18th Airborne Corps units to being used throughout the battle space. This evolution has, however, occurred unevenly and sporadically.[39] The 75th Ranger Regiment began training all nonmedical personnel in TCCC prior to the start of the current conflicts. Lieutenant Colonel Russ Kotwal, the Regimental Surgeon, and his colleagues reported that the incidence of preventable deaths among 419 combat casualties sustained by the 75th Rangers was 3%.[40] This finding stands in dramatic contrast to the 15% to 28% incidence of preventable deaths among U.S. casualties in these conflicts reported in other studies.[21,34,41] Considering the prehospital phase only, the incidence of preventable deaths among fatalities in the 75th Rangers was zero as compared to 24% in the study by Eastridge and coauthors.[34]

The factor common to the two units reported on by Colonels Pennardt[38] and Kotwal[40] is the long-standing practice of teaching TCCC to every combatant so that the most critical lifesaving interventions, like tourniquets, can be accomplished by every one of their unit members. Although observed differences in potentially preventable deaths may be multifactorial, both units with well-documented and extensive TCCC programs throughout the recent conflicts also had the lowest reported incidence of preventable deaths as a result of those conflicts.

TCCC in the U.S. Department of Defense

As a result of the observed success of TCCC training in minimizing preventable combat fatalities, TCCC is now used extensively throughout the U.S. military. USSOCOM[42] mandated TCCC training for its forces in 2005 and, in partnership with the USAISR, established the TCCC Transition Initiative to fast-track TCCC training and equipment to its units.[25] The BUMED-directed review of TCCC[43] conducted in 2006/2007 found that TCCC is now used not only by SOF, but also by all of the conventional forces in the U.S. military, as has been confirmed by other sources.[1,7,8,34,44-48] As of February 2009, the Army is directing that all medical department members undergo predeployment trauma training that includes TCCC.[49]

The Defense Health Board[50] recommended in August 2009 that TCCC be taught to all deploying combatants and to all combatant unit medical providers. **Figure 24-3** contains the

Figure 24-3 Tactical Combat Casualty Care (TCCC) Skill Sets

Skill	All	CLS	CM	CPM
Overview of Tactical Medicine	X	X	X	X
Hemostasis				
Apply Tourniquet	X	X	X	X
Apply Direct Pressure	X	X	X	X
Apply Bandage	X	X	X	X
Apply Combat Gauze	X	X	X	X
Apply Pressure Dressing	X	X	X	X
Apply Combat Ready Clamp, Junctional Emergency Treatment Tool, SAM Junctional Splint			X	X
Casualty Movement Techniques	X	X	X	X
Airway				
Chin Lift/Jaw Thrust Maneuver	X	X	X	X
Nasopharyngeal Airway	X	X	X	X
Recovery Position	X	X	X	X
Sit Up/Lean Forward Airway Position	X	X	X	X
Supraglottic Airway			X	X
Surgical Airway			X	X
Endotracheal Intubation				X
Breathing				
Treat Sucking Chest Wound	X	X	X	X
Needle Thoracostomy		X	X	X
Chest Tube				X
Administer Oxygen			X	X
Intravenous Access and IV Therapy				
Assess for Shock	X	X	X	X
Start IV Line/Saline Lock			X	X
Obtain Intraosseous Access			X	X
IV Fluid Resuscitation			X	X
IV Analgesics (morphine, ketamine)			X	X
Tranexamic Acid			X	X
Administer Blood Products				X
Prevent Hypothermia	X	X	X	X
Penetrating Eye Injuries				
Cover Eye with Rigid Shield	X	X	X	X
Administer Oral Moxifloxacin	X	X	X	X

(Continued on next page)

Figure 24-3 Tactical Combat Casualty Care (TCCC) Skill Sets (*Continued*)

Skill	All	CLS	CM	CPM
Oral and Intramuscular Medications				
Oral Antibiotics	X	X	X	X
Oral Analgesia (non-narcotic)	X	X	X	X
Fentanyl Lozenges			X	X
IM Antibiotics			X	X
IM Ketamine			X	X
IM Morphine			X	X
Fracture Management				
Splinting	X	X	X	X
Traction Splinting		X	X	X
Management of Burns				
Stop the burning process	X	X	X	X
Cover the burned areas	X	X	X	X
Burn Fluid Resuscitation			X	X
Electronic Vital Signs Monitoring				
Electronic Vital Signs Monitoring			X	X

Key

All: All deploying combatants

CLS: Combat lifesaver

CM: Combat medic

CP: Combat paramedic (includes SOF advanced tactical practitioners, I8Ds, PJs, etc.)

Source: Courtesy of Dr. Frank Butler.

recommended skill sets for combat medical personnel, combat lifesavers (nonmedical personnel with extra training in TCCC), and all nonmedical personnel. In March 2009, Dr. Ward Cascells, the Assistant Secretary of Defense for Health Affairs, recommended to the military services that TCCC be used as the standard for training combat medical personnel to manage combat trauma in the tactical prehospital environment.[51] In 2011, this recommendation was repeated by Dr. Cascells's successor, Dr. Jonathan Woodson.[52]

Historically, many lessons learned from military casualty care have found application in civilian trauma care. In recent times, civilian prehospital emergency responders have been called to school shootings, mall shootings, and other terror attacks that present tactical factors similar to those encountered on battlefields. The threat of ongoing hostile fire, treating multiple casualties under cover, and prolonged evacuation times have all come into play. Even in urban settings, getting to, treating, and transporting casualties can require tactics and training outside the parameters of many standard EMS protocols. The mass-casualty incidents at Columbine, Virginia Tech, Tucson, Sandy Hook, the Boston Marathon, and the Washington Navy Yard are cases in point. More widespread adoption of applicable TCCC guidelines into tactical EMS training programs, and other civilian first responder training courses and application of these principles to help care for civilian trauma patients may result in additional lives saved. When applied to active shooter scenarios and other mass-casualty events, TCCC principles may also result in better tactical flow.

Summary

- Combat medical personnel often face multiple challenges in caring for the wounded on the battlefield. These challenges include the threat of hostile fire, working in the dark, multiple casualties, limited medical equipment, and prolonged evacuation times.
- Ignoring the tactical environment when developing battlefield trauma care strategies may increase the number of preventable deaths.
- There are three goals in Tactical Combat Casualty Care (TCCC): (1) Treat the casualty, (2) prevent additional casualties, and (3) complete the mission.
- TCCC is divided into three phases: Care Under Fire, Tactical Field Care, and Tactical Evacuation Care.
- In Care Under Fire, combat medical personnel and casualties are under effective hostile fire, and tactical considerations predominate. In this phase, medical care should be limited to controlling extremity hemorrhage with tourniquets.
- In Tactical Field Care, medical personnel and casualties are not under effective hostile fire. More extensive care can be provided.
- In Tactical Evacuation Care, casualties are transported to a medical treatment facility by aircraft, ground vehicle, or boat. An opportunity exists here to provide additional medical personnel and equipment, raising the level of care that can be delivered.
- The TCCC guidelines are published in the military version of the *Prehospital Trauma Life Support* (*PHTLS*) textbook. They are the only set of battlefield trauma care guidelines to receive the triple endorsement of the American College of Surgeons Committee on Trauma, the National Association of Emergency Medical Technicians, and the U.S. Department of Defense.
- The Committee on Tactical Combat Casualty Care (CoTCCC) updates TCCC guidelines based on ongoing review of the published civilian and military prehospital trauma literature, ongoing interaction with military combat casualty care research laboratories, direct input from experienced combat medical personnel, input from the service medical lessons-learned centers, case reports discussed at the weekly Joint Theater Trauma System process improvement video-teleconferences, and expert opinion from both military and civilian trauma specialists.
- The single most successful TCCC intervention reported to date is the reintroduction of tourniquet use on the battlefield.
- TCCC is now used throughout the U.S. military to train combat medical personnel to manage trauma in the tactical prehospital environment. Adoption of TCCC guidelines into civilian tactical EMS systems is underway, and TCCC principles are now saving lives in those settings as well.

SCENARIO RECAP

You are the only combat medic traveling in a 10-person, four-vehicle convoy through a small village in eastern Iraq. As you pull out on open road at the end of the village, an IED explodes under the second vehicle. There is no follow-up hostile fire, so the unit sets up a secure perimeter. You proceed to assess the three major casualties at the scene.

Casualty 1 is a soldier with femoral arterial bleeding from a large wound on the right thigh, as well as a right hand amputation with blood oozing from the stump. He is conscious and has a good radial pulse.

Casualty 2 is a soldier with a large open head wound in which mangled gray matter is clearly visible. He is unresponsive, and his breathing is agonal.

Casualty 3 is a civilian bystander with penetrating injury to his right lower abdomen. He is conscious and in great pain.

CASEVAC by helicopter is available in 20 minutes, and the flight to the nearest medical treatment facility will take approximately 30 minutes.

SCENARIO SOLUTION

1. What are some of the considerations in managing these casualties that are not present in most civilian settings?
    The factors that the medic must take into consideration in this scenario include:

    - What is the threat of hostile fire?
    - What is the best way to move the casualties to cover?
    - Should the medic attend to the casualties immediately or assist the unit in suppressing hostile fire?
    - Which of the injuries noted are immediately life threatening?
    - What are the most effective interventions for addressing these injuries in this combat setting?
    - What is the threat to evacuation platforms from hostile fire?
    - How long will evacuation take?
    - What type of evacuation platform is best for this situation?

References

1. Butler FK, Blackbourne LH. Battlefield trauma care then and now: a decade of Tactical Combat Casualty Care. *J Trauma Acute Care Surg.* 2012;73(6 Suppl 5):S395–S402.

2. Heiskell LE, Carmona RH. Tactical emergency medical services: an emerging subspecialty in emergency medicine. *Ann Emerg Med.* 1994;23:778–785.

3. Bellamy RF. How shall we train for combat casualty care? *Mil Med.* 1987;152(12):617–621.

4. Baker MS. Advanced trauma life support: is it acceptable stand-alone training for military medicine? *Mil Med.* 1994;159(9):581–590.

5. Butler FK, Hagmann J, Butler EG. Tactical Combat Casualty Care in Special Operations. *Mil Med.* 1996;161(Supp):1–16.

6. Richards TR. Commander, Naval Special Warfare Command. Letter. 1500 Ser 04/0341. April 9, 1997.

7. Butler FK, Holcomb JB, Giebner SD, McSwain NE, Bagian J. Tactical Combat Casualty Care 2007: evolving concepts and battlefield experience. *Mil Med.* 2007;172(S):1–19.

8. Holcomb JB. The 2004 Fitts Lecture: current perspectives on combat casualty care. *J Trauma.* 2005;59:990–1002.

9. Butler FK. Tactical medicine training for SEAL mission commanders. *Mil Med.* 2001;166:625–631.

10. DeLorenzo RA. Medic for the millennium: the U.S. Army 91W healthcare specialist. *Mil Med.* 2001;166(8):685–688.

11. Pappas CG. The Ranger medic. *Mil Med.* 2001;166:394–400.

12. Allen RC, McAtee JM. *Pararescue Medications and Procedures Manual.* Hurlburt Field, FL: Air Force Special Operations Command; 1999.

13. Malish RG. The preparation of a Special Forces company for pilot recovery. *Mil Med.* 1999;164:881–884.

14. Krausz MM. Resuscitation strategies in the Israeli Army. Presentation to the Institute of Medicine Committee on Fluid Resuscitation for Combat Casualties. September 17, 1998.

15. McDevitt I. *Tactical Medicine.* Boulder, CO: Paladin Press; 2001.

16. McSwain NE, Frame S, Paturas JL, eds. *Prehospital Trauma Life Support Manual.* 4th ed. Akron, OH: Mosby; 1999.

17. Butler FK. Tactical combat casualty care: update 2009. *J Trauma.* 2010;69:S10–S13.

18. Grissom CK, Weaver LK, Clemmer TP, Morris AH. Theoretical advantage of oxygen treatment for combat casualties during medical evacuation at high altitude. *J Trauma.* 2006;61:461–467.

19. McSwain NE, Frame S, Salomone JP, eds. *Prehospital Trauma Life Support Manual.* 5th ed. Akron, OH: Mosby; 2003.

20. McSwain NE, Salomone JP, eds. *Prehospital Trauma Life Support Manual.* 6th ed. Akron, OH: Mosby; 2006.

21. Holcomb JB, McMullen NR, Pearse L, et al. Causes of death in Special Operations forces in the Global War on Terror. *Ann Surg.* 2007;245:986–991.

22. Tarpey M. Tactical Combat Casualty Care in Operation Iraqi Freedom. *US Army Med Dept J.* 2005;April–June:38–41.

23. Gresham J. Giving back, again: Master Sgt. Luis Rodriguez and the Tactical Combat Casualty Care Course. In: *Faircount's The Year in Veterans Affairs and Military Medicine: 2005–2006 Edition.* Department of Veterans Affairs: 2006: 136–139.

24. Bottoms M. Tactical Combat Casualty Care—Saving lives on the battlefield. *Tip of the Spear* (Command Publication of the U.S. Special Operations Command). 2006;June:34–35.

25. Butler FK, Holcomb JB. The Tactical Combat Casualty Care transition initiative. *US Army Med Dept J.* 2005;April-June:33–37.

26. Brown BD. Letter of commendation to Army Medical Command. Commander, US Special Operations Command. August 17, 2005.

27. Sohn VY, Miller JP, Koeller CA, et al. From the combat medic to the forward surgical team: the Madigan Model for improving trauma readiness of brigade combat teams fighting the global war on terror. *J Surg Res.* 2007;138:25–31.

28. Holcomb JB, Stansbury LG, Champion HR, Wade C, Bellamy RF. Understanding combat casualty care statistics. *J Trauma.* 2006;60:397–401.

29. Eastridge BJ, Jenkins D, Flaherty S, Schiller H, Holcomb JB. Trauma system development in a theater of war: experiences from Operation Iraqi Freedom and Operation Enduring Freedom. *J Trauma.* 2006;61(6):1366–1372.

30. Beekley AC, Starnes BW, Sebesta JA. Lessons learned from modern military surgery. *Surg Clin N Am.* 2007;87:157–184.

31. Kragh JF, Walters TJ, Baer DJ, et al. Survival with emergency tourniquet use to stop bleeding in major limb trauma. *Ann Surg.* 2009;249:1–7.

32. Kragh JF, Walters TJ, Baer DG, Fox CJ, Wade CE, Salinas J, Holcomb JB. Practical use of emergency tourniquets to stop bleeding in major limb trauma. *J Trauma.* 2008;64:S38–S50.

33. Caravalho J. OTSG Dismounted Complex Blast Injury Task Force; Final Report. June 18, 2011:44–47.

34. Eastridge BJ, Mabry RL, Seguin P, et al. Death on the battlefield (2001–2011): implications for the future of combat casualty care. *J Trauma Acute Care Surg.* 2012;73(6):S431–S437.

35. Mabry R, McManus JG. Prehospital advances in the management of severe penetrating trauma. *Crit Care Med.* 2008;36:S258–S266.

36. Salomone JP. Letter to Assistant Secretary of Defense for Health Affairs. June 10, 2008.

37. Hetzler MR, Ball JA. Thoughts on aid bags: part one. *J Spec Ops Med.* 2008;8(3):47–53.

38. Pennardt A. TCCC in one Special Operations unit. Presentation at CoTCCC Meeting; February 3, 2009.

39. Kotwal R, Butler FK, Edgar E, Shackelford S, Bennett D, Baily JA. Saving lives on the battlefield: an assessment of pre-hospital trauma care in Combined Joint Operating Area—Afghanistan (CJOA-A) Executive Summary. *J Spec Oper Med.* 2013;13(1):77–85.

40. Kotwal RS, Montgomery HR, Kotwal BM, et al. Eliminating preventable death on the battlefield. *Arch Surg.* 2011;146(12):1350–1358.

41. Kelly JF, Ritenhour AE, McLaughlin DF, et al. Injury severity and causes of death from Operation Iraqi Freedom and Operation Enduring Freedom: 2003–2004 versus 2006. *J Trauma.* 2008;64:S21–S27.

42. Brown BD. Special Operations combat medic critical task list. Commander, U.S. Special Operations Command. Letter. March 9, 2005.

43. Bureau of Medicine and Surgery (Navy Surgeon General) Message 111622Z: Tactical Combat Casualty Care training. December 2006.

44. U.S. Marine Corps Message 02004Z: Tactical Combat Casualty Care (TCCC) and Combat Lifesaver (CLS) Fundamentals, Philosophies, and Guidance. August 2006.

45. U.S. Coast Guard Message 221752Z: Tactical Medical Response Program. November 2006.

46. Hostage GM. USSOCOM visit to the Pararescue medical course at Kirtland AFB September 2005. Air Force Education and Training Command. Letter. September 8, 2005.

47. Kiley KC. Operational needs statement for medical simulation training centers for combat lifesavers and Tactical Combat

Casualty Care training. Army Surgeon General. Letter DASG-ZA. September 1, 2005.

48. Blackbourne LH, Baer DG, Eastridge BJ, et al. Military medical revolution: military trauma system. *J Trauma Acute Care Surg.* 2012;73(6 suppl 5):S388–S394.

49. All Army Activities Message 0902031521Z: Mandatory predeployment trauma training for Army medical department personnel. February 3, 2009.

50. Holcomb JB, Wilensky G. Tactical Combat Casualty Care and minimizing preventable deaths in combat casualties. Defense Health Board memorandum. August 6, 2009.

51. Casscells W. Tactical Combat Casualty Care. Assistant Secretary of Defense for Health Affairs memorandum. March 4, 2009.

52. Woodson J. Tactical Combat Casualty Care. Assistant Secretary of Defense for Health Affairs Memorandum. August 23, 2011.

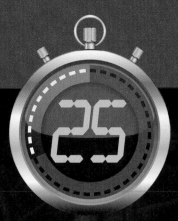

Care Under Fire

CHAPTER OBJECTIVES

At the completion of this chapter, the reader will be able to do the following:

- Discuss the impact of the tactical environment on the management of combat trauma.

- Describe techniques that can be used to quickly move casualties to cover while the unit is engaged in a firefight.

- Explain why spinal immobilization is not a critical need in combat casualties with only penetrating trauma.

- Discuss the rationale for early use of a tourniquet to control life-threatening extremity bleeding during the Care Under Fire phase.

SCENARIO

Your unit is in a five-vehicle convoy moving through a small Iraqi village when a command-detonated improvised explosive device (IED) explodes under the second vehicle. Moderate sniper fire follows and the rest of the convoy is busily engaged in suppressing it. You are a medic in the disabled vehicle, which is not on fire and is right side up. You are not injured and are able to assist. The person next to you has bilateral midthigh traumatic amputations. There is heavy arterial bleeding from the left stump and only mild oozing of blood from the right stump. The casualty is conscious and in moderate pain. What do you do?

1. **What phase of care are you in?**

2. **What is your immediate concern?**

3. **Should you treat the casualty or return fire? Why?**

4. **What is your next action?**

5. **Should you put a tourniquet on the right stump? Why?**

6. **What are your next actions?**

Introduction

As reflected in the Tactical Combat Casualty Care (TCCC) Guidelines for Care Under Fire shown in **Figure 25-1**, very limited medical care should be attempted while the casualty and the unit are under effective hostile fire. Suppression of hostile fire and moving the casualty to a safe position are major considerations at this point. Significant delays for a detailed examination and thorough treatment of all injuries are not advisable while under effective enemy fire.

Casualties who have sustained injuries that are not life threatening and that do not preclude further participation in the fight should continue to assist the unit in suppressing hostile fire. It may also be critical for the combat medical personnel to help suppress hostile fire before attempting to provide care. This can

be especially true in small-unit operations in which friendly fire-power is limited and every weapon in the unit may be needed to prevail.

Moving Casualties in Tactical Settings

In Care Under Fire, the best first step in saving a casualty is usually to control the tactical situation. An axiom of TCCC is that "The best medicine on the battlefield is fire superiority." If hostile fire cannot be effectively suppressed or the unit is unable to break contact with the enemy, it may be necessary to move the casualty to cover. Casualties whose wounds do not prevent them from moving themselves to cover should do so to avoid exposing

Figure 25-1 Basic Management Plan for Care Under Fire

1. Return fire and take cover.
2. Direct or expect casualty to remain engaged as a combatant if appropriate.
3. Direct casualty to move to cover and apply self-aid if able.
4. Try to keep the casualty from sustaining additional wounds.
5. Casualties should be extricated from burning vehicles or buildings and moved to places of relative safety. Do what is necessary to stop the burning process.
6. Airway management is generally best deferred until the Tactical Field Care phase.
7. Stop life-threatening external hemorrhage if tactically feasible:
   • Direct casualty to control hemorrhage by self-aid if able.
   • Use a CoTCCC-recommended tourniquet for hemorrhage that is anatomically amenable to tourniquet application.
   • Apply the tourniquet proximal to the bleeding site, over the uniform, tighten, and move the casualty to cover.

Source: http://www.naemt.org/Libraries/PHTLS%20TCCC/TCCC%20Guidelines%20120917.sflb

the combat medical personnel to unnecessary hazards. If unable to move and unresponsive, the casualty is likely beyond help, and risking the lives of rescuers by subjecting them to enemy fire in an unprotected area at this point in the engagement is usually not warranted.

If a casualty is responsive but unable to move, a rescue plan should be developed, as follows:

1. Determine the potential risk to the rescuers, keeping in mind that rescuers should not move into a zeroed-in position (i.e., where there is effective concentration of enemy fire). Did the casualty trip a booby trap or mine? Where is fire coming from? Is it direct or indirect (e.g., rifle, machine gun, grenade, mortar)? Are there electrical, fire, chemical, water, mechanical, or other environmental hazards?
2. Consider your assets. What can rescuers provide in the way of covering fire, screening, shielding, and rescue-applicable equipment?
3. Make sure all mission personnel understand their role in the rescue and which movement technique is to be used (e.g., drag, carry, rope, stretcher). If possible, let the casualty know what the plan is so that the casualty can assist as much as possible by rolling to a certain position, attaching a dragline to his or her web gear, and identifying hazards.
4. Management of the airway is temporarily deferred until the casualty is safe from hostile fire or other hazards. This minimizes the risk to the rescuer and avoids the difficulty of attempting to manage the airway while dragging the casualty.

The fastest method for moving a casualty is dragging along the long axis of the body by two rescuers (**Figure 25-2**). This drag can be used in buildings, shallow water, snow, and down stairs. It can be accomplished with the rescuers standing or crawling. The use of the casualty's web gear, tactical vest, a dragline, poncho,

clothing, or improvised harness makes the two-person drag easier. However, if those items are not available, then grasping the casualty under the arms is all that is necessary to accomplish this drag. A one-person drag can be used for short distances, but it is more difficult for the rescuer, is slower, and is less controlled (**Figure 25-3**).

The great disadvantage of dragging is that the casualty is in contact with the ground, and this can cause additional injury in rough terrain. Carrying the casualty may be a better option when tactically feasible. The Hawes carry is a one-person technique that allows for rapid movement (**Figure 25-4**). If the casualty can maintain an upright position, the rescuer stands in front of the casualty and squats down. The casualty's arms are moved around the neck of the rescuer and held in place. The rescuer then stands and leans forward, assuming the weight of the casualty, and moves to the desired location. Unlike the

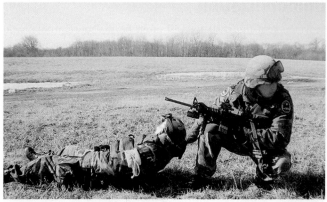

Courtesy of Dr. Mel Otten

Figure 25-3   One-person drag.

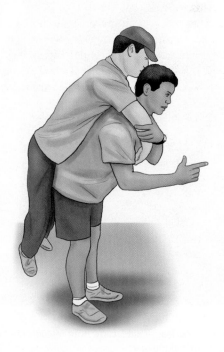

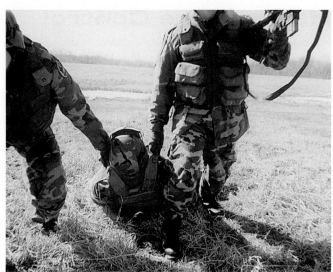

Courtesy of Dr. Mel Otten

Figure 25-2   Two-person drag.

Figure 25-4   Hawes carry.

fireman's carry, which requires greater lifting effort and requires the rescuer to carry a very heavy load in an awkward position, the Hawes carry provides the rescuer greater range of movement and the possibility of being able to use his or her firearm. It also maintains a lower center of gravity for both the casualty and the rescuer, thus minimizing the risk of additional injury from falls during the carry.

Members of SEAL Team THREE devised and use a two-person carry in which one of the casualty's arms is draped over each of the rescuers' shoulders. Each rescuer uses the hand closest to the casualty to lift the casualty by the waist belt. If the casualty is conscious and can hold on to the rescuers' shoulders, the rescuers may use their free arms to employ their weapons if necessary (**Figure 25-5**).

Casualty Movement and Spinal Immobilization

Movement of the casualty will often be the most problematic aspect of providing TCCC.[1] Although a long-standing principle of care in the civilian setting is to perform spinal immobilization prior to moving a trauma patient with a potential spinal injury, this practice should be re-evaluated in the combat setting. Arishita, Vayer, and Bellamy examined the value of cervical spine immobilization in penetrating neck injuries in the Vietnam War and found that in only 1.4% of casualties with penetrating

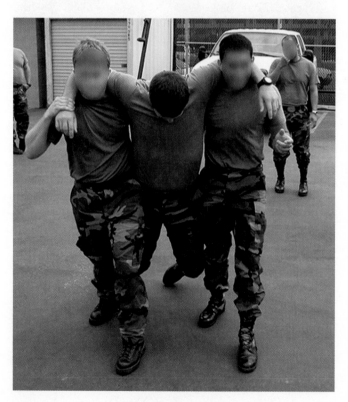

Figure 25-5 SEAL Team THREE carry. Both rescuers are holding the casualty by his belt in the rear.
Source: Courtesy of Dr. Frank Butler.

neck injuries would immobilization of the cervical spine have been of possible benefit.[2] Since the time required to accomplish cervical spine immobilization was found to be 5.5 minutes, even when applied by experienced prehospital care providers, the authors concluded that the potential hazards to both casualty and combat medical personnel outweighed the potential benefit of immobilization.

Kennedy and his coauthors reported similar findings of no cervical spine injuries in 105 victims of gunshot wounds to the head.[3] Other recent papers examining the value of cervical spine immobilization in civilian trauma cases have also found little data to support this practice in trauma victims with only a penetrating mechanism of injury.[4,5]

In casualty scenarios in which the casualty has suffered blunt trauma and is under effective hostile fire (e.g., an ambush in which an improvised explosive device (IED) causes a vehicle to be overturned and the explosion is followed by small arms fire), the combat medic, corpsman, or pararescueman must weigh the risk of injury from hostile fire or vehicle fire secondary to the explosion against the risk of worsening any potential spinal cord injury when making decisions about how and when to move the casualty to cover.

The wounding pattern seen in IED injuries depends on whether the explosion occurred when the casualty was riding in a vehicle (mounted IED attack) or occurred as the casualty stepped on the IED (dismounted IED attack.) The latter mechanism of injury was seen in increasing numbers in Afghanistan during the period of 2010 through 2012, and resulted in an injury pattern referred to as Dismounted Complex Blast Injury (DCBI) (see the Tactical Field Care chapter for more information).[6] Spinal injuries may result from either type of IED attack, and this must be considered when treating IED casualties.[7] With IED injuries, appropriate spinal precautions should be taken as tactically feasible.

Hemorrhage Control

In combat casualties, early control of significant external hemorrhage is the most important intervention. Hemorrhage remains the predominant cause of preventable death in combat fatalities.[8] The renewed focus on prehospital tourniquets to prevent death from extremity hemorrhage as emphasized in TCCC was the single most successful battlefield trauma care innovation to come from the wars in Afghanistan and Iraq. Until recently, combat medical personnel were taught that a tourniquet should be used only as a last resort to control extremity hemorrhage.[9] A study of 2,600 combat fatalities incurred during the Vietnam conflict,[10] and a study of 982 combat fatalities incurred during the early years of conflict in Afghanistan and Iraq[11] reported death rates from extremity hemorrhage of 7.4% and 7.8%, respectively. After the widespread implementation of the tourniquet recommendations from the TCCC guidelines, a recent comprehensive study of 4,596 U.S. combat fatalities from 2001 to 2011 noted that only 2.6% of total combat fatalities resulted from extremity hemorrhage.[12] This dramatic decrease in deaths from extremity hemorrhage resulted from the now ubiquitous fielding of modern tourniquets and aggressive training of all nonmedical personnel on tourniquet application.[9]

Control of significant bleeding from injuries such as scalp lacerations and external torso injuries is also a high priority, but the tactical imperative to maintain fire superiority and to move the casualty to cover dictates that only life-threatening extremity bleeding should warrant any intervention during Care Under Fire. Both the casualty and the other unit members should disregard minor wounds insofar as possible during Care Under Fire, in order to maximize the unit's firepower. If a tourniquet is required during Care Under Fire, the casualty should apply it to himself or herself if at all possible. Tourniquet application should take place under the best cover immediately available to the casualty.

Tourniquets

Failure to use tourniquets continued to result in preventable fatalities at the start of the conflicts in Iraq and Afghanistan. Colonel John Holcomb, then Commander of the U.S. Army Institute of Surgical Research, and his coauthors examined all deaths in Special Operations forces from the start of the Global War on Terrorism in 2001 through November 2004, finding that bleeding from extremity wounds was the cause of 25% of the potentially preventable deaths in combat fatalities.[13] Beekley noted that four of the seven deaths that occurred in a series of 165 casualties cared for at the 31st Combat Support Hospital in Baghdad could have been prevented by the timely use of a tourniquet.[14] Kelly noted 77 deaths from extremity hemorrhage in his study of 982 combat fatalities.[11] Colonel Brian Eastridge found 131 deaths from extremity hemorrhage in his comprehensive study of 4,596 combat fatalities from Afghanistan and Iraq.[8]

As noted above, deaths from extremity hemorrhage can largely be prevented by aggressive use of tourniquets. Tourniquets have been in use on the battlefield for centuries[15] and have been shown to clearly save lives in combat.[16-20] Because of their effectiveness at hemorrhage control and the speed with which they can be applied, tourniquets are the best option for temporary control of life-threatening extremity hemorrhage in the tactical environment. Direct pressure and compression dressings are less desirable than tourniquets in this setting because their application at the point of wounding may result in delays in getting the casualty and the rescuer to cover. Also these interventions provide less definitive control of life-threatening hemorrhage, especially while the casualty is being moved.[21]

Colonel John Kragh's work has confirmed the lifesaving benefit and low incidence of complications from prehospital tourniquet use in combat casualties.[22,23] Tourniquets are most effective in saving lives when applied before the casualty has gone into shock from blood loss.[23] Although tourniquet use has been discouraged by civilian EMS systems in the past because of concern about ischemic damage to the extremity, this has not been found to be a significant problem when tourniquets have been used appropriately during combat operations.[23-25] Tourniquets are used frequently during orthopedic surgical procedures and are relatively safe if left on for less than 2 hours. Prolonged use of a tourniquet can potentially result in the loss of a limb, but saving the life of the casualty must always take precedence if the tourniquet cannot be removed for tactical reasons.

Because of their proven lifesaving value, tourniquets are ubiquitous on the modern battlefield.[12] Several recent papers have called for a re-evaluation of tourniquet use in the civilian prehospital environment as well.[26-30] Note that every combatant on the battlefield should be able to apply a tourniquet to his or her own bleeding extremity or on any unit member that requires one. Hemorrhage control by nonmedical personnel has been a key element in reducing preventable deaths on the battlefield.[31]

Tourniquet Evaluation

There are currently a variety of tourniquets available on the market, and some are more effective than others. In a comparative evaluation of tourniquets available at the time, the U.S. Army Institute of Surgical Research identified three that were 100% effective in stopping arterial blood flow.[32] These were the Combat Application Tourniquet (C-A-T), the SOF Tactical Tourniquet (SOFT-T), and the Emergency and Military Tourniquet (EMT), a pneumatic device. The C-A-T and SOFT-T are both windlass-type devices that are lightweight and relatively inexpensive. These tourniquets can be readily applied to one's own or another's extremity and are rugged, reliable, and small enough to be easily carried. The C-A-T has been designated as an item of individual issue to ground combatants in all services and has proven effective and reliable in the current conflicts[22,23] (**Figure 25-6**).

The other tourniquets found to be effective in the U.S. Army Institute of Surgical Research study may also be useful in some

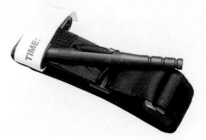

Figure 25-6   Combat Application Tourniquet (C-A-T).
Source: Composite Resources, Inc.

situations. Combat medical personnel experience has found that the SOF Tactical Tourniquet (**Figure 25-7**) may be a better choice if the casualty has large thighs and needs a tourniquet in that location.

The Emergency and Military Tourniquet (**Figure 25-8**) has been found to perform very well in emergency departments,[22] but it is more expensive than the C-A-T. Furthermore, its inflatable cuff may not function if it has had prolonged time in the field or has been exposed to shrapnel strikes.

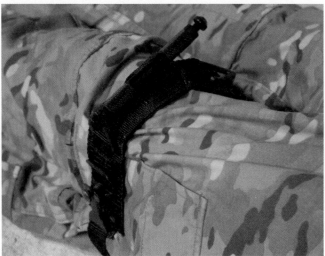

Courtesy of Tactical Medical Solutions.

Figure 25-7 SOF™ Tactical Tourniquet.
Source: Courtesy of Tactical Medical Solutions.

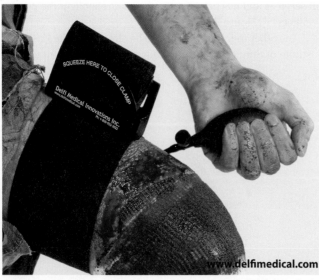

www.delfimedical.com

Courtesy of Delfi Medical Innovations, Inc.

Figure 25-8 Emergency and Military Tourniquet.
Source: Courtesy of Delfi Medical Innovations, Inc.

Tourniquet Application

Tourniquets should be placed clearly proximal to the site of the severe bleeding. They should never be placed directly over a joint. They should also never be placed over a holster or a pocket containing bulky objects that would make tightening the tourniquet more difficult or more painful for the casualty.

During Care Under Fire, tourniquets should be tightened as necessary to stop bleeding from the distal injury. During this phase, time may not permit exposure of the wound, and the tourniquet may have to be placed over the casualty's uniform. Although this is not an ideal application, it is advisable due to the tactical situation and the need to move both casualty and care provider to cover quickly. If bleeding is not controlled with one tourniquet, a second tourniquet should be applied just proximal to the first.

Once time permits in Tactical Field Care, the wound should be exposed and reevaluated, and a replacement tourniquet should be applied directly to the casualty's skin.

The time at which a tourniquet is applied should always be noted on the casualty. This has customarily been done by writing the letter "T" on the casualty's forehead along with the time. This should be done with an indelible ink marker to ensure that this important information does not wash or wipe off. Either the involved extremity or a piece of tape applied to the casualty's chest is an alternative location for noting tourniquet application time. The information should also be recorded on the individual's TCCC Casualty Card. If the casualty has multiple tourniquets with significantly different times of application, this should be noted clearly on the TCCC Casualty Card. See **Figures 25-9** and **25-10** for more information on tourniquet application.

Hemostatic Agents

The requirement to hold direct pressure on the bleeding site after application of a hemostatic agent is tactically infeasible when the casualty and the individual providing care are under

---

Figure 25-9   Tourniquet Application Mistakes

Mistakes to avoid when applying tourniquets include:
- Not using a tourniquet when you should
- Using a tourniquet for minimal bleeding
- Putting the tourniquet on too proximally
- Not making the tourniquet tight enough to effectively stop the bleeding
- Not using a second tourniquet if needed
- Waiting too long to put the tourniquet on
- Periodically loosening the tourniquet to allow blood flow to the injured extremity

Figure 25-10   Tourniquet Tips

All manufactured tourniquets are designed for a single use. A separate group of tourniquets should be used for training, and training tourniquets should not subsequently be issued to individuals for use in combat. Many military units have evolved to a single-tour, single-use policy for tourniquets.

effective hostile fire. Therefore, the use of hemostatic agents during Care Under Fire is not recommended. However, when its application can be achieved in a safer setting, a hemostatic dressing can be a highly effective option for controlling a life-threatening hemorrhage when a tourniquet cannot be applied to the bleeding site. This subject is discussed more fully in the Tactical Field Care chapter.

Airway

No immediate management of the airway should be anticipated during Care Under Fire because of the need to move the casualty to cover as quickly as possible.[1] Since most preventable deaths on the battlefield are caused by hemorrhage, addressing any significant external hemorrhage that may be present will hopefully prevent the casualty from going into hypovolemic shock and requiring airway management. An injury that is severe enough to result in immediate loss of consciousness during Care Under Fire, such as penetrating head trauma, will have a high probability of proving fatal. Airway control should be deferred until Tactical Field Care and until after all major external hemorrhage has been addressed.

Summary

- In Care Under Fire, the need for medical care must be weighed against the need to move to cover and to suppress hostile fire rapidly.
- During Care Under Fire, very limited medical care should be attempted while under effective hostile fire. Suppression of hostile fire and moving the casualty to cover are priorities.
- Casualties who are able to should remain engaged as combatants during Care Under Fire.
- Combat medical personnel may have to help suppress hostile fire before providing care to casualties.
- If the casualty is unable to move and is unresponsive, he or she is likely beyond help. Risking additional lives by exposure to fire in the open in order to move the casualty to cover during Care Under Fire may not be warranted.
- If the casualty is responsive and able to move to cover, he or she should do so immediately.
- If the casualty is responsive but unable to move to cover, a rescue plan should be implemented as outlined in this chapter.
- The fastest method for moving a casualty is dragging him or her along the long axis of the body by two rescuers.
- One-person drags are slower than two-person drags, but have the advantage of exposing only one rescuer to additional risk.
- The Hawes carry can be used by one person and may be useful in some situations.
- A two-person carry used by SEAL Team THREE requires that one of the casualty's arms be draped over each of the rescuers' shoulders with the rescuers grasping the casualty by his or her waist belt. This is a useful option for a two-person carry.
- With penetrating injury to the head or neck, immobilization of the cervical spine during Care Under Fire is not warranted unless blunt injury is present as well.
- In combat casualties with known or possible blunt neck or spine trauma, the first responder must weigh the risk of injury from hostile fire to the casualty and the responder while immobilizing the spine against the risk of causing or worsening a spinal cord injury.
- The wounding pattern of IED injuries is characterized by penetrating injuries superimposed on blast injury from the explosion and possibly blunt injury from motor vehicle trauma. In these settings, injury to the spine is more common and appropriate precautions should be taken when tactical conditions allow.
- Immediate control of extremity hemorrhage with a tourniquet is the most important lifesaving intervention in Care Under Fire and is generally the only medical care that should be undertaken before the casualty is moved to cover.
- Tourniquets save lives in combat when used appropriately. They are most effective when applied before the casualty has gone into shock from blood loss.
- Tourniquets have been shown to be safe when applied for less than 2 hours.

- Two tourniquets have been shown to be 100% effective in stopping arterial blood flow and are recommended for use on the battlefield: the Combat Application Tourniquet (C-A-T), and the SOF Tactical Tourniquet (SOFT-T)
- Tourniquets should be placed proximal to the site of the hemorrhage.
- Tourniquets should never be placed directly over a joint or over pockets containing bulky items.
- The time of tourniquet application should be noted both on the tourniquet itself and on the TCCC Casualty Card.
- The use of hemostatic agents in Care Under Fire is not recommended because of the requirement to hold direct pressure on the bleeding site for 3 minutes after application. This is an unacceptably long period during Care Under Fire.
- Airway management is usually best deferred until Tactical Field Care, and until after major external hemorrhage has been addressed.

SCENARIO RECAP

Your unit is in a five-vehicle convoy moving through a small Iraqi village when a command-detonated IED explodes under the second vehicle. Moderate sniper fire follows and the rest of the convoy is busily engaged in suppressing it. You are a medic in the disabled vehicle, which is not on fire and is right side up. You are not injured and are able to assist. The person next to you has bilateral midthigh traumatic amputations. There is heavy arterial bleeding from the left stump and only mild oozing of blood from the right stump. The casualty is conscious and in moderate pain. What do you do?

SCENARIO SOLUTION

1. **What phase of care are you in?**

   You are in the Care Under Fire phase.

2. **What is your immediate concern?**

   The casualty may exsanguinate quickly from arterial bleeding.

3. **Should you treat the casualty or return fire? Why?**

   You should treat the casualty's extremity hemorrhage. The rest of the convoy is providing suppressive fire, and applying a tourniquet is a fast and easy lifesaving intervention.

4. **What is your next action?**

   Place a tourniquet on the stump of the casualty's left thigh.

5. **Should you put a tourniquet on the right stump? Why?**

   No. The bleeding from the right stump is minimal at this point. Wait until Tactical Field Care, but recheck often.

6. **What are your next actions?**

   Drag the casualty out of the vehicle and move to the best cover. Return fire if needed. Communicate the casualty's status to the team leader.

References

1. Butler FK, Hagmann J, Butler EG. Tactical Combat Casualty Care in Special Operations. *Mil Med.* 1996; 161(Suppl):1–16.

2. Arishita GI, Vayer JS, Bellamy RF. Cervical spine immobilization of penetrating neck wounds in a hostile environment. *J Trauma.* 1989; 29:332–337.

3. Kennedy FR, Gonzalez P, Beitler A, et al. Incidence of cervical spine injury in patients with gunshot wounds to the head. *South Med J.* 1994; 87:621-623.

4. Stuke L, Pons P, Guy J, et al. Prehospital spine immobilization for penetrating trauma—review and recommendations from the Prehospital Trauma Life Support Executive Committee. *J Trauma.* 2011; 71:763–770.

5. Lustenberger T, Talving P, Lam L, et al. Unstable cervical spine fracture after penetrating neck injury: a rare entity in an analysis of 1,069 patients. *J Trauma.* 2011; 70:870–872.

6. Caravalho J. OTSG Dismounted Complex Blast Injury Task Force; Final Report. June 18, 2011:44–47.

7. Comstock S, Pannell D, Talbot M, et al. Spinal injuries after improvised explosive device incidents: implications for Tactical Combat Casualty Care. *J Trauma.* 2011; 71:S413–S417.

8. Eastridge BJ, Mabry R, Seguin P, et al. Pre-hospital death on the battlefield: implications for the future of combat casualty care. *J Trauma Acute Care Surg.* 2012; 73:S431–S437.

9. Butler FK, Blackbourne LH. Battlefield trauma care then and now: a decade of Tactical Combat Casualty Care. *J Trauma Acute Care Surg.* 2012; 73:S395–S402.

10. Maughon JS. An inquiry into the nature of wounds resulting in killed in action in Vietnam. *Mil Med.* 1970; 135:8–13.

11. Kelly JF, Ritenhour AE, McLaughlin DF, et al. Injury severity and causes of death from Operation Iraqi Freedom and Operation Enduring Freedom: 2003–2004 versus 2006. *J Trauma.* 2008; 64:S21–S27.

12. Kotwal RS, Butler FK, Edgar EP, Shackelford SA, Bennett DR, Bailey JA. Saving lives on the battlefield: a joint trauma system review of pre-hospital trauma care in combined joint operating area—Afghanistan (CJOA-A) Executive Summary. *J Spec Oper Med.* 2013; 13(1):77–85.

13. Holcomb JB, McMullen NR, Pearse L, et al. Causes of death in Special Operations Forces in the Global War on Terror. *Ann Surg.* 2007; 245:986–991.

14. Beekley AC, Sebesta JA, Blackbourne LH, et al. Prehospital tourniquet use in Operation Iraqi Freedom: effect on hemorrhage control and outcomes. *J Trauma.* 2008; 64:S28–S37.

15. Mabry RL. Tourniquet use on the battlefield. *Mil Med.* 2006; 171:352–356.

16. Mabry RL, Holcomb JB, Baker A, et al. U.S. Army Rangers in Somalia: an analysis of combat casualties on an urban battlefield. *J Trauma.* 2000; 49:515.

17. Mucciarone JJ, Llewellyn CH, Wightman JM. Tactical Combat Casualty Care in the assault on Punta Paitilla Airfield. *Mil Med.* 2006; 171(8):687–690.

18. Beekley AC, Starnes BW, Sebesta JA. Lessons learned from modern military surgery. *Surg Clin N Am.* 2007; 87:157–184.

19. Tarpey MJ. Tactical combat casualty care in Operation Iraqi Freedom. *U.S. Army Medical Dept J.* April-June 2005:38–41.

20. Tien HC, Jung V, Rizoli SB, Acharya SV, MacDonald JC. An evaluation of Tactical Combat Casualty Care interventions in a combat environment. *J Am Coll Surg.* 2008; 207:174–178.

21. Carey ME. Analysis of wounds incurred by U.S. Army Seventh Corps personnel treated in corps hospitals during Operation Desert Storm, February 20 to March 10, 1991. *J Trauma.* 1996; 40:S165–S169.

22. Kragh JF, Walters TJ, Baer DG, et al. Practical use of emergency tourniquets to stop bleeding in major limb trauma. *J Trauma.* 2008; 64:S38–S50.

23. Kragh JF, Walters TJ, Baer DG, et al. Survival with emergency tourniquet use to stop bleeding in major limb trauma. *Ann Surg.* 2009; 249:1–7.

24. Butler FK, Holcomb JB, Giebner SG, McSwain NE, Bagian J. Tactical Combat Casualty Care 2007: evolving concepts and battlefield experience. *Mil Med.* 2007; 172(S):1–19.

25. Lakstein D, Blumenfeld A, Sokolov T, et al. Tourniquets for hemorrhage control on the battlefield: a four-year accumulated experience. *J Trauma.* 2003; 54:S221–S225.

26. Kalish J, Burke P, Feldman J, et al. The return of tourniquets. *J Em Med Serv.* 2008; 33(8):45–53.

27. Dorlac WC, Debakey ME, Holcomb JB, et al. Mortality from isolated civilian penetrating extremity injury. *J Trauma.* 2005;171:217–222.

28. Doyle GS, Taillac PP. Tourniquets: a review of current use with proposals for expanded prehospital use. *Prehosp Emerg Care.* 2008; 12:241–256.

29. Markov N, Dubose J, Scott D, et al. Anatomic distribution and mortality of arterial injury in the wars in Afghanistan and Iraq with comparison to a civilian benchmark. *J Vasc Surg.* 2012; 56(3):728–736.

30. Butler F, Carmona R. Tactical combat casualty care: from the battlefields of Afghanistan to the streets of America. *Tactical Edge.* Winter 2012.

31. Kotwal RS, Montgomery HR, Kotwal BM, et al. Eliminating preventable death on the battlefield. *Arch Surg.* 2011; 146:1350–1358.

32. Walters TJ, Wenke JC, Greydanus DJ, Kauvar DS, Baer DG. Laboratory evaluation of battlefield tourniquets on human volunteers. U.S. Army Institute of Surgical Research Technical Report 2005–05. September 2005.

SPECIFIC SKILLS

Combat Application Tourniquet (C-A-T®)

C-A-T®: One-Handed Self-Application to an Arm

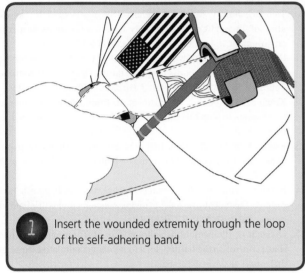

1 Insert the wounded extremity through the loop of the self-adhering band.

Source: Composite Resources Inc.

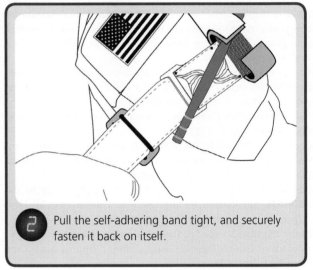

2 Pull the self-adhering band tight, and securely fasten it back on itself.

Source: Composite Resources Inc.

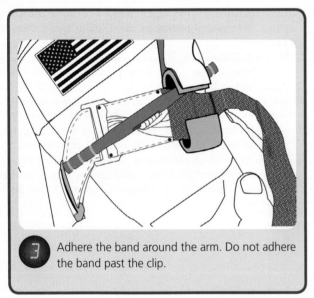

3 Adhere the band around the arm. Do not adhere the band past the clip.

Source: Composite Resources Inc.

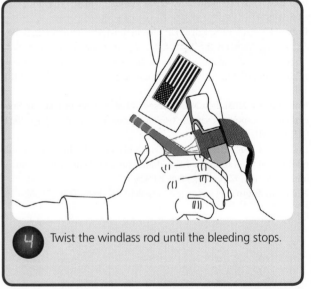

4 Twist the windlass rod until the bleeding stops.

Source: Composite Resources Inc.

SPECIFIC SKILLS

Combat Application Tourniquet (C-A-T®) (continued)

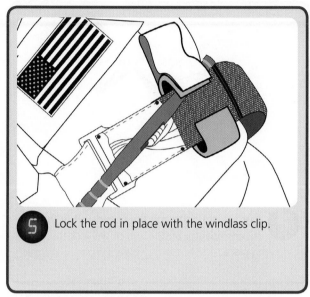

5 Lock the rod in place with the windlass clip.

Source: Composite Resources Inc.

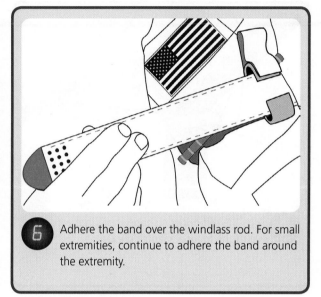

6 Adhere the band over the windlass rod. For small extremities, continue to adhere the band around the extremity.

Source: Composite Resources Inc.

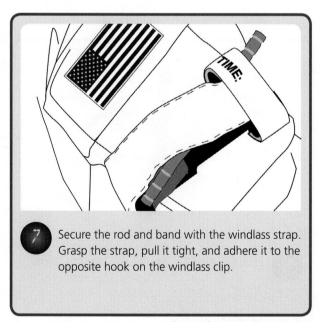

7 Secure the rod and band with the windlass strap. Grasp the strap, pull it tight, and adhere it to the opposite hook on the windlass clip.

Source: Composite Resources Inc.

Combat Application Tourniquet (C-A-T®) (continued)

C-A-T®: Application to a Leg

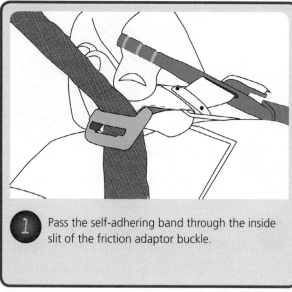

1. Pass the self-adhering band through the inside slit of the friction adaptor buckle.

Source: Composite Resources Inc.

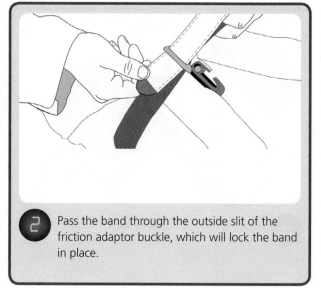

2. Pass the band through the outside slit of the friction adaptor buckle, which will lock the band in place.

Source: Composite Resources Inc.

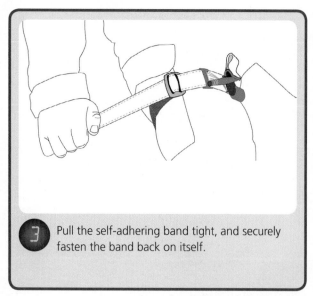

3. Pull the self-adhering band tight, and securely fasten the band back on itself.

Source: Composite Resources Inc.

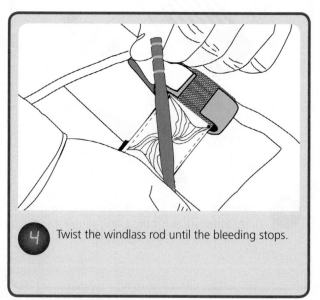

4. Twist the windlass rod until the bleeding stops.

Source: Composite Resources Inc.

Combat Application Tourniquet (C-A-T®) (continued)

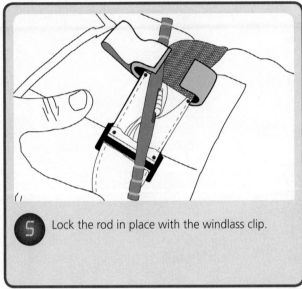

5 Lock the rod in place with the windlass clip.

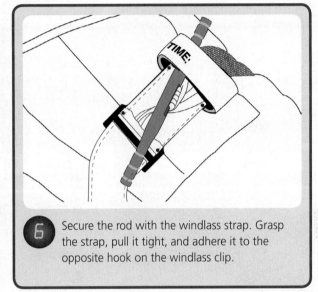

6 Secure the rod with the windlass strap. Grasp the strap, pull it tight, and adhere it to the opposite hook on the windlass clip.

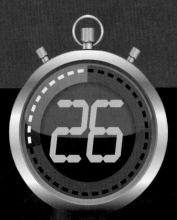
Tactical Field Care

CHAPTER OBJECTIVES

At the completion of this chapter, the reader will be able to do the following:

- Identify the common causes of altered mental status on the battlefield, and state why individuals with altered mental status should be disarmed immediately.

- Discuss the MARCH algorithm for initial care of combat casualties.

- Describe airway control techniques and devices appropriate to the Tactical Field Care phase.

- Discuss the diagnosis and initial treatment of tension pneumothorax on the battlefield.

- Describe the strategy for controlling hemorrhage in Tactical Field Care.

- Describe the recommended procedure for intraosseous access, and state the rationale for its employment.

- Describe the use of tranexamic acid in treating casualties at risk of death from hemorrhage.

- Recite the tactically relevant definition of shock in combat settings, and discuss the prehospital fluid resuscitation of combat casualties in shock.

- Discuss the importance of preventing hypothermia in combat casualties and the preferred methods to accomplish this.

- Describe the management of penetrating eye trauma in a tactical setting.

- Discuss the appropriate use of pulse oximetry in prehospital combat casualty care, and list pitfalls associated with interpretation of pulse oximeter readings.

- Discuss the recommended agents for pain relief in tactical settings.

- Discuss the rationale for early antibiotic intervention in combat casualties, and list the factors involved in selecting antibiotics for use on the battlefield.

- Describe the options for casualty movement in Tactical Field Care.

- Discuss the role of cardiopulmonary resuscitation for combat casualties in the prehospital environment.

- Describe the categories of Tactical Evacuation urgency, and select the appropriate evacuation category for casualties with various injury patterns.

- Describe the recommended Tactical Combat Casualty Care (TCCC) Casualty Card and TCCC After Action Report to be used for documenting TCCC on the battlefield.

- Discuss the importance of communicating calmly and clearly with combat casualties about their injuries.

- Discuss the considerations involved in providing care to wounded hostile combatants.

SCENARIO

While on patrol in the city of Mosul, an infantry platoon comes under small arms fire.

The point man is hit and falls to the ground. The platoon reacts to the contact, rapidly eliminating the ambushing force. The point man is the only casualty in your unit. The platoon leader tells you to take care of the wounded man while the others establish a secure perimeter.

In your rapid initial assessment for life-threatening conditions, you find a gunshot entry wound on the casualty's right upper back. The exit wound is in the right axilla, and there is heavy pulsatile bleeding from it. The casualty is breathing slightly fast. There are no other wounds.

1. **What phase of Tactical Combat Casualty Care (TCCC) are you in?**

2. **What is your immediate concern and how do you address it?**

3. **While addressing your immediate concern, what should you be doing simultaneously?**

4. **What should you do after you finish your first intervention?**

5. **What do you evaluate next?**

6. **Should you treat for a tension pneumothorax? Why?**

7. **What do you want to do after that?**

8. **What interventions come next if the casualty is still in shock?**

9. **What should this casualty's evacuation priority be?**

Introduction

The text in this chapter assumes that life-threatening external hemorrhage was addressed initially during the Care Under Fire phase. If compressible life-threatening hemorrhage is still present as Tactical Combat Casualty Care (TCCC) enters the Tactical Field Care phase, this bleeding should be addressed immediately with an extremity tourniquet, a hemostatic agent, or a junctional tourniquet, as discussed later in this chapter. **Figure 26-1** lists the recommended TCCC guidelines for Tactical Field Care.

Figure 26-1 Basic Management Plan for Tactical Field Care (October 28, 2013)

1. Casualties with an altered mental status should be disarmed immediately.
2. Airway Management
   a. Unconscious casualty without airway obstruction:
      - Chin lift or jaw thrust maneuver
      - Nasopharyngeal airway
      - Place casualty in the recovery position
   b. Casualty with airway obstruction or impending airway obstruction:
      - Chin lift or jaw thrust maneuver
      - Nasopharyngeal airway
      - Allow casualty to assume any position that best protects the airway, to include sitting up.
      - Place unconscious casualty in the recovery position.
      - If previous measures unsuccessful:
      - Surgical cricothyroidotomy (with lidocaine if conscious)
3. Breathing
   a. In a casualty with progressive respiratory distress and known or suspected torso trauma, consider a tension pneumothorax and decompress the chest on the side of the injury with a 14-gauge, 3.25 inch needle/catheter unit inserted in the second intercostal space at the mid-clavicular line. Ensure that the needle entry into the chest is not medial to the nipple line and is not directed towards the heart. An acceptable alternate site is the 4th or 5th intercostal space at the anterior axillary line (AAL).
   b. All open and/or sucking chest wounds should be treated by immediately applying a vented chest seal to cover the defect. If a vented chest seal is not available, use a non-vented chest seal. Monitor the casualty for the potential development of a subsequent tension pneumothorax. If the casualty develops increasing hypoxia, respiratory distress, or hypotension and a tension pneumothorax is suspected, treat by burping or removing the dressing or by needle decompression.
   c. Casualties with moderate/severe TBI should be given supplemental oxygen when available to maintain an oxygen saturation > 90%.
4. Bleeding
   a. Assess for unrecognized hemorrhage and control all sources of bleeding. If not already done, use a CoTCCC-recommended tourniquet to control life-threatening external hemorrhage that is anatomically amenable to tourniquet application or for any traumatic amputation. Apply directly to the skin 2–3 inches above wound.
   b. For compressible hemorrhage not amenable to tourniquet use or as an adjunct to tourniquet removal (if evacuation time is anticipated to be longer than two hours), use Combat Gauze as the hemostatic agent of choice. Combat Gauze should be applied with at least 3 minutes of direct pressure. Before releasing any tourniquet on a casualty who has been resuscitated for hemorrhagic shock, ensure a positive response to resuscitation efforts (i.e., a peripheral pulse normal in character and normal mentation if there is no traumatic brain injury (TBI). If the bleeding site is appropriate for use of a junctional tourniquet, immediately apply a CoTCCC-recommended junctional tourniquet. Do not delay in the application of the junctional tourniquet once it is ready for use. Combat Gauze applied with direct pressure should be used if a junctional tourniquet is not available or while the junctional tourniquet is being readied for use.
   c. Reassess prior tourniquet application. Expose wound and determine if tourniquet is needed. If so, move tourniquet from over uniform and apply directly to skin 2–3 inches above wound. If a tourniquet is not needed, use other techniques to control bleeding.
   d. When time and the tactical situation permit, a distal pulse check should be accomplished. If a distal pulse is still present, consider additional tightening of the tourniquet or the use of a second tourniquet, side by side and proximal to the first, to eliminate the distal pulse.
   e. Expose and clearly mark all tourniquet sites with the time of tourniquet application. Use an indelible marker.
5. Intravenous (IV) access
   - Start an 18-gauge IV or saline lock if indicated.
   - If resuscitation is required and IV access is not obtainable, use the intraosseous (IO) route.
6. Tranexamic Acid (TXA)
   If a casualty is anticipated to need significant blood transfusion (for example: presents with hemorrhagic shock, one or more major amputations, penetrating torso trauma, or evidence of severe bleeding)
   - Administer 1 gram of tranexamic acid in 100 cc Normal Saline or Lactated Ringer's as soon as possible but NOT later than 3 hours after injury.

(Continues on next page)

Figure 26-1 Basic Management Plan for Tactical Field Care (October 28, 2013) (*Continued*)

- Begin second infusion of 1 gm TXA after Hextend or other fluid treatment.

7. Fluid resuscitation

   Assess for hemorrhagic shock; altered mental status (in the absence of head injury) and weak or absent peripheral pulses are the best field indicators of shock.

   a. If not in shock:
      - No IV fluids necessary
      - PO fluids permissible if conscious and can swallow

   b. If in shock:
      - Hextend, 500-mL IV bolus
      - Repeat once after 30 minutes if still in shock.
      - No more than 1000 mL of Hextend

   c. Continued efforts to resuscitate must be weighed against logistical and tactical considerations and the risk of incurring further casualties.

   d. If a casualty with an altered mental status due to suspected TBI has a weak or absent peripheral pulse, resuscitate as necessary to maintain a palpable radial pulse.

8. Prevention of hypothermia

   a. Minimize casualty's exposure to the elements. Keep protective gear on or with the casualty if feasible.

   b. Replace wet clothing with dry if possible. Get the casualty onto an insulated surface as soon as possible.

   c. Apply the Ready-Heat Blanket from the Hypothermia Prevention and Management Kit (HPMK) to the casualty's torso (not directly on the skin) and cover the casualty with the Heat-Reflective Shell (HRS).

   d. If an HRS is not available, the previously recommended combination of the Blizzard Survival Blanket and the Ready Heat blanket may also be used.

   e. If the items mentioned above are not available, use dry blankets, poncho liners, sleeping bags, or anything that will retain heat and keep the casualty dry.

   f. Warm fluids are preferred if IV fluids are required.

9. Penetrating Eye Trauma

   If a penetrating eye injury is noted or suspected:

   a. Perform a rapid field test of visual acuity.

   b. Cover the eye with a rigid eye shield (NOT a pressure patch.)

   c. Ensure that the 400 mg moxifloxacin tablet in the combat pill pack is taken if possible and that IV/IM antibiotics are given as outlined below if oral moxifloxacin cannot be taken.

10. Monitoring

    a. Pulse oximetry should be available as an adjunct to clinical monitoring. All individuals with moderate/severe TBI should be monitored with pulse oximetry.

    b. Readings may be misleading in the settings of shock or marked hypothermia.

11. Inspect and dress known wounds.

12. Check for additional wounds.

13. Analgesia on the battlefield should generally be achieved using one of three options:

Option 1
Mild to Moderate Pain
Casualty is still able to fight
- TCCC Combat pill pack:
  - Tylenol - 650-mg bilayer caplet, 2 PO every 8 hours
  - Meloxicam - 15 mg PO once a day

Option 2
Moderate to Severe Pain
Casualty IS NOT in shock or respiratory distress AND
Casualty IS NOT at significant risk of developing either condition
- Oral transmucosal fentanyl citrate (OTFC) 800 ug
- Place lozenge between the cheek and the gum
- Do not chew the lozenge

Option 3
Moderate to Severe Pain
Casualty IS in hemorrhagic shock or respiratory distress OR
Casualty IS at significant risk of developing either condition
- Ketamine 50 mg IM or IN
Or
- Ketamine 20 mg slow IV or IO
  - Repeat doses q30min prn for IM or IN
  - Repeat doses q20min prn for IV or IO
  - End points: Control of pain or development of nystagmus (rhythmic back-and-forth movement of the eyes)

*Analgesia notes
   a. Casualties may need to be disarmed after being given OTFC or ketamine.

(Continues on next page)

Figure 26-1 Basic Management Plan for Tactical Field Care (October 28, 2013) (*Continued*)

b. Document a mental status exam using the AVPU method prior to administering opioids or ketamine.

c. For all casualties given opiods or ketamine— monitor airway, breathing, and circulation closely

d. Directions for administering OTFC:
   - Recommend taping lozenge-on-a-stick to casualty's finger as an added safety measure OR utilizing a safety pin and rubber band to attach the lozenge (under tension) to the casualty's uniform or plate carrier.
   - Reassess in 15 minutes
   - Add second lozenge, in other cheek, as necessary to control severe pain
   - Monitor for respiratory depression

e. IV Morphine is an alternative to OTFC if IV access has been obtained
   - 5 mg IV/IO
   - Reassess in 10 minutes.
   - Repeat dose every 10 minutes as necessary to control severe pain.
   - Monitor for respiratory depression

f. Naloxone (0.4 mg IV or IM) should be available when using opioid analgesics.

g. Both ketamine and OTFC have the potential to worsen severe TBI. The combat medic, corpsman, or PJ must consider this fact in his or her analgesic decision, but if the casualty is able to complain of pain, then the TBI is likely not severe enough to preclude the use of ketamine or OTFC.

h. Eye injury does not preclude the use of ketamine. The risk of additional damage to the eye from using ketamine is low and maximizing the casualty's chance for survival takes precedence if the casualty is in shock or respiratory distress or at significant risk for either.

i. Ketamine may be a useful adjunct to reduce the amount of opioids required to provide effective pain relief. It is safe to give ketamine to a casualty who has previously received morphine or OTFC. IV Ketamine should be given over 1 minute.

j. If respirations are noted to be reduced after using opioids or ketamine, provide ventilatory support with a bag-valve-mask or mouth-to-mask ventilations.

k. Promethazine, 25 mg IV/IM/IO every 6 hours may be given as needed for nausea or vomiting.

l. Reassess – reassess – reassess!

14. Splint fractures and recheck pulses.

15. Antibiotics: recommended for all open combat wounds
   a. If able to take PO:
      - Moxifloxacin, 400 mg PO one a day
   b. If unable to take PO (shock, unconsciousness):
      - Cefotetan, 2 g IV (slow push over 35 minutes) or IM every 12 hours
        OR
      - Ertapenem, 1 g IV/IM once a day

16. Burns*
   a. Facial burns, especially those that occur in closed spaces, may be associated with inhalation injury. Aggressively monitor airway status and oxygen saturation in such patients and consider early surgical airway for respiratory distress or oxygen desaturation.
   b. Estimate total body surface area (TBSA) burned to the nearest 10% using the Rule of Nines.
   c. Cover the burn area with dry, sterile dressings. For extensive burns (>20%), consider placing the casualty in the Heat-Reflective Shell or Blizzard Survival Blanket from the Hypothermia Prevention Kit in order to both cover the burned areas and prevent hypothermia.
   d. Fluid resuscitation (USAISR Rule of Ten)
      - If burns are greater than 20% of Total Body Surface Area, fluid resuscitation should be initiated as soon as IV/IO access is established. Resuscitation should be initiated with Lactated Ringer's, normal saline, or Hextend. If Hextend is used, no more than 1000 ml should be given, followed by Lactated Ringer's or normal saline as needed.
      - Initial IV/IO fluid rate is calculated as %TBSA x 10cc/hr for adults weighing 40 80 kg.
      - For every 10 kg ABOVE 80 kg, increase initial rate by 100 ml/hr.
      - If hemorrhagic shock is also present, resuscitation for hemorrhagic shock takes precedence over resuscitation for burn shock. Administer IV/IO fluids per the TCCC Guidelines in Section 7.
   e. Analgesia in accordance with the TCCC Guidelines in Section 13 may be administered to treat burn pain.

(*Continues on next page*)

Figure 26-1 Basic Management Plan for Tactical Field Care (October 28, 2013) (*Continued*)

f. Prehospital antibiotic therapy is not indicated solely for burns, but antibiotics should be given per the TCCC guidelines in Section 15 if indicated to prevent infection in penetrating wounds.

g. All TCCC interventions can be performed on or through burned skin in a burn casualty.

17. Communicate with the casualty if possible.
   - Encourage; reassure
   - Explain care

18. Cardiopulmonary resuscitation (CPR).
   Resuscitation on the battlefield for victims of blast or penetrating trauma who have no pulse, no ventilations, and no other signs of life will not be successful and should not be attempted. However, casualties with torso trauma or polytrauma who have no pulse or respirations during TFC should have bilateral needle decompression performed to ensure they do not have a tension pneumothorax prior to discontinuation of care. The procedure is the same as described in Section 3 above.

19. Documentation of Care
   Document clinical assessments, treatments rendered, and changes in the casualty's status on a TCCC Casualty Card (DD Form 1380). Forward this information with the casualty to the next level of care.

*See the Treatment of Burn Casualties in Tactical Combat Casualty Care chapter for discussion of this guideline.

The acronym **MARCH** will help combat medical personnel recall the key initial steps in caring for a combat casualty. The letters refer to the following elements of care:

- **M**—Massive bleeding. Establish immediate control of massive external bleeding with an extremity tourniquet, Combat Gauze, or a junctional tourniquet.
- **A**—Airway. Check the airway and open as needed.
- **R**—Respirations. Treat tension pneumothorax with needle decompression and/or open pneumothorax with a chest seal as needed.
- **C**—Circulation. Assess hemodynamic status and take action as appropriate. Use tranexamic acid, initiate intravenous (IV) or intraosseous (IO) access, and begin fluid resuscitation as needed.
- **H**—Head/Hypothermia. If moderate to severe head injury is present, perform the additional elements of care outlined in this chapter to manage TBI; prevent hypothermia so that the casualty maintains a normal coagulation profile.

The need for tactical situational awareness remains paramount during Tactical Field Care. This is still "outside-the-wire" trauma care, and the threat of hostile fire is still present. Security should be established while care is being rendered. For this reason, another mnemonic recommended for use by combat medical personnel is **S-CAB**:

- **S**—Scene security and situational awareness.
- **C**—Control life-threatening bleeding.
- **A**—Airway. Check the airway and open as needed.
- **B**—Assess Breathing. Treat tension pneumothorax with needle decompression and/or open pneumothorax with a chest seal as needed. "B" also reminds combat medical personnel of blankets to prevent hypothermia.

The casualty should be moved to the best available cover and concealment. Although light discipline is a necessity in conditions of reduced ambient light, a white or red light can be used under cover of a poncho or other cover if this is essential to the care of the casualty. Equipment limitations and environmental extremes are still factors.

Disarming Casualties With Altered Mental Status

Armed combatants with altered mental status pose a serious threat of injury or death to others in their unit if they employ their weapons accidentally or inappropriately. In the combat setting, altered mental status may be due to traumatic brain injury (TBI), shock, and/or analgesic medications. Anyone noted to have an altered mental status should be disarmed immediately, including secondary weapons and explosive devices.[1]

Airway

Airway obstruction on the battlefield is most often due to maxillofacial trauma, which may include both disrupted airway anatomy and bleeding into the airway.

Kelly's autopsy review for causes of death in 982 combat fatalities in Afghanistan and Iraq found that 232 individuals in this cohort died from potentially survivable injuries.[2] Mabry reviewed these findings and determined that 18 (1.8%) of the fatalities with potentially survivable wounds died from airway obstruction. Of note, all 18 had penetrating injury to the face or neck.[3] Nine of these fatalities had injuries to major vascular structures as well; eight had significant airway hemorrhage. Surgical airways were attempted in five cases, but none of these procedures were successful.

Basic Airway Procedures

Unconscious casualties should have their airways opened with the chin-lift or jaw-thrust maneuver.

If spontaneous ventilations are present and there is no airway obstruction, further airway management is best achieved with a nasopharyngeal airway. It is better tolerated than an oropharyngeal airway if the casualty regains consciousness,[4] and a nasopharyngeal airway is less likely to be dislodged during transport.[5] Also, *trismus* (a strong contraction of the jaw muscles) is commonly encountered in head-injured patients, making an oral airway difficult to place. A review of nasopharyngeal airway use on the battlefield found no reported instances of vomiting and aspiration complicating the use of this device in a combat setting.[6] Since the time of that review, one casualty with severe TBI who had vomiting and aspiration with a nasopharyngeal airway in place was identified during one of the Joint Theater Trauma System weekly trauma teleconferences.

Unconscious casualties should be placed in the semi-prone recovery position to prevent aspiration of blood, mucus, or vomitus (**Figure 26-2**).

Advanced Airway Procedures
Endotracheal Intubation

If an airway obstruction develops or persists despite the use of a nasopharyngeal airway, a more definitive airway will be required. The ability of experienced paramedics to perform endotracheal intubation in civilian prehospital settings has been well documented.[7-16] Most studies reported the use of cadaver training, operating room intubations, supervised initial intubations, or a combination of these methods in teaching the skill to paramedics.

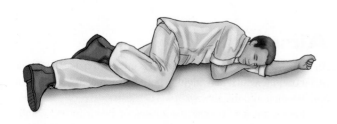

Figure 26-2 Semi-prone recovery position.
Source: Courtesy of MSG Harold Montgomery.

The studies also stressed the importance of continued practice to maintain proficiency.

However, considerations for endotracheal intubation in the battlefield trauma setting are somewhat different[5]:

1. No studies have examined the ability of well-trained but relatively inexperienced combat medical personnel to accomplish endotracheal intubation on the battlefield.
2. Most combat medical personnel have never performed an intubation on a live casualty or even a cadaver.
3. Standard endotracheal intubation techniques entail the use of a tactically compromising white light in the laryngoscope. There was a fatality caused by the use of a white light on the battlefield during an attempted intubation on an Israeli Special Operations mission.[6]
4. Endotracheal intubation may be extremely challenging in casualties with maxillofacial injuries.[17]
5. Esophageal intubation may go unrecognized more easily in the tactical setting, with potentially fatal results for the casualty. In a recent study that included combat medic/corpsman intubations as well as physician and physician-assistant intubations done in prehospital Battalion Aid Station settings, only 22.5% had end-tidal carbon dioxide monitoring confirmation of the correct position for the endotracheal tube.[18]

Endotracheal intubation may be difficult to accomplish even in the hands of more experienced paramedics and even under less austere conditions.[19] One study that examined first-time intubationists trained with mannequin intubations alone noted an initial success rate of only 42% in the ideal setting of the operating room with paralyzed patients.[9] Another study examined intubations performed by basic emergency medical technicians (EMTs) who had been trained in intubation and found that only 53 of 103 patients were successfully intubated.[20] A third paper documented that, even in civilian settings with experienced paramedical personnel, the endotracheal tube was found to be misplaced in 27 of 108 prehospital intubations upon arrival in the emergency department.[21] One report of successful intubations by combat medical personnel used mannequin intubation by just-trained corpsmen as an outcome measure.[22] This may not be an accurate indicator of success under actual battlefield conditions.

The Registry of Emergency Airways Arriving at Combat Hospitals (REACH) study by Adams and his colleagues found a relatively higher success rate in prehospital intubations.[18] However, most of these casualties (81%) were received from Battalion Aid Stations or Forward Surgical Teams where a nurse anesthetist or physician could perform the intubation in somewhat more favorable settings.

Endotracheal intubation in civilian trauma patients is more successful and has fewer complications when it is done with rapid sequence intubation (RSI). Most combat medical personnel, however, do not have initial training or sustainment

CHAPTER 26 Tactical Field Care **687**

training in RSI. Furthermore, without RSI, intubation attempts in a casualty who is not deeply unconscious (a predictor of poor outcomes in combat casualties) will be vigorously resisted by the casualty and should not be attempted.

Supraglottic Airways

Supraglottic airways (e.g., the Laryngeal Mask Airway [LMA], King LT, Combitube) are designed for patients in cardiac arrest or for patients who have been paralyzed but in whom intubation has failed and ventilation is not easily accomplished (can't intubate, can't ventilate). These airways may be difficult to place in all but the most profoundly comatose casualties. These casualties have a very high mortality rate. Whereas previous TCCC recommendations were for the LMA or the Combitube, a recent CoTCCC review of supraglottic airways found that there are presently many supraglottic airways in use and that there was insufficient evidence to identify a single device as being superior to the rest.[23]

Traumatic Airway Obstruction

Airway obstruction in the combat setting typically results from trauma to the face or neck in which blood and/or disrupted anatomy may preclude good visualization of the vocal cords. Conscious casualties with maxillofacial trauma are often able to protect their own airways by the simple act of sitting up and leaning forward so that blood drains out of the mouth instead of down into the airway. This point is reflected in the airway management guideline that calls for the casualty to be allowed to assume whatever position that allows him or her to breathe most easily, including sitting upright if required (**Figure 26-3**). Conscious casualties with maxillofacial trauma should not be forced into a supine position if they are able to breathe more comfortably in the sitting position.

If the sit-up-and-lean-forward position is not feasible or does not provide an acceptable airway, then a surgical airway

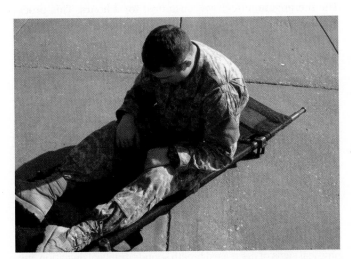

Figure 26-3 Simulated casualty sitting in the tripod position.

Source: Courtesy of MSG Harold Montgomery.

(cricothyroidotomy, cricothyrotomy) is preferable to intubation in these cases, and combat medical personnel should be trained to do surgical airways.[5,17] Cricothyroidotomy has been reported safe and effective in trauma patients,[24] but it is not without complications.[25,26] Even so, cricothyroidotomy provides the best chance for successful airway management in the setting of airway compromise from maxillofacial trauma in tactical settings. Furthermore, it can be performed under local anesthesia with lidocaine in a casualty who is awake.

One of the 12 potentially preventable deaths noted by Colonel John Holcomb, the Commander of the USAISR, and his colleagues[27] was an individual with maxillofacial trauma who was managed with attempted endotracheal intubation instead of a surgical airway. The casualty died from an inadequate airway. The endotracheal tube was found at autopsy to be in a false passage instead of the trachea.

In another case, Macdonald and Tien described a 19-year-old Afghan man with extensive maxillofacial injuries from an improvised explosive device (IED) blast.[28] His respiratory rate was elevated and his oxygen saturation was unsatisfactory even on supplemental oxygen. The medic attending him performed a successful surgical airway with subsequent improvement of the casualty's condition. The medic also performed a needle decompression of a suspected tension pneumothorax. The casualty survived his injuries.

Surgical Airway Training

Surgical airways have been performed successfully in Special Operations units when they are practiced using live tissue models during training.[6] Developing and maintaining this skill is one of the most compelling reasons for combat medical personnel to obtain live tissue training. Note that a surgical airway is NOT indicated simply for unconsciousness when there is no maxillofacial trauma. A nasopharyngeal airway or a supraglottic airway should suffice in those instances unless airway obstruction is noted.

Mabry's analysis of 72 prehospital surgical airways[29] found that (1) 66% of the casualties died, (2) those casualties injured by gunshot wounds to the head or thorax all died, (3) the largest group of survivors had gunshot- or blast-related wounds to the face and/or neck, and (4) the failure rate for the procedure performed by combat medics was 33% compared to 15% for physicians and physician assistants. The latter finding should be evaluated in light of a possible difference in the tactical situations in which combat medics, corpsmen, and pararescuemen (PJs) would have performed the surgical airway (at the point of injury) as opposed to the settings in which the physicians and physician assistants would typically have performed the procedure (at the battalion aid station). Mabry also noted that while the failure rate for surgical airways in the combat setting is three to five times higher than reported in civilian settings, surgical airways in civilian prehospital settings are performed by paramedic-level providers, whereas Army 68-W medics are typically trained to the EMT-Basic level only.

Bennett and coauthors performed a bottom-up review of cricothyroidotomy training at a Naval Hospital and found five specific gap areas in the training[30]: (1) limited anatomic instruction, (2) lack of "hands-on" familiarization with laryngeal anatomy, (3) nonstandardized step-by-step training in the surgical technique involved, (4) anatomically incorrect training manikins, and (5) lack of standardized refresher training frequency. This paper recommended incorporating a step into the training in which students use a marker pen to illustrate on a fellow student exactly where they would make the incision for the cricothyroidotomy. This excellent recommendation adds a bit of adrenalin to the student's learning experience. It is immediately obvious to the instructor if the student locates the incision incorrectly, and that realization, combined with the simulated casualty's awareness of the results, will immediately reinforce either that the anatomy has been mastered or that further instruction is needed.

Thermal or Toxic Gas Injuries to the Airway

Thermal or toxic gas injuries are important considerations in certain tactical situations. These injuries may result in airway edema that can be aggravated by aggressive fluid administration, leading to acute upper airway obstruction. Inhalation injury should be suspected if fire occurs within a confined space or if the casualty has facial burns, singeing of the nasal hairs, or carbonaceous sputum. Sore throat, hoarseness, and wheezing may also be noted. For these casualties, cricothyroidotomy is the airway of choice in the Tactical Field Care phase.

Tension Pneumothorax
Overview

Penetrating trauma is the predominant type of trauma encountered in conventional ground warfare. In a review of fatalities from the Vietnam War, tension pneumothorax was reported as the cause of death in 3% to 4% of the fatally wounded casualties.[31] Prehospital needle decompression may be a lifesaving procedure for these casualties.[5]

Although the common practice of wearing personal protective equipment (body armor) on combat missions has reduced the relative frequency of chest wounds in U.S. combat casualties,[32] chest wounds may still result from bullets or shrapnel impacting near the edge of the body armor and traveling into the chest. Additionally, the potential need to care for both hostile and civilian casualties who were not wearing body armor, and thus were not protected from chest trauma, may require that combat medical personnel treat tension pneumothoraces. The combination of body armor, aggressive needle decompression when indicated, and the use of the longer 3.25-inch needles for needle decompression (as discussed later in this section) has resulted in a decrease in preventable deaths from tension pneumothorax to 0.2% among U.S. combat fatalities as documented in the comprehensive review of combat fatalities

from Afghanistan and Iraq by Colonel Brian Eastridge.[27] This is a decrease of over 90% in this cause of preventable death.

Needle decompression for the initial management of tension pneumothorax has been reported safe and effective in the civilian prehospital setting.[33] A casualty with a penetrating wound to the chest will usually have some degree of pneumothorax as a result of the primary wound. The additional trauma caused by a needle thoracostomy performed on the same side as the chest injury should not significantly worsen the casualty's condition if he or she does not have a tension pneumothorax. This consideration further strengthens the case for the aggressive use of needle decompression in the tactical prehospital setting.[5] Paramedics perform needle decompression of the chest in most civilian emergency medical services (EMS).[5] Combat medical personnel should also be proficient in this technique.

Tube thoracostomy (chest tube) is not recommended for routine use in battlefield trauma care for the following reasons:

1. Chest tubes are not generally needed to provide initial treatment for a tension pneumothorax.
2. Chest tubes are a more difficult and time-consuming intervention for relatively inexperienced medical personnel.
3. Chest tube insertion is more likely to cause additional tissue damage and subsequent infection than needle decompression.

Chest tubes are generally not part of the paramedic's scope of care in civilian EMS settings,[12,16] and no studies were found that address the use of this procedure by combat medical personnel in tactical settings. However, in the case of failure of needle decompression to relieve a suspected tension pneumothorax, simple thoracostomy (creating an opening in the chest wall) or a chest tube may be effective and lifesaving.[34]

Needle decompression with a 14-gauge needle/catheter unit was found to relieve elevated intrapleural pressure rapidly in a swine model of traumatic tension pneumothorax.[35] The therapeutic effect was sustained for 4 hours. This procedure was found to be equivalent to tube thoracostomy with a 32 French chest tube for the 4-hour observation period. The ease and speed of performance and the decreased likelihood of complications make needle decompression the procedure of choice for relieving a tension pneumothorax on the battlefield.

Diagnosing Tension Pneumothorax

A presumptive diagnosis of tension pneumothorax is appropriate when progressively worsening hypoxia, respiratory distress, or shock develops in a casualty with known or suspected torso trauma. Note that penetrating injuries in locations such as the shoulder or the abdomen may also result in pulmonary injury and tension pneumothorax. The battlefield diagnosis of tension pneumothorax should not rely solely on the commonly mentioned physical signs of decreased breath sounds, tracheal deviation, jugular distension, or hyperresonance to percussion. These findings may not always be present and may be difficult to appreciate on the battlefield.

Cannula Length

Cannula length is an important consideration in needle decompression.[36] At the second intercostal space in the midclavicular line, the needle must pass through the pectoral muscles, and in young male military personnel, these muscles can be thick. It is imperative that a needle/catheter unit long enough to reach the thoracic cavity be used in this procedure. Recent studies have noted that the chest wall thickness in many male servicemen may exceed the length of a standard 2-inch (5-centimeter [cm]) needle catheter. Harcke and his colleagues found a mean chest wall thickness of 5.36 cm in 100 autopsy computerized tomography studies of military fatalities.[37] Several of the cases in their autopsy series were noted to have had unsuccessful attempts at needle decompression because the needle/catheter units used for the procedure were too short. The study authors recommended that a 3.25-inch (8-cm) needle/catheter unit be used in order to achieve a 99% success rate of reaching the pleural space.

Other authors have voiced similar concerns.[38,39] In 2006, the U.S. Army Surgeon General directed that needle decompression for soldiers suspected of having a tension pneumothorax should be accomplished using a 3.25-inch (8-cm), 14-gauge needle/catheter unit inserted to the hub.[40] The author of this chapter has found no published reports of death from unrelieved tension pneumothorax in combat casualties since the 3.25-inch (8-cm) catheters were introduced. Even though it may be difficult to appreciate in field settings, if there is no rush of air when the needle is inserted, either it did not go in far enough or no tension pneumothorax was present.

Insertion Site

The needle/catheter unit should be inserted into the second intercostal space at the midclavicular line (2ICS MCL), just over the top of the third rib at a 90-degree angle to the frontal plane of the chest. The needle/catheter unit should be inserted all the way to the hub. The needle should then be removed and the catheter secured to the chest wall. There is no requirement to place a one-way valve or three-way stopcock on the end of the catheter, as air will not enter into the chest cavity in significant amounts through the small bore of the catheter. However, if a tension pneumothorax is present, the increased intrapleural pressure will force air out of the chest through the catheter. Position the casualty in the sitting position if conscious, or in the lateral, recumbent position with the injured side down if unconscious.

Although uncommon, potentially fatal complications may result from needle decompression. These include laceration of the subclavian artery,[41] pulmonary artery injury,[42] cardiac tamponade,[42] and life-threatening hemorrhage.[43] The proximity of the heart and great vessels to the anterior 2ICS MCL approach site imparts great importance to careful technique.[42] A Canadian civilian study of 17 attempted midclavicular line needle decompressions found that 44% were performed too medially.[44] A different study of TCCC interventions in the Canadian armed forces found that seven of seven needle decompressions intended for the second ICS at the midclavicular line were in fact located medial to the midclavicular line.[45] Ensuring that the insertion site for the needle is at or lateral to the nipple line when a midclavicular line insertion site is used will help avoid complications. Additionally, care should be taken to direct the needle perpendicularly to the surface of the chest and not in the direction of the heart and great vessels.

Because of the complications noted at the 2ICS MCL site for needle decompression, some authors have recommended using the third or fourth intercostal space (ICS) at the midaxillary line as an alternate site.[31,38,41] In a report of a series of three patients with life-threatening hemorrhage after needle decompression performed at the second ICS at the midclavicular line, the authors concluded that the procedure could be more safely performed at the fifth ICS at the anterior axillary line (5ICS AAL).[43] The authors noted that the 5ICS AAL site is recommended by Advanced Trauma Life Support (ATLS) for insertion of chest tubes. The fourth or fifth ICS at the anterior axillary line (AAL) is now recommended as an alternate site for needle thoracostomy in the TCCC guidelines.[46] The *Prehospital Trauma Life Support* (*PHTLS*) manual and the U.S. Special Operations Command Combat Trauma Protocols concur with this recommendation. The fifth ICS at the AAL is easily located in young fit males. It lies at the intersection of the nipple line and the lateral border of the pectoralis muscle group.

Reassessment

Any casualty who has undergone needle decompression for relief of a tension pneumothorax must be frequently reassessed. Persistence or recurrence of respiratory distress after needle decompression may occur as a result of any of the following: (1) the respiratory symptoms may have been a manifestation of a condition other than tension pneumothorax—e.g., pulmonary contusion, hemothorax, shock, toxic gas inhalation; (2) inadequate needle length[37]; (3) clotting and/or kinking of the catheter used for decompression; or (4) the airflow through the needle is simply inadequate to match the volume of air escaping from the injured lung into the pleural space.[47]

For more information about needle decompression, see **Figures 26-4** through **26-6**.

Open Pneumothorax

An open pneumothorax ("sucking chest wound") results from an injury that penetrates the chest wall and may or may not include injuries to the underlying lung and pulmonary blood vessels. On the battlefield, these injuries are usually caused by

Figure 26-4   Needle Decompression for Tension Pneumothorax

In two studies comparing needle decompression and tube thoracostomy for tension pneumothorax, Colonel Holcomb and his colleagues[35] reported much greater success with needle decompression than did Colonel Matt Martin and his coauthors.[47] It is worth noting that these two studies used different models of tension pneumothorax. The different outcomes suggest that one of the variables determining outcomes in tension pneumothorax is the rate at which air leaks from the injured lung. If a recurrence of the tension pneumothorax is suspected, the casualty may need repeated needle decompression. If this is unsuccessful, a chest tube may be inserted or a chest tube incision may be made and the pleural space entered with a blunt clamp or a finger, as noted above.[34] In a casualty with nonpenetrating torso trauma, caution must be exercised when considering needle decompression since this procedure could result in a pneumothorax if one is not already present.

Figure 26-5   Needle Decompression in the Field

Case reports of successful relief of tension pneumothorax by combat medical personnel have been noted during the current conflicts in Iraq and Afghanistan, and no major complications from this procedure have been reported.[6]

Figure 26-6   Bilateral Needle Decompression in Traumatic Cardiopulmonary Arrest

Needle decompression has proven lifesaving in some individuals who suffer prehospital cardiopulmonary arrest due to trauma.[48] Bilateral needle decompression should be performed before resuscitation efforts are abandoned when a casualty with torso trauma or polytrauma suffers a prehospital cardiopulmonary arrest.[49]

bullets or shrapnel. Dolley and Brewer describe the pathophysiology of open pneumothorax during World War II noting that an injury penetrating into the pleural space creates a second opening through which air may enter into the thorax.[50] When the casualty inhales, the second traumatic pathway allows air

to enter the pleural cavity that is normally only a potential space while air also travels through the normal pathway to the lungs (via the trachea). The percentage of air that follows the normal pathway is inversely proportional to the size of the defect in the chest wall.

When the chest wall opening is large enough (usually two-thirds or more of the diameter of the trachea) air flows preferentially into the chest cavity via the defect in the chest wall, instead of into the lung via the trachea, as the casualty inhales. (Note: As a point of reference, a nickel is 2 cm in diameter, and the adult trachea is 2.0 to 2.5 cm in diameter.) Air entering through the defect in the chest wall allows the lung on the affected side to collapse (**Figure 26-7**). This prevents normal gas exchange in that lung, causing dyspnea and (potentially) hypoxia and hypercarbia. The risk of death associated with isolated open pneumothorax is not well described, but no fatalities from Afghanistan or Iraq were attributed specifically to open pneumothorax as an isolated injury.[51] Even if an open pneumothorax is not fatal in itself, the resultant impediment to pulmonary gas exchange could contribute to secondary brain injury in casualties with TBI.

The immediate treatment for an open pneumothorax is to seal the opening with an occlusive dressing, thus preventing air from entering the pleural space through the defect in the chest wall. This helps to restore airflow into the lung during inspiration, but it could lead to the development of a tension pneumothorax since there may be an underlying lung injury. In the past, a dressing secured on only three sides was recommended to prevent tension pneumothorax.[52–54] Theoretically, the open side acts as a flutter valve to release any air pressure that may build up in the pleural space, but clinical studies to confirm the efficacy of three-sided dressings have not been performed.

Commercially available vented and un-vented chest seals have been evaluated in a recent animal study for the treatment of

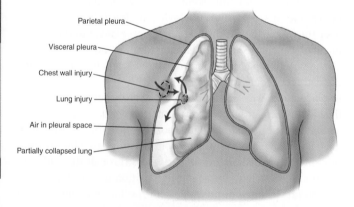

Figure 26-7 Because of the proximity of the chest wall to the lung, it would be extremely difficult for the chest wall to be injured by penetrating trauma and the lung not to be injured. Sealing the hole in the chest wall does not stop any air leakage that may be occurring from the injured lung.

open pneumothorax and prevention of tension pneumothorax.[55] In that study, 200-milliliter (ml) increments of air were injected every 5 minutes into the pleural cavity of swine in whom an open pneumothorax injury had been created until either tension pneumothorax developed or the volume of air injected equaled 100% of the animal's estimated total lung capacity. The authors reported no tension pneumothoraces in the animals treated with vented chest seals (incorporating a one-way valve that allowed air to leave but not to enter the pleural space). Tension pneumothoraces did occur in the animals treated with unvented chest seals.

A vented chest seal, then, is the preferred treatment for an open pneumothorax. If no vented chest seal is available, a non-vented occlusive seal should be used. No matter what dressing or seal is used to close an open chest wound, it is crucial to monitor the casualty for signs of a developing tension pneumothorax. If the casualty is observed to have increasing hypoxia, shock, or respiratory distress, the edge of the chest seal should be lifted (burped) in order to allow the accumulating gas in the pleural space to escape, or the chest should be decompressed using needle decompression. See **Figure 26-8** for advanced treatment of open pneumothorax.

Oxygen Administration

Typically, combat medical personnel do not carry oxygen cylinders into the field as part of their medical loadouts due to the weight of the compressed gas cylinders and the potential for explosions secondary to ballistic damage to the cylinders. However, if oxygen is available during the Tactical Field Care phase, the guidelines for its administration in Tactical Evacuation Care should be followed (see the Tactical Evacuation Care chapter for more details).

Supplemental oxygen is particularly important for casualties who are hypoxic, who are in shock,[56] or who have TBI if oxygen is available in Tactical Field Care. Hypoxia in casualties with TBI is associated with unfavorable outcomes,[57] so casualties with moderate to severe TBI should receive supplemental oxygen when available to maintain their oxygen saturation above 90%. Furthermore, hyperoxia causes cerebral vasoconstriction independently of the effects of hypocapnia, and thereby may help to reduce intracranial pressure.[58,59] Hyperoxia also increases cerebral tissue oxygenation[56] and improves cerebral metabolism in

casualties with severe head injury.[60] For casualties with moderate to severe TBI, supplemental oxygen should be given at the highest inspired fraction of oxygen achievable as early in the continuum of care as possible.[61]

Hemorrhage Control—Tourniquets

Life-threatening extremity hemorrhage should have been previously addressed with a tourniquet in the Care Under Fire phase. The casualty should be reassessed for hemorrhage control during the Tactical Field Care phase. Check for any previously unrecognized sites of significant bleeding and obtain control of any significant bleeding noted. This is followed by a reevaluation of any tourniquets in place. A tourniquet is still the first step to gain control of any life-threatening extremity hemorrhage in locations amenable to tourniquet placement if this has not already been accomplished in the Care Under Fire phase (see **Figure 26-9**).

Hemorrhage control does not stop with the initial tourniquet application. Casualties with tourniquets in place should be rechecked periodically and each time they are moved to ensure that the hemorrhage is still controlled. When time and the tactical situation permit in the Tactical Field Care phase, the wound should be exposed. Wound exposure should be accomplished using trauma shears rather than an unguarded blade to prevent further injury to the extremity. Any tourniquet that was originally placed over the uniform should be replaced with another tourniquet applied directly to the skin 2 to 3 inches proximal to the hemorrhage site.

Pulses distal to every tourniquet should be checked. If a distal pulse is still present, the tourniquet should be tightened or a second tourniquet applied side by side just proximal to the first,[62] and the pulse should be checked again. It is important that the distal arterial blood flow be stopped by the tourniquet. If it is not, a compartment syndrome or expanding hematoma may develop in the limb, creating an avoidable complication for the casualty.[62]

Tourniquet application typically causes the casualty significant pain, but this does not signify incorrect application or that the tourniquet should be discontinued. Pain should be managed with analgesics as appropriate, taking care not to give narcotic

Figure 26-8 Thoracostomy Tube Insertion in Cases of Open Pneumothorax

When time, skills, and circumstances allow, a thoracostomy tube should be placed in the same side of the chest as the open pneumothorax. This is typically accomplished in a medical treatment facility.

Figure 26-9 The Priority of Hemorrhage Control

Hemorrhage control in combat casualties takes precedence over infusing fluids or providing oxygen. Even when treating a casualty who is in obvious shock from his or her wounds, controlling external hemorrhage takes priority over fluid resuscitation.

analgesics to casualties in shock. For casualties with severe tourniquet pain who are in shock, ketamine is the preferred analgesic option.

When evacuation of the casualty is expected to exceed 2 hours and the casualty is not in shock, the possibility of removing the tourniquet and transitioning to another method of hemorrhage control should be considered during Tactical Field Care. If time allows, it may be possible to use hemostatic agents in conjunction with direct pressure, gauze packing, and/or a pressure

bandage to achieve effective hemorrhage control. It is important to note that the tourniquet should not actually be removed from the limb during this process, but slowly loosened after an alternative method of hemorrhage control has been applied. Most importantly, tourniquet removal should not be attempted if the casualty is in shock or if the evacuation time to a medical facility is expected to be 2 hours or less.

Guidelines for tourniquet removal, derived from U.S. Army tourniquet guidelines, are noted in **Figure 26-10**.

Figure 26-10   Tourniquet Tips

Points to Remember

- Damage to the arm or leg is rare if the tourniquet is left on less than 2 hours.
- Tourniquets are often left in place for several hours during surgical procedures.
- In the face of massive extremity hemorrhage, it is better to accept the small risk of damage to the limb than to allow a casualty to bleed to death.

Six Major Tourniquet Mistakes

1. Not using a tourniquet when it should be used
2. Using a tourniquet when it should not be used
3. Putting the tourniquet on too proximally
4. Not tightening the tourniquet well enough
5. Not taking the tourniquet off when possible
6. Periodically loosening the tourniquet to allow intermittent blood flow

Death From Exsanguination

How long does it take to bleed to death from a complete femoral artery and vein disruption?

- Casualties with such an injury are likely to die in about 10 minutes, but some will bleed to death in as little as 3 minutes.

Tourniquet Application

1. Apply without delay for life-threatening extremity bleeding during Care Under Fire.
   - Both the casualty and the person providing care are in serious danger while a tourniquet is being applied during Care Under Fire.
   - The decision regarding the relative risk of further injury versus that of bleeding to death must be made by the person rendering care.
   - *Note*: The lifesaving benefit of a tourniquet is far greater when the tourniquet is applied BEFORE the casualty has gone into shock from the wound.
2. Non-life-threatening bleeding should be ignored until the Tactical Field Care phase.

3. Apply tourniquet proximal to the site of hemorrhage over the uniform during Care Under Fire.
4. Tighten tourniquet until bleeding stops.
5. During Tactical Field Care, expose the wound and reapply the tourniquet directly on the skin 2 to 3 inches proximal to the bleeding site.
6. Check for a distal pulse.
7. Tighten the tourniquet or apply a second tourniquet side by side and just proximal to the first as needed to eliminate the distal pulse.
8. Note the time of tourniquet application.

Removing the Tourniquet

- Remove the tourniquet when direct pressure or hemostatic dressings become feasible and effective, unless the casualty is in shock or the tourniquet has been on for more than 6 hours.
- Only a combat medic, a physician's assistant, or a physician should remove tourniquets.
- Do not remove tourniquet if the distal extremity is gone.
- Do not attempt to remove the tourniquet if the casualty will arrive at a hospital in 2 hours or less after application.

Technique for Removal

1. Apply Combat Gauze as per instructions.
2. Loosen the tourniquet.
3. Apply direct pressure to the bleeding site for 3 minutes.
4. Check for bleeding.
5. If no bleeding, apply pressure dressing over the Combat Gauze.
6. Leave the tourniquet in place but loose.
7. Monitor for bleeding from underneath the pressure dressings.
8. If bleeding does not remain controlled, retighten the tourniquet, remove dressings, and expedite evacuation.

Hemorrhage Control— Hemostatic Agents

Having more time and tactical security during the Tactical Field Care phase allows for more hemorrhage control options. The HemCon dressing and the granular agent QuikClot were the hemostatic agents previously recommended by the CoTCCC based upon their success in controlling severe bleeding in animal models.[63,64] These agents worked effectively,[6,65,66] although some cutaneous burns were reported with QuikClot use.[6,67]

A number of newer hemostatic agents have now become available. These new agents have undergone testing at the U.S. Army Institute of Surgical Research (USAISR).[68] The USAISR studies found the new agents Combat Gauze and WoundStat to be consistently more effective than HemCon and QuikClot. No significant exothermic reaction was noted with either Combat Gauze or WoundStat. Celox was also found to outperform HemCon and QuikClot, although it performed less effectively than WoundStat in the USAISR model of severe femoral bleeding **(Figure 26-11)**. A summary of the relative characteristics of the various hemostatic agents is shown in **Figure 26-12**.

Based on these results, the TCCC guidelines were changed to recommend Combat Gauze **(Figure 26-13)** as the first-line treatment for life-threatening hemorrhage that is not amenable to extremity tourniquet placement. Although WoundStat was more effective, subsequent studies at USAISR demonstrated that WoundStat use resulted in the formation of occlusive thrombi in the injured vessels as well as evidence of toxicity to the endothelial cells.[69] Concern about the implications of these findings for casualties resulted in the discontinuation of its distribution to the U.S. military.

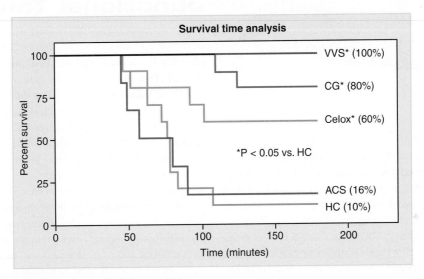

Figure 26-11 Survival time analysis.

Source: Courtesy of Dr. Bijan Kheirabadi.

Hemostatic agent comparison

	QC ACS*	Hem Con	Celox	Woundstat	Combat gauze
Hemostatic efficacy	+	+	+++	++++	++++
Side effect	None	None	Unknown	Yes	None
Ready to use	√	√	√	√	√
Training requirement	+	+	+	+++	++
Lightweight and durable	++	+++	+++	++	+++
2 years shelf life	√	√	√	√	√
Stable in extreme condition	√	√	√	√	√
FDA approved	√	√	√	√	√
Biodegradable	No	No	Yes	No	No
Cost ($)	~ 30	~ 75	~ 25	30-35	~ 25

Figure 26-12 Hemostatic agent comparison.

Source: Courtesy of Dr. Bijan Kheirabadi.

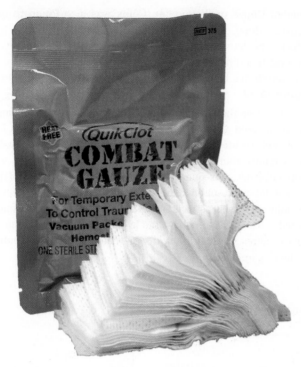

Figure 26-13 Combat Gauze.

Source: Courtesy of Z-Medica.

Combat medical personnel involved in evaluating the options for hemostatic agents voiced a strong preference for a gauze-type agent rather than a powder or granule. This was based on their combat experience of powder or granular agents not working well in wounds in which the bleeding vessel is at the bottom of a narrow wound tract. A gauze-type hemostatic agent is more easily applied in the depth of such wounds. Powder or granular agents also present an ocular hazard when used in windy situations like evacuation by helicopter. They can also be more difficult to remove from wounds than other hemostatic agents when the casualty reaches definitive care. To ensure its effectiveness, Combat Gauze should be applied over the bleeding site with 3 minutes of sustained direct pressure. Simply applying the agents without maintaining pressure is not adequate to achieve the best possible hemostatic effect.[70] Afterward, a pressure dressing can be applied to cover both the wound and the Combat Gauze, and to maintain a degree of pressure.

Combat Gauze is now the most widely used hemostatic dressing on the battlefield.[71] The first report of Combat Gauze used in combat noted a 79% success rate in 14 uses among Israeli Defense Force personnel.[72] Combat Gauze was also found to be effective (93% first attempt, 100% second attempt) in one animal study using a femoral bleeding model even when the animals were acidotic and coagulopathic.[71]

The latest hemostatic dressing technologies are the subjects of ongoing research. A recent study from the Naval Medical Research Unit, San Antonio, found that both Celox Gauze and ChitoGauze produced higher 150-minute survival rates in the standardized USAISR femoral bleeding model than Combat Gauze.[73] Survival was 9 out of 10 (9/10) animals with Celox Gauze, 7/10 with ChitoGauze, 7/10 with Combat Gauze XL, and 6/10 with Combat Gauze. These differences are worthy of note but were not statistically significant. Neither Celox Gauze nor ChitoGauze has yet been tested in the hemostatic safety model developed by Dr. Bijan Kheirabadi, a leading researcher in hemostatic agents at the USAISR.[69] However, chitosan-based hemostatic dressings have been used on the battlefield for almost a decade at this point with no reports of increased rates of adverse events related to these dressings and are currently being considered by the CoTCCC.

Dismounted Complex Blast Injury and Junctional Tourniquets

The pressure-activated IEDs used with increasing frequency by insurgent forces in Afghanistan since 2010 produce an injury complex that has been designated Dismounted Complex Blast Injury (DCBI). This injury pattern is characterized by severe injuries to one or both lower extremities, often accompanied by upper extremity, urogenital, pelvic, and abdominal trauma. Multiple amputations are commonly seen with DCBI.[74] Lower extremity amputations may be quite high, soft-tissue damage is often massive, and control of hemorrhage is often difficult to achieve with tourniquets and Combat Gauze.

The prevalence of DCBI in casualties from Afghanistan has led to the development of devices designed to apply sustained pressure to the large arteries in the groin. One such device is the Combat Ready Clamp (CRoC) **(Figure 26-14)**. The CRoC applies both anterior and posterior pressure to the injured area and has been shown to work well in perfused cadaver and swine models.[75] More recently, the Junctional Emergency Treatment Tool (JETT) and the SAM Junctional Tourniquet (SJT) have also been recommended for use by the CoTCCC **(Figure 26-15)**. If a lower extremity wound is not amenable to tourniquet application and bleeding cannot be controlled by hemostatic agents or pressure dressings, the combat medical personnel should consider immediate application of mechanical direct pressure using one of the three CoTCCC-recommended junctional tourniquets: the CRoC, the JETT, and the SJT. Hemorrhage control should be accomplished as feasible with Combat Gauze and direct pressure while a junctional tourniquet is being readied for use or if there is no junctional tourniquet available.

The Abdominal Aortic & Junctional Tourniquet (AAJT) is another option for junctional hemorrhage control but has a shorter maximum length of application than the three junctional tourniquets listed above **(Figure 26-16)**. The AAJT is also relatively contraindicated in the presence of penetrating abdominal injuries, which often occur in association with junctional bleeding in casualties injured by the dismounted IED attacks currently prevalent in Afghanistan.

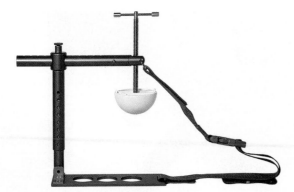

Figure 26-14   Combat Ready Clamp (CRoC).

Source: Courtesy of Combat Medical Systems

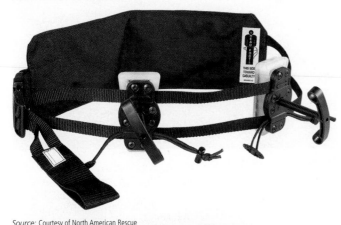

Source: Courtesy of North American Rescue

Figure 26-15   A. Junctional Emergency Treatment Tool (JETT).
B. SAM Junctional Tourniquet (SJT).

Source: Courtesy of SAM Medical Products.

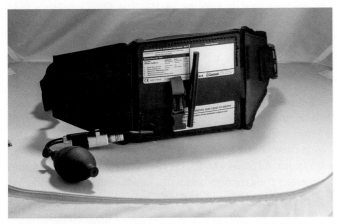

Figure 26-16   Abdominal Aortic & Junctional Tourniquet (AAJT).

Source: Photo by Diane Zahorodny/Chinook Medical Gear

Hemorrhage Control— Direct Pressure

In many cases, control of external hemorrhage can be accomplished by simply applying direct pressure on the bleeding vessel. This is true even for major vessels like the carotid or femoral arteries. However, casualties with life-threatening hemorrhage often bleed to death when direct pressure is the only treatment available to achieve hemostasis. For direct pressure to be effective, it must be applied with both hands using significant force and with the casualty on a surface firm enough to provide effective counterpressure. Typically, direct pressure cannot be effectively applied while the casualty is being moved, even on a hard litter. Additionally, the need to achieve and maintain hemorrhage control with direct pressure makes it impossible for combat medical personnel to perform other interventions for the casualty or to treat other casualties. Lastly, discontinuation of direct pressure to check the status of the bleeding site during transport must be avoided. The direct pressure must be applied without interruption until the casualty reaches a location at which surgical repair of the vessel can be accomplished. For these reasons, tourniquets and hemostatic agents are the favored methods for controlling life-threatening external hemorrhage on the battlefield.

Wounds with minimal external bleeding that do not involve injury to major blood vessels may be dressed with a gauze bandage or simply ignored until the casualty reaches definitive care.

Noncompressible Hemorrhage

For internal hemorrhage from chest and abdominal wounds, the most crucial lifesaving procedure is rapid transport to a facility where definitive surgical control of hemorrhage can be achieved. Internal bleeding may result in shock and subsequent death despite a relatively unimpressive entrance wound. Transport of the casualty with penetrating trauma to the chest or abdomen should be accomplished on an emergent basis. Avoiding platelet-impairing nonsteriodal anti-inflammatory drugs, avoiding overly aggressive prehospital fluid resuscitation, preventing the clotting dysfunction caused by hypothermia, and administering tranexamic acid can improve survival in casualties with noncompressible hemorrhage. These points are discussed further in the relevant sections (Analgesics, Fluid Resuscitation, and Hypothermia Prevention) in this chapter.

Intravenous Access

In civilian trauma care, it is common practice to routinely establish intravenous (IV) access in the prehospital setting for all individuals who have suffered significant trauma. In tactical military settings, this practice has a number of disadvantages. Starting IVs entails costs in both time and equipment. On the battlefield, it is important not to burden combat medical personnel with

Figure 26-17 Intraosseous Vascular Access

The availability of IO vascular access techniques should eliminate the practice of starting IVs on all casualties preemptively in order to avoid the potential difficulties of establishing IV access in a casualty who may later go into shock.

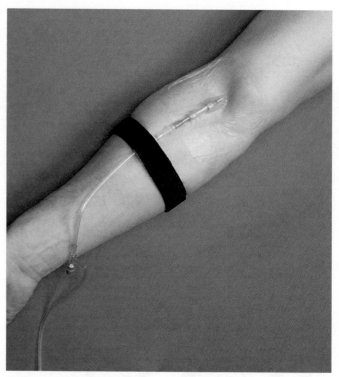

Figure 26-18   Field-capable IV.

Source: Courtesy of North American Rescue.

unnecessary equipment, and not to burden the mission commander with a delay in the unit's tactical flow in order to perform a procedure that is not really needed (see **Figure 26-17**). Intravenous supplies and fluids should be conserved for those casualties with a clear indication for prehospital fluid resuscitation. Only individuals requiring fluid resuscitation for shock and those who need IV medications should have an IV started in TCCC.

Although civilian practice calls for two large-bore (14- or 16-gauge) IV catheters for fluid resuscitation in trauma victims,[4] the 18-gauge catheter is preferred in combat settings because of the relative ease of cannulation compared to that of larger needles.[5] The recommended resuscitation fluid, Hextend, can be administered rapidly through an 18-gauge catheter, and blood products requiring larger cannulae are not typically given during the Tactical Field Care phase.[76,77]

Blood products may be administered in the Tactical Evacuation phase or later at a medical treatment facility (MTF), but field-placed IVs would normally be discontinued in the MTF anyway because of the risk of contamination.[5,78]

Securing Intravenous Lines for Casualty Movement

Intravenous lines started in the field often become dislodged during casualty transport. To address this problem, the 75th Ranger Regiment devised a system for securing IV lines that has proved successful in the field. The first step in their system is insertion of an 18-gauge, 1.25-inch catheter along with a saline lock. The saline lock is then secured by applying a sheet of transparent wound dressing film over the site. Fluids and medications are then given by inserting a second 18-gauge, 1.25-inch needle and catheter through the film dressing and saline lock, then withdrawing the needle. The second catheter is left in place and the IV line secured to the arm with a device that has a circumferential Velcro strap. The transparent film dressing and the line-locking device are common medical tools designed for civilian use. Together they provide for IV access that can withstand rugged handling **(Figure 26-18)**. If the IV line must be discontinued temporarily to facilitate movement on the field, the locking strap, IV line, and second catheter can be quickly disconnected. The first catheter and saline lock remain in place under the film, providing for quick IV access later.

Intraosseous Access

It may be difficult to establish IV access in casualties in shock. An intraosseous (IO) device offers an alternative route for administering fluids and medications in this situation.[79,80] This allows the combat medical personnel to avoid more difficult and invasive techniques such as central venous cannulation or saphenous vein cutdown. Intraosseous access is far easier to obtain than IV access when casualty care is being performed in the dark.

The Pyng FAST1 is the IO device most often used by the U.S. military to date **(Figure 26-19)**. The FAST1 delivers fluid and medications through the bone marrow of the sternal manubrium. Using the sternal notch as a reference point, an adhesive patch is applied that provides a target area for insertion. The device is then aligned with the target, and firm, steady pressure is applied. This action inserts a small, stainless steel tip connected to an infusion tube into the marrow of the manubrium. This technique makes the FAST1 readily applicable in low-light environments.

A clear plastic dome attaches via a Velcro ring, keeping the site clean and visible. The FAST1 device is not spring-loaded, and its configuration renders accidental needle entry into the combat medical personnel's hands unlikely. A disadvantage of the FAST1 is that the casualty's body armor must be removed to insert the device. Doing so makes the casualty more vulnerable to further injury from hostile fire.

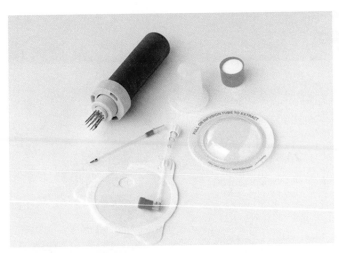

Figure 26-19 Pyng FAST-1®.

Source: Courtesy of Pyng Medical Corp.

The EZ-IO intraosseous infusion system also has been widely used by coalition forces in Iraq and Afghanistan. The original EZ-IO device was not approved for sternal IO access, which was an issue because its original tibial plateau insertion site was not always accessible in combat casualties. However, the EZ-IO system subsequently added needles of various lengths, allowing IO access at the sternum and at six other sites on the proximal humerus, proximal tibia, and distal tibia.

The EZ-IO is small, lightweight, and very easy to use. Both manual and battery-powered versions are available. However, combat medical personnel have noted several disadvantages of the EZ-IO system: the need to construct protection for the infusion needle during transport to prevent accidental disinsertion of the device, significant pain to the casualty when fluids are administered at tibial sites, and loss of potential insertion sites due to extremity trauma. Furthermore, care must be taken not to use a tibial needle at a sternal infusion site. This error has resulted in inadvertent passage of the longer tibial needle through the posterior aspect of the sternum, and infusion of fluid into the mediastinum.[81]

The IO route of vascular access has been used widely in Iraq and Afghanistan and has proven a valuable option for the combat medical personnel.[6,79]

Tranexamic Acid

Noncompressible hemorrhage remains a leading cause of potentially preventable deaths among combat casualties.[2,27,51] The CRASH-2 study examined the effect of **tranexamic acid (TXA)** as an intervention to reduce death from hemorrhage in trauma patients. The study found a small but statistically significant benefit from TXA use. There was no increase in the rate of vascular occlusive events among TXA patients. No unexpected adverse events resulting from TXA use were reported.

Further subgroup analysis of the CRASH-2 data found that the greatest benefit of TXA administration was obtained when the medication was given within 1 hour of injury. Patients receiving TXA within this 1-hour time window had a significantly reduced risk of death from exsanguination. TXA given between 1 and 3 hours postinjury also reduced the risk of death due to bleeding, whereas TXA given more than 3 hours after injury was observed to increase this risk.[82]

The findings of the CRASH-2 study were compelling, but their applicability to the care of combat casualties was uncertain. Different mechanisms of wounding, differences in injury patterns, longer delays to evacuation, and differences in trauma systems made it less than obvious that TXA would provide similar benefits to individuals wounded in combat. The Military Application of Tranexamic Acid in Trauma Emergency Resuscitation (MATTERs) Study was carried out at a Role 3 facility in Afghanistan to investigate the benefit of TXA use in combat casualties.[83] In this series of 896 combat casualties who received blood, mortality in those who received TXA was less than that observed in those who did not, even though those receiving TXA were more seriously injured. In the subgroup of casualties who received massive transfusions, mortality was markedly lower (mortality reduced from 28.1% to 14.4%) in the TXA group compared to the no-TXA group.

The CRASH-2 and MATTERs findings support the use of TXA in combat casualties who are in hemorrhagic shock or at significant risk of it.[84] In TCCC, TXA is indicated for casualties who are anticipated to need significant blood transfusion, such as casualties with hemorrhagic shock, one or more major amputations, penetrating torso trauma, or evidence of severe bleeding. The recommended dose is 1 gram of TXA in 100 cc normal saline or lactated Ringer's, given as soon as possible but NOT later than 3 hours after injury. If evacuation to an MTF is delayed, a second infusion of 1 gm TXA should be administered after Hextend or blood products are administered.

Hemorrhagic Shock

Hemorrhagic shock is a widespread lack of tissue perfusion resulting from blood loss that causes cellular hypoxia, anaerobic metabolism, and decreased cellular energy production. These effects in turn can lead to widespread metabolic dysfunction and death. Hemorrhagic shock is the most common cause of potentially preventable death on the battlefield.[2,51]

The signs classically associated with hemorrhagic (hypovolemic) shock are shown in **Figure 26-20**. However, in austere tactical environments, these signs may be more difficult to appreciate. Combat medical personnel require a fast and reliable clinical indicator of hypovolemic shock. The most useful clinical signs for combat medical personnel to use to identify shock on the battlefield are mental status and radial pulse. The tactically relevant definition of shock is (1) unconsciousness or altered mental status (confused or drowsy) not due to coexisting TBI or drug therapy and/or (2) abnormal (i.e., weak or absent) radial pulse.

Figure 26-20 Classification of Hemorrhagic Shock

	Class I	Class II	Class III	Class IV
Blood loss (ml)	< 750	750–1500	1500–2000	> 2000
Blood loss (% blood volume)	< 15%	15–30%	30–40%	> 40%
Pulse rate	< 100	100–120	120–140	> 140
Blood pressure	Normal	Normal	Decreased	Decreased
Pulse pressure (mm Hg)	Normal or increased	Decreased	Decreased	Decreased
Ventilatory rate	14 to 20	20–30	30–40	> 35
Urine output (ml/hr)	> 30	20–30	5–15	Negligible
CNS/mental status	Slightly anxious	Mildly anxious	Anxious, confused	Confused, lethargic
Fluid replacement	Crystalloid	Crystalloid	Crystalloid and blood	Crystalloid and blood

Source: From American College of Surgeons (ACS) Committee on Trauma. *Advanced Trauma Life Support for Doctors: Student Course Manual.* 8th ed. Chicago, IL: ACS; 2008.

Fluid Resuscitation Strategy in Tactical Settings

Despite its widespread use, the benefit of prehospital fluid resuscitation in trauma patients has not been well established.[7,85–95] ATLS-based civilian trauma courses generally recommend initial fluid resuscitation with 2 liters of a crystalloid solution: either lactated Ringer's or normal saline.

The beneficial effect from crystalloid and colloid fluid resuscitation in hemorrhagic shock has been demonstrated largely in animal models in which the volume of hemorrhage is controlled experimentally and resuscitation is initiated after the hemorrhage has been stopped; these are referred to as "controlled hemorrhage" models.[96,97] Multiple studies using uncontrolled hemorrhagic shock models have found that aggressive fluid resuscitation performed before definitive control of bleeding has been accomplished is associated with either no improvement in survival or increased mortality when compared to no resuscitation or hypotensive resuscitation.[98–104] The vasodilation, increased hydrostatic pressure, and dilution of clotting factors that accompany fluid resuscitation with crystalloids or colloids may interfere with the clotting process at the bleeding site and paradoxically worsen the chance for survival in this setting. However, aggressive fluid resuscitation did improve outcomes for rats with uncontrolled hemorrhagic shock in two studies.[97,105] Both studies used rat tail amputation models, which may not correlate well with uncontrolled hemorrhage on the battlefield from intrathoracic and intra-abdominal injuries. Other studies have noted that fluid resuscitation proved beneficial only after previously uncontrolled hemorrhage was stopped.[106–108]

In studies addressing this issue in trauma patients, one large study of 6,855 trauma casualties found that, although hypotension was associated with a significantly higher mortality rate, the administration of prehospital IV fluids did not reduce this mortality.[102] A retrospective analysis of individuals with ruptured abdominal aortic aneurysms showed a survival rate of 30% for those who were treated with aggressive preoperative colloid fluid replacement, in contrast to a 77% survival rate for those in whom fluid resuscitation was delayed until the time of operative repair.[109] The author of the study strongly recommended that aggressive fluid resuscitation be withheld until after surgical control of the bleeding in patients with this disorder.

Bickell and colleagues published a large, prospective trial that addressed fluid resuscitation in the setting of uncontrolled hemorrhage. The authors studied 598 patients with penetrating torso trauma.[110] They found that aggressive prehospital fluid resuscitation of hypotensive patients with penetrating wounds of the chest and abdomen was associated with a higher mortality rate than that seen in patients for whom aggressive volume replacement was withheld until surgical repair. Further analysis of these data found that this difference was most significant in those casualties with wounds of the chest, with abdominal wounds showing little difference in survival between early and delayed fluid resuscitation.[111] Although confirmation of these findings in other randomized, prospective human studies has not yet been obtained, no human studies were found that demonstrated any definite benefit from large-volume prehospital fluid replacement in casualties with ongoing hemorrhage. Continuing hemorrhage must be suspected in battlefield casualties with penetrating abdominal or thoracic wounds until surgical repair of their injuries has been accomplished.

In light of the studies mentioned above, the recommendation in the original TCCC paper was to withhold aggressive fluid resuscitation from individuals with penetrating torso trauma and uncontrolled hemorrhage.[5] However, at a Special Operations workshop on urban warfare casualties in 1998, there was a clear consensus among the expert panelists that should a casualty with uncontrolled hemorrhage have mental status changes or become unconscious (correlating to systolic blood pressure [SBP] of 50 millimeters of mercury [mm Hg] or less), the casualty should be given enough fluid to resuscitate him or her to the point that mentation improves (correlating to SBP of 70 mm Hg or above). Panel members also stressed the importance of not administering IV fluids in large volumes with the goal of achieving "normal" blood pressure in casualties with penetrating torso wounds, since this could result in disruption of the clot that is hopefully forming at the site of the vascular injury in these casualties.[1]

The combat fluid resuscitation conferences[112] held in 2001 under the sponsorship of the Office of Naval Research and the U.S. Army Medical Research and Materiel Command endorsed the concepts of (1) limited (hypotensive) fluid resuscitation in the setting of uncontrolled hemorrhage and (2) the use of the synthetic colloid Hextend to provide the advantages of lighter weight and smaller volume in the rucksack. Colloids also provide extended intravascular dwell times compared to crystalloids, an important feature when prolonged evacuation times may be involved.

Resuscitation Fluids

Hespan (6% hetastarch in lactated Ringer's) was recommended in the 1996 TCCC paper as a better choice for fluid resuscitation in the Tactical Field Care phase than lactated Ringer's or normal saline.[5] Both lactated Ringer's and normal saline are crystalloids in which the primary osmotically active particle is sodium. Because the sodium ion distributes throughout the entire extracellular fluid compartment, crystalloids move rapidly from the intravascular space to the extravascular space. This shift has significant implications for fluid resuscitation. If a trauma casualty is infused with 1,000 ml of lactated Ringer's, only approximately 200 ml of that volume will remain in the intravascular space 1 hour later.[113–115] This is less of a problem in urban civilian settings because the typical time for transport of the casualty to the hospital in urban trauma systems is less than 15 minutes,[102,116] after which surgical control of hemorrhage can be rapidly achieved and resuscitation with blood products can be accomplished. However, in military settings, where several hours or more may pass before a casualty arrives at an MTF, effective volume resuscitation may be difficult to sustain with crystalloids.

In contrast, the large hetastarch molecule is retained in the intravascular space, and there is no loss of fluid into the interstitium. To the contrary, hetastarch osmotically promotes fluid influx into the vascular space from the interstitium so that an infusion of hetastarch results in an intravascular volume expansion somewhat larger than the volume of fluid infused.[115] This effect is sustained for 8 hours or longer.[117] Although concerns exist about coagulopathies and changes in immune function associated with the use of hetastarch,[118,119] these effects are not seen with infusions of less than 1,500 ml.[120] Hetastarch has been found a safe and effective alternative to lactated Ringer's in resuscitating casualties with controlled hemorrhagic shock.[121,122] Hetastarch

has also been reported to be an acceptable alternative to lactated Ringer's for intraoperative fluid replacement.[123] Hetastarch in saline solution (Hespan) was found in one study to result in increased blood loss compared to the same hetastarch molecule in a balanced electrolyte solution with a lactate buffer and physiologic levels of glucose (Hextend)[124] (**Figure 26-21**).

There are other reasons to prefer hetastarch over crystalloids in tactical settings. Infusion of crystalloids to maintain intravascular volume when surgical control of noncompressible hemorrhage is delayed may result in the need for combat medical personnel to carry large volumes of crystalloid in their rucksacks.[125] This significant burden is tactically undesirable. The expansion of the extravascular fluid space caused by crystalloids may also cause edema and dysfunction in the lungs, the abdomen, the brain, or the muscle compartments of the extremities.[5,125]

The future may provide better options for resuscitation fluids. The Institute of Medicine issued a report in 1999 in which the detrimental immunological effects associated with lactated Ringer's were noted and 7.5% hypertonic saline (HTS) was recommended for initial resuscitation.[126] Many investigators have called for further research to find the optimal resuscitation fluid.[127–141] One promising candidate is hypertonic saline/dextran (HSD). Much of the rationale for recommending HTS was based on human and animal studies that actually studied HSD. The colloid component of this fluid, dextran, may help to increase the intravascular dwell time of the infused HSD volume, in the same way hetastarch does when it is infused in solution. However, HSD is not currently approved by the Food and Drug Administration (FDA) for use in the United States; nor is 7.5% HS. If and when these and additional fluid options become available, the choice of resuscitation fluid in the tactical environment may warrant reconsideration.

Fluid Resuscitation Strategy

How much Hextend solution should be infused to resuscitate a casualty in hemorrhagic shock? Colonel Holcomb[142] proposed a technique of hypotensive fluid resuscitation in the field for casualties in hemorrhagic shock at the 2001 Army/Navy consensus conferences on fluid resuscitation. Whereas the 1996 TCCC guidelines called for Special Operations medics to give 1,000 ml of Hespan to all casualties meeting the requirements for resuscitation, Holcomb proposed that all casualties in shock (defined by

Figure 26-21 Hextend

The Hextend formulation of hetastarch has now been widely used as a front-line resuscitation fluid, and anecdotal reports from combat medical personnel have indicated good and sustained results using hypotensive resuscitation in shock victims.[6]

weak or absent peripheral pulses or altered mental status in the absence of brain injury) be given a 500-ml bolus of Hextend. This should be administered as rapidly as possible using manual pressure on the IV bag or inflatable IV bag cuffs. If no improvement is noted in 30 minutes, the bolus is repeated once. This approach has the following advantages:

1. Better logistics. Not all casualties will require 1,000 ml of Hextend, thus saving fluid and time for other casualties.
2. Decreased rebleeding. Basing the titration of fluids upon a monitored physiologic response may avoid the problem of excessive blood pressure elevation and fatal rebleeding from previously clotted injury sites. The potential for aggressive resuscitation to cause rebleeding at a mean SBP of 94 mm Hg has been demonstrated in animal models of uncontrolled hemorrhage.[143] Interestingly, this recommendation for "hypotensive" resuscitation is reminiscent of similar principles employed in World War II by Beecher.[144]
3. Simplified training. This allows for a single approach to casualties with both controlled and uncontrolled hemorrhage.

Recent Developments in Prehospital Fluid Resuscitation

Recent studies in civilian literature have continued to highlight the uncertain benefits of crystalloids and colloids when used to resuscitate trauma patients prior to blood-component-based therapy.[145-148] The optimal resuscitation of casualties in hemorrhagic shock should be with blood products.[149] Because of the consistent failure of prehospital and emergency department asanguinous fluid administration to show a survival benefit, some trauma systems now initiate definitive resuscitation with plasma and packed red blood cells during transport to the hospital.[145] The British military now uses prehospital blood and plasma on their Medical Emergency Response Team (MERT) evacuation platforms in Afghanistan,[83] and this practice is currently being adopted by U.S. evacuation platforms in Afghanistan. While blood component therapy is not typically available in the Tactical Field Care phase of casualty care, hemostatic resuscitation could be initiated with a dried plasma product. This practice has been recommended by the CoTCCC and the Defense Health Board[150] and is currently being accomplished in Afghanistan by some Special Operations units. This is being done under a treatment protocol, since no FDA-approved dried plasma product is currently available.

Future Research in Fluid Resuscitation

The optimal resuscitation strategy for combat casualties in shock remains a research topic of great importance in battlefield trauma care. Since combat missions do not lend themselves well to the conduct of prospective, randomized, blinded studies on fluid resuscitation, optimal resuscitation strategies will have to be based on the best available evidence from animal studies, evidence found in the civilian prehospital trauma literature, and retrospective studies from combat theaters. Animal models used in studies addressing battlefield fluid resuscitation issues should include a significant delay to surgical repair, simulating the prolonged evacuation times that combat operations often entail.

Care should be taken in extrapolation of the results of resuscitation fluid studies in the civilian sector to the battlefield, since transport times to the hospital in urban areas are usually very short. Additionally, resuscitation studies must address shock in the settings of both controlled and uncontrolled hemorrhage, because of the different physiological considerations in addressing these two clinical conditions. Considering the complexity of this question, definitive studies on fluid resuscitation do not seem imminent, and expert opinion from those knowledgeable in trauma physiology and experienced in trauma care will continue to be critical to defining best practice in combat casualty care.[97,151-153]

Oral Rehydration in Combat Casualties

Trauma surgeons attached to forward-deployed MTFs have noted that many casualties are kept on nothing by mouth (NPO) status for prolonged periods in anticipation of eventual surgery to repair their wounds. With transport delays superimposed on the dehydration often present in combat operations before wounding, these casualties often come to surgery significantly dehydrated. Dehydration adversely affects survival in hypovolemic shock,[1] and the risk of emesis and aspiration was judged to be very low in casualties given only fluids for rehydration.[5] Therefore, oral fluids are recommended for all casualties with a normal state of consciousness and the ability to swallow, including those with penetrating torso trauma **(Figure 26-22)**.

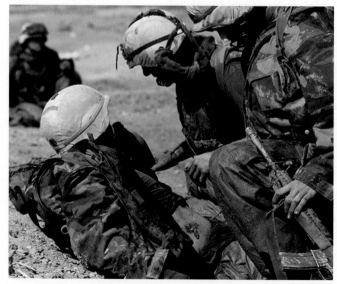

Figure 26-22   Marine with abdominal wound drinking water.
Source: Courtesy of Dr. David Callaway.

Resuscitation of Casualties With Traumatic Brain Injury

The TCCC guidelines call for a modified fluid resuscitation regimen for casualties suffering from both hemorrhagic shock and TBI (**Figure 26-23**). In these casualties, unconsciousness or altered mental status may be caused by either the head injury or the hypovolemic shock. Hypotension in the presence of TBI is associated with a significant increase in mortality.[154] Because of the need to ensure adequate cerebral perfusion pressure, if a casualty with an altered mental status due to suspected TBI has a weak or absent peripheral pulse, resuscitate as necessary to maintain a palpable radial pulse.[155]

Hypothermia and Coagulopathy on the Battlefield

Hypothermia poses a far greater risk to a trauma victim than to an otherwise healthy person. Hypothermia-induced coagulopathy is well described and may occur in a casualty with even mild hypothermia. It results from decreases in platelet function, decreased coagulation cascade enzyme activity, and alterations of the fibrinolytic system.[156,157] Furthermore, the potential for hypothermia in trauma victims is not limited to cold environments; it can occur in warm ambient temperatures as well. Hypovolemic shock results in a decreased ability to produce heat and to maintain normal body temperature. This predisposes shock victims to hypothermia and can contribute to worsening of the hypovolemic state as a result of the ensuing coagulopathy.[158–160]

As many as 66% of civilian trauma patients arrive in emergency departments with core temperatures of less than 36°C (96.8°F), and approximately 80% of casualties who subsequently die from trauma were noted to have a core temperature less than 34°C (93.2°F).[161] In recent years hypothermia has been found to be more prevalent in combat trauma than was previously realized and was found to increase the risk of mortality.[162] Evacuation of a casualty to a medical facility may be delayed for many hours in military settings, increasing the likelihood that hypothermia will complicate trauma management. This problem is exacerbated in helicopter evacuation, in which the casualty is exposed to cooler temperatures at altitude and significant wind chill in an open cabin. The importance of preventing hypothermia in combat casualties was emphasized in a 2006 memo from the Assistant Secretary of Defense for Health Affairs, which noted that body temperature in combat casualties should be maintained as close to 37°C (98.6°F) as possible.[163]

Instituting aggressive steps to prevent hypothermia in casualties is an essential element of care, and simple interventions have proven effective in decreasing the incidence of hypothermia during prolonged evacuations.[164] Because of the physics of heat transfer, it is much easier to prevent hypothermia than to correct it. Therefore, prevention of heat loss should start as soon after wounding as the tactical situation permits. Exposure to the elements should be minimized, and the casualty should be placed on an insulated surface as soon as possible. Protective gear should be kept on or with the casualty, if feasible. After immediately life-threatening issues are addressed, wet clothing should be replaced with dry clothes, if feasible.

The Ready-Heat blanket should be placed on the casualty's chest to provide active warming (**Figure 26-24**), taking care not to place it directly on bare skin to prevent possible burns. The Ready-Heat blanket can provide heating to 40°C (104°F) for up to 8 hours. The casualty should then be wrapped in the Heat-Reflective Shell (HRS). The HRS allows easy access to the casualty for reassessment and possible interventions (e.g., IVs or tourniquets) by means of the Velcro strips down each side. The HRS also utilizes a mummy-like sleeping bag configuration that covers the head, reducing heat loss from the scalp (**Figure 26-25**). Both the Ready-Heat blanket and the HRS are found in the current version of the Hypothermia Prevention and Management Kit (HPMK), which is a commercially available item (**Figure 26-26**). This protective ensemble was shown in U.S. Army Institute of Surgical Research studies to prevent heat loss effectively.[165]

Figure 26-23 Advanced Combat Helmet Padding
An additional note related to TBI: The padding in the Advanced Combat Helmet may become deformed if it is subjected to significant impact force. The helmet padding should be changed as soon as feasible after exposure to significant blunt force.

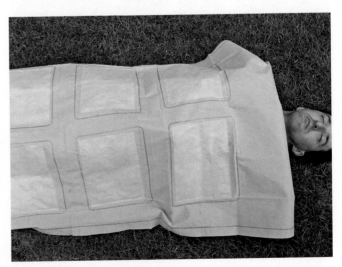

Figure 26-24 Ready-Heat™ blanket.

Source: © Jones and Bartlett Publishers. Ready-Heat Blankets provided courtesy of TechTrade, L.L.C.

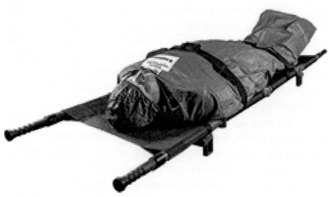

Figure 26-25   Heat Reflective Shell (HRS™)

Source: Courtesy of North American Rescue.

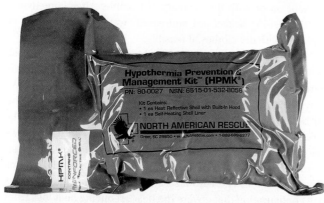

Source: Courtesy of North American Rescue.

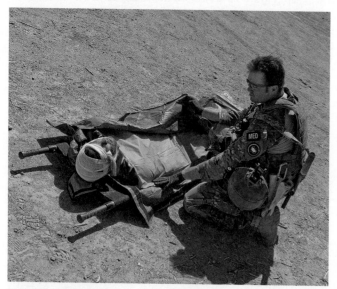

Figure 26-26   Hypothermia Prevention and Management Kit (HPMK).

Source: Courtesy of North American Rescue.

If the HPMK is not available, the previously recommended Blizzard survival blanket/Ready-Heat blanket/Thermo-Lite cap combination can be used, with care taken to prevent helicopter rotor wash from blowing off the cap.[166] If none of these items

is available, then blankets, ponchos, sleeping bags, or other field-expedient materials should be used to keep the casualty warm and dry.

Effective hemorrhage control and fluid resuscitation will help to maintain the casualty's ability to generate heat. Additional measures should be applied as needed throughout Tactical Field Care and Tactical Evacuation Care (**Figure 26-27**), and should be used as far forward in the field as possible. Items 1 to 5 in **Figure 26-27** do not require a power source. Items 6 and 7 are fluid warmers that require power and can deliver heat to the casualty. The items as listed represent a progression of complexity and power requirements that can be used in a layered fashion. Fluid warmers should be considered for any casualty who has hypotension (SBP less than 90 mm Hg), who has received more than 1,000 ml of fluid, or who requires a blood transfusion.

Eye Trauma

When penetrating eye trauma due to shrapnel is suspected, two elements of prehospital care are of paramount importance. The first is to prevent manipulation or additional trauma to the eye that might raise intraocular pressure and result in the expulsion of intraocular contents through the corneal or scleral defect. Protection of the injured eye is best accomplished by taping a rigid shield over the eye. If no rigid eye shield is available, an intact set of protective eyewear may be placed on the casualty and secured in place to protect the eye from further trauma.

Avoid the use of any dressing or bandage that places pressure on a potentially open globe. Pressure dressings are not part of the care of an eye injured in combat and may result in an avoidable permanent loss of vision.

A rapid check of visual acuity should be performed before covering the eye with a shield if the tactical situation permits. A useful field quantification of visual acuity is as follows (from best to worst): (1) can read print, (2) can count the number of fingers

Figure 26-27	**Equipment List for Prevention and Treatment of Hypothermia**

1. TechStyles Thermo-Lite Hypothermia Prevention System Cap
2. Blizzard Survival Blanket, NSN 6532-01-524-6932
3. TechTrade Ready-Heat Blanket, NSN 6532-01-525-4063
4. North American Rescue Heat Reflective Shell
5. North American Rescue Hypothermia Prevention and Management Kit (HPMK), NSN 6515-01-532-8056
6. Thermal Angel, NSN 6515-01-500-3521
7. Belmont FMS 2000, NSN 6515-01-370-5019
8. Bair Hugger, NSN 6530-01-463-6823

held up, (3) can see hand motion, and (4) can see light. Vision should be checked with the other eye closed or covered.

The second important element of care is to prevent the development of posttraumatic **endophthalmitis**, an infection of the anterior and posterior chambers inside the eye. This type of intraocular infection typically has devastating visual results, with only 30% of patients in one study retaining visual acuity greater than or equal to 20/400.[167] *Staphylococcus epidermidis* is the most common pathogen implicated, but *Bacillus cereus* is another very aggressive pathogen often isolated in intraocular infections. The casualty with a penetrating eye injury needs broad spectrum coverage with an antibiotic that has good vitreous penetration. Moxifloxacin 400 milligrams (mg) once a day, given as soon as possible after wounding, is the treatment of choice in the prehospital environment. See **Figures 26-28 – 30** for more information on the field management of penetrating eye injury. The casualty should be evacuated as soon as feasible.

Figure 26-28 Penetrating Eye Injury and Topical Antibiotics

No topical antibiotics (ointments or eye drops) should be used on an unrepaired penetrating injury of the eye.

Figure 26-29 Field Management of Ocular Trauma

These elements of care for eye trauma are consistent with the recommendations in the *Emergency War Surgery Manual* and with the recommendations for managing eye trauma in austere environments found in Dr. Paul Auerbach's textbook, *Wilderness Medicine*, Sixth Edition.[168]

Figure 26-30 Delayed Treatment of Penetrating Eye Injury

In Iraq and Afghanistan, casualties with eye trauma due to intraocular shrapnel or other foreign bodies had no worsening of their visual outcome from delaying the removal of the foreign body for several days as long as aggressive antibiotic therapy was provided, and the penetrating injury to the eye was repaired as soon as possible after the injury was sustained.[169]

Pulse Oximetry

Pulse oximeters are an essential part of the medical kit for combat medical personnel. Although this device has no role during the Care Under Fire phase, pulse oximetry can be a useful tool in the Tactical Field Care and Tactical Evacuation Care phases. Oxygen saturation monitoring should be used in conjunction with other findings from the physical examination to assess for a patent airway and adequate oxygenation. Physical examination is poor at detecting hypoxemia. The presence of central cyanosis—a blue coloration of the tongue and mucous membranes—requires 5 grams per deciliter (g/dl) of desaturated hemoglobin and is an unreliable indicator of hypoxemia, particularly in the presence of hemorrhagic shock. The ability to detect cyanosis is reduced in typical field conditions and is effectively eliminated during night combat operations where the use of white lights is discouraged.

Pulse oximetry should be used for casualties who are unconscious or who have injuries associated with impaired oxygenation (e.g., blast injuries, chest contusion, and penetrating injuries of the chest). It should also be used to monitor casualties with TBI to help ensure that oxygen saturation is maintained at greater than 90%, although supplemental oxygen is typically not available in Tactical Field Care. Hemoglobin oxygen saturation is increasingly considered to be a "fifth vital sign" in trauma care. Combat medical personnel have reported pulse oximetry to be very useful during mass-casualty events.[6]

Casualties exhibiting obvious clinical signs of airway obstruction, tension pneumothorax, or hemorrhage should be managed accordingly, without undue delay to attempt pulse oximetry. When a casualty does have an abnormal pulse oximetry reading, combat medical personnel should reassess the casualty without delay to determine why the reading is abnormal.

Pulse Oximetry Operation

An understanding of the principles of operation involved in pulse oximetry is helpful in understanding the information provided by a pulse oximeter. The goal of pulse oximetry is to measure the ratio of oxygenated hemoglobin to total hemoglobin in arterial blood. This is done by using selected wavelengths of light to determine the oxygen saturation of hemoglobin.[170–176] The light absorption spectrum of oxygenated hemoglobin differs from that of reduced (non-oxygenated) hemoglobin. When two compounds with differing absorption spectra are together in solution, the ratio of their concentrations can be determined from the ratio of the light absorbed at two different wavelengths. From these measurements, the oxygen saturation of arterial blood can be calculated.

An arterial oxygen hemoglobin saturation of 95% or higher indicates that there is an adequate airway and that oxygen is being adequately exchanged in the lungs. Decreases in oxygen saturation may indicate an inadequate airway or pulmonary problems such as a tension pneumothorax, a hemothorax, a sucking chest wound, or a pulmonary contusion. Low hemoglobin oxygen saturations should trigger reassessment of the casualty to

Figure 26-31 Pulse Oximetry and Hypovolemic Shock

Note that good hemoglobin oxygen saturations may be seen in casualties shortly before they go into hypovolemic shock. Pulse oximetry is not useful as an indicator of impending hypovolemic shock.

Figure 26-32 Factors Affecting Readings or Limiting Performance of Pulse Oximeters

Factors Affecting Readings
- Artificially low reading
  - Shock
  - Methemoglobin
  - Cold extremity
- Artificially high reading
  - Carboxyhemoglobin

Factors Limiting Performance
- Inability to obtain or interference with reading
  - Shock
  - Vascular injury
  - Motion artifact
  - Excessive ambient light
  - Skin pigmentation
  - Nail polish or nail coverings
- Pulse oximetry cannot assess:
  - Ventilatory status
  - Oxygen saturations below 83% with same degree of accuracy
- Altitude lowers oxygen saturation in normal individuals as well as casualties unless supplemental oxygen is used.

determine if a lifesaving intervention is indicated (**Figure 26-31**). Identification of low hemoglobin oxygen saturation levels also helps to determine which casualties need urgent evacuation and which casualties will benefit the most from supplemental oxygen if it is available in the Tactical Evacuation Care phase.

Issues With Pulse Oximetry Readings

Pulse oximetry is easily performed, but care must be taken in interpreting the hemoglobin oxygen saturation results displayed by the device. Although pulse oximetry can give accurate estimations of oxygenation, it cannot measure the adequacy of ventilation since it does not measure carbon dioxide in the blood.[177] The absence of an adequate pulse waveform in a casualty in shock makes the readings obtained inaccurate. Poor perfusion is the main cause of failure to obtain a satisfactory signal. **Figure 26-32** lists factors that may affect the readings obtained by pulse oximetry.

Gross movement results in loss of signal, but vibration at frequencies that fall within the possible range of heart rate may lead to erroneous values in pulse oximetry readings. A small (1% to 2%) difference may be seen between a reading taken from a finger and the ear, particularly if the finger is dependent.

Compounds that absorb light at the same wavelengths as oxygenated hemoglobin will result in falsely high readings.[177] The most common and potentially most dangerous of these is **carboxyhemoglobin**, which results from breathing elevated levels of carbon monoxide and causes falsely high saturation readings in a casualty with smoke inhalation or exposure to other sources of carbon monoxide. **Methemoglobin** also interferes with light absorption. Methemoglobinemia may occur in casualties treated with dapsone, primaquine, or other related antimalarials.[179,180] Excessive ambient light may saturate the detector and give erroneous readings.[177] Xenon and infrared lamps are the sources most likely to give problems, but intense daylight as well as fluorescent and incandescent light may also interfere.

Pulse oximetry should not be considered a portable "all-in-one" monitor of oxygenation, pulse rate, rhythm regularity, and overall cardiopulmonary well-being. Overreliance on pulse oximetry may lead to delays in therapy or inappropriate decision making in the field environment. Pulse oximeters, like tourniquets and hemostatic agents, require adequate training to ensure their appropriate use. See **Figures 26-33** and **34** for further considerations pertaining to pulse oximetry.

Figure 26-33 Pulse Oximetry in the Management of TBI

Hypoxemia may worsen outcomes in casualties with moderate/severe TBI. The Brain Trauma Foundation emphasizes the need for all patients with moderate/severe TBI to be monitored with pulse oximetry, and for the arterial hemoglobin oxygen saturation to be maintained at 90% or higher.[178] This recommendation has been added to the TCCC guidelines.[61]

Figure 26-34 Pulse Oximetry During Helicopter Transport

In combat settings, transport of casualties by helicopter is a common cause of decreased hemoglobin oxygen saturation. This decrease is a normal result of the lower partial pressure of oxygen at altitude.

Pain Management in Tactical Settings— Triple Option Analgesia

As in non-combat settings, the preferred analgesic in TCCC depends on the severity of the casualty's pain. Beecher[181] noted in his World War II survey that many men were not in severe pain despite having sustained serious wounds in battle. Obviously, if a casualty's wounds are not significantly painful, no analgesia is required.

Nonsteroidal Anti-inflammatory Drugs

For mild to moderate pain, the preferential cyclooxygenase-2 (COX-2) inhibitor meloxicam (Mobic) is the recommended analgesic. Many analgesics prescribed for mild to moderate pain belong to the NSAID class of medications. Most drugs in this class inhibit platelet function and prolong bleeding time due to their inhibition of cyclooxygenase-1 (COX-1) production.[5,182–184] Analgesic medications that adversely affect platelet function should not be used in a combat setting because platelets are essential to the body's ability to establish hemostasis after a vascular injury.[5] Platelet dysfunction increases the risk of death from hemorrhage in a casualty with significant trauma and bleeding. It is important to note that the adverse effects on clotting ability may persist for a week or more after taking medications such as aspirin or ibuprofen. Medications that decrease platelet function should not be used at all by troops deployed in support of combat operations since these individuals may be called upon to conduct combat missions on very short notice.

Harris and colleagues reported that NSAID use by soldiers at a forward operating base in Afghanistan was prevalent enough to place 75% of the individuals at that base at risk for a self-induced coagulopathy.[185] This is a clear opportunity to improve. Additionally, a recent study noted an increase in mortality in trauma patients taking aspirin.[186] It is important to realize that platelet dysfunction is an important consideration, even for casualties with relatively minor wounds, until they have been evacuated to an MTF or their operating base. The first wounds sustained by a casualty in combat may, unfortunately, not be the last.

Toradol is a medication frequently used in emergency departments for indications such as migraine headaches and severe back pain. Toradol is also an NSAID and inhibits platelet function.[187,188] This medication should be avoided in TCCC and in individuals who may be called upon to conduct combat operations within the next 7 to 10 days.

Meloxicam was chosen as the TCCC NSAID of choice because it is a preferential COX-2 inhibitor and has been documented to spare platelet function.[189,190] It also has an excellent side-effect profile, has proven effective in relieving postoperative pain, and has a 24-hour duration of action.

To augment analgesia and to shorten the time to onset of effect, two tablets of the Tylenol extra-strength formulation of acetaminophen are recommended along with Mobic. This medication provides 8 hours of analgesia through bilayer extended-release caplets. Acetaminophen, like meloxicam, has no adverse effect on platelet function and does not interfere with hemostasis.

In addition to their platelet-sparing qualities, meloxicam and extended-release acetaminophen have the distinct advantage of being nonsedating, which means they do not further impair combat effectiveness. They also avoid the logistical difficulties of controlled medications. Anecdotal experience from casualties in Iraq shows this combination to be very effective in treating pain from minor penetrating soft-tissue injuries.[191,192]

Ideally, these two oral pain medications should be carried by individual combatants as part of a Combat Pill Pack and should be self-administered as soon as feasible after an injury is sustained. This practice should be initiated only after an appropriate program of instruction has been conducted for the unit, and unit personnel have been screened for medication allergies.

Morphine

If the casualty requires more potent pain relief (bone injuries and burns are typically the most painful wounds) and is not in shock or respiratory distress, opioid analgesia should be used. Morphine sulfate remains an excellent choice for analgesia if IV access has been obtained and the casualty is stable from pulmonary and hemodynamic standpoints.[5] The IV route is preferred over the intramuscular (IM) route because of the much more rapid onset of analgesia—several minutes when given IV contrasted to 30 to 60 minutes when given IM.[5] The delayed onset of pain relief makes it difficult to effectively titrate analgesic therapy using IM therapy. The risk of an unintentional overdose of morphine increases if repeated IM injections are given during the time it takes for the initial dose to work.

Oral Transmucosal Fentanyl Citrate

Oral transmucosal fentanyl citrate (OTFC) is recommended when a casualty has severe pain but does not have IV access established. This is a valuable option for combat medical personnel in that starting an IV (1) requires significant time, which is always an important consideration in a time-intensive tactical setting; (2) is a perishable skill that may be difficult to perform for combat medics who do not do it routinely; and (3) is exceedingly difficult to perform at night, even when night vision devices are used.[193]

The use of OTFC was introduced and recommended for battlefield application independently and simultaneously by Colonels Russ Kotwal (the 75th Ranger Regiment Surgeon) and Colonel Kevin O'Connor (the Army Special Missions Unit Surgeon) in 2002. These authors published a retrospective case series documenting that OTFC can provide an alternate means of delivering safe, effective, rapid-onset, and noninvasive pain management in a prehospital combat or austere environment.[191]

Management of the pain of acute combat trauma with OTFC is an off-label use of this medication. An FDA "Black Box" safety warning states that the medication is intended only for cancer patients who are narcotic-tolerant and have breakthrough pain. OTFC has, however, been reported safe and effective for a variety of indications other than breakthrough cancer pain.[194–200] It has also been recommended as a good choice for analgesia in the wilderness environment.[201]

Fentanyl provides effects ranging from analgesia at blood levels of 1 to 2 nanograms per milliliter (ng/ml), to surgical anesthesia and profound respiratory depression at levels of 10 to 20 ng/ml. The maximum serum concentration achieved following a 1,600 microgram (mcg) dose of OTFC was 2.51 ng/ml in clinical efficacy trials.[202] Respiratory depression is reported to occur at serum levels above 2 ng/ml, corresponding to doses greater than 800 mcg. However, an 800-mcg dose of OTFC was found to produce no respiratory depression, even in volunteers with no pain stimulus.[203] Additionally, casualties suffering from combat trauma with severe pain have been noted to tolerate large doses of narcotics without respiratory depression because of the pain's powerful stimulant effect, as long as there is no associated shock.[1]

In a review of the analgesic options available to combat medical personnel in the prehospital battlefield setting, Colonel Ian Wedmore, the Army Surgeon General's Consultant for Emergency Medicine, and his colleagues[192] noted that OTFC "appears to be ideal for administering safe, rapid-onset, oral opiate analgesia in the prehospital austere setting." Kacprowicz and colleagues found that OTFC was "uniquely suited for the management of pain in the combat setting."[204] Over 280 uses of this medication by U.S. combat forces in Iraq and Afghanistan have been documented, and results to date indicate that this medication is safe and effective for use in relieving the pain of combat trauma when used appropriately.[205]

Given the documented safety and efficacy of OTFC in combat trauma, the CoTCCC recommends OTFC for use in casualties who are not in shock or experiencing respiratory distress or judged to be at significant risk for either of those two conditions. The dosage is 800 mcg transbuccally as an initial analgesic dose for any hemodynamically stable casualty who does not otherwise require IV access. As an added safety measure, the simple act of taping the "lozenge-on-a-stick" preparation to the casualty's finger is recommended. Should the casualty inadvertently absorb a dose significant enough to exceed the desired analgesic effect, the resulting somnolence will cause relaxation of the supporting arm. As the arm relaxes, the fentanyl lozenge will be pulled from the casualty's mouth, preventing further absorption.

Most of the experience to date with OTFC on the battlefield has been with the Actiq brand. Other formulations of this medication may have different clinical effects for similar dosages based on variations in bioavailability.

Naloxone

The presence of hemorrhagic shock is a contraindication to opioid analgesics—including both morphine and fentanyl—because of their cardiorespiratory depressant effect. Naloxone must be readily available whenever any narcotic is administered.

Individuals who have received opiates often experience nausea and vomiting, so promethazine (Phenergan), 25 mg, should be given IV or IM as needed to minimize this side effect. Should Phenergan be unavailable or not tolerated by the casualty, ondansetron (Zofran), 4 mg, may be considered as an alternative.

Ketamine

Ketamine is another option for battlefield analgesia[206] (**Figure 26-35**). This agent may be useful in two specific battlefield settings. The first is when the analgesia provided by morphine and/or fentanyl is not adequate and additional analgesic effect is desired. The second is when the casualty is in respiratory distress or hemorrhagic shock.

Ketamine offers prehospital providers the ability to relieve pain without the potential adverse effects of opioids. Opioids should also be administered with caution in casualties who have a high risk of going into shock (e.g., casualties with severe DCBI, penetrating wounds of the chest or abdomen, or pelvic fractures). Hemorrhage is the most common cause of preventable death in the Iraq and Afghanistan conflicts,[51,207] and OTFC or morphine may potentiate hypovolemic shock, which could increase the risk of death in casualties with severe hemorrhage.[206] The hypoxia and hypotension that may be associated with opioid use may also worsen outcomes in TBI.[206] Sedation and nausea are also known side effects of opioids with significant implications for battlefield trauma care.[208]

Because ketamine is highly lipid-soluble, its clinical effects appear within 1 minute of administration when given

Figure 26-35 Battlefield Experience with Ketamine

Respondents in a survey of combat medical personnel conducted by the Naval Operational Medical Lessons Learned Center[219] indicated that IM morphine is the most commonly used battlefield analgesic but rated it less effective than either IV morphine or ketamine. The predominance of IM morphine results mainly from the fact that few combat units other than Special Operations forces have provided OTFC or ketamine to their combat medical personnel. Though ketamine has been used less frequently than morphine and OTFC, it was rated more effective at providing rapid and potent pain relief.[206] Additionally, anecdotal reports in operational settings describe individuals with severe pain refractory to morphine who responded quickly to administration of ketamine.[192]

IV, and within 5 minutes when given IM.[209] It has been used extensively in acute care medicine and has a low frequency of serious adverse effects in doses used for analgesia.[209–213] Ketamine is known for its advantageous effects on hemodynamic stability, airway maintenance, and respiration in comparison to opioids, as well as for its low cost, broad range of clinical applications, ease of storage, and excellent therapeutic index.[214,215] When administered to combat casualties in smaller (analgesic) doses, ketamine does not usually impair airway patency or respiration, and it does not worsen hemorrhagic shock, the leading cause of potentially preventable death on the battlefield.[51,216–218] As the dose-related effect of ketamine transitions from analgesia to anesthesia, **nystagmus** emerges as a side effect of ketamine. The appearance of nystagmus, or the relief of the casualty's pain, should be the end point indicators for ketamine dosage.[206]

Ketamine has been recommended for use on the battlefield by the *Military Advanced Regional Anesthesia and Analgesia Handbook*, the U.S. Special Operations Command Tactical Trauma Protocols, the Army Ranger Medic Protocols, and the *Pararescue Medication and Procedure Handbook*. Recent evidence suggests that low-dose ketamine may also serve as an effective adjunct to opioids and other analgesic agents.[217,220,221]

Ketamine may be administered via intranasal, IM, IO, and IV routes. Intramuscularly, ketamine should be given at a dose of 50 mg, and the dose may be repeated every 30 minutes to 1 hour as necessary to control severe pain or until the casualty develops nystagmus. Ketamine may also be given intranasally at a dose of 50 mg using a nasal atomizer. This dose, too, may be repeated every 30 minutes to 1 hour as necessary to control severe pain or until the casualty develops nystagmus. If IV or IO access has been obtained, ketamine may be given as a 20-mg slow IV/IO push over 1 minute. The casualty should be reassessed in 5 to 10 minutes and repeat IV doses given every 5 to 10 minutes as necessary to control severe pain or, again, until nystagmus appears.

Any casualty receiving ketamine should be monitored for signs of respiratory difficulty or agitation. Ketamine has been reported to cause increased intracranial and intraocular pressure, but the risk of these adverse effects is low and eye injury and mild TBI should not preclude ketamine use in casualties who have moderate to severe pain and in whom opioid use is contraindicated. At higher (anesthetic) doses, the utility of ketamine is limited by undesirable psychomimetic effects (e.g., excessive sedation, cognitive dysfunction, hallucinations and nightmares), but lower doses, like those recommended above, have rarely been associated with adverse effects.[221] In a review of analgesic options for pain relief on the battlefield, Black and McManus[222] extolled the analgesic properties of ketamine administered in doses small enough to avoid anesthesia. They noted that ketamine in these doses produces strong pain relief with a large safety margin. Ketamine may also potentiate the analgesic effects of opioids like morphine and fentanyl, and can help prevent the hyperalgesia sometimes associated with opioid therapy.

In a case series of 13 patients given prehospital ketamine for chemical restraint, Burnett[223] reported a significant incidence of adverse effects, but the mean dose of ketamine administered was much larger than the analgesic dose recommended in TCCC (8 of 13 patients received 500 mg IM in contrast to the 50 mg IM dose recommended here), and all side effects were successfully managed. The authors pointed out that in their EMS system, ketamine is the prehospital drug of choice for chemical restraint in patients with excited delirium syndrome.

Laryngospasm is an infrequently reported side effect of ketamine. If this problem occurs, a brief period of ventilation with a bag-mask will typically resolve it.[223] The frequency of respiratory compromise following procedural sedation and analgesia with ketamine was lower in pediatric patients than with other analgesics, including fentanyl.[224] Anecdotal reports suggest that given the larger diameter of the adult airway, simple airway repositioning is sufficient to relieve airway compromise following ketamine administration.[206]

While the desirable clinical features of ketamine administration (e.g., preservation of spontaneous respiration) are numerous, combat medical personnel must be prepared to deal with its potential side effects.[206] For example, one of the best-known side effects following ketamine administration, is emergence reactions: Patients may make spontaneous utterances and purposeless motions or exhibit agitation. The FDA-approved package insert includes a special note stating that emergence reactions occur in approximately 12% of patients.[225] Although emergence reactions generally occur when higher doses of ketamine than those recommended in this text are used (i.e., anesthetic doses rather than analgesic doses), their management may require active restraint.[226]

In a polytrauma IED blast casualty (i.e., one who may have TBI, a penetrating eye injury, both compressible and noncompressible hemorrhage, and pulmonary injury) with severe pain and contraindications to both opiates and ketamine, which analgesic should be chosen? There are two key points that should be considered in this situation: (1) If the TBI is significant, the casualty is likely to be unconscious and not in need of pain medications. (2) If the casualty is conscious and in pain despite the TBI, ketamine is a better choice than OTFC or morphine. The evidence is currently stronger that opioids (with their attendant side effects of hypotension and hypoxia) are more likely to produce bad outcomes in individuals suffering from both TBI and shock than is ketamine.

Antibiotics

Infections are an important cause of late morbidity and mortality in combat trauma. The need for early administration of antibiotics was recognized over 50 years ago, when Poole[227] observed that:

> . . . the greatest lesson learned from World War II may have been the benefit of the use of penicillin prophylactically in the surgical units closest to the front.

Scott[228] commented after the Korean War:

> In any tactical situation where the casualty cannot reach the aid station until 4 or 5 hours or longer after wounding, antibiotic therapy by the aidman in the field is most desirable.

Early antibiotics are commonly used upon arrival at the emergency department in the treatment of patients with significant trauma. Antibiotics are not used in most civilian prehospital emergency medical systems because of the very short transport times typically encountered in the urban environment. However, definitive care for casualties may be significantly delayed in combat settings due to the longer distances to be covered and tactical constraints on evacuation helicopters and vehicles.[229]

Battlefield antibiotics for combat casualties were proposed in the original TCCC guidelines.[5] Antibiotics must be given as soon as possible after injury to maximize their ability to prevent wound infections. Intramuscular benzylpenicillin started within 1 hour of wounding was found to be effective in preventing streptococcal infections in a swine model of wound infection. If administration was delayed until 6 hours after wounding, however, the medication was not effective.[230] A review of antibiotic use on the battlefield recommended that antibiotics be used if arrival at an MTF was anticipated to be 3 hours or more.[231] However, no evidence was cited in this review to document the efficacy of antibiotics administered beyond the 1-hour period in preventing wound infections.

The importance of early antibiotics has been noted in several reports discussing the battlefield management of combat casualties. Lieutenant Colonel Bob Mabry, a former Special Forces medic and now an emergency medicine physician and Director of the Army EMS Fellowship Program, and his colleagues[32] noted a 15-hour delay before treatment at a forward surgical facility for most of the casualties wounded in the battle of Mogadishu in 1993. The wound infection rate in those casualties was approximately 30%. In contrast, Captain Mike Tarpey, a task force surgeon,[232] reported no infections in the 32 casualties from Task Force 1-15 (Third Infantry Division), which was involved in the drive to Baghdad at the start of the war in Iraq. Early antibiotics were administered on the battlefield and the reported negligible rate of infections was achieved despite casualty evacuation often being delayed on this operation. There were no reports of adverse effects from the use of battlefield antibiotics documented in a 2007 review of TCCC as used on the battlefields of the Global War on Terrorism.[6]

Parenteral (IV or IM) administration of antibiotics is required in casualties who are unconscious or who cannot take medications by mouth due to maxillofacial injuries. It is also required for casualties in shock, in whom the gastrointestinal tract blood flow may be inadequate for absorption of oral medications. Cefotetan was recommended previously because of its broad spectrum of coverage and its 12-hour duration of action. Ertapenem (Invanz) was recommended subsequently by Hospenthal and colleagues as another good antibiotic option because of its once-a-day dosing, excellent coverage, and good safety profile.[231] This recommendation was also endorsed in a more recent review of this topic.[233] Ertapenem should not be mixed or co-infused with other medications because of the potential for crystallization and should not be mixed with diluents containing dextrose (alpha-D-glucose). It may be administered IM if needed.

The logistical burden of carrying, reconstituting, and injecting parenteral medications makes the use of oral antibiotics an attractive alternative when oral administration is possible.[1] In choosing a single antibiotic agent to be the primary oral antibiotic for combat casualties, characteristics such as broad spectrum coverage, minimal side effects, environmental stability, simple and infrequent dosage regimens, and comparatively low cost are all highly desirable. In 2002, O'Connor and Butler proposed the fourth-generation fluoroquinolones gatifloxacin and moxifloxacin as good choices for oral battlefield antibiotics.[229] Gatifloxacin was selected initially based on its lower cost to the military at the time compared to moxifloxacin. Gatifloxacin was later reported to cause disorders of glucose metabolism,[234] so the CoTCCC recommended moxifloxacin as the best replacement oral antibiotic. This choice was endorsed by Hospenthal and his colleagues in 2011.[233]

It is important that the medical leadership in combat units screen their troops for medication allergies when providing their units with prepackaged Combat Pill Packs. For an individual who should not take moxifloxacin or ertapenem, consultation with the unit physician regarding appropriate substitutions is indicated. The unit corpsman, medic, or pararescueman should likewise be aware of any allergies that unit members may have to other medications recommended by the TCCC guidelines.

Casualty Movement

Tactical drag techniques designed to move the casualty to the first point of cover as quickly as possible are described in the Care Under Fire chapter. Because the tactical situation is more controlled in the Tactical Field Care phase, further movement of casualties on the battlefield may be accomplished more easily in this phase The casualty can be disarmed, if indicated, and mission-essential gear distributed to other team members.

If the unit has access to tactical litters, they may be employed at this time. Some of the commonly used tactical litters include the Talon II, the Israeli, the Skedco, and Stokes-type litters. Note that if the casualty will need to be hoisted into a helicopter in the litter, then the litter must be rigid. Either the Skedco or the Stokes basket is better for rough terrain, building interiors, or areas in which the litter must be raised or lowered more than 3 meters (10 feet). These litters can be dragged by two rescuers, if necessary (**Figure 26-36**), rather than carried by four. Folding litters or body bags are other options. The standard Army litter has no good way to restrain the casualty and is difficult to use during movement over rough terrain. The Talon II litter (**Figure 26-37**) has found acceptance in many units, especially in the new vehicle-based lifesaving kits.

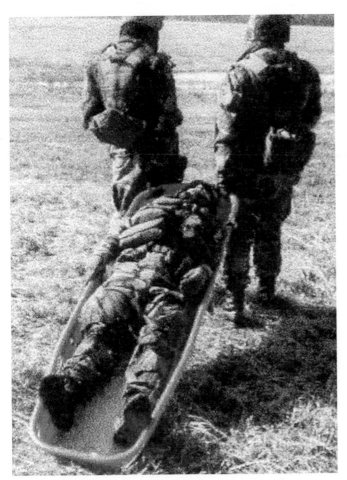

Figure 26-36 Stokes basket drag.

Source: Courtesy of Dr. Mel Otten.

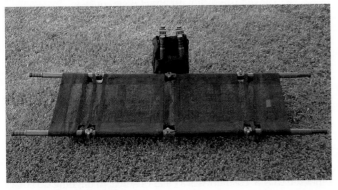

Figure 26-37 Talon II® litter.

Source: Courtesy of Mr. Dom Greydanus.

An improvised litter can be made from a poncho, poncho liner, blanket, field jacket, door, or other field-expedient materials. If the casualty is a victim of blunt trauma and spinal injury is suspected, a rigid litter that provides adequate support to help protect the spinal cord from sustaining secondary injury should be used, if possible. A cervical collar can be improvised from a SAM splint or other material and applied to the casualty before moving. When moving casualties over long distances,

tourniquets, dressings, splints, and IV lines should be checked periodically to ensure they are intact and functioning. Casualties should be protected as much as possible from the elements (e.g., sun, rain, wind, cold, snow, blowing sand, insects) during transport and observed for signs of hypothermia, dehydration, and heat illness.

If no litter is available, the tactical drags and carries described previously in the Care Under Fire phase may be used in Tactical Field Care.

Communicating With the Casualty

Being wounded may generate significant anxiety and fear in the casualty. Talking frankly with the casualty about his or her injuries and offering reassurance by describing the treatments being rendered and emphasizing that everything possible is being done on the casualty's behalf and that he or she will be well cared for will help to counter the casualty's anxiety. This type of communication is just as important on the battlefield as in the MTF and should be a part of the treatment regimen. Be honest about the injuries sustained, but maintain a positive attitude about rescue and treatment.

Cardiopulmonary Resuscitation in Tactical Settings

Cardiopulmonary resuscitation (CPR) was developed to attempt to maintain some level of perfusion and oxygenation in cardiac arrest victims until defibrillation and Advanced Cardiac Life Support measures could be employed. Although CPR may be useful in cardiac patients who have intact anatomy, it will not be successful and is not appropriate for combat casualties still on the battlefield who have sustained trauma severe enough to cause loss of pulse, respirations, and other signs of life.[5,235] Prehospital resuscitation of trauma victims in cardiac arrest is an exercise in futility, even in urban settings where the casualty is close to a trauma center. Branney and colleagues[236] reported only a 2% survival rate (14 of 708) among casualties who underwent thoracotomy after arriving at a hospital emergency department with absent vital signs. Rosemurgy and coauthors reported no survivors in 138 trauma casualties who sustained a prehospital cardiac arrest and for whom CPR was attempted.[237] The authors of that study recommended that CPR for trauma patients in cardiopulmonary arrest not be attempted, even in the civilian prehospital setting, because of the large economic costs and the uniformly unsuccessful results.

Even in individuals with nontraumatic cardiac arrest (i.e., those who have had a sudden cardiac death with no injuries), survival declines rapidly if spontaneous circulation is not promptly restored. Only 2% to 10% of patients with out-of-hospital cardiopulmonary arrest survive to hospital discharge. The chance of survival declines by 10% for every minute that defibrillation is delayed and there is no spontaneous circulation.[238] Even an 8-minute window for defibrillation may be too long.[239] These data are bleak for individuals with cardiac arrest on the battlefield, where early defibrillation cannot be accomplished and where blood loss and severe injuries to vital organs make restoration of spontaneous circulation far more difficult to achieve than in nontraumatic cardiac arrest.

In a battlefield setting, the cost of attempting CPR in casualties with inevitably fatal wounds will be measured in additional lives lost as combat medical personnel are exposed to hostile fire while performing CPR, and care is withheld from casualties with potentially survivable wounds. Successful completion of the unit's mission may also be unnecessarily jeopardized by these efforts. CPR should be considered in the tactical prehospital setting only in the case of selected disorders (such as hypothermia, near-drowning, or electrocution) that have a higher likelihood of responding to CPR than do combat-related injuries such as hemorrhagic shock or severe head trauma resulting in prehospital cardiopulmonary arrest.

Unrecognized tension pneumothorax is one potentially reversible cause of cardiopulmonary arrest in combat casualties. Casualties with torso trauma or polytrauma who have no pulse or respirations during Tactical Field Care should have bilateral needle decompression performed to ensure they do not have a tension pneumothorax prior to discontinuation of care.

Calling for Tactical Evacuation (TACEVAC)

Combat medical personnel caring for a casualty in Tactical Field Care must consider the degree of urgency for the casualty to reach an MTF. The current practice in the Afghanistan theater of operations when requesting evacuation is to categorize casualties using International Security Assistance Force Standard Operating Procedure 312, which follows North Atlantic Treaty Organization (NATO) doctrine. In this classification system, there are three categories:

- A—Urgent. Evacuation within 2 hours (**Figure 26-38**)
- B—Priority. Evacuation within 4 hours
- C—Routine. Evacuation within 24 hours

Figure 26-38   Directed Limit on Evacuation Time for CAT A Casualties

Note that by Secretary of Defense directive, all casualties categorized as CAT A in the Afghanistan theater of operations should be able to be evacuated to an MTF with a surgical capability within 60 minutes from the time that the evacuation mission is approved.

The following lists are offered as suggestions for how different injury patterns should be classified under this system. Note that these are examples only and the evacuation category may need modification based upon the corpsman's, medic's, or PJ's assessment of a particular casualty.

- CAT A—Urgent (Critical, Life-Threatening Injury)
  - Significant injuries from a dismounted IED attack
  - Gunshot wound or penetrating shrapnel to chest, abdomen, or pelvis
  - Any casualty with ongoing airway difficulty
  - Any casualty with ongoing respiratory difficulty
  - Unconscious casualty
  - Casualty with known or suspected spinal injury
  - Casualty in shock
  - Casualty with bleeding that is difficult to control
  - Moderate/severe TBI
  - Burns greater than 20% of total body surface area (TBSA)
- CAT B—Priority (Serious Injury)
  - Isolated, open extremity fracture with bleeding controlled
  - Any casualty with a tourniquet in place
  - Penetrating or other serious eye injury
  - Significant soft-tissue injury without major bleeding
  - Extremity injury with absent distal pulses
  - Burns over 10% to 20% of TBSA
- CAT C—Routine (Mild to Moderate Injury)
  - Concussion (mild TBI)
  - Gunshot wound to an extremity with bleeding controlled without a tourniquet
  - Minor soft-tissue shrapnel injury
  - Closed fracture with intact distal pulses
  - Burns over less than 10% of TBSA

Documenting Tactical Combat Casualty Care

As of this writing, 87% of combat fatalities occur in the prehospital phase of combat casualty care,[51] but only 14% of casualties have prehospital care documented upon arrival at a Role 2 or 3 facility. The lack of adequate documentation of prehospital care rendered to U.S. casualties is a clear obstacle to ongoing CoTCCC and Joint Trauma System efforts to improve that care. This continues to be a requirement gap across the services.[74]

In 2007, a CoTCCC working group was convened to address the lack of prehospital care documentation in the conflicts in Iraq and Afghanistan. At that time, there were over 30,000 casualties from these conflicts, but less than 10% of those casualties' records had any documentation of the care that was provided before the casualty reached an MTF. Unit-level reporting formats were used in almost all cases of successful documentation. It was noted at the conference that, in many instances, those initially providing care were not medical personnel. Documentation of care provided by nonmedical personnel required a format that they could understand and use effectively. Three possible choices for battlefield trauma care documentation were reviewed at the conference. One was the Department of Defense (DoD) paper form 1380, which was most commonly used at the time. Another was the Battlefield Medical Information System—Tactical (BMIS-T)—a personal digital assistant (PDA)-based software program. Neither of these was felt to be the optimal solution for documenting trauma care on the battlefield.

The third option was a casualty card used by the 75th Ranger Regiment. This card was recognized by the working group as an immediate, cost-effective, and easily fielded interim solution. It was developed largely by Ranger medics, had proven easy to use, and was very well accepted by the Rangers and by other Special Operations groups. Using this card, the Regiment had effectively documented the prehospital care provided to almost all of the approximately 450 battle injury and non-battle injury casualties they had sustained in Iraq and Afghanistan at the time of the conference. The data collected were used to create the Ranger Prehospital Trauma Registry, the single best unit-based trauma registry to emerge from these conflicts. This registry, in turn, eventually enabled the most comprehensive study on prehospital care rendered within a combat unit in these two theaters.[240] The Ranger casualty card was recommended by conference attendees, and subsequently endorsed by the CoTCCC, as the preferred method for documenting TCCC on the battlefield.

This "TCCC Casualty Card" was later endorsed by the Defense Health Board[241] and adopted as the standard format for documenting prehospital care by the Department of the Army. The governing Army regulation (AR 40-66 Medical Record Administration and Healthcare Documentation) was amended to permit the TCCC Casualty Card (as DA Form 7656) to become a part of a health record without a medical officer's signature, as required for the old DD 1380 Field Medical Card.

However, the other services did not follow the Army's lead. Consequently, there remained a need for a form acceptable to and used by *all* the services. The Defense Medical Materiel Program Office (DMMPO) noted this need and initiated an effort to develop a single form approved for use across the DoD. That initiative resulted in an updated version of the TCCC Casualty Card developed in 2013 as a joint effort of the CoTCCC, the DMMPO, and the Joint Trauma System.

The 2013 TCCC Casualty Card (**Figure 26-39**) maintains the simple format of the previous TCCC Casualty Card but incorporates a number of modifications that will allow better documentation of prehospital care:

- Includes the casualty Battle Roster Number (to link to the DoD Trauma Registry)
- Better defines the mechanism of injury

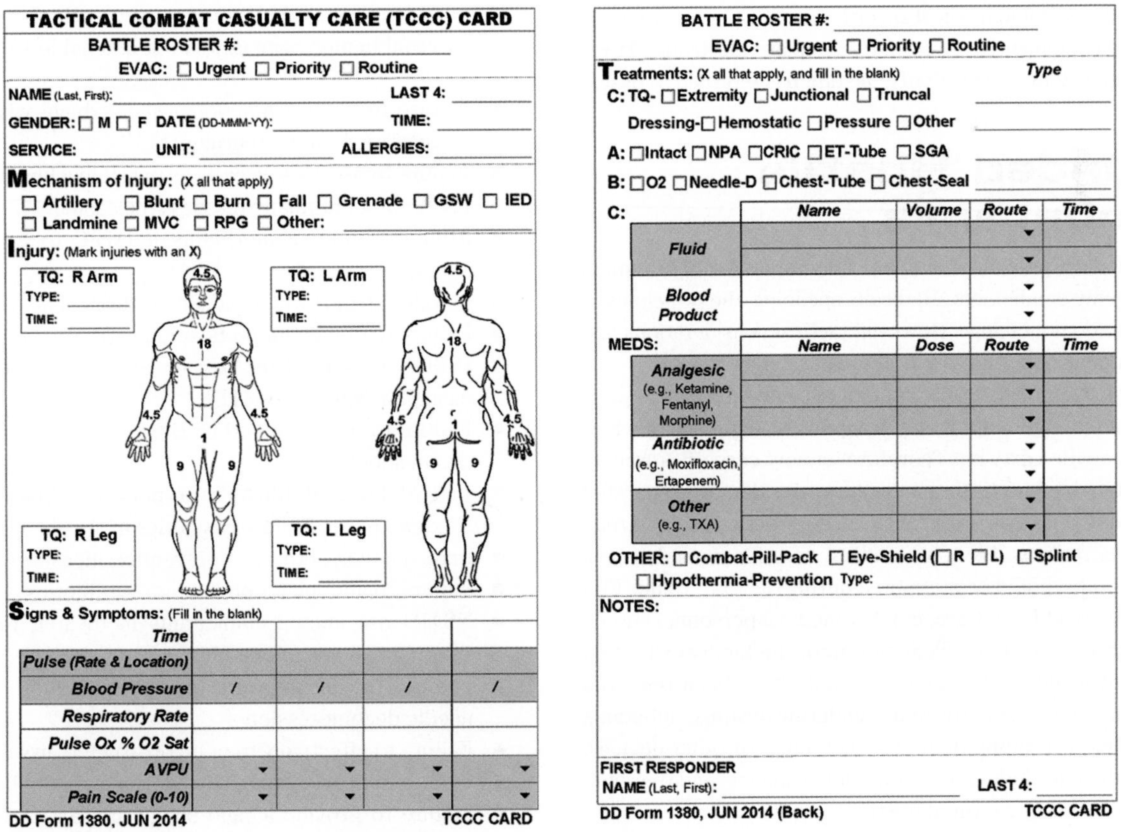

TACTICAL COMBAT CASUALTY CARE (TCCC) CARD

BATTLE ROSTER #: ____
EVAC: ☐ Urgent ☐ Priority ☐ Routine

NAME (Last, First): ____ LAST 4: ____
GENDER: ☐ M ☐ F DATE (DD-MMM-YY): ____ TIME: ____
SERVICE: ____ UNIT: ____ ALLERGIES: ____

Mechanism of Injury: (X all that apply)
☐ Artillery ☐ Blunt ☐ Burn ☐ Fall ☐ Grenade ☐ GSW ☐ IED
☐ Landmine ☐ MVC ☐ RPG ☐ Other: ____

Injury: (Mark injuries with an X)

TQ: R Arm TYPE: ____ TIME: ____
TQ: L Arm TYPE: ____ TIME: ____
TQ: R Leg TYPE: ____ TIME: ____
TQ: L Leg TYPE: ____ TIME: ____

Signs & Symptoms: (Fill in the blank)

Time				
Pulse (Rate & Location)				
Blood Pressure	/	/	/	/
Respiratory Rate				
Pulse Ox % O2 Sat				
AVPU				
Pain Scale (0-10)				

DD Form 1380, JUN 2014 TCCC CARD

BATTLE ROSTER #: ____
EVAC: ☐ Urgent ☐ Priority ☐ Routine

Treatments: (X all that apply, and fill in the blank) Type
C: TQ- ☐ Extremity ☐ Junctional ☐ Truncal ____
Dressing-☐ Hemostatic ☐ Pressure ☐ Other ____
A: ☐ Intact ☐ NPA ☐ CRIC ☐ ET-Tube ☐ SGA ____
B: ☐ O2 ☐ Needle-D ☐ Chest-Tube ☐ Chest-Seal ____

C:	Name	Volume	Route	Time
Fluid				
Fluid				
Blood Product				
Blood Product				

MEDS:	Name	Dose	Route	Time
Analgesic (e.g., Ketamine, Fentanyl, Morphine)				
Analgesic				
Analgesic				
Antibiotic (e.g., Moxifloxacin, Ertapenem)				
Antibiotic				
Other (e.g., TXA)				
Other				

OTHER: ☐ Combat-Pill-Pack ☐ Eye-Shield (☐ R ☐ L) ☐ Splint
☐ Hypothermia-Prevention Type: ____

NOTES:

FIRST RESPONDER
NAME (Last, First): ____ LAST 4: ____

DD Form 1380, JUN 2014 (Back) TCCC CARD

Figure 26-39 2013 TCCC Casualty Card.

Source: Courtesy of USAISR

- Provides improved documentation of tourniquet use
- Adds a section to record the use of junctional tourniquets
- Incorporates a section to document the use of prehospital plasma and blood
- Provides for documentation of the hemoglobin oxygen saturation level
- Adds a section for documentation of the casualty's pain level
- Incorporates a section for supraglottic airway use
- Provides a space for documenting the type of supraglottic airway
- Provides a space for documenting the type of chest seal
- Adds ketamine in the analgesic section
- Incorporates a section for the use of TXA
- Provides a space for documentation of an eye shield
- Provides a space for documentation of Combat Pill Pack usage
- Provides a space for documentation of hypothermia prevention equipment

The TCCC Casualty Card should be completed by the responder who provides the initial point of injury care for each casualty and by all subsequent combat medical personnel. It should be attached to the casualty during the evacuation process. Once the casualty reaches a Level III care facility, the TCCC card should be transcribed by the hospital's patient administration department into the prescribed format to initiate the casualty's longitudinal electronic medical record. The TCCC Casualty Card should be supplemented by a more complete electronic TCCC Casualty After Action Report once the unit has returned to base.

Wounded Hostile Combatants

Combat medical personnel may be called upon to render initial care for enemy combatants. Medically speaking, the principles of trauma care do not change. However, tactical considerations add an extra dimension to the care of these casualties.

Though wounded, enemy personnel may still act as hostile combatants and employ any weapons or explosive devices that they may be carrying. Therefore, enemy casualties remain hostile combatants until they indicate surrender, are separated from all weapons, and are proven to no longer pose a threat. For obvious reasons, then, no medical care for wounded hostile combatants should be attempted during the Care Under Fire phase. In Tactical Field Care, combat medical personnel should not attempt to provide medical care until the tactical situation permits and wounded hostile combatants have been rendered safe by other members of the unit. Rendering hostile combatants safe includes restraining them with flex cuffs or other devices, searching them for hidden weapons and ordnance, and segregating them from other captured hostile combatants.

Once combat medical personnel are sure wounded hostile combatants have been rendered safe, medical care should be provided in accordance with Tactical Field Care guidelines for

U.S. forces. Thereafter, the wounded hostiles should be safeguarded from further injury and sped to the rear as medically and tactically feasible.

Opportunities to Improve

A number of important papers have come out documenting potentially preventable deaths among U.S. combat casualties and offering the opportunity to reinforce training on those interventions that can avoid preventable death.[27,51,207] Additionally, aspects of care that need to be modified or reinforced to ensure optimal combat casualty care are at times identified during weekly trauma teleconferences conducted by the Joint Trauma System.

Recurring issues identified in published studies or in the Joint Trauma System trauma teleconferences that should be emphasized during TCCC training include:

- Failure to control extremity bleeding with a tourniquet
    - Initial tourniquet not adequately tightened
    - No second tourniquet used if indicated
    - No reassessment of the casualty to ensure hemorrhage remains controlled
- Failure to reassess the need for the tourniquet in Tactical Field Care and to attempt to transition to other means of hemorrhage control if the evacuation time is anticipated to be longer than 2 hours
- Failure to use Combat Gauze promptly for significant external hemorrhage that is not amenable to tourniquet use
- Failure to control junctional hemorrhage with Combat Gauze or junctional tourniquets
- Failure to use TXA as early as possible when indicated
- Failure to continually reassess the casualty
- Administration of morphine or OTFC to casualties in shock
- Inability to perform an adequate surgical airway
- Failure to document prehospital care
- Failure to administer oxygen as soon as possible for casualties with severe TBI
- Failure to initiate blood or Hextend therapy for casualties in shock
- Use of lactated Ringer's or normal saline instead of Hextend to resuscitate casualties in shock
- Inadequate hypothermia prevention measures
- Failure to administer prehospital antibiotics
- NSAID use among combatants in theater, resulting in self-induced coagulopathies
- Failure to decompress tension pneumothorax with needle decompression
- Failure to effectively treat an obstructed airway
- Failure to provide adequate analgesia on the battlefield
- Failure to provide a rigid shield and antibiotic for eye injuries
- Use of ocular pressure dressings in casualties with possible penetrating eye injuries

Summary

- Armed combatants with altered mental status should be disarmed immediately.
- Unconscious casualties should have their airways opened initially with the chin-lift or jaw-thrust maneuver.
- Use a nasopharyngeal airway for unconscious patients with spontaneous ventilations and no airway obstruction. It is better tolerated than an oropharyngeal airway if consciousness is regained, and it is less likely to be dislodged.
- Place unconscious casualties in the semi-prone recovery position to help prevent aspiration of stomach contents.
- Allow casualties with maxillofacial trauma to assume whatever position that allows them to breathe most easily, including sitting upright if able.
- A surgical airway is preferable to endotracheal intubation in airway compromise resulting from direct maxillofacial trauma in tactical settings.
- A presumptive diagnosis of tension pneumothorax should be made in the setting of progressively worsening respiratory distress and known or suspected torso trauma.
- Needle decompression should be used to relieve suspected tension pneumothorax in tactical settings.
- When a defect in the chest wall is two-thirds or more of the diameter of the trachea, air will preferentially go into the chest cavity via the opening in the chest wall instead of into the lung via the trachea when the casualty takes a breath. This condition is called an open pneumothorax or sucking chest wound, and it may result in hypoxia.
- Treat an open pneumothorax with a vented occlusive dressing and then monitor the casualty closely for development of a possible tension pneumothorax.
- Reassess sites of previously treated external hemorrhage frequently to ensure that bleeding has not resumed.
- Control of bleeding takes precedence over infusing fluids.
- When time and the tactical situation permit, extremities on which a tourniquet has been applied should be exposed. If life-threatening bleeding is confirmed, the tourniquet should be replaced by another applied directly to the skin 2 to 3 inches proximal to the hemorrhage site.
- After the tourniquet is replaced, check the distal arterial pulse. If still present, tighten the tourniquet or add a second tourniquet if required until the distal pulse is no longer felt.
- Do not attempt to remove a tourniquet if the anticipated evacuation time is less than 2 hours or the casualty is in shock.
- When the anticipated evacuation time exceeds 2 hours and the casualty is not in shock, consider removing the tourniquet and controlling hemorrhage with hemostatic agents and direct pressure.
- Combat Gauze is the hemostatic agent of choice.
- Use the Combat Ready Clamp (CRoC), the Junctional Emergency Treatment Tool (JETT), or the SAM Junctional Tourniquet (SJT) to control junctional hemorrhage.
- Evacuate a casualty with penetrating trauma to the chest or abdomen on an emergent basis, due to the possibility of internal hemorrhage.
- Only individuals in shock or those who need intravenous (IV) medications need to have an IV established. Use an 18-gauge catheter and saline lock for IVs in the field.
- Give tranexamic acid (TXA) as soon as feasible to casualties in or at risk of hemorrhagic shock.
- Once the saline lock is established, secure it with transparent wound-dressing film. Administer fluids by a second needle and catheter through the film dressing. When the infusion is complete, withdraw the needle, leaving the saline lock in place.
- An intraosseous (IO) device is an alternative route for administering fluids when fluid resuscitation is required and IV access cannot be obtained.
- Clinical signs of shock on the battlefield are (1) unconsciousness or altered mental status not due to coexisting traumatic brain injury (TBI) or drug therapy and/or (2) abnormal radial pulse.
- Hextend is the preferred resuscitation fluid on the battlefield because it is retained in the intravascular space for 8 hours or longer, in contrast to lactated Ringer's, which leaves the intravascular space rapidly.
- Casualties in shock should be given a rapid 500-ml bolus of Hextend. The casualty should then be observed for 30 minutes. If there is insufficient clinical improvement, a second 500-ml bolus of Hextend should then be administered in a similar manner.

- Fluids by mouth to prevent dehydration are recommended for all conscious casualties who can take them.
- Casualties with both shock and TBI should receive IV or IO fluids until the radial pulse is restored, which corresponds to a systolic blood pressure of approximately 70 mm Hg.
- To prevent hypothermia and bleeding problems in trauma patients, prevention of heat loss should start as soon as feasible after wounding. Wet clothing should be replaced with dry clothes, and the casualty should be wrapped in a Heat Reflective Shell after a Ready-Heat blanket has been applied to the casualty's torso, outside his or her undershirt.
- In cases of suspected penetrating eye trauma, (1) perform a rapid field test of visual acuity, (2) tape a rigid shield over the eye to prevent further trauma to the eye, and (3) give moxifloxacin 400 mg by mouth as soon as possible to prevent infection inside the eye.
- Never apply a pressure dressing to an eye with a suspected penetrating injury.
- Pulse oximetry should be used in conjunction with physical examination findings to monitor for patent airway and adequate oxygenation. Pulse oximetry is especially important in casualties who are unconscious, who have injuries associated with impaired oxygenation, or who have TBI.
- NSAID analgesic medications that adversely affect platelet function should not be used in combat settings because platelets help the blood to clot when injuries are sustained. Platelet dysfunction increases the risk of bleeding to death. Aspirin and most anti-inflammatory medicines should not be used either for casualties or within a week before possible combat operations.
- For mild to moderate pain resulting from combat wounds, two 7.5-mg tablets of meloxicam are recommended, along with two 650-mg extended-release acetaminophen tablets. These medications have no adverse effect on platelet function, do not interfere with hemostasis, and cause no alterations of mental status.
- Oral transmucosal fentanyl citrate (OTFC) is recommended if the casualty has severe pain but no IV access has been obtained and the casualty is not in shock or respiratory distress or at significant risk of either of these two conditions.
- As an alternative, 5 mg of morphine sulfate IV may be used for severe pain if IV access has already been obtained.
- Morphine and OTFC are contraindicated in the presence of hemorrhagic shock.
- Ketamine, 50 mg IM or intranasally or 20 mg IV, should be used for casualties who have moderate to severe pain but who are in hemorrhagic shock or respiratory distress or are judged to be at significant risk for either condition.
- Antibiotics should be given as soon as possible to any combat casualty with an open wound to help prevent infection.
- IV or IM administration of antibiotics is needed for unconscious casualties.
- Moxifloxacin, 400 mg by mouth, is the recommended antibiotic if the casualty is able to take oral medications. Ertapenem or cefotetan should be used if the casualty requires IV or IM antibiotics.
- Unit medics, corpsmen, PJs, physicians, and physician assistants should screen their troops for allergies and pack alternative antibiotics as needed.
- Litters are typically used to move casualties in the Tactical Field Care phase.
- When moving a casualty long distances, tourniquets, dressings, splints, and IV lines should be checked frequently.
- Reassure and encourage the casualty. Answer questions about his or her injuries honestly, but maintain a positive attitude about rescue and treatment.
- Treat any casualty with polytrauma or torso trauma who subsequently experiences a cardiopulmonary arrest with bilateral needle decompression to relieve a possible undiagnosed tension pneumothorax.
- Cardiopulmonary resuscitation for trauma casualties with no pulse, no respirations, and no other signs of life should not be attempted in the Tactical Field Card phase, except in cases of hypothermia, near-drowning, or electrocution.
- Document the casualty's injuries and the care rendered on the TCCC Casualty Card, and forward it with the casualty to the next echelon of care.
- Enemy casualties remain hostile combatants until they indicate surrender, are separated from their weapons, have been searched and secured, and are proven to no longer pose a threat. After that has been done, they should receive the same treatment that would be rendered to U.S. forces according to the guidelines in this chapter.

SCENARIO RECAP

While on patrol in the city of Mosul, an infantry platoon comes under small arms fire.

The point man is hit and falls to the ground. The platoon reacts to the contact, rapidly eliminating the ambushing force. The point man is the only casualty in your unit. The platoon leader tells you to take care of the wounded man while the others establish a secure perimeter.

In your rapid initial assessment for life-threatening conditions, you find a gunshot entry wound on the casualty's right upper back. The exit wound is in the right axilla, and there is heavy pulsatile bleeding from it. The casualty is breathing slightly fast. There are no other wounds.

SCENARIO SOLUTION

1. **What phase of TCCC are you in?**

   You are in the Tactical Field Care phase.

2. **What is your immediate concern and how do you address it?**

   Your immediate concern is the life-threatening hemorrhage from the right axillary wound. Expose the wound. Pack a Combat Gauze dressing into the wound. Hold firm direct pressure with both hands for a minimum of 3 minutes.

3. **While addressing your immediate concern, what should you be doing simultaneously?**

   While holding direct pressure, you talk to the casualty, checking both airway and mental status and providing reassurance. While you are doing this, you note that the casualty becomes drowsy.

4. **What should you do after you finish your first intervention?**

   You check for other sources of external bleeding. You find none and the axillary bleeding is controlled.

5. **What do you evaluate next?**

   After confirming that there is no other significant external bleeding, you check his airway and breathing. You notice that his airway is clear, but his breathing is deep and rapid and appears labored.

6. **Should you treat for a tension pneumothorax? Why?**

   Yes—the casualty has a chest wound, has labored breathing, and is in shock. You perform a needle decompression of the right chest and note the hiss of escaping air. His breathing becomes slower and easier.

7. **What do you want to do after that?**

   After treating the tension pneumothorax, check the left radial pulse (not the right because of his wound). It is not palpable.

8. **What interventions come next if the casualty is still in shock?**

   Start an IV or IO and administer TXA followed by Hextend.

9. **What should this casualty's evacuation priority be?**

   Call for a "CAT A—Urgent" evacuation.

References

1. Butler FK, Hagmann JH, Richards DT. Tactical management of urban warfare casualties in special operations. *Mil Med.* 2000;165(4)(suppl):1–48.

2. Kelly JF, Ritenour AE, McLaughlin DF, et al. Injury severity and causes of death from Operation Iraqi Freedom and Operation Enduring Freedom: 2003–2004 versus 2006. *J Trauma.* 2008;64(2)(suppl):S21-S26.

3. Mabry RL, Edens JW, Pearse L, Kelly JF, Harcke H. Fatal airway injuries during Operation Enduring Freedom and Operation Iraqi Freedom. *Prehosp Emerg Care.* 2010;14(2):272–277.

4. Alexander RH, Proctor HJ, eds. *ATLS for Doctors Student Manual.* Chicago, IL: American College of Surgeons; 1993.

5. Butler FK, Hagmann J, Butler EG. Tactical combat casualty care in special operations. *Mil Med.* 1996;161(suppl):3–16.

6. Butler FK, Holcomb JB, Giebner SD, McSwain NE, Bagian J. Tactical combat casualty care 2007: evolving concepts and battlefield experience. *Mil Med.* 2007;172(11)(suppl):1–19.

7. Smith JP, Bodai BI. The urban paramedic's scope of practice. *JAMA.* 1985;253(4):544–548.

8. Sladen A. Emergency endotracheal intubation: who can—who should? *Chest.* 1979;75(5):535–536.

9. Stewart RD, Paris PM, Winter PM, Pelton GH, Cannon GM. Field endotracheal intubation by paramedical personnel. Success rates and complications. *Chest.* 1984;85(3):341–345.

10. Jacobs LM, Berrizbeitia LD, Bennet B, Madigan C. Endotracheal intubation in the prehospital phase of emergency medical care. *JAMA.* 1983;250(16):2175–2177.

11. Pointer JE. Clinical characteristics of paramedics' performance of endotracheal intubation. *J Emerg Med.* 1988;6(6):505–509.

12. Lavery RF, Doran J, Tortella BJ, Cody RP. A survey of advanced life support practices in the United States. *Prehosp Disaster Med.* 1992;7(2):144–150.

13. DeLeo BC. Endotracheal intubation by rescue squad personnel. *Heart Lung.* 1977;65:851–854.

14. Trooskin SZ, Rabinowitz S, Eldridge C, McGowan D, Flancbaum L. Teaching endotracheal intubation using animals and cadavers. *Prehosp Disaster Med.* 1992;7(2):179–182.

15. Stewart RD, Paris PM, Pelton GH, Garretson D. Effect of varied training techniques on field endotracheal intubation success rates. *Ann Emerg Med.* 13(11):1032–1036.

16. Cameron PA, Flett K, Kaan E, Atkin C, Dziukas L. Helicopter retrieval of primary trauma patients by a paramedic helicopter service. *Aust N Z J Surg.* 1993;63(10):790–797.

17. Zajtchuk R, Jenkins DP, Bellamy RF, Quick CM, Moore CC. Combat casualty care guidelines for Operation Desert Storm. Washington, DC: Office of the Army Surgeon General; 1991.

18. Adams BD, Cuniowski PA, Muck A, DeLorenzo RA. Registry of emergency airways arriving at combat hospitals. *J Trauma.* 64(6):1548–1554.

19. Reinhart DJ, Simmons G. Comparison of placement of the laryngeal mask airway with endotracheal tube by paramedics and respiratory therapists. *Ann Emerg Med.* 1994;24(2):260–263.

20. Stratton SJ, Kane G, Gunter CS, et al. Prospective study of manikin-only versus manikin and human subject endotracheal intubation training of paramedics. *Ann Emerg Med.* 1991;20(12):1314–1318.

21. Katz SH, Falk JL. Misplaced endotracheal tubes by paramedics in an urban emergency medical services system. *Ann Emerg Med.* 2001;37(1):32–37.

22. Calkins MD, Robinson TD. Combat trauma airway management: endotracheal intubation versus laryngeal mask airway versus Combitube use by Navy SEAL and Reconnaissance combat corpsmen. *J Trauma.* 1999;46(5):927–932.

23. Dickey NW. Supraglottic Airway Use in Tactical Evacuation Care 2012–06. Defense Health Board Memorandum. September 17, 2012. http://health.mil/dhb/recommendations/2012/2012-06.pdf. Accessed July 29, 2013.

24. Salvino CK, Dries D, Gamelli R, Murphy-Macobobby M, Mashall W. Emergency cricothyroidotomy in trauma victims. *J Trauma.* 1993;34(4):503–505.

25. McGill J, Clinton JE, Ruiz E. Cricothyrotomy in the emergency department. *Ann Emerg Med.* 1982;11(7):361–364.

26. Erlandson MJ, Clinton JE, Ruiz E, Cohen J. Cricothyrotomy in the emergency department revisited. *J Emerg Med.* 1989;7(2):115–118.

27. Holcomb JB, McMullin NR, Pearse L, et al. Causes of death in Special Operations Forces in the global war on terrorism. *Ann Surg.* 2007;245(6):986–991.

28. MacDonald JC, Tien HC. Emergency battlefield cricothyrotomy. *CMAJ.* 2008;178(9):1133–1135.

29. Mabry R. An analysis of battlefield cricothyrotomy in Iraq and Afghanistan. *J Spec Oper Med.* 2012;12(1):17–23.

30. Bennett B, Cailteux-Zevallos B, Kotora J. Cricothyroidotomy bottom-up training review: battlefield lessons learned. *Mil Med.* 2011;176(11):1311–1319.

31. McPherson JJ, Feigin DS, Bellamy RF. Prevalence of tension pneumothorax in fatally wounded combat casualties. *J Trauma.* 2006;60(3):573–578.

32. Mabry RL, Holcomb JB, Baker AM, et al. United States Army Rangers in Somalia: an analysis of combat casualties on an urban battlefield. *J Trauma.* 2000;49(3):515–528.

33. Warner KJ, Copass MK, Bulger EM. Paramedic use of needle thoracostomy in the prehospital environment. *Prehosp Emerg Care.* 2008;12(2):162–168.

34. Jones R, Hollingsworth J. Tension pneumothoraces not responding to needle thoracentesis. *J Emerg Med.* 2002;19(2):176–177.

35. Holcomb JB, McManus JB, Kerr ST, Pusateri AE. Needle versus tube thoracostomy in a swine model of traumatic tension hemopneumothorax. *Prehosp Emerg Care.* 2009;13(1):18–27.

36. Britten S, Palmer SH, Snow TM. Needle thoracocentesis in tension pneumothorax: insufficient cannula length and potential failure. *Injury.* 1996;27(5):321–322.

37. Harcke HT, Pearse LA, Levy AD, Getz JM, Robinson SR. Chest wall thickness in military personnel: implications for needle thoracentesis in tension pneumothorax. *Mil Med.* 172(12):1260–1263.

38. Zengerink I, Brink PR, Laupland KB, et al. Needle thoracostomy in the treatment of tension pneumothorax in trauma patients: what size needle? *J Trauma.* 2008;64(1):111–114.

39. Givens ML, Ayotte K, Manifold C. Needle thoracostomy: implications of computed tomography chest wall thickness. *Acad Emerg Med.* 2004;11(2):211–213.

40. Kiley KC. Management of Soldiers with Tension Pneumothorax. US Army Surgeon General Memorandum. August 25, 2006.

41. Riwoe D, Poncia H. Subclavian artery laceration: a serious complication of needle decompression. *Emerg Med Australas.* 2011;23(5):651–653.

42. Butler KL, Best IM, Weaver L, Bumpers HL. Pulmonary artery injury and cardiac tamponade after needle decompression of a suspected tension pneumothorax. *J Trauma.* 2003;54(3):610–611.

43. Rawlins R, Brown KM, Carr CS, Cameron CR. Life-threatening haemorrhage after anterior needle aspiration of pneumothoraces: a role for lateral needle aspiration in emergency decompression of spontaneous pneumothorax. *Emerg Med J.* 2003;20(4):383–384.

44. Netto F, Shulman H, Rizoli S, et al. Are needle decompressions for tension pneumothoraces being performed appropriately for appropriate indications? *Am J Emerg Med.* 2008;26(5):597–602.

45. Tien HC, Jung V, Rizoli SB, Acharya SV, MacDonald JC. An evaluation of Tactical Combat Casualty Care interventions in a combat environment. *J Am Coll Surg.* 2008;207(2):174–178.

46. Dickey N. Needle Decompression of Tension Pneumothorax—Tactical Combat Casualty Care Recommendations 2012–5. Defense Health Board Memorandum. July 7, 2012. http://health.mil/dhb/recommendations/2012/2012–05.pdf. Accessed June 13, 2013.

47. Martin M, Satterly S, Inaba K, Blair K. Does needle thoracostomy provide adequate and effective decompression of tension pneumothorax? *J Trauma Acute Care Surg.* 2012;73(6):1412–1417.

48. Mistry N, Bleetman A, Roberts KJ. Chest decompression during the resuscitation of patients in prehospital traumatic cardiac arrest. *Emerg Med J.* 2009;26(10):738–740.

49. Dickey NW, Jenkins D. Needle Decompression of Tension Pneumothorax and Cardiopulmonary Resuscitation Tactical Combat Casualty Care Guidelines Recommendations 2011–8. Defense Health Board Memorandum. October 11, 2011. http://www.health.mil/dhb/recommendations/2011/2011–08.pdf. Accessed June 13, 2013.

50. Dolley F, Brewer L. Chest Injuries. *Ann Surg.* 1942:116(5):668–686.

51. Eastridge BJ, Mabry RL, Seguin P, et al. Death on the Battlefield (2001–2011): implications for the future of combat casualty care. *J Trauma Acute Care Surg.* 2012;73(6)(suppl 5):S431-S437.

52. Szul AC, Davis LB, Maston BG, Wise D, Sparacino LR, eds. *Emergency War Surgery.* Third United States Revision. Washington, DC: The Borden Institute; 2004.

53. McSwain NE, Salome JP, Pons PT, eds. *Prehospital Trauma Life Support.* 6th ed. St Louis, MO: Mosby; 2006:280.

54. Hodgetts TJ, Hanian CG, Newey CG. Battlefield first aid: a simple, systematic approach for every soldier. *J R Army Med Corps.* 1999;145(2):55–59.

55. Kheirabadi BS, Terrazas IB, Koller A, et al. Vented versus unvented chest seals for treatment of pneumothorax and prevention of tension pneumothorax in a swine model. *J Trauma Acute Care Surg.* 2013;75(1):150–156.

56. Grissom CK, Weaver LK, Clemmer TP, Morris AH. Theoretical advantage of oxygen treatment for combat casualties during medical evacuation at high altitude. *J Trauma.* 2006;61(2):461–467.

57. Chi JH, Knudson MM, Vassar MJ, et al. Prehospital hypoxia affects outcome in patients with traumatic brain injury: a prospective multicenter study. *J Trauma.* 2006;61(5):1134–1141.

58. Floyd TF, Clark JM, Gelfand R, et al. Independent cerebral vasoconstrictive effects of hyperoxia and accompanying arterial hypocapnia at 1 ATA. *J Appl Physiol.* 2003;95(6):2453–2461.

59. Tisdall MM, Taylor C, Tachtisidis I, Leung TS, Elwell CE, Smith M. The effect of cerebral tissue oxygenation index of changes in the concentrations of inspired oxygen and end-tidal carbon dioxide in healthy adult volunteers. *Anesth Analg.* 2009;109(3):906–913.

60. Tolias C, Reinert M, Seiler R, Gilman C, Scharf A, Bullock MR. Normobaric hyperoxia-induced improvement in cerebral metabolism and reduction in intracranial pressure in patients with severe head injury: a prospective historical cohort-matched study. *J Neurosurg.* 2004;101(3):435–444.

61. Dickey NW. Management of Traumatic Brain Injury in Tactical Combat Casualty Care 2012–04. Defense Health Board Memorandum. July 26, 2012. http://health.mil/dhb/recommendations/2012/2012–04.pdf. Accessed July 11, 2013.

62. Kragh JF, Walters TJ, Baer DG, et al. Practical use of emergency tourniquets to stop bleeding in major limb trauma. *J Trauma.* 2008;64(2)(suppl):S38-S49.

63. Pusateri AE, Modrow HE, Harris RA, et al. Advanced hemostatic dressing development program: animal model selection criteria and results of a study of nine hemostatic dressings in a model of severe large venous hemorrhage and hepatic injury in swine. *J Trauma.* 2003;55(3):518–526.

64. Alam HB, Uy GB, Miller D, et al. Comparative analysis of hemostatic agents in a swine model of lethal groin injury. *J Trauma.* 2003;54(6):1077–1082.

65. Rhee P, Brown C, Martin M, et al. QuikClot use in trauma for hemorrhage control: case series of 103 documented uses. *J Trauma.* 2008;64(4):1093–1099.

66. Wedmore I, McManus JG, Pusateri AE, Holcomb JB. A special report on the chitosan-based hemostatic dressing: experience in current combat operations. *J Trauma.* 2006;60(3):655–658.

67. McManus J, Hurtado T, Pusateri A, Knoop KJ. A case series describing thermal injury resulting from zeolite use for hemorrhage control in combat operations. *Prehosp Emerg Care.* 2007;11(1):67–71.

68. Kheirabadi BS, Edens JW, Terrazas IB, et al. Comparison of new hemostatic granules/powders with currently deployed hemostatic products in a lethal model of extremity arterial hemorrhage in swine. *J Trauma.* 2009;66(2):316–326.

69. Kheirabadi B, Mace J, Terrazas I, et al. Safety evaluation of new hemostatic agents, smectite granules, and kaolin-coated gauze in a vascular injury wound model in swine. *J Trauma.* 2010;68(2):269–278.

70. Watters JM, Van PY, Hamilton GJ, Sambasivan C, Differding JA, Schreiberet. Advanced hemostatic dressings are not superior to gauze for care under fire scenarios. *J Trauma.* 2011;70(6):1413–1419.

71. Causey MW, McVay DP, Miller S, Beekley A, Martin M. The efficacy of Combat Gauze in extreme physiologic conditions. *J Surg Res.* 2012;177(2):301–305.

72. Ran Y, Hadad E, Daher S, et al. QuikClot Combat Gauze for hemorrhage control in military trauma: January 2009 Israel Defense Force experience in the Gaza Strip—a preliminary report of 14 cases. *Prehosp Disaster Med.* 2010;25(6):584–588.

73. Rall JM, Cox JM, Songer A, et al. Naval Medical Research Unit San Antonio. Comparison of novel hemostatic gauzes to QuikClot Combat Gauze in a standardized swine model of uncontrolled hemorrhage. Technical Report 2012–22. March 23, 2012. http://www.medicalsci.com/files/tccc_rall_new_hemostatic_gauzes_namru-sa_tr_2012–22.pdf. Accessed July 15, 2013.

74. Caravalho J. Dismounted Complex Injury Task Force. Report of the Army Dismounted Complex Injury Task Force. June 18, 2011. http://www.armymedicine.army.mil/reports/DCBI%20Task%20Force%20Report%20(Redacted%20Final).pdf?. Accessed July 15, 2013.

75. Dubick MA, Kragh JF, eds. U.S. Army Institute of Surgical Research. Evaluations of the Combat Ready Clamp to control bleeding in human cadavers, manikins, swine femoral artery hemorrhage model and swine carcasses. UUSAISR Institutional Report June 2012. http://www.dtic.mil/cgi-bin/GetTRDoc?AD=ADA569685. Accessed July 15, 2013.

76. Aeder MI, Crowe JP, Rhodes RS, Schuck JM, Wolf WM. Technical limitations in the rapid infusion of intravenous fluids. *Ann Emerg Med.*1985;14(4):307–310.

77. Hoelzer MF. Recent advances in intravenous therapy. *Emerg Med Clin North Am.* 1986;4(3):487–500.

78. Lawrence DW, Lauro AJ. Complications from IV therapy: results from field-started and emergency department-started IVs compared. *Ann Emerg Med.* 1988;17(4):314–317.

79. Dubick MA, Holcomb JB. A review of intraosseous vascular access: current status and military application. *Mil Med.* 2000;165(7): 552–559.

80. Calkins MD, Fitzgerald G, Bentley TB, Burris D. Intraosseous infusion devices: a comparison for potential use in special operations. *J Trauma.* 2000;48(6):1068–1074.

81. Harcke HT, Mazuchowski E. Feedback to the field: perforation of the sternum by an intraosseous infusion device. Defense Medical Material Program Office Website. https://www.dmsb.mil/refDocs/F2TF/F2TF_6_Perforation_of_Sternum_by_IO_Device.pdf. Accessed May 13, 2014.

82. CRASH-2 collaborators, Roberts I, Shakur H, et al. The importance of early treatment with tranexamic acid in bleeding trauma patients: an exploratory analysis of the CRASH-2 randomized controlled trial. *Lancet.* 2011;377(9771):1096–1101.

83. Morrison JJ, Dubose JJ, Rasmussen TE, Midwinter MJ. Military Application of Tranexamic Acid in Trauma Emergency Resuscitation (MATTERs) Study. *Arch Surg.* 2012;147(2):113–119.

84. Dickey NW, Jenkins D. Defense Health Board Recommendation for the Addition of Tranexamic Acid to the Tactical Combat Casualty Care Guidelines. Defense Health Board Memorandum. September 23, 2011. http://health.mil/dhb/recommendations/2011/2011–06.pdf. Accessed July 17, 2013.

85. Krausz MM. Controversies in shock research: hypertonic resuscitation—pros and cons. *Shock.* 1995;3(1):69–72.

86. Smith JP, Bodai BI, Hill AS, Frey CF. Prehospital stabilization of critically injured patients: a failed concept. *J Trauma.* 1985;25(1):65–70.

87. Dronen SC, Stern S, Baldursson J, Irvin C, Syverud S. Improved outcome with early blood administration in a near-fatal model of porcine hemorrhagic shock. *Am J Emerg Med.* 1992;10(6): 533–537.

88. Chudnofsky CR, Dronen SC, Syverud SA, Hedges JR, Zink BJ. Early versus late fluid resuscitation: lack of effect in porcine hemorrhagic shock. *Ann Emerg Med.* 1989;18(2):122–126.

89. Bickell WH. Are victims of injury sometimes victimized by attempts at fluid resuscitation? *Ann Emerg Med.* 1993;22(2):225–226.

90. Chudnofsky CR, Dronen SC, Syverud SA, Zink BJ, Hedges JR. Intravenous fluid therapy in the prehospital management of hemorrhagic shock: improved outcome with hypertonic saline/6% dextran 70 in a swine model. *Am J Emerg Med.* 1989;7(4):357–363.

91. Kaweski SM, Sise MJ, Virgilio RW. The effect of prehospital fluids on survival in trauma patients. *J Trauma.* 1990:30(10):1215–1218.

92. Deakin CD, Hicks IR. AB or ABC: prehospital fluid management in major trauma. *J Accid Emerg Med.* 1994;11(3):154–157.

93. Krausz MM, Bar-Ziv M, Rabinovici R, gross D. "Scoop and run" or stabilize hemorrhagic shock with normal saline or small-volume hypertonic saline? *J Trauma.* 33(1):6–10.

94. Kowalenko J, Stern S, Dronen S, Wang X. Improved outcome with hypotensive resuscitation of uncontrolled hemorrhagic shock in a swine model. *J Trauma.* 1992;33(3):349–353.

95. Kramer GC, Perron PR, Lindsey DC, et al. Small-volume resuscitation with hypertonic saline dextran solution.*Surgery.* 1986;100(2):239–247.

96. Krausz MM, Klemm O, Amstislavsky T, Horovitz M. The effect of heat load and dehydration on hypertonic saline solution treatment on uncontrolled hemorrhagic shock. *J Trauma.* 1995;38(5):747–752.

97. Krausz MM, Horn Y, Gross D. The combined effect of small volume hypertonic saline and normal saline solutions in uncontrolled hemorrhagic shock. *Surg Gynecol Obstet.* 174(5):363–368.

98. Gross D, Landau EH, Klin B, Krausz MM. Treatment of uncontrolled hemorrhagic shock with hypertonic saline solution. *Surg Gynecal Obstet.* 1990;170(2):106–112.

99. Stern SA, Dronen SC, Birrer P, Wang X. Effect of blood pressure on hemorrhage volume and survival in a near-fatal hemorrhage model incorporating a vascular injury.*Ann Emerg Med.* 1993;22(2):155–163.

100. Bickell WH, Bruttig SP, Millnamow GA, O'Benar J, Wade CE. Use of hypertonic saline/dextran versus lactated Ringer's solution as a resuscitation fluid after uncontrolled aortic hemorrhage in anesthetized swine. *Ann Emerg Med.* 1992;21(9):1077–1085.

101. Dontigny L. Small-volume resuscitation. *Can J Surg.* 1992;35(1):31–33.

102. Gross D, Landau EH, Assalia A, Krausz MM. Is hypertonic saline resuscitation safe in 'uncontrolled' hemorrhagic shock? *J Trauma.* 1988;28(6):751–756.

103. Shaftan GW, Chiu CJ, Dennis C, Harris B. Fundamentals of physiological control of arterial hemorrhage. *Surgery.* 1965;58(5):851–856.

104. Milles G, Koucky CJ, Zacheis HG. Experimental uncontrolled arterial hemorrhage. *Surgery.* 1966;60(2):434–442.

105. Sindlinger JF, Soucy DM, Greene SP, Barber AE, Illner H, Shires GT. The effects of isotonic saline volume resuscitation in uncontrolled hemorrhage. *Surg Gynecol Obstet.* 1993;177(6):545–550.

106. Landau EH, Gross D, Assalia A, Krausz MM. Treatment of uncontrolled hemorrhagic shock by hypertonic saline and external counterpressure. *Ann Emerg Med.* 1989;18(10):1039–1043.

107. Rabinovici R, Krausz MM, Feurstein G. Control of bleeding is essential for a successful treatment of hemorrhagic shock with 7.5 per cent sodium chloride solution. *Surg Gynecol Obstet.* 1991;173(2):98–106.

108. Landau EH, Gross D, Assalia A, Feigin E, Krausz MM. Hypertonic saline infusion in hemorrhagic shock treated by military antishock trousers (MAST) in awake sheep. *Crit Care Med.* 21(10):1554–1562.

109. Crawford ES. Ruptured abdominal aortic aneurysm. *J Vasc Surg.* 1991;13(2):348–350.

110. Bickell WH, Wall MJ, Pepe PE, et al. Immediate versus delayed fluid resuscitation for hypotensive patients with penetrating torso injuries. *N Engl J Med.* 1994;331(17):1105–1109.

111. Wall MJ. Audiovisual presentation at the 53rd annual meeting of the American Association for the Surgery of Trauma. New Orleans, LA. 1994.

112. Champion HR. Combat fluid resuscitation: introduction and overview of conferences. *J Trauma.* 2003;54(5)(suppl):S7-S12.

113. Rainey TG, Read CA. The pharmacology of colloids and crystalloids. In: Chernow B, ed. *The Pharmacologic Approach to the Critically Ill Patient.* 2nd ed. Baltimore, MD: Williams & Wilkins; 1988:219–240.

114. Carey JS, Scharschmidt BF, Culliford AT, Greenlee JE, Scott CR. Hemodynamic effectiveness of colloid and electrolyte solutions for replacement of simulated operative blood loss. *Surg Gynecol Obstet.* 1970;131(4):679–686.

115. Marino PL. Colloid and crystalloid resuscitation. In Marino, PL. *The ICU Book.* Malvern, PA: Williams & Wilkins; 1991:205–216.

116. Strauss RG. Review of the effects of hydroxyethyl starch on the blood coagulation system. *Transfusion*. 1981;21(3):299–302.

117. Mortelmans Y, Merckx E, van Nerom C, et al. Effect of an equal volume replacement with 500cc 6% hydroxyethyl starch on the blood and plasma volume of healthy volunteers. *Eur J Anesthesiol*.1995; 12(3):259–264.

118. Napolitano LM. Resuscitation following trauma and hemorrhagic shock: is hydroxyethyl starch safe? *Crit Care Med*. 1995;23(5):795–797.

119. Dalrymple-Hay MB, Aitchison R, Collins P, Sekhar M, Colvin B. Hydroxyethyl starch induced acquired von Willebrand's disease. *Clin Lab Haematol*. 1992;14(3):209–211.

120. Via D, Kaufman C, Anderson D, Stanton K, Rhee P. Effect of hydroxyethyl starch on coagulopathy in a swine model of hemorrhagic shock resuscitation. *J Trauma*. 2001;50(6):1076–1082.

121. Shatney CH, Deepika K, Militello PR, Majerus TC, Dawson RB. Efficacy of hetastarch in the resuscitation of patients with multisystem trauma and shock. *Arch Surg*. 1983;118(7):804–809.

122. Falk JL, O'Brien JF, Kerr R. Fluid resuscitation in traumatic hemorrhagic shock. *Crit Care Clin*. 1992;8(2):323–340.

123. Ratner LE, Smith GW. Intraoperative fluid management. *Surg Clin North Am*. 1993;73(2):229–241.

124. Gan TJ, Bennett-Guerrero E, Phillips-Bute B, et al. Hextend, a physiologically balanced plasma expander for large volume use in major surgery: a randomized phase III clinical trial. Hextend Study Group. *Anesth Analg*. 1999;88(5):992–998.

125. Pearce FJ, Lyons WS. Logistics of parenteral fluids in battlefield resuscitation. *Mil Med*. 1999;164(9):653–655.

126. Pope A, French G, Longnecker DE, eds. Fluid resuscitation. State of the Science for Treating Combat Casualties and Civilian Injuries. Washington, DC: National Academy Press; 1999.

127. Rhee P, Koustova E, Alam HB. Searching for the optimal resuscitation method: recommendations for the initial fluid resuscitation of combat casualties. *J Trauma*. 2003;54(5)(suppl):S52-S62.

128. Rhee P, Burris D, Kaufmann C, et al. Lactated Ringer's solution resuscitation causes neutrophil activation after hemorrhagic shock. *J Trauma*. 1998;44(2):313–319.

129. Burris D, Rhee P, Kaufmann C, et al. Controlled resuscitation for uncontrolled hemorrhagic shock. *J Trauma*. 1999;462:216–223.

130. Deb S, Martin B, Sun L, et al. Resuscitation with lactated Ringer's in rats with hemorrhagic shock induces immediate apoptosis. *J Trauma*. 1999;46(4):582–588.

131. Sun L, Ruff P, Austin B, et al. Early up-regulation of intercellular adhesion lolecule-1 and vascular cell adhesion molecule-1 expression in rats with hemorrhagic shock and resuscitation. *Shock*. 1999;11(6):416–422.

132. Rhee P, Wang D, Ruff P, et al. Human neutrophil activation and increased adhesion by various resuscitation fluids. *Crit Care Med*. 2000;28(1):74–78.

133. Alam HB, Sun L, Ruff P, Austin B, Burris D, Rhee P. E- and P-selectin expression depends on the resuscitation fluid used in hemorrhaged rats. *J Surg Res*. 2000;94(2):145–152.

134. Alam HB, Austin B, Koustova E, Rhee P. Resuscitation-induced pulmonary apoptosis and intracellular adhesion molecule-1 expression in rats are attenuated by the use of Ketone Ringer's solution. *J Am Coll Surg*. 2001;193(3):255–263.

135. Deb S, Sun L, Martin B, et al. Lactated ringer's solution and hetastarch but not plasma resuscitation after rat hemorrhagic shock is associated with immediate lung apoptosis by the up-regulation of the Bax protein. *J Trauma*. 2000;49(1):47–53.

136. Rhee P, Morris J, Durham R, et al. Recombinant humanized monoclonal antibody against CD18 (rhuMAb CD18) in traumatic hemorrhagic shock: results of a phase II clinical trial. Traumatic Shock Group. *J Trauma*. 2000;49(4):611–619.

137. Lieberthal W, Fuhro R, Alam H, et al. Comparison of a 50% exchange-transfusion with albumin, hetastarch, and modified hemoglobin solutions. *Shock*. 2002;7(1):61–69.

138. Gushchin V, Stegalkina S, Alam HB, et al. Cytokine expression profiling in human leukocytes after exposure to hypertonic and isotonic fluids. *J Trauma*. 2002;52(5):867–871.

139. Koustova E, Stanton K, Gushchin V, et al. Effects of lactated Ringer's solutions on human leukocytes. *J Trauma*. 2002;52(5):872–878.

140. Alam HB, Stegalkina S, Rhee P, Koustova E. cDNA array analysis of gene expression following hemorrhagic shock and resuscitation in rats. *Resuscitation*. 2002;54(2):195–206.

141. Alam H, Koustova E, Stanton K, Burris D, Rich N, Rhee P. Effect of different resuscitation strategies on neutrophil activation in a swine model of hemorrhagic shock. *Resuscitation*. 60(1):91–99.

142. Holcomb JB. Fluid resuscitation in modern combat casualty care: lessons learned from Somalia. *J Trauma*. 2003;54(suppl 5): S46-S51.

143. Sondeen J, Coppes VG, Holcomb JB. Blood pressure at which rebleeding occurs after resuscitation in swine with aortic injury. *J Trauma*. 2003;54(suppl 5):S110-S117.

144. Beecher HK. *Resuscitation and Anesthesia for Wounded Men: The Management of Traumatic Shock*. Springfield, IL: Charles C. Thomas; 1949.

145. Haut ER, Kalish BT, Cotton BA, et al. Prehospital intravenous fluid administration is associated with higher mortality in trauma patients: a National Trauma Data Bank analysis. *Ann Surg*. 2011;253(2):371–377.

146. Ley E, Clond M, Srour M, et al. Emergency department crystalloid resuscitation of 1.5 L or more is associated with increased mortality in elderly and nonelderly trauma patients. *J Trauma*. 2011;70(2):398–400.

147. Lissauer ME, Chi A, Kramer ME, Scalea TM, Johnson SB. Association of 6% hetastarch resuscitation with adverse outcomes in critically ill trauma patients. *Am J Surg*. 2011;202(1):501–508.

148. Duke MD, Guidry C, Guice J, et al. Restrictive fluid resuscitation in combination with damage control resuscitation: time for adaptation. *J Trauma Acute Care Surg*. 2012;73(3):674–678.

149. Holcomb, JB. Optimal use of blood products in severely injured trauma patients. *Hematol Am Soc Hematol Educ Program*. 2010;2010:465–469.

150. Dickey NW, Jenkins D, Butler FK. Use of Dried Plasma in Prehospital Battlefield Resuscitation 2011–04. Defense Health Board Memorandum. August 8, 2011. http://health.mil/dhb/recommendations/2011/2011–04.pdf. Accessed August 13, 2013.

151. DeBakey ME. *General Surgery*. Washington, DC: US Government Printing Office; 1956. *Surgery in World War II*; vol 2.

152. Churchill ED. *Surgeon to Soldiers: Diary and Records of the Surgical Consultant, Allied Forces Headquarters. WWII*. Philadelphia, PA: Lippincott; 1972.

153. Eastridge BJ, Jenkins D, Flaherty S, Schiller H, Holcomb JB. Trauma system development in a theater of war: experiences from Operation Iraqi Freedom and Operation Enduring Freedom. *J Trauma*. 2006;61(6):1366–1373.

154. Manley G, Knudson MM, Morabito D, et al. Hypotension, hypoxia, and head injury: frequency, duration, and consequences. *Arch Surg*. 2001;136(10):1118–1123.

155. Lednar WM, Poland GA, Holcomb JB, Butler FK. Recommendations Regarding the Tactical Combat Casualty Care Guidelines on Fluid Resuscitation. Defense Health Board Memorandum. December 10, 2010. http://health.mil/dhb/recommendations/2010/2010–06.pdf. Accessed August 13, 2013.

156. Wolberg AS, Meng ZH, Monroe DM 3rd, Hoffman M. A systematic evaluation of the effect of temperature on coagulation enzyme activity and platelet function. *J Trauma.* 2004;56(6):1221–1228.

157. Watts DD, Trask A, Soeken K, Perdue P, Dols S, Kaufmann C. Hypothermic coagulopathy in trauma: effect of varying levels of hypothermia on enzyme speed, platelet function, and fibrinolytic activity. *J Trauma.* 1998;44(5):846–854.

158. Peng RY, Bongard FS. Hypothermia in trauma patients. *J Am Coll Surg.* 1999;188(6):685–696.

159. Fries D, Innerhofer P, Schobersberger W. Coagulation management in trauma patients. *Curr Opin Anaesthesiol.* 2002;15(2):217–223.

160. Carr ME Jr. Monitoring of hemostasis in combat trauma patients. *Mil Med.* 2004;169(suppl 12):11–15.

161. Joint Theater Trauma System Clinical Practice Guideline. Hypothermia prevention, monitoring, and management. http://www.usaisr.amedd.army.mil/assets/cpgs/Hypothermia_Prevention_20_Sep_12.pdf. Published September 12, 2012. Accessed August 14, 2013.

162. Arthurs Z, Cuadrado D, Beekley, et al. The impact of hypothermia on trauma care at the 31st combat support hospital. *Am J Surg.* 2006;191(5):610–614.

163. Winkenwerder W. Defense-wide Policy on Combat Trauma Casualty Hypothermia Prevention and Treatment. Assistant Secretary of Defense for Health Affairs Memorandum. February 16, 2006. http://www.health.mil/libraries/HA_Policies_and_Guidelines/06–005.pdf. Accessed August 14, 2013.

164. Husum H, Olsen T, Murad M, Wisborg T, Gilbert M. Preventing post-injury hypothermia during prolonged prehospital evacuation. *Prehosp Disaster Med.* 2002;17(1):23–26.

165. Allen PB, Salyer SW, Dubick MA, Holcomb JB, Blackbourne LH. Preventing hypothermia: comparison of current devices used by the U.S. Army with an in vitro warmed fluid model. *J Trauma.* 2010;69(suppl):S154-S161.

166. Lednar WM, Poland GA, Holcomb JB, Butler FK. Tactical Combat Casualty Care Guidelines on the Prevention of Hypothermia. Defense Health Board Memorandum. December 10, 2010. http://health.mil/dhb/recommendations/2010/2010–05.pdf. Accessed August 14, 2013.

167. Kressloff MS, Castellarin AA, Zarbin MA. Endophthalmitis. *Surv Ophthalmol.* 1998;43(3):193–224.

168. Butler FK. The eye in the wilderness. In: Auerbach PS, ed. *Wilderness Medicine.* 6th ed. St. Louis, MO: Mosby; 2012

169. Colyer MH, Weber ED, Weichel ED, et al. Delayed intraocular foreign body removal without endophthalmitis during Operations Iraqi Freedom and Enduring Freedom. *Ophthalmology.* 2007;114:1439–1447.

170. Schnapp LM, Cohen NH. Pulse oximetry. Uses and abuses. *Chest.* 1990;98(5):1244–1250.

171. Hanning CD, Alexander-Williams JM. Pulse oximetry: a practical review. *BMJ.* 1995;311(7001):367–370.

172. Moran RF, Clausen JL, Ehrmeyer SS, Feil M, Van Kessel Al, Eichhorn JH. Oxygen content, hemoglobin oxygen, "saturation," and related quantities in blood: terminology, measurement, and reporting. National Committee for Clinical Laboratory Standards 1990; C25-P:10:1–49.

173. Huch A, Huch R, Konig V, et al. Limitations of pulse oximetry. *Lancet.* 1988;1(8581):357–358.

174. Hansen JE, Casaburi R. Validity of ear oximetry in clinical exercise testing. *Chest.* 1987;91(3):333–337.

175. Ries AL, Prewitt LM, Johnson JJ. Skin color and ear oximetry. *Chest.* 1989;96(2):287–290.

176. Shapiro BA, Crane RD. Blood gas monitoring: yesterday, today, and tomorrow. *Crit Care Med.* 1989;17(6):573–581.

177. Davidson JA, Hosie HE. Limitations of pulse oximetry: respiratory insufficiency—a failure of detection. *BMJ.* 1993;307(6900):372–373.

178. Badjatia N, Carney N, Crocco TJ, et al. Brain Trauma Foundation; BTF Center for Guidelines Management. Guidelines for the prehospital management of traumatic brain injury. 2nd edition. *Prehosp Emerg Care.* 2008;12(suppl 1):S1-S52.

179. Trillo RA Jr, Aukburg S. Dapsone-induced methemoglobinemia and pulse oximetry. *Anesthesiology.* 1992;77(3):594–596.

180. Sin DD, Shafran SD. Dapsone- and primaquine-induced methemoglobinemia in HIV-infected individuals. *J Acquir Immune Defic Syndr Hum Retrovirol.* 1996;12(5):477–481.

181. Beecher HK. Pain in men wounded in battle. *Bull US Army Med Dep.* 1946;5:445–454.

182. Vonkeman HE, van de Laar MA. Nonsteroidal anti-inflammatory drugs: adverse effects and their prevention. *Semin Arthritis Rheum.* 2010;39(4):294–312.

183. Van Ryn J, Kink-Eiband M, Kuritsch I, et al. Meloxicam does not affect the antiplatelet effect of aspirin in healthy male and female volunteers. *J Clin Pharmacol.* 2004;44(7):777–784.

184. Knijff-Dutmer EA, Kalsbeek-Batenburg EM, Koerts J, van de Laar MA. Platelet function is inhibited by non-selective non-steroidal anti-inflammatory drugs but not by cyclooygenase-2-selective inhibitors in patients with rheumatoid arthritis. *Rheumatology (Oxford).* 2002;41(4):458–461.

185. Harris M, Baba R, Nahouraii R, Gould P. Self-induced bleeding diathesis in soldiers at a FOB in south eastern Afghanistan. *Mil Med.* 2012;177(8):928–929.

186. Ivascu FA, Howells GA, Junn FS, Bair HA, Bendick PJ, Janczyk RJ. Predictors of mortality in trauma patients with intracranial hemorrhage on preinjury aspirin or clopidogrel. *J Trauma.* 2008;65(4):785–788.

187. Singer AJ, Mynster CJ, McMahon BJ. The effect of IM ketorolac tromethamine on bleeding time: a prospective, interventional, controlled study. *Am J Emerg Med.* 2003;21(5):441–443.

188. Greer IA. Effect of ketorolac tromethamine on hemostasis. *Pharmacotherapy.* 1990;10(6, pt 2):71S-76S.

189. Rinder HM, Tracey JB, Souhrada M, Wang C, Gagnier RP, Wood CC. Effects of meloxicam on platelet function in healthy adults: a randomized, double-blind, placebo-controlled trial. *J Clin Pharmacol.* 2002;42(8):881–886.

190. de Meijer A, Vollaard H, de Metz M, Verbruggen B, Thomas C, Novakova I. Meloxicam, 15 mg/day, spares platelet function in healthy volunteers. *Clin Pharmacol Ther.* 1999;66(4):425–430.

191. Kotwal RS, O'Connor KC, Johnson TR, Mosely DS, Meyer DE, Holcomb JB. A novel pain management strategy for combat casualty care. *Ann Emerg Med.* 2004;44(2):121–127.

192. Wedmore IS, Johnson T, Czarnik J, Hendrix S. Pain management in the wilderness and operational setting. *Emerg Med Clin North Am.* 2005;23(2):585–601, xi-xii.

193. Schwartz RB, Charity BM. Use of night vision goggles and low-level light source in obtaining intravenous access in tactical conditions of darkness. *Mil Med.* 2001;166(11):982–983.

194. Lind GH, Marcus MA, Mears SL, et al. Oral transmucosal fentanyl citrate for analgesia and sedation in the emergency department. *Ann Emerg Med*. 1991;20(10):1117–1120.

195. Gauna AA, Kang SK, Triano ML, Swatko ER, Vanston VJ. Oral transmucosal fentanyl citrate for dyspnea in terminally ill patients: an observational case series. *J Palliat Med*. 2008;11(4):643–648.

196. Collado F, Torres LM. Association of transdermal fentanyl and oral transmucosal fentanyl citrate in the treatment of opioid naive patients with severe chronic noncancer pain. *J Opioid Manag*. 2008;4(2):111–115.

197. Mahar PJ, Rana JA, Kennedy CS, Christopher NC. A randomized clinical trial of oral transmucosal fentanyl citrate versus intravenous morphine sulphate for initial control of pain in children with extremity injuries. *Pediatric Emerg Care*. 2007;23(8):544–548.

198. MacIntyre PA, Margetts L, Larsen D, Barker L. Oral transmucosal fentanyl citrate versus placebo for painful dressing changes: a crossover trial. *J Wound Care*. 2007;16(3):118–121.

199. Aronoff GM, Brennan MJ, Pritchard DD, Ginsberg B. Evidence-based oral transmucosal fentanyl citrate (OTFC) dosing guidelines. *Pain Med*. 2005;6(4):305–314.

200. Landy SH. Oral transmucosal fentanyl citrate for the treatment of migraine headache pain in outpatients: a case series. *Headache*. 2004;44(8):762–766.

201. Weiss EA. Medical considerations for the wilderness and adventure travelers. *Med Clin North Am*. 1999;83(4): 885–902, v-vi.

202. U.S. Food and Drug Administration (FDA) Center for Drug Evaluation and Research. NDA 20–747: Clinical Pharmacology and Biopharmaceutics Review of Actiq (Oral Transmucosal Fentanyl Citrate). Rockville, MD: FDA; 1997. http://www.accessdata.fda.gov/drugsatfda_docs/label/2011/20747orig1s029rems.pdf. Accessed August 15, 2013.

203. Lee M, Kern SE, Kisicki JC, Egan TD. A pharmacokinetic study to compare two simultaneous 400 microg doses with a single 800 microg dose of oral transmucosal fentanyl citrate. *J Pain Symptom Manage*. 2003;26(2):743–747.

204. Kacprowicz R, Johnson T, Mosely D. Fentanyl for pain control in special operations. *J Spec Oper Med*. 2008;8(1):48–53.

205. Wedmore IS, Kotwal RS, McManus JG, et al. Safety and efficacy of oral transmucosal fentanyl citrate for prehospital pain control on the battlefield. *J Trauma Acute Care Surg*. 2012;73(6)(suppl 5):S490-S495.

206. Dickey N. Prehospital use of ketamine in battlefield analgesia 2012–03. Defense Health Board Memorandum. March 8, 2012. http://health.mil/dhb/recommendations/2012/2012-03.pdf. Accessed August 14, 2013.

207. Kelly JF, Ritenour AE, McLaughlin DF, et al. Injury severity and causes of death from Operation Iraqi Freedom and Operation Enduring Freedom: 2003–2004 versus 2006. *J Trauma*. 2008;64(2)(suppl):S21-S26.

208. Jennings PA, Cameron P, Bernard S, et al. Morphine and ketamine is superior to morphine alone for out-of-hospital trauma analgesia: a randomized controlled trial. *Ann Emerg Med*. 2012;59(6):497–503.

209. Alonso-Serra HM, Weslet K; National Association of EMS Physicians Standards and Clinical Practices Committee. Prehospital pain management. *Prehosp Emerg Care*. 2003;7(4):482–488.

210. Cherry DA, Plummer JL, Gourlay GK, Coates KR, Odgers CL. Ketamine as an adjunct to morphine in the treatment of pain. *Pain*. 1995;62(1):119–121.

211. Howes MC. Ketamine for paediatric sedation/analgesia in the emergency department. *Emerg Med J*. 2004;21(3):275–280.

212. Porter K. Ketamine in prehospital care. *Emerg Med J*. 2004;21(3): 351–354.

213. Jennings PA, Cameron P, Bernard S. Ketamine as an analgesic in the pre-hospital setting: a systematic review. *Acta Anaesthiol Scand*. 2011;55(6):638–643.

214. Gaydos SJ, Webb CM, Walters PL, King MR, Wildzunas RM. Comparison of the Effects of Ketamine and Morphine on the Performance of Representative Military Tasks. U.S. Army Aeromedical Research Laboratory Report No. 2010–17. http://www.dtic.mil/cgi-bin/GetTRDoc?AD=ADA528747. Published August 2010. Accessed August 14, 2013.

215. Craven R. Ketamine. *Anaesthesia*. 2007;62(suppl 1):48–53.

216. White PF, Way WL, Trevor AJ. Ketamine-its pharmacology and therapeutic uses. *Anesthesiology*. 1982;56(2):119–136.

217. Subramaniam K, Subramaniam B, Steinbrook RA. Ketamine as adjuvant analgesic to opioids: a quantitative and qualitative systematic review. *Anesth Analg*. 2004;99(2):482–495.

218. Porter K. Ketamine in prehospital care. *Emerg Med J*. 2004; 21(3):351–354.

219. Naval Operational Medical Lessons Learned Center. Combat Medical Personnel Evaluation of Battlefield Trauma Care Equipment Initial Report. November 2011http://www.medicalsci.com/files/jan_2012_newsletter_final.pdf. Accessed August 14, 2013.

220. Schmid RL, Sandler AN, Katz J. Use and efficacy of low-dose ketamine in the management of acute postoperative pain: a review of current techniques and outcomes. *Pain*. 1999;82(2):111–125.

221. Buvanendran A, Kroin J. Multimodal analgesia for controlling acute postoperative pain. *Curr Opin Anesthesiol*. 2009;22(5):588–593.

222. Black IH, McManus J. Pain management in current combat operations. *Prehosp Emerg Care*. 2009;13(2):223–227.

223. Burnett AM, Salzmann JG, Griffith KR, Kroeger B, Frascone RJ. The emergency department experience with prehospital ketamine: a case series of 13 patients. *Prehosp Emerg Care*. 2012;16(4):553–559.

224. Roback MG, Wathen JE, Bajaj L, Bothner JP. Adverse events associated with procedural sedation in a pediatric emergency department: a comparison of common parenteral drugs. *Acad Emerg Med*. 2005;12(6):508–513.

225. Ketamine Hydrochloride Injection, USP [package insert]. Lake Forest, IL: Bioniche Pharma USA LLC; 2008

226. Guldner GT, Petinaux B, Clemens P, Foster S, Antoine S. Ketamine for procedural sedation and analgesia by nonanesthesiologists in the field: a review for military health care providers. *Mil Med*. 2006;171(6):484–490.

227. Poole LT. Army progress with penicillin. *Br J Surg*. 1944;32(125): 110–111.

228. Scott R Jr. Care of the battle casualty in advance of the aid station. Medical Science Publication No. 4, Volume 1. US Army Medical Department Office of Medical History website. http://history.amedd.army.mil/booksdocs/korea/recad1/ch1–4.html. Accessed August 15, 2013.

229. O'Connor K, Butler F. Antibiotics in tactical combat casualty care 2002. *Mil Med*. 2003;168(11):911–914.

230. Mellor SG, Cooper GJ, Bowyer GW. Efficacy of delayed administration of benzylpenicillin in the control of infection in penetrating soft tissue injuries in war. *J Trauma*. 1996;40(suppl 3):S128–S134.

231. Hospenthal DR, Murray CK, Anderson RC, et al. Guidelines for prevention of infection after combat-related injuries. *J Trauma*. 2008;64(3)(suppl):S211–S220.

232. Tarpey MJ. Tactical Combat Casualty Care in Operation Iraqi Freedom. *US Army Med Dep J.* April-June 2005;38–41.

233. Hospenthal DR, Murray CK, Andersen RC, et al. Guidelines for the prevention of infections associated with combat-related injuries: 2011 update: endorsed by the Infectious Diseases Society of America and the Surgical Infection Society. *J Trauma.* 2011;71 (2 Suppl 2):S210–234.

234. Yamada C, Nagashima K, Takahashi A, et al. Gatifloxacin acutely stimulates insulin secretion and chronically suppresses insulin biosynthesis. *Eur J Pharmacol.* 2006;553(1–3):67–72.

235. Battistella FD, Nugent W, Owings JT, Anderson JT. Field triage of the pulseless trauma patient. *Arch Surg.* 1999;134(7):742–745.

236. Branney SW, Moore EE, Feldhaus KM, Wolfe RE. Critical analysis of two decades of experience with postinjury emergency department thoracotomy in a regional trauma center. *J Trauma.* 1988;45(1):87–94.

237. Rosemurgy AS, Norris PA, Olson SM, Hurst JM, Albrink MH. Prehospital traumatic cardiac arrest: the cost of futility. *J Trauma.* 1993;35(3):468–473.

238. Wieneke H, Konorza T, Breuckmann F, Reinsch N, Erbel R. Automatic external defibrillator—mode of operation and clinical use (in German). *Dtsch Med Wochenschr.* 2008;133(42):2163–2167.

239. De Maio VJ, Stiell IG, Wells GA, Spaite DW; Ontario Prehospital Advanced Life Support Study Group. Optimal defibrillation response intervals for maximum out-of-hospital cardiac arrest survival rates. *Ann Emerg Med.* 2003;42(2):242–250.

240. Kotwal RS, Butler FK, Edgar EP, Shackelford SA, Bennett DR, Bailey JA. Saving lives on the battlefield: a Joint Trauma System review of pre-hospital trauma care in Combined Joint Operating Area—Afghanistan (CJOA-A) Executive Summary. *J Spec Oper Med.* 2013;13(1):77–85.January 30, 2013. http://www.stormingmedia.us/44/4473/A447375.html. Accessed August 28, 2013.

241. Wilensky G, Holcomb J. Tactical Combat Casualty Care and Minimizing Preventable Fatalities in Combat. Defense Health Board Memorandum. August 6, 2009. http://health.mil/dhb/recommendations/2009/2009–05.pdf. Accessed August 27, 2013.

SPECIFIC SKILLS

Hemorrhage Control

Combat Gauze

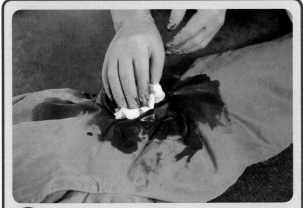

1. Expose the injury by opening or cutting away the casualty's clothing. If possible, remove excess blood from the wound while preserving any clots that may have formed. Locate the source of the most active bleeding.

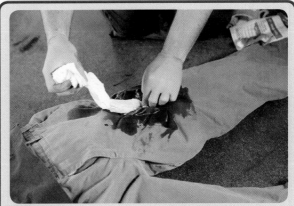

2. Remove the Combat Gauze from its sterile package and pack it tightly into the wound directly over the site of the most active bleeding. More than one gauze package may be required to control the hemorrhage. Combat Gauze may be repacked or adjusted in the wound to ensure proper placement.

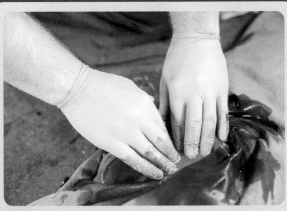

3. Quickly apply pressure until bleeding stops. Hold continuous pressure for at least 3 minutes. Reassess to ensure bleeding is controlled. Combat Gauze may be repacked or a second gauze used if initial application fails to provide hemostasis.

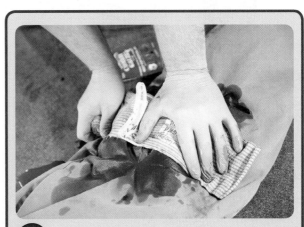

4. Leave Combat Gauze in place. Wrap to effectively secure the dressing in the wound. Although the Emergency Trauma Bandage is shown in this picture, the wound may be secured with any compression bandage, Ace wrap, roller gauze, or cravat.

SPECIFIC SKILLS

Pyng FAST-1®

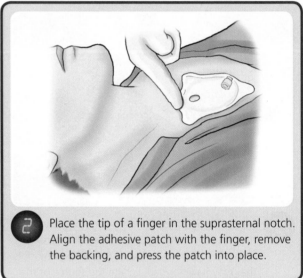

1 Prepare the site using aseptic technique.

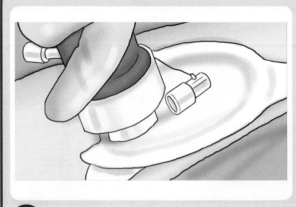

2 Place the tip of a finger in the suprasternal notch. Align the adhesive patch with the finger, remove the backing, and press the patch into place.

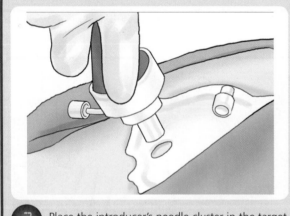

3 Place the introducer's needle cluster in the target opening, holding the introducer perpendicular to the manubrium. Keep forearm and wrist in line with the introducer.

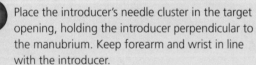

4 Apply steadily increasing pressure until the introducer releases.

SPECIFIC SKILLS

Pyng FAST-1® (continued)

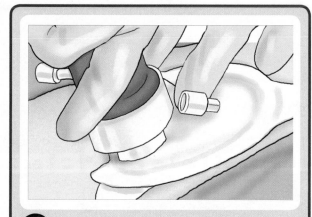

5 Remove the introducer by pulling straight back. Cover the introducer's needle cluster with the supplied plastic safety cap.

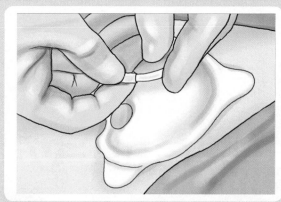

6 Connect the infusion tube to the tube on the target patch. Assure patency by using a syringe to aspirate marrow.

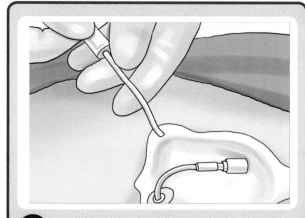

7 Connect the IV line to the target patch tube. Open the IV line to assure free flow. Be sure to flush the IO line with 10 ml of fluid to clear the bone plug from the device.

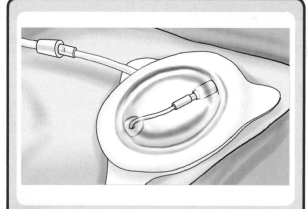

8 Place the protective dome over the target patch and connected tubes. It is held in place by a Velcro ring.

CHAPTER

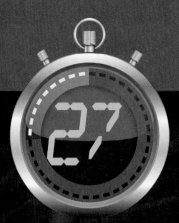

27

Tactical Evacuation Care

CHAPTER OBJECTIVES

At the completion of this chapter, the reader will be able to do the following:

- Delineate the scope of Tactical Evacuation (TACEVAC) Care and its inclusion of both Casualty Evacuation (CASEVAC) and Medical Evacuation (MEDEVAC).

- Describe the additional interventions and modified management strategies that may be indicated during TACEVAC given the increased stability of the circumstances and the additional personnel

and equipment that should be available in the Tactical Evacuation phase as compared to Tactical Field Care.

- Define the indications for transfusions in the field, and discuss the requirement to do so under protocol.

- Describe the management of wounded hostile combatants during TACEVAC.

SCENARIO

You are a medic aboard a MEDEVAC Blackhawk that has landed in a secure landing zone (LZ) in the mountains of southeastern Afghanistan to extract a Ranger who has multiple shrapnel wounds from a rocket-propelled grenade (RPG) blast. The LZ altitude is 6,000 feet, and the ambient temperature is 64°F (18°C). The casualty, who has been stabilized by the platoon medic, is able to converse normally and has a tourniquet over his uniform on his upper right thigh. His right shirt sleeve is missing, and there is a pressure dressing around his right upper arm. There is a saline lock in his left antecubital fossa.

The platoon medic tells you that the casualty lost a lot of blood from his thigh wound and was drowsy and confused before the tourniquet was applied 30 minutes ago. He received 500 milliliters of Hextend, to which he responded well, and has been stable since. The wound with the pressure dressing was packed with Combat Gauze underneath. He has taken moxifloxacin 400 milligrams by mouth and has an 800-microgram fentanyl lozenge in his right cheek. He has been drinking water from his canteen.

1. **What are your considerations for the care of this casualty during the 30-minute helicopter flight back to the Combat Support Hospital?**

2. **What do you do first?**

3. **What do you do next?**

4. **Should you start an intravenous (IV) line through the saline lock in anticipation of the need for a second bolus of Hextend?**

5. **Should you remove the tourniquet?**

6. **Should you remove the fentanyl lozenge?**

7. **What else do you want to do?**

8. **Is there anything else to attend to during the flight to the Combat Support Hospital?**

Introduction

The term **Casualty Evacuation**, or "CASEVAC," is used to describe the unregulated movement of casualties from the point of wounding to the first point of advanced medical care (a Role 2 Forward Surgical Team or higher). CASEVAC platforms are typically armed tactical assets that bear no Red Cross markings. These are often aircraft, vehicles, or boats of opportunity. During the drive on Baghdad in Operation Iraqi Freedom, some casualties were moved to the rear on tanks because use of Medical Evacuation aircraft and vehicles was not feasible given the tactical circumstances.

The term **Medical Evacuation**, or "MEDEVAC," refers to medically regulated casualty movement using dedicated medical evacuation platforms (ground vehicles, rotary wing aircraft, etc.). These are crewed by medical attendants and often have more medical treatment equipment available than nonmedical assets. MEDEVAC platforms are predesignated assets that bear Red Cross markings and no offensive weaponry such as rockets or missiles. MEDEVAC movements may include both clearing casualties from the battlefield and moving casualties between medical treatment facilities.

Since casualty movement following Tactical Field Care may be either CASEVAC or MEDEVAC, the third phase of care in Tactical Combat Casualty Care (TCCC) is designated Tactical Evacuation (TACEVAC) to encompass both types of platforms.

In contrast, the term **aeromedical evacuation** is typically used to describe the aeromedical transfer of casualties between medical treatment facilities in theater or to the Role 4 hospital in Landstuhl. Aeromedical evacuation is beyond the scope of TCCC, but will be discussed in the Aeromedical Evacuation in a Combat Theater chapter. **En route care** is a more general term that includes all of the above types of casualty transport.

Evacuation of the wounded from the battlefield using ground, air, or maritime platforms presents an opportunity to bring in additional medical equipment and personnel. This allows for the expanded monitoring and therapeutic measures outlined in the TCCC Guidelines for the TACEVAC phase **(Figure 27-1)**. For example, the TACEVAC provider may have at his or her disposal more options for airway management, fluid resuscitation, and prevention of hypothermia than were available in Care Under Fire or Tactical Field Care. As noted in the 2012 TCCC update paper[1]:

> Recent reviews of this topic have offered the possibility for significant improvements in care through providing evacuation providers trained to at least the critical care flight paramedic level, ensuring that blood and plasma are available for casualties in hemorrhagic shock, using the most capable evacuation platforms available, ensuring TCCC training for all evacuation providers, and having advanced airway options, intravenously administered medications, and other interventions routinely available for critical casualties.[2-7]

The survival advantage has been found to be the greatest, as would be expected, in the subset of casualties with severe but not overwhelming injuries.[5]

The order of the elements of care in TACEVAC listed in Figure 27-1 presupposes that life-threatening hemorrhage has been successfully addressed previously in the casualty's care. If this is not the case, then hemorrhage control should take first precedence in TACEVAC as well.

Figure 27-1　Basic Management Plan for Tactical Evacuation* Care (October 28th, 2013)

1. Airway Management
   a. Unconscious casualty without airway obstruction:
      - Chin lift or jaw thrust maneuver
      - Nasopharyngeal airway
      - Place casualty in the recovery position
   b. Casualty with airway obstruction or impending airway obstruction:
      - Chin lift or jaw thrust maneuver
      - Nasopharyngeal airway
      - Allow casualty to assume any position that best protects the airway, to include sitting up.
      - Place unconscious casualty in the recovery position.
      - If above measures unsuccessful:
        - Supraglottic airway or
        - Endotracheal intubation or
        - Surgical cricothyroidotomy (with lidocaine if conscious).
   c. Spinal immobilization is not necessary for casualties with penetrating trauma.
2. Breathing
   a. In a casualty with progressive respiratory distress and known or suspected torso trauma, consider a tension pneumothorax and decompress the chest on the side of the injury with a 14-gauge, 3.25 inch needle/catheter unit inserted in the second intercostal space at the midclavicular line. Ensure that the needle entry into the chest is not medial to the nipple line and is not directed towards the heart. An acceptable alternate site is the 4th or 5th intercostal space at the anterior axillary line (AAL).
   b. Consider chest tube insertion if no improvement and/or long transport is anticipated.
   c. Most combat casualties do not require supplemental oxygen, but administration of oxygen may be of benefit for the following types of casualties:
      - Low oxygen saturation by pulse oximetry
      - Injuries associated with impaired oxygenation
      - Unconscious casualty
      - Casualty with TBI (maintain oxygen saturation > 90%)
      - Casualty in shock
      - Casualty at altitude
   d. All open and/or sucking chest wounds should be treated by immediately applying a vented chest seal to cover the defect. If a vented chest seal is not available, use a non-vented chest seal. Monitor the casualty for the potential development of a subsequent tension pneumothorax. If the casualty develops increasing hypoxia, respiratory distress, or hypotension and a tension pneumothorax is suspected, treat by burping or removing the dressing or by needle decompression.
3. Bleeding
   a. Assess for unrecognized hemorrhage and control all sources of bleeding. If not already done, use a CoTCCC-recommended tourniquet to control life-threatening external hemorrhage that is anatomically amenable to tourniquet application or for any traumatic amputation. Apply directly to the skin 2–3 inches above wound.
   b. For compressible hemorrhage not amenable to tourniquet use or as an adjunct to tourniquet removal (if evacuation time is anticipated to be longer than two hours), use Combat Gauze as the hemostatic agent of choice. Combat Gauze should be applied with at least 3 minutes of direct pressure. Before releasing any tourniquet on a casualty who has been resuscitated for hemorrhagic shock, ensure a positive response to resuscitation efforts (i.e., a peripheral pulse normal in character and normal mentation if there is no TBI.) If the bleeding site is appropriate for use of a junctional tourniquet, immediately apply a CoTCCC-recommended junctional tourniquet. Do not delay in the application of the junctional tourniquet once it is ready for use. Combat Gauze applied with direct pressure should be used if a junctional tourniquet is not available or while the junctional tourniquet is being readied for use.

(Continues on next page)

Figure 27-1   Basic Management Plan for Tactical Evacuation* Care (October 28th, 2013) (*Continued*)

c. Reassess prior tourniquet application. Expose wound and determine if tourniquet is needed. If so, move tourniquet from over uniform and apply directly to skin 2–3 inches above wound. If a tourniquet is not needed, use other techniques to control bleeding.

d. When time and the tactical situation permit, a distal pulse check should be accomplished. If a distal pulse is still present, consider additional tightening of the tourniquet or the use of a second tourniquet, side-by-side and proximal to the first, to eliminate the distal pulse.

e. Expose and clearly mark all tourniquet sites with the time of tourniquet application. Use an indelible marker.

4. Intravenous (IV) access
   a. Reassess need for IV access.
      - If indicated, start an 18-gauge IV or saline lock
      - If resuscitation is required and IV access is not obtainable, use intraosseous (IO) route.

5. Tranexamic Acid (TXA)
   If a casualty is anticipated to need significant blood transfusion (for example: presents with hemorrhagic shock, one or more major amputations, penetrating torso trauma, or evidence of severe bleeding):
   - Administer 1 gram of tranexamic acid in 100 cc Normal Saline or Lactated Ringers as soon as possible but NOT later than 3 hours after injury.
   - Begin second infusion of 1 gm TXA after Hextend or other fluid treatment.

6. Traumatic Brain Injury (TBI)
   a. Casualties with moderate/severe TBI should be monitored for:
      - Decreases in level of consciousness
      - Pupillary dilation
      - SBP should be >90 mmHg
      - O2 sat > 90
      - Hypothermia
      - PCO2 (If capnography is available, maintain between 35–40 mmHg)
      - Penetrating head trauma (if present, administer antibiotics)
      - Assume a spinal (neck) injury until cleared.
   b. Unilateral pupillary dilation accompanied by a decreased level of consciousness may signify impending cerebral herniation; if these signs occur, take the following actions to decrease intracranial pressure:
      - Administer 250 cc of 3% or 5% hypertonic saline bolus.

- Elevate the casualty's head 30 degrees.
- Hyperventilate the casualty.
   a. Respiratory rate 20
   b. Capnography should be used to maintain the end-tidal CO_2 between 30–35
   c. The highest oxygen concentration (FIO_2) possible should be used for hyperventilation.

Notes:
- Do not hyperventilate unless signs of impending herniation are present.
- Casualties may be hyperventilated with oxygen using the bag-valve-mask technique.

7. Fluid resuscitation
   Reassess for hemorrhagic shock (altered mental status in the absence of brain injury and/or change in pulse character.) If (BP) monitoring is available, maintain target systolic BP 80–90 mmHg.
   a. If not in shock:
      - No IV fluids necessary.
      - PO fluids permissible if conscious and can swallow.
   b. If in shock and blood products are not available:
      - Hextend 500-mL IV bolus
      - Repeat after 30 minutes if still in shock.
      - Continue resuscitation with Hextend or crystalloid solution as needed to maintain target BP or clinical improvement.
   c. If in shock and blood products are available under an approved command or theater protocol:
      - Resuscitate with 2 units of plasma followed by packed red blood cells (PRBCs) in a 1:1 ratio. If blood component therapy is not available, transfuse fresh whole blood. Continue resuscitation as needed to maintain target BP or clinical improvement.
   d. If a casualty with an altered mental status due to suspected TBI has a weak or absent peripheral pulse, resuscitate as necessary to maintain a palpable radial pulse. If BP monitoring is available, maintain target systolic BP of at least 90 mmHg.

8. Prevention of hypothermia
   a. Minimize casualty's exposure to the elements. Keep protective gear on or with the casualty if feasible.
   b. Replace wet clothing with dry if possible. Get the casualty onto an insulated surface as soon as possible.
   c. Apply the Ready-Heat Blanket from the Hypothermia Prevention and Management Kit (HPMK) to the casualty's torso (not directly on the skin) and cover the casualty with the Heat-Reflective Shell (HRS).

(*Continues on next page*)

Figure 27-1 Basic Management Plan for Tactical Evacuation* Care (October 28th, 2013) *(Continued)*

d. If an HRS is not available, the previously recommended combination of the Blizzard Survival Blanket and the Ready Heat blanket may also be used.

e. If the items mentioned above are not available, use poncho liners, sleeping bags, or anything that will retain heat and keep the casualty dry.

f. Use a portable fluid warmer capable of warming all IV fluids including blood products.

g. Protect the casualty from wind if doors must be kept open.

9. Penetrating Eye Trauma

If a penetrating eye injury is noted or suspected:

a. Perform a rapid field test of visual acuity.

b. Cover the eye with a rigid eye shield (NOT a pressure patch).

c. Ensure that the 400 mg moxifloxacin tablet in the combat pill pack is taken, if possible, and that IV/IM antibiotics are given as outlined below if oral moxifloxacin cannot be taken.

10. Monitoring

Institute pulse oximetry and other electronic monitoring of vital signs, if indicated. All individuals with moderate/severe TBI should be monitored with pulse oximetry.

11. Inspect and dress known wounds if not already done.

12. Check for additional wounds.

13. Analgesia on the battlefield should generally be achieved using one of three options:

Option 1

Mild to Moderate Pain
Casualty is still able to fight
- TCCC Combat pill pack:
- Tylenol - 650-mg bilayer caplet, 2 PO every 8 hours
- Meloxicam - 15 mg PO once a day

Option 2

Moderate to Severe Pain
Casualty IS NOT in shock or respiratory distress AND
Casualty IS NOT at significant risk of developing either condition
- Oral transmucosal fentanyl citrate (OTFC) 800 ug
- Place lozenge between the cheek and the gum
- Do not chew the lozenge

Option 3

Moderate to Severe Pain
Casualty IS in hemorrhagic shock or respiratory distress OR

Casualty IS at significant risk of developing either condition
- Ketamine 50 mg IM or IN
Or
- Ketamine 20 mg slow IV or IO
  - Repeat doses q30min prn for IM or IN
  - Repeat doses q20min prn for IV or IO
  - End points: Control of pain or development of nystagmus
    (rhythmic back-and-forth movement of the eyes)

*Analgesia notes

a. Casualties may need to be disarmed after being given OTFC or ketamine.

b. Document a mental status exam using the AVPU method prior to administering opioids or ketamine.

c. For all casualties given opioids or ketamine – monitor airway, breathing, and circulation closely

d. Directions for administering OTFC:
- Recommend taping lozenge-on-a-stick to casualty's finger as an added safety measure OR utilizing a safety pin and rubber band to attach the lozenge (under tension) to the patients uniform or plate carrier.
- Reassess in 15 minutes
- Add second lozenge, in other cheek, as necessary to control severe pain
- Monitor for respiratory depression

e. IV Morphine is an alternative to OTFC if IV access has been obtained
- 5 mg IV/IO
- Reassess in 10 minutes.
- Repeat dose every 10 minutes as necessary to control severe pain.
- Monitor for respiratory depression

f. Naloxone (0.4 mg IV or IM) should be available when using opioid analgesics.

g. Both ketamine and OTFC have the potential to worsen severe TBI. The combat medic, corpsman, or PJ must consider this fact in his or her analgesic decision, but if the casualty is able to complain of pain, then the TBI is likely not severe enough to preclude the use of ketamine or OTFC.

h. Eye injury does not preclude the use of ketamine. The risk of additional damage to the eye from using ketamine is low and maximizing the casualty's chance for survival takes precedence if the casualty is in shock or respiratory distress or at significant risk for either.

(Continues on next page)

Figure 27-1 Basic Management Plan for Tactical Evacuation* Care (October 28th, 2013) (Continued)

i. Ketamine may be a useful adjunct to reduce the amount of opioids required to provide effective pain relief. It is safe to give ketamine to a casualty who has previously received morphine or OTFC. IV Ketamine should be given over 1 minute.

j. If respirations are noted to be reduced after using opioids or ketamine, provide ventilatory support with a bag-valve-mask or mouth-to-mask ventilations.

k. Promethazine, 25 mg IV/IM/IO every 6 hours may be given as needed for nausea or vomiting.

l. Reassess – reassess – reassess!

14. Reassess fractures and recheck pulses.

15. Antibiotics: recommended for all open combat wounds

   a. If able to take PO:
   - Moxifloxacin, 400 mg PO once a day

   b. If unable to take PO (shock, unconsciousness):
   - Cefotetan, 2 gm IV (slow push over 3-5 minutes) or IM every 12 hours,
   or
   - Ertapenem, 1 gm IV/IM once a day

16. Burns**

   a. Facial burns, especially those that occur in closed spaces, may be associated with inhalation injury. Aggressively monitor airway status and oxygen saturation in such patients and consider early surgical airway for respiratory distress or oxygen desaturation.

   b. Estimate total body surface area (TBSA) burned to the nearest 10% using the Rule of Nines.

   c. Cover the burn area with dry, sterile dressings. For extensive burns (>20%), consider placing the casualty in the Heat-Reflective Shell or Blizzard Survival Blanket from the Hypothermia Prevention Kit in order to both cover the burned areas and prevent hypothermia.

   d. Fluid resuscitation (USAISR Rule of Ten)
   - If burns are greater than 20% of Total Body Surface Area, fluid resuscitation should be initiated as soon as IV/IO access is established. Resuscitation should be initiated with Lactated Ringer's, normal saline, or Hextend. If Hextend is used, no more than 1000 ml should be given, followed by Lactated Ringer's or normal saline as needed.
   - Initial IV/IO fluid rate is calculated as %TBSA x 10cc/hr for adults weighing 40–80 kg.
   - For every 10 kg ABOVE 80 kg, increase initial rate by 100 ml/hr.
   - If hemorrhagic shock is also present, resuscitation for hemorrhagic shock takes precedence over resuscitation for burn shock. Administer IV/IO fluids per the TCCC Guidelines in Section 7.

   e. Analgesia in accordance with TCCC Guidelines in Section 13 may be administered to treat burn pain.

   f. Prehospital antibiotic therapy is not indicated solely for burns, but antibiotics should be given per TCCC guidelines in Section 15 if indicated to prevent infection in penetrating wounds.

   g. All TCCC interventions can be performed on or through burned skin in a burn casualty.

   h. Burn patients are particularly susceptible to hypothermia. Extra emphasis should be placed on barrier heat loss prevention methods and IV fluid warming in this phase.

17. The Pneumatic Antishock Garment (PASG) may be useful for stabilizing pelvic fractures and controlling pelvic and abdominal bleeding. Application and extended use must be carefully monitored. The PASG is contraindicated for casualties with thoracic or brain injuries.

18. CPR in TACEVAC Care

   a. Casualties with torso trauma or polytrauma who have no pulse or respirations during TACEVAC should have bilateral needle decompression performed to ensure they do not have a tension pneumothorax. The procedure is the same as described in section 2 above.

   b. CPR may be attempted during this phase of care if the casualty does not have obviously fatal wounds and will be arriving at a facility with a surgical capability within a short period of time. CPR should not be done at the expense of compromising the mission or denying lifesaving care to other casualties.

19. Documentation of Care

   Document clinical assessments, treatments rendered, and changes in the casualty's status on a TCCC Casualty Card (**DD Form 1380**). Forward this information with the casualty to the next level of care.

*The new term "Tactical Evacuation" (TACEVAC) includes both Casualty Evacuation (CASEVAC) and Medical Evacuation (MEDEVAC) as defined in Joint Publication 4–02.

**See the Treatment of Burn Casualties in Tactical Combat Casualty Care, for discussion of this guideline.

Airway

The opportunity to carry additional equipment and work in a more secure environment allows for an expanded range of therapeutic airway interventions. Endotracheal intubation and supraglottic airways (SGAs)[8–10] are all potentially feasible airway alternatives in this phase if the nasopharyngeal airway is insufficient to manage the airway. SGAs may be especially useful in the subset of patients who are unconscious, but have no direct maxillofacial trauma that results in airway obstruction.[11] Schwartz and colleagues reported success in performing endotracheal intubation with the aid of night-vision goggles.[12] Most airway fatalities in combat are related to maxillofacial trauma, and airway problems in this setting may be best managed by allowing the casualty to maintain the sit-up-and-lean-forward position, as mentioned in the Tactical Field Care chapter, unless requirements for spinal immobilization preclude this option. A surgical airway remains a valuable option if the individual providing care has the requisite skill and the other measures previously described have failed or are not feasible.[13]

Decreased pressure at altitude will result in an increase in the volume of gas enclosed in spaces with flexible walls, such as air-filled cuffs in endotracheal tubes and SGAs. Saline should be used to inflate cuffs on devices used in casualties who will be transported in unpressurized aircraft. Medical providers on evacuation aircraft should check to ensure that this has been done, and relieve any altitude-related overpressure in cuffs that may have been filled with air by ground medics. Note that SGAs such as the I-Gel that have a gel-filled cuff do not require venting at altitude.

Breathing

Any gas trapped in the pleural space will also expand at altitude, thus increasing the risk of a tension pneumothorax. Casualties with chest trauma should be watched for respiratory distress, hypoxia, and/or hypotension with a high index of suspicion for tension pneumothorax. This is especially true for any casualty who has been treated for a sucking chest wound or has already been treated with needle thoracostomy. The use of vented chest seals as now recommended by TCCC should help to reduce the risk of tension pneumothorax in sucking chest wounds that have been treated with a chest seal.

Oxygen is often available on TACEVAC platforms. Many casualties do not require supplemental oxygen, but some conditions may warrant its use. Casualties with injuries that impair ventilation (unconsciousness) or gas exchange (inhalation injury or exposure to smoke or toxic fumes), casualties with blunt or penetrating pulmonary injury, casualties in shock, or any casualty with low oxygen saturation on pulse oximetry may benefit from supplemental oxygen.[14] Casualties being transported by air should be monitored for a drop in oxygen saturation due to the lower oxygen partial pressures at altitude.

As noted in the Tactical Field Care chapter, hypoxia in casualties with traumatic brain injury (TBI) is associated with unfavorable outcomes,[15] so casualties with moderate to severe TBI should be given supplemental oxygen, when available, to maintain an oxygen saturation of greater than 90%. Furthermore, hyperoxia causes cerebral vasoconstriction independently of the effects of hypocapnia and therefore may help to reduce intracranial pressure.[16,17] Hyperoxia has also been shown to increase cerebral tissue oxygenation[17] and to improve cerebral metabolism in casualties with severe head injury.[18–20] For casualties with moderate to severe TBI, then, supplemental oxygen should be given at the highest inspired fraction of oxygen achievable as early in the continuum of care as possible.[21]

Bleeding

Hemorrhage is the leading cause of preventable death in combat casualties.[22] Early and definitive control of external hemorrhage using TCCC principles has been shown to produce dramatic reductions in preventable deaths.[23] The TACEVAC phase usually offers an opportunity to reassess the casualty in a more controlled and stable environment. Assessment of wounds and hemorrhage control should be a priority in this phase as it may be the first opportunity to fully assess the severity and extent of wounds managed rapidly during the Care Under Fire and Tactical Field Care phases. To the extent possible, all areas of the casualty's body should be examined for additional wounds, and the adequacy of hemorrhage control measures previously employed should be reassessed. The same principles of hemorrhage control should be employed, including the use of tourniquets and Combat Gauze.

In the TACEVAC phase, it is appropriate to reassess for the continued need of a tourniquet to achieve or maintain hemorrhage control. As noted previously, the presence of shock or an anticipated time of 2 hours or less from tourniquet placement until arrival at a medical treatment facility are contraindications to tourniquet removal in the field. If tourniquet removal is indicated, the wound should be exposed and Combat Gauze should be applied with direct pressure as outlined in the Tactical Field Care chapter. If a tourniquet remains necessary, it should be removed from over the uniform after replacing it with another tourniquet applied directly to the skin 2 to 3 inches above the wound.

As time and the tactical situation permit, a distal pulse check should be accomplished. If there is ongoing hemorrhage or a persistent distal pulse, the tourniquet should be tightened or a second tourniquet applied just proximal to the first.

The TACEVAC phase may also provide the first opportunity to employ junctional hemorrhage control devices as discussed in the Tactical Field Care chapter.[21,24,25]

Tranexamic Acid

Administration of tranexamic acid (TXA) has been shown to confer a survival benefit in bleeding patients. TXA should be administered as soon as possible when indicated, but not more than 3 hours after the injury was sustained.[26–28] The indications and directions for use are outlined in the Tactical Field Care chapter.

Fluid Resuscitation

Recent experience in resuscitating severely injured casualties who require massive transfusions (10 or more units of packed red blood cells [PRBCs]) has shown that infusing freshly thawed plasma and PRBCs in a 1:1 ratio increases survival.[29-33] Early (within the first 6 hours after injury) administration of freshly thawed plasma is critical to maximize casualty survival.[24] This practice (known as Damage Control Resuscitation (DCR)) helps to restore clotting factors lost due to bleeding and to improve coagulation status as well as to restore oxygen-carrying capability.[29,34-37]

Fluid resuscitation recommendations for TACEVAC were updated in 2010. For casualties who are in shock, the resuscitation option of choice is plasma and PRBCs administered in a 1:1 ratio, when use of these products is logistically feasible.[38,39] Both PRBCs and plasma are now routinely carried by the British Medical Emergency Rescue Teams (MERTs). PRBCs are carried and used by U.S. Air Force Pararescue teams (PEDRO) and by some U.S. Army MEDEVAC (DUSTOFF) units.[40] For many casualties, use of these products has improved hemodynamic stability during transport. The use of PRBCs and whole blood has a good safety profile in the deployed setting.[33]

Although the literature on DCR often discusses the use of platelets in addition to PRBCs and plasma, the use of platelets in the prehospital setting is not feasible given the blood-banking techniques currently present in theater. Blood component therapy initiated in the TACEVAC phase may be a factor in the increased survival noted in critically injured casualties in two studies on TACEVAC care and survival.[5,6] Decreased use of crystalloids in resuscitation has been associated with improved outcomes.[41,42]

In order to administer blood component therapy safely and effectively, the following elements must be in place:

1. Obtaining PRBCs and plasma for transport into prehospital settings must be logistically feasible in the area of operations.
2. A protocol must be in place that has been coordinated with the appropriate blood-banking facilities and approved by both theater and unit medical leadership.
3. Combat medical personnel must be well trained in the transfusion protocol.

The details of the protocol may vary depending on the maturity of the theater, service guidelines, the specific tactical scenario(s) envisioned, and the blood-banking logistics in the area of operations. In general, though, the following items should be addressed:

- Training of combat medical personnel in the protocol
- Documentation of this training
- Retraining interval
- Determination of which blood products will be used (PRBCs, plasma)
- Ratio of plasma and platelets to PRBC units infused
- Blood type (ABO and Rh) compatibility issues

- Transport container to be used
- Transport container handling instructions
- Storage temperature requirements
- Storage temperature documentation requirements
- Disposition of unused units upon return of containers
- Maximum time allowed for transport in a container
- Number and types of units to be transported
- Indications for transfusion
- Procedure for transfusion
- Equipment required
- Pretransfusion check of units
- Protective equipment required
- Transfusion rate
- Transfusion pressure
- Warming of units
- Monitoring during transfusion
- End points of resuscitation
- Management of transfusion reactions
- Documentation of transfusion

If plasma and PRBCs are not available, hypotensive resuscitation with Hextend should be carried out with an initial 500-mL bolus, followed by a second bolus in 30 minutes if clinically indicated, as outlined in the Tactical Field Care chapter.[39] If necessary, resuscitation may be continued with crystalloid solutions or additional Hextend in a casualty who has already received two 500-ml boluses of Hextend. Both Hextend and crystalloids replace intravascular volume but do not replace oxygen-carrying capacity or clotting factors. They also contribute to dilutional coagulopathy.

Combat medical personnel should always recognize the importance of hypotensive resuscitation in the setting of uncontrolled hemorrhage and avoid over-resuscitation. Blood pressure monitoring will typically be present on TACEVAC platforms. Regardless of the fluids used, resuscitation should be titrated to a target systolic blood pressure (BP) of 80 to 90 milliliters of mercury (mm Hg). If the casualty has sustained a TBI, however, the target systolic BP is at least 90 mm Hg.[39]

Electronic Monitoring

Casualty assessment is typically difficult inside TACEVAC platforms due to high noise and vibration levels and the need to avoid using lights at night for tactical safety reasons. For instance, helicopter transport impairs or precludes the ability of combat medical personnel to auscultate the lungs[43,44] and even to palpate the carotid pulse.[45] To provide for reliable assessment of the casualty's status during transport under such conditions, electronic monitoring should be available in this phase of TCCC. Electronic monitoring systems capable of reporting BP, heart rate, pulse oximetry, and capnography are commercially available and should be used during TACEVAC for seriously injured casualties. As an example, the presence of an esophageal intubation will need to be determined by a decrease in oxygen saturation or an absence of expired carbon dioxide since it will be impossible to hear breath sounds inside a noisy aircraft or vehicle.

A national sample of 250 air transport agencies reported that more than 75% of these agencies monitored oxygenation and ventilation during transport.[46] The significant effect of altitude on oxygenation **(Figure 27-2)** must be considered when interpreting pulse oximetry readings while operating in mountainous regions and during aircraft evacuation in airframes with unpressurized cabins.[47,48]

Traumatic Brain Injury in TACEVAC Care

Prevention of hypoxia and hypotension is especially important in casualties with TBI because these conditions may result in secondary injury to the traumatized brain. Casualties with moderate to severe TBI should be monitored carefully for:

- Decreases in level of consciousness
- Pupillary dilation
- Systolic BP maintained at greater than 90 mm Hg
- Oxygen saturation maintained at greater than 90%
- Hypothermia
- Partial pressure of carbon dioxide maintained within 35 to 40 mm Hg (if capnography is available)

If penetrating head trauma is present, antibiotics should be administered. Combat medical personnel should assume a cervical spine injury, until cleared, in TBI casualties when the mechanism of injury includes blunt trauma.[20]

Unilateral pupillary dilation accompanied by a decreased level of consciousness may signify impending cerebral herniation; if these signs occur, take the following actions to decrease intracranial pressure:

- Administer 250 cc of 3% or 5% hypertonic saline bolus.
- Elevate the casualty's head 30 degrees.
- Hyperventilate the casualty.
- Maintain a respiratory rate of 20 if capnography is not available.
- If capnography is available, maintain the end-tidal carbon dioxide between 30 and 35 mm Hg

Altitude	Oxygen Saturation
Sea level	97%
5000 feet	96%
8000 feet	93%
12,000 feet	86%

Figure 27-2 Approximate Pulse Oximetry Values for Healthy Volunteers at Altitude

Source: Courtesy of Dr. Frank Butler

Note that the highest oxygen concentration (FiO_2) possible should be used for hyperventilation. Do not hyperventilate casualties unless signs of impending herniation are present. Casualties may be hyperventilated with oxygen using a bag-mask.

Prevention of Hypothermia

Efforts to minimize heat loss should continue during TACEVAC Care. Given the potential for heat loss due to wind chill and the lower temperatures encountered at altitude, the casualty must be aggressively protected against cold stress during evacuation. Hypothermia may occur rapidly in conditions that expose the casualty to water, wind, and cold surfaces, such as the floor of a vehicle or aircraft in cooler environments **(Figure 27-3)**. Even in warm ambient temperatures, it is possible for the casualty to become significantly hypothermic if appropriate measures to preserve core temperature are not employed. Hypothermia prevention measures are discussed in the Tactical Field Care chapter. Casualties in shock are at increased risk of hypothermia since they are not able to generate body heat at a normal rate.

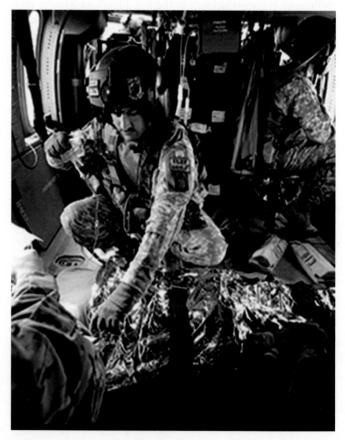

Figure 27-3 If helicopter doors stay open during flight, wind could cause casualties to become hypothermic during transport.

Source: U.S. Navy photo by Petty Officer Daniel Gay.

Analgesia

The use of appropriate analgesics should be continued in the TACEVAC phase of care. Remember that medications that impair platelet function should not be used in combat casualties. Oral transmucosal fentanyl citrate is a good option when the casualty is not in shock.[49,50] Remember also that opioids are contraindicated in casualties in hemorrhagic shock or with respiratory difficulty. Ketamine is a good option for casualties whose pain is severe but in whom opioids should not be used.[51]

Casualty Movement

Conventional litters should be available during TACEVAC. The casualty should be made as comfortable as possible on a litter and kept warm and dry. If an improvised litter is used, it should be padded, and any field-expedient materials used to treat the casualty should be replaced with conventional splints, tourniquets, and dressings as soon as feasible.

Cardiopulmonary Resuscitation During TACEVAC

The prognosis for trauma patients with prehospital cardiac arrest is very poor. As noted in the Tactical Field Care chapter, casualties with torso trauma or polytrauma who lose their pulse or respirations during TACEVAC should have bilateral needle decompression performed to ensure they do not have a tension pneumothorax.

Cardiopulmonary resuscitation (CPR) may be attempted during this phase of care if the casualty does not have obviously fatal wounds and will be arriving at a facility with a surgical capability within a short period of time. CPR should not be done at the expense of compromising the mission or denying lifesaving care to other casualties.[52]

If the evacuation platform has the appropriate personnel and equipment, resuscitative thoracostomy may be indicated if the casualty has a cardiopulmonary arrest during transport. A recent study noted that of 29 patients who arrested en route, 13 (44.8%) had a transient return of spontaneous circulation, with three 30-day survivors (10.3%).[53]

Care for Wounded Hostile Combatants

In the TACEVAC phase, the principles of care are the same for wounded hostile combatants as for coalition forces AFTER the prisoner security measures described in the Tactical Field Care chapter have been accomplished. The rules of engagement may dictate the evacuation process for wounded hostile combatants, but proper prisoner-handling procedures must be maintained throughout, with particular attention to restraint and security. Remember that each hostile combatant in custody represents a potential threat not only to combat medical personnel, but to the entire unit. Speed wounded enemy combatants to the rear as fast as medically and tactically feasible.

In an era in which hostile forces routinely use suicide bomber tactics, the concealment of improvised explosive devices (IEDs) on hostile combatant casualties or even on apparently friendly local national casualties is an additional concern. This has led some evacuation units to require that all noncoalition casualties be searched thoroughly for IEDs before they are loaded onto an evacuation platform.[54]

Summary

- Additional medical equipment and personnel should be provided in the Tactical Evacuation (TACEVAC) phase. This allows for an enhanced level of medical care compared to Care Under Fire and Tactical Field Care.
- Casualties with torso trauma should be monitored for respiratory distress with a high index of suspicion for tension pneumothorax. Expansion of intrapleural gas due to the lower pressure at altitude may result in a tension pneumothorax.
- Casualties with injuries that interfere with breathing, or who have a low oxygen saturation on pulse oximetry, or those who are in shock should be given oxygen during TACEVAC, if it is available.
- During the TACEVAC phase, a thorough examination for additional wounds should be performed. The adequacy of hemorrhage control measures previously employed should be reassessed and replaced or enhanced as needed.
- Fluid resuscitation should be continued as needed with the goal of maintaining a palpable peripheral pulse and normal mentation. If electronic blood pressure (BP) monitoring is available, resuscitate to a systolic BP of 80 to 90 mm HG.
- Plasma and packed red blood cells (PRBCs) administered in a 1:1 ratio should be used in this phase of care, if logistically feasible.

- Blood products, if used, must be administered by combat medical personnel trained in blood transfusion and under a preapproved protocol.
- Electronic monitoring systems capable of reporting BP, heart rate, pulse oximetry, and capnography should be used during evacuation.
- If a casualty with traumatic brain injury (TBI) is unconscious and has a weak or absent peripheral pulse, resuscitate as necessary to maintain a systolic BP of at least 90 mm Hg.
- Altitude significantly affects oxygenation in aircraft with unpressurized cabins, and this should be considered when interpreting pulse oximetry readings.
- Casualties with moderate to severe TBI should be monitored carefully for signs of impending cerebral herniation, and steps should be taken to lower intracranial pressure if decreasing level of consciousness and unilateral papillary dilation are noted.
- Casualties should be aggressively protected against hypothermia during evacuation.
- Proper prisoner-handling procedures should be maintained throughout the treatment and evacuation of wounded hostile combatants.
- All noncoalition casualties should be searched thoroughly for improvised explosive devices (IEDs) before being loaded onto an evacuation platform.

SCENARIO RECAP

You are a medic aboard a MEDEVAC Blackhawk that has landed in a secure LZ in the mountains of southeastern Afghanistan to extract a Ranger who has multiple shrapnel wounds from an RPG blast. The LZ altitude is 6,000 feet, and the ambient temperature is 64°F (18°C). The casualty, who has been stabilized by the platoon medic, is able to converse normally and has a tourniquet over his uniform on his upper right thigh. His right shirt sleeve is missing, and there is a pressure dressing around his right upper arm. There is a saline lock in his left antecubital fossa.

The platoon medic tells you that the casualty lost a lot of blood from his thigh wound and was drowsy and confused before the tourniquet was applied 30 minutes ago. He received 500 milliliters of Hextend, to which he responded well, and has been stable since. The wound with the pressure dressing was packed with Combat Gauze underneath. He has taken moxifloxacin 400 milligrams by mouth, and has an 800-microgram fentanyl lozenge in his right cheek. He has been drinking water from his canteen.

SCENARIO SOLUTION

1. **What are your considerations for the care of this casualty during the 30-minute helicopter flight back to the Combat Support Hospital?**

   This casualty is now apparently stable, but had been noted to be in hemorrhagic shock earlier.

2. **What do you do first?**

   You check all the pressure dressings and see no signs of bleeding from these wounds. You ensure that there are no other sites of major bleeding.

3. **What do you do next?**

   You next confirm that he is responsive; he answers questions appropriately and has a good radial pulse.

4. **Should you start an intravenous (IV) line through the saline lock in anticipation of the need for a second bolus of Hextend?**

   Yes, it is probably a good idea to start an IV line through the saline lock. You can run crystalloid at a keep-vein-open rate to keep the line open.

5. Should you remove the tourniquet?

No, you should not remove the tourniquet. Even though pressure dressings over Combat Gauze are present on the distal wounds, you will risk further bleeding by releasing the tourniquet's pressure, and the casualty will be at the emergency department within 2 hours of the tourniquet's application. It is better at this point not to remove the tourniquet. If feasible, you may replace it with another tourniquet applied directly to the skin 2 to 3 inches proximal to the site of the bleeding.

6. Should you remove the fentanyl lozenge?

You should remove the fentanyl lozenge, since the casualty was previously in shock. If the casualty's pain level requires analgesia, ketamine is a better analgesic option in casualties who are in or at risk for hemorrhagic shock.[50] Opiates may cause cardiorespiratory depression and must be used with caution in casualties who have recently been hypotensive or who are in danger of going into shock.

7. What else do you want to do?

You also want to establish electronic monitoring of the casualty. You place a pulse oximeter from the PROPAC on board the helicopter on a finger of the casualty's left hand. Pulse rate is 100 beats per minute, and oxygen saturation is 90%.

8. Is there anything else to attend to during the flight to the Combat Support Hospital?

Yes, you should be concerned about this level of oxygen saturation, but this decrease in oxygen saturation is likely due to the altitude. You will keep a careful eye on this during the flight. Administer supplemental oxygen as needed to maintain an oxygen saturation of 90% or higher. You should also keep the casualty warm during the flight to the Combat Support Hospital.

References

1. Butler FK, Blackbourne LH. Battlefield trauma care then and now: a decade of Tactical Combat Casualty Care. *J Trauma Acute Care Surg.* 2012;73(suppl):S395–S402.

2. Mabry RL. Memorandum for Record, United States Central Command Joint Theater Trauma System, After Action Report for MEDCOM Tasker 1039.01C, February 7, 2011. http://www.michaelyon-online.com/images/pdf/bm_oef_jtts_medevac_medical_director_aar__3.pdf. Accessed May 7, 2013.

3. Caravalho J. OTSG Dismounted Complex Blast Injury Task Force: Final Report. June 18, 2011:44–47.

4. Mabry R, Apodaca A, Penrod J, Orman J, Gerhardt R. Impact of critical care trained flight paramedics on casualty survival during helicopter evacuation in the current war in Afghanistan. *J Trauma Acute Care Surg.* 2012;73(suppl): S32–S37.

5. Morrison JJ, Oh J, Dubose JJ, O'Reilly DJ, et al. En-route care capability from point of injury impacts mortality after severe wartime injury. *Ann Surg.* 2013;257:330–334.

6. Apodaca A, Olson CM, Bailey J, Butler FK, Eastridge BJ, Kuncir E. Performance improvement evaluation of forward aeromedical evacuation platforms in Operation Enduring Freedom. *J Trauma Acute Care Surg.* 2013;75(2 Suppl 2):S157–S163.

7. Dickey N, Jenkins D, Butler F. Tactical Evacuation Care improvements within the Department of Defense. Defense Health Board Memo. August 8, 2011. http://health.mil/dhb/recommendations/2011/2011–03.pdf. Accessed May 7, 2013.

8. Martin SE, Ochsner G, Jarman RH, et al. Use of the laryngeal mask airway in air transport when intubation fails. *J Trauma.* 1999;47(2):352–357.

9. Joo HS, Kapoor S, Rose DK, Naik VN. The intubating mask airway after induction of general anesthesia versus awake fiber optic intubation in patients with difficult airways. *Anesth Analg.* 2001;92(5):1342–1346.

10. Blostein PA, Koestner AJ, Hoak S. Failed rapid sequence intubation in trauma patients: esophageal-tracheal Combitube is a useful adjunct. *J Trauma.* 1998;44:534–537.

11. Dickey N. Supraglottic airway use in Tactical Evacuation Care. Defense Health Board Memo. September 17, 2012. http://health.mil/dhb/recommendations/2012/2012–06.pdf. Accessed May 7, 2013.

12. Schwartz RB, Gillis WL, Miles RJ. Orotracheal intubation in darkness using night vision goggles. *Mil Med.* 2001;166:984–986.

13. Fortune JB, Judkins DG, Scanzaroli D, et al. Efficacy of prehospital surgical cricothyrotomy in trauma patients. *J Trauma.* 1997;42(5):832–836.

14. Grissom CK, Weaver LK, Clemmer TP, Morris AH. Theoretical advantage of oxygen treatment for combat casualties during medical evacuation at high altitude. *J Trauma.* 2006;61(2):461–467.

15. Chi JH, Knudson MM, Vassar MJ, et al. Prehospital hypoxia affects outcome in patients with traumatic brain injury: a prospective multicenter study. *J Trauma.* 2006;61(5):1134–1141.

16. Floyd T, Clark J, Gelfand R, et al. Independent cerebral vasoconstrictive effects of hyperoxia and accompanying arterial hypocapnia at 1 ATA. *J Appl Physiol.* 2003;95(6):2453–2461.

17. Tisdall M, Taylor C, Tachtisidis I, et al. The effect of cerebral tissue oxygenation index of changes in the concentrations of inspired oxygen and end-tidal carbon dioxide in healthy adult volunteers. *Anesth Analg.* 2009;109(3):906–913.

18. Tolias C, Reinert M, Seiler R, et al. Normobaric hyperoxia-induced improvement in cerebral metabolism and reduction in intracranial pressure in patients with severe head injury: a prospective historical cohort-matched study. *J Neurosurg.* 2004;101(3):435–444.

19. Tolias CM, Kumaria A, Bullock MR. Hyperoxia and traumatic brain injury. *J Neurosurg.* 2009;110(3):607–609.

20. Dickey N. Management of traumatic brain injury in Tactical Combat Casualty Care. Defense Health Board Memo. July 26, 2012. http://health.mil/dhb/recommendations/2012/2012–04.pdf. Accessed May 7, 2013.

21. Dickey N, Jenkins D. Combat Ready Clamp addition to the Tactical Combat Casualty Care Guidelines. Defense Health Board Memo. September 23, 2011.http://health.mil/dhb/recommendations/2011/2011–07.pdf. Accessed May 7, 2013.

22. Eastridge BJ, Mabry R, Seguin P, et al. Pre-hospital death on the battlefield: implications for the future of combat casualty care. *J Trauma Acute Care Surg.* 2012;73:S431–S437.

23. Kotwal RS, Montgomery HR, Kotwal BM, et al. Eliminating preventable death on the battlefield. *Arch Surgery.* 2011;146:1350–1358.

24. Tovmassian RV, Kragh JF, Dubick MA, Baer DG, Blackbourne LH. Combat Ready Clamp medic technique. *J Spec Ops Med.* 2012;12:72–78.

25. Dubick M, Kragh JF. Evaluation of the Combat Ready Clamp to control bleeding in human cadavers, manikins, swine femoral artery hemorrhage model and swine carcasses. U.S. Army Institute of Surgical Research Technical Report. June 2012.

26. Dickey N, Jenkins D. Recommendations regarding the addition of tranexamic acid to the Tactical Combat Casualty Care Guidelines. Defense Health Board Memo. September 23, 2011. http://health.mil/dhb/recommendations/2011/2011–06.pdf. Accessed May 7, 2013.

27. Morrison JJ, Dubose JJ, Rasmussen TE, Midwinter MJ. Military application of tranexamic acid in trauma emergency resuscitation study (MATTERs). *Arch Surg.* 2012;147(2):113–119.

28. CRASH-2 Collaborators. The importance of early treatment with tranexamic acid in bleeding trauma patients: an exploratory analysis of the CRASH-2 randomized controlled trial. *Lancet.* 2011;377: 1096–1101.

29. Holcomb JB, Wade CE, Michalek JE, et al. Improved plasma and platelet to red blood cell ratios improves outcome in 466 massively transfused civilian trauma patients. *Ann Surg.* 2008;248(3):447–458.

30. Streets CG. Lessons from the battlefield in the management of major trauma. *Br J Surg.* 2009;96(8):831–832.

31. Hess JR, Holcomb JB. Transfusion practice in military trauma. *Transfus Med.* 2008;18(3):143–150.

32. Beekley AC, Starnes BW, Sebesta JA. Lessons learned from modern military surgery. *Surg Clin N Am.* 2007;87(1):157–184.

33. Borgman MA, Spinella PC, Perkins JG, et al. The ratio of blood products transfused affects mortality in patients receiving massive transfusions at a combat support hospital. *J Trauma.* 63(4):805–813.

34. Zink KA, Sambasivan CN, Holcomb JB, Chisholm G, Schreiber MA. A high ratio of plasma and platelets to packed red blood cells in the first 6 hours of massive transfusion improves outcomes in a large multicenter study. *Am J Surg.* 2009;197(5):565–570.

35. Holcomb JB, Spinella PC. Optimal use of blood in trauma patients. *Biologicals.* 2010;38(1):72–77.

36. Holcomb JB. Damage control resuscitation. *J Trauma.* 2007;62: S36–S37.

37. Holcomb JB. Optimal use of blood products in severely injured trauma patients. *Hematology.* 2010;2010:465–469.

38. Hetzler MR, Risk G. Damage control resuscitation for the Special Forces medic: simplifying and improving prolonged trauma care: parts one and two. *J Spec Oper Med.* 2009;9(3):14–21, 53–62.

39. Lednar WM, Poland GA, Holcomb JB, Butler FK. Recommendations regarding the Tactical Combat Casualty Care Guidelines on fluid resuscitation. Defense Health Board Memo. December 10, 2010. http://health.mil/dhb/recommendations/2010/2010–06.pdf. Accessed May 7, 2013.

40. Kotwal RS, Butler FK, Edgar EP, Shackelford SA, Bennett DR, Bailey JA. Saving lives on the battlefield: a joint trauma system review of pre-hospital trauma care in combined joint operating area—Afghanistan (CJOA-A) Executive Summary. *J Spec Oper Med.* 2013;13(1):77–85.

41. Duke MD, Guidry C, Guice J, et al. Restrictive fluid resuscitation in combination with damage control resuscitation: time for adaptation. *J Trauma Acute Care Surg.* 2012;73:674–678.

42. Morrison CA, Carrick MM, Norman MA, et al. Hypotensive resuscitation strategy reduces transfusion requirements and severe postoperative coagulopathy in trauma patients with hemorrhagic shock: preliminary results of a randomized controlled trial. *J Trauma.* 2011:70:652–663.

43. Fromm RE Jr, Varon J. Air medical transport. *J Fam Pract.* 1993;36(3):313–318.

44. Fromm RE Jr, Dellinger RP. Transport of critically ill patients. *J Intensive Care Med.* 1992;7(5):223–233.

45. Hunt RC, Carroll RG, Whitley TW, Bryan-Berge DM, Dufresne DA. Adverse effect of helicopter flight on the ability to palpate carotid pulses. *Ann Emerg Med.* 1994;24(2):190–193.

46. Perez L, Klofas E, Wise L. Oxygenation/ventilation of transported intubated adult patients: a national survey of organizational practices. *Air Med J.* 2000;19(2):55–58.

47. Pilmanis AA. USSOCOM Biomedical Initiatives Steering Committee interim report. August 2004 (unpublished data).

48. Luks AM, Swenson ER. Pulse oximetry at high altitude. *High Alt Med Biol.* 2011;12:109–119.

49. Kotwal R, O'Connor KC, Johnson TR, Mosely DS, Meyer DE, Holcomb JB. A novel pain management strategy for combat casualty care. *Ann Emerg Med.* 2004;44:121–127.

50. Wedmore IS, Kotwal RS, McManus JG, et al. Safety and efficacy of oral transmucosal fentanyl citrate for prehospital pain control on the battlefield. *J Trauma Acute Care Surg.* 2012;73:S490–S495.

51. Dickey N. Prehospital use of ketamine in battlefield analgesia. Defense Health Board Memo. March 8, 2012. http://health.mil/dhb/recommendations/2012/2012–03.pdf. Accessed May 8, 2013.

52. Dickey N. Needle decompression of tension pneumothorax—Tactical Combat Casualty Care recommendations 2012–5. Defense Health Board Memo. July 7, 2012

53. Morrison J, Poon H, Rasmussen T, et al. Resuscitative thoracotomy following wartime injury. *J Trauma Acute Care Surg.* 2013;74(3):825–829.

54. Kotwal RS, Butler FK, Edgar EP, Shackelford SA, Bennett DR, Bailey JA. Saving lives on the battlefield: a joint trauma system review of pre-hospital trauma care in combined joint operations area—Afghanistan (CJOA-A). Final report of the U.S. Central Command Pre-Hospital Trauma Care Assessment Team dated 30 January 2013. http://www.jsomonline.org/PDFs/CENTCOM%20Prehospital%20Final%20Report%20130130.pdf. Accessed May 8, 2013.

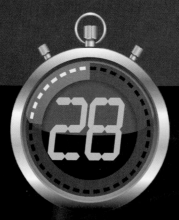
Scenarios

CHAPTER OBJECTIVES

At the completion of this chapter, the reader will be able to do the following:

- Apply and adapt the tenets of Tactical Combat Casualty Care (TCCC) to the care of casualties in the context of realistic combat scenarios.

Introduction

From the lessons learned in the wars in Vietnam, Iraq, and Afghanistan, we now recognize that the leading causes of preventable combat-related deaths are hemorrhage, airway obstruction, and tension pneumothorax.[1-6] The most recent data from Iraq and Afghanistan found that hemorrhage accounted for 90.9% of preventable prehospital deaths (with truncal being the most common site, followed by junctional and extremity hemorrhage), airway obstruction accounted for 7.9% of preventable deaths, and tension pneumothorax was responsible for the remaining 1.1%.[3]

Beyond intervening to prevent imminent death, there are a number of combat casualty care conditions requiring immediate attention to reduce suffering, morbidity, and disability.[7-11] Care for these includes shock management, analgesia, infection prophylaxis, spinal cord protection, traumatic brain injury treatment, and hypothermia prevention. Ensuring the best outcome for the casualty requires that life threats and the other conditions previously listed be addressed rapidly, often within the first few minutes after wounding. Combat medical personnel are critical to this effort.

Combat medical personnel are charged with rapid decision making, immediate action, and competent technical performance under a wide range of challenging, austere, and dangerous conditions. To illustrate the performance of casualty care in the combat environment, several scenarios will be presented in this chapter. Each scenario presents some of the unique features of the combat environment and describes the key medical assessments and interventions performed by combat medical personnel. The scenarios are themed in such a way that the focus is on a defined set of clinical problems. Not every Tactical Combat Casualty Care (TCCC) principle is highlighted in every scenario; rather the scenarios are intended to illustrate how combat medical personnel must combine good medicine with good small unit tactics to optimize the care provided to each casualty on the battlefield.

The text in this chapter is not intended to suggest that the answers provided are the only acceptable answers. Other answers may turn out to be just as good or better, depending on the evolving tactical circumstances.

SCENARIO 1 – GUNSHOT WOUND ON NIGHT PATROL

You are a medic operating in Afghanistan as part of a combat element on a nighttime direct action mission. While moving by foot along the edge of a cultivated field at night, one man of your four-person team is shot and falls into an irrigation ditch. You and your uninjured teammates take immediate cover and begin returning fire. You call to the wounded man, asking how badly he is hit. He responds, telling you that he has been shot in the left leg just above the knee. He is under effective cover but cannot move.

1. **What do you know about the wounded man already?**
   He is alert enough to speak coherently, so he probably has an acceptable blood pressure and his airway is open.

2. **What do you want to know next?**
   You need to determine how badly he is bleeding and whether he has other injuries. Fire from four hostiles is keeping you and the other two team members very busy, and you cannot leave your cover without getting shot yourself. While you and your other teammates continue the firefight, you ask the casualty if he can tell how much blood is coming out of the wound. He tells you he cannot tell, but his leg is really messed up and he can feel blood on the trousers of his uniform. You ask him if he has been hit anywhere else. He says he does not think so, but his leg really hurts.

3. **What do you do next?**
   You tell the casualty to put a tourniquet on his leg and then get back in the fight if he can. In Care Under Fire, the best thing a medic can do for the casualty and the rest of the team may be to take cover and return fire **(Figure 28-1)**. If a medic gets killed trying to get to a casualty, he has done the casualty, the rest of the team, and himself no good. In a situation like this one, the overriding concern is suppression of enemy fire, and every gun, including the medic's and the casualty's, may be needed. Casualties who are able should remain engaged in the firefight and/or the prosecution of the mission. This casualty was trained and equipped to apply a tourniquet to his own leg. Because his wound was at a site where a tourniquet could be effectively applied above it, he was able to address potentially life-threatening extremity hemorrhage via self-aid. Both he and the medic were able to remain under cover and involved in the fight. In this way, the risk of further injury to the casualty, the medic, and the other members of the team was minimized.

   After several minutes of intense fighting, your team eliminates all hostile fire, and you are able to tend to the casualty. You find him lying on his back in two inches of muddy water at the bottom of the irrigation ditch. He is alert and oriented, but in great pain. He has a strong radial pulse. He tells you again that the gunshot wound to his left leg is his only injury. When you cut open his trousers leg, there is an open fracture of his femur. His pain is so great, he stops you from doing a sweep of his leg.

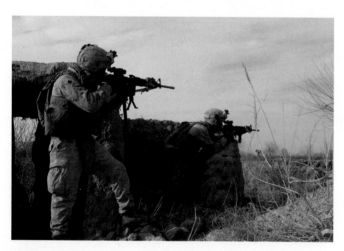

Figure 28-1 Cover and return fire are the priorities in the Care Under Fire phase.
Source: Courtesy of Lance Cpl James Clark/U.S. Marine Corps

4. **What is the greatest tactical need at this point?**
   Your team needs to call for an extract. Since it is difficult to move the casualty and the four hostiles are now neutralized, you elect to call for an evacuation at your current location.

5. **What do you need to do for the casualty?**
   Ensure hemorrhage control, rule out other injuries, provide pain relief, administer antibiotics, prepare him to move, and protect him from hypothermia.

6. **How do you do all that?**
You cannot use a light because the enemy may be nearby, and he will not let you sweep his leg. Since you cannot see or feel well enough to assess for sites of bleeding and amount of blood lost, or to determine if he is still bleeding, you elect to place a second tourniquet higher on his left thigh. You sweep everything other than his left leg and find no other injuries. His clinical status has not changed.

   You give him the moxifloxacin from his Combat Pill Pack and stick one 800-microgram (mcg) oral transmucosal fentanyl citrate (OTFC) lozenge in his cheek. You gently place a large dressing over the entire wounded area. You splint the casualty's left leg alongside his right. You check to make sure both tourniquets are still tight and in place. The casualty's clinical status has not changed—he is alert and still in severe pain—so you give him a second OTFC lozenge in his other cheek.

   You have elected to leave his body armor on since you may get into another firefight, so you put a Ready Heat Blanket over him just below the bottom edge of his armor, placing it on top of his t-shirt to prevent direct contact with the skin, and cover him with the Heat Reflective Shell.

7. **What does the casualty need more than anything else at this point?**
He needs continued control of his bleeding and expedited evacuation.

8. **What should you be doing for him until he gets to more advanced care?**
Continue to monitor his clinical status. You notice that he is drowsy.

9. **What is the most significant possible cause of a decline in mental status in this casualty?**
Ongoing blood loss

10. **What else do you want to know?**

   - Pulse character? His radial pulse is now rapid and weak.
   - Tourniquets okay? They are both still in place, but you suspect that the wound is still bleeding.
   - Breathing okay? His breathing is slightly rapid but not labored.

11. **What is most likely happening?**
The casualty is going into hemorrhagic shock.

12. **What makes you think so?**

   - Mental status and radial pulse character have deteriorated.
   - Even though the tourniquets look okay, you suspect continued bleeding.
   - Breathing is slightly rapid.
   - 1,600 mcg of OTFC is not that large of a dose for a young, healthy male in acute pain. It is unlikely that this amount could have caused the change in mental status observed in this casualty.
   - Hemorrhage is the number one cause of preventable combat death.

13. **What do you do?**
You tighten both tourniquets.

14. **What else?**
Because this casualty will need significant blood transfusion due to his hemorrhagic shock, you infuse 1 gram (gm) of tranexamic acid (TXA) in 100 cubic centimeters (cc) of normal saline (NS). It is difficult to start intravenous (IV) therapy at night, so you place a sternal intraosseous (IO) device.

15. **What next?**
Next you resuscitate the casualty with 500 milliliters (ml) of Hextend. Ten minutes after the Hextend bolus, the casualty is a little less drowsy and his radial pulse is a little stronger. You check the tourniquets, and they are still in place and tight. You can detect no bleeding.

16. **What next?**
You complete the TCCC casualty card while waiting for the evac helicopter to arrive.

SCENARIO 2 – ROCKET-PROPELLED GRENADE ATTACK IN AN URBAN ENVIRONMENT

While you are on patrol in an urban environment, your squad comes under small arms fire and rocket-propelled grenade (RPG) attack. The point man and a second man are hit. The squad reacts to the contact, rapidly eliminating the ambushing hostiles. There are no other casualties. A secure perimeter is established, and the squad leader instructs you to take care of the casualties.

You move to Casualty 1 and quickly perform a primary assessment for life-threatening injuries. His mental status is normal and his breathing is rapid but unlabored. You discover a gunshot wound with a small hole that is likely the entrance on his right upper back and what appears to be a larger exit wound in his right armpit. You see pulsatile bleeding from that wound.

1. **What is your immediate concern?**
    The bleeding is life threatening. A lifesaving intervention is urgently needed.

2. **How do you handle it?**
    You immediately expose the area, pack Combat Gauze into the wound, and hold direct pressure for 3 minutes. While you are performing these actions, you are talking to the casualty in order to check both his airway and his mental status. After 3 minutes, the external bleeding appears controlled, so you build a pressure dressing over the Combat Gauze. This dressing also covers the entrance wound.

    You notice the casualty is more anxious and short of breath. You recheck for other sources of bleeding and find none. Suddenly, the casualty becomes unresponsive. His left radial pulse is not palpable. His breathing grows very rapid and shallow.

3. **What do you think is going on?**
    Given the location of the chest wound and the sudden decompensation, you suspect a tension pneumothorax.

4. **What are you going to do about it?**
    You perform a needle decompression of the right chest and hear the soft hiss of escaping air. The casualty becomes conscious again and you note improvement in the rate and depth of his respirations.

5. **What next?**
    Recheck the casualty's pulse. The radial pulse is now normal.

6. **What next?**
    You move to Casualty 2, who reports that he was hit on his right side. He denies loss of consciousness, and his mental status is normal. He complains of shortness of breath and appears anxious. Upon examination, the only injury you find is a shrapnel wound in the midaxillary line on his right side at nipple level. The wound is about the size of a quarter. A piece of shrapnel apparently slipped between the plates of his armor. Sucking and hissing sounds are coming from the wound.

7. **What is the diagnosis?**
    Open pneumothorax (or sucking chest wound)

8. **How can you help this man?**
    You apply a vented chest seal over the wound and the casualty's breathing quickly improves.

9. **What else do you want to know?**

    - Exit wound? You can't find one.
    - Cardiovascular status? He is alert and oriented, and his radial pulses are strong.
    - Neurologic status? He is alert and oriented, he moves all his extremities, and he has no gross sensory abnormalities.
    - Other injuries? You find none.

Medical Evacuation (MEDEVAC) for the two casualties is requested from headquarters. In anticipation of a helicopter evacuation **(Figure 28-2)**, you prepare the casualties for flight, including saline locks, antibiotics, and analgesia.

10. Which analgesic would you use?
Casualty 1 is not complaining of severe pain, so you elect to defer analgesic medications. You use ketamine for Casualty 2 because he has an injury that might impair respiration.

You place them in Hypothermia Prevention and Management Kits (HPMKs) to ensure that the cold environment of helicopter flight does not induce hypothermia. You plan to remind the flight paramedic to keep the doors closed during the flight if possible.

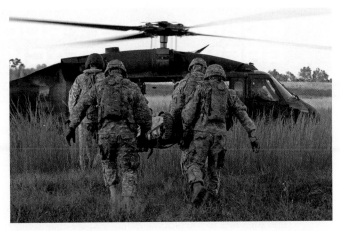

Figure 28-2 Evacuation by air requires special considerations.
Source: Courtesy of Kimberly Lamb, U.S. Army.

11. What do you do next?
You complete TCCC casualty cards while waiting for the evac helicopter to arrive.

The casualties are picked up by an Army DUSTOFF helicopter. Immediately after takeoff, the casualty with the back-to-right axillary gunshot wound develops sudden-onset shortness of breath and hypoxemia as measured by pulse oximetry. The flight paramedic recalls Boyle's law, by which gas expands at altitude, thus potentially causing air trapped in the pleural space to expand and convert a simple pneumothorax to a tension pneumothorax. She responds by immediately inserting a second needle for decompression. The casualty's condition improves immediately.

12. What should the flight paramedic do now?
Continue to monitor both casualties' respirations, blood pressure, and oxygen saturation as well as watch for any signs of external hemorrhage.

The DUSTOFF unit delivers both casualties to the Role 3 medical treatment facility and communicates their clinical histories to the emergency medical staff.

SCENARIO 3 – ROCKET-PROPELLED GRENADE ATTACK DURING A CONVOY

You are riding with a squad in the back of a cargo Humvee along a road at the outskirts of a small Afghani village. When you stop at an intersection, a lone attacker located about 50 meters away takes aim with an RPG and fires the rocket. The warhead explodes against the right front wheel. The vehicle sustains moderate damage to its right side and veers into a concrete barrier. Small flames erupt from the engine compartment.

Everyone in the vehicle is shaken, but all are alert and responsive at first and scramble to exit the vehicle. You grab your rifle and medical kit and hit the ground running. However, the front right passenger makes it only a few meters from the Humvee and then falls to the ground. Before you are able to reach cover, the unit begins to take small arms fire from several locations.

1. **What should you do to help the casualty who is lying out in the open?**
Do your best to eliminate hostile fire. Minimize unit exposure to hostile fire.

2. **What can you do at this point to protect the casualty from being shot?**
Eliminate hostile fire and direct the casualty to move to the nearest cover.

You drop behind cover that gives you a hasty fighting position and start firing back at the enemy. The casualty takes cover behind the Humvee. After a 5-minute firefight, hostile fire is eliminated. The squad sets up a perimeter, and the squad leader gives you the go-ahead to care for the casualty. Because there may still be a risk of sniper fire, you want to relocate the casualty to cover behind a low stone wall nearby. He is still alert but in acute respiratory distress and is unable to walk at this point.

3. **How do you move him?**
You use the one-person drag.

4. **Why do you choose this method?**

   ■ You do not have help since the other squad members are providing security.
   ■ The ground you have to cross is fairly smooth.
   ■ You can stabilize the casualty's cervical spine (blunt trauma) by cradling his head and neck with your forearms.

In your initial assessment, you find the casualty has a disfigured right zygomatic arch and a broken jaw, and there is blood in his mouth. You note swelling, bruising, and abrasions over the right side of his neck. There is no obvious life-threatening external bleeding. He is not talking and does not respond to questions about neck pain. He responds to deep pain with barely audible moaning. His radial pulse is strong. His breathing is shallow, slow, and sonorous. Opening his body armor and blouse, you observe that the rise and fall of his chest are symmetrical, but there is little excursion.

5. **What is your primary concern?**
The casualty may still be breathing spontaneously, but his respiratory effort is weak. The disrupted anatomy and bleeding from injuries to his lower face and neck could be blocking his airway.

6. **What do you do?**
The casualty's clinical status and the mechanism of his injuries make it impossible to rule out a spinal injury. Taking care to keep his neck stable, you do a chin lift and notice that the casualty's respirations get a little deeper. Next, you inset a nasopharyngeal airway. The casualty's breathing is still weak and noisy. His oxygen saturation is 65%.

7. **What next?**
   You judge that the casualty does not yet have an adequate airway and elect to do a cricothyroidotomy. As you perform this procedure **(Figure 28-3)**, you give the squad leader the information he needs for a 9-line MEDEVAC request. He lets you call over one of the Combat Lifesavers in the squad to help you out. After the procedure is performed, the casualty becomes alert and his oxygen saturation improves to 94%. You secure the cricothyrotomy tube. Your squad leader tells you to prepare for MEDEVAC by helicopter in 30 minutes.

8. **What else do you want to do for this casualty?**
   Stabilize his cervical spine.

9. **How do you do that?**
   You do not have a cervical collar (C-collar) with you, so you use manual in-line stabilization. The MEDEVAC helicopter will have a C-collar and spine board.

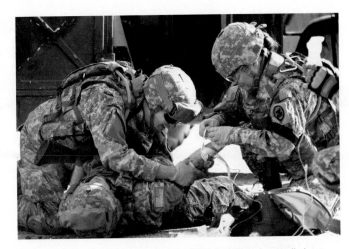

Figure 28-3 Addressing acute breathing problems is usually best deferred until the Tactical Field Care or Tactical Evacuation Care phase.
Source: Courtesy of U.S. Army Medical Department.

10. **What else should you consider?**

    - Rule out unrecognized bleeding? You have another squad member check for bleeding and he finds find none.
    - TXA? Not indicated because the radial pulse is normal.
    - IV/IO fluids? Not indicated at this point.
    - Hypothermia prevention? Yes, this is very important.
    - Analgesia? The casualty cannot speak but appears uncomfortable and indicates "yes" when asked if he is in pain. You give him 50 milligrams of ketamine intramuscularly (IM).
    - Antibiotics? Yes, you administer 1 gm of ertapenem IM.

11. **What next?**
    You complete the TCCC casualty card while waiting for the evac helicopter to arrive.
    When the MEDEVAC helicopter arrives, you, the Combat Lifesaver, and the flight paramedic place the casualty on a spine board and apply a C-collar. You brief the flight paramedic on the casualty's course so far and give him the casualty's TCCC card.

SCENARIO 4 – DISMOUNTED IMPROVISED EXPLOSIVE DEVICE ATTACK

You are a medic in a 12-man Marine squad moving into a small village. One patrol member steps on a pressure-plate activated improvised explosive device (IED). Three patrol members are injured. Unhurt members of the patrol form a protective perimeter around the casualties. There is no follow-on hostile fire, at least for the moment.

1. **What phase of care are you in right now?**
   You are in the Tactical Field Care phase because there is no incoming fire at present, but the patrol is alert for any hostile fire that may ensue.

2. **What do you do first?**
   You perform a rapid assessment of the casualties. Casualty 1 is obviously dead from a devastating head wound. Casualty 2 has multiple small fragment wounds to the back of his arms and legs, and to his buttocks, but there is no obvious major hemorrhage. He is alert and oriented. Casualty 3 has sustained a traumatic amputation of his left leg just below the hip, with additional pelvic and inguinal wounds. He is bleeding heavily from multiple points in and around the amputation site. He is agitated, making loud but incomprehensible sounds, and is weakly thrashing about with his remaining extremities.

3. **How do you begin caring for the casualties?**
   You divide the labor. You direct a squad Combat Lifesaver to evaluate the casualty with the shrapnel wounds, Casualty 2. You take Casualty 3, the casualty with the amputation, and apply a tourniquet above the amputation site **(Figure 28-4)**.

4. **Whose Combat Application Tourniquet are you using?**
   One of your own. You would normally use the casualty's, but you are in a real hurry and do not have time to inspect the casualty's tourniquet to make sure it was not damaged in the blast.

5. **Where do you apply it?**
   You apply the tourniquet as high on the femoral stump as you can. You continue to tighten the tourniquet but cannot get a good purchase on the stump, and there is still significant bleeding, from both the amputation site and the inguinal wound.

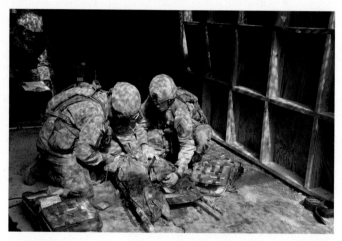

Figure 28-4   Traumatic amputations require the application of a tourniquet.
Source: Courtesy of Lori Newman/U.S. Army.

6. **What now?**
   You break out your Combat Gauze and, with help from another patrol member, apply it to the bleeding sites with 3 minutes of firm direct pressure. The bleeding is still not controlled.

7. **What next?**
   You break out your Combat Ready Clamp (CRoC) and quickly assemble it. You apply the CRoC to the casualty's right groin and achieve control of the hemorrhage.
   The squad sends in the 9-line MEDEVAC request and alerts them of the RPG hazard in the nearby village. The squad is then directed to move the casualties on foot to a landing zone (LZ) in an open area 1 kilometer away from the village.
   Casualty 2 takes his Combat Pill Pack. He continues to be a functioning unit member and assists with the mission. However, Casualty 3 is now conscious but confused. His radial pulse is not palpable and his carotid pulse is thready and rapid.

8. **What is the most likely diagnosis for Casualty 3?**
   Hemorrhagic shock

9. **What treatment do you provide Casualty 3?**

You place a sternal IO device and infuse 1 gm of TXA in 100 cc of normal saline, flush the IO line, and follow that with a 500-cc bolus of Hextend. When the bolus is in, the casualty's carotid pulse gets a little stronger, and his radial pulse is now palpable. He is alert but confused. He is breathing adequately and is not complaining of pain at the moment.

10. **Now that you have IO access, are there other meds you would give?**

Yes, IV antibiotics via slow IV push.

11. **What further care is required?**

Place a pulse oximeter on Casualty 3. His oxygen saturation is 95%. The mission commander gives the order to move out for the designated LZ. The deceased casualty is moved with a two-person drag. Casualty 3 is moved using a three-person carry. The Marines carrying Casualty 3 monitor the site of the previous hemorrhage to ensure that it does not begin to bleed again. The other five patrol members provide security during the movement to the LZ.

The patrol arrives at the LZ. The helicopter is 10 minutes out. It has been about 45 minutes since the first bolus of Hextend went in, and Casualty 3's status is the same.

12. **What next?**

You infuse a second 500-ml bolus of Hextend into Casualty 3.

13. **What else do you want to do?**

You thoroughly reassess Casualty 2 and Casualty 3 and find no new conditions requiring immediate treatment. You place Casualty 3 in an HPMK after rechecking to ensure that his previous hemorrhage remains controlled.

14. **What next?**

You complete TCCC casualty cards while waiting for the evac helicopter to arrive.

15. **In addition to monitoring for continued hemorrhage control, what is Casualty 3 likely to need during the 20-minute MEDEVAC flight?**

He may need further fluid resuscitation, preferably with plasma and packed red blood cells if available. High-flow supplemental oxygen should be started using a reservoir mask. If his mental status continues to improve and pain becomes an issue, he may need ketamine.

SCENARIO 5 – FAST-ROPING CASUALTY IN AN URBAN ENVIRONMENT

A 14-man Special Operations assault team fast-ropes from a helicopter hovering about 25 meters (80 feet) above the ground for a building assault in a high-threat urban environment. On exiting, one of the last members of the team loses his grip and falls to the ground **(Figure 28-5)**. The helicopter, unable to loiter at the scene or evacuate the casualty, departs quickly with its escort gunship. You, one of two medics on the team, attend immediately to the casualty. The mission commander instructs the rest of the team to form a defensive perimeter. There are hostiles all around you in the streets, and the unit begins to take sporadic fire from several directions. The casualty is unconscious.

1. **What is the first priority?**
Provide cover for the team, including the casualty.

2. **Why?**
There are many armed hostiles in street crowds all around you. It is unlikely that the team can eliminate all hostile fire. The best way to deal with injuries is to prevent them, so the team takes cover behind a nearby low wall.

3. **How do you move the casualty?**
You and the team member move him using a two-man carry, taking care to minimize head and neck movement.

4. **The low wall provides effective cover from incoming fire. What phase of care are you in?**
You are in the Tactical Field Care phase, but a very high-risk version of it.

5. **What do you do next?**
Safely behind cover, you begin your assessment of the casualty. He is still unresponsive; you find no signs of external hemorrhage. He has a patent airway, adequate breathing, and a strong radial pulse. You note bilateral open femur fractures and are aware of the high incidence of spinal and pelvic fractures in high falls. While maintaining improvised cervical stabilization, you remove his weapons, helmet, and body armor to facilitate your examination. Your further assessment reveals symmetrical and responsive pupils and ecchymosis at the left mastoid area (Battle's sign). The casualty remains unresponsive. You place a pulse oximeter on his finger; his oxygen saturation is 94%.

6. **What is the diagnosis?**
Traumatic brain injury due to blunt trauma, and bilateral open femur fractures. You cannot rule out spinal injury, and he may have noncompressible abdominal or thoracic hemorrhage.

You inform the team leader of the urgency of the casualty's condition. The team leader reports back that the mission has been altered to accommodate the casualty and four armored Humvees have been dispatched for evacuation. Their estimated time of arrival is 15 minutes. Two of the vehicles have litters, but one of the team members finds a door nearby and you use it as an improvised rigid litter so that you can minimize the time required on-scene once the vehicles arrive.

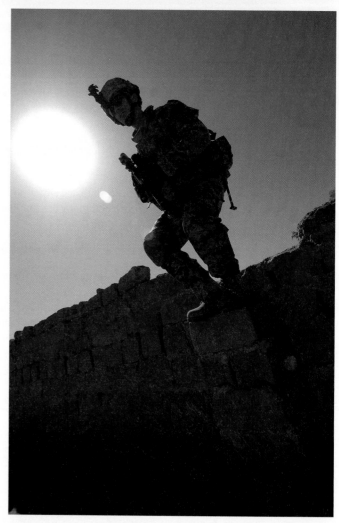

Figure 28-5 Not all combat-related trauma involves weapons. Falls represent an important mechanism of injury on the battlefield.
Source: Courtesy of Sgt. Timothy Kingston/US Army.

7. **What do you do next?**

   While continuing to monitor him, you apply the C-collar that you thought to bring for this type of mission, and you insert a nasopharyngeal airway. (Note that a field-expedient cervical collar can also be made from a SAM splint.) You then insert a saline lock.

8. **Does the casualty need any meds?**

   Because of the high probability of noncompressible hemorrhage in a fall of this magnitude, you elect to administer TXA. The casualty remains unconscious, so he does not need analgesics. He has open femur fractures, so you administer IV antibiotics after the TXA is in.

9. **What do you do next?**

   The door effectively splints the femur fractures after you secured his legs to the door with tactical tape and covered the wounds with sterile dressings. You put a Ready Heat Blanket over the casualty's t-shirt and place him into a Heat Reflective Shell. You then put his helmet back on and lay his body armor over him.

   The vehicles were due to arrive 10 minutes ago but have not yet done so. The team members continue to maintain security and minimize incoming hostile fire.

10. **What next?**

    You reassess the casualty and note his respirations have become very shallow and the left pupil is now dilated. He remains unresponsive.

11. **What is happening clinically with this casualty?**

    Cerebral herniation

12. **What can you do about it?**

    You have no oxygen in TFC. You use a bag-mask device to ventilate the casualty. Capnography is not available, so you use a ventilation rate of 20 breaths/minute. You elevate the head of the improvised rigid litter 30 degrees. You would give 250 ml of 3% saline IV if you had it, but you do not. You monitor his oxygen saturation with a pulse oximeter, and it remains above 90%.

13. **What next?**

    You complete the TCCC casualty card while waiting for the evac vehicles to arrive.

    The vehicles arrive shortly thereafter. You have unit members help you carefully move the casualty into the vehicles and secure the improvised litter as best you can. Everyone else mounts up in the other vehicles, and the convoy moves out.

References

1. Gerhardt RG, Mabry RL, De Lorenzo RA, Butler FK. Fundamentals of combat casualty care. In: Savitsky E, Eastridge B. *Combat Casualty Care—Lessons Learned from OEF and OIF*. Fort Detrick, MD: Borden Institute; 2011.

2. Butler FK Jr, Blackbourne LH. Battlefield trauma care then and now: a decade of Tactical Combat Casualty Care. *J Trauma Acute Care Surg.* 2012;73(6 suppl 5):s395-s402.

3. Eastridge BJ, Mabry RL, Seguin P, Cantrell J, et al. Death on the battlefield (2001–2011): implications for the future of combat casualty care. *J Trauma Acute Care Surg.* 2012;73(6 Suppl 5):s431-s437.

4. Kotwal RS, Montgomery HR, Mechler KK. A prehospital trauma registry for Tactical Combat Casualty Care. *J Spec Oper Med.* 2011;11(3):127-128.

5. Pannell D, Brisebois R, Talbot M, Trottier V, et al. Causes of death in Canadian Forces members deployed to Afghanistan and implications on Tactical Combat Casualty Care provision. *J Trauma.* 2011;71(5 Suppl 1):S401-S407.

6. Deal VT, McDowell D, Benson P, Iddins B, et al. Tactical Combat Casualty Care February 2010. Direct from the Battlefield: TCCC lessons learned in Iraq and Afghanistan. *J Spec Oper Med.* 2010;10(3):77-119.

7. Committee on Tactical Combat Casualty Care, Defense Health Board, U.S. Department of Defense: Tactical Combat Casualty Care Guidelines. September 17, 2012. Washington, DC.

8. Gerhardt RG, Adams BD, De Lorenzo RA, et al. Panel synopsis: pre-hospital combat health support 2010: what should our azimuth be? *J Trauma.* 2007;62(6 Suppl):S15-S16.

9. Adams BD, Cuniowski PA, Muck A, De Lorenzo RA. Registry of emergency airways at combat hospitals. *J Trauma.* 2008;64(6):1548-1554.

10. Bell RS, Vo AH, Neal CJ, et al. Military traumatic brain and spinal column injury: a 5-year study of the impact blast and other military grade weaponry on the central nervous system. *J Trauma.* 2009;66(4 Suppl 5):S104-S111.

11. Morrison JJ, Dubose JJ, Rasmussen TE, Midwinter MJ. Military Application of Tranexamic Acid in Trauma Emergency Resuscitation (MATTERs) Study. *Arch Surg.* 2012;147(2):113-119.

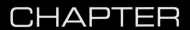
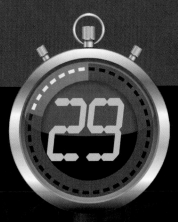

CHAPTER **29**

Aeromedical Evacuation in a Combat Theater

CHAPTER OBJECTIVES

At the completion of this chapter, the reader will be able to do the following:

- Define the terms Casualty Evacuation (CASEVAC), Medical Evacuation (MEDEVAC), Tactical Evacuation (TACEVAC), and aeromedical evacuation.

- State the difference between a casualty and a patient in the aeromedical evacuation chain.

- Discuss the limitations on combat casualty care imposed by the environment of a rotary-wing platform.

- Recognize techniques and procedures to ensure safety during rotary-wing evacuation.

- Discuss the concepts and requirements of en route care.

- Specify the common stressors of aeromedical evacuation, and discuss the effects and management of each.

SCENARIO

You are the senior flight nurse in an aeromedical evacuation team on board a MEDEVAC C-130 assigned to transfer a patient from the Role 3 hospital in Kandahar, Afghanistan, to Craig Joint Theater Hospital in Bagram. As the aircraft makes its final approach, it comes under small arms fire. Two of the team members are wounded. Casualty 1 has sustained a gunshot wound to his right inguinal area with heavy bleeding. Casualty 2 has an injury to her left thigh with pulsatile bleeding. The aircraft banks away from the approach and there is no further incoming fire.

1. What phase of Tactical Combat Casualty Care (TCCC) are you in?

2. You now need to do two things simultaneously. What are they?

3. What do you do next?

Introduction

History of Aeromedical Casualty Movement

The concept of moving combat casualties by air has been recognized since the early days of aviation. The first recorded movement of combat casualties by air is thought to have occurred in 1870 during the Franco-Prussian War. At the siege of Paris, 160 wounded French soldiers were flown out over the Prussian lines in hot-air balloons.[1] Limited attempts at movement of casualties by air occurred during World War I and through the 1920s and 1930s.

Large-scale casualty movement by air did not occur until World War II, during which more than 1.4 million casualties were moved by air, with only 46 deaths occurring in flight.[1] It must be noted that the majority of these flights originated in rear staging areas for hospital-treated casualties who had been transported from the battlefield by the more traditional means of ground evacuation. Aeromedical evacuation from the battlefield was not readily practiced during World War II because of the limitations of the fixed-wing aircraft of the era.

The development of rotary-wing aircraft in the mid-1940s opened dramatic new capabilities for evacuation of the injured combatant. The first movement of a casualty by helicopter occurred in Burma in 1944.[2] During the Korean War, more than 17,700 casualties were flown by the newly introduced rotary-wing aircraft, many directly from the battle zone.[1] The introduction of a helicopter evacuation system in the Korean conflict is often credited as the most important reason for the improved survival rate among combat casualties seen during this conflict.

The rotary-wing evacuation system developed further during the Vietnam War. By 1967, more than 94,000 casualties had been flown out of combat zones by helicopters like the venerable UH-1.[3] The comparative success of the Vietnam evacuation system led to its widespread adaptation by civilian programs within the continental United States (CONUS), beginning in the mid-1970s. The majority of current civilian "Life Flight" programs trace their

roots to the experience provided by the military aeromedical evacuation units during the conflicts in Korea and Vietnam.[1,4]

En Route Care

The introduction of rotary-wing evacuation aircraft sparked the recognition that a variety of missions may be involved in the movement of casualties: from the point of wounding, through the initial resuscitation, to the final point of care. Recent experience gained from aeromedical evacuation during Operation Iraqi Freedom and Operation Enduring Freedom has significantly increased the understanding and appreciation of the aeromedical evacuation process. The most significant of these revisions is the recognition of the role of continuous, high-intensity medical care throughout the continuum of care, from the point of wounding to the point of final definitive care and rehabilitation. Aeromedical evacuation is a continuum of care, usually associated with some form of transportation or movement (rotary-wing, fixed-wing, or other), while medical care is ongoing. The term *en route care* is employed to encompass and characterize this seamless continuum of medical care from the point-of-injury (by field medics, battalion aid station surgeons, etc.), through theater facilities (Role 3 Combat Support Hospital [CSH], theater hospital), and onward to CONUS facilities (medical treatment facilities [MTFs], rehabilitation centers, Veteran's Administration [VA] centers).

The Committee on Tactical Combat Casualty Care (CoTCCC) revised the definitions of its third phase of care to reflect operational, doctrinal, logistical, and medical concerns. The phrase Tactical Evacuation (TACEVAC) combines Casualty Evacuation (CASEVAC) and Medical Evacuation (MEDEVAC) operations into a spectrum of continuous en route care from the point of wounding to the first MTF. Although doctrinal differences exist among the service branches regarding terminology and definitions of phases of care, for purposes of the following discussion, casualty movement may be described as follows:

1. CASEVAC: Evacuation of a casualty from the battlefield to an MTF using tactical platforms (i.e., vehicles not

dedicated to medical missions). CASEVAC assets are owned by line commanders and are an integral part of combat missions. They are designed accordingly, with armor and offensive weaponry such as crew-served automatic weapons, rockets, and missiles.

2. MEDEVAC: Evacuation of a casualty from the battlefield to an MTF, or from one MTF to another within the tactical theater, using dedicated medical assets, usually marked with a red cross. These evacuation assets are not part of the offensive forces; they are part of the casualty care plan. MEDEVAC assets may be rotary-wing or fixed-wing aircraft, such as the C-130, that are dedicated to medical missions.

3. TACEVAC: En route care from the battlefield to a theater Role 2 or Role 3 MTF, including both CASEVAC and MEDEVAC.

4. Aeromedical evacuation: A term most commonly utilized by the U.S. Air Force to designate the movement of a patient from a point of care within the theater to a more rearward location, such as regional hospital or CONUS. Traditionally, this phase of movement has employed fixed-wing jet aircraft such as the C-17.

In practice, the lines separating CASEVAC, MEDEVAC, and aeromedical evacuation are blurred at times because doctrine, circumstances, and medical care require flexibility **(Figure 29-1)**. In recent years, prehospital care capabilities across all phases of casualty care and movement have significantly improved, reflecting advancements in medical technology, pharmacology, and casualty management doctrine. In theaters such as Afghanistan, where the evacuation system is well established, the transport distances are relatively short, and there is definitive air superiority, it is common for a U.S. combat casualty to be evacuated by helicopter within 30 minutes of injury, be at a forward surgical facility or a combat support hospital within 30 minutes, and be on the way back to CONUS within 48 hours of wounding.

When Does a Casualty Become a Patient?

In the process of aeromedical evacuation, a wounded soldier is considered a casualty until he or she reaches the first point of definitive medical care. Once entered into the medical care system, the casualty is considered a "patient" (although this section uniformly uses "casualty").

Tactical Evacuation (TACEVAC) Care

Principles

Although CASEVAC, MEDEVAC, and aeromedical evacuation can all involve the transport of casualties by air, they may be functionally very different. In CASEVAC, casualties are moved from the point of injury to a place of initial surgical care. In most cases, this is a relatively short transport accomplished by rotary-wing aircraft, although it can be conducted using ground vehicles or watercraft. TACEVAC aircraft must frequently fly into the Forward Edge of the Battle Area (FEBA) and may come under enemy fire. The aircraft used in this mission may be tactical aircraft that are designated for a single mission (aircraft of opportunity) or may have a secondary CASEVAC role designated during premission planning. When the tactical situation allows, dedicated aircraft designed and equipped for medical missions (e.g., an air ambulance) may be used for MEDEVAC **(Figure 29-2)**.

Casualties needing evacuation from the field are, by definition, recently injured, and may be quite unstable. Essential care must be focused on lifesaving maneuvers that enhance survival while minimizing additional risk to the casualty, the unit's mission, and the evacuation crew. Tactical imperatives to accomplish the mission or prevent further casualties may impose severe limitations on medical capabilities during TACEVAC. It is desirable to keep ground time in the forward area to a minimum; therefore, most CASEVAC/MEDEVAC care is delivered during flight in a

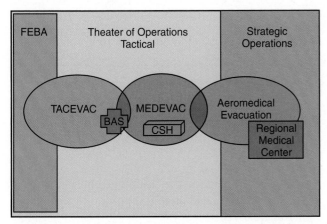

Figure 29-1 Schematic representation of the continuum of evacuation.

Source: Courtesy of Stephen Giebner, MD

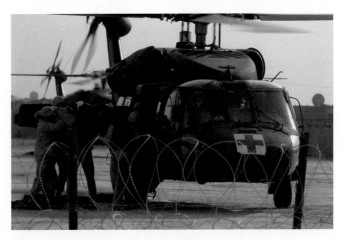

Figure 29-2 UH-60 Black Hawk MEDEVAC helicopter.

Source: Courtesy of SPC Algernon E, Crawley, Jr/ U.S. Department of Defense

noisy, turbulent, and crowded environment, very different from a hospital trauma bay. Excellent tactical flying and premission planning are essential to keep the aircraft, crew, and casualties safe. As discussed in the Tactical Field Care chapter, consideration must be given to whether the medical needs of the casualty justify the additional risk and tactical exposure that an urgent TACEVAC mission may generate for the casualty's unit as well as for the TACEVAC platform and its crew. Alternative modes of evacuation (e.g., ground or water) and the impact of delayed transport should be included in the decision-making process.[5]

Medical Care

TACEVAC operations typically occur after the Care Under Fire and Tactical Field Care phases, and may allow for increased opportunities for intervention. Hemorrhage control, airway management, respiratory support as needed, intravenous (IV) access, treatment of shock, hypothermia prevention, and relief of pain continue to be the core of treatment during TACEVAC. Once underway in a TACEVAC platform, the challenges imposed by limited space, a very high noise level, low light conditions, shock and vibration due to platform movement, and ongoing combat conditions often continue to make optimal trauma care difficult. Equipment used during TACEVAC should be lightweight and robust enough to withstand the rugged environment.

In the setting of nighttime tactical conditions, light sources should be minimized, and subdued light (e.g., Phantom light, Petzl light) or infrared light sources (in conjunction with night vision devices) should be used. White lights should be avoided because of their adverse impact on the crew's vision and because they may provide a targeting profile for the enemy. TACEVAC providers should be practiced in medical care techniques in darkened conditions while underway in tactical vehicles and aircraft.

Preparation of Casualty

The principles of casualty preparation for TACEVAC fall under the same guidelines as discussed in the Care Under Fire and Tactical Field Care chapters. For TACEVAC by air, a landing zone should be prepared in accordance with standard guidance (Figure 29-3). Helicopters are vulnerable to hostile fire, and minimizing casualty transfer time is essential to optimizing the chance of survival for both the casualty and the aircraft.

Helicopter safety is critical in TACEVAC operations. Engine-running onloads and offloads are the norm, and rotors will be turning. It is imperative that everyone who assists in loading patients on and off helicopters be familiar with rotary-wing operational procedures under all conditions.

Casualties should have eye and ear protection, as should all members of the loading crew. Most helicopters should be approached from the nose or the sides. Personnel should never enter the rotor disc area (the area under the rotor blades) unless they have been cleared to enter by the helicopter crew. If the helicopter is on a slope, personnel should approach and depart from the downslope side.[1,5]

Figure 29-3 Preparation for CASEVAC by Air

1. Determine the number of casualties to be moved, the requirement for movement by helicopter, and the urgency of the movement; evaluate the tactical situation.
   - Note that in some cases, it is faster and safer to move casualties by ground than by air.
   - Not all casualties require urgent evacuation.
   - The tactical situation may preclude evacuation by air (e.g., heavy enemy fire).
   - Environmental conditions, such as darkness, bad weather, or lack of a suitable landing zone, may prevent evacuation by air.
2. Locate and mark a suitable helicopter landing zone (HLZ) or pickup site. The HLZ should be as flat as possible, with even terrain and no surrounding large trees, wires, or tall structures.
   - The HLZ should be a minimum of 30 meters (100 feet) in diameter, or larger if a CH-47 or MH-53 will be landing.
   - Mark (or prepare to mark) the HLZ as per protocol (VS-17 panels, smoke, chemical lights, strobe lights, vehicle lights).
   - If possible, have a wind indicator (wind sock or ribbon on stick) just outside the HLZ, easily visible to the pilot.
   - In a tactical situation, keep the HLZ as inconspicuous as possible to prevent the enemy from zeroing in on it.
3. Prepare the casualties for flight.
   - If possible, perform any urgent medical procedures, such as hemorrhage control, airway or breathing interventions, or starting IV lines, while still on the ground.
   - Move the casualties near the HLZ, and stage them perpendicular to the line of approach/departure of the aircraft, but well outside the HLZ.
   - Protect the casualties' ears with earplugs. Protect the casualties' eyes with goggles. Litter bearers should have earplugs and goggles in place.
4. Load the casualties.
   - Do not approach the helicopter until the crew has seen you and given you positive clearance to approach the aircraft.

(Continues on next page)

Figure 29-3 Preparation for CASEVAC by Air (*Continued*)

- Do not approach the rear of the aircraft unless you are specifically directed to go there by the aircraft crew. (The CH-46, CH-47, and CH/MH-53 have rear loading ramps, and you will probably be directed to load casualties there. Do not approach from the rear of an H-60 or any other helicopter with a tail rotor.)

- Load the casualties as directed by the aircraft crew.
- Minimize the time that the aircraft is on the ground.
- As soon as loading is complete, exit the rotor disc area and clear the HLZ.

Figure 29-4 Standard Nine-Line MEDEVAC Request

Line 1: Location of Casualty and Helicopter Landing Zone (HLZ)

Location can be given in grid coordinates, latitude/longitude, or any other system that is clearly understood by all parties. In hostile areas the HLZ coordinates should be encrypted to prevent enemy forces ascertaining the location of the HLZ.

Line 2: Radio Frequency and Call Sign

Radio the frequency and call sign of the unit requesting the MEDEVAC. Again, in hostile situations this should be encrypted.

Line 3: Evacuation Precedence

- A = Urgent
- B = Urgent/surgical
- C = Priority
- D = Routine
- E = Convenience

Each letter is preceded by the number of casualties in each category. For example, "3 ALPHA, 2 BRAVO, 1 CHARLIE" means there are three urgent casualties, two urgent surgical casualties, and 1 priority casualty requiring MEDEVAC.

Line 4: Special Equipment Requests

This line requests specialized extraction or medical equipment.
- A = None
- B = Hoist required
- C = Extraction equipment required
- D = Ventilator required

Line 5: Numbers of Litter and Ambulatory Patients

- L = Litter casualties
- A = Ambulatory casualties

Each category is preceded by the number of casualties. For example, "3 LIMA, 2 ALPHA" means three litter casualties and two ambulatory casualties require MEDEVAC.

Line 6: Evacuation Site Security

This indicates the level of hostile threat in the area.
- N = No threat
- P = Possible enemy troops in the area
- E = Enemy troops in the area
- X = Hot HLZ, armed escort needed

Line 7: Marking of Evacuation Site

- A = Colored panels (VS-17 panel)
- B = Pyrotechnic signals
- C = Smoke
- D = No designation
- E = Other means of designation

Line 8: Casualty Nationalities and Combat Status

- A = U.S. Military
- B = U.S. Civilian
- C = Non-U.S. Military
- D = Non-U.S. Civilian
- E = Enemy prisoner of war

Line 9: NBC/Terrain Specifics

- N = Nuclear
- B = Biologic
- C = Chemical

Describe any terrain features that may help the crew locate the HLZ from the air or that may affect their approach, such as trees, electrical wires, or sloping terrain.

Calling for TACEVAC

A standard method of calling for a TACEVAC is the nine-line evacuation request **(Figure 29-4)**. Other methods are also used, but regardless of the method, it should be specified during premission planning so that everyone involved in the operation is familiar with the chosen format.

MTF-to-MTF MEDEVAC

The term MEDEVAC also applies to the movement of a patient from one MTF to another MTF within the theater—for example, the movement of a casualty from a Role 2 Forward Resuscitative Surgical Team to a Role 3 Combat Support Hospital. MEDEVAC also describes the movement of a patient from a Combat Support Hospital or other MTF to a regional staging facility theater air hub, or other aeromedical staging facility.

MTF-to-MTF MEDEVAC operations may involve either rotary-wing or fixed-wing tactical aircraft **(Figure 29-5)**. As the duration of medical missions extends sufficiently to require the use of fixed-wing aircraft, the considerations for MEDEVAC missions more closely reflect those discussed next for aeromedical evacuation.

Aeromedical Evacuation

Doctrine and Principles

In aeromedical evacuation, patients who have received appropriate medical care and are stable (or stabilized) are flown relatively long distances in fixed-wing aircraft. Some aircraft used for aeromedical evacuation, like the C-130, are capable of dirt-strip operations, but in most cases a fixed airfield is necessary. Aeromedical evacuation aircraft may occasionally be at risk from enemy fire, but usually not to the same extent as rotary-wing TACEVAC aircraft. Duration of flight (and, thus, length of in-flight medical care) is usually longer in aeromedical evacuation than in TACEVAC flights. It is not unusual for these missions to last 10 to 12 hours.

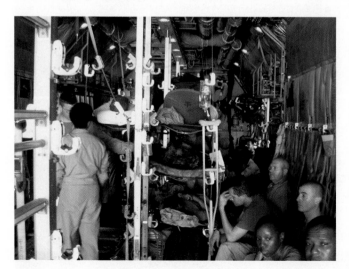

Figure 29-5 En route care during MEDEVAC.
Source: Courtesy of Dr. Jay Johannigman

The medical support crew of an aeromedical evacuation mission usually consists of persons specifically trained in the requirements and challenges of the flight environment. A typical crew consists of two flight nurses and three aeromedical technicians. Physicians are not normally part of an aeromedical evacuation crew. Flight nurses and aeromedical evacuation technicians are trained regarding altitude physiology, nursing considerations in the aeromedical evacuation environment, aircraft power and oxygen systems, emergency procedures, aeromedical evacuation aircraft configuration, and survival. The standard aeromedical evacuation crew can be pared down or augmented as required.

Role of Critical Care Air Transport Team

The medical experiences of recent military operations have significantly challenged portions of conventional aeromedical evacuation doctrine. The fluidity of the battle space and the mobility of maneuvering forces have put increasing emphasis on a medical capability that is equally fluid. Traditional aeromedical evacuation doctrine provided for the movement of a stable casualty who had received extensive care at an advanced facility (Role 3). It has become increasingly apparent that tactical combat considerations as well as evolving medical support doctrine will emphasize the capability to move "stabilized" casualties (i.e., those who have undergone Damage Control Resuscitation and Damage Control Surgery) at theater medical facilities but are not yet "stable." For the purposes of this discussion, a "stabilized" casualty is defined as a casualty with:

- Hemorrhage controlled
- Shock treated
- Airway controlled
- Fractures splinted

The development of the Critical Care Air Transport Team (CCATT) arose from the need to provide en route care for stabilized, but not necessarily stable, casualties from forward locations **(Figure 29-6)**. A CCATT is composed of an intensivist-trained physician (anesthesia, surgery, emergency medicine, or pulmonary medicine), a critical care nurse, and a respiratory therapist. The CCATT's equipment is self-contained and self-carried **(Figure 29-7)** and can facilitate care for three critically ill intubated patients or a total of six critical patients. All of the medical equipment that a CCATT carries has been tested and approved for use in flight.

A CCATT functions to augment a standard aeromedical evacuation team and provides extended capability to far-forward locations via the provision of continuous en route intensive care. This concept ensures that the critically ill casualty may be moved rearward without degrading the capabilities of the forward medical units. CCATTs may be co-located at aeromedical evacuation hubs, theater hospitals, or other rearward locations. CCATTs are moved forward with the airframe and aeromedical crew as medical circumstances dictate. A CCATT may be effectively employed to provide continuous critical care from the battlefield rearward to CONUS, thus ensuring seamless en route care.

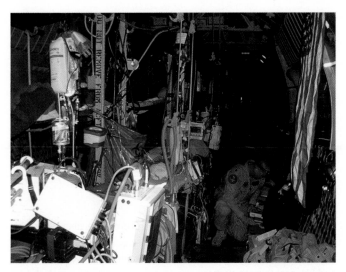

Figure 29-6 Critical Care Air Transport Team (CCATT) evacuation.
Source: Courtesy of Dr. Jay Johannigman

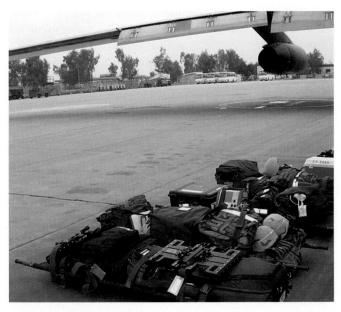

Figure 29-7 CCATT equipment load.
Source: Courtesy of Dr. Jay Johannigman

Additional Specialized Teams

Other specialized aeromedical transport teams are available as needed. For example, the U.S. Army's Burn Special Medical Augmentation Response Team (SMART) is based out of the Institute of Surgical Research at the San Antonio Military Medical Center. Burn SMART specializes in the transport of critically injured burn casualties, multiple-trauma casualties with burns, and victims of chemical blister agents.

During Operation Iraqi Freedom and Operation Enduring Freedom, a specialized pulmonary CCATT team was stationed at Landstuhl Regional Medical Center and was available with advanced pulmonary rescue equipment, including extracorporeal devices to maintain oxygenation.

Stressors of Aeromedical Evacuation

During air transport, casualties may be exposed to a variety of environmental stressors that may adversely affect their medical outcome and complicate the provision of care. These elements are collectively referred to as the "stressors of flight." Stressors common to both rotary-wing and fixed-wing aircraft may include elevated ambient-noise levels, vibration, decreased atmospheric pressure, hypoxia, dehydration, and thermal stress.[1,4-6]

Ambient Noise

High levels of ambient noise can damage hearing and make situational awareness pertaining to the casualty difficult. It is important that both the casualty and the medical personnel providing care have hearing protection, like earplugs, headset, or flight helmet. It is virtually impossible to hear breath sounds or take a manual blood pressure (BP) reading in a helicopter, and it is difficult in most fixed-wing aircraft, making electronic monitoring technology a requisite for optimal care. Hearing protection makes these tasks even more difficult. Recent advances have introduced wireless headsets to facilitate crew communication and provide hearing protection.

Vibration

Vibration is a recognized stressor that results in physical fatigue and poses challenges to the provision of ongoing medical care. Vibration impairs the evaluation of a casualty in flight by compromising physical examination (e.g., pulse and BP detection), and in some instances by interfering with electronic monitoring equipment. In preparation for long-duration aeromedical evacuation flights, it is desirable to establish redundant means of monitoring casualties and their vital signs (e.g., electronic BP monitoring as well as an arterial line to measure BP if indicated; pulse oximetry and mechanical spirometer to monitor ventilation).

The combination of vibration, turbulence, low light conditions, and limited space creates extremely challenging working conditions for the medical crew providing casualty care. It is possible to accomplish most medical procedures in flight; however, it will be more challenging than performing the same procedure on the ground. If possible, medical procedures such as starting IV lines, applying splints or dressings, and performing airway procedures (e.g., endotracheal intubation) should be accomplished before flight.[4,5] If a particular potential problem (e.g., unstable airway) is a concern, it is prudent to address this issue aggressively before transport rather than midway through flight at altitude and in the dark.[4] With this in mind, it is important for medical personnel to err on the side of over-preparation before aeromedical evacuation.

Decreased Atmospheric Pressure

Since the inception of aviation, it has been recognized that as an aircraft ascends in altitude, the ambient atmospheric pressure decreases. Boyle's law states that, for a given amount of gas, pressure and volume are inversely proportional. In practical terms, this means that as an aircraft ascends to altitude, any gas trapped in the body or in a closed space will either expand in volume or, if expansion is not possible, will create a pressure differential that may result in pressure-related injury, or **barotrauma**. Conversely, as the aircraft descends, ambient pressure increases and trapped gas in a space that is able to change in its dimensions will decrease in volume.

For example, if a (theoretically perfectly elastic) balloon contains 1 liter of gas at sea level (ambient pressure = 760 milliliters of mercury [mm Hg]), that balloon will expand in volume to 2 liters at 18,000 feet (5,486 meters [m]) above sea level (ambient pressure = 380 mm Hg).[1,4] Most fixed-wing aircraft are pressurized, meaning that the pressure inside the aircraft cabin (cabin altitude) is maintained at a higher level than the outside ambient pressure. This pressurization decreases pressure-related effects as the aircraft ascends and descends. However, most aircraft cannot maintain sea-level pressure up to their typical cruising altitudes. For example, the C-130 can maintain sea-level cabin pressure only up to an altitude of about 18,000 feet.[7] Even commercial aircraft routinely have cabin altitudes of 6,000 to 8,000 feet (1,829 to 2,438 m) when at cruising altitude.[1,4] Most helicopters are not pressurized, so the aircraft altitude and the cabin altitude are the same.

Boyle's law can have potentially disastrous consequences for casualties during aeromedical evacuation. Care must be taken to provide adequate means of decompression for the medically relevant closed spaces of the human body. Gas trapped in distensible spaces in the body such as the intestines, the middle ear, or the chest will expand as altitude increases and contract as altitude decreases. A casualty with a simple pneumothorax at low altitude may develop a life-threatening tension pneumothorax as the gas in the chest expands on ascent. Therefore, a pneumothorax must be appropriately treated with a decompressive device, such as a chest tube, before flight. The presence of an untreated pneumothorax is one of the few absolute contraindications to aeromedical evacuation.[6] MEDEVAC may be possible without a chest tube if the helicopter maintains a low altitude; however, the medical personnel should monitor the casualty carefully and be prepared to perform a needle decompression if signs or symptoms of a tension pneumothorax appear.

Gas in the intestines, ears, and sinuses will usually find a means of decompression during ascent. On descent, however, air must be added to the middle ear and sinuses to prevent ear and sinus "squeeze." If the patient is unconscious, has injury to the maxillofacial area, or has other pathology (e.g., cold), ventilation of the middle ears and sinuses may be difficult. Comatose or semiconscious patients may become combative as a result of pain from occult ear or sinus squeeze. Appropriate management of patients at risk for these events may include the administration of nasal decongestants (e.g., phenylephrine nasal spray) before flight.[4-6]

Gas-filled bladders on medical equipment are also affected by changes in atmospheric pressure. On ascent, gas in endo-

tracheal tube cuffs, IV pressure bags, air splints, military antishock trousers (MAST), and similar devices will expand. This can increase pressure on tissues enough to cause damage. On descent, volume will decrease. Medical personnel should avoid the use of air splints in flight if possible. MAST and IV pressure bags should be closely monitored and air added or removed as necessary.[4-6] Endotracheal tube cuff volume must be monitored with great care during ascent and descent. Even minor volume changes can lead to pressure necrosis of the trachea or air leakage around the cuff.

Altitude Hypoxia

As an aircraft ascends and the ambient pressure decreases, the partial pressure of oxygen in the air decreases. Therefore, as altitude increases, the number of oxygen molecules available to the body in each breath decreases, and measures must be undertaken to prevent hypoxia.[1,4-6] For a healthy individual, altitude hypoxia is usually not significant below altitudes of 10,000 feet (3,048 m). For casualties with respiratory compromise or pre-existing anemia, however, altitude hypoxia may pose a significant problem at much lower altitudes.

Altitude hypoxia is readily treated by the provision of supplemental oxygen.[1,4] Not all trauma casualties will need oxygen during flight, especially if the cabin altitude is maintained at or below 10,000 feet (3,048 m). Monitoring with pulse oximetry is the preferred way to determine the need for supplemental oxygen, allowing medical personnel to titrate oxygen delivery. Patients with significant traumatic brain injuries (Glasgow Coma Scale less than 12) may suffer secondary brain injury from hypoxia. The occurrence of hypoxia in the head-injured patient is associated with worsening of outcomes. Supplemental oxygen should be utilized as needed to maintain an oxygen saturation greater than 90% in these patients.

Dehydration

A problem unique to pressurized aircraft is the low relative humidity of the cabin environment. Cold, low-pressure air from outside the aircraft is compressed, heated, and vented into the cabin to provide pressurization. This process results in cabin air with negligible water-vapor content. Relative humidity in an aircraft cabin at cruising altitude can be as low as 10% to 20%.[6] The extremely low ambient humidity of the aircraft results in increased insensible water loss from both the casualty and the medical crew. The casualty must be kept adequately hydrated, as must medical personnel and flight crew.

Burn casualties are especially susceptible to insensible water loss because of the compromised dermal barrier. Specific care should be exercised to prevent thermal and fluid losses as well as to monitor intravascular volume and hydration status in the burn casualty during evacuation.

Figure 29-8 Plan for Hypothermia Prevention as Casualty Is Moved to the Rear

At ROLE 1 utilize:
1. Ready Heat Blanket
2. Heat Reflective Shell

At ROLE 2 utilize:
1. Ready Heat Blanket
2. Heat Reflective Shell
3. IV fluid warmers (e.g., ENFLOW or Belmont Buddy Lite)
4. Bair Hugger

At ROLE 3 utilize:
1. Ready Heat Blanket
2. Heat Reflective Shell
3. Bair Hugger
4. Belmont FMS 2000

On any evacuation platform utilize:
1. Ready Heat Blanket
2. Heat Reflective Shell
3. IV fluid warmers (e.g., ENFLOW or Belmont Buddy Lite)

Thermal Stressors

As an aircraft ascends, the ambient temperature decreases. Most helicopters and fixed-wing aircraft have heating systems, but it frequently becomes cold in the aircraft, particularly on long-duration flights. In Operation Iraqi Freedom, medical evacuation crews were often challenged by severe extremes of both cold (flight operations) and heat (onload/offload ground operations). Medical personnel should carefully package and prepare casualties so that appropriate thermal control and casualty comfort may be maintained through a wide range of temperatures.

A coherent hypothermia prevention and reversal strategy is required during premission planning. A layered approach should be used, taking into account weight, cube, power requirements, clinical effectiveness, and practicality **(Figure 29-8)**. All devices used to prevent hypothermia should be capable of employment on any evacuation platform.

Electronic Equipment Considerations

Electronic monitoring equipment offers significant opportunity to increase the situational awareness pertaining to the patient during en route care movement. However, it is critical for the safety of both the casualty and the flight crew that all such electronic equipment be tested and approved for use in the aeromedical environment. Aircraft electronic systems may interfere with monitors, giving rise to false readings or inoperative equipment. Of equal if not greater concern, electronic monitoring equipment may interfere with aircraft systems.[1,4] This is particularly true in rotary-wing platforms, in which medical monitors may be only inches from critical flight avionics equipment. For this reason, all electronic aeromedical equipment must be tested before use in flight. This type of testing for fixed-wing aircraft is performed by the U.S. Air Force at the 311th Human Systems Wing, Brooks City-Base, Texas. Similar testing on rotary-wing aircraft is performed by the U.S. Army at Fort Rucker, Alabama.

Patient Movement Regulation

Aeromedical evacuation is a more formal, measured process than TACEVAC. In most cases, aeromedical evacuation is arranged after the patient has been admitted and treated at a field medical facility. The sending medical unit initiates the process through the generation of a Patient Movement Request (PMR). The PMR is subsequently routed through the Patient Movement Requirement Center (PMRC). The PMRC validates the PMR (basically finds the best-fit transportation option to meet the casualty's clinical needs) and hands the PMR to the theater Air Mobility Operations Control Center (AMOCC), which tasks the aircraft and crews to perform the mission.[8]

Patients are classified into one of three movement priority categories based upon the assessed medical conditions and requirements for further care: routine (can be moved as aircraft are available), priority (must be moved within 72 hours), or urgent (must be moved within 24 hours). All casualties moved by aeromedical evacuation must be cleared for flight by a flight surgeon. The flight surgeon is responsible for assisting the medical team with considering and clearing the patient in preparation for flight. This clearance requires recognition of the stressors of the hypobaric environment and includes consideration of conditions such as the evolution of trapped gas (e.g., pneumothorax, retro-bulbar orbital air, pneumocephalus) and preparation for the stressors of flight. This may be accomplished by discussing the case with the theater validating flight surgeon by radio or phone if a flight surgeon is not available locally.[8]

Under usual circumstances, casualties moved via routine aeromedical evacuation must be stable. If critical or stabilized casualties need to be flown, a special transport team such as a CCATT may be requested to assist in the movement process.

Summary

- The term en route care is employed to encompass and characterize a seamless continuum of medical care from the point-of-injury, through theater facilities, and onward to CONUS facilities.
- Although doctrinal differences exist among the service branches regarding terminology and definitions of phases of care, casualty movement in TCCC may be described as follows:

  1. CASEVAC: Evacuation of a casualty from the battlefield to an MTF using tactical platforms.
  2. MEDEVAC: Evacuation of a casualty from the battlefield to an MTF, or from one MTF to another within the tactical theater, using dedicated medical assets, usually marked with a red cross.
  3. TACEVAC: En route care from the battlefield to a theater Role 2 or Role 3 MTF, including both CASEVAC and MEDEVAC.
  4. Aeromedical evacuation: A term most commonly utilized by the U.S. Air Force to designate the movement of a patient from a point of care within the theater to a more rearward location, such as regional hospital or CONUS.

- In the process of aeromedical evacuation, a wounded soldier is considered a casualty until he or she reaches the first point of definitive medical care. Once entered into the medical care system, the casualty is considered a "patient."

SCENARIO RECAP

You are a flight nurse in an aeromedical evacuation team on board a MEDEVAC C-130 assigned to transfer a patient from the Role 3 hospital in Kandahar, Afghanistan, to Craig Joint Theater Hospital in Bagram. As the aircraft makes its final approach, it comes under small arms fire. Two of the team members are wounded. Casualty 1 has sustained a gunshot wound to his right inguinal area with heavy bleeding. Casualty 2 has an injury to her left thigh with pulsatile bleeding. The aircraft banks away from the approach and there is no further incoming fire.

SCENARIO SOLUTION

1. What phase of TCCC are you in?

You are now in the TACEVAC phase of care. The incoming fire has ceased and you will be transported in your aircraft to an MTF.

2. You now need to do two things simultaneously. What are they?

Both casualties have external hemorrhage that may be lethal if not quickly controlled. You apply a tourniquet to Casualty 2's left thigh while directing an aircrew member to hold Combat Gauze with direct pressure to the bleeding inguinal wound on Casualty 1.

3. What do you do next?

After ensuring that the tourniquet has stopped Casualty 2's bleeding, you move to apply a junctional tourniquet to provide more definitive control of Casualty 1's inguinal bleeding.

An important point in this scenario is that anyone can become a casualty in a combat zone and anyone may need to provide lifesaving battlefield trauma care to another team member.

References

1. Bagian JP, Allen RC. Aeromedical transport. In: Auerbach PS, ed. *Wilderness Medicine*. 4th ed. St. Louis, MO: Mosby; 2004.

2. Golbey SB. Dust off. *AOPA Pilot*. 1987;30:46.

3. Neel S. Army aeromedical evacuation procedures in Vietnam: implications for rural America. *JAMA*. 1968;204(4):309–313.

4. Hurd WW, Jernigan JG. *Aeromedical Evacuation: Management of Acute and Stabilized Patients*. New York, NY: Springer-Verlag; 2003.

5. DeLorenzo RA, Porter RS. *Tactical Emergency Care: Military and Operational Out-of-Hospital Medicine*. Upper Saddle River, NY: Prentice-Hall; 1999.

6. U.S. Air Force. *Air Force Instruction 41–307: Aeromedical Evacuation Patient Considerations and Standards of Care*. August 20, 2003. http://static.e-publishing.af.mil/production/1/af_sg/publication/afi41-307/afi41–307.pdf. Accessed September 3, 2013.

7. U.S. Air Force. Technical Order 1C-130H-1. C-130H Flight Manual. 2002.

8. U.S. Air Force. Access to the aeromedical evacuation system. Air Mobility Command Pamphlet 11–303. November 2000.

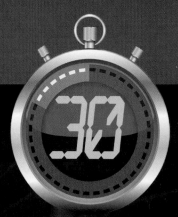

CHAPTER 30

Joint Trauma System

CHAPTER OBJECTIVES

At the completion of this chapter, the reader will be able to do the following:

- State the ultimate vision of the Joint Trauma System.

- List the components of the Joint Trauma System.

- Describe the five roles of injury care in the contemporary military model of combat trauma care.

SCENARIO

Your platoon is on a mounted patrol in Helmand Province, about 100 miles west of Kandahar, when the second vehicle in the convoy is attacked by a roadside improvised explosive device (IED). Upon securing the scene, you identify and treat the only serious casualty, who received multiple fragment wounds to his right extremities and torso. The casualty is evacuated by helicopter to the Combat Support Hospital in Kandahar, and your platoon returns to base. Twenty-four hours later, your Commanding Officer requests an update on the casualty's whereabouts and condition.

1. **Which medical treatment facility (MTF) would you contact first?**

2. **This facility informs you that your casualty was MEDEVACed out of theater 12 hours ago after damage control surgery. He was in stable condition when he left. To which MTF would you direct your next call?**

3. **You find out that your casualty is no longer in the intensive care unit but is on a ward in stable condition. He is scheduled for evacuation to San Antonio Military Medical Center (SAMMC) in 48 hours. There, he will receive convalescent and rehabilitative care. What level medical facility is SAMMC?**

Introduction

Trauma care has evolved from a synergistic relationship between the military and civilian medical environments for the past two centuries.[1-3] Modern battlefield concepts of triage, evacuation, and tiered implementation of battlefield medical care were developed by Baron Dominique Jean Larrey during the Napoleonic era (1797–1815). During the American Civil War (1860–1865), military physicians realized the need for prompt attention to the wounded, early debridement and amputation to mitigate the effects of tissue injury and infection, and evacuation of the casualty from the battlefield. World War I (1914–1917) saw further advances in the concept of evacuation and the development of echelons of medical care.

During World War II (1939–1945), blood transfusion and resuscitative fluids were widely introduced into the combat environment, and surgical practice was improved to care for wounded soldiers. Drawing on his World War II experiences, Dr. Michael DeBakey noted that wars have always promoted advances in trauma care due to the concentrated exposure of military hospitals to large numbers of casualties during a relatively short span of time. Furthermore, this wartime medical experience fostered a fundamental desire to improve outcomes by improving practice.[4] During the Vietnam War, more highly trained combat medic personnel treating casualties at the point of wounding and prompt aeromedical evacuation decreased battlefield mortality even further.[5]

In the civilian realm, in 1966 the National Academy of Sciences (NAS) published "Accidental Death and Disability: The Neglected Disease of Modern Society," noting trauma to be one of the most significant public health issues faced by the United States. Concomitant with advances on the battlefield and the conclusions of the NAS was the formal development of civilian trauma centers. In 1976, the American College of Surgeons produced the first iteration of injury care guidelines, titled "Hospital Resources for the Optimal Care of the Injured Patient."[6] The concepts promoted therein rapidly evolved into the development of formal, integrated trauma systems. Trauma centers and trauma systems in the United States have had a remarkable impact on improving outcomes of injured patients, reducing mortality by up to 15% in mature systems.[2,5,7-19]

Despite the successes of civilian trauma systems, military medicine had not yet adopted this concept. Reports from Operation Desert Shield and Desert Storm in 1992 highlighted a number of opportunities to improve in the area of military trauma systems. Inadequacies were formally noted in both preparation and delivery of trauma care in the combat environment.[3,20-22] Shortly following the terrorist attacks of September 11, 2001, the United States once again had vast numbers of soldiers committed to armed conflict. In order to mimic civilian trauma system outcome successes, the **Joint Theater Trauma System (JTTS)** was conceptualized as a deployable medical asset incorporating a systematic and integrated approach to better organize and coordinate battlefield trauma care. It was designed to minimize morbidity and mortality and optimize the ability to provide essential care required for combat injuries. The more global, overarching **Joint Trauma System (JTS)** was promulgated as a natural progression of these efforts to extend the care and outcome effects across the entire spectrum of combat casualty care from point of injury through rehabilitation. The mantra of the JTS is to improve battlefield trauma care by enabling the right patient, at the right place, and the right time, to receive the right care ("R4") (**Figure 30-1**).

This chapter will assist combat medical personnel in understanding how prehospital trauma management is incorporated into the broader context of the military trauma care system.

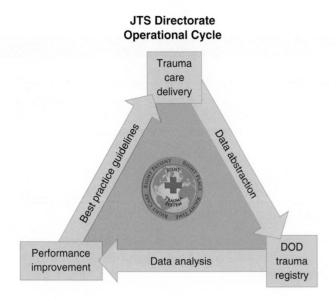

Figure 30-1 Joint Trauma System operational cycle.
Source: Courtesy of Dr. Brian Eastridge, COL, MC, USA (Ret); inset logo Courtesy of USAISR.

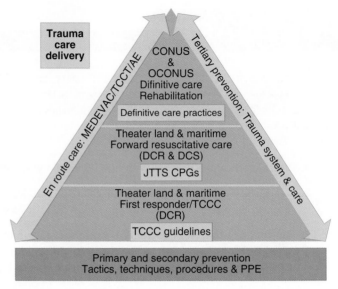

Figure 30-2 Joint Trauma System combat casualty care delivery paradigm.
Source: Courtesy of Dr. Brian Eastridge, COL, MC, USA (Ret).

The Joint Trauma System and the Department of Defense Trauma Registry

The ultimate vision of the JTS is that every soldier, marine, sailor, or airman injured on the battlefield or in the theater of operations has the optimal chance for survival and maximal potential for functional recovery. To attain this vision, the missions of the JTS include the following:

- Improve organization and delivery of trauma care
- Improve communication among combat medical personnel in the evacuation chain to ensure continuity of care and access to patient care data
- Develop and populate the Department of Defense Trauma Registry (DoDTR) in order to capture and report battlefield injury demographics, evaluate care provided, and document outcomes
- Provide a common vehicle to collect, store, and analyze battlefield casualty data for the entire Department of Defense (DOD), and incorporate all trauma-relevant data throughout the entire continuum of care
- Enable a joint strategic and tactical medical research program in support of the warfighter by providing a structured and comprehensive trauma database
- Facilitate movement, collection, and sharing of theater combat casualty data across all roles of care and all the services

- Evaluate and recommend new equipment or medical supplies for use in theater to improve efficiency, support clinical innovation, reduce cost, and improve outcomes
- Facilitate medical performance improvement to promote real-time, data-driven clinical process improvements and improved outcomes
- Develop and maintain evidence-supported clinical practice guidelines
- Identify combat casualty care training requirements
- Maintain currency of trauma care and systems

The components of the JTS system, modeled after successful civilian counterparts, include prevention, prehospital care, acute injury care, evacuation, and rehabilitation (**Figure 30-2**).[23] To further develop the trauma system process, it was incumbent upon the system to foster focused education, leadership and communication, quality improvement/performance improvement, research, and information systems (**Figure 30-3**). The development of a joint trauma registry, the DoDTR, supported system needs such as data-based command decision making, performance improvement, and research to reduce morbidity and mortality.

Prevention

Data from the DoDTR are shared with numerous military organizations to help optimize battlefield injury prevention measures. Data relating to demographics, mechanism of injury, wounding patterns, and evacuation are analyzed to develop better warrior protective material solutions, improve prehospital injury mitigation strategies, and optimally allocate medical and evacuation resources to the battlefield.

Core Functions and Services

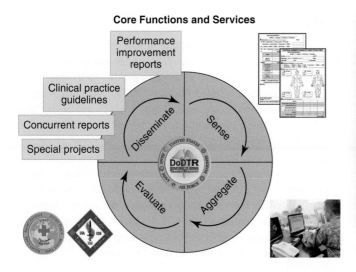

Figure 30-3 Joint Trauma System core functions.
Source: Courtesy of Dr. Brian Eastridge, COL, MC, USA (Ret); inset logo Courtesy of USAISR; inset photo Courtesy of Medical Communications for Combat Casualty Care/U.S. Army.

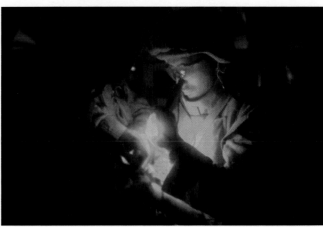

Figure 30-4 A Navy corpsman treats a wounded Marine at night.
Source: Courtesy of U.S. Department of Defense

Battlefield Injury Care Capabilities

Military doctrine supports a battlefield trauma care continuum made manifest by multiple coexistent roles of triage, treatment, and evacuation dissimilar to the civilian trauma system. The current military combat casualty care paradigm consists of five discrete roles of injury care. The basic tenets of the tiered roles of battlefield injury care are aggressive stabilization, resuscitation, staged treatment, and evacuation of the wounded to progressively higher roles of care. This paradigm is designed to improve injury outcomes while being sensitive to the realities of the resource-constrained environment of operations.

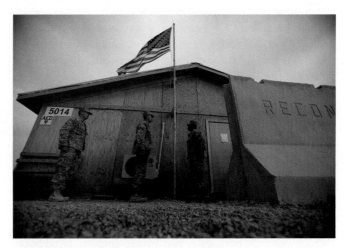

Figure 30-5 A Battalion Aid Station is a Role 1 facility.
Source: Courtesy of Sgt. Bryan Peterson/DVIDS.

Role 1 (Prehospital)

Role 1 care can be stratified into two categories: field care and Role 1 medical treatment facility (MTF) care. Role 1 field care begins with Tactical Combat Casualty Care (TCCC) as delivered by a varying combination of self-aid, buddy aid, and treatment by a **Combat Lifesaver**, followed in most cases by care being rendered by a combat medic, corpsman, or more highly trained Special Operations medic or pararescueman (PJ) (**Figure 30-4**). These combat medical personnel, utilizing the concepts of TCCC, have had a substantial impact on the case fatality rate among those injured in combat in modern contingency operations.[24,25]

Role 1 MTF care, often referred to as battalion aid station care, is provided in aid stations that have the capability to maneuver with the operational line units they support (**Figure 30-5**). These stations are staffed by medical technicians and a physician or a physician's assistant. They function out of tent-based deployable medical systems, fixed facilities of opportunity, or vehicles. Care at this resource-constrained role

is mainly limited to TCCC and/or Advanced Trauma Life Support (ATLS), including establishment of endotracheal intubation, surgical airway management, administration of intravenous fluids and antibiotics, and splint stabilization of wounds and fractures. The goal of medical management at Role 1 facilities is to return less severely injured casualties to duty and to expeditiously treat more severely injured casualties and then evacuate them to the most appropriate MTF in the continuum of care.

Role 2 (Acute MTF Care)

Role 2 facilities and capabilities vary by service. The two basic elements of Role 2 medical treatment facilities are a treatment unit with patient holding capacity and a small surgical element that has the capability to perform lifesaving resuscitative surgery for short bursts at high operational tempo (**Figure 30-6**). The surgical component must be small enough to be mobile, but still have the resource capacity to maintain patient intake, surgical

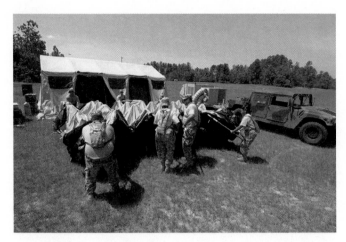

Figure 30-6   U.S. Army's 628th Forward Surgical Team assembles its Role 2 facility during an exercise.
Source: Courtesy of U.S. Department of Defense

stabilization, and postoperative critical care for limited periods of time. Because of the innately resource-constrained forward deployed environment, surgical procedures undertaken at Role 2 facilities are often damage control: temporizing procedures to protect life and limb.

Role 3

Role 3 facilities are the most robust of in-theater medical treatment facilities (**Figure 30-7**). Though not fully deployed in current contingency operations, Role 3 medical treatment facilities offer a fuller complement of hospital and provider resources. Capabilities at Role 3 facilities extend beyond resuscitative surgery to encompass a broad range of surgical subspecialties including neurosurgery, oral and maxillofacial surgery, cardiothoracic surgery, burn care, and plastic surgery. In addition, Role 3 units have anesthesiologists, intensivists, and emergency medicine providers to augment surgical resources. Another substantial capability at these facilities is the provision of extended intensive care services supported by nursing professionals.

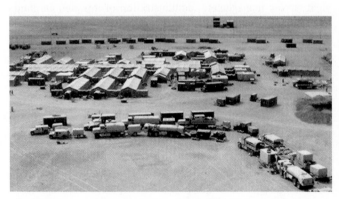

Figure 30-7   A deployed Role 3 Army Combat Support Hospital.
Source: Courtesy of U.S. Department of Defense

Role 4

Role 4 care is provided outside the active theater of operations and can be divided into two distinct entities—those outside the continental United States (OCONUS) (**Figure 30-8**) and those within the continental United States (CONUS). Definitive surgical therapy outside the combat zone is typically initiated at the Role 4 MTF. For the last 12 years of U.S. conflict in the Middle East, the Role 4 MTF has been the Landstuhl Army Regional Medical Center in Germany. However, it should be mentioned that improved paradigms of prehospital care, damage control resuscitation, surgical intervention strategies, and improved techniques for evacuation of combat casualties have markedly decreased the interval between wounding and arrival at a Role 4 MTF. As a result, many injured casualties still require stabilizing or temporizing surgical procedures and intensive care management at Role 4 facilities.

Role 5

Definitive surgery, convalescent, restorative, and rehabilitative care are usually provided at Role 5 facilities within CONUS, such as Walter Reed National Military Medical Center or San Antonio Military Medical Center (**Figure 30-9**).

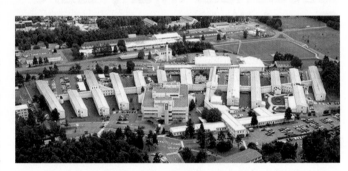

Figure 30-8   Landstuhl Regional Medical Center is a Role 4 facility located in Germany.
Source: Courtesy of U.S. Department of Defense

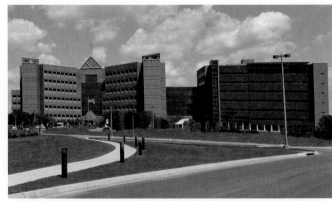

Figure 30-9   San Antonio Military Medical Center is a CONUS Role 5 facility located in San Antonio, Texas.
Source: Courtesy of U.S. Department of Defense

Evacuation

Evacuation of combat casualties progresses through a well-established continuum. Evacuation from the point of wounding can occur by ground, but in the current operational environment in Afghanistan, it usually entails transport by helicopter. Casualty evacuation (CASEVAC) refers to the movement of a casualty to an MTF by nonmedical combatant aircraft or ground vehicles. CASEVAC missions are often conducted using platforms of opportunity.

Medical evacuation (MEDEVAC) refers to the aeromedical transport of injured casualties with well-defined en route medical capability from the point of injury to the first MTF or between MTFs within theater. MEDEVAC platforms are dedicated medical assets. Strategic aeromedical evacuations from the theater to the Role 4 facility in Landstuhl are accomplished by fixed-wing Air Force aircraft. High-risk trauma patients are transported by Critical Care Air Transport Teams (CCATTs) with augmented medical resources to ensure the best possible outcomes.

Continuum of Care

As the global combat trauma system of the DOD, the JTS provides a continuum of care for the battlefield casualty that can spread over thousands of miles and bridge multiple roles of medical care, coordinating both the care delivered and patient movement (**Figure 30-10**). Data-driven real-time performance improvement initiatives within the JTS have led to remarkable improvement in combat injury outcomes.[26]

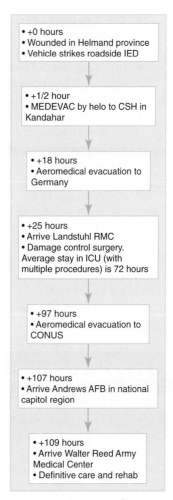

- +0 hours
- Wounded in Helmand province
- Vehicle strikes roadside IED

- +1/2 hour
- MEDEVAC by helo to CSH in Kandahar

- +18 hours
- Aeromedical evacuation to Germany

- +25 hours
- Arrive Landstuhl RMC
- Damage control surgery. Average stay in ICU (with multiple procedures) is 72 hours

- +97 hours
- Aeromedical evacuation to CONUS

- +107 hours
- Arrive Andrews AFB in national capitol region

- +109 hours
- Arrive Walter Reed Army Medical Center
- Definitive care and rehab

Figure 30-10 Typical evacuation timeline in a mature theater of operations.
Source: Courtesy Dr. Stephen Giebner

Summary

- The basic tenets of the Joint Trauma System (JTS) are early and definitive control of external hemorrhage, aggressive stabilization, resuscitation, staged treatment, and evacuation of the wounded to progressively higher levels of care.
- The five discrete roles of injury care within the JTS are designed to optimize injury outcomes while operating within resource constraints.
- Role 1 field care begins with Tactical Combat Casualty Care (TCCC) as provided initially by self-aid and typically progresses through a sequence of buddy aid to Combat Lifesaver treatment to more advanced care by a combat medic, corpsman, or more highly trained Special Operations medic.
- Role 1 medical treatment facility (MTF) care is provided in facilities like Battalion Aid Stations that are typically staffed by medical technicians and a physician or a physician's assistant. They function out of tent-based deployable medical systems, fixed facilities of opportunity, or vehicles. Care at this level is mainly limited by resource constraints to TCCC and/or Advanced Trauma Life Support (ATLS).
- Role 2 facilities consist of treatment units with some patient holding capacity and a small surgical element to perform lifesaving resuscitative surgery for short bursts at a high operational tempo. Surgical procedures undertaken at Role 2 facilities are usually damage control: temporizing procedures to protect life and limb.

- Role 3 facilities offer capabilities beyond resuscitative surgery, which may include neurosurgery, oral and maxillofacial surgery, cardiothoracic surgery, burn surgery, and plastic surgery. These units also have anesthesiologists, intensivists, nursing staff, and emergency medicine providers.
- Role 4 care is provided outside the active theater of operations, and can be divided into two distinct entities—outside the continental United States (OCONUS) or within (CONUS). Definitive surgical therapy outside the combat zone is typically initiated at the Role 4 MTF.
- Improved care at Roles 1 through 3 facilities and greater evacuation capabilities have markedly decreased the interval between wounding and arrival at a Role 4 facility. As a result, many casualties still require stabilization, temporizing surgical procedures, and intensive care management at Role 4 facilities.
- Definitive surgery, convalescent, restorative, and rehabilitative care are usually provided at Role 5 facilities within CONUS, such as Walter Reed National Military Medical Center or San Antonio Military Medical Center.
- The functions of the JTS are facilitated by the DoDTR, providing for system needs such as data-based command decision making, performance improvement, and research to reduce morbidity and mortality.
- Data from the DoDTR are analyzed to develop better warrior protective material solutions, to improve prehospital injury mitigation strategies, and to optimally allocate medical and evacuation resources to the battlefield.
- The continuum of care for combat casualties is spread over thousands of miles and multiple levels of medical care. The JTS provides for coordination of patient care and movement across this continuum, with the goal of producing the optimal chance for survival and maximal potential for functional recovery.

SCENARIO RECAP

Your platoon is on a mounted patrol in Helmand Province, about 100 miles west of Kandahar, when the second vehicle in the convoy is attacked by a roadside IED. Upon securing the scene, you identify and treat the only serious casualty, who received multiple fragment wounds to his right extremities and torso. The casualty is evacuated by helicopter to the Combat Support Hospital in Kandahar, and your platoon returns to base. Twenty-four hours later, your Commanding Officer requests an update on the casualty's whereabouts and condition.

SCENARIO SOLUTION

1. **Which medical treatment facility (MTF) would you contact first?**

   The Combat Support Hospital at Kandahar

2. **This facility informs you that your casualty was MEDEVACed out of theater 12 hours ago after damage control surgery. He was in stable condition when he left. To which MTF would you direct your next call?**

   The Role 4 facility that receives casualties from the Afghan theater—in this case, Landstuhl Regional Medical Center in Germany

3. **You find out that your casualty is no longer in the intensive care unit but is on a ward in stable condition. He is scheduled for evacuation to San Antonio Military Medical Center (SAMMC) in 48 hours. There, he will receive convalescent and rehabilitative care. What level medical facility is SAMMC?**

   Role 5

References

1. Tracy E. Combining military and civilian trauma systems: the best of both worlds. *Top Emerg Med*. 2005;27:170–175.

2. Trunkey DD. History and development of trauma care in the United States. *Clin Orthop Relat Res*. 2000;(374):36–46.

3. Trunkey DD. In search of solutions. *J Trauma*. 2002;53(6):1189–1191.

4. DeBakey ME. History, the torch that illuminates: lessons from military medicine. *Mil Med*. 1996;161(12):711–716.

5. Hoff WS, Schwab CW. Trauma system development in North America. *Clin Orthop Relat Res*. 2004;(422):17–22.

6. American College of Surgeons. Hospital resources for optimal care of the injured patient. Prepared by a Task force of the Committee on Trauma of the American College of Surgeons. *Bull Am Coll Surg*. 1979;64(8):43–48.

7. Demetriades D, Kimbrell B, Salim A, et al. Trauma deaths in a mature urban trauma system: is "trimodal" distribution a valid concept? *J Am Coll Surg*. 2005;201(3):343–348.

8. Jurkovich GJ, Mock C. Systematic review of trauma system effectiveness based on registry comparisons. *J Trauma*. 1999;47(3 Suppl):S46–S55.

9. Mann NC. Assessing the effectiveness and optimal structure of trauma systems: a consensus among experts. *J Trauma*. 1999;47(3 Suppl):S69–S74.

10. Mann NC, Mullins RJ. Research recommendations and proposed action items to facilitate trauma system implementation and evaluation. *J Trauma*. 1999;47(3 Suppl):S75–S78.

11. Mann NC, Mullins RJ, MacKenzie EJ, Jurkovich GJ, Mock CN. Systematic review of published evidence regarding trauma system effectiveness. *J Trauma*. 1999;47(3 Suppl):S25–S33.

12. Mullins RJ. A historical perspective of trauma system development in the United States. *J Trauma*. 1999;47(3 Suppl):S8–S14.

13. Mullins RJ, Mann NC. Population-based research assessing the effectiveness of trauma systems. *J Trauma*. 1999;47(3 Suppl):S59–S66.

14. Mullins RJ, Mann NC. Introduction to the Academic Symposium to Evaluate Evidence Regarding the Efficacy of Trauma Systems. *J Trauma*. 1999;47(3 Suppl):S3–S7.

15. Mullins RJ, Veum-Stone J, Hedges JR, et al. Influence of a statewide trauma system on location of hospitalization and outcome of injured patients. *J Trauma*. 1996;40(4):536–545, discussion 545–546.

16. Nathens AB, Jurkovich GJ, Rivara FP, Maier RV. Effectiveness of state trauma systems in reducing injury-related mortality: a national evaluation. *J Trauma*. 2000;48(1):25–30, discussion 30–31.

17. O'Keefe GE, Jurkovich GJ, Copass M, Maier RV. Ten-year trend in survival and resource utilization at a level I trauma center. *Ann Surg*. 1999;229(3):409–415.

18. Trunkey DD. Trauma care systems. *Emerg Med Clin North Am*. 1984;2(4):913–922.

19. West JG, Williams MJ, Trunkey DD, Wolferth CC Jr. Trauma systems. Current status—future challenges. *JAMA*. 1988;259(24):3597–3600.

20. Operation Desert Storm: Full Army Medical Capability Not Achieved. Washington, DC: GAO/NSIAD-92-175; 1992.

21. War Time Medical Care: DOD Is Addressing Capability Shortfalls, but Challenges Remain. Washington, DC: GAO/NSIAD-96-224; 1996.

22. War Time Medical Care: Personnel Requirements Still Not Resolved. Washington, DC: GAO/NSIAD-96-173; 1996.

23. American College of Surgeons. *Resources for the Optimal Care of the Injured Patient: 1999*. Chicago, IL: American College of Surgeons; 1999:135.

24. Eastridge BJ, Mabry R, Seguin P, et al. Pre-hospital death on the battlefield: implications for the future of combat casualty care. *J Trauma Acute Care Surg*. 2012;73:S431–S437.

25. Kotwal RS, Montgomery HR, Kotwal BM, et al. Eliminating preventable death on the battlefield. *Arch Surg*. 2011;146:1350–1358.

26. Blackbourne LH, Baer DG, Eastridge BJ, et al. Military medical revolution: military trauma system. *J Trauma Acute Care Surg*. 2012;73(6 suppl 5):S388–S394.

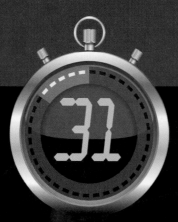

CHAPTER 31

Triage in Tactical Combat Casualty Care

CHAPTER OBJECTIVES

At the completion of this chapter, the reader will be able to do the following:

- List the casualty categories used in battlefield triage and describe each.

- Identify the physiologic parameters of most importance in battlefield triage, and state how they are used to gauge a casualty's need for lifesaving intervention (LSI) and the probability of survival.

- Given the physiologic data of primary interest on a casualty, place the casualty in the proper triage category.

SCENARIO

You are the only medic doing triage at a mass-casualty incident and are at least an hour from the closest surgical facility.

1. The first casualty you assess has a gunshot wound through his right chest and obvious difficulty breathing. He can communicate with you appropriately. His radial pulse, though rapid, is strong. What is his initial triage category?
   A Minimal
   B Delayed
   C Immediate
   D Expectant

2. The second casualty you see has multiple chest and abdominal fragment wounds, no radial pulse, barely palpable carotid pulse, and shallow intermittent breathing. He is unresponsive. What is his initial triage category?
   A Minimal
   B Delayed
   C Immediate
   D Expectant

3. Which of the two casualties would you treat first?
   A Casualty 1
   B Casualty 2

4. After the first casualty has undergone needle decompression of his tension pneumothorax, his breathing returns to normal, his radial pulse is strong and no longer rapid, and he can converse normally though with some pain. What is his new triage category?
   A Minimal
   B Delayed
   C Immediate
   D Expectant

Introduction

Triage is a system of sorting and categorizing casualties formalized by Baron Dominique Jean Larrey, the surgeon-in-chief of the Napoleonic armies between 1797 and 1815. During this time, Baron Larrey initiated a system of battlefield stabilization, tourniquet use, and subsequent rapid evacuation to definitive care. He established a rule for the triage of war casualties: treating the wounded according to the seriousness of their injuries and urgency of need for medical care, regardless of rank or nationality.[1] Similarly, modern battlefield triage is a process for sorting casualties into groups based on their need for, or likely benefit from, immediate medical treatment **(Figure 31-1)**. It is an iterative process whereby casualties are prioritized for treatment and evacuation, performed at every level of care.

Figure 31-1 Triage Categories

To be effective, triage requires appropriate categorization of casualties. These categories determine priority for treatment and evacuation. The four categories of tactical triage are:

- *Minimal:* Casualties in this category are often referred to as the "walking wounded." Although these patients may appear to be in bad shape at first, it is their physiologic state that tells the true story. These casualties have minor injuries (e.g., small burns, lacerations, abrasions, or small fractures) that can usually be treated with self-aid or buddy aid. These casualties should be utilized for mission requirements (e.g., scene security), to help treat and/or transport the more seriously wounded, or put back into the fight.
- *Delayed:* This category includes those wounded who are likely to need surgery, but whose general condition permits delay in surgical treatment without unduly endangering the life, limb, or eyesight of the casualty. Sustaining treatment will be required (e.g., oral or intravenous fluids, splinting, administration of antibiotics, and pain control), but can

(Continues on next page)

Figure 31-1   Triage Categories (*Continued*)

possibly wait. Examples of casualties in this category include those with no evidence of shock who have large soft-tissue wounds, fractures of major bones, intra-abdominal and/or thoracic wounds, and burns to less than 20% of total body surface area.

- *Immediate:* This category includes those casualties who require an immediate lifesaving intervention and/or surgery. Put simply, if medical attention is not provided, they will die. The key to successful triage is to locate these individuals as quickly as possible. Casualties do not remain in this category for an extended period of time. They are either found, triaged, and treated, or they die! Hemodynamically unstable casualties with airway obstruction, chest or abdominal injuries, massive external bleeding, or shock deserve this classification.
- *Expectant:* Casualties in this category have wounds that are so extensive, that even if they were the sole casualty and had the benefit of optimal medical resources, their survival would be highly unlikely. Even so, expectant casualties should not be neglected. They should receive comfort measures and pain medication if possible, and they deserve retriage as appropriate. Examples of expectant casualties are the unresponsive with injuries such as penetrating head trauma with obvious massive damage to the brain.

Triage in Tactical Combat Casualty Care

The realities of combat dictate that battlefield triage must take place in an environment limited in resources for treatment and transport. The treatment and evacuation priorities of combat casualties across the phases of Tactical Combat Casualty Care (TCCC) are outlined in the Tactical Field Care and Tactical Evacuation Care chapters. Triage of casualties during TCCC merely establishes priority of care and order of movement, not whether treatment will be provided or what treatment is indicated **(Figure 31-2)**. Effective triage may dictate that some casualties do not receive immediate treatment and are returned to the fight.

Figure 31-2   Triage in TCCC

Triage in the Care Under Fire Phase
1. Get the casualties who are not clearly dead to cover, if possible.
2. Control life-threatening extremity hemorrhage.
3. Continue with the mission/fight.

Triage in the Tactical Field Care Phase
1. Perform an initial rapid assessment of the casualty for triage purposes. This should take no more than 1 minute per casualty.
2. If a casualty can walk, he or she will probably do well, if there is no significant internal or external hemorrhage and/or difficulty with airway/breathing.
3. Perform immediate lifesaving interventions (LSIs) as indicated, such as applying a tourniquet for life-threatening extremity hemorrhage, using Combat Gauze or junctional hemorrhage control devices for life-threatening external hemorrhage at a site where a tourniquet cannot be applied, or performing needle decompression of a tension pneumothorax. Move rapidly.
4. Reverse treatment from airway-breathing-circulation (ABC) to circulation-breathing-airway (CBA). The majority of preventable deaths on the battlefield are the result of failure to control external hemorrhage. It does no good to ensure a patent airway when the casualty has lost too much blood to survive.
5. Talk to the casualty while checking the radial pulse. If the casualty can talk easily, obeys commands and has a strong radial pulse, then the casualty has an excellent chance of survival, if there is no ongoing internal or external hemorrhage. This casualty is usually in the minimal or delayed category.

(Continues on next page)

Figure 31-2 Triage in TCCC (*Continued*)

6. If the casualty obeys commands, but has a weak or absent radial pulse, the casualty is at increased risk of dying and may benefit from an immediate LSI. This casualty is in the immediate category.

7. If the casualty does not obey commands AND has a weak or absent radial pulse, the casualty has a markedly increased chance of dying (greater than 92%) and may benefit from an immediate LSI. This casualty is in the immediate or possibly expectant category depending upon resource constraints and evacuation time.

8. Prepare casualties to move out of the area. Prevent hypothermia.

Triage in the Tactical Evacuation Phase
1. Triage the casualties again. Categories and treatment requirements can and will change.
2. Use any advanced diagnostic equipment available at this level to assist in triage.
3. Soft-tissue injuries are common and may look bad but do not kill unless associated with shock.
4. Bleeding from most extremity wounds should be controllable with a tourniquet or hemostatic dressing. Tactical Evacuation delays should not increase mortality if bleeding is fully controlled.
5. Casualties who are in shock should be evacuated as soon as possible.
6. Casualties with penetrating wounds of the chest who have respiratory distress unrelieved by needle decompression of the chest should be evacuated as soon as possible. If available, place a chest tube.
7. Casualties with penetrating wounds of the chest or abdomen who are in shock have a high risk of dying and should be evacuated as soon as possible.
8. Casualties with blunt or penetrating trauma to the face associated with difficulty breathing should immediately receive definitive airway control and should be evacuated as soon as possible.
9. Casualties with blunt or penetrating wounds of the head in which there is obvious massive brain damage and unconsciousness are unlikely to survive with or without emergent evacuation.
10. Casualties who have blunt or penetrating wounds to the head in which the skull has been penetrated but are still conscious should be evacuated as soon as possible.
11. Casualties with penetrating wounds of the chest or abdomen who are not in shock at their 15-minute evaluation have a moderate risk of developing late shock from slowly bleeding internal injuries. They should be carefully monitored and evacuated as soon as feasible.

Proper triage aids the combat medical personnel in deciding which casualties have the greatest probability of survival and in weighing the casualties' relative needs for a lifesaving intervention (LSI), thus determining priority and urgency for treatment and evacuation. Using a standardized approach to the triage of combat casualties will help combat medical personnel correctly segregate, treat, and prioritize evacuation in the shortest possible time.[2] Triage ensures the greatest care for the greatest number and the maximal utilization of medical personnel, equipment, and facilities, especially in a mass-casualty incident. Improved triage leads to improved survival. To be maximally effective, the most experienced combat medical personnel available should perform initial triage and direct treatment. He or she is generally the one most familiar with the natural course of injuries, knows best when treatment is futile or emergently indicated, and is best able to identify those casualties who can be returned to battle. The senior provider should direct other resources (Combat Lifesavers, first aid providers) to assist with immediate treatment and movement to a Casualty Collection Point (CCP) or evacuation platform.

Combat Triage Decision Algorithm

Currently, most civilian triage algorithms utilize physiologic and anatomic criteria because these are readily assessable at the point of injury and provide insight as to a casualty's current status and likely outcome.[3-5] Accuracy in triage depends upon using only those criteria shown to predict outcomes and the need for immediate intervention. These criteria include a cursory evaluation, the physiologic status, and anatomic criteria. The purpose of the cursory evaluation is to rapidly detect those casualties with minor injuries and those mortally wounded.

Physiologic Status

The next step, an assessment of physiologic criteria, is intended to allow for rapid identification of critically injured patients by assessing the casualty's level of consciousness (Glasgow Coma Scale) and measuring the casualty's vital signs (systolic blood pressure and respiratory status).[3,6-8] These criteria demonstrate high predictive value for severe injury. Multiple peer-reviewed articles published since 2006 support this process for triage in the civilian sector.[9–12]

Because the austere and often hazardous tactical environment precludes the use of sophisticated monitoring equipment, battlefield evaluation relies upon simple assessment tools. For triage in tactical situations, two criteria are highly predictive of outcomes: the casualty's ability to follow simple commands (from the motor component of the Glasgow Coma Scale) and the character and rate of the radial pulse (used as a surrogate for systolic blood pressure). Based on these criteria and other published data, a triage decision algorithm has been developed for TCCC **(Figure 31-3)**.[3–8,13–15]

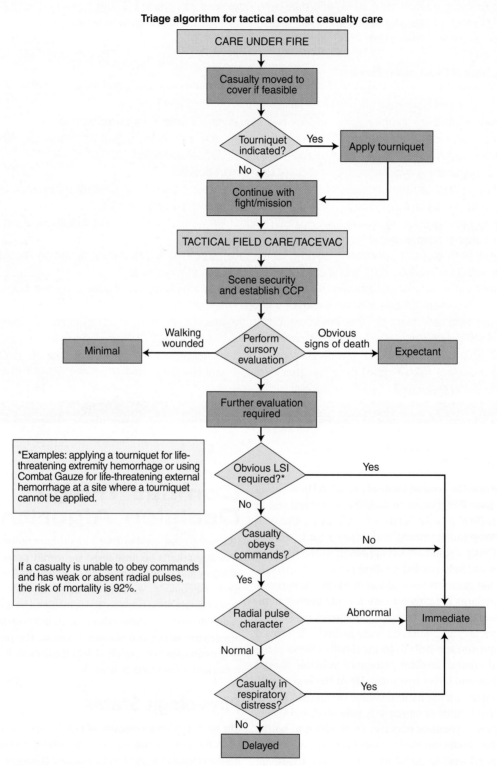

Figure 31-3 Triage algorithm for TCCC.

Source: Courtesy of Dr. John Holcomb

Unless there is significant external hemorrhage, airway or breathing difficulty, or a gunshot wound to the torso, the ability to ambulate usually places a casualty initially into the minimal category, whereas obvious signs of death will place a casualty in the expectant category. For those casualties not falling into either of these categories, further assessment is required. All casualties requiring an LSI are placed initially in the immediate category. However, once the LSI is performed, a casualty must be retriaged. Again, triage is a continuous process and frequent reassessment is required—a casualty may move from one category to another at each assessment.

The combat medical personnel performing triage should talk to the casualty while checking the casualty's radial pulse. If the casualty obeys commands and has a normal radial pulse, then he or she has a greater than 95% chance of survival. Following this step, the casualty should be visually assessed for respiratory distress. A respiratory rate of less than 10 or greater than 30 breaths per minute, or the need for ventilatory support, identifies the casualty as seriously injured.[6] If a casualty can obey commands, possesses a strong radial pulse, is in no respiratory distress, and has no significant external hemorrhage, then the casualty should be placed initially in the delayed category.

Anatomic Criteria

In civilian trauma care, using physiologic and anatomic criteria alone for triage of patients may result in a high degree of undertriage, or assigning patients to a lower-than-actual risk category. Inclusion of special considerations when assessing the need for transport to advanced trauma care can reduce that problem.[16] This need for special assessment considerations also applies to combat trauma. For instance, certain casualties may have normal physiologic criteria but have an anatomic injury that might require the highest level of care. Combat medical personnel should maintain a low threshold for early intervention and evacuation if any of the following injuries are identified[6]:

- Serious penetrating injuries to head, neck, torso, and extremities proximal to elbow or knee
- Chest wall instability or deformity
- Two or more proximal long-bone fractures
- Crushed, degloved, mangled, or pulseless extremity
- Amputation proximal to wrist or ankle
- Pelvic fractures (consider internal hemorrhage)

- Open or depressed skull fractures
- Paralysis

Mechanism of injury is also an independent predictor of mortality and functional impairment of blunt trauma victims.[16,17] Falls greater than 20 feet, high-risk vehicle crashes, and exposure to blasts are attended by a great risk of severe trauma. Serious injury and the need for rapid evacuation to definitive care should be anticipated.

Planning and Protection

In preparing for combat, with its propensity for mass-casualty incidents, many factors must be considered during mission planning and rehearsed in training to ensure mission accomplishment and proper care of our soldiers **(Figure 31-4)**. Environment, mission, and timeline are critical factors that will affect the way triage is executed. How and where will the triage area and CCP be set up and security maintained? What are the evacuation assets available and the response time frame?

While performing triage, it is important to remember to protect one's self and other rescuers as well as preventing further harm to the casualties. Those responsible for triage must remember at all times that triage is not definitive treatment and constant reassessment is needed to identify casualties who may have deteriorated or improved.

Figure 31-4 Pearls for Mass-Casualty Triage

- Secure the area and ensure scene safety.
- Establish the scene commander and medical director.
- Establish Command Post (CP), Casualty Collection Point(s) (CCPs), and routes of access.
- Estimate initial number and severity of casualties.
- Identify additional hazards (e.g., smoke; nuclear, biologic, chemical [NBC]).
- Assign initial triage categories.
- Perform required lifesaving interventions.
- Retriage with an extended secondary assessment as time permits.

Summary

- Triage is a process for sorting casualties into groups based on their need for, or potential benefit from, medical treatment.
- The most experienced combat medical personnel should perform initial triage because they are the most familiar with the natural course of injuries and know best when treatment will likely be futile.
- There are four triage categories: minimal, delayed, immediate, and expectant.
- Further evaluation is required for those casualties who do not fall into the minimal or expectant category.
- The minimal category includes those with minor injuries that can usually be cared for with self-aid or buddy aid.
- The ability to ambulate places a casualty immediately into the minimal category, unless there is significant external hemorrhage, airway or breathing difficulty, or a penetrating wound to the torso.
- If a casualty can obey commands, possesses a strong radial pulse, and is in no respiratory distress, the casualty should be placed in the minimal or delayed category.
- The delayed category includes those wounded who may need surgery but whose general condition permits delay in surgical treatment without unduly endangering the life or limb of the casualty, though some sustaining treatment will probably be required.
- The immediate category includes those who require an immediate LSI and/or surgery.
- All casualties requiring an LSI are placed initially in the immediate category, and once the LSI is performed, the casualty must be retriaged.
- The expectant category includes those with wounds that are so extensive that, even with optimal treatment, their survival would be highly unlikely.
- Obvious signs of death will place a casualty in the expectant category.
- Triage is a continuous process. Frequent reassessment is needed to identify casualties who may have deteriorated or improved.
- Triage is not definitive treatment.

SCENARIO RECAP

You are the only medic doing triage at a mass-casualty incident and are at least an hour from the closest surgical facility.

SCENARIO SOLUTION

1. The first casualty you assess has a gunshot wound through his right chest and obvious difficulty breathing. He can communicate with you appropriately. His radial pulse, though rapid, is strong. What is his initial triage category?

   C. Immediate

2. The second casualty you see has multiple chest and abdominal fragment wounds, no radial pulse, barely palpable carotid pulse, and shallow intermittent breathing. He is unresponsive. What is his initial triage category?

   C. Immediate

3. Which of the two casualties would you treat first?

   A. Casualty 1

4. After the first casualty has undergone needle decompression of his tension pneumothorax, his breathing returns to normal, his radial pulse is strong and no longer rapid, and he can converse normally, though with some pain. What is his new triage category?

   B. Delayed

References

1. Bodemer CW. Baron Dominique Jean Larrey, Napoleon's surgeon. *Bull Am Coll Surg*. 1982;67(7):18–21.

2. Baxt WG, Jones G, Fortlage D. The trauma triage rule:a new, resource-based approach to the prehospital identification of major trauma victims. *Ann Emerg Med*. 1990;19(12):1401–1406.

3. Butler FK, Hagmann J, Butler EJ. Tactical combat casualty care in special operations. *Mil Med*. 1996;161(Suppl):3–15.

4. Ekblad GS. Training medics for the combat environment of tomorrow. *Mil Med*. 1990;155:232–234.

5. Centers for Disease Control and Prevention. Guidelines for field triage of injured patients:Recommendations of the National Expert Panel on Field Triage. *MMWR*. 2009;58(RR-1):1–35.

6. Centers for Disease Control and Prevention. Guidelines for field triage of injured patients:Recommendations of the National Expert Panel on Field Triage. *MMWR*. 2012;61(RR-1):1–20.

7. Meredith W, Rutledge R, Hansen A, et al. Field triage of trauma patients based upon the ability to follow commands:a study in 29,573 injured patients. *J Trauma*. 1995;38(1):129–135.

8. McManus J, Yershov A, Ludwig D, et al. Radial pulse character relationships to systolic blood pressure and trauma outcomes. *Prehosp Emerg Care*. 2005;9:423–428.

9. Cherry RA, King TS, Carney DE, Bryant P, Cooney RN. Trauma team activation and the impact on mortality. *J Trauma*. 2007;63:326–30.

10. Edelman DA, White MT, Tyburski JG, Wilson RF. Post-traumatic hypotension:should systolic blood pressure of 90–109 mmHg be included? *Shock*. 2007;27:134–138.

11. Codner P, Obaid A, Porral D, Lush S, Cinat M. Is field hypotension a reliable indicator of significant injury in trauma patients who are normotensive on arrival to the emergency department? *Am Surg*. 2005;71:768–771.

12. Lipsky AM, Gausche-Hill M, Henneman PL, et al. Prehospital hypotension is a predictor of the need for an emergent, therapeutic operation in trauma patients with normal systolic blood pressure in the emergency department. *J Trauma*. 2006;61:1228–1233.

13. Garner A, Lee A, Harrison K, Shultz C. Disaster medicine/domestic preparedness. *Ann Emerg Med*. 2001;38(5):541–548.

14. Holcomb J, Niles S, Miller C, Hinds D, Duke J, Moore F. Prehospital physiologic data and lifesaving interventions in trauma patients. *Mil Med*. 2005;170(1):7–13.

15. Eastridge B, Salinas J, McManus J, et al. Field Triage Score (FTS):development and validation of a simple and practical prehospital triage instrument. (Submitted to the *Journal of Trauma*, 2010—in review.)

16. Brown JB, Stassen NA, Bankey PE, Sangosanya AT, Cheng JD, Gestring ML. Mechanism of injury and special consideration criteria still matter:an evaluation of the National Trauma Triage Protocol. *J Trauma*. 2011;70:38–44, discussion 44–45.

17. Haider AH, Chang DC, Haut ER, Cornwell EE, Efron DT. Mechanism of injury predicts patient mortality and impairment after blunt trauma. *J Surg Res*. 2009;153:138–142.

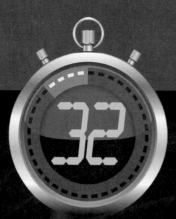

CHAPTER 32

Injuries from Explosives

CHAPTER OBJECTIVES

At the completion of this chapter, the reader will be able to do the following:

- List the five categories of mechanism of explosion-related injury and give examples of each category.

- Describe how explosion-related injuries differ from other types of injuries.

- Discuss the precautions that responders to explosive blast incidents need to take.

- Describe the major wounding effects of explosives and types of treatment typically required.

SCENARIO

While on foot patrol on a rural road, one member of a five-member team triggers an improvised explosive device (IED). One casualty is dead, two have minor injuries, and one has sustained significant blast injuries to his lower torso and right lower extremity. You are providing medical care to the team.

1. **What are the tactical considerations in this situation?**

Introduction

A contemporary understanding of injury from explosives is essential for all providers of emergency care in both military and civilian settings. Medical personnel need to understand the pathophysiology of injury caused by the improvised explosive devices (IEDs) so widely used by insurgents and terrorists. As Lemonick cautions us:

> Because of the increasing risk of terrorist IED attacks on civilians, non-military health care providers must become familiar with the characteristics of explosives and of explosions and of the nature of the injuries they may inflict.[1]

Explosions occur in homes, primarily due to gas leaks or fires. Explosions are an occupational hazard of many industries, including mining, demolition, chemical manufacture, fuel transport and refining, and grain storage. Industrial explosions result from chemical spills, fires, faulty equipment maintenance, or electrical/machinery malfunctions and may produce toxic fumes, building collapse, secondary explosions, falling debris, and large numbers of casualties. However, as a whole, unintentional explosions are responsible for relatively few injuries and deaths (e.g., 151 in the United States in 2005[2]) compared with the large numbers of injuries and deaths produced by explosives used by terrorists and military adversaries.

Explosives are the predominant cause of combat injury and death. In the postmaneuver insurgency phase in Iraq, explosives accounted for about 60% of injuries to American combatants.[3] Between 2001 and 2009, the majority of U.S. troop deaths (72%) were caused by explosions.[4] In Afghanistan, the number of IED events (IEDs detected, disarmed, or detonated) increased more than 80% between 2009 and 2011 (from 9,300 to 16,800) and totaled 14,500 as of mid-December 2012.[5] IEDs caused an average of 46% of all U.S. troop deaths in Afghanistan over the past 5 years,[6] and according to the Joint Improvised Explosive Device Defeat Organization (JIEDDO), they were responsible for 63% of all U.S. casualties in Iraq and Afghanistan in 2011.[7]

Insurgents and terrorists worldwide are increasingly using bombs, especially IEDs, against civilian targets as well. In 2011, a reported 10,283 terrorist attacks took place throughout the world, injuring almost 45,000 people and causing 12,533 deaths,

of which 51% were civilians.[8] Almost half (43%) of the attacks and most (75%) of the deaths were caused by bombings, including suicide bombings, with IEDs implicated in most cases.[8] The reason for such widespread and increasing use of IEDs is that these devices are inexpensive, are made from easily obtained materials (such as ammonium nitrate, which is derived from a common agricultural fertilizer and used in 70% of IEDs in Afghanistan[5]), and result in the devastating havoc that focuses international exposure on the attackers' cause.

Explosive attacks typically result in mass-casualty incidents (MCIs). For example, the 1995 attack on the Murrah Building in Oklahoma City killed 168 and injured 518. Suicide bomb attacks in Israel, which occur both in open areas and confined spaces (such as buildings or buses), have produced limited mass-casualty events on a regular basis. However, most recently, countries such as Afghanistan, Iraq, Pakistan, Somalia, and Nigeria have been the sites of terrorist attacks that result in mass casualties.[8]

At present, although the United States is not typically exposed to as many explosive attacks as other countries, explosion-related incidents reported to the U.S. Bomb Data Center totaled 5,219 in 2011 (more than 14 per day), an almost 38% increase over 2004 (**Figure 32-1**).[9] Between January and September 2011, 367 homemade bomb attacks occurred in the United States.[10]

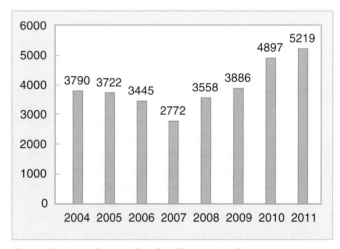

Figure 32-1   Explosion-Related Incidents, United States, 2004–2011.

Source: Reproduced from Bureau of Alcohol, Tobacco, Firearms and Explosives: Fact sheet. U.S. Bomb Data Center. http://www.atf.gov/publications/factsheets/factsheet-us-bomb-data-center.pdf. Accessed January 11, 2013

According to the Director of JIEDDO, Army Lieutenant General Michael Barbero:

> If we think [attacks with improvised devices are] going to go away after Iraq and Afghanistan, we're dreaming. ... Their popularity among criminals, narcotics traffickers and terrorists continues to grow, aided by the [online] spread ... of bomb-making technology.[10]

Because both civilian and military responders may be called upon during an explosive attack on civilian populations, all health care providers need to be familiar with their roles during these increasingly frequent occurrences, and to be aware of and able to prevent or mitigate the attacks against first responders that often accompany terrorist bombings.[8]

Overview

Injuries from explosions differ significantly from injuries due to other mechanisms and are more complex than those typically seen in civilian practice. The most important differences are:

- *Explosions cause injury by multiple mechanisms.* Unlike vehicular injury (blunt trauma) and injuries from bullets (ballistic/gunshot), which apply relatively simple mechanisms to transfer energy to the human body, an explosion causes energy to be transferred in complex and multiple fashions. Energy from explosions is primarily designed to propel fragments (primary and secondary) at high velocity. Thus, the most significant cause of injury is multiple fragment wounds. However, primary blast overpressure, whole or partial body translocation, injury from building collapse (including crush injury), and injury from fireball and dust inhalation can all play a part in the complex anatomic and physiologic dysfunction inflicted on the body by an explosion.
- *Explosions cause multiple injuries.* Unlike other mechanisms, survivors of explosive blasts tend to have multiple injuries involving numerous anatomic areas and organs.
- *Explosions have multiple etiologies.* For example, when a vehicle is hit by an IED, the initial set of forces is a result of the explosion. However, the vehicle may be translocated and forcibly inverted or vectored into a tree or culvert, causing multiple blunt injuries that accompany penetrating wounds. Personal protective devices worn by vehicle occupants may modify these injuries.

Further, the rate at which blast overpressure couples energy to the body is much higher than, for instance, energy coupling in a motor vehicle crash. This can cause unique tissue distortions and malfunctions.

Training of medical care professionals, from first responders to definitive care providers, in blast injury management is severely lacking. Also lacking is knowledge of the effects of combinations of multiple fragment injuries and blast overpressure on tissue reaction and implications for treatment. This chapter will acquaint the reader with contemporary practice and knowledge of this current health care imperative.

Explosive Agents
Categories

Explosives fall into one of two categories based on velocity of detonation: low explosives and high explosives. IEDs may be made of high or low explosives, or a combination of both.[11]

Low Explosives

When activated, low explosives (e.g., dynamite, gunpowder) change relatively slowly from a solid to a gaseous state, in an action more characteristic of deflagration (burning) than of detonation. Low explosives, which include pipe bombs and pure petroleum-based bombs such as Molotov cocktails, lack the highly compressed blast wave and shattering effect (brisance) that define high explosives.[11] Injuries caused by low explosives typically include fragment and thermal injuries, not the primary blast injuries that are often associated with high explosives.[12]

High Explosives

High explosives react almost instantaneously in that they detonate rather than deflagrate, and their detonation velocity greatly exceeds the speed of sound.[12] The initial explosion creates an immediate rise in pressure, creating a shock wave that travels outward at supersonic speed (3,000 to 8,000 meters/second [10,000 to 26,000 feet/second]). The shock wave is the leading front and an integral component of the blast wave, which is created upon the rapid release of enormous amounts of energy, with subsequent propulsion of fragments, generation of environmental debris, and often intense thermal radiation.

High explosives are frequently used in military ordnance and IEDs. Their sharp, shattering effect (brisance) can pulverize bone and soft tissue, create blast overpressure injuries (barotrauma), and propel primary and secondary fragments and debris at ballistic speeds. With conventional high explosives, the blast wave decays very rapidly and is significantly affected by the environment. The rapid change in pressure and the duration of depressurization affect the severity of resultant primary blast injury.

The power of an explosive for military demolitions is expressed as its **relative effectiveness (RE) factor**, which is calculated based on its detonating velocity relative to that of trinitrotoluene (TNT) (which has an RE factor of 1.00).[13] **Rate of detonation**, given in feet per second, and RE factors for typical high explosives used in IEDs are shown in (**Figure 32-2**).[14] A sampling of high explosives currently in use is given in (**Figure 32-3**).

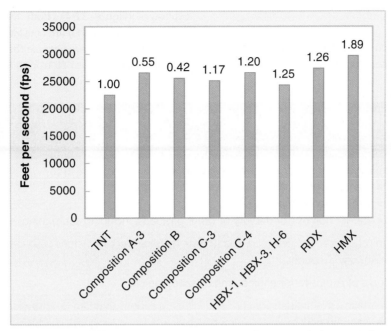

Figure 32-2 Velocity of Detonation and Relative Effectiveness (RE) Factors of Typical High Explosives Used in IEDs[14]

Source: Data from: U.S. Navy Salvage Engineer's Handbook, Volume 1 (Salvage Engineering). U.S. Navy Salvor's Handbook. S0300-A8-HBK-010. 1997.

Figure 32-3 Sample of High Explosives Currently in Use[15-18]

Name Abbreviated	Expanded	Description
TNT	Trinitrotoluene	Conventional explosive; "TNT equivalent" is used as a measure of energy released from other explosives
AN	Ammonium nitrate	Often mixed with fuel oil; used in the 1995 Oklahoma City bombing
Tetryl	2,4,6 tetranitro-N-methylaniline	Used as a booster; placed next to detonator
Nitroglycerin	—	A liquid, unstable high explosive used as a component of dynamite
RDX	Cyclotrimethylenetrinitramine, $C_3H_6N_6O_6$	Second in strength to nitroglycerin among common explosive substances
PETN	Pentaerythritol tetranitrate	One of the strongest known high explosives
Semtex	PETN plus RDX	General purpose, odorless plastic explosive
HMX	Cyclotetramethylene tetranitramine	Highest energy, mass-produced solid explosive made in the United States; a component of plastic-bonded explosives and rocket propellants; used as a high-explosive burster charge
TATP	Triacetone triperoxide	One of the most sensitive explosives (i.e., to impact, temperature change, friction); suspected agent in 2005 London bombings and suicide bomb attacks in Israel
EGDN	Ethylene glycol dinitrate	A liquid explosive typically found in dynamite explosives such as those used in the 2004 Madrid bombings

Types

Because this manual is focused on combat medical personnel, the primary emphasis in this chapter is on antipersonnel, not industrial, explosives (**Figure 32-4**). Both manufactured and improvised explosive devices (IEDs) are considered, with an emphasis on the latter because they have become the principal wounding agent of current conflicts[19,20] and of terrorists and insurgents.

Figure 32-4 Classifications of Major Explosive Weapons Currently in Use[21]

Class	Description
Air-dropped bombs	Explosive weapons dropped from aircraft, including: ■ General purpose/high-explosive (GP/HE) bombs ■ Penetration bombs ■ Carrier bombs (for delivery of other payloads, including submunitions)
Booby traps	Explosive weapons designed to detonate by unsuspecting victims (also known as "victim-activated" explosive weapons)
Demolition charges	Blocks of explosive for engineering or sabotage use
Grenades	Small explosive antipersonnel or antivehicle weapons that can be thrown or fired, including: ■ Hand grenades (blast, fragmentation) ■ Anti-armor ■ Rifle ■ Spin-stabilized
Explosive projectiles	Explosive projectiles fired through a barrel after ignition of a propellant, including: ■ Armour-piercing high explosive (APHE) ■ High-explosive anti-tank (HEAT) ■ High-explosive fragmentation (HE frag) ■ High-explosive "squash head" (HESH) ■ Carrier (for delivery of other payloads such as submunitions)
IEDs	Explosive weapons of any class (e.g., grenade, bomb) that are not mass produced (although they may use mass-produced components), including: ■ Person-borne (suicide) bombs ■ Vehicle-borne IEDs (VBIEDs) ■ Roadside IEDs
Land mines	Victim-activated explosive devices, including: ■ Antipersonnel mines ■ Antivehicle mines
Missiles	Explosive devices with propulsion and guidance systems, including: ■ Air-to-air missiles ■ Air-to-surface missiles ■ Anti-tank guided missiles ■ Surface-to-air missiles (static, mobile, portable) ■ Surface-to-surface missiles
Mortars	Indirect fire weapons that are often muzzle-loaded, including: ■ High explosives ■ Carriers for delivery of other payloads such as submunitions
Rockets	Unguided munitions with propulsion systems, including: ■ Air-launched rockets ■ Artillery rockets ■ Rocket-propelled grenades (RPGs)

(Continues on next page)

Figure 32-4 Classifications of Major Explosive Weapons Currently in Use[21] (*Continued*)	
Class	**Description**
Submunitions	Smaller explosive weapons delivered by carrier bombs, projectiles, or mortar bombs (often "cluster munitions"), including: ■ Anti-armor ■ High-explosive fragmentation ■ Dual-purpose improved conventional munitions (DPICM)
Underwater devices	These include: ■ Depth charges ■ Limpet mines ■ Naval mines ■ Torpedoes

Manufactured explosives refer to mass-produced, military-issued/tested weapons (e.g., land mines, mortars, grenades), whereas IEDs refer to devices made in small batches or adapted from existing weapons.[11] Of the three classes of conventional antipersonnel land mines (static, bounding, and horizontal spray), the static mine is most common throughout the world, and its mechanism of injury is unique.

The line between manufactured and improvised explosive devices blurs when manufactured explosives are adapted for use as IEDs, as described by Keller:

> Terrorists … find it stunningly easy to obtain artillery shells, missile warheads, mortar rounds, and other high explosives for quick conversion to IEDs …. The terrorists simply rig them with cheap RF [radiofrequency] detonators and bury them where military convoys or other targets of opportunity are likely to pass by. When the targets are in range, they trigger the explosives with radio signals from cell phones, garage-door openers, or other easily obtained devices.[22]

Manufactured Explosives

Manufactured explosives include grenades (including rocket-propelled grenades, the most widely used anti-tank weapon in the world), rocket launchers fitted with thermobaric or explosive fragmentation antipersonnel warheads,[23] and antipersonnel mines.[24]

Enhanced blast weapons (EBWs) are a type of manufactured explosive that originated with the military. EBWs are incorporated into munitions that range from small grenades to large rockets, and are a likely threat to military personnel in stabilization and peacekeeping operations.[25] The primary mechanism of injury of EBWs is blast overpressure, with secondary and tertiary effects similar to those of conventional bombs. EBWs may also create a vacuum effect, which can cause suffocation.[26] EBWs are increasingly deployed with thermobaric (TBX) and/or fuel–air explosives (FAEs), which generate significant thermal output and may contain toxic materials. An example is the Russian RPO-A, which may contain the carcinogen isopropyl nitrate.[26]

Advanced thermobaric weapons (also known as vacuum bombs) come in all sizes, from small, slide-action grenade launchers to long-range, multiple-barrel rocket launchers (MBRLs). An RPG-7 may be equipped with the thermobaric TBG-7V round, which "shreds and incinerates everyone within a 30-foot radius of where it detonates."[27] These weapons are especially effective in urban environments because they can propagate around, into, under, and over objects, and their effects are magnified in enclosed spaces.[28]

Improvised Explosive Devices

The most common weapons in insurgency and terrorist warfare are IEDs (**Figure 32-5**). These weapons are designed to increase the range of damage by propelling high-velocity, preformed fragments a greater distance and introducing a variety of wounding agents. An IED consists of an armoring/firing switch, a power source, a detonator, and a main charge (explosive or incendiary), and it can be triggered by a timer that can be set well in advance of the detonation, by remote control, or—in the case of suicide bomb attacks—by the assailant at the scene.[23] Primitive IEDs can be made from everyday items such as fertilizer and batteries, but most use a small amount of military- or industrial-grade explosive to trigger a larger amount of lower-grade material (e.g., materials contained in gas cylinders). In the 1983 bombing of the U.S. Marine barracks in Lebanon, a truck carrying cylinders of compressed gas and 90 kilograms (kg; 200 pounds) of explosives collapsed a seven-story building, killing 241 U.S. military personnel.[29]

IEDs range in sophistication from simple pipe bombs to truck bombs containing thousands of kilograms of TNT equivalent.[30] They are categorized by the U.S. Technical Support Working Group (TSWG) based on size and destructive potential (**Figure 32-6**).[23]

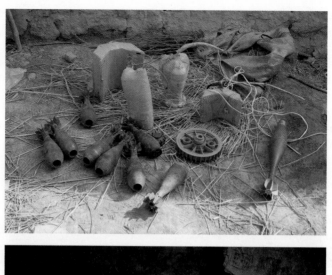

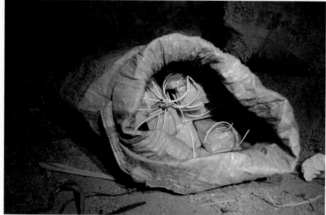

Figure 32-5   IEDS found in Afghanistan[31,32]

Source: A. Courtesy isafmedia. License link: https://creativecommons.org/licenses/by/2.0/deed.en; B. Image by Corporal Barry Lloyd RLC; ©Crown Copyright 2014

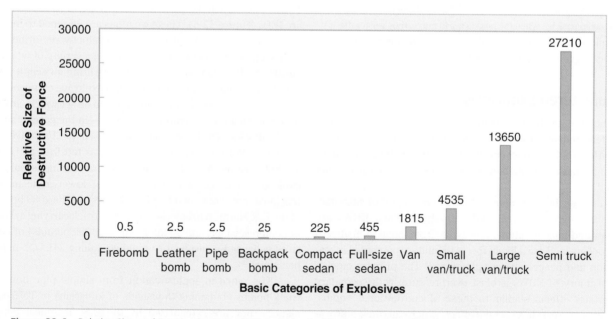

Figure 32-6   Relative Size trand Destructive Force (TNT-equivalent) of Basic Categories of Explosives[23]

Source: Data from: Sullivan JP, Bunker RJ, Lorelli EJ, et al. Jane's Unconventional Weapons Response Handbook. Alexandria, VA: Jane's Information Group; 2002

IEDs are the preferred weapon of insurgents. In Iraq, with its modern system of paved roads, and where soldiers typically travel by vehicle, military-grade ordnance was, and is, being modified into IEDs for use in roadside attacks.[33] During the worst period of the Iraq war, approximately 50 IED attacks, mainly roadside attacks, occurred each day.[34] In more rural Afghanistan, which has few highways and paved roads, soldiers are more often on foot and are typically targeted with homemade IEDs using fertilizer components from Pakistan.[33]

IEDs may be victim-operated (e.g., mines and booby traps); operated on a time delay (including pipe and vehicle bombs); command-operated (triggered by the user); projected (launched like a rocket or mortar); or operated with a combination of firing methods (time-delay plus backup is common).[23] The panic and disruption associated with IEDs may also be caused by hoax IEDs and false (misreported) IEDs.[23] IED technology used in Iraq includes electronic triggering sensors and explosively formed projectiles (EFPs), which are explosive-filled pipes sealed with a cone-shaped metal cap that, upon detonation, is propelled at a speed high enough to penetrate and shatter both armor and the vehicle compartment.[35] Another type of IED frequently used in Iraq is the "sticky IED," or IEDs attached to magnets and attached to the bottom of vehicles.[34] In Afghanistan, on the other hand, IEDs are currently simpler devices that use fertilizer and crude triggers, contain less metal (making them harder to detect), and are less lethal compared to those used in Iraq.[36]

Positioning techniques used to maximize IED damage include coupling/daisy chaining (linking multiple IEDs together) and boosting (stacking IEDs underground to minimize detection and increase the force of the blast).[37,38] Other common practices are packing IEDs with fragments such as nuts, bolts, ball bearings, nails, and pieces of concrete (a frequent phenomenon in suicide bomb attacks in Israel).[39] IEDs are often camouflaged (e.g., to look like garbage along the side of the road) or hidden under rocks, in animal carcasses, etc., and may be detonated using direct wiring, remote devices such as doorbells, or radio control, or by being thrown (e.g., from an overpass onto a vehicle) or launched.[40] Often, decoy devices are placed in plain sight so vehicles will stop near live, hidden IEDs.

Factors that Worsen Outcomes

The potency of an explosive device against a target can be increased in a variety of ways, as summarized in **Figure 32-7**.[41] The primary factors that influence outcomes include magnitude of and distance from the explosion, explosion within a confined space, and building collapse.[42,43] Fragments, which may be primary (i.e., part of the explosive device itself) or secondary (generated from the environment—e.g., glass, vehicle, or building debris), are the main cause of injury and death. Although proximity to the point of detonation clearly increases the risk of fragment injury, fragments are propelled great distances and can cause injury at distances far beyond the reach of blast overpressure.[43]

Figure 32-7   Prognostic Factors for Terrorist Bombings[44–46]

Category	Factor	Description
Agent	Type of explosive used	
	Amount of explosive used	The greater the TNT-equivalent of an explosive, the greater its wounding potential
	Magnitude of explosion	A primary wounding factor
	Secondary effects of debris or shrapnel	Constitute most explosion-related injuries
	Presence of flame or hot gases	Burn injuries
	Presence of dust or smoke	Inhalation injuries or asphyxiation
Location	Presence of a barrier between victim and explosion	Does not mitigate primary blast but may reduce exposure to fragments
	Urban or remote setting	Influences emergency response factors
	Indoors or in contained space	Significantly more injuries and deaths than in open-space explosions; increased rates of tympanic membrane rupture and blast lung
	Building collapse	Crush injuries
	Entrapment under debris	Crush injuries
	Propulsion of victim and subsequent blunt trauma	Blunt injuries

(Continues on next page)

Figure 32-7 Prognostic Factors for Terrorist Bombings[44–46] (*Continued*)

Category	Factor	Description
Victim	Distance from explosion	The closer to the point of detonation, the more severe the injury magnitude and type of injury
	Body position during explosion	Those positioned perpendicular to blast wave are impacted more severely than those positioned horizontally
	Anatomic site of injury	Depends on above factors
Emergency response	Triage efficiency	Improves survival
	Reduced time to treatment	Improves survival
	Immediate presence of surgeons	Improves survival

When an explosion occurs in an enclosed space, blast waves bouncing off structures collide with the primary blast wave, significantly increasing the damaging potential of the pressure waves. Further, in buildings or vehicles with fire-suppression systems, toxic gases may be released.[30] In the 1995 Oklahoma City bombing, 82% of injuries and 87% of deaths occurred inside the building, compared to 18% injuries and 5% deaths occurring outside the building.[47,48] In the 1996 Khobar Towers bombing, almost all of the injuries and deaths occurred among individuals who had been in the building or on a balcony.[49] Detonation of a bomb on a bus or inside a vehicle is a prime example of how terrorists use a confined space to cause maximum injury to tight clusters of casualties through penetration by metal fragments from disintegrating vehicle parts. The vast increase in injury severity and mortality associated with this technique is illustrated in **Figure 32-8**, which shows severe injuries (expressed as an Injury Severity Score greater than 15 or 16) and deaths associated with open-air and bus bombings in two Israeli studies.

Bombs detonated near or inside buildings often cause them to collapse (80% of the deaths in Oklahoma City were caused by collapse of the building structure rather than by the explosion itself), creating a high probability of secondary and tertiary injury effects. **Figure 32-9** shows the mechanism of blast-induced structural weakening and collapse. Structural collapse produces large numbers of casualties both inside and outside the structure, with increased frequency of inhalation and crush injury.[51]

Secondary explosions may be created by FAEs that disperse and ignite a spray of aerosol fuel, or cluster bombs, which distribute "bomblets" that explode over a wider area. The term *secondary explosions* also refers to a second round of explosions targeted at rescuers and responders assembling at the scene or to when the initial blast sets off additional explosions. Secondary attacks may also be initiated by snipers. Thus, it is important to exercise caution when approaching the scene of a blast to rule out the possibility of secondary attacks. To prevent further injuries, bystanders should be instructed to

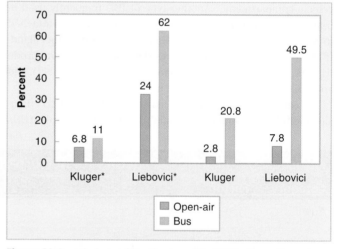

Figure 32-8 Injuries and Deaths Associated With Open-Air and Enclosed-Space (Bus) Explosions[42,50]

Source: Data from: Kluger Y. Bomb explosions in acts of terrorism—Detonation, wound ballistics, triage, and medical concerns. Isr Med Assoc J. 2003;5(4):235–240 and Leibovici D, Gofrit ON, Stein M, et al. Blast injuries: bus versus open-air bombings—a comparative study of injuries in survivors of open-air versus confined-space explosions. J Trauma. 1996;41(6):1030–1035.

vacate the area.[52] The Centers for Disease Control and Prevention warns:

> Although most terrorist IED attacks outside war zones target civilians or symbols of authority and usually involve a single device, some are designed specifically to target emergency response personnel. The most common tactics involve using secondary or tertiary devices in tiered or sequential attacks intended to kill or maim response personnel after they arrive on the scene of an initial IED incident.[53]

Patterns of Injury

Explosions produce patterns of injury different from other types of trauma with respect to demographics of patients, distribution and

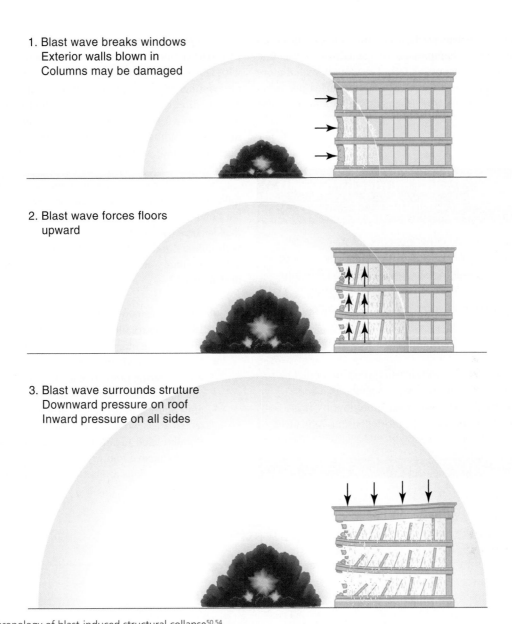

1. Blast wave breaks windows
   Exterior walls blown in
   Columns may be damaged

2. Blast wave forces floors
   upward

3. Blast wave surrounds struture
   Downward pressure on roof
   Inward pressure on all sides

Figure 32-9 Chronology of blast-induced structural collapse[50,54]

Source: Reproduced from Primer to Design Safe School Projects in Case of Terrorist Attacks and School Shootings. FEMA 428/BIPS-07/January 2012. US Department of Homeland Security, Federal Emergency Management Agency: Buildings and Infrastructure Protection Series, p. 4–9, Department of Homeland Security Web site. http://www.dhs.gov/xlibrary/assets/st/bips07_428_schools.pdf. Accessed January 29, 2013.

severity of injury, and frequent occurrence of injuries in several body regions or multiple injuries in the same body region.

When compared with patients injured via other types of trauma (e.g., gunshot wounds), victims of terrorist bombs are primarily in the age range of 15 to 44 years,[55] have more severe injuries, require more surgical intervention, and have three times the rate of mortality.[56,57]

After exposure to an explosive device, most casualties with lethal injuries die immediately. Although the large majority of survivors do not have life-threatening injuries, 10% to 15% of casualties have critical injuries and may be saved with appropriate management.[47,58,59] An analysis of 3,357 casualties of terrorist bombings worldwide yielded specific patterns of injury, as outlined in **Figure 32-10**.[57]

Comparison of patterns of injury in terrorist bombing victims versus trauma patients whose injuries were attributed to other causes revealed that terrorist bombing victims had increased incidence of severe injury (29% vs. 10%, **Figure 32-11**), with subsequent increased use of intensive care centers, prolonged hospital length of stay, more surgical interventions, and increased hospital mortality.[60] Approximately half of all initial casualties needed medical care within the first hour after the explosion. Those with minor injuries often bypassed prehospital care providers and went directly to the closest hospitals, where they often arrived before those who were more seriously injured.[52]

Although most survivable injuries occur from fragments, many injuries from explosive devices result from multiple etiologies of injury, each compounding the condition to make the total effect more difficult for the body to handle.

Combined/multiple injuries—including primary blast, penetrating fragment, crush, burn, and inhalation injuries—occur often, especially in urban warfare environments or in urban terrorist bombings. A comparison of casualties in the first and second phases of Operation Iraqi Freedom revealed more deaths, higher injury severity, more major injuries per casualty, and more casualties with fragment wounds in the latter phase.[61,62]

Compared with non-terror-related trauma, civilian victims of terrorist bombings are generally more seriously injured, with more body regions injured (see **Figure 32-11**). For example, victims of suicide bomb attacks exhibit a characteristic combination of blunt injury, burns, and numerous penetrating injuries with extensive soft-tissue damage,[63–65] with typical injuries including penetrating injuries to the head, extremities, and torso, as well as burns, open fractures, and blast lung.[66,67]

Whereas bomb injuries in military personnel previously followed a pattern characteristic of fragment injury and civilian bomb injuries were distinguished by the addition of materials such as nails or bolts, the widespread use of IEDs against both military and civilian targets is now common. Differences between military and civilian casualties of bomb blasts include the following[68]:

- Military casualties are more likely to be healthy males, 18 to 35 years old, whereas civilian casualties are more often young, old, or female and may be in poor health.
- Unlike their civilian counterparts, military casualties are often wearing protective gear, reducing the risk of head and upper torso injury. This can result in devastating limb injuries in casualties in whom wounds in the protected areas would have been fatal.
- Bombs used against military targets are typically high-explosive military ordnance, whereas bombs used against civilians are both low- and high-explosive IEDs.

Figure 32-10   Typical Injuries in Terrorist Bombings[57]

- Wounds tend to be either noncritical soft-tissue or skeletal injuries, or critical, with little middle ground.
- Head injuries predominate among fatalities (50% to 70%).
- Most head injury survivors (98.5%) have noncritical injuries.
- Head injuries are disproportionate to exposed total body surface area.
- Most trauma victims with blast lung die immediately.
- Survivors have a low incidence of abdominal and chest wounds, burns, traumatic amputations, and blast lung, although specific mortalities are high (10% to 40%).

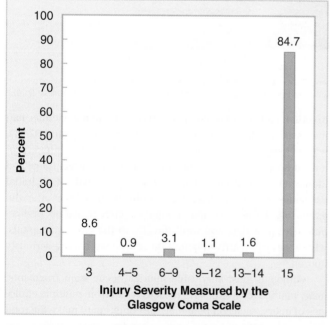

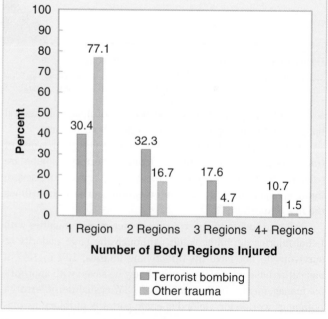

Figure 32-11   Patterns of injury in terrorist bombings: injury severity (left) and number of body regions injured (right).[67]

Source: Data from: Frykberg ER. Medical management of disasters and mass casualties from terrorist bombings: How can we cope? J Trauma. 2002;53(2):201–212.

Certain patterns of injury have emerged from Iraq and Afghanistan as a result of explosive devices used in a particular manner in certain tactical situations. For example, an explosive device detonated under a Humvee can produce massive injury to sitting occupants, including severe pelvic injury as a result of secondary fragmentation from the vehicle itself. Likewise, explosive devices detonated at the roadside will often injure the front-seat passenger who is riding with an arm and leg outside the vehicle, weapon at the ready. This results in injuries to the right arm, right leg, and face, with little injury to the other occupants.

In Afghanistan, a new injury trend was identified in 2010, which is on the rise in dismounted patrols. This pattern, known as dismounted complex blast injury (DCBI), is characterized by a combination of high lower-extremity amputation, pelvic and genital injuries, and injuries to the spine.[69]

Triage

Accurate triage is essential in effective, timely matching of casualty need and available resources. In a tactical setting, this requires an accurate assessment of the urgency of the casualties' needs. In general, uncontrolled hemorrhage and emergence of shock, as evidenced by vanishing radial pulse, require urgent treatment. However, if the bleeding can be stopped and resuscitation is seen to be effective in maintaining a radial pulse and a conversational level of consciousness, evacuation can be delayed for a limited period.

Mass-casualty triage presents different problems especially when related to explosions. As previously discussed, the distribution of injuries from a bomb explosion is normally a significant number of lightly wounded casualties and a significant number of deaths, with a smaller number of high-risk casualties requiring urgent medical treatment. The natural flow of individuals accessing a medical care system is often such that the "walking wounded" and lesser-injured casualties arrive at the emergency facility first, thus impeding access to care for the more critically injured casualties who follow. Therefore, it is essential that triage decisions be repeated and confirmed at every level of care so that overtriage and undertriage can be minimized.[70]

Overtriage is the assignment of unnecessarily high priority to lesser-injured individuals. Although this ensures prompt access to care, overtriage may deluge the health care system and allocate resources away from those who might be in desperate need. Overtriage can result in increased preventable mortality for casualties with an Injury Severity Score greater than 15 (moderate injury).[63] Overtriage following explosions is often self-directed. Thus, it is vital to establish an outer perimeter around hospital facilities so that floods of patients with minor injuries cannot gain access to resources that should be reserved for the most severely injured that follow. Undertriage clearly should be avoided to ensure that more severely injured casualties receive prompt access to care.

Triage for MCIs (bomb attacks and other types) is performed with a focus on providing an acceptable quality of care to minimize morbidity and mortality with limited resources.[71,72] This means identifying from among the minimally wounded, dead, and expectant casualties the small subset of casualties with critical injuries who have a chance of survival and focusing scarce personnel and resources on them. This challenge, and that of identifying casualties at risk for occult injuries, can more effectively be met with a thorough understanding of the mechanics and patterns specific to explosion-related injury.[58] For example, understanding that explosions in confined spaces (e.g., vehicles) cause more primary blast effects, lung damage, and penetrating injuries than explosions in open areas will raise the index of suspicion for these types of injuries when encountering victims of confined-space explosions. It is important to keep in mind that survivors of blast explosions not initially considered critically injured should nonetheless be monitored in order to identify subtle signs of deterioration that may indicate the need for immediate care.[58]

Further, with the complex injuries often sustained by blast victims (e.g., devastating multi-mechanistic injuries to more than one body region or multiple injuries in the same body area), it is more important than ever to triage these blast victims for transport to the highest available level of care. This fundamental tenet of civilian trauma systems[73] is becoming increasingly prioritized in the military arena.[74]

Taxonomy

Blast injury is a generalized term often used to refer to various injuries caused by an explosive device. However, it is important to differentiate among these injuries because they vary according to injury category. Injuries from explosions are generally classified as primary, secondary, tertiary, quaternary, and quinary after the injury taxonomy described in Department of Defense Directive 6025.21E[75] (**Figure 32-12**),[76] as follows:

- Primary injuries, resulting from the blast wave or overpressure, which cause direct tissue damage or primary blast injury; unique to high explosives
- Secondary injuries, in which ballistic wounds are produced by missiles or primary fragments from the exploding weapon (shrapnel, preformed, and unformed fragments) and secondary fragments, or projectiles, from the environment (e.g., debris, vehicular metal)
- Tertiary injuries, caused by propulsion of casualties onto the ground or into solid objects and structural collapse with concomitant crush and blunt trauma
- Quaternary injuries, including burns and toxicities from fuel, metals, septic syndromes from soil, and environmental contamination
- Quinary injuries, such as those caused by radiation, chemicals, or biologic agents—i.e., from radiation-enhanced explosives ("dirty bombs")

Although these categories are useful ways to think about explosion-related injuries, it is important to note that these

Figure 32-12 Blast-Injury Categories[75]

Effects	Impact	Mechanism of Injury	Typical Injuries
Primary	Direct blast effects (over- and underpressurization)	Produced by contact of blast shockwave with body Stress and shear waves occur in tissues Waves reinforced/reflected at tissue density interfaces Gas-filled organs (lungs, ears, etc.) at particular risk	Tympanic membrane rupture Blast lung Eye injuries Concussion Traumatic amputation in foot-activated IEDs
Secondary	Projectiles propelled by explosion	Ballistic wounds produced by: • Primary fragments (pieces of exploding weapon), or • Secondary fragments (environmental fragments, e.g., glass)	Penetrating injuries Traumatic amputations Concussion Lacerations
Tertiary	Propulsion of body onto hard surface or object, or propulsion of objects onto individuals	Whole body translocation Crush injuries caused by structural damage and building collapse	Blunt injuries Crush syndrome Compartment syndrome Concussion
Quaternary	Heat and/or combustion fumes	Burns and toxidromes from fuel, metals Septic syndromes from soil and environmental contamination	Burns Inhalation injury Asphyxiation
Quinary	Additives such as radiation or chemicals (e.g., dirty bombs)	Contamination of tissue from: • Bacteria, radiation, or chemical agents, or • Allogenic bone fragments	Variety of health effects, depending on agent

injuries often occur in combination.[46] The greatest diagnostic challenges for clinicians at all levels of care in the aftermath of explosions are the large numbers of casualties and multiple penetrating injuries.[66,77]

Assessment and Management by Blast Injury Category

Plans for scene assessment and security must be worked out in advance, with the first priority being to ensure scene safety and ensure lack of persistence of a threat. This is particularly important in the tactical or terrorist environment in which a small explosion can draw combatants into the field of a large explosion or to sniper fire. It is a well-known tactic of terrorists to attract security and health care personnel into the environment and then explode a second device or begin a secondary attack.

As in any medical emergency, combat medical personnel responding to the scene of an explosive blast should employ standard operating procedures of assessment and initial management consisting of aggressive and definitive control of external hemorrhage, clearing the airway, promoting breathing, splinting fractures, etc. Because bomb explosions typically constitute an MCI, mass-casualty principles of triage and treatment should be used, with rapid evacuation to a medical facility as the primary objective.[78]

In this section, each injury category is described and guidelines for assessment and management are given as needed. A summary of typical explosion-related injuries by organ system is given in **Figure 32-13**. General principles to aid in management of blast victims include the following[1]:

- Early mortality is caused primarily by multiple trauma, then by trauma to the head, thorax, and abdomen.[79–81]
- Effective triage and prompt medical attention to those whose survival depends on it are essential. This effort entails delaying care for those with minor injuries and minimizing care for those with likely lethal injuries, such as those with burns approaching 100% of total body surface area or those in cardiac arrest.[1,47,76]
- Initial history and physical exam should include the elements listed in **Figure 32-14**.

It is predominantly with primary blast injury that assessment and care will differ because it is only at the scene of an explosion that combat medical personnel will encounter such

Figure 32-13 Summary of Typical Blast Injuries by Organ System[11]

System	Injury/Condition
Auditory	Tympanic membrane rupture, ossicular disruption, cochlear damage, foreign body implantation
Face and eye	Facial fracture, perforated globe, foreign body, air embolism
Respiratory	Blast lung, hemothorax, pneumothorax, pulmonary contusion/hemorrhage, arteriovenous fistulas (source of air embolism), airway epithelial damage, aspiration pneumonitis, sepsis
Digestive	Bowel perforation, hemorrhage, ruptured liver or spleen, sepsis, mesenteric ischemia from air embolism
Circulatory	Cardiac contusion, myocardial infarction from air embolism, shock, vasovagal hypotension, peripheral vascular injury, other air embolism-induced injury
Central nervous system	Concussion, closed and open brain injury, stroke, spinal cord injury, air embolism-induced injury
Renal	Renal contusion, laceration, acute renal failure due to rhabdomyolysis, hypotension, and hypovolemia
Extremity	Traumatic amputation, fractures, crush injuries, compartment syndrome, burns, cuts, lacerations, acute arterial occlusion, air embolism-induced injury

Figure 32-14 Components of Rapid Assessment of Blast Victims[1,47,79,80]

History		Physical
Symptoms	Circumstances	Blood in external ear or nose
Deafness	Close proximity to blast	Cyanosis
Tinnitus	Enclosed-space explosion	Hemoptysis
Earache	Entrapment	Cough
Nausea	Crush	Rales
Retrograde amnesia	Compartment syndrome	Rhonchi
	Comorbid conditions	Abdominal tenderness, rigidity, guarding
	Underwater or undergrtound	

injuries. Fortunately, dominant primary blast injury in survivors is not common. The secondary through quinary injuries described here, although characteristic of explosive blast, are also exhibited in other trauma, and, therefore, care will not differ for these injuries. As stated previously, the predominant issue with explosions is fragment injury and multisystem, multi-etiology injury.

Primary Blast Injury

Primary blast injury results from interaction of the blast wave with the body or tissue to produce stress and shear waves (**Figure 32-15**). The strongest blast wave that can allow for a high probability of survival lasts a few milliseconds and has a peak pressure of approximately 300 pounds per square inch (psi).[30] Overpressure injury most often occurs in areas in which tissue densities change (e.g., tympanic membrane, lung air–tissue interfaces, or heart fluid–muscle interface).

The degree of primary blast-induced damage to the body is dependent on the intensity of the blast overpressure, which, in turn, depends on the size of the explosive,[82] proximity of the victim to the point of detonation, and whether or not the victim was in an enclosed space.[50,83] Backpack bombs, for example, have a range of serious injury of 10 to 30 meters (33 to 98 feet),

Figure 32-15 Characteristics of Stress and Shear Waves

Stress Waves	Shear Waves
• High frequency • Supersonic, longitudinal pressure waves • Create high local forces with small, rapid distortions • Produce microvascular injury • Are reinforced/reflected at tissue interfaces, thereby enhancing injury potential, especially in gas-filled organs such as the lungs, ears, and intestines • Cause injury via pressure differentials across delicate structures (e.g., alveoli), rapid compression/re-expansion of gas-filled structures, and reflection of the tension wave (a component of the compressive stress wave) at the tissue–gas interface • Cause mucosal/submucosal damage and serosal injury that may represent full-thickness damage	• Low frequency • Transverse waves with a lower velocity and longer duration that cause asynchronous movement of tissues • Degree of damage depends on extent to which the asynchronous motions overcome inherent tissue elasticity, resulting in tearing of tissue and possible disruption of attachments.

passenger vehicle bombs have a range of 450 to 840 meters (1,476 to 2,756 feet), and large-scale truck bombs have a range of 1,150 to 1,980 meters (3,773 to 6,496 feet).[52] After an attack in which conventional high explosives are used, few victims close to the epicenter of the explosion will survive with life-threatening primary blast injury (rates of 0.1% to 2% have been reported[82,83]) because most will have typically been killed by fragments and fire.[84]

Peak overpressures inside enclosed, blast-loaded vehicles typically exceed the threshold for unprotected ear damage but stay below the threshold for blast lung injuries. Because unprotected ear damage pressure levels are very low (5 psi, see **Figure 32-16**), hearing-based crew safety requirements are not appropriate. At present, it is not clear whether hearing threshold values are below that for neurologic injury.

Underwater Explosions

In water, the body reacts very differently to pressure waves and is more susceptible to injury. Close to the explosion, there is a very rapid, high-pressure wave front. At greater distances, the waveform more closely approximates the low-frequency, continuous waveform. Water is approximately 800 times denser than air and approximately 10,000 times less compressible. A diver in shallow water or at the surface will receive not only the direct blast wave from the explosion, but also the reflected waves from the surface or seabed and any surrounding structures (**Figure 32-17**). Explosions underwater are estimated to be three times stronger than their counterparts on land,[46,86] and the deeper the subject is immersed, the greater the effect of the blast. Pulmonary hemorrhage is the most frequent injury related to underwater blast, followed by injury to the susceptible gas-filled intestines.

Assessment and Management

Knowledge of the characteristics of blast physics and primary blast injury is helpful for effective initial evaluation, triage, and treatment of casualties with suspected primary blast injury.

In severe blast injury, immediate death typically occurs, which may be attributed to a characteristic triad of physiologic responses to the primary blast overpressure: (1) bradycardia, (2) apnea, and (3) hypotension.[89] Immediate death has also been attributed to massive air embolism, which results from disruption of the alveolar wall and adjacent pulmonary capillaries with air emboli, primarily affecting cerebral and coronary vessels. In immediate survivors, dysrhythmias, signs of neurologic injury, and retinal artery air emboli have been noted.

In survivors, primary blast injury can present with no outward signs of trauma or may present as perforated eardrums, ocular trauma, flash burns, traumatic amputation, or acute dyspnea.[67,90] Patients with these signs and symptoms may at first appear stable but may deteriorate quickly.

Blast testing has revealed thresholds of injury for organs classified as (1) air-containing (lung, eardrum, gastrointestinal [GI] tract, larynx, trachea); (2) liver and spleen; and (3) kidney, pancreas, and gallbladder.[30] The first group is the most vulnerable, exhibiting the first signs of injury at the lowest threshold, followed by the second, and then the third group.[30] Of the air-containing organs, the tympanic membrane is the most frequent site of injury, followed by the lungs.

Use of the Trendelenburg position is not recommended for casualties of blast explosions because it may increase the risk of coronary air embolus. Immediate therapy is supplemental oxygen, with hyperbaric oxygen being the definitive treatment of systemic air embolus (although this is rarely available or clinically practical). Alveolar–venous fistulas are thought to resolve in 24 hours but must be considered a continuing risk in casualties who require

Figure 32-16 Short-Duration Pressure Effects From Blasts on Unprotected Persons[85]

Pressure (psi)	Effect		
	Eardrum Rupture	Lung Injury	Death
5	Possible		
15	50% chance		
30–40	Almost certain	Possible	
80		50% chance	
100–200			Possible
130–180			50% chance
200–250			Almost certain

psi, pounds per square inch

positive-pressure ventilation, especially with application of positive end-expiratory pressure (PEEP) typically used for hypoxic pathophysiology.[91]

Tympanic Membrane Rupture

The auditory system is very susceptible to blast and is the site of the most frequently detected blast injury.[92] Immediate, but often temporary, blast-induced deafness often occurs, which heightens anxiety and impedes communication; deafness may be permanent or may resolve within hours. Sensorineural hearing loss associated with high-pitched tinnitus frequently occurs immediately after a blast.

The tympanic membrane is the functional structure injured at the lowest pressure by blasts and, thus, may assist in detecting other primary blast effects. Higher overpressures may result in permanent hearing loss.[92] The presence of tympanic membrane rupture has traditionally been used as a marker of primary blast injury, although its absence does not absolutely rule out lung injuries.[92–94] The incidence of tympanic membrane rupture increases with proximity to the epicenter and when the explosion occurs in an enclosed space.[90]

Perforation of the eardrum (in the anteroinferior part of the pars tensa) is the most common physical finding and may occur at pressures as low as 5 to 15 psi.[95,96] Deafness, tinnitus, and vertigo may indicate rupture and should heighten suspicion of it in the event that the tympanic membrane cannot be visualized.

Examination of casualties with blast injury should include otoscopic identification of tympanic membrane rupture. Absence of rupture may lower (but not eliminate) the index of suspicion for primary blast injury, except when the casualty exhibits abdominal pain, dyspnea, or respiratory distress.

Treatment of ruptured tympanic membrane is not a priority. Signs and symptoms include hearing loss and bleeding from the ears. The diagnosis may be confirmed by visualizing the eardrum with an otoscope. A large proportion (50% to 80%) of ruptured tympanic membranes heal spontaneously.[97]

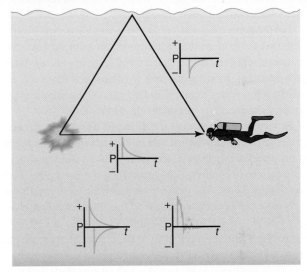

Superimposition of direct- and surface-reflected blast waves

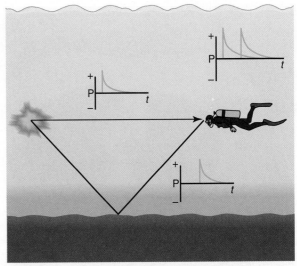

Superimposition of direct- and bottom-reflected blast waves

Figure 32-17 Blast effects on a diver in shallow water[87,88]

Source: Reproduced from: Cudahy E, Parvin S. The Effects of Underwater Blast on Divers. Naval Submarine Medical Research Laboratory. NSMRL Report 1218

Although not a priority for treatment, auditory injury should be addressed within 24 hours and the auditory canal cleaned of all debris. However, probing or irrigating the auditory canal should be avoided. When the ear is full of contaminated debris, antibiotic eardrops should be administered.

With respect to the outer ear, traumatic blast amputation of an ear or earlobe has been shown to be almost uniformly associated with fatal injury.[98]

Pulmonary Injury

The lung is the second-most susceptible organ to primary blast injury.[99] Increased overpressure increases pulmonary damage, with overpressures of 200 psi uniformly fatal in open-air blasts.[87] Blast injury to the lungs is the most common cause of injury and death from the primary blast effect alone, although it occurs with variable frequency, ranging from 7% to 39% in several studies.[71,93,100] The effect of body armor in preventing the pulmonary effects of primary blast continues to be discussed.[99]

The pulmonary sequelae of blast wave exposure are collectively referred to as *blast lung*. Although it occurs rarely among survivors,[101] blast lung is an often-fatal combination of acute respiratory distress (dyspnea/apnea), bradycardia, and hypotension subsequent to a blast exposure.[11] Patients with blast lung may exhibit hypoxemia and hemoptysis and may require endotracheal intubation.

Reflection of stress waves at rigid interfaces of the lungs causes paramediastinal, peribronchial, and subpleural tissue disruption and hemorrhage. Primary blast effect on the chest wall also produces a classic pattern of contusion and hemorrhage on the surface of the lungs (**Figure 32-18**). The index of suspicion for blast lung (if combat medical personnel have access to this information) at charge sizes of 1, 10, and 100 kg (2.2, 22, and 222 pounds) of TNT equivalent would occur at distances from the charge of approximately 3.5, 7.5, and 37.5 meters (11.5, 24.6, and 123 feet), respectively, for blasts close to ground level. This is a general guideline that may be especially useful when casualties have multiple injuries.[90]

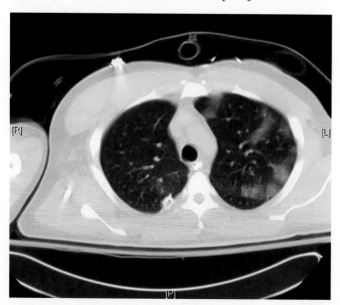

Figure 32-18 Classic pattern of blast on lungs.
Source: Courtesy of H.R. Champion

Among survivors of primary blast injury, clinical manifestations may be present immediately[102,103] or may have a delayed onset of 24 to 48 hours.[104] Bleeding from the ears is a sign of possible blast lung or hollow organ injury.[105] Intrapulmonary hemorrhage and focal alveolar edema result in frothy, bloody secretions and lead to ventilation–perfusion mismatch, increased intrapulmonary shunting, and decreased compliance. Hypoxia results from increased work of breathing, pathophysiologically similar to pulmonary contusions induced by other mechanisms of nonpenetrating thoracic trauma.[106] Other injuries may include pneumothorax, hemothorax, subcutaneous and mediastinal emphysema, pneumoperitoneum, and tension pneumoperitoneum.[107,108]

Primary blast injury to the lung may not be immediately apparent, yet may require complex ventilatory and fluid management and support.[52] Recommended guidelines for care include the following:

1. Monitor for frothy secretions and respiratory distress.
2. Monitor early for hemodynamic parameters.
3. Provide oxygen if available:
   - Use high-frequency ventilation, with liberal hypercapnea.
   - Limit peak inspiratory pressures, because elevated pressures increase the risk of air embolism or pneumothorax.[51]
4. Carefully manage fluid administration, avoiding fluid overload; although the ideal fluid for resuscitation in blast injury is not known, the following guidelines are recommended:
   - Optimize preload without overload.
   - Use crystalloid, with or without colloid.
   - Consider using recombinant factor VIIa as an adjuvant therapy in casualties with obvious pulmonary hemorrhage.
   - In most cases, avoid resuscitating to a mean arterial pressure greater than 60 millimeters of mercury (mm Hg).
5. Continually monitor the casualty because edema is a common sequela in casualties with lung damage. If pneumothorax begins to develop, employ a tube thoracostomy immediately.
6. Consider a prophylactic tube thoracostomy if casualties must be evacuated by air or when close observation is impractical.
7. Do not remove impaled objects. Shorten impaled objects to facilitate transport, and then wrap them carefully to prevent movement before surgical exploration.
8. If traumatic brain injury (TBI) is present, prevent/minimize hypercapnia to avoid intracranial hypertension.

The role of antibiotics and corticosteroids is not currently defined.

Gastrointestinal Tract Injuries

Although much less common than massive lethal injuries, ear and lung injuries, and penetrating fragment injury, primary blast injury to the intestines does occur, and casualties should be examined and monitored for delayed perforation or presentation of this condition. A review of U.S. Army collective animal data indicates that primary blast injury to the GI tract is as prevalent as pulmonary injuries in free-field blasts,[109] and when multiple detonations occur in a complex environment (i.e., inside a structure), the GI tract appears more susceptible to injury.[110] A review of the literature on terrorist bombings between 1996 and 2002 revealed that intestinal perforation was the most common type of primary blast injury to the abdomen,[56] primarily occurring in suicide bombings (both in open air and in enclosed spaces).[111] Victims of underwater blasts are at greater risk of GI injury than lung injury, especially with partial submersion.[112]

The lower GI tract is often filled with gas. The ileocecal area is most susceptible to primary blast injury, and the small intestine is generally spared. Blast-induced rapid compression and decompression damage the stomach wall, often creating a rupture that leads to peritonitis, hemorrhage, bleeding and devascularizing injury, and submucosal to transmural injury. Multifocal intramural hematoma is the characteristic injury, which begins in the submucosa and extends with increasing severity to become a large, transmural confluent hematoma that may involve the mesentery and vascular supply. Serosal injury should always be considered indicative of transmural injury.[113]

Symptoms include nausea and vomiting; pain in the abdomen, rectum, and testes; straining/inability to urinate or defecate; and, rarely, hematemesis. In primary blast with pulmonary injury, free-air and even tension pneumoperitoneum without intestinal injury have been reported.

Intestinal perforation, which is considered a closed injury, is common, but open injuries may occur as well. Signs and symptoms, which may be hard to discern in the immediate postblast period, may include pain in the abdomen, rectum, and testes. Treatment does not differ from treatment of GI injuries resulting from other mechanisms.[114]

Abdominal Injuries

A recent review of the literature on abdominal injury from primary blast revealed that, although the incidence was highly variable (1% to 33%, and as high as 69% in underwater blasts), and less frequent than abdominal injury from fragments, it has a high risk of morbidity and death.[115] Reasons for this include the fact that issues may present days or weeks after injury (e.g., perforation of a GI mural hematoma).[113] Most affected are the terminal ileum and cecum.[115] British combat casualty data (2003 to 2008) showed that vascular injuries to the abdomen and thorax were extremely rare (occurring in 2% of casualties who did not return to duty) but 100% fatal.[116]

Traumatic Brain Injury

TBI is a major cause of death in bomb attacks, accounting for 71% of early deaths and 52% of later deaths.[57] Between 2001 and 2009, TBI was the primary cause of death (83%) among U.S. combat casualties with injuries deemed nonsurvivable.[4] Lethal

TBI is often caused by secondary and tertiary effects, but significant histologic damage and central nervous system dysfunction can occur with the primary blast overpressure.[117] Casualties may present with periods of loss of consciousness, agitation, excitability, and irrational behavior. Moderate and severe TBI are incapacitating. Long-term sequelae and coexistent posttraumatic stress disorder (PTSD) have also been associated with TBI from primary blast mechanisms,[118] especially with repeated exposures.[119,120]

The evidence is becoming clear that large numbers of previously unrecognized TBIs are occurring in military personnel from IED blasts in Iraq and Afghanistan (Stone JR, Bass CR, Helm G, unpublished data, 2008).[78,121] Between 2000 and the third quarter of 2012, more than 260,000 U.S. service members suffered a TBI, with the incidence of mild TBI comprising 76.4% and increasing with much greater frequency than any other category (moderate, severe, penetrating) of TBI (2000 to 2011 data shown in **Figure 32-19**).[122] A test series evaluating the effects of high-rate mechanical insults alone found evidence of brain injury in large animal specimens for short-duration blasts that do not result in fatal pulmonary injuries.[99] However, the etiology, mechanistic basis, and detailed progression of such brain injuries remain obscure and easily confused with other diagnoses.

Visible wounds or obvious penetration of the skull may indicate "conventional" or penetrating TBIs, which are easily diagnosed. In the blast etiology of blunt head trauma, the initial high-pressure shock wave is followed closely by a gust of displaced air filling the vacuum. These extreme fluctuations in pressures, which may be 1,000 times greater than atmospheric pressure,[30] may cause concussion, loss of consciousness, loss of vision, deafness, and neurologic and cognitive deficits.[3] Shear and stress waves of the primary blast may cause concussion, hemorrhage, edema, diffuse axonal injury, and formation of gas emboli leading to infarction.[123]

Signs and symptoms of TBI may include loss of consciousness, acute headache, amnesia, confusion, and disorientation.[124] In the past, researchers had difficulty differentiating mild TBI from

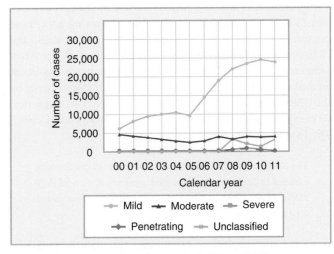

Figure 32-19 TBI incidence by severity (2000 to 2011).

Source: Data from: Armed Forces Surveillance Center, 2013

psychological trauma,[125–128] but more recent studies have been able to document physical damage to the brain in animal studies.[117,129–131]

Immediate treatment of TBI does not differ for blast-related injuries and includes immediate attention to hemorrhage control, securing of the airway, judicious fluid resuscitation, and attention to other immediately life-threatening injuries in an effort to prevent hypoxia and hypotension (and thus secondary brain injury).

Further efforts to detect and record TBI are described in **Figures 32-20** and **32-21**.

Solid Organ Injuries

Injuries to the liver, spleen, adrenal glands, kidneys, and testicles have all been reported in underwater blasts,[135] although solid-organ injury is less common in air blasts. These injuries are probably caused by shear forces and present similarly to solid organ injury resulting from blunt trauma. Gallbladder, renal pelvis, and bladder injury secondary to primary blast have rarely been recorded, most likely because of their fluid contents.[136] These injuries present like hemorrhagic shock and should be treated accordingly.

Traumatic Amputation

Traumatic amputation resulting from a primary blast has traditionally been a marker of injury severity with few survivors.[98,137] However, in recent years data show both improved survivability and increased severity in the form of more casualties losing multiple limbs. In the 2005 London train bombings, 24.5% of those with traumatic amputations survived.[138] Analysis revealed that survival in several cases was associated being seated instead of standing because (1) seated victims were far enough away from the explosion to avoid receiving an incident pressure high enough to be fatal, but the pressure was magnified by the solid surface of the bench to create enough force to sever a limb; and (2) the legs of the seated victims were as much as a half meter (1.5 feet) closer to the explosion than the chest.[138]

Combat casualty data show that in 2009, casualties evacuated to higher levels of care included 86 amputees (largely attributed to IED attacks), with 63 having one limb amputated and 23 having multiple amputations. The following year, these numbers had risen to 187 amputees, with 115 having single and 72 having multiple limbs amputated. In its final report, the Army Dismounted Complex Injury Task Force presented the results of an evaluation of 111 blast-related fatalities in 2010 conducted by the Office of the Armed Forces Medical Examiner. In that series, 68 (61%) had multiple limbs amputated, up from 28% in 2007.[70] The Task Force noted:

> The ATO's [Afghanistan Theater of Operations] most dramatic changes in 2010 were the increased numbers of bilateral thigh amputations, triple and quadruple amputations, and associated genital injuries.[70]

Land mine explosions often cause traumatic amputations via the primary blast shock wave,[139] which fractures the bone before the limb is amputated by the blast wind.[41] The levels of

Figure 32-20   MACE

Short- or long-term transient cognitive decrement associated with mild TBI is of significant concern in combat. Mild TBI can result from blunt head trauma or exposure to blast overpressure. To assess the impact of these exposures, the Department of Defense has fielded the Military Acute Concussion Evaluation (MACE).[132] Updated in 2012, the MACE is a tool for small-unit commanders and medics to assess cognitive function following incidents to help evaluate immediate fitness for continued combatant function in a tactical setting.

Figure 32-21   The Breacher Study

Mild TBI due to blast injury may initially be asymptomatic (loss of consciousness need not be present for mild TBI to occur[133]), but may cause cognitive and performance decrements with the passage of time, especially in the event of repeated exposures. As reported by Sharon Weinberger in *Nature*, the Defense Advanced Research Projects Agency (DARPA) and the Office of Naval Research sponsored a study to research this phenomenon in Marines who use explosives to gain access to buildings. Results indicate that these individuals, known as *breachers*, have neurologic deficits that are associated with long-term, repeated exposure to explosive blast events.[134] In the article, Ms. Weinberger noted the release of the Pentagon's initial guidance on screening for TBI, including the mandatory assessment for TBI of any person exposed to a blast within 50 meters.

amputation following explosions are counterintuitive; instead of occurring through joints as one might imagine, they tend to occur approximately 4 to 6 inches (10 to 13 centimeters) proximal or distal to the joint surfaces. In cases of traumatic amputation in a surviving casualty, the injury should be treated symptomatically.

Secondary Injury

Most injuries in explosions are from fragments. Fragment munitions are frequently designed to generate multiple small preformed fragments that weigh 1 to 2 grams and are 2 to 3 mm in diameter, whereas others may have larger fragments that weigh as much as 20 grams. Both lighter- and heavier-weight varieties have initial velocities of 1,500 meters/second (5,000 feet/second) that decelerate rapidly (especially in the presence of large, irregularly shaped fragments).

Secondary fragment injuries are caused by energy transfer and the velocity of the projectile and are the most common injuries sustained in bomb explosions. Fragments take the form of both the exploding pieces of the bomb itself and the shattered pieces of glass, wood, etc., from the environment,[44] frequently including metal from disintegrating vehicle interiors. Environmental debris such as glass, splinters, soil, and various structural particles are major causes of multiple fragment wounds (**Figure 32-22**). Glass is the most ubiquitous wounding agent among environmental fragments. For example, in the 1996 Khobar Towers bombing, 88% of injuries were caused by glass, especially from windows and patio doors.[49]

Magnitude of injury is thought to depend more on the inherent tissue characteristics of the affected organ than on the projectile itself, with clinical impact and priority of treatment determined by the tissue or organ involved. For example, the presence of numerous extremity wounds does not usually have high associated morbidity or mortality, whereas wounds of the eyes or thorax are much more likely to be immediately disabling or life threatening, respectively.

The threat of injury from fragments exceeds that of the blast wave by a factor of 100. Therefore, in a free-field environment, a casualty is unlikely to be affected by blast overpressure within ranges that usually result in potentially survivable fragment injury. For example, in an open-space detonation of a 155-mm (200-pound/91-kg) shell, death from primary blast and fragments, as well as eardrum rupture, is likely to occur within 50 feet (15 meters [m]) of the detonation. At 80 feet (24 m), death from fragments is likely. At 130 feet (40 m), fragment injury and temporary hearing-threshold shift is likely, and at distances as far as 1,800 feet (549 m), fragment injury is still possible.

A diagram of projected injuries from terrorist bombs ranging from small bombs packed in luggage to large truck bombs

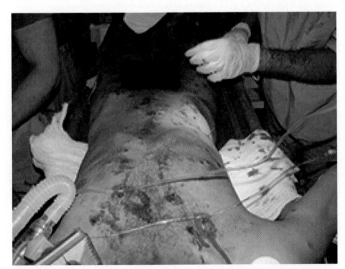

Figure 32-22 Fragmentation injury from environmental debris.
Source: Courtesy of Maj. Scott Gering, Operation Iraqi Freedom

shows that most injuries will be caused by glass fragments as well as structural collapse (**Figure 32-23**).[54] Fragment throw distance and blast overpressure are both a function of casing material thickness and net explosive weight. However, in a free-field environment, in which there are no structures to block the propagation of casing fragments, the dominant injury mechanism from a cased weapon is always fragment penetration.

Assessment and Management

Multiple Injuries

Fragment injuries from explosive blasts differ from other penetrating injuries in the type and quantity of penetrating agents, which often occur across multiple body regions. Ideally, each fragment injury would be treated as a specific injury based on its size, severity, and location. General treatment guidelines can be found in other chapters; however, the unique aspect of explosive injuries is the massive number of individual injuries that can occur, making individualized treatment for each wound difficult, if not impossible, in certain settings (**Figure 32-24**). General principles must apply, with attention to airway, control of bleeding, resuscitation, immobilization, and splinting.

For military personnel, the abdomen and chest have a greatly reduced incidence of secondary penetrating injury because they are protected by body armor. However, fragments can enter laterally and below the body armor and in junctions between the torso, arms, neck, and legs. Penetrating wounds entering the torso from explosions must be managed in the same way as any other penetrating injury, treating respiratory distress and shock as needed. The chest must be evaluated for penetration and pneumohemothorax. Abdominal wounds should be dressed with a view to providing definitive therapy within 8 hours, or if shock occurs from hemorrhage, treatment must be provided as a matter of extreme urgency. In the absence of body armor, significant fragment injury can occur, with as many as 30 or 40 fragments lacerating the body. In the field, it is often difficult to ascertain which, if any, of these fragments have penetrated the torso.

Penetrating fragment wounds of the abdomen and thorax are no different than other penetrating wounds, except that the number of pieces of metal and the small size of visceral injuries demand meticulous attention to detail. Almost all penetrating thoracic wounds can be successfully managed by tube thoracostomy. In the event that wounds are grossly contaminated, as is common, standard infection prophylaxis protocols should be followed.

Limb Injuries

Limbs are the body areas most often injured in explosions. In combat, limb injury accounts for 70% of injuries. Such injuries vary from minor to massive and may include multiple amputations and near-amputations. A focal explosive force is exerted by antipersonnel mines, which often injure the limbs with a combination of primary and secondary blast. Such injuries can be

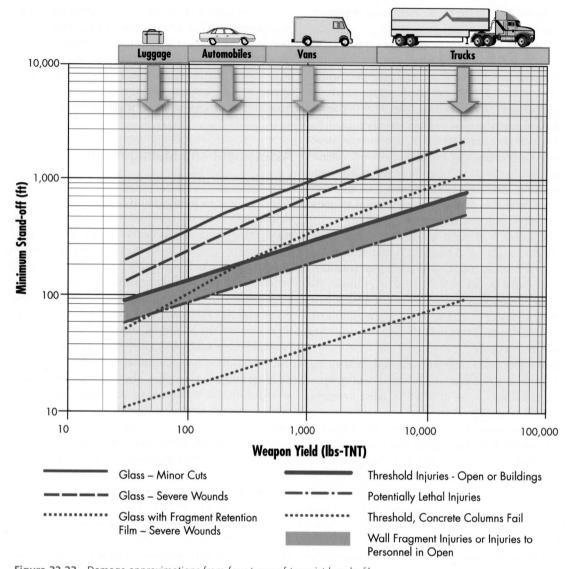

Figure 32-23   Damage approximations from four types of terrorist bombs.[54]

Source: Reproduced from Reference Manual to Mitigate Potential Terrorist Attacks Against Buildings. FEMA 426. Figure 4-2, p239. December 2003. http://www.fema.gov/pdf/plan/prevent/rms/428/fema428_ch4.pdf

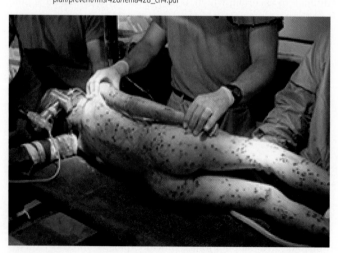

Figure 32-24   Multiple fragment wounds from a cluster bomblet.

Source: Courtesy of Maj. Scott Gering, Operation Iraqi Freedom

devastating, especially if contaminated with dirt or other debris, causing tremendous pain and often requiring emergency hemostatic maneuvers, including application of tourniquets and pressure dressings. Scene and initial therapy should usually involve tourniquet(s) to stop hemorrhage. Definitive treatment for such injuries must include thorough debridement, often to the point of completing amputation of seriously injured limbs. Injuries from exploding mines are extremely serious, with a combination of primary and secondary blast wounds in localized body areas. Mine injuries often require extensive, staged treatment and transfusions.

Casualties with long-bone fractures should be managed with temporary splinting to prevent further soft-tissue damage, minimize further neurovascular compromise and bleeding,[140,141] and reduce pain. No attempt should be made to reduce or manipulate fractures. Current practice is to apply a transport external fixator at Level II and transport to Level III.

All open or compound fractures should be immobilized and covered with bulky sterile dressings, followed by administration of systemic, broad-spectrum antibiotics. Tetanus prophylaxis or booster injections should be given during initial treatment.

All war wounds are contaminated by soil, clothing, and skin, whereas low-velocity fragmentation wounds are minimally contaminated with debris. Bacterial contamination is common in fragmentation wounds,[142] although infection is uncommon in small, low-velocity extremity wounds. Standard protocol should be followed.

Injuries to the Eye

Although the eyes are extremely resistant to primary blast injury, they are vulnerable to secondary and tertiary mechanisms, with resultant penetrating trauma. The most significant injuries to the eyes are caused by explosions that produce shattered glass or tiny metal fragments. Most injuries can be prevented by wearing eye protection. Secondary blast injuries include corneoscleral lacerations, orbital fractures, hyphema, lid lacerations, traumatic cataracts, optic nerve injury, serous retinitis, and rupture of the globe. A high proportion of these injuries are caused by minute (1- to 2-mm) fragments entering the eye, causing damage that can result in blindness. As many as 10% of all survivors of blast injury have significant eye injuries from projectile perforation, with symptoms that may include pain, irritation, sensation of a foreign body, changes in visual acuity, swelling, and contusions.[11] Among survivors of the September 11, 2001, attacks on the World Trade Center, 26% had ocular injuries attributed to smoke, dust, fumes, and debris.[143]

Ocular injuries can occur with all categories of mines. The primary mechanism of injury involves the products of detonation and environmental fragments and debris, which cause penetrating ocular wounds.[144]

Injuries to the eye should be treated as follows:

- Cover the eye with a rigid shield that does not place pressure on the eye.
- In cases in which the globe is exposed, consider provisional repair of eyelid laceration.
- Emergency enucleation is not advised.
- Do not remove objects penetrating the eye at the scene; cover the eye with a paper cup or other clean object that will not exert pressure on the globe.
- Treat chemical burns (such as those sustained from car battery acid) with at least 60 minutes of irrigation using sterile saline or the cleanest water available.
- If toxic substance release is suspected, wear eye protection such as polycarbonate goggles.

Tertiary Injury

Tertiary injuries, which result when a casualty is propelled into a hard surface or a hard surface is propelled onto a casualty, are the second most common type of injury among survivors of bomb attacks.[86] These injuries include closed head injuries, blunt trauma to the abdomen and thorax, spinal injury, fractures of the extremities, and less-severe injuries such as dislocations, sprains, and strains.[49] The presence of rib fractures should increase suspicion of tertiary or quaternary injury to the thorax. Muscle, bone, and solid-organ injury are much more likely to result from the tertiary and quaternary effects of the blast than from the blast wave alone.[91]

Crush injuries and compartment syndrome are tertiary injuries that frequently accompany structural collapse. Compartment syndrome, initiated by the buildup of pressure in myofascial compartments, is an acute condition that can cause loss of limb, paralysis, or death. Damage to muscle groups causes swelling, ultimate constriction by the unyielding fascia, compression on and reduced supply of oxygen and nutrients to nerves and blood vessels, and ultimately cell death.[145] Irreversible tissue death can occur in as few as 4 hours, depending on the location of injury and the compartmental pressure. Compartment syndrome is distinguished by its localized effects from crush syndrome, which has systemic effects.

Spinal injury may result when a patient is propelled onto a hard surface, shattering vertebrae. In Afghanistan, spinal injuries have increased due to roadside bombs that propel the military's Mine Resistant Ambush Protected (MRAP) vehicles into the air, throwing the occupants against the interior, causing damage to spinal columns (including crush injuries), concussions, and broken bones of the feet and ankles.[146] This phenomenon was the catalyst for redesigning the seats in MRAP vehicles to absorb the blast (blast mitigation seats) or to float above the floor and hull to isolate it from blast effects (suspended seats) and increase the headroom.[147]

Assessment and Management

Tertiary mechanisms may result in blunt injuries such as head and spinal cord trauma, and if structural collapse occurs, compartment syndrome or crush syndrome may result.

Compartment Syndrome

In compartment syndrome, the damaged muscle swells (creating pressure within its inelastic sheath), becomes ischemic, continues swelling, increases compartment pressures, decreases tissue perfusion, and further increases ischemia. Left untreated, compartment syndrome causes local tissue necrosis, which may lead to paralysis, amputation, and death, and also presages development of crush syndrome. Compartment syndrome usually involves the extremities but occasionally involves the buttocks[148,149] and abdominal muscles (e.g., rectus).[150] The most characteristic sign of compartment syndrome is pain out of proportion to visible injury. Other signs include pain when the affected muscles are stretched, tension and swelling involving the gluteal or rectus abdominis muscles, and absence of pulses in the affected area (**Figure 32-25**).

Figure 32-25 The Five Ps of Compartment Syndrome

Pain out of proportion to the injury
Pain with passive stretching
Pressure, tension, or swelling
Paresthesia, or loss of feeling, below affected area
Pulselessness, usually in late stages

Field management of compartment syndrome should include the following:

- Administration of high-flow oxygen
- Splinting when long transport times are anticipated
- Expeditious transport to definitive care
- Fluid resuscitation
- Analgesia

No ice or elevation should be used. U.S. Army Reserve protocol for management of compartment syndrome includes performance of field fasciotomy.[145] Fasciotomy is the only definitive treatment for a patient with compartment syndrome.

Crush Syndrome

Crush syndrome occurs when the muscle is damaged, causing cell disruption, ischemia and leakage, and vascular compression of and reduced blood supply to tissues. Cell death occurs in muscle tissue after approximately 4 hours without blood. The lethality of crush syndrome is related to reperfusion, whereby toxins are released into the body. Oliguric renal failure, the most severe endpoint of crush syndrome, also causes potassium accumulation in addition to that released from damaged muscle. An illustrative case of crush syndrome involved a woman pinned for 12 hours in the wreckage after a train derailment in 1987. Although she remained conscious and oriented and her vital signs were stable, shortly after she was extricated, she went into cardiac arrest and died.[145]

Indicators of crush syndrome include compression for 1 hour or longer; involvement of large muscle mass; no pain in area of compression; shock; clammy, cool, pale skin; rapid, weak pulse; and no pulses or capillary refill.[145]

Treatment of crush syndrome includes the following:

- Maintenance of hydration and alkalization[151]
- Fluid therapy that maintains renal perfusion without fluid overload
- Airway management, including protection from dust
- Oxygenation
- Maintenance of body temperature
- Rapid transport to definitive care
- Maintenance of circulation
- Treatment of shock
- Fluid resuscitation

- Cardiac monitoring
- Analgesia
- Expeditious extrication

In most circumstances, immediately before extrication, the casualty should be given a 1- to 2-liter bolus of normal saline or lactated Ringer's solution and 2 ampules of sodium bicarbonate.[145]

Spinal Injury

If signs and symptoms of spinal cord injury (e.g., numbness, inability to move or breathe independently, neck or back pain) are present, the cervical spine should be stabilized if the tactical situation allows, since injuries from explosives entail the potential of spinal fractures from tertiary blast effects. Spinal injury should also be assumed in a casualty who is unconscious from blast-related trauma. Often, however, stabilization may have to be delayed until a secure environment is obtained and preparations can be made for immediate evacuation to definitive neurosurgical support.

Quaternary Injury

Quaternary injuries include burns, inhalation injury, and asphyxiation resulting from fire or fumes. The flash (fireball) produced by the detonation of an explosion can reach temperatures greater than 3,000°C (5,432°F).[59] IEDs are the primary cause of burn injuries in recent conflicts and most often affect the head and hands (i.e., areas not covered by body armor or fire-resistant uniforms).[152] Almost one-fifth (17%) of surviving casualties of terrorist bomb attacks have sustained burns in addition to their other injuries.[153]

Common substances causing inhalation injury after an explosion are smoke, nitrogen oxides, cyanide, phosgene, carbon monoxide, and heavy metal fumes. Inhalation injury occurs primarily in conjunction with fires or structural collapse. In the 1993 World Trade Center bombing, for example, almost all survivors had smoke inhalation, a result of the ensuing fires and prolonged evacuation.[58] In the subsequent World Trade Center attack in 2001, half of immediate survivors had inhalation injury caused by fires and dust from the building collapse.[58]

Assessment and Management

Burns after an explosion should be treated as any other burn wounds. For field treatment guidelines, see the chapter titled Treatment of Burn Casualties in Tactical Combat Casualty Care.

Quinary Injury

Quinary injuries include those caused by release of toxic (chemical, biologic, or radioactive) agents or by introduction of foreign bodies that have the potential to transmit disease. In suicide bomb attacks, fragments of body parts from the assailant or other bombing casualties may become projectiles, embedding in the bodies of victims and increasing the risk for transmission of blood-borne disease agents such as hepatitis B virus and human immuno-deficiency virus (HIV).[98] Of six such cases in the medical literature, two resulted from suicide bombings; in one, embedded bone fragments tested positive for hepatitis B.[154–156]

Chemical agents may come in contact with skin or be inhaled and cause early effects such as coughing, itching, and eye inflammation. It may be difficult to tell if a chemical agent has been released, because it may be odorless and cause no initial symptoms. Classifications of chemical agents include the following:

- *Nerve agents.* These are quickly absorbed through the skin and mucous membranes and cause an almost immediate, often lethal, reaction.[157] Signs and symptoms of nerve agent poisoning include pinpoint pupils, muscular twitching, unexplained nasal secretion, salivation, tightness of the chest, shortness of breath, or nausea and abdominal cramps. These signs and symptoms call for immediate intramuscular injection of 2 mg of atropine, combined if possible with oxime.[158] Indications of the presence of nerve agents such as sarin gas or soman are advanced respiratory failure or victims who are dead but have no apparent major injuries.[11,157]
- *Blister/vesicant agents.* These agents burn and blister on contact and cause damage to the mucous membranes of the respiratory tract when inhaled. Of particular importance to note is that some blister agents (e.g., mustard gas or phosgene) have a latent symptom-free period that may last 2 to 6 hours.[158–160]
- *Choking agents.* Signs and symptoms of exposure to choking agents (e.g., phosgene and chlorine) may include coughing, choking, tightness in the chest, vomiting, headache, and lacrimation. However, as with some blister agents, no symptoms may be evident immediately following exposure.[158]

Thus, in addition to dealing with the usual traumatic injuries expected from an explosive event, you may also be faced with victims who, after treatment for minor injuries at the site, may develop subsequent toxic, potentially lethal effects.[157]

Theoretically, drug-resistant bacteria (e.g., methicillin-resistant *Staphylococcus aureus* [MRSA]) could also be disseminated by an explosive device. If a biologic agent (e.g., anthrax or ricin) is released, no immediate signs of illness will be apparent. As with some chemical agents, biologic agents have an initial symptom-free incubation period, which may last days instead of hours, depending on the agent.[157] Thus, it may not be possible to tell if such an agent has been released in an explosion, especially in the midst of the ensuing debris, dust, and fire.[158]

Contamination of an explosive with radioactive material results in radiation exposure that varies with the size and sophistication of the explosive, the type of material, weather conditions, and speed of evacuation from the scene.[161]

A noted quinary effect of explosions is the phenomenon of "human remains shrapnel," in which a bone fragment from the assailant (usually a suicide bomber) pierces the skin of a victim.[162] Management of injuries from bone projectiles depends on whether the bone belongs to the patient (autogenic fragment) or came from someone else (allogenic fragment). Autogenic bone penetration typically presents as an open fracture that is managed as any open fracture. Penetration by allogenic fragments, however, carries the risk of transmitting bloodborne diseases such as HIV or hepatitis B.[156] The latter are treated in a standard fashion, but PPE must be worn and the receiving facility must be notified.

Assessment and Management

Nerve Agents and Radioactive Material

Removal of shoes and clothing will reduce contamination by 90%, and particulate contaminants on the skin and hair can be washed off. Internal contaminants are not transmissible.[161] Antidotes are available for certain nerve agents (e.g., sarin gas).

Blister Agents

Treatment of casualties with blister agent exposure includes the following:

- Decontaminating affected areas
- Rinsing eyes
- Applying topical steroid creams and sprays
- Preventing secondary infection and pneumonia
- Administering analgesia

Choking Agents

Treatment of casualties with choking agent exposure may include the following[163]:

- Decontaminating affected areas
- Rinsing eyes with normal saline or water for at least 3 minutes
- Monitoring hemoglobin oxygen saturation.
- Administering oxygen as rapidly as possible
- If pulmonary edema is present, administering PEEP oxygen, diuretics, or bronchodilators

Lessons for first responders from the 1995 release of sarin gas in the Tokyo subway system included the following[164]:

- Wear PPE.
- Stand upwind and uphill of the toxic cloud.
- Communicate with victims remotely (e.g., via bullhorn) until the toxic agent is identified.
- Wait for the hazardous materials team.

Until the agent has been identified, responders should treat exposed persons as dictated by their conditions (e.g., chemical burns, pulmonary edema, cardiorespiratory failure, neurologic damage, shock).[165]

Combination Injuries

In their 2007 summary of lessons learned from explosive attacks, Harrisson, Kirkman, and Mahoney noted the appearance in professional jargon of the term "multidimensional injury" to refer to the great complexity and severity of blast injury due to trauma involving multiple body regions and organs.[4141]

Owen-Smith, discussing the complexity of blast wounds in a 1979 article on bomb blast injuries, observed, "These injury characteristics, which are not normally seen in routine trauma care, create difficult surgical challenges in triage decision making and treatment."[87]

Explosion-related injuries frequently occur in combinations of mechanisms and injury types/categories. Commonly seen penetrating combat injuries include soft-tissue fragment wounds, high-velocity penetration, blast injuries (mutilating or nonmutilating), and/or bilateral and multiple injuries that result from explosive devices, including IEDs. The cumulative effect of multiple injuries upon mortality has been estimated at approximately 15% as each additional viscus is injured.[166] Devastating injuries to multiple areas of the body are characteristic of IED attacks. In two studies of military IED casualties, 13% to 51% had a combination of primary and secondary injuries.[167–169]

In several studies of terrorist bomb attacks, a majority of the victims had injuries that fell in more than one of the above categories.[170–174] Almogy and his coauthors[175] reviewed injuries from suicide bombings in 2004, noting that the injury pattern is most commonly characterized by multiple blunt and penetrating injuries of varying severity spread over a large surface area.

Another type of explosive that typically causes both primary and secondary injury is the land mine. The stress waves produced by the blast can propagate as far as the midthigh, with demyelination of nerves occurring 30 cm (1 foot) above the most proximal area of tissue injury. This effect, combined with fragments from the device, soil, and footwear, produces the classic land mine injury of complete tissue destruction distally, associated with traumatic amputation at the midfoot or distal tibia (**Figure 32-26**). Proximal to the variable level of amputation, there is complete stripping of tissue from the bony structures and separation of fascial planes contaminated with soil, debris, microorganisms, and pieces of the device, footwear, and clothing.

Associated penetrating injury to the contralateral limb and perineum is common.[176] Land mine injuries occur in three distinct patterns: (1) severe lower extremity, perineal, and genital injuries caused by contact with a buried mine; (2) less severe lower extremity injury, less traumatic amputation, and often head, thoracic, and abdominal injuries caused by a proximity-device explosion; and (3) severe head, face, and upper extremity injuries resulting from mine handling or clearing.[177]

Combined blast and penetrating injuries are almost always the most life threatening, and the basic principles of the ABCs should always be followed when dealing with multiple injuries.

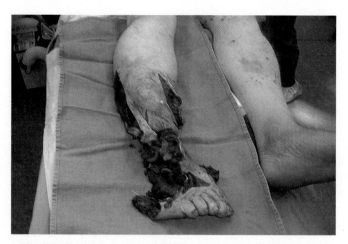

Figure 32-26 Classic pattern of land mine injury to the lower leg with radiographs.
Source: Courtesy of H.R. Champion

Special Considerations

Personal Protection

Because of the initial symptom-free period after exposure to some toxic agents, it may not be possible to ascertain that chemical or biologic contamination has occurred. Thus, combat medical responders may inadvertently be exposed directly (e.g., in the case of choking agents such as phosgene) or via contact with casualties.[159] Thus, in a bombing incident with suspected chemical or biologic agents, PPE should be worn that is commensurate with the suspected agent, degree of hazard, and individual role at the scene.[178]

Another protective measure that should be taken when responding to the scene of a bomb attack is to avoid, insofar as is possible, secondary bomb attacks that are often set to go off when responders arrive at the scene.[179] Avoidance tactics include (1) not moving or handling any suspected item; (2) not operating radios, cell phones, or other electronic devices that may trigger a detonator; (3) being aware of the fact that explosives are often placed near flammable materials; and (4) staying alert for suspicious individuals.[23]

Casualties with retained, unexploded ordnance should be transported in the position found so as not to change the missile orientation; they always should be grounded to the airframe if evacuated by air. Such casualties should be isolated, and, in an MCI, they should be treated last because the removal of ordnance is time-consuming, and surgeons must attend to other casualties before placing themselves at risk. Closed-chest massage or defibrillation should never be attempted in these casualties, and during removal, any equipment emanating electrical energy, heat, vibrations, or sonic waves (e.g., electrocautery, ultrasound, blood warmers, power instruments) should not be used. These casualties should be placed in a protected area away from the main hospital, and all personnel in the immediate area should use body armor or explosive ordnance disposal (EOD) equipment. EOD personnel should be involved before removal to help identify the round and fuse. A plain radiograph will help in planning the operative removal

Figure 32-27   Guidelines for Removal of Ordnance From Casualties[180]

- Notify explosive ordnance disposal (EOD) team.
- Do not use cardiopulmonary resuscitation (CPR) or electric shock.
- Isolate casualty in a protected area (sandbagged bunker).
- Ensure protective equipment is available for medical personnel.
- Do not use cautery, power equipment, or blood warmers.
- Avoid vibration, change in temperature, and change in missile orientation.
- Use plain radiography, not computed tomography (CT) or ultrasound.
- Perform only minimal anesthesia; anesthesia provider leaves after induction.
- Ensure surgeon and assistant (EOD) are only personnel present during removal.
- Remove ordnance without changing its orientation, and hand over to EOD.
- Move casualty to operating theater for definitive procedure.

of the unexploded ordnance and will not cause the round to explode. Anesthesia should be restricted to the minimum required and should be used in such a manner that the anesthesia provider need not be present during removal of the ordnance.

The only personnel required during removal should be the surgeon and an assistant, ideally EOD personnel. The round should be removed "en bloc" without touching the missile with metal instruments. Every effort should be employed by the surgeon to maintain the orientation of the missile until it is removed from the area by EOD. **Figure 32-27** outlines the basic guidelines for removal of ordnance.[180]

Psychological Considerations

The vast majority of casualties, as well as health care personnel, typically sustain psychological damage as the result of their ordeal. Reactions range from acute stress reaction to acute stress disorder to posttraumatic stress disorder (PTSD). All casualties exhibiting decreased awareness, acute anxiety, dissociative symptoms (including a sense of time distortion), or other stress-related symptoms must be provided with screening for mild TBI and survivor counseling, utilizing social work, chaplain, and psychiatric resources as needed.

Summary

- Explosive devices are the most common source of injury in both military and terrorist settings and can produce devastating casualties in small and large numbers.
- Mass-casualty explosion-related events, once the sole province of the battlefield hospital, now threaten the urban hospital, the civilian trauma surgeon, and health systems throughout the world.
- All combat medical personnel and providers need to bear the burden of preparing for influxes of overwhelming numbers of casualties with primary blast and penetrating wounds, as well as burns and crush injuries.
- It is important that combat medical personnel:
  1. Understand the nature of the explosive weapons that are causing death and serious injuries with increasing frequency
  2. Recognize the physiologic consequences of these weapons of war and terror
  3. Are prepared to provide care that will save lives and reduce morbidity

SCENARIO RECAP

While on foot patrol on a rural road, one member of a five-member team triggers an IED. One casualty is dead, two have minor injuries, and one has sustained significant blast injuries to his lower torso and right lower extremity. You are the person providing medical care.

SCENARIO SOLUTION

1. **What are the tactical considerations in this situation?**
   a. Will an ambush or sniper fire follow?
   b. Is there a second device?
   c. Should the team set security and treat the casualties in place?
   d. Where is the nearest effective cover? Is that cover safe?

There is no immediate follow-on hostile fire. You and the other uninjured man use a two-man drag to move the seriously injured casualty to cover, stabilizing his neck as best you can. You pass by a derelict truck and elect to gather in a shallow depression behind a small mound of rocks and dirt. The uninjured man and the casualties with minor injuries set a perimeter, and you begin to treat the seriously wounded man.

2. **Why did you bypass the derelict truck?**

It was the most obvious cover, so it was also a likely place for a second IED.

3. **What will you do initially for this casualty?**

Identify and stop life-threatening bleeding. You quickly cut off the casualty's trousers. His right foot is missing and his right lower leg is badly mangled. There are multiple large, bleeding wounds high on his right thigh, and there are several wounds in his perineum and right buttocks. You apply a Combat Ready Clamp (CRoC) to his right inguinal region, and that seems to control the severe bleeding from his thigh. He is breathing spontaneously, has a palpable radial pulse, and is unresponsive. The uninjured man is calling in for reinforcement and MEDEVAC. Estimated time of arrival is 20 minutes. You have taken no sniper fire so far.

4. **Does the casualty need fluids?**

You stopped the life-threatening bleeding, and his radial pulse is present, so his mental status decrement is probably due to TBI from blast injury. IV fluid therapy is not indicated at this time, and it may make blast lung (if present) worse.

5. **Do you need to attain IV access?**

Yes. Medications are warranted, and he may well need fluid resuscitation before you get him to the emergency department. You cannot rule out internal bleeding from penetrating torso injury at this point, and you must be prepared to prevent hypotension in this casualty with a TBI. You place a sternal IO device and attach an IV setup. The casualty's status is unchanged.

6. **What next?**

Administer 1 gm of tranexamic acid in 100 cc normal saline IO followed by ertapenem 1 gm IO.

7. **With respect to blast as the source of the casualty's injuries, is his TBI a primary or secondary blast injury?**

You carefully remove his helmet and examine his head. You find no indication of either penetrating or blunt trauma. His TBI is probably a primary blast injury.

8. **Should you be concerned about other primary blast injuries?**

Yes. The casualty is breathing normally at this time, his breath sounds are clear, and he is oxygenating well at 98%. Nevertheless, his respiratory status must be closely monitored throughout evacuation. You also find that both his tympanic membranes are ruptured.

9. **Is C-spine stabilization indicated?**

Yes. The casualty is breathing spontaneously, but you cannot test for sensation or mobility. Spinal cord injury cannot be ruled out, even though you believe his TBI to be primary (vs. secondary or tertiary) blast injury.

10. **What else?**

Check for uncontrolled bleeding and other injuries. Insert a nasopharyngeal airway. Check his eyewear, lids, and visible parts of his globes. Monitor pulse oximetry values. Dress all known wounds. Check for burns. Keep him warm. Continue to monitor closely.

11. **What else would you like to do while waiting for MEDEVAC?**

Document injuries, care rendered, and response to treatment on a TCCC Casualty Card.

References

1. Lemonick DM. Bombings and blast injuries: a primer for physicians. *Am J Clin Med*. 2011;8(3):134–140.

2. Hall HR Jr. Deaths due to unintentional injury from explosions. National Fire Protection Association. http://www.arfireprevention.org/pdf/Deaths_Due_to_Unintentional_Injury_from_Explosions.pdf. Published April 2009. Accessed April 30, 2014.

3. Eshel D. IED blast related brain injuries: The silent killer. Defense Update. http://www.defense-update.com/analysis/analysis_270507_blast.htm. Updated June 6, 2010. Accessed April 30, 2014.

4. Eastridge BJ, Hardin M, Cantrell J, et al. Died of wounds on the battlefield: causation and implications for improving combat casualty care. *J Trauma*. 2011;71(suppl):S4-S8.

5. Bosker AJ; Joint Improvised Explosive Device Defeat Organization. Cooperative engagement with Pakistan needed to counter IED networks in Afghanistan. https://www.jieddo.mil/news_story.aspx?ID=1502. Published December 13, 2012. Accessed April 30, 2014.

6. Livingston IS, O'Hanlon M; Brookings Institution. Afghanistan Index. http://www.brookings.edu/~/media/Programs/foreign%20policy/afghanistan%20index/index20120918.pdf. Published September 18, 2012. Accessed April 30, 2014.

7. Porter G. How the U.S. quietly lost the IED war in Afghanistan. Inter Press Service. http://www.ipsnews.net/2012/10/how-the-u-s-quietly-lost-the-ied-war-in-afghanistan/. Published October 9, 2012. Accessed April 30, 2014.

8. National Counterterrorism Center. 2011 Report on Terrorism. Information available as of March 12, 2012. http://www.fas.org/irp/threat/nctc2011.pdf. Accessed April 30, 2014.

9. Bureau of Alcohol, Tobacco, Firearms and Explosives. Fact sheet. U.S. Bomb Data Center. http://www.atf.gov/publications/factsheets/factsheet-us-bomb-data-center.html. Accessed January 11, 2013.

10. Vanden Brook T. IED attacks increase outside of Afghanistan, Iraq. *USA Today*. October 19, 2011. http://usatoday30.usatoday.com/news/military/story/2011–10–19/ied-use-increasing/50831988/1. Accessed April 30, 2014.

11. Centers for Disease Control and Prevention. CDC Emergency Preparedness and Response: Explosions and blast injuries: a primer for clinicians. http://emergency.cdc.gov/masscasualties/explosions.asp. Accessed April 30, 2014.

12. Brevard SB, Champion H, Katz D. Weapons effects. In: Savitsky E, Eastridge B, eds. *Combat Casualty Care: Lessons Learned from OEF and OIF*. Fort Detrick, MD: Borden Institute; 2012.

13. Global Security.org. Explosives. http://www.globalsecurity.org/military/systems/munitions/explosives.htm. Updated July 7, 2011. Accessed April 30, 2014.

14. *U.S. Navy Salvage Engineer's Handbook*. Vol 1 (Salvage Engineering). S0300-A8-HBK-010. 1997. http://wetlands.simplyaquatics.com/d/14936–1/sehv1.pdf. Accessed April 30, 2014.

15. GlobalSecurity.org. Explosives—compositions. http://www.globalsecurity.org/military/systems/munitions/explosives-compositions.htm. Updated July 7, 2011. Accessed April 30, 2014.

16. GlobalSecurity.org. Booster explosives. http://www.globalsecurity.org/military/systems/munitions/explosives-booster.htm. Updated July 7, 2011. Accessed April 30, 2014.

17. GlobalSecurity.org. Explosives—nitramines. http://www.globalsecurity.org/military/systems/munitions/explosives-nitramines.htm. Updated July 7, 2011. Accessed April 30, 2014.

18. Ostmark H, Wallin S, Pettersson A, Oser H. Real-time detection of IED explosives with laser ionization mass spectrometry. In: Schubert H, Rimski-Korsakov A, eds. *Stand-off Detection of Suicide Bombers and Mobile Subjects*. NATO Security Through Science Series. Netherlands: Springer; 2006.

19. Wade AL, Dye JL, Mohrle CR, Galarneau MR. Head, face, and neck injuries during Operation Iraqi Freedom II: results from the U.S. Navy-Marine Corps Combat Trauma Registry. *J Trauma*. 2007;63: 836–840.

20. Gondusky JS, Reiter MP. Protecting military convoys in Iraq: an examination of battle injuries sustained by a mechanized battalion during Operation Iraqi Freedom II. *Mil Med*. 2005;170: 546–549.

21. Moyers R. *Explosive Violence: The Problem of Explosive Weapons*. Landmine Action Website. http://www.landmineaction.org/resources/Explosive%20violence.pdf. Published August 11, 2009. Accessed April 30, 2014.

22. Keller J. A COTS response to the IED threat. Military Aerospace and Electronics Website. http://www.militaryaerospace.com/articles/print/volume-17/issue-11/departments/trends/a-cots-response-to-the-ied-threat.html. Published November 1, 2006. Accessed April 30, 2014.

23. Sullivan JP, Bunker RJ, Lorelli EJ, et al. *Jane's Unconventional Weapons Response Handbook*. Alexandria, VA: Jane's Information Group; 2002.

24. Horrocks CL. Blast injuries: biophysics, pathophysiology and management principles. *J R Army Med Corps*. 2001;147(1):28–40.

25. Murray SB, Anderson CJ, Zhang F, et al. Force protection against enhanced blast. Report No. DRDC-Suffield-SL-2006–174. Defense Research and Development Canada Website. http://cradpdf.drdc-rddc.gc.ca/PDFS/unc53/p526381.pdf. Published January 1, 2006. Accessed April 30, 2014.

26. Bean JR. Enhanced blast weapons and forward medical treatment. *Army Med Dept J*. 2004;April-June:48–51.

27. Wilson J. Weapons of the insurgents. *Popular Mechanics*. 2004;(March):64–70.

28. Phillips YY, Richmond DR. Primary blast injury and basic research: a brief history. In: Bellamy RF, Zajtchuk R, eds. *Conventional Warfare: Ballistic, Blast, and Burn Injuries*. Washington, DC: Office of the Surgeon General, Department of the Army; 1989:221–240.

29. Dugdale-Pointon T. Terrorist weapons: bombs (IEDs). Military History Encyclopedia on the Web Website. http://www.rickard.karoo.net/articles/weapons_terrorbomb.html. Published August 27, 2003. Accessed April 30, 2014.

30. Stuhmiller JH. Blast injury: translating research into operational medicine. In: Santee WR, Friedl KE, eds. *Military Quantitative Physiology: Problems and Concepts in Military Operational Medicine*. Washington, DC: Office of the Surgeon General, Department of the Army; 2008:267–302.

31. Thompson M. Protecting the troops from "underbody threats" with lighter armor. *Time* U.S. Website. http://nation.time.com/2012/11/06/protecting-the-troops-from-underbody-threats-with-lighter-armor/. Published November 6, 2012. Accessed April 30, 2014.

32. Haleem A. Taliban's home-made IED proves challenging to NATO. The Hindu Website. http://www.thehindu.com/opinion/op-ed/talibans-homemade-ied-proves-challenging-to-nato/article615820.ece. Updated September 6, 2010. Accessed April 30, 2014.

33. Murray W. IED detection/defeat. Special Operations Technology. 2012;10(5).

34. McEvers K. "Sticky IED" attacks increase in Iraq. NPR News Website. http://www.npr.org/2010/12/03/131774133/Iraqi-Insurgents-Use-IEDs-To-Target-Iraqis. Published December 3, 2010. Accessed April 30, 2014.

35. Anderson J, Fainaru S, Finer J. Bigger, stronger homemade bombs now to blame for half of U.S. deaths. *Washington Post* Website.

http://www.washingtonpost.com/wp-dyn/content/article/2005/10/25/AR2005102501987.html. Published October 26, 2005. Accessed April 30, 2014.

36. Neptune M, Quexada D. Analysis. Afghan IEDs have been somewhat different than those perfected in Iraq. United for Peace of Pierce County Website. http://www.ufppc.org/us-a-world-news-mainmenu-35/9500-analysis-afghan-ieds-have-been-somewhat-different-than-those-perfected-in-iraq.html. March 31, 2010. Accessed May 30, 2014.

37. GlobalSecurity.org. Improvised explosive devices (IEDs)/booby traps. http://www.globalsecurity.org/military/intro/ied.htm. Updated May 7, 2011. Accessed April 30, 2014.

38. Wilson C. Improvised explosive devices in Iraq: effects and countermeasures. CRS Report for Congress. Congressional Research Service. U.S. Department of State Website. http://www.fpc.state.gov/documents/organization/57512.pdf. Published November 23, 2005. Accessed April 30, 2014.

39. Bala M, Shussman N, Rivkind AI, et al. The pattern of thoracic trauma after suicide terrorist bombing attacks. *J Trauma.* 2010;69(5): 1022–1029.

40. GlobalSecurity.org. Improvised explosive devices (IEDs)—Iraq. http://www.globalsecurity.org/military/intro/ied-iraq.htm. Updated May 7, 2011. Accessed April 30, 2014.

41. Harrisson SE, Kirkman E, Mahoney P. Lessons learnt from explosive attacks. *J R Army Med Corps.* 2007;153(4):278–282.

42. Kluger Y. Bomb explosions in acts of terrorism—detonation, wound ballistics, triage, and medical concerns. *Isr Med Assoc J.* 2003;5(4):235–240.

43. Champion HR, Holcomb JB, Young LA, Wade CE. Injuries from explosions: physics, biophysics, pathology, and research focus needs. *J Trauma.* 2009;66(5):1468–1477.

44. Arnold JL, Tsai M-C, Halpern P, et al. Mass-casualty, terrorist bombings: epidemiological outcomes, resource utilization, and time course of emergency needs, Part I. *Prehosp Disaster Med.* 2003;18(3): 220–234.

45. Stuhmiller JH, Phillips YY, Richmond DR. The physics and mechanism of primary blast injury. In: Bellamy RF, Jenkins DP, Zajtcjuk JT, et al., eds. *Conventional Warfare: Ballistic, Blast, and Burn Injuries.* Washington, DC: Office of the Surgeon General; 1991:241–250.

46. Briggs SM, Brinsfield KH. *Advanced Disaster Medical Response.* Boston, MA: Harvard Medical International Trauma & Disaster Institute; 2003.

47. Mallonee S, Shariat S, Stennies G, et al. Physical injuries and fatalities resulting from the Oklahoma City bombing. *JAMA.* 1996;276(5): 382–387.

48. Prendergast J. Oklahoma City aftermath. *Civil Eng.* 1995;65:40–45.

49. Thompson T, Brown S, Mallonee S, Sunshine D. Fatal and non-fatal injuries among U.S. Air Force personnel resulting from the terrorist bombing of the Khobar Towers. *J Trauma.* 2004;57(2):208–215.

50. Leibovici D, Gofrit ON, Stein M, et al. Blast injuries: bus versus open-air bombings—a comparative study of injuries in survivors of open-air versus confined-space explosions. *J Trauma.* 1996;41(6): 1030–1035.

51. Halpern P, Tsai M-C, Arnold JL. Mass-casualty, terrorist bombings: implications for emergency department and hospital emergency response. Part II. *Prehosp Disaster Med.* 2003;18(3):235–241.

52. Centers for Disease Control and Prevention. After a terrorist bombing: health and safety information for emergency care providers. CDC Website. http://www.bt.cdc.gov/masscasualties/pdf/afterbombing-msgs-ECP.pdf. Published October 22, 2008. Accessed April 30, 2014.

53. National Counterterrorism Center. IED targeting of first response personnel—tactics and indicators. NCTC 2012–34a. Public Intelligence Website. http://info.publicintelligence.net/NCTC-FirstResponderIEDs.pdf. Published August 7, 2012. Accessed April 30, 2014.

54. U.S. Department of Homeland Security, Federal Emergency Management Agency. *Primer to Design Safe School Projects in Case of Terrorist Attacks and School Shootings.* Buildings and Infrastructure Protection Series, pp. 4–9. Department of Homeland Security Website. http://www.dhs.gov/xlibrary/assets/st/bips07_428_schools.pdf. Published January 2012. Accessed April 30, 2014.

55. Peleg K, Aharonson-Daniel L, Michael M, et al. Patterns of injury in hospitalized terrorist victims. *Am J Emerg Med.* 2003;21(4): 258–262.

56. Bala M, Rivkind AI, Zamir G, et al. Abdominal trauma after terrorist bombing attacks exhibits a unique pattern of injury. *Ann Surg.* 2008;248(2):303–309.

57. Frykberg ER, Tepas JJ III. Terrorist bombings: lessons learned from Belfast to Beirut. *Ann Surg.* 1988;208(5):569–576.

58. Quenemoen LE, Davis YM, Malilay J, et al. The World Trade Center bombing: injury prevention strategies for high-rise building fires. *Disasters.* 1996;20(2):125–132.

59. Marshall TK. Injury by firearms, bombs, and explosives: explosion injuries. In: Tedeschi CG, Eckert WG, eds. *Forensic Medicine: A study in Trauma and Environmental Hazards.* Vol 1. Mechanical Trauma. Philadelphia, PA: Saunders; 1977.

60. Kluger Y, Peleg K, Daniel-Aharonson L, et al. The special injury pattern in terrorist bombings. *J Am Coll Surg.* 2004;199(6):875–879.

61. Brethauer SA, Chao A, Chambers LW, et al. Invasion versus insurgency: U.S. Navy/Marine Corps forward surgical care during Operation Iraqi Freedom. *Arch Surg.* 2008;143(6):564–569.

62. Kelly JF, Ritenour AE, McLaughlin DF. Injury severity and causes of death from Operation Iraqi Freedom and Operation Enduring Freedom: 2003–2004 versus 2006. *J Trauma.* 2008;64(2)(suppl):S21-S27.

63. Almogy G, Belzberg H, Mintz Y, et al. Suicide bombing attacks: update and modifications to the protocol. *Ann Surg.* 2004;239(3):295–303.

64. Aschkenasy-Steuer G, Shamir M, Rivkind A, et al. Clinical review: the Israeli experience—conventional terrorist and critical care. *Crit Care.* 2005;9(5):490–499.

65. Almogy G, Rivkind AI. Surgical lessons learned from suicide bombing attacks. *J Am Coll Surg.* 2006;202(2):313–319.

66. Wade CE, Ritenour AE, Eastridge BJ, et al. Explosion injuries treated at combat support hospitals in the Global War on Terrorism. In: Elsayed NM, Atkins JL, eds. *Explosion and Blast-Related Injuries: Effects of Explosion and Blast From Military Operations and Acts of Terrorism.* Burlington, MA: Elsevier Academic Press; 2008:41–72.

67. Almogy G, Mintz Y, Zamir G, et al. Suicide bombing attacks: can external signs predict internal injuries? *Ann Surg.* 2006;243(4):541–546.

68. Davis TE, Lee CY. Asymmetric war (terrorism) and the epidemiology of blast trauma. U.S. Department of Health & Human Services. Greater New York Hospital Association Website. http://www.gnyha.org/ResourceCenter/NewDownload/?id=67&type=1. Published November 3, 2005. Accessed May 30, 2014.

69. Dismounted Complex Blast Injury Task Force. Dismounted complex blast injury. Army Medicine Website. http://armymedicine.mil/Documents/DCBI-Task-Force-Report-Redacted-Final.pdf. Published June 18, 2011. Accessed April 30, 2014.

70. Frykberg ER. Medical management of disasters and mass casualties from terrorist bombings: How can we cope? *J Trauma.* 2002;53(2):201–212.

71. Levi L, Michaelson M, Admi H, et al. National strategy for mass-casualty situations and its effects on the hospital. *Prehosp Disaster Med*. 2002;17(1):12–16.

72. Hamblin DL. Learning to treat terrorist attack victims. *Ortho Today Int*. 2008;11(3):16.

73. Hodgetts T, Smith J. Essential role of prehospital care in the optimal outcome from major trauma. *Emerg Med*. 2000;12(2):103–111.

74. Clarke JE, Davis PR. Medical evacuation and triage of combat casualties in Helmand Province, Afghanistan: October 2010–April 2011. *Mil Med*. 2012;177(11):1261–1266.

75. Department of Defense Directive 6025.21E: Medical Research for Prevention, Mitigation, and Treatment of Blast Injuries. Defense Technical Information Website. http://www.dtic.mil/whs/directives/corres/pdf/602521p.pdf. Published July 5, 2006. Accessed April 30, 2014.

76. DePalma RG, Burris DG, Champion HR, Hodgson MJ. Blast injuries. *N Engl J Med*. 2005;352(13):1335–1342.

77. Beekley AC, Starnes BW, Sebesta JA. Lessons learned from modern military surgery. *Surg Clin N Am*. 2007;87(1):157–184.

78. Warden DL, French L. Traumatic brain injury in the war zone. *N Engl J Med*. 2005;353(6):633–634.

79. Stewart C. Blast injuries: preparing for the inevitable. Emergency Medicine Practice. EB Medicine Website. http://www.ebmedicine.net/topics.php?paction=showTopic&topic_id=18. Published April 2006. Accessed April 30, 2014.

80. Sasser SM, Hunt RC. Clinician Outreach and Community Activity (COCA) Conference Call. Bombings: injury patterns and care. CDC Training & Continuing Education Online system. Centers for Disease Control and Prevention Website. http://emergency.cdc.gov/masscasualties/bombings_injurycare.asp. Published August 3, 2010. Accessed May 30, 2014.

81. Mines M, Thach A, Mallonee S, et al. Ocular injuries sustained by survivors of the Oklahoma City bombing. *Ophthalmology*. 2000;107(5):837–843.

82. Persaud R, Hajioff D, Wareing M, Chevretton E. Otological trauma resulting from the Soho nail bomb in London, April 1999. *Clin Otolaryngol Allied Sci*. 2003;28(3):203–206.

83. Gondusky JS, Reiter MP. Protecting military convoys in Iraq: an examination of battle injuries sustained by a mechanized battalion during Operation Iraqi Freedom II. *Mil Med*. 2005;170(6):546–549.

84. Katz E, Ofek B, Adler J, et al. Primary blast injury after a bomb explosion in a civilian bus. *Ann Surg*. 1989;209(4):484–488.

85. Avidan V, Hersch M, Armon Y, et al. Blast lung injury: clinical manifestations, treatment, and outcome. *Am J Surg*. 2005;190(6):926–931.

86. Ciraulo DL, Frykberg ER. The surgeon and acts of civilian terrorism. *J Am Coll Surg*. 2006;203(6):942–950.

87. Owen-Smith M. Bomb blast injuries: in an explosive situation. *Nurs Mirror*. 1979;149(13):35–39.

88. Cudahy E, Parvin S. The Effects of Underwater Blast on Divers. Naval Sub-marine Medical Research Laboratory. NSMRL Report 1218. Rubicon Foundation Website. http://archive.rubicon-foundation.org/xmlui/bitstream/handle/123456789/7518/ADA404719.pdf?sequence=108. Published August 2, 2001. Accessed April 30, 2014.

89. Guy RJ, Glover MA, Cripps NP. The pathophysiology of primary blast injury and its implications for treatment. Part I. The thorax. *J R Nav Med Serv*. 1998;84(2):79–86.

90. Almogy G, Luria T, Richter E, et al. Can external signs of trauma guide management? Lessons learned from suicide bombing attacks in Israel. *Arch Surg*. 2005;240(4):390–393.

91. Guy RJ, Kirkman E, Watkins PE, Cooper GJ. Physiologic responses to primary blast. *J Trauma*. 45(6):983–987.

92. Ritenour AE, Wickley A, Ritenour JS, et al. Tympanic membrane perforation and hearing loss from blast overpressure in Operation Enduring Freedom and Operation Iraqi Freedom wounded. *J Trauma*. 2008;65(2 suppl):S174-S178.

93. Mellor SG. The relationship of blast loading to death and injury from explosion. *World J Surg*. 1992;16(5):893–898.

94. Peters P. Primary blast injury: an intact tympanic membrane does not indicate the lack of a pulmonary blast injury. *Mil Med*. 2011;176(1):110–114.

95. Jensen JH, Bonding P. Experimental pressure induced rupture of the tympanic membrane in man. *Acta Otolarygol*. 1993;113(1):62–67.

96. Kerr AG. Blast injury to the ear: a review. *Rev Environ Health*. 1987;7(1–2):65–79.

97. Kerr AG, Byrne JE. Concussive effects of bomb blast on the ear. *J Laryngol Otol*. 1975;89(2):131–143.

98. Stein M, Hirshberg A. Medical consequences of terrorism: the conventional weapon threat. *Surg Clin North Am*. 1999;79(6):1537–1552.

99. Bass C, Rafaels KA, Salzar RS. Pulmonary injury risk assessment for short-duration blasts. *J Trauma*. 2008;65(3):604–615.

100. Mellor SG, Cooper GJ. Analysis of 828 servicemen killed or injured by explosion in Northern Ireland 1970–84: the Hostile Action Casualty System. *Br J Surg*. 1989;76(10):1006–1010.

101. Cooper GJ. Protection of the lung from blast overpressure by thoracic stress wave decouplers. *J Trauma*. 1996;40(3 suppl):105S-110S.

102. Caseby NG, Porter MF. Blast injury to the lungs: clinical presentation, management and course. *Injury*. 1976;8(1):1–12.

103. Leibovici D, Gofrit ON, Shapira SC. Eardrum perforation in explosion survivors: is it a marker of pulmonary blast injury? *Ann Emerg Med*. 1999;34(2):168–172.

104. Coppel DL. Blast injuries of the lungs. *Br J Surg*. 1976;63(10):735–737.

105. EMS Continuing Education Online. Blast injuries. University Hospitals (Cleveland, OH) Website. http://www.emsconedonline.com/pdfs/EMT-%20BLAST%20INJURIES-Trauma.pdf. Updated March 5, 2009. Accessed January 31, 2013.

106. Cohn SM. Pulmonary contusion: review of the clinical entity. *J Trauma*. 1997;42(5):973–979.

107. Arnold L, Halperin P, Tsai MC, Smithline H. Mass-casualty terrorist bombings: a comparison of outcomes by bombing type. *Ann Emerg Med*. 2004;43(2):263–273.

108. Oppenheim A, Pizov R, Pikarsky A, et al. Tension pneumoperitoneum after blast injury: dramatic improvement in ventilatory and hemodynamic parameters after surgical decompression. *J Trauma*. 1998;44(5):915–917.

109. Johnson DL, Yelverton JT, Hicks W, Doyal R. Blast overpressure studies with animals and man: non-auditory damage risk assessment for simulated weapons fired from an enclosure. http://www.dtic.mil/dtic/tr/fulltext/u2/a280435.pdf. Published November 15, 1993. Accessed April 30, 2014.

110. Stuhmiller LM, Ho KH, Stuhmiller JH. Health hazards assessment for blast overpressure exposures. Defense Technical Information Center Website. http://www.dtic.mil/cgi-bin/GetTRDoc?AD=ADA303649. Published November 1995. Accessed April 30, 2014.

111. Paran H, Neufeld D, Shwartz I, et al. Perforation of the terminal ileum induced by blast injury: delayed diagnosis or delayed perforation? *J Trauma*. 1996;40(3):472–475.

112. Harmon JW, Haluszka M. Care of blast-injured casualties with gastrointestinal injuries. *Mil Med*. 1983;148(7):586–588.

113. Cripps NP, Cooper GJ. Risk of late perforation in intestinal contusions caused by explosive blast. *Br J Surg.* 1997;84(9):1298–1303.

114. Blast related injuries. *FMST Student Manual—2008 Web Edition.* United States Marine Corps Field Medical Training Battalion, Camp Lejeune. Operational Medicine Website http://www.operationalmedicine.org/TextbookFiles/FMST_20008/FMST_1424.htm. Accessed April 30, 2014.

115. Owers C, Morgan JL, Garner JP. Abdominal trauma in primary blast injury. *Br J Surg.* 2011;98(2):168–179.

116. Stannard A, Brown K, Benson C, et al. Outcome after vascular trauma in a deployed military trauma system. *Br J Surg.* 2011;98(2):228–234.

117. Kocsis JD, Tessler A. Pathology of blast-related brain injury. *J Rehab Res Dev.* 2009;46(6):667–672.

118. Trudeau DL, Anderson J, Hansen LM, et al. Findings of mild traumatic brain injury in combat veterans with PTSD and a history of blast concussion. *J Neuropsychiatry Clin Neurosci.* 1998;10(3):308–313.

119. Moore B. Blast injuries—a prehospital perspective. *J Emerg Prim Health Care.* 2006;4(1):1–13. http://ro.ecu.edu.au/cgi/viewcontent.cgi?article=1190&context=jephc. Accessed April 30, 2014.

120. Ruff RL, Riechers RG 2nd, Wang XF, et al. A case-control study examining whether neurological deficits and PTSD in combat veterans are related to episodes of mild TBI. *BMJ Open.* 2012;2(2):e000312.

121. Armonda RA, Bell RS, Vo AH, et al. Wartime traumatic cerebral vasospasm: recent review of combat casualties. *Neurosurgery.* 2006;59(6):1215–1225.

122. DoD worldwide numbers for TBI. Defense and Veterans Brain Injury Center Website. http://www.dvbic.org/dod-worldwide-numbers-tbi. Updated February 10, 2012. Accessed April 30, 2014.

123. Taber KH, Warden DL, Hurley RA. Blast-related traumatic brain injury: what is known? *J Neuropsychiatry Clin Neurosci.* 2006;18(2):141–145.

124. Rutland-Brown W, Langlois JA, Nicaj L, et al. Traumatic brain injuries after mass-casualty incidents: lessons from the 11 September 2001 World Trade Center attacks. *Prehosp Disast Med.* 2007;22(3):157–164.

125. Mott FW. The effects of high explosives upon the central nervous system. *Lancet.* 1916;1:441–449.

126. Fabing HD. Cerebral blast syndrome in combat soldiers. *Arch Neurol Psychiatry.* 1947;57(1):14–57.

127. Cramer F, Paster S, Stephenson C. Cerebral injuries due to explosion waves, cerebral blast concussion; a pathological, clinical and electroencephalographic study. *Arch Neurol Psychiatry.* 1949;61(1):1–20.

128. Macleod AD. Shell shock, Gordon Holmes and the Great War. *J R Soc Med.* 2004;97(2):86–89.

129. Cernak I, Savic J, Malicevic Z, et al. Involvement of the central nervous system in the general response to pulmonary blast injury. *J Trauma.* 1996;40(3 suppl):S100-S104.

130. Cernak I, Wang Z, Jiang J, et al. Ultrastructural and functional characteristics of blast injury-induced neurotrauma. *J Trauma.* 2001;50(4):695–706.

131. Cernak I, Wang Z, Jiang J, et al. Cognitive deficits following blast injury-induced neurotrauma: possible involvement of nitric oxide. *Brain Inj.* 2001;15(7):593–612.

132. Military Acute Concussion Evaluation (MACE) Pocket Cards. Defense and Veterans Brain Injury Center Website. http://www.dvbic.org/material/military-acute-concussion-evaluation-mace-pocket-cards. Accessed January 30, 2013.

133. Xydakis MS, Ling GS, Mulligan LP, et al. Epidemiologic aspects of traumatic brain injury in acute combat casualties at a major military medical center: a cohort study. *Ann Neurol.* 2012;72(5):673–681.

134. Weinberger S. Bombs' hidden impact: the brain war. *Nature.* 2011;477:390–393.

135. Huller T, Bazini Y. Blast injuries of the chest and abdomen. *Arch Surg.* 1970;100(1):24–30.

136. Rossle R. Pathology of blast effects. In: *German Aviation Medicine in World War II.* Vol 2. Washington, DC: U.S. Government Printing Office; 1950:1260–1273.

137. Hadden WA, Rutherford WH, Merrett JD. The injuries of terrorist bombing: a study of 1532 consecutive patients. *Br J Surg.* 1978;65(8):525–531.

138. Patel H, Dryden S, Gupta A, Ang SC. Pattern and mechanism of traumatic limb amputations after explosive blast: experience from the 07/07/05 London terrorist bombings. *J Trauma.* 2012;73(1):276–281.

139. Hull JB, Cooper GJ. Pattern and mechanism of traumatic amputation by explosive blast. *J Trauma.* 1996;40(3 suppl):S198-S205.

140. Abarbanell NR. Prehospital midthigh trauma and traction splint use: recommendations for treatment protocols. *Am J Emerg Med.* 2001;19(2):137–140.

141. Wood SP, Vrahas M, Wedel SK. Femur fracture immobilization with traction splints in multisystem trauma patients. *Prehosp Emerg Care.* 2003;7(2):241–243.

142. Hill PF, Edwards DP, Bowyer GW. Small fragment wounds: biophysics, pathophysiology and principles of management. *J R Army Med Corps.* 2001;147(1):41–51.

143. Rapid assessment of injuries among survivors of the terrorist attack on the World Trade Center—New York City, September 11, 2001. *MMWR.* 2002;51(1):1–5.

144. Dalinchuk MM, Lalzoi MN. [Eye injuries in explosive mine wounds.] [Article in Russian]. *Voen Med Zh.* 1989;8:28–30.

145. Bittenbender C. Compartment syndrome versus crush syndrome: the difference between each and their respective prehospital treatments. Talk presented at: National Collegiate EMS Foundation 10th Annual Conference; February 21–23, 2003; Arlington, VA. http://www.ncemsf.org/about/conf2003/lectures/bittenbender_crush.pdf. Accessed April 30, 2014.

146. Zoroya G. Spinal injuries up among troops. *USA Today.* November 4, 2009. http://usatoday30.usatoday.com/news/world/2009-11-03-afghanistan-ieds_N.htm. Accessed April 30, 2014.

147. Kauchak M. Land mines and IEDs are dangerous for the damage they cause with fragmentation but the more critical element is the ability to mitigate the energy to transfer of the blast to the seat occupant. *Special Oper Tech.* 2008;6(8).

148. Brumback RJ. Traumatic rupture of the superior gluteal artery, without fracture of the pelvis causing compartment syndrome of the buttock. A case report. *J Bone Joint Surg Am.* 1990;72(1):134–137.

149. Su WT, Stone DH, Lamparello PJ, Rockman CB. Gluteal compartment syndrome following elective unilateral iliac artery embolization. *J Vasc Surg.* 2004;39(3):672–675.

150. O'Mara MS, Semins H, Hathaway D, Caushaj PF. Abdominal compartment syndrome as a consequence of rectus sheath hematoma. *Am Surg.* 2003;69(11):975–977.

151. Abassi ZA, Hoffman A, Better OS. Acute renal failure complicating muscle crush injury. *Semin Nephrol.* 1998;18(5):558–565.

152. Kauvar DS, Wolf SE, Wade CE, et al. Burns sustained in combat explosions in Operations Iraqi and Enduring Freedom (OIF/OEF explosion burns). *Burns.* 2006;32(7):853–857.

153. Aharonson-Daniel L, Klein Y, Peleg K. Suicide bombers form a new injury profile. *Ann Surg*. 2006;244(6):1018–1023.

154. Liebner ED, Weil Y, Gross E, et al. A broken bone without a fracture: traumatic foreign bone implantation resulting from a mass-casualty bombing. *J Trauma*. 2005;58(2):388–390.

155. Braverman I, Wexler D, Oren M. A novel mode of infection with hepatitis B: penetrating bone fragments due to the explosion of a suicide bomber. *Isr Med J*. 2002;4(7):528–529.

156. Wong JM, Marsh D, Abu-Sitta G, et al. Biological foreign body implantation in victims of the London July 7th suicide bombings. *J Trauma*. 2006 60(2):402–404.

157. Hanson D. Car bomb response. Cover report: disaster preparedness/terrorism response. EMS World Website. http://www.emsworld.com/article/10324195/car-bomb-response. Published February 1, 2005. Accessed April 30, 2014.

158. Types of chemical weapons. Federation of American Scientists Website. http://www.fas.org/programs/ssp/bio/chemweapons/cwagents.html. Published April 23, 2010. Accessed April 30, 2014.

159. Chemical and biological attacks, detection, and response FAQ. KI4U. Inc. Website. http://www.ki4u.com/chemical_biological_attack_detection_response.htm. Updated January 1, 2011. Accessed April 30, 2014.

160. Emergency preparedness and response: chemical categories. Centers for Disease Control and Prevention (CDC) Website. http://www.bt.cdc.gov/agent/agentlistchem-category.asp. Updated April 8, 2013. Accessed April 30, 2014.

161. DeGarmo B. Radiological terrorism. Saint Louis University School of Public Health Website. bioterrorism.slu.edu/bt/products/ahec_rad/ppt/Dirty%20Bomb.ppt. April 22, 2003. Accessed April 30, 2014.

162. Singer P, Cohen J, Stein M. Conventional terrorism and critical care. *Crit Care Med*. 2005;33(1 suppl):S61-S65.

163. Factsheet on chemical and biological warfare agents: choking agent: CG. http://www.cbwinfo.com/Chemical/Pulmonary/CG.shtml. Accessed January 31, 2013.

164. Committee on Confronting Terrorism in Russia. High-impact terrorism: proceedings of a Russian-American workshop. Washington, DC: 2002, National Academy Press; 2002.

165. Centers for Disease Control and Prevention, Strategic Planning Workgroup. Chemical and biological terrorism: strategic plan for preparedness and response. MMWR. 2000;49:1–14.

166. Wolff LH, Giddings WP, Childs SB, et al. Time lag and the multiplicity factor in abdominal injuries. In: DeBakey ME, ed. Surgery in World War II. Vol. 2, General Surgery. Washington, DC: Office of the Surgeon General, Department of the Army; 1955:103—117.

167. Cernak I, Savic J, Ignjatovic D, Miodrag J., Jevtic M. Blast injury from explosive munitions. J Trauma. 1999;47(1):96—103.

168. Chambers LW, Green DJ, Gillingham BL, et al. The experience of the U.S. Marine Corps' surgical shock trauma platoon with 417 operative combat casualties during a 12 month period of Operation Iraqi Freedom. J Trauma. 2006;60(6):1155—1164.

169. Chambers LW, Rhee P, Baker BC, et al. Initial experience of U.S. Marine Corps Forward Resuscitative Surgical System during Operation Iraqi Freedom. Arch Surg. 2005;140(1):26—32.

170. Ad-El DD, Eldad A, Mintz Y, et al. Suicide bombing injuries: the Jerusalem experience of exceptional tissue damage posing a new challenge for the reconstructive surgeon. Plast Reconstr Surg. 2006;118(2):383–387.

171. Aharonson-Daniel L, Waisman Y, Dannon YL, Peleg K. Epidemiology of terror-related versus non-terror-related traumatic injury in children. Pediatrics. 2003;112(4):e280—e284. http://www.pediatricsdigest.mobi/content/112/4/e280.full.pdf. Accessed May 3, 2012.

172. Aschkenasy-Steuer G, Shamir M, Rivkind A, et al. Clinical review: the Israeli experience: conventional terrorism and critical care. *Crit Care*. 2005;9(5):490–499.

173. Almogy G, Rivkind AI. Surgical lessons learned from suicide bombing attacks. J Am Coll Surg. 2006;202(2):313—319.

174. Bala M, Wilner D, Keidar A, et al. Indicators of the need for ICU admission following suicide bombing attacks. Scand J Trauma Resusc Emerg Med. 2012;20:19–24.

175. Almogy G, Belzberg H, Mintz Y, et al. Suicide bombing attacks: update and modifications to the protocol. Ann Surg. 2004;239(3):295—303.

176. Trimble K, Clasper J. Antipersonnel mine injury: mechanism and medical management. *J R Army Med Corps*. 2001;147(1):73–79.

177. Coupland RM, Korver A. Injuries from antipersonnel mines: the experience of the International Committee of the Red Cross. BMJ. 1991;303(6816):1509–1512.

178. Cox RD. Hazmat: personal protective equipment. Medscape Web site. http://emedicine.medscape.com/article/764812-overview#aw2aab6b5. Updated March 18, 2011. Accessed December 30, 2012.

179. Erich J. Extreme EMS: training for terrorism response. Emerg Med Serv. 2003;32(3):60–62.

180. Lein B, Holcomb J, Brill S, et al. Removal of unexploded ordnance from patients: a 50-year military experience and current recommendations. Mil Med. 1999;164(3):163–165.

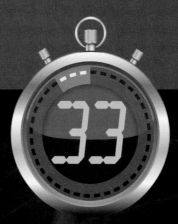

CHAPTER 33

Treatment of Burn Casualties in Tactical Combat Casualty Care

CHAPTER OBJECTIVES

At the completion of this chapter, the reader will be able to do the following:

- Describe the Rule of Nines for estimation of burn size.

- Describe the modern classification system for burn depth.

- Use the U.S. Army Institute of Surgical Research (USAISR) Rule of Ten to calculate initial fluid resuscitation rate for an adult burn victim.

- Discuss the prehospital management of severe burn injuries.

SCENARIO

You are a medic assigned to an infantry platoon. Your unit is on a patrol in eastern Afghanistan when an improvised explosive device (IED) detonates underneath your vehicle, causing it to catch fire. Three soldiers are injured in this incident. After the area is secured, you begin to assess the casualties.

Soldier 1 is a 21-year-old male who is alert, following commands, and walking around. He has sustained burns to his whole face, the lower half of both arms, and the lower part of both legs except for his feet. He has no other visible injuries. His radial pulse is 110 beats/min and strong, and his respiratory rate is 18 breaths/min. He weighs 70 kilograms (kg; 154 pounds).

Soldier 2 is a 27-year-old platoon sergeant who is confused and disoriented. His left foot is severely mangled and bleeding badly. He has burns to the lower right arm, left hand, and left lower leg. His radial pulse is strong at 135 beats/min, and he is breathing quickly. He weighs 75 kg (165 pounds).

Soldier 3 is a 20-year-old male who has partial traumatic amputations of both legs below the knees and is losing a lot of blood. He is completely unresponsive. There are burns to his face, both arms, both legs, and the lower third of his anterior and posterior torso. His radial pulses are not palpable, but he is breathing spontaneously, though slowly. He weighs 90 kg (198 pounds).

1. **What is the triage category for each of these casualties?**

2. **What is the initial management of each casualty?**

3. **What is the extent of burn for each casualty (percentage of total body surface area [%TBSA])?**

4. **Calculate the initial fluid resuscitation, and describe how you will monitor the effectiveness of the resuscitation.**

Introduction

Burn injuries impact about 5% to 10% of combat casualties. It is difficult to care for patients with burns under normal circumstances, but the treatment of casualties with burns during combat and deployment missions is fraught with additional challenges. Combat medical personnel not only must adapt to the combat environment but must also ensure that casualties receive the best care from the point of injury until their arrival at their final destination.

During recent conflicts, the U.S. armed forces have devised a global evacuation system that is unparalleled in the history of combat medicine. U.S. armed forces have the capability to transport casualties from the battlefield to the continental United States (CONUS) in as little as 48 hours, delivering high-quality medical care throughout the evacuation chain. Significant advancements have been made in the care of casualties with burns since the start of Operation Iraqi Freedom (OIF) and Operation Enduring Freedom (OEF). Lessons learned during these conflicts have been analyzed and improvements implemented in real time. The predeployment training that is provided to combat medics, nurses, physicians, and other medical personnel is essential to ensuring that they are equipped to deliver the best care to our wounded warriors.

Primary Assessment

Combat medical personnel evaluating casualties with thermal injuries should make sure they do not become casualties themselves as a result of entering an environment that is unsafe. For example, they should don proper protective equipment before entering a chemically contaminated environment, or ensure that the power is shut off before touching the casualty if the injury is a result of contact with an electrical source.

Prehospital assessment of the casualty with thermal injuries is similar to that of any injured patient. Once all significant external bleeding is controlled, the acronym ABCDE—which stands for Airway, Breathing, Circulation, neurologic Disability, and Expose/Environment—is appropriate for casualties with burn injuries. A combination of burns and non-burn injuries must be considered in combat casualties. Examples include blast and burn injuries in explosions, blunt injuries and burns in motor vehicle collisions involving fires or falls/jumping from burning structures, and injuries resulting from falling debris in a burning structure. The combination of burn and non-burn injuries results in a synergistic increase in mortality.[1]

Airway

The casualty should be assessed immediately for the need for intubation. This is especially important in casualties with findings suggestive of inhalation injury. These findings include facial burns, carbonaceous sputum, stridor, hoarseness, or cough. Direct thermal injury to the face, or a large total body surface area burn resulting in generalized edema, can make intubation extremely challenging. Casualties with burn injuries may also require intubation due to decreased mental status, which may be caused by low oxygen levels in a fire environment, inhalation of toxic gases, head injury, or hypovolemic shock. Securing the endotracheal tube (ET tube) in casualties with facial burns is critical to prevent catastrophic airway loss, since adhesive tape typically does not stick to burned skin. Therefore, cotton ties ("umbilical tape"), or other devices for securing the ET tube all the way around the head and neck, are required.

Some casualties with burn injuries are at increased risk of cervical spine injury. These individuals include those who have sustained motor vehicle collisions, falls, high-voltage electric injuries, or blast injury. In these casualties, cervical spine stabilization is important.

Breathing

Assessment of bilateral breath sounds and pulse oximetry (Spo_2) follow airway evaluation. Processes in combat casualties that may compromise either the airway or breathing include hemothorax, pneumothorax, rib fractures, and pulmonary contusion. The presence of an inhalation injury may cause delayed respiratory failure.

Burning compounds can release a variety of chemicals. Fires involving wood, charcoal, natural gas, petroleum, or similar compounds release carbon monoxide. Carbon monoxide impairs the ability of hemoglobin to carry oxygen and can cause symptoms of decreased oxygenation ranging from nausea and headache to myocardial infarction, mental status changes, and death. It binds powerfully with hemoglobin, turning the blood bright red and producing misleading (i.e., not low) SaO_2 readings. Therefore, casualties with suspected carbon monoxide poisoning should receive 100% oxygen until a measurement of the carboxyhemoglobin level can be obtained in the emergency department.

Fires involving materials like plastics and foam may release cyanide. Cyanide gas is also a chemical warfare agent. Cyanide compromises the cells' ability to use oxygen. No rapid test exists for diagnosis of cyanide poisoning. Symptoms include loss of consciousness, hypotension, and respiratory arrest. Cyanide poisoning is treated with intravenous (IV) hydroxocobalamin (e.g., Cyanokit), a form of high-dose vitamin B_{12}.

Full-thickness burns across the chest can impair breathing by a straightjacket-like effect. These patients will be difficult to ventilate with a bag-mask device and may suffer cardiopulmonary arrest. In this situation, immediate chest escharotomy (by a qualified provider) is required to create room for the chest to expand.

Circulation

Bleeding from non-burn injuries may occur in combination with burns in combat trauma. In a casualty with burn injuries and bleeding, the source of the hemorrhage should be identified and the bleeding controlled with direct pressure using Combat Gauze, tourniquets, and/or junctional hemorrhage control devices as described in the Tactical Field Care chapter.

After bleeding is controlled, peripheral IV catheters should be placed to initiate fluid resuscitation. Placing an IV line through unburned skin is preferable; placing it through burned skin is acceptable, if necessary. An intraosseous (IO) device may be placed if IV access cannot be obtained. All lines should be secured with tape, gauze, Coban, or suture to prevent inadvertent removal during transport.

Casualties with deep, circumferential burns of an extremity can lose blood flow as swelling develops beneath the burns. Monitor pulses in these extremities, and elevate them on pillows or blankets to slow the swelling process. Loss of pulses may indicate severe shock (requiring immediate fluid resuscitation) or may be the result of a tourniquet-like effect of the circumferential burns (requiring rapid transport to a medical treatment facility for surgical release of the burns).

Disability

A brief assessment of the casualty for any gross neurologic deficits should be performed. A decreased level of consciousness (LOC) is abnormal even after a large burn, unless something else is wrong with the casualty. Decreased LOC in casualties with burn injuries is commonly associated with asphyxiation or traumatic brain injury (TBI). Asphyxiation can occur in the fire environment as oxygen levels drop and carbon dioxide levels rise. Alternatively, casualties may inhale toxic gases (i.e., carbon monoxide or cyanide).

Casualties with burn injuries should also be evaluated for motor deficits consistent with spinal cord injury. Casualties suffering high-voltage electrical injuries can be thrown from the power source and may sustain concomitant spinal trauma.

Expose/Environment

Any burning material, such as clothing, should be removed immediately. Dry chemicals should be brushed off; all chemically injured areas should undergo copious decontamination with water. This is particularly critical for casualties with acid or alkali exposure to the eyes. All burned areas should be exposed. Jewelry should be removed from all fingers because of the risk of swelling.

There may be a role for immediate cooling of thermal burns with cold water. However, this application should be limited in duration (3 to 5 minutes) and extent, since casualties with burn injuries are at high risk of hypothermia.

During transport, hypothermia should be prevented by wrapping burn wounds in dry gauze and placing the casualty in a Heat Reflective Shell after the primary assessment is complete. Vehicles or aircraft used for evacuation should be warmed during transport, if possible.

After the primary assessment is performed, reassessment of each portion of the ABCDEs should be repeated as deemed necessary. Caring for casualties suffering thermal and other traumas is a dynamic process, and they can deteriorate rapidly. The secondary assessment is performed by examining the casualty from head to toe. A history of the events surrounding the injury should be obtained from the casualty and any witnesses whenever possible. The casualty's medical history, medications, allergies, last meal, and any other pertinent information should also be sought. Fluid resuscitation should be begun as soon as IV/IO access is established (a detailed discussion will appear later in the chapter). When available, analgesia following Tactical Combat Casualty Care guidelines should be administered to treat the significant pain that can accompany burn wounds.

Physical Characteristics of the Burn Wound

The skin is the largest organ system in the human body. It is composed of two layers: the epidermis and the dermis. The thickness of the skin varies from region to region of the body, with the skin being thinnest at the eyelids and thickest on the soles. Skin thickness also varies based on age and gender.[2] The skin protects the body against fluid and electrolyte loss, infection, and radiant energy. It allows the body to maintain a constant interior temperature in response to changes in the environment and activity. These vital functions are impaired by burns.

Types of Burns

Thermal Burns

The mechanisms of burn injury that can be seen on the battlefield include thermal, chemical, and electrical. Thermal injury is by far the most common, involving direct damage to skin and underlying structures by heat.[3] Thermal injury can result from contact with open flames, scalds from hot liquids, blast from explosive/incendiary devices, or direct contact with a heated object causing coagulation necrosis of the skin. Factors that affect the depth of a burn include the temperature of the heat source, duration of exposure, age of the casualty, and location of the burn (variations in skin thickness throughout the body can alter the depth of the burn injury).

Chemical Burns

Chemical burns are caused by exposure to alkalis (bases), acids, petroleum products, or chemical munitions.[4] These burns can be lethal when systemic absorption of the chemical occurs or a large area of skin is injured. The severity of the injury is dependent upon the concentration of the chemical, the type of chemical, and the duration of the exposure.[5] The final extent of tissue damage from a chemical burn is difficult to assess immediately after exposure because absorption of a chemical deposited on the skin may continue for hours. The key to chemical injury treatment is rapid and thorough decontamination.

The majority of chemical compounds are removed by wiping off any dry material and irrigating the exposed areas with water. Hydrofluoric acid, commonly used in oil refining and industrial cleaning agents, binds serum calcium and can lead to hypocalcemia and tetany. In addition to irrigation with water, areas burned by hydrofluoric acid should be covered with 2.5% calcium gluconate gel (mix calcium gluconate with a lubricant like Surgilube).

White phosphorus is an incendiary agent used in some munitions. It is also found in fertilizers, pesticides, and fireworks. Above 86°F (30°C), white phosphorus ignites spontaneously when in contact with air, producing a yellow flame and white smoke in the wound bed. To prevent spontaneous ignition, the wound should be immediately immersed in water or saline and then placed in water- or saline-soaked dressings.

Furthermore, phosphate may be absorbed into the body. Phosphate binds with calcium, causing potentially life-threatening reduction in the level of calcium in the blood (hypocalcemia) and/or hyperphosphatemia as early as 1 hour after a burn injury. The casualty's electrocardiogram and calcium levels should be monitored.[4]

Electrical Injury

Electrical injury is classified as low voltage or high voltage. Low-voltage injuries result from exposure to power sources less than 1,000 volts. Most wall sockets and residential electrical wiring are low voltage—220 volts or less depending on the country. Low-voltage electrical injuries may cause arrhythmias in addition to burns.

High-voltage power sources are greater than 1,000 volts. High-tension wires are common high-voltage sources. High-voltage electrical injuries may result in occult injuries in addition to burns. For example, muscle can be severely damaged. Muscle breakdown can lead to rhabdomyolysis, kidney failure, and arrhythmias. Rhabdomyolysis should be suspected in the presence of dark red urine, even if red blood cells are absent on microscopic exam. Aggressive fluid resuscitation is the treatment for rhabdomyolysis.

High-voltage sources also tend to project a casualty away from the power source, causing blunt trauma, which may include fractures of any portion of the spine. Any victim of high-voltage injury should be evaluated for blunt trauma and should be transported with spinal precautions.

Burn Depth

Superficial Burn

Burn depth is classified by the depth of injury (**Figure 33-1**). A **superficial burn** injures only the epidermis. Skin integrity remains intact. These burns are painful and erythematous without blistering or open wounds. An example of a superficial burn is sunburn. Rapid wound healing occurs (less than 1 week) without scarring. These burns are not included in the calculation of total body surface area burned.

Partial-Thickness Burn

A partial-thickness burn destroys the epidermis and part of the dermis but does not extend through the entire dermis. A **superficial partial-thickness burn** causes destruction of the epidermis and the upper dermis. These wounds tend to be bright red to mottled in appearance and are wet to the touch. Blisters are commonly seen in superficial partial-thickness burns. Severe pain is caused by exposure of dermal nerve endings to air. It is important to leave blisters intact in the field because they act as a temporary "field dressing" for the injury. These burns tend to weep fluid, contributing to volume loss. Additionally, casualties may become hypothermic due to saturated dressings that may require frequent changes. These wounds tend to heal spontaneously with

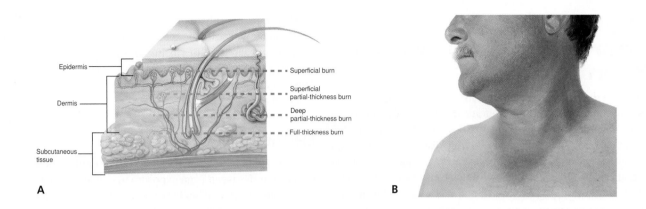

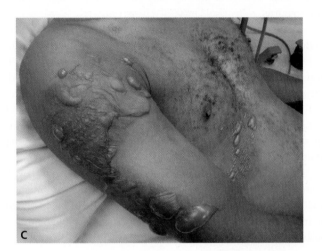

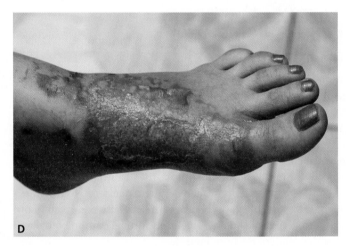

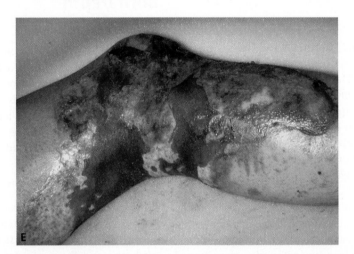

Figure 33-1 **A.** Illustration demonstrating burn depth in relation to skin structures. **B.** Superficial burn. **C.** Superficial partial-thickness burn. **D.** Deep partial-thickness burn. **E.** Full-thickness burn.

Source: **B.** © Suzanne Tucker/ShutterStock, Inc. **C.** Courtesy of Rhonda Beck. **D.** © OlegD/ShutterStock, Inc. **E.** © John Radcliffe Hospital / Science Source.

minimal scarring in 1 to 2 weeks, as long as adequate wound care is implemented.

Of greater concern are **deep partial-thickness burns**. These burns involve complete destruction of the epidermis and most of the dermis. Wounds are characteristically dark red to yellowish-white in color, are minimally blanching, are slightly moist, and exhibit decreased sensation to skin prick. Blisters are uncommon in burns of this depth. Pain is minimal due to destruction of pain fibers in the dermis. Blood flow to areas with deep partial-thickness burns is compromised, allowing for increased risk of infection and wound conversion to full-thickness injury. Wound healing may take weeks to months with increased risk of hypertrophic scarring if treated nonoperatively. Excision and grafting is commonly warranted to expedite wound healing in these casualties.

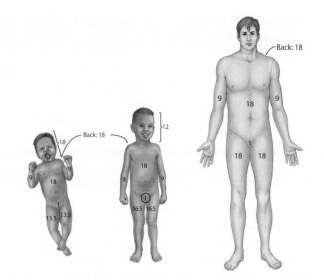

Figure 33-2 The Rule of Nines for burn area estimation.

Full-Thickness Burn

Full-thickness burns are characterized by injury of the epidermis, dermis, and underlying skin structures (hair follicles and glands). The burned tissue appears charred or whitish in color, is dry and leathery, and is insensate. Thrombosed blood vessels may be visible. This eschar is a potent stimulator of the inflammatory response and is a medium for microorganism growth. These burns do not heal readily, and there is a high risk of hypertrophic scarring if they are not excised but are instead allowed to close by contraction.

Subdermal Burn

Subdermal burns extend through subcutaneous tissue into fascia, muscle, and even bone. Fatality rates among victims of these burns (unless small in area) are high. For survivors, the extensive damage associated with subdermal burns often leads to severe functional impairment or amputation. These casualties will require specialized burn care and reconstructive surgery.[5]

Burn Size

The estimation of burn size is an important step in burn care. Most importantly, it helps with determining the volume of fluid required to resuscitate the casualty. Burn size is expressed as a percentage of total body surface area (%TBSA). Superficial burns are not included in the measurement of %TBSA. Burn injuries on adults should be initially mapped in the field using the "Rule of Nines," a method that assigns percentages (9% to major regions) to different areas of the body[6] (**Figure 33-2**). This mapping technique must be modified for use in children, whose heads occupy a larger portion of the body and whose lower extremities occupy a smaller portion. The Lund and Browder chart is a more detailed burn diagram suitable for use in hospitals (**Figure 33-3**).[7]

Region	%
Head	
Neck	
Ant. Trunk	
Post. Trunk	
Right arm	
Left arm	
Buttocks	
Genitalia	
Right leg	
Left leg	
Total burn	

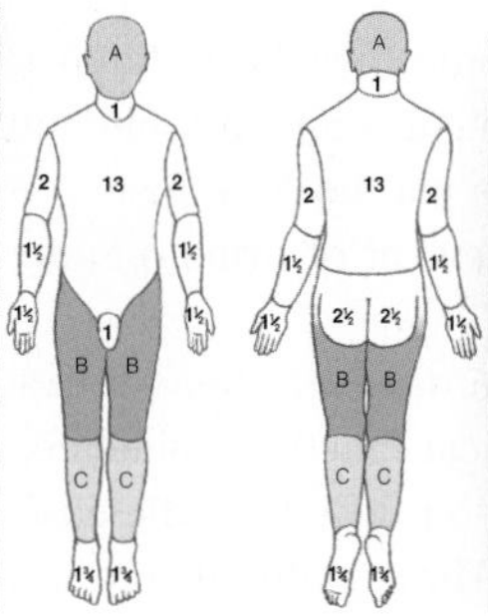

Age (years)	A (½ of head)	B (½ of one thigh)	C (½ of one leg)
0	9½	2¾	2½
1	8½	3¼	2½
5	6½	4	2¾
10	5½	4¼	3
15	4½	4½	3¼
Adult	3½	4¾	3

Relative percentages of body surface area affected by growth

Figure 33-3 Lund and Browder burn area map.

Fluid Resuscitation for Burn Injury

Burn injury involving approximately 20% TBSA or more results in massive fluid shifts. These fluid shifts can cause hypovolemic shock during the first 48 hours after a burn injury. Delayed or inadequate replacement of volume results in poor tissue perfusion and possibly death. Over-resuscitation, in contrast, may cause complications related to edema, including abdominal and extremity compartment syndromes or even death. The goal of fluid resuscitation after a severe burn injury is to replace the losses with just enough fluid to maintain adequate tissue perfusion throughout the 48-hour period following injury.

There are several formulas for estimating how much fluid to give the casualty in this situation. For example, IV fluid can be given at a rate based on the modified Brooke formula: total volume to be infused over the first 24 hours = 2 (milliliters) ml × weight in kilograms (kg) × TBSA, with one-half administered over the first 8 hours postburn and one-half over the second 16 hours. To simplify this calculation, the U.S. Army Institute of Surgical Research (USAISR) Burn Center advocates the USAISR Rule of Ten formula for adult patients (**Figure 33-4**).

Figure 33-4 The USAISR Rule of Ten

1. Estimate the burn size to the nearest 10%.
2. %TBSA × 10 = Initial fluid rate (for ADULT patients weighing 40 to 80 kg).
3. For every 10 kg ABOVE 80 kg, increase the rate by 100 ml/hr.
4. Titrate to a urine output of 30 to 50 ml/hr.

To illustrate, if one is faced with resuscitating three patients with varying burn sizes of 30%, 50%, and 70%, initial fluid rates of 300, 500, and 700 ml/hr of fluid, respectively, would be initiated.[8]

Lactated Ringer's solution is the preferred fluid for resuscitation of burn victims, but resuscitation can be initiated with normal saline or Hextend. If Hextend is used, no more than 1,000 ml should be given, followed by lactated Ringer's or normal saline as needed.

Optimal care requires adjusting the lactated Ringer's rate each hour, with the goal of maintaining a urine output of 30 to 50 ml/hr in adults—no more and no less. Insertion of a Foley catheter and hourly measurement of urine output, fluid input, and vital signs are required.

In an effort to help standardize care, the Joint Trauma System published a Burn Care Clinical Practice Guideline, including a Burn Flow Sheet to help better document the casualty's resuscitation during evacuation. These materials are available at all Role 3 facilities and on the USAISR website: http://www.usaisr.amedd.army.mil/clinical_practice_guidelines.html.[9]

Pediatric Casualties

Children require proportionally larger volumes of IV fluid than adults with similar-sized burns. The "Rule of Ten" is designed for *adults only* and thus should not be utilized when treating children. For pediatric casualties, the following formula should be used: Total volume of lactated Ringer's to infuse over the first 24 hours postburn = 3 ml × weight in kg × %TBSA. Give one-half of this over the first 8 hours and one-half over the second 16 hours.[10]

Additionally, very young children and infants may be unable to maintain their glucose levels during periods of stress. They should receive 5% dextrose in one-half normal saline ($D_5$1/2NS) at a standard maintenance rate *in addition* to the burn resuscitation fluids using the following formulas:

- 0 to 10 kg: 4 ml/kg/hr
- 10 to 20 kg: 40 ml/hr + 2 ml/kg/hr
- Greater than 20 kg: 60 ml/hr + 1 ml/kg/hr

Special Circumstances

It is important to realize that the presence of multiple trauma, inhalation injury, or electric injury will often augment fluid needs. Blood loss resulting in massive transfusion may dominate the fluid resuscitation requirements in casualties with both burns and non-burn injuries. In cases where sufficient IV fluids are not available, oral or nasogastric tube resuscitation can be used to resuscitate casualties with burns of up to about 30% TBSA.[9] An oral resuscitation fluid can be prepared by adding 8 teaspoons of sugar and 1 teaspoon of salt to each liter of clean potable water.[11]

Wound Care

Many factors affect the treatment of casualties with burn injuries on the battlefield including availability of medical evacuation, capabilities of the medical treatment facility, training of combat medical personnel, and external tactical threats. Regardless, clinical outcomes will be determined to a large extent by the quality of medical treatment provided in the theater of operations. Therefore, predeployment training in courses such as the American Burn Association's Advanced Burn Life Support (ABLS) course, the Department of Defense's Joint Forces Combat Trauma Management Course (JFCTMC), and the Emergency War Surgery (EWS) course are critical for relaying the basic knowledge needed to treat this special population of casualties. The physical appearance of burn injuries can be distracting and may cause inexperienced combat medical personnel to overlook other less obvious injuries. Therefore, early emphasis must be placed on identifying and treating all life-threatening injuries. This becomes particularly important for casualties injured by improvised explosive devices (IEDs).

Care Under Fire Phase

During the Care Under Fire Phase, the most important aspect of care is to separate the casualty from the source of burn injury and immediately stop the burning process. Stopping the burning process may be accomplished by applying a nonflammable liquid, having the casualty drop and roll, smothering the flames with a blanket, or using any other expedient means available.

Tactical Field Care Phase

In the Tactical Field Care phase, burns should be covered with dry, sterile dressings. After appropriate lifesaving interventions are accomplished, casualties with extensive burns may be placed in the Heat Reflective Shell, which will both cover the burned areas with a clean material and help to prevent hypothermia. Combat medical personnel should then calculate the burn area as described earlier, remembering that superficial burns are not included in this calculation.

Fluid resuscitation, if needed to prevent burn shock (greater than 20% TBSA), should be initiated as soon as IV/IO access is established. Resuscitation for hemorrhagic shock, if present, takes precedence over burn resuscitation and should be administered per TCCC guidelines for shock.

Analgesia in accordance with TCCC guidelines should be administered as needed for burn pain. Antibiotic therapy in the field for burn wounds alone is not recommended, but antibiotics may be given per TCCC guidelines if indicated to prevent infection in penetrating wounds.

Tactical Evacuation Care Phase

The key to successful treatment of casualties with burn injuries is urgent transport to definitive care. Care of the casualty with burn injuries in the Tactical Evacuation Care phase is similar to that in the Tactical Field Care phase except that additional emphasis should be placed on hypothermia prevention.

Medical Treatment Facility

At the Role 2b Forward Surgical Team or Role 3 Combat Support Hospital, fluid resuscitation is continued and initial wound care is performed in addition to addressing other life-threatening injuries. The surgical management of burn wounds in deployed settings focuses on cleansing the wounds and preventing compartment syndrome. Burn wounds should be cleansed with chlorhexidine gluconate (Hibiclens) solution, removing all surface debris and contamination.

Patients with circumferential deep burns of the extremities are at risk of edema causing constriction of blood flow. To prevent this, a surgeon makes an incision into the burned skin (escharotomy) along the medial and lateral lines of the limb (**Figure 33-5**).

After debridement, burn wounds should be dressed with topical antimicrobial agents to prevent infection. There are a variety of topical agents that can be used, including silver sulfadiazine cream, 11% mafenide acetate cream, and 5% mafenide acetate solution.[13] Silver-impregnated nylon dressings are an alternative (**Figure 33-6**). These dressings are easy to apply and may not have to be changed for 3 to 5 days (if the wounds are clean). Burned extremities (especially upper extremities) should be elevated to reduce edema.

Fire can also cause eye injuries, so irrigation with sterile water or saline is performed to remove any debris from the eye, and the corneas are examined with a Wood's lamp.

Evacuation of Patients With Burns

In comparison with previous conflicts, U.S. military medical care during the recent conflicts in Iraq and Afghanistan has been characterized by rapid aeromedical evacuation. The average time elapsed from point of injury in these theaters to arrival in CONUS is 96 hours. All attempts are made to evacuate patients with burns as expeditiously as possible, but severe respiratory and hemodynamic compromise can delay transport. Most of these patients have been stabilized and their burn resuscitation has been completed by the time they arrive at the U.S. Army Burn Center at the USAISR in Texas. Patients with severe burn injury or respiratory status that precludes conventional mechanical ventilation may require transatlantic aeromedical evacuation by the USAISR Burn Flight Team (**Figure 33-7**).

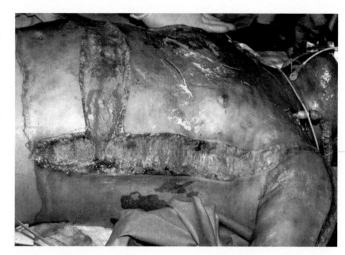

Figure 33-5 Escharotomies.
Source: Courtesy U.S. Army Burn Center.

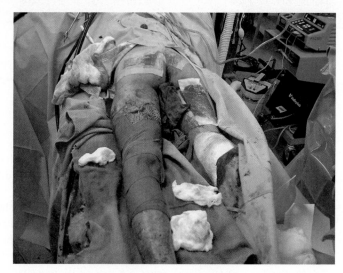

Figure 33-6 Silver-impregnated nylon dressings.
Source: Courtesy U.S. Army Burn Center.

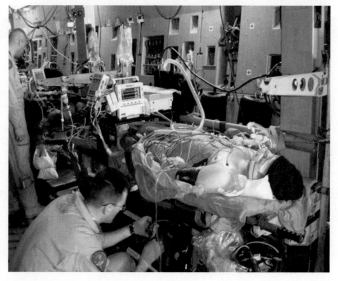

Figure 33-7 U.S. Army Burn Flight Team transport setup.
Source: Courtesy U.S. Army Burn Center.

Casualties are rarely triaged to the expectant category on the basis of burn size. Patients with a TBSA exceeding 95% have survived with a good quality of life.[12]

U.S. Army Institute of Surgical Research Burn Flight Team

The USAISR Burn Flight Team (BFT) was created in the 1950s and was instrumental in evacuating patients with burns from Vietnam. Since that time, the BFT has been activated for both humanitarian and wartime missions. The BFT consists of five personnel: a burn surgeon, a registered nurse, a licensed practical nurse, a respiratory technician, and an operations non-commissioned officer (NCO).

The BFT typically transports patients with greater than 40% TBSA burns, with inhalation injury, and/or with both burns and multiple non-burn injuries from combat trauma. These patients may also require special ventilator support. The BFT usually transports patients on C-17 or C-121 aircraft and relies on U.S. Air Force Aeromedical Evacuation Squadrons for logistical support. Since 2003, the BFT has conducted over 90 missions and has evacuated over 350 combat casualties to the U.S. Army Burn Center.[14]

Summary

- The proper management of the thermally injured combat casualty requires a unique set of skills.
- The primary assessment is key to identifying life-threatening injuries and beginning lifesaving therapies.
- Burn depth is gauged as superficial, superficial partial thickness, deep partial thickness, full thickness, or subdermal.
- Burn size is expressed as a percentage of total body surface area (%TBSA). In adults, TBSA is estimated using the Rule of Nines.
- A knowledge of basic burn wound care is imperative in a deployed environment.
- In the field, burns should be covered with dry, sterile dressings.
- The ability to determine the total burn surface area and an understanding of burn resuscitation is crucial so that care of the casualty is not delayed.
- Initial fluid therapy, if needed to prevent burn shock in adults, is calculated using the Rule of Ten. Lactated Ringer's solution is the fluid of choice for resuscitation of casualties with burn injuries.
- The care that burn casualties receive in the early stages of their injury will largely determine their outcomes.

SCENARIO RECAP

You are a medic assigned to an infantry platoon. Your unit is on a patrol in eastern Afghanistan when an IED detonates underneath your vehicle, causing it to catch fire. Three soldiers are injured in this incident. After the area is secured, you begin to assess the casualties.

Soldier 1 is a 21-year-old male who is alert, following commands, and walking around. He has sustained burns to his whole face, the lower half of both arms, and the lower part of both legs except for his feet. He has no other visible injuries. His radial pulse is 110 beats/min and strong, and his respiratory rate is 18 breaths/min. He weighs 70 kg (154 pounds).

Soldier 2 is a 27-year-old platoon sergeant who is confused and disoriented. His left foot is severely mangled and bleeding badly. He has burns to the lower right arm, left hand, and left lower leg. His radial pulse is strong at 135 beats/min, and he is breathing quickly. He weighs 75 kg (165 pounds).

Soldier 3 is a 20-year-old male who has partial traumatic amputations of both legs below the knees and is losing a lot of blood. He is completely unresponsive. There are burns to his face, both arms, both legs, and the lower third of his anterior and posterior torso. His radial pulses are not palpable, but he is breathing spontaneously, though slowly. He weighs 90 kg (198 pounds).

SCENARIO SOLUTION

1. What is the triage category for each of these casualties?

Soldier 3 is in the immediate category since he cannot walk or talk, and immediate lifesaving intervention is indicated. Soldier 2 has an altered mental status and is hemorrhaging from an extensive wound. His radial pulse is still palpable, but fast. His mental status decrement may be due to traumatic brain injury or blood loss that may be compensated for the moment. He should be placed in the immediate category. Soldier 1 is walking, talking, and obeying commands, but has serious burn injury. He is in the delayed category.

2. What is the initial management of each casualty?

- Soldier 3 initially needs tourniquets on both legs, an IV or IO bolus of Hextend, cricothyroidotomy, ventilatory support with a bag-mask device, tranexamic acid (TXA), cervical-spine stabilization, and antibiotics.
- Soldier 2 should have a tourniquet placed above his injured left foot, IV or IO access established, and cervical-spine stabilization. You should anticipate his near-term need for a definitive airway and fluid resuscitation for hemorrhagic shock. IV antibiotics are indicated, and if he should need fluid resuscitation, he will also need TXA.
- Soldier 1 may soon need significant analgesia. His airway should be assessed and frequently rechecked for patency.

3. What is the extent of burn for each casualty (%TBSA)?

With deductions for the back of the head and the amputations, the calculated burn surface area for Soldier 3 is about 70%, for Soldier 2 is about 15%, and for Solider 1 is about 31%.

4. Calculate the initial fluid resuscitation, and describe how you will monitor the effectiveness of the resuscitation.

- For Soldier 3, calculated burn resuscitation is:
  - 70% TBSA × 10 = 700 ml/hr
  - Add 100 ml/hr for the extra 10 kg over 80 kg = 800 ml/hr
  - Monitor urine output and adjust fluids to achieve and maintain 30 to 50 ml/hr.
- The TBSA for Soldier 2 is 15%, so resuscitation for burn fluid shift, per se, is not indicated.
- For Soldier 1, TBSA is 31%, so rounded to the nearest ten, 30 × 10 = 300 ml/hr. He weighs 70 kg, so the initial rate is not increased. Urine output should be monitored hourly and fluid rate adjusted as needed to maintain 30 to 50 ml/hr.

Note: All three of these casualties should have their burn wounds dressed after secondary assessment, and soldiers 2 and 3 should be given supplemental oxygen as soon as it becomes available in the evacuation process. They should also be protected from hypothermia.

References

1. Santaniello JM, Luchette FA, Esposito TJ, et al. Ten year experience of burn, trauma, and combined burn/trauma injuries comparing outcomes. *J Trauma*. 2004;57(4):696–700.

2. Bishop JF. Burn wound assessment and surgical management. *Crit Care Nurs Clin N Am*. 2004;16(1):145–177.

3. National Burn Repository 2005 Report. American Burn Association Website. http://www.ameriburn.org/NBR2005.pdf. Accessed May 4, 2014.

4. Barillo DJ, Cancio LC, Goodwin CW. Treatment of white phosphorus and other chemical burn injuries at one burn center over a 51-year period. *Burns*. 2004;30(5):448–452.

5. American Burn Association. *Advanced Burn Life Support Course Provider Manual*. Chicago, IL: American Burn Association; 2001.

6. Knaysi GA, Crikelair GF, Crosman B. The rule of nines: its history and accuracy. *Plast Reconstr Surg*. 1968;41(6):560–563.

7. Lund CC, Browder NC. The estimation of areas of burn. *Surg Gynecol Obstet*. 1944;79(4):352–358.

8. Chung KK, Salinas J, Renz EM, et al. Simple derivation of the initial fluid rate for the resuscitation of severely burned adult combat casualties: in silico validation of the rule of ten. *J Trauma*. 2010;69(suppl 1):S49–S54.

9. Chung KK, Blackbourne LH, Wolf SE, et al. Evolution of burn resuscitation in Operation Iraqi Freedom. *J Burn Care Res*. 2006;27(5):606–611.

10. Pham TN, Cancio LC, Gibran NS. American Burn Association practice guidelines: burn shock resuscitation. *J Burn Care Res*. 2008;29(1):257–266.

11. Cancio LC, Kramer GC, Hoskins SL. Gastrointestinal fluid resuscitation of thermally injured patients. *J Burn Care Res*. 2006;27:561–569.

12. White CE, Renz EM. Advances in surgical care: management of severe burn injury. *Crit Care Med*. 2008;36(7 suppl.):S318–S324.

13. Borden Institute. *Emergency War Surgery: The Third United States Revision*. Fort Dietrich, MD: Borden Institute; 2004.

14. Renz EM, Cancio LC, Barillo DJ, et al. Long range transport of war-related burn casualties. *J Trauma*. 2008;64(2 suppl):S136–S145.

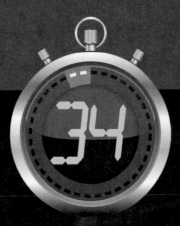

CHAPTER 34

Casualty Response Planning in Tactical Combat Casualty Care

CHAPTER OBJECTIVES

At the completion of this chapter, the reader will be able to do the following:

- Identify the core components of a medical threat assessment.

- List six sources of medical intelligence suitable for premission planning.

- Discuss the importance of alternate planning.

- List the five types of mission rehearsals and define each.

- Discuss the site characteristics of a good casualty collection point.

Introduction

The tactical environment encompasses the actions of armed personnel who are actively engaged in or directly maneuvering to kill or capture one another, or seize one another's terrain or assets. It is the part of the battlefield where every resource is limited, and nothing is truly secure or safe. Environmental factors like topography or weather influence the battle and can make or break the day. The fighting may include anything from exchanges over a few hundred meters to hand-to-hand combat. Decisions and actions are measured in seconds. The outcome of any battle may be judged a success, a disaster, or anything in between.

Both realistic training and actual combat operations will inevitably result in casualties. Tactical casualty scenarios can range from one casualty to dozens, with degrees of trauma from minor to massive, and is usually a mix of these. The tactical situation or prosecution of the mission may overrule medical decisions. Time is usually critical for the mission and for the casualties.

Trauma care is optimized by minimizing the time between wounding and treatment with a level of care sufficient to the injury sustained. This capability is dependent upon the availability of adequate equipment and supplies, and the knowledge and skills necessary to perform the inherent tasks. Tactical leaders can significantly reduce the number of casualties who are killed in action or die of their wounds by simply positioning optimal medical capability in close proximity to the point of wounding. Survival of the combat casualty lies primarily in the hands of the person who initiates treatment. Managing casualty response, including contingency planning, casualty collection points, and tactical evacuation, is a tactical leader's task; supplying medical expertise throughout the casualty's care, both while on the battlefield and during evacuation from it, is a combat medic's task.

Casualty Response System

Both tactical leaders and tactical medical advisors must be intimately familiar with the tactics, techniques, and procedures involved in the implementation of a **Casualty Response System**. This is not a medical system; instead, it is a tactical system of tiered casualty management that integrates the expertise of nonmedical and medical personnel in order to achieve the best possible outcomes for both the mission and the casualties.

In the tactical environment, anyone has the potential to be a "first responder." Therefore, all who engage in combat operations must understand the basic tenets of Tactical Combat Casualty Care (TCCC). If all personnel are well versed in appropriate levels of TCCC, they will be able to provide casualty care collectively as a team, while minimizing interference with the unit's tactical flow during combat operations. In warfare, the majority of all combat deaths have historically occurred prior to casualties receiving advanced trauma care.

Training

Actions conducted in training equate to actions conducted in combat. Implementing a Casualty Response System should be viewed as a battle drill. It should be integrated into all combat training exercises and rehearsed to the greatest extent possible. If rehearsals are performed to standard, the novelty of a real casualty will be mitigated. Realistic training will save lives on the battlefield. Safety is paramount, but risk reduction in training should not be purchased with preventable death in combat.

Training should be conducted to standard and not to time. The basics of casualty management can be mastered through repetition and conditioning, and as in any serious training regimen, discipline precludes shortcuts. The more conditioned an individual and a team become through training, the more likely they will achieve optimal outcomes for their casualties on the battlefield. The true success of a Casualty Response System will be defined by a team's ability to successfully prosecute the mission while minimizing morbidity and mortality.

Focus on the Possible

In planning and training for combat casualty management, the focus should be on the possible, not the impossible. Essentially, there are three groups of casualties that will be encountered. In the first group, no matter what you do, the wounded will live. In the second group, no matter what you do, they will die. In the third group, if you do the right thing, at the right time, your treatment will make the difference between life and death or between greater and lesser disability. The Casualty Response System should focus its efforts on this third group, as there is a much greater probability of positively affecting their outcomes.

Decisions in tactical casualty management should not be made by persons far removed from the fighting. The Casualty Response System should be a flattened organization with decentralized decision making that empowers first responders, tactical leaders, and combat medical personnel at all levels. When those who must implement the system far forward also direct its operation far forward, they are likely to invest in realistic casualty management training in order to become more efficient and effective at and near the point of injury. Ultimately, this will equate to lives saved.

Medical Planning

Medical planning in line units relies heavily on the experience and knowledge of unit physician assistants and senior medics. *All* tactical medics, from the most junior to the most senior, should become skilled medical planners. Effective medical planning requires that the medical planner be well integrated into the unit's (company/battalion/brigade/regimental) mission planning staff. Many medical issues that arise during tactical planning are regulated, decided, or solved by other members of the staff, including the S3 (Operations), S3 (Air), S4 (Logistics), Commanders, Executive Officers, First Sergeants, and Platoon Sergeants. Good working relationships and effective communications must be maintained for successful medical planning.

Medical planners must be fluent in the unit's tactical planning sequences (compressed or deliberate) and have a good understanding of the role they play therein. Medical planners should be involved as early as possible in planning sequences for *all* training exercises and real-world contingencies. It is a good idea for medical planners to make a planning checklist and timeline of planning events or milestones for every exercise and operation.

A medical plan should include an overall casualty response plan in which every unit member has a role. When a casualty occurs, it is not just the combat medic's problem; it is a tactical problem that must be planned for and solved by the entire unit. Units should integrate a casualty response phase into all of their tactical battle drills. Unit members and leadership must be well versed in the casualty response plan.

Combat medical personnel have a tendency to focus on providing critical patient care once they begin treating casualties and, as such, may not be able to maintain sufficient situational awareness to execute the casualty response plan. The unit must be able to execute the casualty response plan around the medic while the medic treats the wounded.

Predeployment Requirements

The unit should conduct predeployment medical training and casualty response drills during training exercises. The time to ponder what can be done during the Care Under Fire phase is not when real bullets are flying. A comprehensive medical skills training program will enable units to prepare for casualties sustained in combat operations. Individual operators should be trained in first responder TCCC skills and equipped appropriately long before launching on the combat mission. A unit that conducts TCCC skills training for individual operators and integrates

Figure 34-1 The 75th Ranger Regiment

The 75th Ranger Regiment has seen extensive combat action while conducting direct-action combat operations in Afghanistan beginning in October 2001 and Iraq beginning in March 2003. From these dates to March 2010, the Regiment sustained a total of 419 battle injuries—180 during 8.5 years in Afghanistan and 239 during 7 years in Iraq. These numbers include 387 wounded in action, 28 killed in action, and 4 who later died of their wounds. Notable throughout this time frame is that the Regiment has had *no* Level I prehospital medically preventable combat deaths.

Source: Kotwal, Russ S., Montgomery, Harold R. et al (2011). Eliminating Preventable Death on the Battlefield. Archives of Surgery, 146(12). Copyright © 2011 American Medical Association. All rights reserved.

casualty response drills into unit exercises will reduce preventable combat deaths **(Figure 34-1)**.

Medical Threat Assessment

The medical planner must assess all medical threats the unit may face during the operation. This assessment includes environmental health hazards as well as specific threats from enemy weapons systems. Through the medical threat assessment, the medical planner will identify preventive measures the unit can employ to minimize these threats. Once the preventive measures appropriate to the mission have been selected, medical planners must be prepared to make recommendations to unit commanders, leaders, and members on how to employ them. The overall goal is to have healthy operators ready to perform a mission, to keep them healthy during the mission, and to bring healthy operators back home.

Identify the Area of Operations (AO)

The medical planner must develop a clear understanding of medical threats and assets in the countries, regions, and environments in which the operation will be conducted. The locations of targets, staging bases, etc., must be known in order to adequately plan for medical threats. The most important area to assess is the target area. This is the area or region in which the unit will be conducting tactical missions. The host country or staging area must also be evaluated. This is the secure region used as a base of operations. The threats here may or may not be the same as those of the target area.

Identify Medical Intelligence and Health Threats

Medical intelligence is a key component of all training and contingency operations. Information on hazardous plants and animals, prevalent diseases, required immunizations and chemoprophylaxis, climatology, and medical and hospital capabilities in the areas involved should be gathered. The National Center for Medical Intelligence (NCMI) is a primary source for medical intelligence. NCMI collects and disseminates information on disease occurrence, medical capabilities, health services, and environmental health hazards specific to regions around the world. The Internet address for the NCMI is https://www.intelink.gov/ncmi/index.php (Common Access Card required). Some other sources for medical intelligence available online are:

- Centers for Disease Control and Prevention (CDC): http://www.cdc.gov/
- U.S. Department of State, Bureau of Consular Affairs: http://travel.state.gov/travel/travel_1744.html
- World Health Organization (WHO): http://www.who.int/en/
- U.S. Army Public Health Command: http://phc.amedd.army.mil/

The medical planner must also maintain an awareness of the unit's medical readiness status. A review of immunization and health records should be conducted well before the operation begins.

The types of enemy weapons the unit may encounter, including chemical and biologic weapons, must also be determined. The medical planner should make recommendations to prevent and treat the injuries these weapons may inflict, such as the use of body armor, chemoprophylaxis, or protective masks.

Higher Headquarters Orders and Guidelines

Higher Headquarters Medical Guidelines and Requirements

The operational headquarters will often publish specific guidelines regarding casualty evacuation and hospitalization as well as preventive medicine requirements in its operations orders (OPORDs). The medical planner must determine if unit members will have to take medications before, during, and after the mission to prevent illnesses such as malaria. A key question that must be asked is, "Does the unit need to change anything from their normal procedures to meet higher headquarters requirements?"

Requests for Information (RFI)

Medical planners should be familiar with the processes for requesting updates to dated information about disease or environmental threats. Sources for such periodic reports and publications may lie within the chain of command or may be external, such as international health organizations. Maps, imagery, and information on medical facilities in the staging or target areas may also be needed.

Determine Medical Assets

On a given operation, the unit will be supported by its internal medical assets. External medical personnel, equipment, or units may also be attached as needed. A thorough understanding of all medical assets assigned to the mission is crucial. This includes the proper unit designations or names, number of personnel by specialty, treatment and evacuation capabilities, logistical requirements, task organization, and command and control. It is important to ensure that all external medical assets are well connected into the unit's structure operationally, logistically, and administratively.

Evacuation Assets

There are two basic types of evacuation conducted during combat operations: Casualty Evacuation (CASEVAC) and Medical Evacuation (MEDEVAC). CASEVAC implies the use of nonmedical platforms to evacuate casualties. These mission platforms are ground vehicles, watercraft, or aircraft typically used by the unit for infiltration, exfiltration, or resupply. These vehicles do not usually have combat medical personnel or equipment onboard unless previously assigned in the operational plan. These assets are more suited for routine evacuation of nonemergent casualties, but pre-staged combat medical personnel and equipment can facilitate the treatment and transport of the more seriously wounded. Medical planners should plan for the use of CASEVAC assets as much as possible, as these assets are often the most readily available for rapid evacuation. Furthermore, these vehicles are usually armed and, thus, are better prepared to conduct evacuation while the fight with the enemy is ongoing.

MEDEVAC refers to the use of dedicated medical platforms whose primary mission is the evacuation of casualties. Most often conducted by aircraft, MEDEVAC can also be carried out using medically staffed and equipped frontline ambulances (FLAs). MEDEVAC platforms are usually assigned to a regulated region, are not under the direct control of the tactical unit, and must be requested through operational channels. Controllers in operations centers receive MEDEVAC requests and launch or divert MEDEVAC assets as required on a prioritized basis.

Unit medical planners should determine the casualty evacuation assets that will likely be needed to support the unit's mission, whether by air, ground, or water. Assets should be matched to the expected needs in premission planning.

Requesting Evacuation

MEDEVAC requests are normally transmitted using the standard North Atlantic Treaty Organization (NATO) Nine-Line MEDEVAC Request Format **(Figure 34-2).**

The MEDEVAC request provides controllers in operations centers with the critical information needed to launch and manage MEDEVAC platforms. CASEVAC requests can be tailored specifically to the unit mission and operating area but typically consist of the first five lines of a MEDEVAC request. This works for CASEVAC platforms since they are normally already part of the tactical operation, and the drivers have a clear understanding of the battle space through previous coordination and ongoing communications.

Familiarization With Evacuation Assets

In premission planning, there are key questions that must be answered concerning CASEVAC and MEDEVAC. How many and what type of platforms are available? What are the capabilities, limitations, and restrictions of the platforms? Are air evacuation assets capable of hoist or high-angle extractions? What medical equipment is on board each platform? Who are the assigned combat medical personnel and to what levels are they trained?

Figure 34-2 MEDEVAC Request Format*

Line	Item	Brevity Codes
1	Location/Grid	Grid
2	Frequency and Call Sign of Requesting Unit	FM freq Call sign
3	Number of Patients by Precedence	A—Urgent B—Urgent surgical C—Priority D—Routine E—Convenience
4	Special Equipment Needed	A—None B—Hoist C—Extraction equipment D—Ventilator
5	Number of Patients by Type (Litter and Ambulatory)	L—Number of litter patients A—Number of ambulatory patients
6 (Wartime)	Security at Pickup Site (Wartime)	N—No enemy troops in area P—Possibly enemy troops in area E—Enemy troops in area (use caution) X—Enemy troops in area (armed escort required)
6 (Peacetime)	Number and Type of Wounded, Injured, or Ill	Description of each
7	Method of Marking Pickup Site	A—Panels B—Pyrotechnic signal C—Smoke signal D—None E—Other (specify)
8	Patient Nationality and Status	A—U.S. military B—U.S. civilian C—Non-U.S. military D—Non-U.S. civilian E—Enemy prisoner of war
9 (Wartime)	NBC Contamination (Wartime)	N—Nuclear B—Biologic C—Chemical
9 (Peacetime)	Terrain Description (features in and around the landing site)	

*Use lines 1–5 for precoordinated CASEVAC requests using organic assets.

Source: Reproduced from the Ranger Medic Handbook, © William Donovan

Rehearsals With External Assets

The unit's leaders and combat medical personnel should coordinate face to face with external evacuation personnel prior to mission execution to ensure a clear understanding of procedures by all personnel. If possible, live rehearsals with evacuation assets should be conducted to prepare for smooth handover of casualties. Unit operators should practice with the evacuation platforms as aid-and-litter teams. During the real evacuation of a wounded and bleeding casualty is not the time to learn how to secure a litter inside an aircraft.

Surgical and Area Medical Support Assets

The medical treatment facilities to which combat casualties will be transported should be identified and their capabilities and capacities (especially surgical) documented. With this knowledge, medical planners can predict how many of what type of casualties could overwhelm a given facility, and casualty flow can be directed accordingly. Furthermore, casualties can be routed directly to facilities with greater capabilities if dictated by the severity of their injuries. For casualties with severe injuries, evacuation to a fully capable combat support hospital has been found to produce better outcomes than evacuation to a treatment facility with limited surgical and intensive care capabilities if the evacuation times are comparable.

It is highly desirable to visit the supporting medical facilities to gain an understanding of their physical layouts and unique equipment. Face-to-face coordination with appropriate staff personnel is most important. Also, unit medical personnel must know how to follow up with the unit casualties, as commanders will require serial reports on their status.

Deployed troops will suffer routine illnesses and noncombat injuries that may require medical attention exceeding the combat medic's scope of practice. Area medical support assets are those facilities that provide medical services other than combat trauma care to meet these needs. Established policies and procedures for operators' routine medical care at area medical support facilities should be conveyed to unit leaders and medical personnel.

Primary and Alternate Planning

As with all military operations, the unit and the medical planner should always have backup plans. A unit should never launch on a combat mission with only one planned means of casualty evacuation, for example. In this instance, alternatives for all possible routes of evacuation (e.g., air, ground, water) should be written into the medical plan. Alternate receiving facilities should be identified in case mass-casualty situations occur or conditions prohibit evacuation to primary facilities. Additionally, weather and environmental conditions can have detrimental effects on preplanned evacuation operations that can be mitigated by a good alternate plan.

Tactical Medical Support Plan Development

Understand the Tactical Commander's Plan

Medical planners must understand the overall scheme of maneuver of the forces arrayed on the battlefield in order to develop a good medical support plan for expected casualties. This understanding is gained by attending all of the operations planning meetings

and ensuring that medical operations are well synchronized into the tactical plan. Tactical plans may evolve rapidly, so the medical planner must keep abreast of changes and should participate in course of action development to determine if the various options can be supported medically.

Estimate Casualties

Both medical and tactical planners should predict where casualties are likely to occur and develop casualty management and evacuation plans for all phases of the operation (infiltration, assault, clear/secure, consolidation, exploitation, defense, and exfiltration). Computer-based planning tools such as the Medical Course of Action Tool (MCOAT) can assist medical planners in forecasting attrition during military operations. Other key elements to consider are the layout of the target and template of enemy positions as projected by intelligence and operations staffs. Understanding the commander's tactical plan will indicate how best to develop the medical support plan.

Casualties should be expected and planned for in all phases of the tactical operation. The following questions will help develop casualty management plans:

- Where on the target is it anticipated that casualties will be sustained?
- What types of injuries are expected based on the type of operation and enemy weapons?
- Where are the most critical locations for unit medics to be positioned?
- Do you need to task organize the medical team to separate locations or to separate fighting elements?
- Where does the unit need to establish **casualty collection points (CCPs)** based on the expectations of casualties?
- What evacuation methods should be considered?
- Where are the nearest helicopter landing zones (HLZs) or ambulance exchange points (AXPs) to high-casualty areas?
- Where should medical assets or augmentation be staged?
- How will casualties be moved from point to point on the target prior to evacuation from the target?

The casualty estimation also includes projecting Disease and Non-battle Injury (DNBI), the potential for non-battle-related illness and injury calculated from known medical threats, unit activities, previous events, and individual health profiles. DNBI includes trauma such as parachute landing injuries that do not occur as a result of combat. The MCOAT can assist with casualty estimations for injuries of this type.

Issue Initial Medical Planning Guidance to Subordinates

Medical planners should constantly disseminate information to subordinate elements and junior combat medical personnel.

Information provided should be as comprehensive as possible consistent with operational security considerations. Guidance on crafting medical plans should include the medical threat analysis, medical assets, copies of higher OPORDs or operational plans (OPLANs), and information that will assist subordinates with medical planning at their level. Guidance from above helps junior combat medical personnel better prepare themselves and their equipment for tactical operations.

Determine Casualty Flow From Target to Hospitalization

If possible, casualty flow should be planned from the point of injury all the way back to admission to a medical facility in the Continental United States (CONUS). However, in an established combat theater, a casualty may be admitted, treated and even released from an intermediate facility between the battlefield and CONUS **(Figure 34-3)**. At a minimum, combat medical personnel should always have a detailed understanding of the casualty flow up to two levels above their units in the chain of evacuation, including patient regulating, casualty accountability, and hospitalization requirements. For example, a platoon medic should have a good understanding of where a casualty goes after leaving the CCP or battalion aid station.

There are several issues that need to be addressed and questions answered in order to establish casualty flow:

- To what location(s) will the unit's casualties be evacuated?
- Will evacuation to and from CCPs be conducted by ground, air, or water assets?
- How will evacuation be conducted to **casualty transload points**?
- What are the distances and times of travel?
- Will the expected casualties be able to make it that far? If not, which parts of the medical support plan need to be corrected?
- Who will evacuate the casualties?
- Will medical assets be properly positioned to ensure continuity of care?

Determine Key Locations

Key locations for medical assets are determined based upon the casualty estimation and the commander's tactical assault plan:

- Where should the CCP be located?
- Where should patient exchanges (HLZs, AXPs) be located?
- Where are the projected fighting positions, blocking positions, roadblocks, and checkpoints?
- Where will Command and Control be located?
- Who will be in charge of each key location?
- Are both primary and alternate locations for all medical functions within the medical support plan established?
- What are the planned ground movement routes?

Establish the Tactical Medical Support Plan

The medical support plan can be developed alongside tactical plans, but often it is difficult to lock in the medical support plan until tactical planners have settled on the preferred course of action. The tactical portion of the medical support plan should include the following elements:

1. The distribution, task organization, and tactical movement (infiltration/exfiltration) of medical elements, all synchronized with each other and the overall tactical plan
2. The casualty flow plan from point of injury through evacuation to a medical treatment facility, including primary and secondary evacuation routes, methods, and modes (aid and litter, air, ground, water)
3. Primary and alternate sites for CCPs, casualty evacuation points (CEPs), HLZs, and possible casualty exchange points (CXPs)
4. A medical communications plan (Will medical nets be required? Will combat medical personnel carry radios? How will casualty information and evacuation requests be relayed from element to element?)

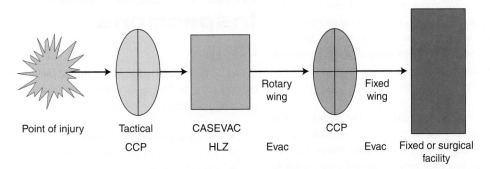

Figure 34-3 Casualty flow from target to hospitalization.

Source: Reproduced from the Ranger Medic Handbook, © William Donovan

5. A medical resupply plan if the operation will continue for a length of time
6. Plans for the management of wounded hostile combatants and noncombatant casualties

Air Tactical Evacuation Plan

The following information should be gathered in the formulation of a tactical air evacuation plan:

- What aircraft types will be used, and what is the maximum casualty load of each type?
- How will the casualties be loaded and are there any patient packaging requirements?
- Are there specific loading procedures and approach procedures to the aircraft?
- What is medical capability aboard each aircraft (equipment and personnel)?
- Is any special casualty management equipment required?
- Can the aircraft deliver prepackaged medical resupply bundles?
- What are the request procedures and who is the launch authority?
- What are the landing requirements (landing zone dimensions, markings required, and special equipment required)?

Ground Tactical Evacuation Plan

There are two major sections of a ground tactical evacuation plan. The first section is comprised of those actions required to move casualties within the target area. This section applies even if moving casualties to an aircraft extraction point. The other section describes the actions required to evacuate casualties from the target area to a medical facility by ground vehicles. The security of the ground element is a critical aspect of moving casualties within or out of the target area. The unit must ensure that a fighting element will protect the evacuation asset from enemy attack.

Ground tactical evacuation at the objective consists of moving casualties from their points of injury to CCPs or evacuation points. Aid-and-litter teams should be formed by nonmedical personnel within the fighting elements. These personnel should be trained and equipped to conduct this secondary mission prior to launching the tactical mission. Vehicles of opportunity such as abandoned or captured enemy vehicles on the target can be used to move casualties. For instance, in an airport seizure, the unit could use baggage carts to move casualties.

Planning for evacuation by ground from the objective to a medical facility incorporates the same kind of information as planning for air evacuation, except for questions unique to land vehicles. However, one critical aspect of ground evacuation is

determining whether the unit will conduct the evacuation using its own assets or call upon another unit.

Medical Communications

The Tactical Medical Support Plan includes a plan for medical communications. In formulating the medical communication plan, the following should be considered:

- Will all combat medical personnel have radios? If not, how will the radios be assigned among them?
- Will combat medical personnel be able to contact a higher-level care provider for guidance?
- What types of radios will be used?
- What communications security requirements will be in effect?
- How will medical Command and Control be delineated?
- What will the medical call signs be?
- Which frequencies will be assigned to medical elements?
- Which frequencies will be assigned to the evacuation assets?
- Who will be responsible for reporting casualties, to whom, and in what format?

Medical Resupply Requirements and Methods

Medical planners must first develop a thorough understanding of the unit's normal medical equipage, supplies, load plans, and premission shortages. For the tactical medical support plan, determinations are made regarding the equipment and supplies that will be initially carried into the target, and a further plan established for a first and second echelon of resupply. For exercises, Class VIII (medical supply) accounts at medical treatment facilities near the training area can be established. Though not normally a unit function, tactical medical planners should also understand the acquisition and availability of blood products, special vaccines, antidotes, and antivenins as required.

Briefs, Rehearsals, and Precombat Inspections

Briefs

Typically, the OPORD at all levels should include the tactical medical support plan. The medical brief for the tactical medical support plan should include at a minimum:

- All identified health threats
- An overview of the Casualty Response System
- Casualty flow

- Key locations (CCPs, HLZs, AXPs, etc.)
- Requesting procedures (CASEVAC, MEDEVAC, assistance, resupply)
- Medic call signs and frequencies
- Tracking and reporting casualties

Rehearsals

Rehearsals allow unit members to familiarize themselves with the briefed plan and to visualize the expected action. Depending on the level and repetition of rehearsal, unit members can develop a thorough familiarity with the sequence of events that will be executed. A rehearsal should be conducted as a scripted event that lays out the operational plan in a sequence of overlapping events. Contingencies and complications can be injected to assess unit member reactions and to practice alternate plans.

Full dress rehearsals provide the most detailed understanding of the operation and involve all unit members executing their expected tasks, flowing through the expected timeline of the event. A full dress rehearsal is essentially a military field exercise—a training event preparing for the real event at a location with a similar layout. Obviously, full dress rehearsals are the most time- and resource-intensive and cannot be done for short-notice or compressed operational timelines.

A *reduced force rehearsal* involves only key leadership of subordinates and operational units. Although such rehearsals are less time- and resource-consuming, they are dependent on leaders driving nearly all actions.

Terrain model rehearsals, also known as rock drills or sandbox drills, use miniature depictions of the operational area. Historically, terrain model rehearsals are probably the most commonly used method for rehearsal of military operations. A terrain model can be as simple as sticks and rocks arranged on the ground or as elaborate as scale models of buildings and vehicles. Though miniaturized, a terrain model can provide unit members with a reasonable visualization of the objective and the operational area. Leaders at all levels should use the model to rehearse their missions with subordinates.

Map rehearsals can be used virtually anywhere, using actual maps or sketches of operational areas. Similar to a terrain model, a map rehearsal provides visualization of the objective, but with limits. A map rehearsal usually involves a small number of people who must squeeze together to see the map, and symbols are often used to depict objects and units. Map rehearsals are best left to the most time-sensitive or austere situations, when elaborate exercises or terrain models are simply not possible.

A *radio* or *communications rehearsal*, also known as a COMMEX, is a combination of testing communications systems and unit members running through the sequence of events through radio calls. For the communications equipment tests, using the same equipment, same frequencies, and same distances specified in the operational plan will provide the unit with the best insight into whether their equipment will function as needed. If possible, line-of-sight obstacles such as buildings or terrain should be interposed between radios to exactly replicate conditions at the target. For the sequence of event radio calls, the unit should utilize an execution checklist that prescribes a specific sequence of events and deviations with specific code words so that unit members know something has been completed or complicated.

If possible, the unit should exercise the Casualty Response System by rehearsing expected and possible actions on the objective such as:

- First responder drills
- Squad casualty response drills (Care Under Fire, TACEVAC request and loading)
- Aid-and-litter team drills
- CCP operations (assembly, security and movement, casualty movement, CCP markings, vehicle parking, link-up procedures, casualty tracking and recording, triage, treatment and management of casualties)
- Mass-casualty plan
- COMMEX—communications exercise/radio test
- Casualty tracking/accountability

Precombat Inspections

Every combat unit should conduct precombat inspections (PCIs) prior to launching on a mission. PCI is conducted from the lowest leadership levels to the highest; no one should ever be exempted. Medically, this process includes:

- Individual unit members
  - First aid kits
  - Individual preventive medicine (e.g., water purification, chemoprophylaxis)
- Squad casualty response kit
  - Team first responder bags
  - Evacuation equipment (e.g., Skedco, litters)
  - Vehicle-mounted aid bags
- Medic aid bags (pack and/or reconfigure as required)
  - Select appropriate aid bag system for mission requirements.
  - Ensure packing list agrees with recommended stockage.
- Resupply packages (pack and/or reconfigure per mission requirements)
  - Reconfigure in accordance with mission specifics (ground, air, etc.).
  - Utilize bundles or pull-off configuration as required.
  - Pre-position as required with aircraft and vehicles or at staging base with logistics teams.
- Medic individual equipment (e.g., weapon, night vision device, radio, mission-specific gear)
- Evacuation assets (e.g., quads, vehicles)

Casualty Collection Point Operations

Checklist for the Establishment and Operation of Tactical CCPs

CCP Site Selection

- Should be reasonably close the fight
- Should be located near areas where casualties are likely to occur
- Must provide cover and concealment from the enemy
- Should be inside a building or on hardstand (an exclusive CCP building limits confusion)
- Should have access to evacuation routes (foot, vehicle, or aircraft)
- Should be proximal to "lines of drift" or paths across terrain that are the most likely to be used when going from one place to another (These are paths of least resistance that offer the greatest ease while taking into account obstacles and modes of transit on the objective.)
- Should be adjacent to tactical choke points (breeches, HLZs, etc.)
- Should avoid natural or enemy choke points
- Should be an area providing passive security (inside the perimeter)
- Should have good drainage
- Should be accessible to evacuation assets
- Should be expandable if casualty load increases

CCP Operational Guidelines

- First Sergeant (1SG) or Platoon Sergeant (PSG) is responsible for casualty flow and everything outside the CCP.
    - Provides for CCP structure and organization (color coded with ChemLights)
    - Maintains command and control and battlefield situational awareness
    - Controls aid-and-litter teams and provides security
    - Strips, bags, tags, organizes, and maintains casualties' tactical gear outside the treatment area
    - Is accountable for tracking casualties and equipment into and out of CCP and reports to higher command
    - Moves casualties through CCP entrance/exit choke point, which should be marked with an infrared ChemLight
- Combat medical personnel are responsible for everything inside the CCP.
    - Triage officer sorts and organizes casualties at choke point into appropriate treatment categories.
    - Medical officers and medics organize medical equipment and supplies and treat casualties.
    - EMTs, first responders, and aid-and-litter teams assist with treatment and packaging of casualties.
- Minimal casualties should remain with original element or assist with CCP security if possible.
- KIAs (Soldiers, Sailors, Airmen, or Marines killed in action) should remain with original element.

Guidelines for Establishing CCP Inside a Building

- Ensure building is cleared and secured.
- Enter and assess the building prior to receiving casualties.
    - Use largest rooms.
    - Consider litter/Skedco movement (Can you do it in the area?).
    - Determine whether separate rooms for treatment categories are available.
    - Determine location of choke point/triage.
    - Minimize congestion.
- Remove/relocate furniture or obstructions.
- Color code rooms to treatment categories (mark doors, etc.).

CCP Duties and Responsibilities

Tactical Medics

- Triage, treat, monitor, and package.
- Delegate treatment.
- Request assistance from other medical or unit assets.
- Provide guidance and recommendations to leadership on casualty management and evacuation.

Unit Leadership and Medical Planners

- Establish and secure CCPs.
- Provide assistance to medics with augmentation and direct aid-and-litter teams.
- Gather and distribute casualty equipment and sensitive items.
- Ensure accountability and reporting to higher authority.
- Request evacuation and establish CASEVAC or MEDEVAC link-up points.
- Manage KIA remains.

General Guidelines for CCP Personnel

- Maintain security.
- Maintain command and control.
- Maintain appropriate medical treatment.
- Maintain situational awareness.
- Maintain organization.
- Maintain control of equipment and supplies.
- Maintain accountability.

General CCP Layout Templates

Figures 34-4 through **34-9** depict common configurations for CCPs.

After Action Review

After each operation, an assessment of the unit's conduct from beginning to end is conducted to gather all possible lessons. The following questions provide a basic topic list for the After Action Review:

- Was the mission executed as planned?
- What went right?

- What went wrong?
- What could have been done better?
- What could be fixed by planning/preparation?
- What could be fixed by training?
- What could be fixed by equipment modification?
- What "Sustains and Improves" can be identified in each phase of the operation?

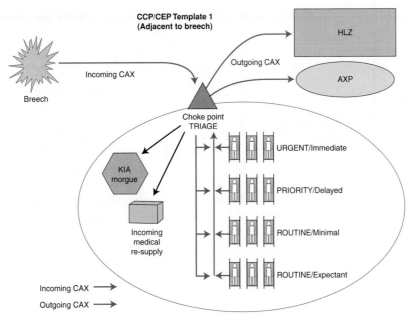

Figure 34-4 CCP/CEP Template 1: Adjacent to breech.

Source: Reproduced from the Ranger Medic Handbook, © William Donovan

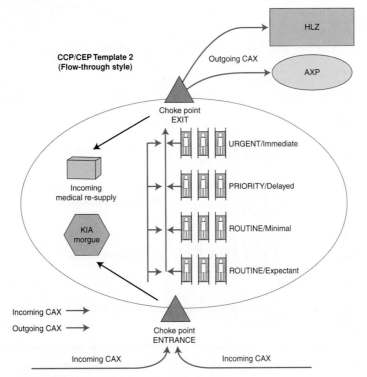

Figure 34-5 CCP/CEP Template 2: Flow-through style.

Source: Reproduced from the Ranger Medic Handbook, © William Donovan

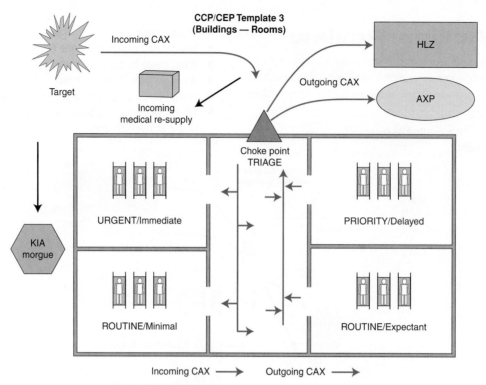

Figure 34-6 CCP/CEP Template 3: Building—rooms.

Source: Reproduced from the Ranger Medic Handbook, © William Donovan

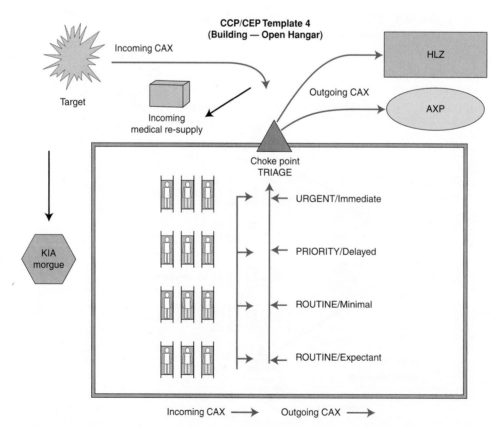

Figure 34-7 CCP/CEP Template 4: Building—open hangar.

Source: Reproduced from the Ranger Medic Handbook, © William Donovan

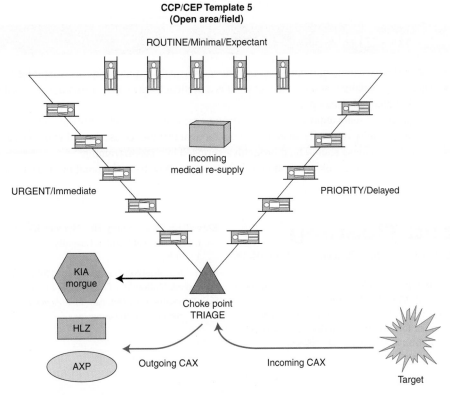

Figure 34-8   CCP/CEP Template 5: Open area/field.
Source: Reproduced from the Ranger Medic Handbook, © William Donovan

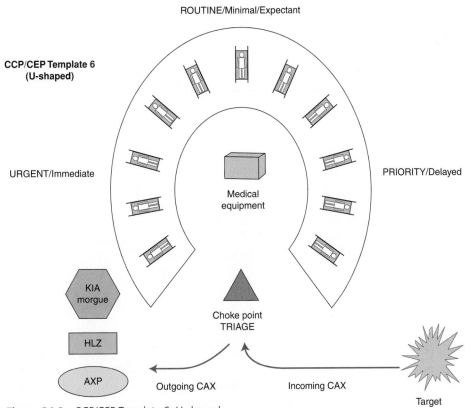

Figure 34-9   CCP/CEP Template 6: U-shaped.
Source: Reproduced from the Ranger Medic Handbook, © William Donovan

Summary

- Suboptimal casualty outcomes can be reduced through casualty response planning, training, and rehearsals.
- Directing casualty response management is a tactical leader's task; providing medical expertise is a task for combat medical personnel.
- An integrated team approach to casualty management can directly translate into significant reduction in the casualty fatality rate and can minimize the tactical turbulence associated with taking casualties.
- Casualty response should be thoroughly exercised in mission training.
- Premission medical planning should cover casualty flow from the point of injury to definitive care.

Suggested Reading

Center for Army Lessons Learned. Medical Planning Newsletter 04–18, December 2004.

Dupuy TN. *Attrition: Forecasting Battlefield Casualties and Equipment Losses in Modern War.* Falls Church, VA: Nova; 1995.

Kotwal RS, Meyer DE, O'Connor KC, et al. Army Ranger casualty, attrition, and surgery rates for airborne operations in Afghanistan and Iraq. *Aviat Space Environ Med.* 2004;75(10):833–840.

Kotwal RS, Montgomery HR, Mechler KK. A prehospital trauma registry for Tactical Combat Casualty Care. *J Spec Oper Med.* 2011;11(3): 127–128.

Kotwal RS, Montgomery HR, Hammesfahr JF. *Ranger Medic Handbook.* 3rd ed. Midlothian, TX: CielAzul Publications; 2007.

U.S. Department of Defense. *U.S. Army Ranger Handbook.* New York, NY: Skyhorse Publishing; 2006.

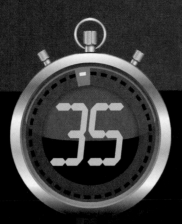
Medical Support of Urban Operations

CHAPTER OBJECTIVES

At the completion of this chapter, the reader will be able to do the following:

- List and describe the four distinct levels of urban battle space.

- Describe the effects of urban terrain on communications, navigation, and logistics in combat operations.

- Discuss the injury patterns likely to be encountered during urban operations.

- Discuss adjustments in medical support that should be anticipated for urban combat operations.

SCENARIO

Your platoon is patrolling the streets of Mogadishu on foot when you are suddenly attacked at an intersection by multiple hostiles firing from the street ahead and from windows above. The platoon quickly takes cover in the lobby of an abandoned, shot-up apartment building. Two rocket-propelled grenades (RPGs) strike the outside of the wall you and two others are kneeling behind, collapsing the wall. The legs of the soldier beside you are trapped by reinforced concrete and cinder blocks. The casualty is alert but in great pain.

The platoon's fire forces the hostiles back. The lobby is secured and you have good cover from sniper fire. Your platoon leader calls for vehicular extraction; the estimated time of arrival (ETA) is 40 minutes. You are the medic, and you have three casualties to care for.

- Casualty 1 has a massive wound to the right side of his head. Heavily disrupted brain tissue is visible. He is unresponsive, has no palpable carotid pulse, and is not breathing.
- Casualty 2 is the soldier trapped by the fallen rubble. He is screaming in pain and asking for help to get his legs free. His radial pulse is strong and rapid. Two platoon members are digging him out.
- Casualty 3 has a fragment wound to the left side of the neck and mandible, with heavy bleeding from his neck wound. He is leaning forward with blood draining out of his mouth, holding direct pressure on his neck wound with his hand. He is alert and responds to instructions but cannot talk.

1.   What do you do?

> The future of warfare lies in the streets, sewers, high-rise buildings, industrial
> parks and the sprawl of houses, shacks and shelters that form the broken
> cities of our world.
>
> —Ralph Peters[1]

Introduction

Warfare in cites is inevitable. Historically, military planners have sought to avoid combat in cities, preferring to isolate, bypass, or avoid them. Urban combat places tremendous demands on resources and manpower, often resulting in large numbers of casualties. Nevertheless, some of the most intense battles in history have occurred in and around urban areas. Stalingrad, Achen, Manila, Hue, Sarajevo, Mogadishu, Grozny, Fallujah—the very names of these cities conjure images of brutal, house-to-house combat.

Since the fall of the Berlin Wall and the end of the Cold War, many new and different threats have emerged. Global terrorism, international criminal activity, the illegal drug trade, and regional despotisms such as Iran and North Korea have replaced the monolithic Soviet military as challenges to the security of the United States. Rogue nations and shadowy international terrorist groups like Al-Qaeda, lacking the resources to fight a conventional war against the United States or other Western powers, instead seek battles that exploit weaknesses in conventional military power while emphasizing their own strengths. During these **asymmetric conflicts**, the tactics of terrorism, insurgency, and unconventional guerilla warfare are commonly used by a weaker opponent against a stronger conventional force. The rapidly urbanizing developing world will likely be the setting for many of these future conflicts.

Cites have historically been "centers of gravity" during war. They serve as control points—centers of finance, population, and industry. If current demographic trends continue, by 2015 more than 500 cities will have populations greater than 1 million. By 2025, more than 85% of the world's population will live in and around cities.

The modern spectrum of urban conflict is vast; from the Battle of Stalingrad in World War II to the 1992 Los Angeles riots, there have been an estimated 1.6 million casualties. U.S. military forces must be prepared to fight a determined enemy in the urban environment. General Charles Krulak, a former Commandant of the U.S. Marine Corp, described a "three block war" wherein U.S. armed forces would conduct humanitarian assistance, peacekeeping operations, and intense, highly lethal urban combat in separate parts of the same city.[2]

This chapter provides an overview of planning considerations for combat medical personnel supporting urban operations. Characteristics of the urban battlefield, an overview of the likely types of casualties, and training and planning considerations will be discussed. It is difficult to develop specific tactics, techniques, and procedures (TTPs) applicable to all combat medical personnel who may fight in a city. No one-size-fits-all solution is available. In future urban battles, nonmedical personnel and combat medical personnel alike will be required to quickly adapt to the current mission, terrain, and situation.

Urban Terrain

The *United States Marine Corp Manual on Military Operations in Urban Terrain, MCWP 3-35.3*, and the *Joint Publication 3-06, Doctrine for Joint Urban Operations*, are both excellent references for planning urban operations and for descriptions of tactical considerations encountered in urban terrain.

The urban battlefield is a three-dimensional, 360-degree battle space encompassing great variations in terrain. A single city may include deep, dense "urban canyons" with large blocks of tall, multistoried buildings with hundreds of rooms and corridors; large blocks of industrial areas with factories and warehouses; and sprawling suburban residential areas. Each of these elements has distinctive characteristics that present unique challenges.

The *United States Marine Corps Manual on Military Operations in Urban Terrain* divides the urban battle space into four distinct levels:

1. The *subterranean level* consists of sewers, tunnels, networks, subway systems, and underground garages. Forces can move unobserved beneath an enemy to attack the enemy's rear or flank. Subterranean systems in large cities may be extensive (e.g., the New York City subway system or the London Underground).
2. The *street level* may include broad avenues and highways or narrow backstreets and alleys. Generally this level provides a rapid avenue of approach, but it also channelizes combatants, making them vulnerable to ambush **(Figure 35-1)**. Confined on either side by buildings and structures, the street level can be easily blocked by obstacles such as rubble or disabled vehicles.
3. The *building level* provides numerous locations for cover and concealment, serving as a vertical barrier to attacking forces while providing multiple fighting positions for defenders. The many rooms and windows of multistory

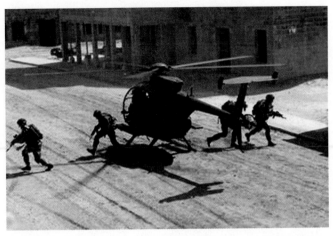

Figure 35-2 Helicopters provide rapid means of infiltration into the urban battlefield but are vulnerable to small arms fire, rocket-propelled grenades, and surface-to-air-missiles.
Source: Courtesy of U.S. Department of Defense

structures offer a variety of positions for snipers while the upper floors provide excellent locations for anti-armor weapons to be fired down onto vehicles, exploiting weaknesses in their armor.

4. The *air level* can serve as a high-speed avenue of approach for the insertion and extraction of forces. Aircraft are vulnerable to man-made obstacles on buildings and rooftops such as power lines, antennae, and radio towers. Aircraft are also subject to small arms and anti-aircraft fire from buildings and rooftops **(Figure 35-2)**. Aircraft ambushes in urban areas, conducted successfully in the past against U.S. forces in Mogadishu and Russian forces in Chechnya, make urban air operations difficult and dangerous.

It is likely that on the modern urban battlefield, combat will take place on all these levels simultaneously.

Characteristics of Urban Combat

Urban operations are characterized by intense small-unit, infantry engagements. Fighting takes place at close range and is often hand to hand **(Figure 35-3)**. Because of the three-dimensional nature of the battlefield and the density of numerous man-made structures, troops are often dispersed into small teams.

This greater dispersion of forces makes it difficult for leaders to see and control their forces. Difficulties in communication increase chaos and confusion. Troops fighting in built-up areas require strong small-unit leaders who possess a high level of situational awareness, flexibility, and initiative.

Operations in built-up areas are manpower-, resource-, and time-intensive. Whereas military planners normally recommend a three to one (3:1) friendly force versus hostile force

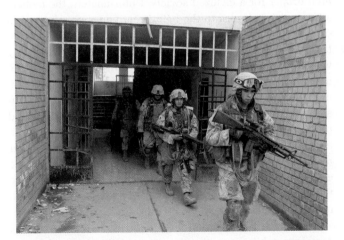

Figure 35-1 The concrete and masonry construction of walls, streets, and buildings form "bullet funnels."
Source: Courtesy of LCpl James J. Vooris/US Marine Corps/Official DoD Photo

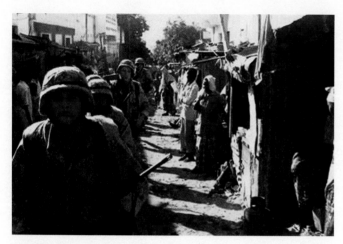

Figure 35-3 The close-quarter nature of urban combat places significant psychological stress on combatants.

Source: Courtesy of U.S. Department of Defense

manpower ratio to conduct offensive operations, urban operations may require a 5:1 ratio. In one war-game scenario conducted by the U.S. Marine Corps titled Urban Canyon, it was estimated that a dense city "core" area 20 by 20 square blocks with 20- to 60-story buildings would require 49 infantry battalions and 10 days to clear, having assumed only 10 seconds would be spent clearing each room. An operation of this scale would require every squad of infantry in the U.S. Army and Marine Corps.

Radio communications are often degraded by steel and concrete structures. Troops operating in the subterranean level may have no communication capability outside their immediate area. Poor electronic communications combined with the greater dispersion and isolation of forces increases the risk of friendly fire casualties.

Navigation in cities may be challenging. Many cities in developing countries lack organized urban planning. As a result, many areas lack street signs and are poorly mapped. Physical factors that interfere with radio communications may also render global positioning systems unreliable. Overhead imagery and human intelligence are crucial for accurate navigation.

The highly intense nature of urban warfare places extraordinary demands on logistical support systems. Requirements for ammunition, fuel, water, food, and medical supplies are significantly higher than for a conventional rural battle. Support troops and supply trains are targeted as they try to deliver food, water, and ammunition to forces in urban combat. Lightly armed logistics and support units may not be able to deliver supplies to areas near intense fighting. Delivery by heavy armored vehicle or by hand may be required, making resupply difficult. Logistics demands are further increased by the requirement to provide humanitarian relief during the course of the fighting.[3]

Armored vehicles are vulnerable to ambush if not supported by infantry,[4,5] so traditional heavy weapons such as armor and artillery may be of limited use for fighting in cities. For example, during the early stages of the Russian conflict in Chechnya,

the Russian 131st Brigade lost 20 of its 26 tanks and 102 of its 120 armored personnel carriers. Its commander and almost 1,000 officers and men died, and 74 were taken prisoner. The Chechens allowed the armored columns, unsupported by dismounted infantry, to enter the city and lured them into narrow, confined streets. Small groups of Chechen fighters with anti-tank rockets then attacked the lead and rear vehicles. The columns, effectively isolated from friendly forces and immobilized, were then methodically destroyed.

The Chechens also used "three-tiered" ambushes, directing fire from positions in basements, street-level windows, upper stories, and rooftops simultaneously. Their positions in the subterranean and upper floors were out of the elevation and depression ranges of the Russian guns.[4] Rockets were fired down onto the tanks and armored personnel carriers, exploiting the relatively thin armor of the tops of these vehicles.

During the battle of Stalingrad, the Soviet forces maintained their lines in close opposition to the Germans', sometimes as near as 50 meters. This tactic not only placed constant psychological stress on the German forces, who feared constant close-range attack, but also negated their substantial air superiority. Chechen forces fighting in Grozny adopted similar tactics.

Restrictive Rules of Engagement

Civilian populations encountered in urban warfare may be armed and hostile, such as those encountered by U.S. Army Rangers in Somalia in October of 1993, or they may simply be innocents caught in the crossfire. Insurgents and terrorists will likely blend in with civilian populations, making target discrimination difficult and increasing the likelihood of unintentional civilian injuries.

U.S. forces and our allies operate with restrictive rules of engagement (ROEs) reflecting morals and values considered proper for a civilized society. Unfortunately, the tactical advantage often goes to the belligerent party who disregards or actively endangers the safety of civilians. Civilians may be targeted or held hostage on an urban battlefield by an enemy wishing to create a humanitarian crisis or to manipulate the media. Shocking images of maimed and dead women and children, burned homes, and mourning families are disproportionately featured by media outlets. This practice is manipulated by hostile forces, who may stage and time attacks on military or civilian targets to maximize media exposure in order to degrade popular and political support for the conflict. The effects of the media coverage during combat operations, and the need to respond to it, are often variables in the decision making of senior military and political leaders.

The unacceptability of high U.S. casualty rates to the American public is another important political consideration. The first Persian Gulf War created a (perhaps false) perception that military operations, relying on high-technology equipment, can be conducted cleanly without casualties or collateral damage.[6]

Casualties

Casualty rates in mid- to high-intensity urban operations are higher than in most conventional operations. The types of injuries encountered in urban fighting vary according to the weapons and tactics used by the combatants, though several trends can be identified. In operations where armored vehicles were used extensively, such as the Battle for Grozny during the Russian campaign in Chechnya, injury from fragments and blasts are common, reflecting the use of anti-tank munitions, explosive shells from tanks, mortars, artillery, and land mines. Where troops operate in dismounted formations, gunshot wounds from machine guns and assault rifles produce the most serious casualties. During Operation Iraqi Freedom (OIF) and Operation Enduring Freedom (OEF), enemy forces used improvised explosive devices (IEDs) to initiate ambushes, resulting in a mix of mutilating blast injuries and penetrating trauma.

Snipers are a common and significant threat when fighting in urban areas **(Figure 35-4)**. Urban terrain provides the sniper numerous hiding sites and cover for moving from one position to the next. The sniper can engage at much closer ranges, increasing accuracy. The vulnerable anterior head, face, and neck are often hit. In Chechnya, snipers prevented rapid medical evacuation, and the wounded frequently could not be moved until nightfall.[3]

Penetrating Injury

Body armor is critical for survival on the urban battlefield. Contemporary body armor (with front and back plates) used in OEF and OIF has greatly reduced thoracic and upper abdominal injuries. However, improvements in armor for the head and torso have paradoxically resulted in an increased number of severe extremity injuries such as traumatic amputations. U.S. Army Rangers fighting in Somalia experienced nearly 60% fewer fatal chest injuries compared to those suffered during the Vietnam War. The incidence of fatal abdominal wounds was not significantly different from the Vietnam War because missiles entered through the hips, groin, and abdomen below the area covered by armor. Lethal head injury rates were the same.[7] Future innovations in body armor should make it stronger, lighter, and cooler, while adding coverage to vulnerable areas such as the face, groin, and pelvis.

Other individual protective equipment such as eye protection, gloves, and knee and elbow pads will prevent injury as combatants fight through streets and buildings strewn with rubble. The current emphasis on eye protection during OEF/OIF has saved the sight of many U.S. service members.

Blunt Trauma

Although penetrating wounds from small arms and blasts produce the greatest number and severity of injuries, severe blunt trauma injury must be anticipated in urban combat. Soldiers fall while climbing up and down buildings. Explosive munitions create numerous unstable structures that crush and trap victims. Vehicle crashes, a result of hostile fire or operator fatigue, produce injuries like those seen daily on American highways **(Figure 35-5)**.

Tools used during peacetime urban search and rescue operations, such as pry bars, jacks, ropes, and cutting tools, are needed to extricate wounded soldiers from wrecked vehicles and collapsed structures. Search and rescue is difficult and dangerous enough in a peacetime environment. Locating and rescuing soldiers trapped in collapsed structures during combat is an incredible challenge **(Figure 35-6)**.

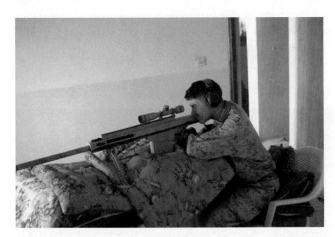

Figure 35-4 On the urban battlefield, snipers are able to engage targets at much closer ranges, increasing lethality.

Source: Courtesy of U.S. Department of Defense

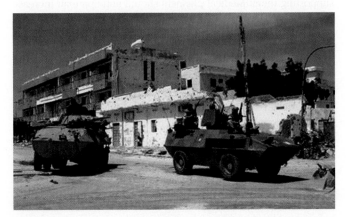

Figure 35-5 Troops mounted on vehicles while fighting in urban areas are not only vulnerable to penetrating and blast injuries, but also to blunt trauma from vehicular accidents.

Source: Courtesy of U.S. Department of Defense

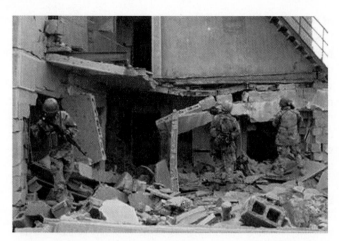

Figure 35-6 Buildings and other structures are subject to collapse when targeted by explosive munitions. Locating and extracting casualties trapped in these structures during a battle is extremely difficult and dangerous.

Source: Courtesy of U.S. Department of Defense

Psychological Injury

The intense nature of urban combat may produce more psychological casualties than conventional operations produce. The Russians experienced more psychiatric casualties while fighting in Chechnya than in their war in Afghanistan. The Russian troops were generally poorly trained conscripts who fought under horrendous conditions. Psychiatric screening of Russian troops who served in Chechnya revealed that 72% suffered some type of psychological disorder such as insomnia, lack of motivation, anxiety, fatigue, or hypochondriacal fixation.[8] While these findings may not be applicable to the professional, well-trained U.S. forces, they do reflect the conditions experienced during intense urban combat. Combat at close range, the constant threat of sniper fire and hidden IEDs, shadowy enemies mixed into the civilian population, and prolonged exposure to the dead and dying require a regular rotation of not only combat troops but also the medical personnel supporting them. Medical planners should anticipate an increase in combat stress casualties and augment units with mental health professionals trained to treat combat stress disorders.

Civilian Casualties

Large numbers of civilian casualties may be encountered. Medical planners must anticipate the need to care for them. In some instances, civilians can be directed to current and existing local health care facilities. In others, especially in extremely poor countries, large numbers of injured civilians may quickly overwhelm U.S. military medical capabilities and impede their ability to support troops. A clear plan for civilian casualty care must be in place before hostilities begin.

Combat medical personnel anticipating battlefield trauma should also be prepared to manage pediatric and geriatric trauma, tropical diseases, nutritional diseases, and poorly managed chronic medical conditions like diabetes.

Medical Preparation for Urban Combat

Wide dispersal of personnel in small units decreases direct access to casualties by combat medical personnel. Medics will be spread thin and may not be able to reach a wounded soldier only a few meters away during intense fighting. They may also be quickly overwhelmed by multiple casualties. Units fighting in cities must be very well trained in self-aid and buddy aid[9] using the principles of Tactical Combat Casualty Care (TCCC).

A robust individual first aid kit should include a functional and easily applied field tourniquet, a field dressing, a hemostatic agent, and the medications recommended by the Committee on Tactical Combat Casualty Care (CoTCCC). Units receiving more advanced medical training, such as Special Operations Forces, could further augment individual first aid kits in accordance with their higher level of training.

Units fighting in cities should augment their organic medical capabilities at all levels **(Figure 35-7)**. For instance, since moving casualties over broken, irregular terrain is difficult and hazardous to the casualty, an aid-and-litter team should be designated for each infantry squad. Team members should receive additional medical training with emphasis on TCCC, and each team should be issued a robust squad medical kit including lightweight litters. Support personnel at company and battalion level can be trained in TCCC and serve as additional litter teams.[9] Mounted troops should have an advanced medical kit in every vehicle in case the primary medical vehicle is disabled or destroyed. Combat medical personnel should be placed at strong points, at key positions, and with isolated units.

Aid stations and Forward Surgical Teams (FSTs) should be located as far forward as possible, in locations that provide adequate cover, security, and vehicle access, such as an underground parking garage or basement.[3] Medical support personnel present easy "soft" targets for enemy forces fighting an asymmetric conflict. If medical personnel are to be located well forward, they must be able to provide appropriate security and they must possess the same battlefield awareness and survival skills as nonmedical personnel.

Figure 35-7 Medical augmentation for Russian forces in Grozny.

During combat in and around Grozny, the Russians augmented each maneuver company with a physician's assistant and each battalion with a physician and an ambulance company. Surgeons, anesthetists, and additional nurses manned the regimental medical post.[10]

CHAPTER 35 Medical Support of Urban Operations **843**

Evacuation

Evacuating casualties from the urban battlefield is difficult and time-consuming. Casualties may have to be carried by hand to a secure consolidation point. As discussed earlier, it may take hours to move a litter patient a few hundred yards over broken, exposed terrain covered by enemy fire. Unarmored vehicles and ambulances are likely to be targeted as they evacuate casualties. Even armored vehicles are vulnerable. The M113 Armored Personnel Carrier was called a "death trap" for evacuation of casualties during the 1982 conflict in Beirut.[5] These vehicles were attacked from the upper floors of buildings with rocket-propelled grenades (RPGs) that penetrated the thinner armor on the top of the vehicle. Vehicles with heavy armor such as the battle tank were used successfully to evacuate casualties during the Battle of Beirut[5] and by U.S. Marines fighting the Battle for Hue during the Tet Offensive in Vietnam. The fighting in Grozny[11] and Mogadishu[12] proved the need for an armored ambulance resistant to small arms and RPG fire that can maneuver over rubble-strewn streets. The U.S. Army's new Stryker combat vehicle ambulance may fill this need.

Helicopter evacuation is more dangerous during urban conflict than during conventional operations. The density of urban structures and the proximity of hostile combatants allow few landing zones. Even when a physically adequate landing zone is available, it is likely to be covered by enemy fire from rooftops and upper floors. Helicopters have been downed by small arms fire during numerous urban battles. RPGs, Stingers, and machine gun fire have proven effective in disabling moving aircraft in both Afghanistan and Iraq. During the Russian fighting in Grozny, the wounded were normally evacuated to the regimental medical post by armored ambulance. Evacuation by helicopter was used far less than in the Russo-Afghani conflict, especially after several MEDEVAC helicopters were lost to enemy fire.[10]

Infectious Disease

Infectious disease is a major threat during urban conflicts. In many areas of the developing world where future conflicts are likely to occur, there is poor public health infrastructure, contaminated water supplies, poor sanitation, and high levels of endemic disease. A military conflict will overwhelm the meager health and sanitation infrastructures of large, poverty-stricken cities within the developing world **(Figure 35-8)**.

Humanitarian crises generated by armed conflict in these settings can be massive and may endanger tactical and strategic aims. Soldiers interacting with civilians and enemy prisoners could be exposed to endemic diseases such as tuberculosis, malaria, and leishmaniasis. Sexually transmitted diseases such as gonorrhea, syphilis, hepatitis, and human immunodeficiency virus (HIV) also pose a serious risk to soldiers if they interact socially with locals. Barrier and personal protective measures should be provided as a force health protection measure.[8] Disease vectors such as rats, lice, ticks, and mosquitoes as well as feral animals and unburied bodies present additional public health hazards.

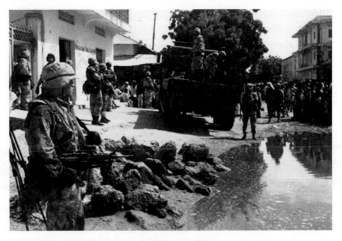

Figure 35-8 Sanitation may be nonexistent in areas affected by urban conflict.
Source: Courtesy of U.S. Department of Defense

Potable Water

Potable water is scarce. Troops engaged in urban and mountainous operations can potentially consume up to 5 to 6 quarts (4.7 to 5.7 liters) per day (about 20 to 24 eight-ounce glasses), depending on the soldier's level of physical activity and the weather conditions. As the weather warms, daily consumption can be expected to increase substantially. Less active troops will need to drink about 5 to 7 quarts (4.7 to 6.6 liters) per day, and more active troops, 7 to 9 quarts (6.6 to 8.5 liters) per day. Supplying frontline troops with enough water during urban combat is difficult. Logistics units may not be able to deliver enough water near intense fighting. Water resupply may have to be carried by hand or by armored vehicle, severely limiting quantity and consuming valuable manpower. Thirsty troops may be tempted to drink from local sources that may be heavily contaminated by infectious diseases like hepatitis, intestinal parasites, or industrial waste. In one Russian brigade in Chechnya, 15% of the unit was sick with hepatitis at one time due to contaminated water.[13]

The Future

The end of the Cold War left the United States as the sole remaining superpower, with no other nation able to match American might on a conventional battlefield. Future struggles will likely see U.S. forces drawn into cities as terrorists, criminals, regional despots, and rogue nations seek to engage and bog U.S. forces down in asymmetric battles intended to erode national will. Military and medical planners will continue to struggle to appropriately train and equip U.S. forces in the face of finite resources; to minimize friendly and innocent civilian casualties while isolating and destroying the enemy; to both prevent and mitigate complex humanitarian crises; and to manage intense and often one-sided media scrutiny, all while holding true to the mores and ethics of our military and our society. Tactical and even strategic success in future urban conflicts may well be determined by the thoughtful, deliberate, and proactive execution of medical support.

As stated by Ralph Peters, urban environments are[1]:

. . . the post-modern equivalent of jungles and mountains—citadels of the dispossessed and irreconcilable. A military unprepared for urban operations across a broad spectrum is unprepared for tomorrow.

Summary

- Urban combat can involve action on four levels: subterranean, street, building, and air.
- Urban operations are characterized by intense small-unit infantry engagements and are manpower-, resource-, and time-intensive. Navigation, communication, and logistics are all more difficult.
- In urban environments, engagements are often at close range due to the wide variety and ready availability of cover and concealment. Closer engagement allows for more accurate fire.
- Insurgents and terrorists can blend in with the civilian populations. Civilians may be innocents caught up in the conflict, or may be armed and hostile.
- Casualty rates are higher in urban as opposed to conventional operations. Penetrating, blunt, and blast trauma should be expected and planned for. Psychological casualty rates may also be higher.
- Medical planning for support of urban operations should include preparations for civilian casualties, complex ground evacuation, infectious diseases, poor sanitation, and advanced first responder care training and equipage.

SCENARIO RECAP

Your platoon is patrolling the streets of Mogadishu on foot when you are suddenly attacked at an intersection by multiple hostiles firing from the street ahead and from windows above. The platoon quickly takes cover in the lobby of an abandoned, shot-up apartment building. Two RPGs strike the outside of the wall you and two others are kneeling behind, collapsing the wall. The legs of the soldier beside you are trapped by reinforced concrete and cinder blocks. The casualty is alert but in great pain.

The platoon's fire forces the hostiles back. The lobby is secured and you have good cover from sniper fire. Your platoon leader calls for vehicular extraction; the ETA is 40 minutes. You are the medic, and you have three casualties to care for.

- Casualty 1 has a massive wound to the right side of his head. Heavily disrupted brain tissue is visible. He is unresponsive, has no palpable carotid pulse, and is not breathing.
- Casualty 2 is the soldier trapped by the fallen rubble. He is screaming in pain and asking for help to get his legs free. His radial pulse is strong and rapid. Two platoon members are digging him out.
- Casualty 3 has a fragment wound to the left side of his neck and mandible, with heavy bleeding from his neck wound. He is leaning forward with blood draining out of his mouth, holding direct pressure on his neck wound with his hand. He is alert and responds to instructions but cannot talk.

SCENARIO SOLUTION

1. **What do you do?**

You must first decide where to begin.

2. **Who should you treat first and why?**

First treat Casualty 3 because he may bleed to death in the next few minutes and the best lifesaving intervention can be applied quickly. Casualty 1 is dead, and you can do nothing further for Casualty 2 until he is freed.

While you are applying Combat Gauze to the neck wound of Casualty 3, you note an open fracture of the jaw, which is slowly oozing dark red blood. You stop the external bleeding, but the patient continues to lean forward with blood dripping from his mouth.

3. **What do you do next?**

Check for other wounds. There are none.

4. **Does he need an IV?**

Yes. You controlled the bleeding before he went into shock, so he doesn't need IV fluid resuscitation at this point, but he probably shouldn't try to swallow antibiotic pills. Antibiotics can be given intramuscularly, but he may have already lost significant blood volume and may lose more during evacuation, so you elect to start an IV.

You place a field-appropriate IV line and give cefotetan, 2 grams IV (slow push over 3 to 5 minutes).

5. **What else do you want to do?**

Provide analgesia, if needed. Either morphine or ketamine can be given via the IV if pain is severe. Monitor the casualty's breathing after analgesics are given.

6. **Should you lay the casualty down?**

No

7. **Why not?**

He is maintaining a patent airway on his own. If he is forced to lie on his back, the blood now dripping from his mouth may drain into his airway.

8. **If the casualty becomes unconscious, what should you do?**

Unconsciousness may be from either airway obstruction or blood loss. First place him in the rescue position and listen for continued spontaneous respiration while you look quickly to determine if heavy bleeding has resumed. Address any life-threatening hemorrhage, then attend to his airway. A pulse oximeter may help to identify hypoxia, if present.

9. **Even if the casualty breathes on his own in the rescue position, you would probably have to secure his airway to transport him while unconscious. How would you do it?**

Cricothyroidotomy

At this point, the enemy's fire remains ineffective. Casualty 2 has just been freed from the rubble. He is still complaining loudly of great pain in his legs, and his radial pulse is strong. You remove his boots and socks and cut his pant legs open. His left lower leg has been badly crushed, and there is diffuse oozing of blood over the calf. There is gross instability and crepitance at the midtibial level. His left foot looks normal when you take off his boot, and the dorsalis pedis pulse is normal. He cannot, however, feel your touch on his foot or wiggle his toes. His right calf is badly bruised diffusely, but skeletal, vascular, and neurologic exams of the right lower leg and foot are normal.

10. **What do you do first?**

You check him carefully for other injuries, and find none.

(Continues on next page)

11. What do you do next?

Dress and splint the left lower leg. You reassess vascular and neurologic status, which are unchanged.

12. What else does he need?

Administer moxifloxacin and oral transmucosal fentanyl citrate.

13. What about an IV?

He doesn't need one at this point, but a saline lock wouldn't hurt since you have time and security.

Your platoon leader has called for reinforcements and tactical evacuation for the casualties. The ETA is 50 minutes. Your platoon is keeping the hostiles at bay.

14. What do you do during this interval?

You should repeatedly reassess the casualties, and you might want to dress the head wound of the deceased. Ensure the casualties are protected from hypothermia.

References

1. Peters R. Our soldiers, their cities. *Parameters U.S. Army War Coll Q.* 1996;26(1):43–50.

2. Krulak CC. The three block war: fighting in urban areas. *Vital Speech Day.* 1997;139.

3. Grau LW, Thomas TL. "Soft Log" and the concrete canyons: Russian urban combat logistics in Grozny. *Marine Corps Gazette.* 1999;Oct:67–75.

4. Grau LW. Changing Russian urban tactics: the aftermath of the battle for Grozny. *INSS Strateg Forum.* 1995;38.

5. Yheskel B. *Military Operations in Urbanized Terrain (MOUT), Medical Aspects, Lebanon War 1982—A Case Study.* Bethesda, MD: Uniformed Services University of the Health Sciences; 1985.

6. Akers FH, Singleton GB. *Task Force Ranger: A Case Study Examining the Application of Advanced Technologies in Modern Urban Warfare.* Oak Ridge, TN. National Security Program Office, Oak Ridge Y-12 Plant; 2000.

7. Mabry RL, Holcomb JB, Baker AM, et al. U.S. Army Rangers in Somalia. *J Trauma.* 2000;49:515–528.

8. Novikov VS. The psychophysiological support of the combat activities of servicemen. *Voen Med Zh.* 1996;317(4):37–40.

9. Grau LW, Gbur CJ. Mars and Hippocrates in Megapolis: urban combat and medical support. *Army Med Dept J.* 2003;Jan/Feb/Mar:19-26.

10. Grau LW, Jorgensen WA. Handling the wounded in a counter-guerrilla war: the Soviet/Russian experience in Afghanistan and Chechnya. *Army Med Dept J.* 1998;Jan/Feb:2-10.

11. Savvin Y. Za zhizni voinov [For the lives of warriors]. *Armeyskiy sbornik [Army Digest].* 1995;45.

12. Butler FK, Hagmann JH, Richards DT. Tactical management of urban warfare casualties in special operations. *Mil Med.* 2000;165(suppl 4): 1–48.

13. Grau LW, Jorgensen WA. Viral hepatitis and the Russian War in Chechnya. *Army Med Dept J.* 1997;May/Jun:2-5.

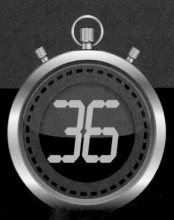

Ethical Considerations for the Combat Medic

It is the duty of any military force to wage war, and in the absence of war, to prepare for it.

General Douglas MacArthur[1]

Ethics in Conflict

War is prosecuted by killing people and destroying things. It ends when the enemy capitulates or is totally annihilated, whichever comes first. We are charged as combat medics to render care in order to relieve pain and suffering, to friend and foe alike. This seems a paradox, especially in the Special Operations setting where the combat medic is also a belligerent. In fact, it is not. Although some argue that combat itself is so highly unethical as to defy attempts to apply ethical precepts, some cultures have had specific ethical principles for engaging in combat.[2]

The focus of every soldier in combat, medic or not, should be support of his or her fellow warriors in completion of their primary mission. Once the tactical situation is secure, attention can be turned to those in need of care. The practical sense of this approach is borne of the historical fact that those with medical expertise in hostile engagements are always a small minority. If the medic becomes a casualty, the quality of care in the local theater drops dramatically. Therefore, it is clear that for the sake of those who might benefit from his or her attention, the medic should predicate his or her actions on the tactical situation. Articles 12 and 13 of the First Geneva Convention of 1949 dictate that the wounded should be cared for in the order of severity of their wounds without regard to their status as friendly or hostile.[3] This is not to suggest that a medic should abandon his or her duty to his or her mission to tend enemy wounded before the immediate fight has ended.

In every war—save some specific battles—succor, however meager, has been afforded surviving enemy combatants. The first war in which medical care and transport of wounded was organized and standardized was the War Between the States. Both sides had high morbidity and mortality rates, and tragically, both sides were American. Over 400,000 were wounded and over 204,000 killed.[4] Both sides had Surgeons General and Medical and Ambulance Corps. In 1863, at the height of that terrible war, Major General J. E. B. Stuart issued Cavalry Tactic, General Order number 26:

> The Ambulance Corps alone will be allowed to remove the wounded, and all will bear in mind that our first duty to our wounded is to win the victory.[5]

Well said. The goal of combat medical personnel should be to give aid to as many who need it as possible within the limits of time available and the tactical situation. It is not necessary to hate one's enemy in order to kill him or to love him in order to treat his wounds. It is simply expeditious and proper to remember your duty to your country, your comrades-in-arms, and your fellow man, and apply your talent, skills, and training as the opportunity presents.

Ethics in Triage

Triage and treatment require judgment and decisiveness to be maximally effective.

The principles and ethics of triage for medical personnel are discussed at length in Chapter 7 of Part I of the *Textbook of Military Medicine*.[2] This historical review gives much food for thought on those factors influential in the formation of ethical precepts. In part it reads:

> In ordinary emergency situations the most seriously ill might be allowed to die so that limited medical resources can be devoted to salvaging the lives and limbs of the seriously injured. In combat settings, this might be carried a step further in rendering care first to those most likely to carry out the combat mission, that is, the lightly wounded combat stress casualties. The military is mission driven and resource scarce, and this creates ethical dilemmas in terms of individual survival. Differing perspectives on impairment result in a conflict between putting the mission first versus the risk of increased morbidity. The principle of military triage holds that individual soldiers' interests can be sacrificed when necessary either for the medical welfare of other soldiers or to further military goals. Yet, triage and different degrees of risk taking by certain groups is less than fully analogous. When triage takes place, no group is singled out on the basis of some pre-existing characteristic that subjects some to a greater risk of morbidity or death.

Ethics, like judgment, can be taught but not guaranteed.

Ethics and Prisoners of War

Incarceration, isolation, and even physical restraints are methods sometimes necessary to deny the enemy opportunity to continue hostile acts. These are not to be misconstrued as acts of torture or abuse. Admiral Raphael Semmes captured or sank 67 enemy vessels with the single unescorted ship he commanded during the War Between the States, a record that stands unbroken. He took many prisoners, including wounded. When the tactical situation dictated (i.e., more prisoners than crew to guard them), he put them in irons. Since his side lost and he had been extraordinarily effective as a Confederate naval commander, the victorious government of the North charged him after the war with being a "privateer" (pirate) during the war. Many of his former prisoners were called to testify during his several-month-long trial. Not a single one alleged mistreatment or torture despite the irons and meager rations for weeks when shipboard rations were short. He was completely exonerated.[6] When applied, the Golden Rule is truly golden.

Summary

Merriam-Webster's Collegiate Dictionary defines ethics as "a set of moral principles" and "the principles of conduct governing an individual or a group."[7] The history of the application of principles of conduct, moral and otherwise, among humans fills many volumes. Those ethics range from "Kill 'em all and let God sort 'em out" to "Treat friend and foe with equal love and kindness." It is not the purpose of this text to dictate a particular ethic but to remind military caregivers that those who may someday sit in judgment of their actions will certainly use a set of values in assessing the appropriateness of those actions.

References

1. McArthur D. Public Address 1949. In: Taylor RL, Rosenbach WE, eds. *Military Leadership: In Pursuit of Excellence.* 4th ed. Boulder, CO: Westview Press; 2000.

2. Department of the Army. *The Textbook of Military Medicine.* Washington, DC: Borden Institute, Office of the Surgeon General, U.S. Army; 1994.

3. International Committee of the Red Cross. Convention (1) for the Amelioration of the Condition of the Wounded and Sick in Armed Forces in the Field. http://www.icrc.org/ihl.nsf/full/365? opendocument. Accessed April 18, 2013.

4. Kuz JE, Bengston BP. *Orthopaedic Injuries of the Civil War: An Atlas of Orthopaedic Injuries and Treatments During the Civil War.* Kennesaw, GA: Kennesaw Mountain Press; 1996:10.

5. McClellan HB. General Orders, No. 26, Hdqrs. Cav. Div., Army Northern VA, July 30, 1863. In: Commander United States War Department. *The War of the Rebellion: A Compilation of the Official Records of the Union and Confederate Armies.* Washington, DC: Government Printing Office; 1880-1901: Series 1, vol XXVII, Part III, 1055. http://ebooks.library.cornell.edu/cgi/t/text/pageviewer-idx?c=moawar; cc=moawar;idno=waro0045;node=waro0045%3A2;view=image; seq=1057;size=100;page=root. Accessed April 19, 2013.

6. Spencer WF. *Raphael Semmes: The Philosophical Mariner.* Tuscaloosa, AL: University of Alabama Press; 1997.

7. *Merriam-Webster's Collegiate Dictionary.* 11th ed. Springfield, MA: Merriam-Webster; 2007.

Glossary

ABD An abbreviation for "army battle dressing."

abuse The willful infliction of injury, unreasonable confinement, intimidation, or cruel punishment resulting in physical or psychological harm or pain, or the withholding of services that would prevent these events.

acetylcholine A chemical that functions as a neurotransmitter, released at the end of nerve cells to transmit a nervous system impulse.

acid A chemical substance that has a pH less than 7 and that will neutralize an alkali.

acidosis Accumulation of acids and decreased pH of the blood.

active strategy When referring to injury prevention, prevention steps that require the active participation of the individual—e.g., wearing a helmet.

acute mountain sickness A constellation of symptoms that result from travel to high altitude (usually above 8,000 feet [2,400 meters]).

acute respiratory distress syndrome (ARDS) Respiratory insufficiency as a result of damage to the lining of the capillaries and alveoli in the lung, leading to the leakage of fluid into the interstitial spaces and alveoli.

acute radiation syndrome (ARS) The physiologic consequences of whole-body radiation; characterized initially by acute nausea and vomiting, followed by damage to the bone marrow (hematologic syndrome), the gastrointestinal tract, and the cardiovascular/central nervous system.

acute tubular necrosis (ATN) Acute damage to the renal tubules, usually due to ischemia associated with shock.

advance directive A written declaration that describes end-of-life treatment wishes and appoints medical decision makers in the event that the patient is unable to make a medical decision for himself or herself. The two types of written advance directives most often encountered are a living will and a medical power of attorney.

aerobic metabolism Oxygen-based metabolism; the body's principal combustion process; the most efficient process for the production of cellular energy.

aeromedical evacuation The transfer of casualties between medical treatment facilities within a theater of operations or from a theater to a Role 4 hospital.

aerosol Solid particles and liquid particles that are suspended in air.

afterload The pressure against which the left ventricle must pump out (eject) blood with each beat.

After-Action Review (AAR) A structured review for analyzing what happened, why it happened, and how it can be done better.

air density As used in this text, the property of organs having approximately the same weight and density as air—e.g., lung tissue.

air-purifying respirator (APR) A device that uses a filter, canister, or cartridge to remove contaminants from ambient air that passes through the air-purifying component and makes the air safe to breathe.

alpha particle A particle emitted during the decay of a radioactive material; consists of two protons and two neutrons, thus giving the particle a positive charge.

alveoli The terminal air sacs of the respiratory tract where the respiratory system meets the circulatory system and gas exchange occurs.

anaerobic metabolism Metabolism not using oxygen; an inefficient process for the production of cellular energy.

anaphylactic shock A life-threatening allergic reaction, usually characterized by hives (urticaria), shortness of breath and wheezing, and cardiovascular collapse.

anastomosis A connection between two structures such as two blood vessels or adjacent bowel.

anhidrosis The absence of sweating.

anisocoria Inequality of pupil size.

antecedent Something that occurred earlier in time.

anterior cord syndrome Damage to the anterior portion of the spinal cord, usually as a result of bony fragments or pressure on spinal arteries.

aortography An x-ray study of the aorta in which a radio-opaque contrast material is injected into the circulatory system to show the aorta.

apnea The absence of breathing.

apoptosis A process of cell death in which a programmed series of events leads to the death of a cell without causing inflammation.

appendicular skeleton That portion of the skeleton that includes the shoulders and arms as well as the pelvis and legs.

aqueous A system that is water-based or in which water is the solvent.

arachnoid mater (arachnoid membrane) Spiderweb-like transparent membrane between the dura mater and the pia mater; the middle of the three meningeal membranes surrounding the brain.

aspiration pneumonitis Inflammation and pneumonia caused by inhaling gastric contents or vomitus.

assist control (A/C) ventilation A form of mechanical ventilation; breaths may be assisted by the ventilator if the patient triggers the device by adequately attempting to breathe in or will automatically occur if the patient does not breathe.

Asymmetric conflict A conflict between nations or groups that have disparate military capabilities and strategies, and during which, each attempts to exploit the other's characteristic weaknesses.

atelectasis Collapse of alveoli or part of the lung.

atherosclerosis A narrowing of the blood vessels; a condition in which the inner layer of the artery wall thickens while fatty deposits build up within the artery.

atlas The first cervical vertebra (C1); the skull perches upon it.

atropine A chemical that competitively inhibits the effect of acetylcholine at parasympathetic nerve endings; anticholinergic medication; used to treat victims of nerve agent poisoning.

austere environment A setting in which resources, supplies, equipment, personnel, transportation, and other aspects of the physical, political, social, and economic environments are extremely limited.

autonomic nervous system The part of the central nervous system that directs and controls the involuntary functions of the body.

autonomy A competent adult patient's right to direct his or her own health care free from interference or undue influence.

autoregulation The biologic process of detecting change within the system and adjusting for that change; in the circulatory system, the process of maintaining a constant blood flow as blood pressure changes.

awareness level In hazardous materials training, the basic level of knowledge a responder should have, involved recognition of an incident, isolation and protection from exposure, and

notification that the incident is happening.

axial loading The force acting on or applied to the long axis of an object; typically refers to force applied to the spine from the head downward; may also result from the weight of the body being applied to the lower part of the spine, as would occur in a fall from a height landing on the feet.

axis The second cervical vertebra (C2); its shape allows for the wide possible range of rotation of the head. Also, an imaginary line that passes through the center of the body.

bag-mask device A mechanical ventilation device consisting of a self-inflating bag made of plastic or rubber and several one-way valves; squeezing the bag results in positive-pressure ventilation through a mask or endotracheal tube. May be used with or without supplementary oxygen.

baroreceptor A sensory nerve ending that is stimulated by changes in blood pressure. Baroreceptors are found in the walls of the atria of the heart, vena cava, aortic arch, and carotid sinus.

barotrauma Injury caused by pressure differential, especially to the closed cavities in the body such as the middle ear or the lung.

basal level Baseline or minimal level.

basal metabolic rate The number of calories the body burns while at rest, resulting in heat production as a by-product of metabolism.

base A chemical with a pH greater than 7; dissolves in water and releases hydroxide ions or accepts hydrogen ions; causes liquefaction necrosis of tissue.

basilar skull fracture A fracture of the floor of the cranium.

behavioral regulation (and physiologic thermoregulation) An individual's

conscious response to environmental thermal change and the physical actions taken to keep warm or cool.

beneficence An ethical term that means "to do good"; requires prehospital care providers to act in a manner that maximizes the benefits and minimizes the risks to the patient.

beta particle A high-speed or high-energy electron emitted from radioactive decay.

biologic agent A bacterium, virus, or toxin that can be used as a weapon of mass destruction.

blast lung injury (BLI) Results from exposure to high-order explosive blast overpressure wave; lung damage varies from scattered petechiae to contusions and pulmonary hemorrhage.

blast overpressure Pressure exceeding normal atmospheric pressure that results from a high-order explosive detonation.

blast wave A sharply defined wave front of increased pressure that propagates outward from the center of an explosion.

blast wind The result of the sudden displacement of air from an explosion.

blind nasotracheal intubation A technique of inserting an endotracheal tube through the nares into the trachea without visualizing the larynx and vocal cords.

blister agent A chemical that creates burnlike injuries; used as a weapon of mass destruction.

blunt trauma Nonpenetrating trauma caused by a rapidly moving object that impacts the body.

bradypnea Abnormally slow breathing rate; usually less than 12 breaths per minute.

brain stem The stemlike part of the brain that connects the cerebral hemispheres with the spinal cord.

bronchioles The small divisions of the bronchial tubes through which air passes to the alveoli.

Brown-Séquard syndrome A condition caused by penetrating injury that involves hemitransection of the spinal cord; only one side of the cord is involved.

capillary The smallest type of blood vessel. These minute blood vessels are only one cell wide, allowing for diffusion and osmosis of oxygen and nutrients through the capillary walls.

capnography (end-tidal carbon dioxide) The method of measuring and monitoring the partial pressure of carbon dioxide in a sample of gas. It can correlate to the arterial partial pressure of carbon dioxide ($PaCO_2$).

carboxyhemoglobin Hemoglobin on which the sites usually bound to oxygen are bound to carbon monoxide. Carboxyhemoglobin does not function reversibly as an oxygen carrier.

cardiac output The volume of blood pumped by the heart (reported in liters per minute).

cardiac tamponade Compression of the heart from an accumulation of fluid in the pericardium surrounding the heart; in the case of trauma, the fluid is usually blood; the accumulation of fluid prevents normal blood return to the heart by compressing the heart, thus impairing circulation.

cardiogenic shock Shock that results from failure of the heart's pumping activity; causes can be categorized as either intrinsic, a result of direct damage to the heart itself, or extrinsic, related to a problem outside the heart.

Care Under Fire A phase of combat casualty care when casualties, combat medical personnel and their units are under effective hostile fire. The care that can be delivered is very limited.

Casualty Evacuation (CASEVAC) The unregulated movement of casualties from the point of wounding to the first point of advanced medical care using armed tactical vehicles.

casualty collection point (CCP) A specified location within a tactical area of operation that is used for the assembly, triage, treatment, preparation for transport, and subsequent evacuation of combat casualties.

casualty response system The tactical plans and resources within a military unit that provides for the continued treatment and movement of casualties as part of the unit's battle plan.

Casualty Transload Point (CTP) A specified location where casualties are transferred from one mode of medical evacuation to another.

cataract A condition of the eye in which the lens becomes progressively more opaque and blocks and distorts light entering the eye and blurs vision.

catecholamines A group of chemicals produced by the body that work as important nerve transmitters. The main catecholamines made by the body are dopamine, epinephrine (also called adrenalin), and norepinephrine. They are part of the body's sympathetic defense mechanism used in preparing the body to act.

caudad Toward the tail (coccyx).

cavitation The act of forcing tissues of the body out of their normal position; to cause a temporary or permanent cavity (e.g., when the body is struck by a bullet, the acceleration of particles of tissue away from the missile produces an area of injury in which a large temporary cavity occurs).

cellular respiration The use of oxygen by the cells to produce energy.

central cord syndrome Damage to the central portion of the spinal cord that usually occurs with hyperextension of the cervical area; characterized by weakness or paralysis of the upper extremities but not the lower extremities.

central neurogenic hyperventilation Pathologic rapid and shallow ventilatory pattern associated with head injury and increased intracranial pressure.

cerebellum A portion of the brain that lies beneath the cerebrum and behind the medulla oblongata and is concerned with coordination of movement.

cerebral perfusion pressure The amount of pressure needed to maintain cerebral blood flow; calculated as the difference between the mean arterial pressure (MAP) and the intracranial pressure (ICP).

cerebral vascular resistance The resistance to blood flow that must be overcome in order to push blood through the blood vessels in and around the brain.

cerebrospinal fluid (CSF) A fluid found in the subarachnoid space and dural sheath; acts as a shock absorber, protecting the brain and spinal cord from jarring impact.

cerebrum The largest part of the brain; responsible for the control of specific intellectual, sensory, and motor functions.

chemical energy The energy, usually in the form of heat, that results from the interaction of a chemical with other chemicals or human tissue.

chemoreceptor A sensory nerve ending that is stimulated by and reacts to certain chemical stimuli; located outside of the central nervous system. Chemoreceptors are found in the large arteries of the thorax and neck, the taste buds, and the olfactory cells of the nose.

chemosis A watery swelling of the covering (conjunctiva) of the eye.

chilblains Red or purple skin lesions on the skin that are itchy and painful and appear after cold exposure, particularly in patients with poor underlying circulation.

choke A constriction in the barrel of a shotgun to decrease the amount of pellet spread after firing.

chokes ("the chokes") A form of decompression sickness characterized by cough, substernal chest pain, cyanosis, dyspnea, shock, and cardiopulmonary arrest.

cilia Hairlike processes of cells that propel foreign particles and mucus from the bronchi.

cingulate herniation A condition in which the cingulate gyrus along the medial surface of the cerebral hemispheres is forced under the falx, usually as a result of hemorrhage or edema, causing injury to the medial cerebral hemispheres and the midbrain.

circumferential burn A burn that encompasses an entire body part such as the arm, leg, or chest.

classic heatstroke A disorder that results from exposure to high humidity and high temperature, characterized by elevated body temperature above 104°F (40°C) and neurologic abnormalities (altered mental status).

closed fracture A fracture of a bone in which the overlying skin is not interrupted.

coagulative necrosis The type of tissue damage that results from acid exposure; the damaged tissue forms a barrier that prevents deeper penetration of the acid.

coagulopathy Impairment in the normal blood-clotting capabilities.

cold zone A geographic area that is free from contamination from a hazardous material.

cold-induced diuresis Increased urine production as a result of peripheral vasoconstriction from exposure to cold.

cold-induced vasodilation (CIVD) Physiologic response that occurs once an extremity has been cooled to 50°F (10°C) in an effort to provide some protection from the cold.

combat lifesaver A nonmedical soldier who provides lifesaving measures as a secondary mission as his/her primary (combat) mission allows. The Combat Lifesaver may also assist the combat medic in providing care and preparing casualties for evacuation when the Combat Lifesaver has no other combat duties to perform. Combat Lifesaver training is a bridge between the self-aid/buddy-aid (first aid) training given to all soldiers during basic training and the medical training given to the combat medic.

command The first component of the incident command system, responsible for all incident oversight and management. It is the only position in the incident command system that must always be staffed.

command staff The public information officer, safety officer, and liaison officer; they report directly to the incident commander.

commission A purposeful act.

commotio cordis Sudden cardiac dysrhythmia, often fatal, that results from a blow to the anterior chest or sternum.

compartment syndrome The clinical findings noted from ischemia and compromised circulation that can occur from vascular injury causing hypoxia of muscles in an extremity compartment. The cellular edema produces increased pressure in a closed fascial or bony compartment.

competence (1) A legal term referring to a person's general ability to make good decisions for himself or herself; (2) the ability, skill, knowledge, and qualification to do something successfully.

complete cord transection Complete damage and severing of the spinal cord; all spinal tracts are interrupted, and all normal neurologic functions distal to the site are lost.

comprehensive emergency management The steps needed to manage an incident, consisting of four components: mitigation, preparation, response, and recovery.

compressibility The ability to be deformed by the transfer of energy.

compression The type of force involved in impacts resulting in a tissue, organ, or other body part being squeezed between two or more objects or body parts.

compression injury An injury caused by severe crushing and squeezing forces; may occur to the external structure of the body or to the internal organs.

conduction The transfer of heat between two objects in direct contact with each other.

confidentiality The obligation of health care providers to not share patient information that is disclosed to them within the patient–provider relationship to anyone other than those the patient has authorized, other medical professionals involved in the patient's care, and agencies responsible for processing state and/or federally mandated reporting.

conjunctiva The clear (usually) mucous membrane that covers the sclera (white part of the eye) and lines the eyelids.

contact wound The type of wound that occurs when the muzzle of a gun touches the patient at the time of discharge, resulting in a circular entrance wound, often associated with visible burns, soot, or the imprint of the muzzle.

contrecoup injury An injury to parts of the brain located on the side opposite that of the primary injury.

convection The transfer of heat from the movement or circulation of a gas or liquid, such as the heating of water or air in contact with a body, removing that air (such as by wind) or water, and then having to heat the new air or water that replaces what left.

cord compression Pressure on the spinal cord caused by swelling, bone fragments, or hematoma, which may result in tissue ischemia and, in some cases, may require decompression to prevent a permanent loss of function.

cord concussion The temporary disruption of the spinal cord functions distal to the site of a spinal cord injury.

cord contusion Bruising or bleeding into the tissue of the spinal cord, which may also result in a temporary loss of cord functions distal to the injury.

cord laceration An injury that occurs when spinal cord tissue is torn or cut.

core temperature (1) The temperature at which vital organs are maintained and function best; (2) the measured temperature of the deep structures and organs of the body.

cornea The dome-shaped transparent outer portion of the eye that covers the pupil and colored iris.

coup injury An injury to the brain located on the same side as the point of impact.

cranial vault The space within the skull or cranium.

crepitus A crackling sound made by bone ends grating together.

Critical Incident Stress Management (CISM) A group of intervention strategies used to help prevent and manage stress after an incident.

Cushing's phenomenon The combination of increased arterial blood pressure and the resultant bradycardia that can occur with increased intracranial pressure.

cyanosis Blue coloring of skin, mucous membranes, or nail beds indicating unoxygenated hemoglobin and a lack of adequate oxygen levels in the blood; usually secondary to inadequate ventilation or decreased perfusion.

dead space The amount of space that contains air that never reaches the alveoli to participate in the critical gas exchange process.

debridement The removal, usually surgically, of dead or damaged tissue.

decerebrate posturing Characteristic posture that occurs when a painful stimulus is introduced; the extremities are stiff and extended and the head is retracted. One of the forms of pathologic posturing (response) commonly associated with increased intracranial pressure.

decomposition A state of decay or rotting.

decompression sickness A group of disorders that result from the effects of increased pressure on gases in a diver's body.

decontamination Reduction or removal of hazardous chemical, biologic, or radiologic agents.

decorticate posturing A characteristic pathologic posture of a patient with increased intracranial pressure; when a painful stimulus is introduced, the patient is rigidly still with the back and lower extremities extended while the arms are flexed and fists clenched.

deep frostbite Freezing of tissue that affects skin, muscle, and bone.

delayed primary closure Delayed suturing of a wound for 48 to 72 hours to allow any swelling to go down and to ensure that there are no signs of infection.

denuded Having the covering or surface layer removed.

dependent lividity The settling or pooling of blood in the lowest lying portions of a deceased body.

dermatome The sensory area on the body for which a nerve root is responsible. Collectively, they allow the body areas to be mapped out for each spinal level and to help locate a spinal cord injury.

dermis The layer of skin just under the epidermis made up of a framework of connective tissues containing blood vessels, nerve endings, sebaceous glands, and sweat glands.

designated incident facility An assigned location where specific incident command system functions are performed; for example, incident command is located at the incident command post.

devitalized Lifeless or dead.

diaphragm The dome-shaped muscle that divides the chest and abdomen and that functions as part of the breathing process.

diastole Ventricular relaxation (ventricular filling).

digital (tactile) intubation A technique for nonvisualized endotracheal intubation that involves the provider placing his or her fingers into the patient's mouth and throat to guide the placement of the endotracheal tube.

distraction The pulling apart of two structures—e.g., pulling apart the fractured components of a bone or part of the spine.

distributive shock Shock that occurs when the vascular container enlarges without a proportional increase in fluid volume.

diverter A device on a shotgun to spread the pellets into a wider, horizontal path when fired.

Don Juan syndrome The pattern of injury that often occurs when victims fall or jump from a height and land on their feet. Bilateral calcaneus (heel bone) fractures are often associated with this syndrome. After the feet land and stop moving, the body is forced into flexion as the weight of the still-moving head, torso, and pelvis come to bear. This can cause compression fractures of the spinal column in the thoracic and lumbar areas.

dorsal root The spinal nerve root responsible for sensory impulses.

drowning The process of experiencing respiratory impairment from submersion/immersion in liquid; may or may not result in death.

DUMBELS A mnemonic that represents the constellation of symptoms associated with the muscarinic effects of nerve agent toxicity (diarrhea, urination, miosis, bradycardia, bronchorrhea, bronchospasm, emesis, lacrimation, salivation, sweating).

dura mater The outer tough membrane covering the spinal cord and brain; the outer of the three meningeal layers. Literally means "tough mother."

dynamic pressure The component of an explosion that is directional and felt as a blast wind.

dysarthria Difficulty speaking.

dysbarism The changes that result physiologically as a result of changes in ambient environmental pressure.

ecchymosis A bluish or purple irregularly formed spot or area resulting from a hemorrhagic area below the skin.

eclampsia A syndrome in pregnant women that includes hypertension, peripheral edema, and seizures; also called toxemia of pregnancy.

edema A local or generalized condition in which some of the body tissues contain an excessive amount of fluid; generally includes swelling of the tissue.

edentulism The absence of teeth.

elasticity The ability to stretch.

electrical energy The result of movement of electrons between two points.

endophthalmitis Inflammation of the interior of the eye often due to infection secondary to penetrating injury.

endotracheal tube A plastic tube that is inserted into the trachea to ensure an open airway and used to assist a patient to breathe.

en route care Care provided to casualties during any type of casualty movement.

environmental temperature The thermal temperature of the air surrounding an individual.

epidermis The outermost layer of the skin, which is made up entirely of dead epithelial cells with no blood vessels.

epidural hematoma Arterial bleeding that collects between the skull and dura mater.

epidural space Potential space between the dura mater surrounding the brain and the cranium. Contains the meningeal arteries.

epiglottis A leaf-shaped structure that acts as a gate or flapper valve and directs air into the trachea and solids and liquids into the esophagus.

epinephrine A chemical released from the adrenal glands that stimulates the heart to increase cardiac output by increasing the strength and rate of contractions.

epithelial Any tissue that covers a surface or lines a cavity.

eschar Thick scab of dead tissue, often resulting from a burn.

escharotomy An incision made into an eschar to allow the tissues underlying the tough, leathery damaged skin created by severe burns to expand as they swell.

esophagus The muscular tube that connects the mouth to the stomach.

eucapnic state A condition in which the blood carbon dioxide level is within a normal range.

eupnea Normal, unlabored, quiet breathing or respiration.

evaporation Change from liquid to vapor.

event phase The moment of the actual trauma.

evisceration A condition in which a portion of the intestine or other abdominal organ is displaced through an open wound and protrudes externally outside the abdominal cavity.

exercise-associated hyponatremia (EAH) A life-threatening condition associated with excessive consumption of water (1.5 quarts [1.4 liters] or greater per hour) during prolonged activities leading to marked lowering of the sodium concentration in blood.

exercise-associated hyponatremic encephalopathy (EAHE) A life-threatening condition of cerebral edema resulting from lowered sodium concentration in blood from excessive consumption of water (1.5 quarts [1.4 liters] or greater per hour) during prolonged activities.

exertional heatstroke (EHS) A condition of elevated body temperature usually in males working or exercising in the heat and humidity, characterized by pale, sweaty skin, elevated body temperature, and altered mentation.

exsanguination Total loss of blood volume, producing death.

external respiration The transfer of oxygen molecules from the atmosphere to the blood.

extracellular fluid All body fluid that is not contained within cells.

extramural (extraluminal) pressure Pressure in the tissue surrounding the vessel.

extreme altitude An elevation higher than 18,045 feet (5,500 meters).

face-to-face intubation A technique for endotracheal intubation in which the endotracheal tube is inserted orally while the intubator is facing the patient instead of being located at the usual location above the head of the patient.

falx A vertical fold of the thick dura that separates the two halves of the cerebrum of the brain.

fascia A flat band of tissue that separates different layers; a fibrous band of tissue that encloses muscle.

field exercise A training event that involves the actual execution and performance of the community disaster-response plan.

finance/administration section The section responsible for all costs and financial actions of the incident.

first death peak The first of three peaks that occur with death from trauma; results from massive injury or rapid exsanguination; can be minimized by preventive measures.

first-degree frostbite Epidermal injury limited to skin that had brief contact with cold air or metal; involved skin appears white or as yellowish plaque; there is no blister or tissue loss; skin thaws quickly, feels numb, and appears red with surrounding edema; healing occurs in 7 to 10 days.

flail chest A chest with an unstable segment produced by multiple ribs fractured in two or more places or including a fractured sternum.

flail sternum A variation of flail chest that involves fracture of the ribs on both sides of the sternum, allowing the sternum to float freely.

flat bone A thin, flat, and compact bone, such as the sternum, ribs, and scapulae.

fontanelle The soft, membranous space between the unfused bones of an infant's skull; often referred to as the "soft spot."

foramen A small opening; plural is *foramina*.

foramen magnum The opening at the base of the skull through which the medulla oblongata passes.

fourth-degree burn A burn injury that involves all layers of the skin, as well as the underlying fat, muscles, bone, or internal organs.

fourth-degree frostbite A freezing injury that involves the skin, underlying tissue, muscle, and bone.

fragmentation The breaking up of an object to produce multiple parts or shrapnel.

frostbite The freezing of body tissue as a result of exposure to freezing or below-freezing temperatures.

full-thickness (third-degree) burn A burn to the epidermis, dermis, and subcutaneous tissue (possibly deeper). Skin may look charred or leathery.

galea aponeurotica A tough, thick layer of tissue underneath the scalp that covers the cranium.

gamma ray A ray of high-energy electromagnetic radiation released as a result of radioactive material decay.

grand mal seizure A generalized seizure that involves loss of consciousness and muscle contractions; also known as tonic-clonic seizure.

group training Disaster response training directed at specific response groups.

Haddon Matrix A table that shows the interaction of host, agent, and environmental factors in an incident.

heat acclimatization A process of increasing tolerance to exposure to heat.

heat stress index The combination of ambient temperature and relative humidity.

heatstroke An acute and dangerous reaction to heat exposure characterized by high body temperature and altered mental status.

heat syncope Fainting or lightheadedness after standing for prolonged periods in a hot environment; results from vasodilation and venous blood pooling in the legs, causing low blood pressure.

heat tetany A rare and self-limited condition that results from hyperventilation due to acute exposure to short, intense heat conditions.

hemiparesis Weakness limited to one side of the body.

hemiplegia Paralysis on one side of the body.

hemorrhagic shock Hypovolemic shock resulting from blood loss.

hemothorax Blood in the pleural space.

high altitude An elevation above 5,000 to 11,480 feet (1,500 to 3,500 meters).

high-altitude cerebral edema (HACE) A life-threatening complication of brain swelling that results from travel to high altitude (usually above 8,000 feet [2,400 meters]).

high-altitude pulmonary edema (HAPE) A life-threatening complication of fluid accumulating in the lungs that results from travel to high altitude (usually above 8,000 feet [2,400 meters]).

high explosive A type of explosive designed to detonate and release its energy very quickly; capable of producing a shock wave, or overpressure phenomenon, which can result in primary blast injury.

homeostasis A constant, stable internal environment; the balance necessary to maintain healthy life processes.

homeotherm A warm-blooded animal.

hot zone The geographic area of highest contamination from a hazardous material; only specially trained and equipped workers may enter this area.

hydrofluoric acid A type of acid; exposure to even small amounts can lead to life-threatening lowering of the serum calcium levels and cardiac dysrhythmias.

hypercarbia An increased level of carbon dioxide in the body.

hyperchloremic acidosis A type of metabolic acidosis (decrease in blood pH) associated with an increase in the amount of chloride ion in the blood; may result from the administration of large amounts of normal saline.

hyperextension Extreme or abnormal extension of a joint; a position of maximum extension. Hyperextension of the neck is produced when the head is extended posterior to a neutral position and can result in a fracture or dislocation of the vertebrae or in spinal cord damage in a patient with an unstable spine.

hyperflexion Extreme or abnormal flexion of a joint. A position of maximum flexion. Increased flexion

of the neck can result in a fracture or dislocation of the vertebrae or in spinal cord damage in a patient with an unstable spine.

hyperkalemia Increased blood potassium.

hyper-rotation Excessive rotation.

hypertension A blood pressure greater than the upper limits of the normal range; generally considered to exist if the patient's systolic pressure is greater than 140 mm Hg.

hypertonic saline Any solution of sodium chloride in water with a concentration of sodium chloride greater than physiologic saline, which is 0.9% sodium chloride, the same as body fluid.

hyphema A collection of blood in the anterior chamber of the eye, between the clear cornea and the colored iris.

hypobaric hypoxia Hypoxia caused by the decrease in atmospheric pressure and the partial pressure of oxygen at increasingly higher altitudes.

hypochlorite solution A solution used in the production of household bleaches and industrial cleaners.

hypoperfusion Inadequate blood flow to cells with properly oxygenated blood.

hypopharynx The lower portion of the pharynx that opens into the larynx anteriorly and the esophagus posteriorly.

hypothalamus The area of the brain that functions as the thermoregulatory center and the body's thermostat to control neurologic and hormonal regulation of body temperature.

hypothermia A condition characterized by core body temperature below normal range, usually between 78°F and 90°F (26–32°C).

hypoventilation Inadequate ventilation when minute volume falls below normal.

hypovolemic shock Shock caused by loss of blood or fluid.

hypoxia (hypoxemia) Deficiency of oxygen; inadequate available oxygen. Lack of adequate oxygenation of the lungs due to inadequate minute volume (air exchange in the lungs) or a decreased concentration of oxygen in the inspired air. Cellular hypoxia is inadequate oxygen available to the cells.

iatrogenic Caused by the treatment.

ICS general staff The chiefs of each of the four major sections of the incident command system (ICS): operations, planning, logistics, and finance/administration.

immersion A condition occurring when water has splashed or washed over the face and airway, allowing for drowning to occur by aspiration.

immersion foot A nonfreezing cold exposure injury caused by prolonged immersion of extremities in wet and moisture that is cool to cold; also referred to as trench foot.

impact phase The phase of the disaster cycle that involves the actual incident or disaster.

incident action plan (IAP) A continuously updated outline of the overall strategy, tactics, and risk management plans developed by the incident commander or the incident command system staff.

incident command post (ICP) The location at which incident command functions are performed.

incident command system (ICS) A system that defines the chain of command and organization of the various resources that respond during a disaster.

incident commander (IC) The individual responsible for all aspects of a response to an incident, including developing incident objectives, managing all incident operations, setting priorities, and defining the incident command system organization for the particular response; the IC position will always be filled.

incisura (tentorial incisura) Opening in the tentorium cerebelli at the junction of the midbrain and the cerebrum. The brain stem is inferior to the incisura.

incomplete cord transection Partial transection of the spinal cord in which some tracts and motor/sensory functions remain intact.

independent learning Studying on one's own.

inferior vena cava A major vein that carries deoxygenated blood from the lower half of the body back to the heart.

inhalation The process of drawing air into the lungs.

injury A harmful event that arises from the release of specific forms of physical energy or barriers to normal flow of energy.

injury process Similar to disease, a process involving a host, an agent (in the case of injury the agent is energy), and an environment or situation that allows the host and agent to interact.

inner perimeter A geographic boundary at a hazardous incident surrounding the area of highest danger and potential lethality.

insensible loss The unmeasured loss of water and heat from exhaled air, skin, and mucous membranes.

integrated communications A communications system that allows all responders at an incident to communicate with supervisors and subordinates.

intentional injury Injury associated with an act of interpersonal or self-directed violence.

intercostal muscles The muscles located between the ribs that connect the ribs to one another and assist with breathing.

intermediate-range wound A penetrating gunshot wound that occurs at a distance of approximately 6 to 18 feet (1.8 to 5.5 m).

intermittent mandatory ventilation (IMV) A form of mechanical ventilation that delivers a set rate and tidal volume to patients.

internal (cellular) respiration The movement or diffusion of oxygen molecules from the red blood cells into the tissue cells.

interstitial fluid The extracellular fluid located between the cell wall and the capillary wall.

intervertebral foramen A notch through which nerves pass in the inferior lateral side of the vertebra.

intracellular fluid Fluid within the cells.

intracranial pressure The pressure exerted against the inside of the skull by brain tissue, blood, and cerebrospinal fluid; usually less than 15 mm Hg in adults and 3 to 7 mm Hg in children.

intramural (intraluminal) pressure The pressure exerted against the inside of the walls of blood vessels by the intravascular fluids and blood pressure cycle.

involuntary guarding Rigidity or spasm of the abdominal wall muscles in response to peritonitis.

ionization The process by which a molecule becomes charged by gaining or losing an electron.

ipsilateral On the same side.

iris The colored portion of the eye that contains the adjustable opening of the pupil.

ischemic sensitivity The sensitivity of the cells of a tissue to the lack of oxygen before cell death occurs.

Joint Theater Trauma System (JTTS) A system established to provide CENTCOM theaters of operation (OEF and OIF) with care and movement of casualties through treatment facilities providing increasing levels of trauma care from the point of wounding on the battlefield to rehabilitation in the United States.

Joint Trauma System (JTS) A system deployed by the DOD to provide any theater of operation anywhere in the world with care and movement of casualties through treatment facilities providing increasing levels of trauma care from the point of wounding in the area of operation to rehabilitation in the United States.

justice That which is fair or just; in medicine, usually refers to how medical resources are distributed with regard to health care.

kill zone The area of greatest risk in a hazardous incident; the area within the inner perimeter.

kinematics The process of looking at the mechanism of injury of an incident to determine what injuries are likely to have resulted from the forces and motion and changes in motion involved; the science of motion.

kinetic energy (KE) Energy available from movement. Function of the weight of an item and its speed: $KE = 1/2$ of the mass $\times$ the velocity squared.

kyphosis A forward, humplike curvature of the spine commonly associated with the aging process. Kyphosis may be caused by aging, rickets, or tuberculosis of the spine.

lactated Ringer's (LR) An intravenous crystalloid solution that is isotonic with blood and used to replenish circulating volume and electrolytes; contains water, sodium, chloride, calcium, potassium, and lactate.

laryngeal mask airway (LMA) An airway management device; the distal end that is inserted into the patient's mouth is shaped like an oval mask to cover the supraglottic structures and isolate the trachea to allow for air passage.

larynx The structure located just above the trachea that contains the vocal cords and the muscles that make them work.

law of conservation of energy A law of physics stating that energy cannot be created or destroyed but only changed in form.

Lewisite An oily liquid used as a chemical weapon to produce burnlike blisters; it is a blister agent (vesicant).

liaison officer A command staff member who assists or coordinates with multiple agencies; serves as an intermediary between the incident commander and outside agencies.

Lichtenberg's figure A branching or fernlike reddish skin marking that is painless and results from being struck by lightning.

ligament A band of tough, fibrous tissue connecting bone to bone.

liquefaction necrosis The type of tissue injury that occurs when an alkali damages human tissue; the base liquefies the tissue, which allows for deeper penetration of the chemical.

living will A form of advance directive that expresses a patient's end-of-life treatment wishes, such as whether mechanical ventilation, CPR, dialysis, or other types of life-prolonging or life-sustaining treatments are desired; generally does not go into effect until the patient lacks decision-making capacity and has been certified by a health care professional, usually a doctor, to be either terminally ill or permanently unconscious.

logistics section The section responsible for providing all services, equipment, and facilities for the incident.

logistics section chief The position responsible for directing the logistics function for the incident commander.

long bones Femur, humerus, ulna, radius, tibia, and fibula.

long-range wound A penetrating gunshot wound that occurs at a distance greater than 18 feet (5.5 m).

low explosive A type of explosive that changes relatively slowly from a solid or liquid to a gaseous state (in an action more characteristic of burning than of detonation); because they release their energy much more slowly, low explosives do not produce blast overpressure.

maceration Softening of the skin as a result of exposure to constant moisture; the skin turns white and breaks down, and can easily become infected.

maculopapular rash A skin rash characterized by areas of reddish discoloration (macules) in association with small, raised bumps (papules).

magnesium A highly flammable chemical element used to make incendiary weapons; also an essential electrolyte in human physiology.

mammalian diving reflex A reflex that occurs with submersion in cold water (less than 70°F [21°C]) resulting in rapid slowing of the body's metabolism, spasm of the larynx, shunting of blood from the periphery to the heart and brain, and a marked decrease in heart and respiratory rate.

manually triggered (oxygen-powered) device An oxygen-powered ventilation device powered by pressurized oxygen, triggered manually to deliver a breath; may cause gastric distension and pulmonary barotrauma.

mass-casualty incident (MCI) An incident (such as a plane crash, building collapse, or fire) that produces a large number of victims from one mechanism, at one place, and at the same time; also referred to as multiple-casualty incident.

mass-casualty incident (MCI) response The postevent actions taken to minimize damage, morbidity, and mortality resulting from the incident.

mean arterial pressure (MAP) The average pressure in the vascular system, estimated by adding one-third of the pulse pressure to the diastolic pressure.

mechanical energy The energy that an object contains when it is in motion.

mediastinum The middle of the thoracic cavity containing the heart, great vessels, trachea, main bronchi, and esophagus.

Medical Evacuation (MEDEVAC) The medically regulated movement of casualties using dedicated medical evacuation vehicles.

medical power of attorney (MPOA) An advance directive document used by competent adults to appoint someone to make medical decisions for them in the event that they are unable to make such decisions for themselves. Unlike living wills, MPOAs go into effect immediately anytime a patient is incapable of making his or her own decision, regardless of pre-existing condition, and become inactive again when/if the patient regains decision-making capacity.

medulla (medulla oblongata) Part of the brain stem. The medulla is the primary regulatory center of autonomic control of the cardiovascular system.

meninges Three membranes that cover the brain tissue and the spinal cord; the dura mater, arachnoid, and pia mater.

methemoglobin Hemoglobin in which the iron has been oxidized to the ferric state by ionic bonding. Methemoglobin does not function reversibly as an oxygen carrier.

midbrain The portion of the brain stem located above the pons; contains nerve pathways that go between the cerebrum and the medulla oblongata and contains centers for visual and auditory reflexes.

minute ventilation See *minute volume*.

minute volume The amount of air exchanged each minute; calculated by multiplying the volume of each breath (tidal volume) by the number of breaths per minute (rate).

mitigation In emergency medicine, a reduction in the loss of life and property by lessening the impact of disasters.

MTWHF A mnemonic that represents the constellation of symptoms associated with stimulation of nicotinic receptors, usually after nerve agent exposure; MTWHF stands for mydriasis (rarely seen), tachycardia, weakness, hypertension, hyperglycemia, fasciculations.

mucocutaneous Made up of or pertaining to both skin and mucous membranes.

multisystem trauma patient A patient with injury to more than one body system.

muscarinic site An acetylcholine receptor found primarily in smooth muscle and glands.

myocardial hypertrophy An increase in the heart's muscle mass and size.

myoglobin A protein found in muscle that is responsible for giving muscle its characteristic red color.

myoglobinuria The release of myoglobin into the bloodstream in considerable amounts, causing a reddish or tea-colored urine, toxicity to the kidneys, and kidney failure.

nasopharyngeal airway An airway that is placed in the nostril and follows the floor of the nasal cavity directly posterior to the nasopharynx in order to lift the tongue off of the back of the pharynx and open the airway. This airway is commonly tolerated by patients with a gag reflex.

nasopharynx The upper portion of the airway, situated above the soft palate.

neural arches Two curved sides of the vertebrae.

neurogenic "shock" Shock that occurs when a cervical spine injury damages the spinal cord above where the nerves of the sympathetic nervous system exit, thus interfering with the normal vasoconstriction and leading to vasodilitation and decreased blood pressure.

neutral position The position of a joint that allows for maximal movement; neither flexed nor extended.

Newton's first law of motion A fundamental law of physics stating that a body at rest will remain at rest, and a body in motion will remain in motion unless acted on by an outside force.

Newton's second law of motion A fundamental law of physics stating that the acceleration of an object is directly proportional to the magnitude of the force applied, in the same direction as the force applied, and inversely proportional to the mass of the object.

Newton's third law of motion A fundamental law of physics stating that for every action, there is an equal and opposite reaction.

nicotinic site An acetylcholine receptor found primarily in skeletal muscle.

nitrogen mustard An oily chemical used as a chemical weapon to produce burnlike blisters; can also damage the respiratory tract, gastrointestinal tract, and bone marrow; blister agent;

vesicant; also used as an anticancer medication.

nonfreezing cold injury (NFCI) A syndrome resulting from damage to peripheral tissues, caused by prolonged (hours to days) exposure to wet/cold; also called immersion foot and trench foot.

nonmaleficence An ethical principle that obligates the medical provider to not take actions that may harm the patient or place the patient in harm's way.

norepinephrine A chemical released by the sympathetic nervous system that triggers constriction of the blood vessels to reduce the size of the vascular container and bring it more closely into proportion with the volume of the remaining fluid.

normal saline An intravenous crystalloid solution comprised of water and sodium and chloride in a concentration of 0.9%.

nystagmus An involuntary, rapid, rhythmic movement of the eyes.

obtunded A condition in which the patient's mental capacity is dulled or diminished; mild to moderate decreased level of consciousness with impaired sensory perception.

oculomotor nerve The third cranial nerve; controls pupillary constriction and certain eye movements.

omentum A fold of peritoneum that covers and connects the stomach to other intra-abdominal organs.

omission The failure to act.

oncotic pressure Pressure that determines the amount of fluid within the vascular space.

open fracture A fracture of a bone in which the skin is broken.

open globe A penetrating injury to the eye; injury that involves the full thickness of the cornea or the sclera of the eye.

open pneumothorax (sucking chest wound) A penetrating wound to the chest that causes the chest wall to be opened, producing a preferential pathway for air moving from the outside environment into the thorax.

operations level In hazardous materials training, the level of knowledge and training that a responder should have when involved in the response to and control of an incident involving chemical spills or release.

operations section The section responsible for all tactical operations at the incident.

operations section chief The position responsible for managing all operations activities in the incident command system.

oropharyngeal airway An airway that, when placed in the oropharynx superior to the tongue, holds the tongue forward to assist in maintaining an open airway; used only in patients with no gag reflex.

oropharynx The central portion of the pharynx lying between the soft palate and the upper portion of the epiglottis.

orotracheal intubation A method of securing an open and patent airway that involves insertion of a plastic tube through the mouth into the trachea.

osmosis The movement of water (or other solvent) across a membrane from an area that is hypotonic to an area that is hypertonic.

osteophytosis The development of bony outgrowths, usually along joints, particularly of the spine; also referred to as bone spurs.

osteoporosis A loss of normal bone density with thinning of bone tissue and the growth of small holes in the bone. The disorder may cause pain (especially in the lower back), frequent broken bones, loss of body height,

and various poorly formed parts of the body. Commonly a part of the normal aging process.

out-of-hospital do not resuscitate (DNR) An order given by a physician to ensure that prehospital care providers do not perform CPR on a terminally ill patient at home, or in some other community or nonclinical setting, against the patient's wishes.

outer perimeter The geographic boundary that defines the "safe zone" where no threat should exist at a hazardous incident.

overpressure phenomenon The sudden increase in atmospheric pressure or shock wave that occurs in proximity to the detonation of a high explosive.

oxygen delivery The process of oxygen transfer from the atmosphere to the red blood cells (RBCs) during ventilation and the transportation of these RBCs to the tissues via the cardiovascular system.

oxygenation The process of providing, treating, or enriching with oxygen.

paradoxical pulse A condition in which the patient's systolic blood pressure drops more than 10 to 15 mm Hg during each inspiration, usually due to the effect of increased intrathoracic pressure such as would occur with tension pneumothorax or from pericardial tamponade.

parasympathetic nervous system The division of the nervous system that maintains normal body functions.

parenchyma The essential or functional cells or elements of an organ.

paresthesia Abnormal skin sensations that include tingling, "pins and needles," burning, prickling, and crawling.

parietal pleura A thin membrane that lines the inner side of the thoracic cavity.

partial-thickness (second-degree) burn A burn that involves both the epidermis and the dermis. Skin presents with reddened areas, blisters, or open, weeping wounds.

passive strategy In injury prevention, a prevention method that requires no action on the part of the individual— e.g., vehicle air bags.

patent airway An open, unobstructed airway of sufficient size to allow for normal volumes of air exchange.

patient care report (PCR) The written report documenting the prehospital care provided to a patient; includes the history, assessment, prehospital interventions, reassessment, and patient response to treatment.

peak overpressure The maximum value of pressure experienced at a given location at the moment a blast wave from a high explosive reaches the location.

pediatric trauma score (PTS) A clinical scoring system based on clinical information that is predictive of severity of injury and can be used for triage decision making.

pelvic ring The round shape that comprises the pelvis; made up of the ilium, ischium, pubis, sacrum, and coccyx; also referred to as the pelvic girdle.

penetrating trauma Trauma that results when an object penetrates the skin and injures underlying structures. Generally produces both permanent and temporary cavities.

percutaneous Occurring through the skin—e.g., a needlestick.

percutaneous transtracheal ventilation (PTV) A procedure in which a 16-gauge or larger needle through which the patient is ventilated is inserted directly into the lumen of the trachea through the cricothyroid membrane, or directly through the tracheal wall.

pericardiocentesis A procedure that involves insertion of a needle into the pericardial space to remove accumulated blood or fluid.

periorbital ecchymosis See *raccoon eyes*.

periosteum The thick layer of connective tissue that covers the surface of bones, except for the joint surfaces.

peritoneal space The space in the anterior abdominal cavity that contains the bowel, spleen, liver, stomach, and gallbladder. The peritoneal space is covered by the peritoneum. Also referred to as the peritoneal cavity.

peritoneum The lining of the abdominal cavity.

peritonitis Inflammation of the peritoneum.

pharynx The throat; a tubelike structure that is a passage for both the breathing and digestive tracts. Oropharynx-area of the pharynx posterior to the mouth; nasopharynx-area of the pharynx beyond the posterior nares of the nose.

physician orders for life-sustaining treatment (POLST) An advance directive that allows for the acceptance or refusal of a wide variety of life-sustaining treatments, such as CPR, medical nutrition and hydration, and ventilator support, and allows prehospital care providers to access an active physician order regarding the end-of-life wishes of the terminally ill and frail elderly.

physiologic reserve The excess functional capacity of an organ or organ system.

physiologic thermoregulation The process by which the body's temperature is controlled; involves dilation and constriction of blood vessels to help remove or conserve body heat.

pia mater A thin vascular membrane closely adhering to the brain and spinal cord and proximal portions of the nerves; the innermost of the three meningeal membranes that cover the brain.

planning section The ICS section responsible for the collection and evaluation of information related to the incident.

planning section chief The ICS position responsible for collecting and evaluating information and assisting in planning with the incident commander.

pneumothorax An injury that results in air in the pleural space; commonly producing a collapsed lung. A pneumothorax can be open with an opening through the chest wall to the outside or closed resulting from blunt trauma or a spontaneous collapse.

positive end-expiratory pressure (PEEP) The pressure in the lungs above atmospheric pressure at the end of expiration; also refers to a ventilatory technique to assist breathing in which an increased amount of pressure is applied to the lungs at the end of expiration to increase the amount of air remaining in the lungs and enhance gas exchange.

postevent phase The phase beginning as soon as the energy from the crash is absorbed and the patient is traumatized; the phase of prehospital care that includes response time, Golden Period, and transport time.

posttraumatic endophthalmitis Infection of the intraocular contents, usually as a result of penetrating trauma to the eye.

posttraumatic stress disorder (PTSD) A mental health condition that results from exposure to a horrific or terrifying event and leads to flashbacks to the incident, nightmares, anxiety, and uncontrollable thoughts about the incident.

powered air-purifying respirator (PAPR) A protective respiratory device that draws ambient air through a filter canister and delivers it under positive pressure to a facemask or hood.

pre-event phase/precrash phase The phase that includes all of the events that precede an incident (e.g., ingestion of drugs and alcohol) and conditions that predate the incident (e.g., acute or pre-existing medical conditions). This phase includes injury prevention and preparedness.

preference The manner in which the principle of care is achieved in the time given and by the prehospital care provider available.

preload The volume and pressure of the blood coming into the heart from the systemic circulatory system (venous return).

preparedness A step of comprehensive emergency management that involves identifying, in advance of an incident, the specific supplies, equipment, and personnel that would be needed to manage an incident, as well as the specific action plan that would be taken if an incident were to occur.

presbycusis A condition characterized by a gradual decline in hearing.

primary blast injury (PBI) An injury that is caused by exposure to the blast overpressure wave from the detonation of a high explosive (e.g., pulmonary bleeding, pneumothorax, perforation of the gastrointestinal tract).

primary contamination Exposure to a hazardous substance at its point of release.

primary hypothermia A decrease in body temperature that occurs when healthy individuals are unprepared for overwhelming acute or chronic cold exposure.

principle An element that must be present, accomplished, or ensured by the health care provider in order to optimize patient survival and outcome; also refers to the four ethical concepts of autonomy, nonmaleficence, beneficence, and justice.

principlism The use of the four ethical principles of autonomy, nonmaleficence, beneficence, and justice, which provide a framework for one to weigh and balance the benefits and burdens of treating a specific patient in order to do what is in the patient's best interest.

privacy The right of patients to control who has access to their personal health information.

prodrome (predisaster) phase (warning phase) The phase in the disaster cycle in which a specific event has been identified as inevitably going to occur and in which specific steps can be taken to mitigate the effects of the ensuing events.

profile A penetrating object's initial size and the degree of change in size that occurs at the time of impact.

psychogenic "shock" A temporary neurogenic shock as a result of psychological stress (fainting).

public health impact of injury The totality of the impact of injury on the health of the public; includes deaths, injury, disability, and financial considerations.

public information officer (PIO) The ICS command staff officer responsible for interacting with the public and media and distributing information.

pulmonary contusion A bruising of the lungs; can be secondary to blunt or penetrating trauma.

pulse oximeter A device that measures arterial oxyhemoglobin saturation. The value is determined by measuring the absorption ratio of red and infrared light passed through the tissue.

pulse pressure (1) The increase in pressure (surge) that is created as each new bolus of blood leaves the left ventricle with each contraction; (2) the difference between the systolic and diastolic blood pressures (systolic pressure minus diastolic pressure equals pulse pressure).

pulseless electrical activity A condition characterized by organized electrical activity on cardiac monitoring without an associated palpable pulse.

quaternary blast injury An injury from a blast or explosion that includes burns and toxicities from fuel, metals, trauma from structural collapse, septic syndromes from soil, and environmental contamination.

quaternary effect See *quaternary blast injury*.

quiescence (interdisaster period) The time in between disasters or mass-casualty incidents during which risk assessment and mitigation activities are undertaken and when plans for the response to likely events are developed, tested, and implemented.

quinary blast injury A hyperinflammatory state in blast victims thought to result from bacteria, chemicals, or radioactive materials added to the explosive device and released upon detonation.

raccoon eyes (periorbital ecchymosis) Contusion or ecchymotic area around each eye, limited by the orbital margins; may result from direct trauma to the orbit or from basilar skull fracture.

radiation The direct transfer of energy from a warm object to a cooler one by infrared radiation.

radiation dispersion device (RDD) A conventional explosive with a radionuclide (radioactive material) attached that is detonated to disperse the radioactive material.

radiation energy Any electromagnetic wave that travels in rays and has no physical mass to it.

rapid sequence intubation (RSI) A method of patient intubation that includes pharmacologic adjuncts for sedation and muscle relaxation.

rate of detonation The rate at which the detonation/combustion wave travels through the explosive material usually reported in feet or meters per second.

rebound tenderness A physical examination finding that occurs by pressing deeply on the abdomen and then quickly releasing the pressure, causing more severe pain when the abdominal pressure is suddenly released.

recovery (reconstruction) phase The period during the disaster cycle that addresses the community's resources to endure, emerge, and rebuild from the effects of the disaster through the coordinated efforts of the medical, public health, and community infrastructure (physical and political); this period is usually the longest, lasting months, and perhaps years, before a community fully recovers.

red blood cell (RBC) A disc-shaped cell that contains hemoglobin to carry oxygen to the organs and cells of the body.

relative effectiveness (RE) factor The power of an explosive substance relative to that of TNT.

remote assessment A process by which tactical operators and providers gather information without revealing their position or intent to the hostile force; includes remote observation with binoculars, remote acoustic surveillance, and thermal imaging.

rescue (emergency or relief) phase The period during the disaster cycle immediately following the impact, during which response occurs and appropriate management and intervention can save lives.

resource management Agreements and procedures that enable local, state, and federal agencies to work together under one command during a large-scale incident.

respiration The total ventilatory and circulatory processes involved in the exchange of oxygen and carbon dioxide between the outside atmosphere and the cells of the body. Sometimes in medicine limited to meaning breathing and the steps in ventilation.

reticular activating system (RAS) The central nervous system control center responsible for maintaining the level of consciousness and alertness.

retroperitoneal space The space in the posterior abdominal cavity that contains the kidneys, ureters, bladder, reproductive organs, inferior vena cava, abdominal aorta, pancreas, a portion of the duodenum, colon, and rectum.

retroperitoneum See *retroperitoneal space.*

rhabdomyolysis The breakdown of muscle tissue with the release of intracellular muscle components into the circulation.

rifling Grooves on the inside of the barrel that spin a single missile (bullet) in a stable flight pattern toward the target.

rigor mortis The temporary stiffening and rigidity of muscles and joints that occurs after death; typically begins within 2 to 4 hours of death and lasts approximately 36 to 48 hours.

riot control agent A chemical agent used to rapidly and briefly disable those exposed to it by causing irritation to the skin, mucous membranes, lungs, and eyes.

sacral spine (sacrum) Part of the spinal column below the lumbar spine containing the five sacral vertebrae (S1–S5), which are connected by immovable joints to form the sacrum. The sacrum is the weight-bearing base of the spinal column and is also a part of the pelvic girdle.

safety officer The ICS command staff officer who is responsible for monitoring, assessing, and ensuring the safety of emergency personnel.

SAMPLE history A mnemonic to remember the components of the history; stands for symptoms, allergies, medication, past medical and surgical history, last meal, and events leading up to the injury.

sclera The dense, fibrous, white outer layer of the eyeball.

second death peak The second of three peaks that occur with death from trauma; occurs within minutes to a few hours after injury; can be minimized by rapid prehospital assessment, treatment, and transport.

second-degree frostbite A freezing injury due to cold exposure that involves the epidermis and superficial dermis; initially appears similar to first-degree injury, but frozen tissues are deeper; after thawing, results in superficial skin blisters surrounded by erythema and edema; there is no permanent loss of tissue; healing occurs in 3 to 4 weeks.

secondary blast injury Injury that results from shrapnel, flying debris, and bomb fragments; typically causes penetrating ballistic injury.

secondary contamination Exposure to a hazardous substance after it has been carried away from the point of origin by a victim, a responder, or a piece of equipment.

secondary hypothermia A decrease in body temperature as a consequence of a patient's systemic disorder, including hypothyroidism, hypoadrenalism, trauma, carcinoma, and sepsis.

secondary impact syndrome The sudden deterioration in neurologic status in patients who have sustained a concussion and then have a second concussion before the symptoms from the first one have fully resolved.

self-aid The provision of medical care to one's self after sustaining an injury.

self-contained breathing apparatus (SCBA) A personal protective device consisting of a mask and portable supply of air, used in environments that are oxygen-deficient or pose a risk of toxic inhalation.

self-contained underwater breathing apparatus (SCUBA) A portable breathing device for underwater use, consisting of a mask with connecting tubes to a tank of compressed air.

senescence The process of aging.

sepsis Infection that has spread to involve the entire body.

septic shock Shock resulting from locally active hormones due to widespread systemic infection, causing damage to the walls of blood vessels, producing both peripheral vasodilation and leakage of fluid from the capillaries into the interstitial space.

sequela An aftereffect or complication of a disease or injury; plural is *sequelae.*

sesamoid bone A bone, usually small and round, located within tendons.

shear Change-of-speed force resulting in a cutting or tearing of body parts.

shear force Energy applied to the body that tends to move an organ or part of the body in one direction while the adjacent part moves in a different direction or remains fixed in place.

shock A widespread lack of tissue perfusion with oxygenated red blood cells that leads to anaerobic metabolism and decreased energy production.

shock front The boundary between the blast overpressure wave created by a high explosive detonation and normal atmospheric pressure.

shock wave See *shock front.*

short bones Metacarpals, metatarsals, phalanges.

simple pneumothorax The presence of air within the pleural space.

simulation A form of training that involves the imitation, enactment, or representation, verbally or with models, of the management of an incident or patient.

single command A command structure in which a single individual is responsible for all of the strategic objectives of the incident. Typically used when an incident is within a single jurisdiction and is managed by a single discipline.

single-system trauma patient A patient who has experienced trauma that involves injury to only one body system.

sniffing position A slightly superior anterior position of the head and neck to optimize ventilation as well as the view during endotracheal intubation.

solar keratitis Burns to the cornea of the eye that result from exposure to ultraviolet light, commonly as a result of reflection off of snow; also referred to as snow blindness.

solid density Tissue density consistent with bone.

span of control In an incident command system, the number of subordinates who report to one supervisor at any level within the response organization;

in most situations, one person can effectively supervise only three to seven people or resources.

specialist level In hazardous materials incidents, an individual who is trained to provide command and support skills.

spinal shock An injury to the spinal cord that results in a temporary loss of sensory and motor function.

spinal stenosis Narrowing of the spinal canal.

spinous process The tail-like structure on the posterior region of the vertebrae.

sprain An injury in which ligaments are stretched or even partially torn.

spray The dispersal pattern of pellets fired from a shotgun.

spread See *spray.*

staging area A predetermined area where resources, equipment, and personnel can be located safely and at the ready for assignment.

START triage algorithm A method of evaluating patients and assigning priority for treatment and transport during a mass-casualty incident; involves evaluating the respiratory status, perfusion status, and mental status of the patient.

status epilepticus A life-threatening condition in which a seizure persists for greater than 5 minutes or in which two or more seizures occur without a period of wakening in between.

steady-state metabolism A condition of stable cellular, organ, and body function.

stellate wound A star-shaped wound.

stipple Multiple small dots resulting from gun powder from point-blank gunshot wounds.

stopping distance The distance over which a moving object comes to a stop; a measure of how quickly energy is dissipated or transferred.

stress wave A supersonic, longitudinal pressure wave that (1) creates high local forces with small, rapid distortions; (2) produces microvascular injury; and (3) is reinforced and reflected at tissue interfaces, thereby enhancing injury potential, especially in gas-filled organs such as the lungs, ears, and intestines.

stroke volume The volume of blood pumped out by each contraction (stroke) of the left ventricle.

subarachnoid hemorrhage (SAH) Bleeding into the cerebrospinal fluid-filled space beneath the arachnoid membrane.

subconjunctival hemorrhage Bleeding found between the clear conjunctiva covering the eye and the white sclera.

subcutaneous emphysema Accumulation of air in the soft tissues of the body.

subcutaneous (or hypodermis) layer The layer of skin just under the dermis that is a combination of elastic and fibrous tissue as well as fat deposits.

subdural hematoma A collection of blood between the dura mater and the arachnoid membrane.

sublimation A process in which solids emit vapors, bypassing the liquid state.

subluxation A partial or incomplete dislocation.

submersion A situation where the entire body goes completely under water.

sulfur mustard An oily, clear to yellow-brown liquid that can be aerosolized by a bomb blast or a sprayer; a vesicant or blister agent used as a weapon of mass destruction.

superficial (first-degree) burn A burn to the epidermis only; red, inflamed, and painful skin.

superficial frostbite A freezing injury due to cold exposure that affects the skin and subcutaneous tissues, resulting in clear blisters when rewarmed.

superior vena cava A major vein that carries deoxygenated blood from the upper portion of the body back to the heart.

supplied air respirator (SAR) A personal protective device consisting of a mask and source of air that is not carried by the responder; used in environments that are oxygen-deficient or pose a risk of toxic inhalation.

supraglottic airway An airway device inserted blindly into the mouth and pharynx; designed to isolate the trachea from the esophagus; none of these devices provide a complete seal of the trachea, so the risk of aspiration is lowered but not completely prevented.

surgical cricothyrotomy A procedure to open a patient's airway that is accomplished by making an incision into the cricothyroid membrane in the neck to open the airway into the trachea.

surveillance The process of collecting data within a community, usually for infectious diseases.

sutural bones The flat bones that make up the skull.

sympathetic nervous system The division of the nervous system that produces the fight-or-flight response.

systemic vascular resistance The amount of resistance to the flow of blood through the vessels. It increases as the vessel constricts. Any change in lumen diameter or vessel elasticity can influence the amount of resistance.

systolic blood pressure Peak blood pressure produced by the force of the contraction (systole) of the ventricles of the heart.

tachypnea An increased breathing rate.

Tactical Casualty Care (TCC) The emergency medical care provided in a hazardous or tactical situation.

Tactical Emergency Medical Support (TEMS) An out-of-hospital system of care dedicated to enhancing the probability of special operations law enforcement mission success, reducing mission medical liability and risk, and promoting public safety.

Tactical Evacuation Care A phase of combat casualty care in which casualties are transported to a medical facility in an aircraft, ground vehicle or boat. Additional combat medical personnel and equipment on the evacuation platform may allow an increased level of care during transport.

Tactical Field Care A phase of combat casualty care in which the casualty and combat medical personnel and their units are not under effective hostile fire. The care that can be provided is limited by the knowledge and skill of the combat medical personnel and the equipment they have with them on the battlefield.

tamponade The closure or blockage of a wound or blood vessel; also the compression of the heart by the accumulation of blood or fluid in the pericardium.

technician level In hazardous materials incidents, an individual trained to work within the hazardous area and stop the release of hazardous materials.

tendon A band of tough, inelastic, fibrous tissue that connects a muscle to bone.

tension pneumothorax A condition in which the air pressure in the pleural space exceeds the outside atmospheric pressure and cannot escape, the affected side becomes hyperinflated, compressing the lung on the involved side and shifting the mediastinum to the opposite side to partially collapse the other lung; usually progressive and is an imminently life-threatening condition.

tentorial incisura See *incisura*.

tentorium cerebelli (tentorium) An infolding of the dura that forms a covering over the cerebellum. The tentorium is a part of the floor of the upper skull just below the brain (cerebrum).

tertiary blast injury An injury that occurs from an explosion when the victim becomes a missile and is thrown against some object; injuries, usually blunt, are similar to those sustained in ejections from vehicles, in falls from significant heights, or when the victim is thrown against an object by the force wave resulting from an explosion.

thermal energy Energy associated with increased temperature and heat.

thermal equilibrium The transfer of heat from a warmer object to a colder object in an effort to create the same temperature between them.

thermal gradient The difference in temperature (high vs. low temperature) between two objects.

thermite An incendiary compound that consists of powdered aluminum and iron oxide that burns furiously at 3,600°F (1,982°C) and scatters molten iron.

thermoregulatory center The area of the brain (hypothalamus) that controls body temperature.

third death peak The third of three peaks that occur with death from trauma; occurs several days or weeks after the initial injury, usually caused by sepsis and organ failure.

third-degree frostbite A freezing injury due to cold exposure that involves the epidermis and dermis layers; skin is frozen with restricted mobility; after tissue thaws, skin swells and develops blood-filled blister (hemorrhagic bulla), indicating vascular trauma to deep tissues; skin loss occurs slowly, leading to mummification and sloughing; healing is slow.

tidal volume The normal volume of air exchanged with each ventilation. About 500 ml of air is exchanged between the lungs and the atmosphere with each breath in a healthy adult at rest.

tonsillar herniation The process by which the brain is pushed down toward the foramen magnum and pushes the cerebellum and medulla ahead of it, causing damage and, ultimately, death.

total lung capacity The total volume of air in the lungs after a forced inhalation.

toxidrome A collection of clinical signs and symptoms that suggest exposure to a certain class of chemical or toxin.

tracheal shift Movement or displacement of the trachea away from the midline of the neck.

tranexamic acid (TXA) A medicine that impedes the dissolution of fibrin, the essential protein in the formation of blood clots. It is given to trauma victims to help prevent hemorrhage.

transesophageal echocardiography A technique of performing ultrasound of the heart using an ultrasound probe inserted into the esophagus.

transmission-based PPE The personal protective equipment used, in addition to standard precautions, to prevent transmission of disease; includes aerosol, contact, and droplet precautions.

transmural pressure Difference between the pressure inside a blood vessel and the pressure outside the vessel.

transverse process A protuberance at each side of a vertebra near the lateral margins.

trauma chin lift A maneuver used to relieve a variety of anatomic airway obstructions in patients who are breathing spontaneously; accomplished by grasping the chin and lower incisors and then lifting to pull the mandible forward.

trauma jaw thrust A maneuver that allows opening of the airway with little or no movement of the head and cervical spine; the mandible is thrust forward by placing the thumbs on each zygomatic arch and placing the index and long fingers under the mandible and at the same angle, thrusting the mandible forward.

traumatic asphyxia Blunt and crushing injuries to the chest and abdomen with marked increase of intravascular pressure, producing rupture of the capillaries; characterized by a purplish discoloration of the skin of the upper torso and face along with petecchiae of the skin.

traumatic rhabdomyolysis See *rhabdomyolysis.*

trench foot A nonfreezing cold exposure injury caused by prolonged immersion of extremities in wet and moisture that is cool to cold; also referred to as immersion foot.

triage French word meaning "to sort"; a process in which a group of patients is sorted according to their priority of need for care. When only several patients are involved, triage involves assessing each patient, meeting all of the patients' highest priority needs first, and then moving to lower priority items. In a mass-casualty incident with a large number of patients involved, triage is done by determining both urgency and potential for survival.

triage officer A trained individual who oversees the process of assigning injury severity categories and prioritization of treatment and transport.

tumble An end-over-end motion. Bullets commonly tumble when resistance is met by the leading edge of the missile.

uncal herniation The process by which an expanding mass (usually hemorrhage or swelling) along the convexity of the brain pushes the medial portion of the temporal lobe downward through the tentorium that supports the cerebrum, causing damage to the brain stem.

uncus The medial portion of the temporal lobe.

unified command (UC) An ICS command structure in which the incident commanders of all of the various agencies responding to an event work together to manage the incident.

unintentional injury An injury that was unplanned and did not involve intent to harm.

unity of command An incident command system management concept in which each responder has only one direct supervisor.

vapor A solid or liquid in a gaseous state, usually visible as a fine cloud or mist.

ventilation Movement of air into and out of the lungs through the normal breathing process; the mechanical process by which air moves from the atmosphere outside the body through the mouth, nose, pharynx, trachea, bronchi, and bronchioles, and into and out of the alveoli. To ventilate a patient is to provide positive-pressure inspirations with a ventilating device, such as a bag-mask device, and then alternately allowing time for passive exhalation to occur; used in patients who are apneic or who cannot provide adequate ventilation for themselves.

vertebral foramen Hole or opening in the bony structure of the vertebrae through which blood vessels and nerves pass.

very high altitude Elevation levels between 11,480 to 18,045 feet (3,500 to 5,500 meters).

vesicant A chemical agent such as sulfur mustard and lewisite used as a weapon of mass destruction; also referred to as blister agent because these agents create an injury that is visually similar to a burn.

vestibular folds The false vocal cords that direct airflow through the vocal cords.

vestibular nuclei The areas of the brain from which the vestibular nerves responsible for balance arise.

viscera The internal organs of the body.

visceral pleura A thin membrane that covers the outer surface of each lung.

vitreous humor The clear, jelly-like material that fills the eye behind the lens and maintains the eyeball's round shape.

volatility The likelihood that solids or liquids will vaporize into a gaseous form at room temperature.

voluntary guarding An assessment finding in which the patient tenses the abdominal muscles when the provider palpates a tender area of the abdomen.

warm zone A geographic area of diminished contamination from a hazardous material and the location for the contamination reduction corridor where exposed patients are decontaminated by the hazardous materials team.

water density Organs that have a tissue density similar to that of water— e.g., liver, spleen, muscle.

weapon of mass destruction A chemical, biologic, radiologic, or explosive agent designed to create significant damage and large numbers of casualties.

white blood cell A nearly colorless blood cell in the circulation responsible for responding to invading microorganisms.

white phosphorus An incendiary agent used in the production of munitions.

work of breathing The physical work or effort performed in moving the chest wall and diaphragm to breathe.

years of potential life lost (YPLL) An estimate of the impact of an injury calculated by subtracting age at death from a fixed age of the group under examination, usually 65 or 70 years or the life expectancy of the group.

zone of coagulation The region of greatest tissue destruction in a full-thickness burn; the tissue in this zone is *necrotic* (dead) and is not capable of tissue repair.

zone of hyperemia The outermost zone in a full-thickness burn; has minimal cellular injury and is characterized by increased blood flow secondary to an inflammatory reaction initiated by the burn injury.

zone of stasis The region next to the zone of coagulation; blood flow to this region is stagnant and the cells in this zone are injured, but not irreversibly. If they are subsequently deprived of the delivery of oxygen or blood flow, these viable cells will die and become necrotic. Timely and appropriate burn care will preserve blood flow and oxygen delivery to these injured cells.

Index

autonomy, 40, 41
  advance directives, 42
  privacy and confidentiality, 41
  truth telling, 41–42
autoregulation, 263
  of cerebral blood flow, 263–264
autoregulatory mechanism, 264
avoidance tactics, 804
AVPU, 143, 143*f*, 439
axial loading, 296
axial unloading, 303
axis, 292, 293*f*

B

Babinski reflex, 266
Bacillus anthracis, 529
backpack bombs, 793
bacterial contamination, 801
bag-mask device, 170, 188, 202
  two-provider method, 202–203
bag-mask ventilation, 435
  use of correct-sized, 437
BAL. *See* British anti-lewisite
Ball, Justin, 660
Banks, Sam, 8
Barbero, Michael, 782
baroreceptors, 339
barotrauma, 517, 610–613, 760
  signs, symptoms, and treatment, 617*f*
basal level, 546
basal metabolic rate, 545, 563
bases, 424
basilar skull fractures, 273
Battle of Bull Run, 7
battlefield injury care
  Role 1 (prehospital), 767, 767*f*
  Role 2 (acute MTF care), 767–768, 768*f*
  Role 3 facilities, 768, 768*f*
  Role 4 facilities, 768, 768*f*
  Role 5 facilities, 768, 768*f*
battlefield medical care, 765
Battlefield Medical Information System—
  Tactical (BMIS-T), 711
battlefield trauma care
  in Iraq and Afghanistan, 659–660
  TCCC-based training, 658–659
Battle's sign, 273
Beck's triad, 351
bee sting, 647–648

behavioral regulation, 545
bellows effect, 97
bends, 614
beneficence, 40, 42–43
benzodiazepines, 283, 395
beta-adrenergic blocking agents, 231
beta blockers, 467
beta burn, 534
beta-particle radiation, 534, 537
BFT. *See* Burn Flight Team
bilateral needle decompression, in
  traumatic cardiopulmonary
  arrest, 690*f*
bimodal patient transport, 521
biologic agents, 511, 527–533
  precautions, 529*f*
biologic WMD agents, classification of, 527*f*
birdshot, 105, 106*f*
"Black Box" safety warning, 706
Black Death, 530
blast-induced structural collapse,
  chronology of, 789*f*
blast-induced structural weakening,
  mechanism of, 788
blast injuries, 107–110, 790
  assessment and management, 782,
    792–793
    combination injuries, 804
    primary blast injury, 793–798
    quaternary injury, 802
    quinary injury, 802–804
    secondary injury, 798–801
    tertiary injury, 801–802
  blast waves and body, 108
  categories, 109*f*, 519*f*, 791, 792*f*
  examination of casualties with, 795
  explosion-related injuries, 108–109
  injury from fragments, 109–110
  to lungs, 796
  multi-etiology injury, 110
  physics of blast, 108
blast lung, 796
blast lung injury (BLI), 520*f*
blast overpressure, 108
blast testing, 794
blast victims
  components of rapid assessment of,
    792, 793*f*
  principles to aid in management of, 792

blast wave, 108, 516, 517*f*
blast wind, 108, 519
bleeding, 682*f*, 728*f*–729*f*, 732, 744
bleeding, primary survey, 141–143
BLI. *See* blast lung injury
blind nasotracheal intubation (BNTI),
  181, 281
blister agents, 425, 803
blisters, 409*f*, 815, 817
blocking therapy, 538
blood-borne pathogens, 128–130
blood-clotting cascade, 66, 67*f*
blood-clotting system, 233
blood-glucose measurement, 270
blood, hemodynamic response, 59–60
blood pressure
  aortic disruption, 353*f*
  vital signs of shock, 229–230
blood substitutes, 240
blood vessels, cardiovascular response,
  59
blown pupil, 266
Blue Star of Life, 8
blunt cardiac injury, 349–350
blunt cardiac rupture, 350
blunt force injury, 340
blunt head trauma, 797
blunt injury, 276
blunt trauma, 76, 78–98, 261, 841, 841*f*,
  842*f*
  abdomen, 97–98
  abdominal trauma, 367
  defined, 76
  falls, 92–93
  head, 94
  injuries, 366
  mechanical principles, 79
  neck, 94–95
  spinal trauma, 298–299
  sports injuries, 93
  thorax, 95–97
BMIS-T. *See* Battlefield Medical
  Information System—Tactical
BNTI. *See* blind nasotracheal intubation
board splint, 391*f*
body armor, 841
bomb injuries, 790
bomb threats (safe evacuation distances),
  124*f*

head trauma, 282–283
heat-related illness, 582–584
high-altitude illness, 629–630
lightning injury, 629
musculoskeletal trauma, 400
patient, 159
pediatric trauma, 450, 452
recreational scuba-related diving
    injuries, 629
shock, 244–245
spinal trauma, 311
thoracic trauma, 356–357
promethazine, 706
prone/semi-prone patient, 318–319
prophylactic tube thoracostomy, 796
PSG. *See* Platoon Sergeant
psychogenic "shock," 64
psychological injury, 842
psychological response, to disasters,
    503–504
PTS. *See* Pediatric Trauma Score
PTSD. *See* posttraumatic stress disorder
PTV. *See* percutaneous transtracheal
    ventilation
public health impact of injury, 21, 26–27
public information officer (PIO), 497
PubMed, 44*f*
pulmonary contusions, 340, 342
pulmonary hemorrhage, 794
pulmonary injury, 796
pulmonary overinflation barotrauma,
    612–613
pulmonary overpressurization syndrome
    (POPS), 612
pulmonary sequelae of blast wave
    exposure, 796
pulmonary system, thorax, 104
pulmonary volumes/relationships, 339*f*
pulse, 227
    circulatory status, 142
pulse oximeters, 190–191, 190*f*, 225, 703
pulse oximetry, 145, 340
    issues with readings, 704, 704*f*
    operation, 703–704
    values of, 734*f*
pulse pressure, 58
pulse rate, vital signs of shock, 229
pulseless electrical activity (PEA), 157,
    350

pulseless ventricular tachycardia, 158
pulselessness, 398
pupil, 152*f*
pupil constriction, 152*f*
pupil dilation, 152*f*
pupillary inequality, 272
Pyng FAST1, 696, 697*f*, 724–725
pyramidal fracture, 275

Q

quaternary blast injuries, 109*f*, 519*f*, 520
quaternary effects, 520
quaternary injuries, 790, 792*f*, 802
quiescence/interdisaster period, 489
quinary blast injuries, 108, 109*f*
quinary injuries, 790, 792*f*, 793, 802–804

R

Raccoon eyes, 451*f*
radiation, 545
    exposure to, 422
radiation burns, 422–423
radiation catastrophes, medical effects
    of, 534–537
radiation dispersion devices (RDDs), 534
radiation energy, 16
radiation exposure, treatment and
    decontamination for, 538*f*
radio communications, 840
radio/communications rehearsal, 831
radioactive materials, 803
radioiodine, 538
radiologic disasters, 533–538, 534*f*
radionuclide, 533
Rami fractures, 389
range, 105
Ranger casualty card, 711
Ranger Regiment, 825*f*
rapid extrication, 324–328
    vs. short device for seated patient, 309
rapid response, initial fluid bolus, 244
rapid sequence intubation (RSI), 182–184,
    182*f*–183*f*, 443*f*, 686–687
    protocol, 281
rapid wound healing, 815
rate of detonation, 782
RBCs. *See* red blood cells
RDDs. *See* radiation dispersion devices
RE. *See* relative effectiveness

Ready-Heat blanket, 701, 701*f*
rear-impact collisions, 83
rebound tenderness, 369
recompression therapy, 616*f*
reconstruction phase, 489
recovery, 490
recovery phase, 489
red blood cells (RBCs), 50, 476
reduced force rehearsal, 831
reflective clothing, 117–118
reflective cones, 118
rehearsals, 831
relative effectiveness (RE), 783*f*
    factor, 782
relative hypovolemia, 63, 297
relief of anxiety, 395
relief phase, 489
requests for information (RFI), 826
rescue, 489
rescue plan, Care Under Fire, 669
rescue throw lines, 603*f*
research, prehospital care, 43
    EMS literature, reading, 43
    evaluation, steps in, 44–45
    evidence, types of, 43–44
resource management, 496
respiration, 336
respiratory rate, 140
respiratory system, 164–166, 165*f*
    airway and, 50–54, 51*f*
    organs of, 165*f*
response, 490
response time, 5
restrictive rules of engagement (ROEs),
    840
resuscitation, 145–146
resuscitation fluids, 699
reticular activating system, 261
retroperitoneal space, 363, 365*f*
retroperitoneum, 271
reverse squeeze, 611–613
Revised Trauma Score (RTS), 439
RFI. *See* requests for information
rhabdomyolysis, 582, 815
rhinorrhea, 525
rib fractures, 341
rifles, 105
rifling, 105
right heart, 58

fluid resuscitation strategy with, 701, 701*f*

management of suspected, 284*f*

pediatric trauma, 445–446

pulse oximetry, management of, 704*f*

in TACEVAC Care, 729*f*, 734

traumatic cardiopulmonary arrest, 156–158

bilateral needle decompression in, 690*f*

traumatic rhabdomyolysis, 398

traumatic shock

classification of, 219

types of, 219–224, 219*f*

traumatic subarachnoid hemorrhage (tSAH), 280

treatment area, 503

trench foot, 567

Trendelenburg position, 237

trendelenburg position, use of, 794

triage, 131, 773, 791–792

categories of, 773*f*–774*f*

disaster management, 499, 499*f*

ethics in, 849

explosions and WMD, 514

field triage scheme, 153–154

planning and protection, 777, 777*f*

scene, 130–134

in TCCC, 774–775, 774*f*–775*f*

triage algorithm, for TCCC, 776*f*

triage and initial stabilization, 493, 499*f*

Triage Decision Scheme, 153–154

triage officer, 499

triage systems, 514

trinitrotoluene (TNT), 782

trismus, 686

Trunkey, Donald, 5, 9

truth telling, 41–42

tSAH. *See* traumatic subarachnoid hemorrhage

TSWG. *See* U.S. Technical Support Working Group

tube thoracostomy, 347–348, 348*f*, 688

tumble, 99

turbinates, 150*f*, 165*f*

2-PAM chloride, 525

two-person drag, 669, 669*f*

two-provider method, 202–203

2004 Madrid terrorist bombing, 502*f*

TXA. *See* tranexamic acid

tympanic membrane rupture, 108–109, 795–796

type I DCS, 614, 618*f*

type II DCS, 614, 618*f*

U

UH-60 Black Hawk MEDEVAC helicopter, 755*f*

ultraviolet (UV) rays, 642–643

umbilicus level, 294

uncal herniation, 265

uncontrolled hemorrhage, 241

uncontrolled hemorrhagic shock models, 698

uncus, 265

Understanding Combat Casualty Care Statistics (Holcomb), 660

undertriage, 153

underwater devices, 785*f*

underwater explosions, 794

unequal pupils, 152*f*

unified command, 494

unified command system, 125

unilateral pupillary dilation, 734

unintentional injury, 4, 4*f*, 19

unit leadership, 832

unit-level reporting formats, 710

unity of command, 495

unprotected persons, short-duration pressure effects from blasts on, 794, 795*f*

unstable spinal column injury, 296

up-and-over path, 80–81

upper airway, 164

sounds, 171

upper respiratory tract, 165*f*

upward streamer, 593

urban combat

characteristics of, 839–840, 840*f*

medical preparation for, 842–843

restrictive rules of engagement, 840

urban environment

fast-roping casualty in, 750–751, 750*f*

rocket-propelled grenade attack in, 744–745, 745*f*

urban operations, casualties, 841–842

urban terrain, 839, 839*f*

urinary catheter, 159

U.S. Air Force Aeromedical Evacuation Squadrons for logistical support, 820

U.S. Army Institute of Surgical Research (USAISR), 659, 693

Rule of Ten, 817, 818*f*

U.S. Army Institute of Surgical Research (USAISR) Burn Center, 817

U.S. Army Institute of Surgical Research Burn Flight Team, 819, 819*f*, 820

U.S. Army's 628th forward Surgical Team, 768*f*

U.S. Food and Drug Administration (FDA), 236, 524

U.S. Special Operations Command (USSOCOM), 657

U.S. Technical Support Working Group (TSWG), 785

USAISR. *See* U.S. Army Institute of Surgical Research

USAISR Burn Center. *See* U.S. Army Institute of Surgical Research Burn Center

USSOCOM. *See* U.S. Special Operations Command

uvula, 165*f*

V

vacuum bombs. *See* advanced thermobaric weapons

vacuum mattress splint, 301, 302*f*

vacuum splint, 391*f*

vacuum splint application, 331–333

Valium, 526

valvular disruption, 65, 223

valvular rupture, 350

vapor, 522

varicella, 531, 532*f*

variola major, 531

variola minor, 531

vascular access, 444

shock management, 237–238

vascular system, thorax, 104–105

vasoconstriction, 61, 169, 220

vasogenic shock. *See* distributive shock

vasovagal "shock," 64

vecuronium, 185*f*

vehicle incompatibility, 86